Shorter Oxford Textbook of Psychiatry

FIFTH EDITION

Michael Gelder
Paul Harrison
and
Philip Cowen

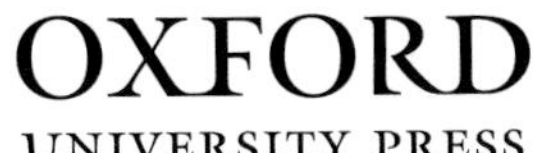
UNIVERSITY PRESS

OXFORD
UNIVERSITY PRESS

Great Clarendon Street, Oxford OX2 6DP

Oxford University Press is a department of the University of Oxford.
It furthers the University's objective of excellence in research, scholarship, and education by publishing worldwide in

Oxford New York

Athens Auckland Bangkok Bogotá Buenos Aires Calcutta
Cape Town Chennai Dar es Salaam Delhi Florence Hong Kong Istanbul
Karachi Kuala Lumpur Madrid Melbourne Mexico City Mumbai
Nairobi Paris São Paulo Singapore Taipei Tokyo Toronto Warsaw

with associated companies in Berlin Ibadan

Oxford is a registered trade mark of Oxford University Press
in the UK and in certain other countries

Published in the United States
by Oxford University Press Inc., New York

First published 2006

British Library Cataloguing in Publication Data

Data available

Library of Congress Cataloguing in Publication Data

Gelder, Michael G.
Shorter Oxford textbook of psychiatry / Michael Gelder, Philip Cowen, Paul Harrison. - 5th ed.
Includes bibliographical references and index.
1. Psychiatry. I. Cowen, Philip. II. Harrison, P. J. (Paul J.), 1960- III. Title.
[DNLM: 1. Mental Disorders. 2. Psychiatry. WM 140 G315s 2006]
RC454.G42 2006 616.89-dc22 2005033086

ISBN 0 19 856896 7 (Hbk: alk. paper) 978 0 19 856896 4
ISBN 0 19 856667 0 (Pbk: alk. paper) 978 0 19 856667 0

10 9 8 7 6 5 4 3 2 1

Typeset by EXPO Holdings Sdn Bhd, Malaysia
Printed in Great Britain
on acid-free paper by
Ashford Colour Press Ltd, Gosport, Hampshire

Preface to the fifth edition

This fifth edition has been revised thoroughly to take account of new research and changes in clinical practice since the publication of the previous edition. In this work of revision, we have been greatly assisted by colleagues who have advised us about individual chapters. We are grateful to these advisors, whose names are listed on p. ix.

We have made one change to the order of chapters. In all previous editions, classification was considered after assessment. In this edition, we have reversed the order on the grounds that classification, and diagnosis, have to be understood before a full assessment can be made. In all chapters, we have made more use of lists and tables to present information in a concise and easily remembered way. For readers who wish to know more, we have provided references throughout the text as well as suggestions for further reading at the end of each chapter. For the first time, we have included references to sources on the Internet, such as the Cochrane Collaboration and National Institute for Clinical Excellence; these will be freely available to many readers, including those working in the British National Health Service, and accessible to other readers through libraries or by individual subscription. More extensive information about all the topics in this book will be found in its companion volume, the *New Oxford Textbook of Psychiatry*, a comprehensive multi-authored work of reference.

This is the first edition to have been written without Richard Mayou, who has retired. We pay tribute to his important contributions to the success of all previous editions, through his broad knowledge of psychiatry and especially of its interface with general medicine. We also record with great sadness the recent death of Dennis Gath, one of the original authors of this book. His wide scholarship and unsurpassed clarity of expression played an essential role in the original success of the book, and we have attempted to preserve these values in the present edition.

In writings about psychiatry, the terms psychiatric disorder, mental disorder, and mental illness are used widely and, for the most part, interchangeably. We have followed this common practice, regarding them as generally equivalent and using whichever term seems best fitted to the context in which it appears.

Finally we thank Valerie West and Linda Carter for their considerable help in the preparation of the reference list, and in proof reading.

MG
PC
PJH
November 2005

Contents

Chapter advisors

We wish to thank the following colleagues who advised us about the revision of the major parts of the book:

Kathryn Abel
Senior Lecturer, Department of Psychiatry, University of Manchester

Christopher Bass
Consultant Liaison Psychiatrist, Department of Psychological Medicine, John Radcliffe Hospital, Oxford; Honorary Clinical Senior Lecturer, University of Oxford

Zubin Bhagwagar
Clinical Lecturer, Department of Psychiatry, University of Oxford

David Clark
Professor of Psychology, Institute of Psychiatry, King's College London

John Cooper
Emeritus Professor of Psychiatry, University of Nottingham

Shoumitro Deb
Clinical Professor of Neuropsychiatry and Learning Disability, Department of Psychiatry, Division of Neuroscience, University of Birmingham, Queen Elizabeth Hospital, Birmingham

Anke Ehlers
Professor of Experimental Psychopathology, Institute of Psychiatry, London

Christopher Fairburn
Wellcome Principal Research Fellow and Professor of Psychiatry, University of Oxford

Seena Fazel
Consultant in Forensic Psychiatry, Oxfordshire Mental Healthcare NHS Trust

Simon Fleminger
Consultant Neuropsychiatrist, Maudsley Hospital, London

Gillian Forrest
Formerly, Consultant Child and Adolescent Psychiatrist, Park Hospital for Children, Oxford; Honorary Clinical Senior Lecturer, University of Oxford

Hamid Ghodse
Director of the International Centre for Drug Policy, St Georges Hospital Medical School, London

Ian Goodyer
Professor of Child and Adolescent Psychiatry, Cambridge University; Honorary Consultant Child Psychiatrist, Department of Child Psychiatry, Douglas House, Cambridge

Keith Hawton
Professor of Psychiatry, University of Oxford; Director, University of Oxford Centre for Suicide Research, Warneford Hospital Oxford

Michael Hobbs
Consultant Psychiatrist in Psychotherapy, Oxfordshire Mental Health Trust; Medical Director, Oxfordshire and Berkshire Mental Health NHS Trusts; Honorary Clinical Senior Lecturer, University of Oxford

Tony Hope
Professor of Medical Ethics and Director of the Ethox Centre, University of Oxford

Robin Jacoby
Professor of Old Age Psychiatry, Department of Psychiatry, University of Oxford

Max Marshall
Professor of Community Psychiatry, Manchester University; Honorary Consultant Psychiatrist and Medical Director, Lancashire Care NHS Trust

Steve Pearce
Consultant Psychiatrist in Psychotherapy, and Progamme Director, Complex Needs Service, Warneford Hospital, Oxford; Honorary Clinical Senior Lecturer, University of Oxford

Roz Shafran
Wellcome Research Career Development Fellow, Department of Psychiatry, University of Oxford

Michael Sharpe
Professor of Psychological Medicine and Symptoms Research, School of Molecular and Clinical Medicine, University of Edinburgh; Honorary Consultant in Psychological Medicine to NHS Lothian

Matthew Taylor
Research Fellow, Department of Psychiatry, University of Oxford

Sarah Welch
Consultant in Substance Misuse, Gloucestershire Partnership NHS Trust

Kevan Wylie
Consultant in Sexual Medicine and Psychosexual Therapy, Porterbrook Clinic, Sheffield; Consultant Andrologist, Royal Hallamshire Hospital, Sheffield

CHAPTER 1

Symptoms and signs of psychiatric disorders

Chapter contents

Psychiatrists require two distinct capacities. One is the capacity to collect clinical data objectively and accurately by history-taking and examination of the mental state, and to organize the data in a systematic and balanced way. The other is the capacity for intuitive understanding of each patient as an individual. When the psychiatrist exercises the first capacity, he draws on his clinical skills and knowledge of clinical phenomena; when he exercises the second capacity, he draws on his knowledge of human nature and experience with former patients to gain insights into the patient he is now seeing. Both capacities can be developed by listening to patients, and by learning from more experienced psychiatrists. A textbook can provide the information and describe the procedures necessary to develop the first capacity. The focus of this chapter on the first capacity does not imply that intuitive understanding is unimportant, but simply that it cannot be learnt directly or solely from a textbook.

Skill in examining patients depends on a sound knowledge of how symptoms and signs are defined. Without such knowledge, the psychiatrist is liable to misclassify phenomena and thereby make inaccurate diagnoses. For this reason, this chapter is concerned with the definition of the key symptoms and signs of psychiatric disorders. Having elicited a patient's symptoms and signs, the psychiatrist needs to decide how far these phenomena fall into a pattern that has been observed in other patients. In other words, he decides whether the clinical features conform to a recognized syndrome. He does this by combining observations about the patient's present state with information about the history of the condition. The value of identifying a syndrome is that it helps to predict prognosis and to select an effective treatment. It does this by directing the psychiatrist to the relevant body of accumulated knowledge about the causes, treatment, and outcome of similar patients. Diagnosis and classification are discussed in the next chapter, and also in each of the chapters dealing with the various psychiatric disorders. Chapter 3 discusses *how* to elicit and interpret the symptoms described in this chapter, and how to integrate the information in order to arrive at a syndromal diagnosis, since this in turn is the basis for a rational approach to management and prognosis.

As much of the present chapter consists of definitions and descriptions of symptoms and signs, it may be less easy to read than those that follow. It is suggested that the reader might approach it in two stages. The first reading would be applied to the introductory sections and to a general understanding of the more frequently observed phenomena. The second reading would focus on details of definition and the less common symptoms and signs, and might be done best in conjunction with an opportunity to interview a patient exhibiting them.

General issues

Before individual phenomena are described, some general issues will be considered concerning the methods of studying symptoms and signs, and the terms used to describe them.

Psychopathology

The study of abnormal states of mind is known as **psychopathology**. The term embraces two distinct approaches to the subject: **descriptive** and **experimental**. This chapter is concerned almost exclusively with the former; the latter is introduced here but discussed in later chapters.

Descriptive psychopathology

Descriptive psychopathology is the objective description of abnormal states of mind avoiding, as far as possible, preconceived ideas or theories, and limited to the description of conscious experiences and observable behaviour. It is sometimes also called **phenomenology** or **phenomenological psychopathology** although the terms are not in fact synonymous, and phenomenology has additional meanings (Berrios, 1992).

The aim of descriptive psychopathology is to elucidate the essential qualities of morbid mental experiences and to understand each patient's experience of illness. It therefore requires the ability to elicit, identify, and interpret the symptoms of psychiatric disorders, and as such is a key element of clinical practice; indeed it has been described as 'the fundamental professional skill of the psychiatrist' (Sims, 2003).

The most important exponent of descriptive psychopathology was the German psychiatrist and philosopher, Karl Jaspers. His classic work, *Allgemeine Psychopathologie* (*General psychopathology*), first published in 1913, still provides the most complete account of the subject, with the seventh edition available in an English translation by Hoenig and Hamilton (Jaspers, 1963). Sims (2003) provides a more readable and up to date text, and a briefer introduction to Jaspers' views can be found in Jaspers (1968).

Experimental psychopathology

This approach seeks to explain abnormal mental phenomena as well as to describe them. One of the first attempts was **psychodynamic psychopathology**, originating in Freud's psychoanalytic investigations (see p. 89). It explains the causes of abnormal mental events in terms of mental processes of which the patient is unaware (they are 'unconscious'). For example, Freud explained persecutory delusions as being evidence, in the conscious mind, of activities in the unconscious mind, including the mechanisms of repression and projection (see p. 309).

Subsequently, experimental psychopathology has focused on empirically measurable and verifiable, conscious, psychological processes, using experimental methods such as cognitive and behavioural psychology and functional brain imaging. For example, there are cognitive theories of the origin of delusions, panic attacks, and depression. Though experimental psychopathology is concerned with the causes of symptoms, it is usually conducted in the context of the syndromes in which the symptoms occur. Thus, its findings are discussed in the chapter covering the disorder in question.

Terms and concepts used in descriptive psychopathology

Symptoms and signs

In general medicine, there is a clear definition of, and separation between, a symptom and a sign. In psychiatry, the situation is different. There are few 'signs' in the medical sense (apart from the motor abnormalities of catatonic schizophrenia, or the physical manifestations of anorexia nervosa), with most diagnostic information coming from the history and observations of the patient's appearance and behaviour. Use of the word 'sign' in psychiatry is therefore less clear, and two different uses may be encountered. First, it may be used to refer to a feature noted by the observer rather than something spoken by the patient (e.g. a patient who appears to be responding to a hallucination). Second, it may refer to a group of symptoms that the observer interprets in aggregation as a sign of a particular disorder. In practice, the phrase 'symptoms and signs' is often used interchangeably with 'symptoms' (as we have done in this chapter), to refer collectively to the phenomena of psychiatric disorders, without a clear distinction being drawn between the two words.

Subjective and objective

In general medicine, subjective and objective are used as counterparts of symptoms and signs respectively, with objective being defined as something observed directly by the doctor (e.g. meningism, jaundice) – even though, strictly speaking, it is a subjective judgment on his part as to what has been observed.

In psychiatry, the terms have broadly similar meanings as in medicine, though with a blurring between them, just as there is for symptoms and signs. 'Objective' refers to features observed during an interview, i.e. the patient's appearance and behaviour. The term is usually used when the psychiatrist wants to compare this with the patient's description of symptoms. For example, in evaluation of depression, complaints of low mood and tearfulness are **subjective** features, whereas observations of poor eye contact, psychomotor retardation, and crying, are **objective** ones. If both are present, the psychiatrist might record 'subjective *and* objective evidence of depression', with the combination providing stronger evidence than either alone. However, if the patient's behaviour and manner in the interview appear entirely normal, she records 'not objectively depressed', despite the subjective complaints. It is then incumbent on the psychiatrist to explore the reasons for the discrepancy and to decide what diagnostic conclusions she should draw. As a rule, objective signs are accorded greater weight. Thus, the psychiatrist may diagnose a depressive disorder if there is sufficient evidence of this kind, even if the person denies the subjective experience of feeling depressed; conversely, she may question the significance of complaints of low mood, however prominent, if there are none of the objective features associated with the diagnosis.

Form and content

When psychiatric symptoms are described, it is useful to distinguish between form and content, a distinction best explained by an example. If a patient says that, when he is alone, he hears voices calling him a homosexual, the **form** of the experience is an auditory hallucination (see below) whilst the **content** is the statement that he is homosexual. Another person might hear voices saying that she is about to be killed; again the form is an auditory hallucination but the content is different. A third person might experience repeated intrusive thoughts that he is homosexual but realizes that these are untrue. The content is the same as that of the first example (concerning homosexuality) but the form is different.

Form is often critical when making a diagnosis; from the examples above, the presence of a hallucination indicates (by definition) a psychosis of one kind or another, whereas the third example suggests obsessive–compulsive disorder. Content is less diagnostically useful, but can be very important in management; for example, the content of a delusion may suggest that the patient could attack a supposed persecutor. It is also the content not the form that is of concern to the patient, whose priority will be to discuss the persecution and its implications, and who may be irritated by what seem irrelevant questions about the form of the belief. The psychiatrist must be sensitive to this difference in emphasis between the two parties.

Primary and secondary

With regard to symptoms, the terms primary and secondary are often used, but unfortunately with two different meanings. The first meaning is **temporal**, simply referring to which occurred first. The second meaning is **causal**, whereby primary means 'arising directly from the pathological process', and secondary means 'arising as a reaction to a primary symptom'. The two meanings often coincide since symptoms that arise directly from the pathological process usually appear first. However, although subsequent symptoms are often a reaction to the first symptoms, they are not always of this kind, for they too may arise direct from the pathological process. The terms primary and secondary are used more often in the temporal sense because this usage does not involve an inference about causality. However, many patients cannot say in what order their symptoms appeared. In such cases, when it seems likely that one symptom is a reaction to another, for example, that a delusion of being followed by persecutors is a reaction to hearing accusing voices, it is called secondary (using the word in the causal sense). The terms primary and secondary are also used, in a causal sense, in the description of syndromes.

Understanding and explanation

Jaspers (1913) contrasted two forms of understanding when applied to symptoms. The first, called *verstehen* (understanding) is the attempt to appreciate the patient's subjective experience: what does it feel like? This important skill requires intuition and empathy. The second approach is *erklaren* (explanation), which accounts for events in terms of external factors; for example, the patient's low mood can be 'explained' by her recent redundancy. The latter approach requires knowledge of psychiatric aetiology.

The significance of individual symptoms

Psychiatric disorders are diagnosed when a defined group of symptoms (a syndrome) is present. Almost any single symptom can be experienced by a healthy person; even hallucinations, often regarded as a hallmark of mental disorder, are sometimes experienced transiently by healthy people. An exception is that an isolated delusion is generally considered to be evidence of psychiatric disorder if it is definite and persistent (see Chapter 13). In general, however, the finding of a single symptom is not evidence of psychiatric disorder but an indication for a thorough and, if necessary, repeated search for other symptoms and signs of psychiatric disorder. The dangers of not adhering to this principle are exemplified by the study of Rosenhahn (1973). Eight 'patients' presented with the complaint that they heard the words 'empty, hollow, thud' being said out loud. All eight were admitted and diagnosed with schizophrenia, despite denying all other symptoms and behaving entirely normally. This study also illustrates the importance of descriptive psychopathology, and of having reliable diagnostic criteria (Chapter 2), as fundamental aspects of psychiatry.

The patient's experience

Symptoms and signs are only part of the subject matter of psychopathology. It is concerned also with the patient's experience of illness, and the way in which psychiatric disorder changes his view of himself, his hopes for the future, and his view of the world. This may be seen as one example of the understanding (*verstehen*) mentioned above. A depressive disorder may have a very different effect on a person who has lived a satisfying and happy life and has fulfilled his major ambitions, and a person who has had many previous misfortunes but has lived on hopes of future success. To understand this aspect of the patient's experience of psychiatric disorder, the psychiatrist has to understand him in the way that a biographer understands his subject. This way of understanding is sometimes called the life-story approach. It is not something that can be readily assimilated from textbooks; it can be learnt best by taking time to listen to patients. The psychiatrist may be helped by reading biographies or works of literature that provide insights into the ways in which experiences throughout life shape the personality, and help explain the diverse ways in which different people respond to the same events.

Cultural variations in psychopathology

Symptoms are similar in their form in widely different cultures. However, there are cultural differences in the symptoms that are revealed to doctors; for example, people from the Indian subcontinent are less likely than Europeans to report low mood when they have a depressive disorder, and more likely to report somatic symptoms. The content of symptoms also differs between cultures. For example, people from some African cultures may have delusions concerned with evil spirits, a subject that is observed infrequently among Europeans. Cultural differences also affect the person's subjective experience of illness, and therefore influence one's understanding (in the sense used above) of it (Fabrega, 2000). In some cultures, the effects of psychiatric disorder are ascribed to witchcraft, a belief that adds to the patient's distress. In others, mental illness is so greatly stigmatized that it may be a bar to marriage. In such a culture the effect of illness on the patient's view of herself and her future will be very different from the effect on a patient living in a society that is more tolerant of mental disorder.

Descriptions of symptoms and signs

Disturbances of emotion and mood

Much of psychiatry is concerned with abnormal emotional states, particularly disturbances of mood and other emotions, especially anxiety. Before describing the main symptoms of this kind, it is worth clarifying two areas of terminology which may cause confusion, in part because their usage has changed over the years.

First, 'mood' can either be used as a broad term to encompass all emotions (e.g. 'anxious mood'), or in a more restricted sense to mean the emotion which runs from depression at one end to mania at the other. The former usage is now uncommon. The latter usage is emphasized by the fact that in current diagnostic systems, 'mood disorders' are those in which depression and mania are the defining characteristics, whereas disorders defined by anxiety or other emotional disturbances are categorized separately. In this section, features common to both 'mood' and 'other emotions' are described first, before the specific features of anxiety, depression, and mania are discussed separately.

The second point concerns the term **affect**. The word is now usually used interchangeably with mood, in the more limited meaning of the latter word. Hence, 'his affect was normal'; 'he has an affective disorder'. However, in the past, the words had different nuances of meaning; mood referred to a prevailing and prolonged state, whereas affect was linked to a particular aspect or object, and was more transitory.

Emotions and mood may be abnormal in three ways:

1. Its nature may be altered;
2. It may fluctuate more or less than usual; and
3. It may be inconsistent with the patient's thoughts or actions or with his current circumstances.

Changes in the nature of emotions and mood

These can be towards anxiety, depression, elation, or irritability and anger. Any of these changes may be associated with events in the person's life, but they may arise without an apparent reason. They are usually accompanied by other symptoms and signs. For example, an increase of anxiety is accompanied by autonomic overactivity and increased muscle tension, and depression is accompanied by gloomy preoccupations and psychomotor slowness.

Changes in the way that emotions and mood vary

Emotions and mood vary in relation to the person's circumstances and preoccupations. In abnormal states, the variations may be greater or less than normal. Increased variation is called **lability** of mood; extreme variation is sometimes called **emotional incontinence**.

Reduced variation is called **blunting** or **flattening**. These terms have been used with subtly different meanings, but are now usually used interchangeably. It usually occurs in depression and schizophrenia. Severe flattening is sometimes called **apathy** (note the difference from the layman's meaning of the word).

Incongruity of emotion

Emotion can also vary in a way that is not in keeping with the person's circumstances and thoughts, and is called **incongruous** or **inappropriate**. For example, a patient may appear to be in high spirits and laugh when talking about the death of his mother. Such incongruity must be distinguished from the embarrassed laughter that indicates that the person is ill at ease.

Clinical associations of emotional and mood disturbances

Disturbances of emotions and mood are seen in essentially all psychiatric disorders. They are the central feature of mood disorders and anxiety disorders. They are common also in eating disorders, substance-induced disorders, delirium, dementia, and schizophrenia.

Anxiety

Anxiety is a normal response to danger but is abnormal when its severity is out of proportion to the threat of danger or when it outlasts the threat. Anxious mood is closely coupled with somatic and autonomic components, and with psychological ones. All can be thought of as equivalent to the preparations for dealing with danger seen in other mammals, ready for flight from, avoidance of, or fighting with, a predator. Mild-to-moderate anxiety enhances most kinds of performance, but high levels interfere with it.

The anxiety response is considered further in Chapter 9; here, its main components are summarized as follows:

- *Psychological.* The essential feelings of dread and apprehension are accompanied by restlessness, narrowing of attention to focus on the source of danger, worrying thoughts, increased alertness (with insomnia), and irritability.
- *Somatic.* Muscle tension and respiration increase. If these changes are not followed by physical activity, they may be experienced as muscle tension tremor, or the effects of hyperventilation (e.g. dizziness).
- *Autonomic.* Heart rate and sweating increase, the mouth becomes dry, and there may be an urge to urinate or defecate.
- *Avoidance of danger.* A phobia is a persistent, irrational fear of a specific object or situation. Usually there is also a marked wish to avoid the object, though this is not the always the case, e.g. fear of illness (hypochondriasis). The fear is out of proportion to the objective threat, and is recognized as such by the person experiencing it. Phobias include animate objects, natural phenomena, and situations. Phobic people feel anxious not only in the presence of the object or situation but also when thinking about it (**anticipatory anxiety**). Phobias are discussed further in relation to anxiety disorders on p. 183.

Clinical associations

Phobias are common among healthy children, becoming less frequent in adolescence and adult life. Phobic symptoms occur in all kinds of anxiety disorder but are the major feature in phobic disorders.

Depression

Depression is a normal response to loss or misfortune, when it may be called grief or mourning. Depression is abnormal when it is out of proportion to the misfortune, or is unduly prolonged. Depressed mood is closely coupled with other changes, notably a lowering of self-esteem, pessimistic or negative thinking, and a reduction or loss of the experience of pleasure (**anhedonia**). A depressed person has a characteristic expression and appearance, with turned corners of the mouth, a furrowed brow, and a hunched, dejected posture. The level of arousal is reduced in some depressed patients (**psychomotor retardation**) but increased in others with a consequent feeling of restlessness or agitation. The psychopathology of depression is discussed further in Chapter 11.

Clinical associations

Depression can occur in any psychiatric disorder. It is the defining feature of mood disorders, and commonly occurs in schizophrenia, anxiety, obsessional–compulsive disorder, eating disorders, and in substance-induced disorders. It can also be a manifestation of an organic disorder.

Elation

Happy moods have been studied less than depressed mood. Elation is an extreme degree of happy mood which, like depression, is coupled with other changes including increased feelings of self-confidence and well-being, increased activity, and increased arousal. The latter is usually experienced as pleasant but sometimes as an unpleasant feeling of restlessness. Elation occurs most often in mania and hypomania.

Irritability and anger

Irritability is a state of increased readiness for anger. Both irritability and anger may occur in many kinds of disorder so that they are of little value in diagnosis. They are, however, of great importance in risk assessment and risk management, since they may result in harm to others and self (Chapter 3). Irritability may occur in anxiety disorders, depression, mania, dementia, and drug intoxication.

Disturbances of perception

Specific kinds of perceptual disturbance are symptoms of severe psychiatric disorders. It is therefore important to be able to identify these symptoms, and distinguish them from the other, much less significant and common alterations in sensory experience which occur. We thus describe perceptual phenomena in some detail.

Perception and imagery

Perception is the process of becoming aware of what is presented through the sense organs. It is not a direct awareness of data from the sense organs because these data are acted on by cognitive processes that reassemble them and extract patterns. Perception can be attended to or ignored, but it cannot be terminated by an effort of will.

Imagery is the awareness of a percept that has been generated within the mind. Imagery can be called up and terminated by an effort of will. Images are experienced as lacking the sense of reality that characterizes perception so that a healthy person can distinguish between images and percepts. A few people experience **eidetic imagery**, visual imagery so intense and detailed that it has a 'photographic' quality akin to a percept, though in other ways it differs from a percept. Imagery is generally terminated when perception starts. Occasionally, imagery persists despite the presence of percept (provided this is weak and unstructured). This sort of imagery is called **pareidolia**.

Percepts may alter in intensity and in quality. Anxious people may experience sensations as more intense than usual; for example, a person may be unusually sensitive to noise. In mania, perceptions seem more vivid than usual. Depressed patients may experience perceptions as dull and lifeless.

Illusions

Illusions are misperceptions of external stimuli. They occur when the general level of sensory stimulation is reduced and when attention is not focused on the relevant sensory modality. For example, at dusk the outline of a bush may be perceived at first as that of a man, though not when attention is focused on the outline. Illusions occur also when the level of consciousness is reduced, as in delirium, even if illumination is normal. In both a healthy state and in delirium, illusions are more likely when the person is anxious. Thus in a dark lane a frightened person is more likely than a calm person to misperceive the outline of a bush as that of a man.

Hallucinations

A **hallucination** is a percept experienced in the absence of an external stimulus to the corresponding sense organ. It differs from an illusion in being experienced as originating in the outside world or from within the person's body (rather than as imagined). Hallucinations cannot be terminated at will.

Hallucinations are generally indications of significant psychiatric disorder, and specific types of hallucination are characteristic of different disorders, as outlined below. However, hallucinations occur occasionally in healthy people, usually when falling asleep (**hypnagogic hallucinations**) or on waking (**hypnopompic hallucinations**). These two types of hallucination may be either visual or auditory, the latter sometimes as the experience of hearing one's name called. Such hallucinations are common in narcolepsy (see p. 373). Some recently bereaved people experience hallucinations of the dead person. Hallucinations can occur after sensory deprivation, in people with blindness or deafness of peripheral origin, occasionally in neurological disorders affecting the visual pathways, in epilepsy (Chapter 14), and in the Charles Bonnet syndrome (p. 515).

Types of hallucination

Hallucinations can be described in terms of their complexity and their sensory modality (Table 1.1). The term **elementary hallucination** refers to experiences such as bangs, whistles, and flashes of light; **complex hallucination** refers to experiences such as hearing voices or music, or seeing faces and scenes.

Auditory hallucinations may be experienced as noises, music, or voices. Voices may be heard clearly or indistinctly; they may seem to speak words, phrases, or sentences. They may seem to address the patient directly (**second-person hallucinations**) or talk to one another referring to the patient as 'he' or 'she' (**third-person hallucinations**). Sometimes patients say that the voices anticipate what they are about to think a few moments later. Sometimes the voices seem to speak the patient's thoughts as he is thinking them (***Gedankenlautwerden***) or to repeat them immediately after he has thought them (***écho de la pensée***).

Visual hallucinations may also be elementary or complex. The content may appear normal or abnormal in size; hallucinations of dwarf figures are sometimes called **lilliputian**. Occasionally, patients describe the experience of visual hallucinations located outside the field of vision, usually behind the head (**extracampine hallucinations**).

Olfactory and gustatory hallucinations are frequently experienced together. The smells and tastes are often unpleasant.

Tactile hallucinations, sometimes called **haptic** hallucinations, may be experienced as sensations of being touched, pricked, or strangled. Sometimes they are felt as movements just below the skin, which the patient may attribute to insects, worms, or other small creatures burrowing through the tissues. **Hallucinations of deep sensation** may be experienced as feelings of the viscera being pulled upon or distended, or of sexual stimulation or electric shocks.

An **autoscopic hallucination** is the experience of seeing one's own body projected into external space, usually in front of oneself, for short periods. The experience is reported occasionally by healthy people in situations of sensory deprivation, when it is called an out-of-body experience, or after a near-fatal accident or heart attack when it has been called a near-death experience. Rarely, the experience is accompanied by the conviction that the person has a double (*Doppelganger*).

Reflex hallucination is a rare phenomenon in which a stimulus in one sensory modality results in a hallucination in another; for example, music may provoke visual hallucinations.

TABLE 1.1 Descriptions of hallucinations

According to complexity
◆ elementary
◆ complex
According to sensory modality
◆ auditory
◆ visual
◆ olfactory and gustatory
◆ somatic (tactile and deep)
According to special features
◆ auditory
◆ second-person
◆ third-person
◆ *Gedankenlautwerden*
◆ *écho de la pensée*
◆ visual
◆ extracampine
Autoscopic hallucinations
Reflex hallucinations
Hypnagogic and hypnopompic hallucinations

Clinical associations of hallucinations

Hallucinations occur in diverse disorders, notably schizophrenia, severe mood disorder, organic disorders, and dissociative states. Therefore, the finding of hallucinations does not itself help much in diagnosis. However, the following kinds of hallucination do have important diagnostic implications:

- **Auditory hallucination.** Only clearly heard voices (not noises or music) have diagnostic significance. Third-person hallucinations (introduced above) are associated strongly with schizophrenia. Such voices may be experienced as commenting on the patient's intentions (e.g. 'he wants to make love to her') or actions (e.g. 'she is washing her face'), or may make critical comments. Second-person auditory hallucinations (i.e. which appear to address the patient) do not point to a particular diagnosis, but their content and the patient's reaction to it may do so. Thus, voices with derogatory content (e.g. 'you are a failure, you are wicked'), suggest severe depressive disorder, especially when the patient accepts them as justified. In schizophrenia, the patient more often resents such comments. Voices which anticipate, echo, or repeat the patient's thoughts also suggest schizophrenia.
- **Visual hallucinations** should always raise the possibility of an organic disorder, although they occur also in severe affective disorders, schizophrenia, and dissociative disorder. The content of visual hallucinations is of little significance in diagnosis. Autoscopic hallucinations also raise suspicion of an organic disorder, such as temporal lobe epilepsy.
- **Hallucinations of taste and smell** are infrequent. They may occur in schizophrenia, severe depressive disorders, and temporal lobe epilepsy, and in tumours affecting the olfactory pathways.
- **Tactile and somatic hallucinations** are suggestive of schizophrenia, especially if they are bizarre in content or interpretation. The sensation of insects moving under the skin (**formication**) occurs in people who abuse cocaine.

Pseudohallucinations

This term refers to experiences that are similar to hallucinations but do not meet all the requirements of the definition, nor have the same implications. The word has two distinct meanings, which correspond to two of the ways in which an experience can fail to meet the criteria for a 'true' hallucination. In the first meaning, pseudohallucination is a sensory experience that differs from a hallucination in not seeming to the patient to represent external reality, being located within the mind rather than in external space. In this way pseudohallucinations resemble imagery though, unlike imagery, they cannot be dismissed by an effort of will. In the second meaning, the sensory experience appears to originate in the external world, but it seems unreal. For a more detailed discussion, see Hare (1973) and Taylor (1981).

Both definitions of pseudohallucination are difficult to apply clinically because patients can seldom describe their experiences in adequate detail. In any event, it is usually sufficient to decide whether a perceptual experience is a 'true' hallucination or not, since it is only the former which carry diagnostic significance. If it is not a hallucination, the experience should be described, but need not be labelled as one or other kind of pseudohallucination.

Abnormalities in the meaning attached to percepts

A **delusional perception** is a delusion arising directly from a normal percept. This is sometimes erroneously considered a perceptual disturbance, but is really a disorder of thought, and thus discussed in the next section.

Disturbances of thoughts

Disturbances of thoughts and thought processes are amongst the most diagnostically significant symptoms in psychiatry. As with disturbances of perception, therefore, this area of descriptive psychopathology merits relatively detailed description. It covers two kinds of phenomena:

1. *Disturbance of thoughts* themselves. That is, a change in the nature of individual thoughts. The category of delusion is particularly important. Disturbances of thought are covered in this section.
2. *Disturbance of the thinking process* and the linking together of different thoughts; this may affect the speed or the form of the relationship between thoughts. These phenomena are covered in the next section.

Delusions

A **delusion** is a belief that is firmly held on inadequate grounds, is not affected by rational argument or evidence to the contrary, and is not a conventional belief that the person might be expected to hold given her educational, cultural and religious background. This definition is intended to separate delusions, which are cardinal symptoms of severe psychiatric disorder (specifically, of psychosis), from other kinds of abnormal thoughts and from strongly held beliefs found among healthy people. There are several problems with the definition, summarized in Box 1.1, but it suffices as a starting point to discuss delusions in more detail.

Although not part of the definition, another characteristic feature of delusions is that they have a marked effect on the person's feeling and actions – in the same

BOX 1.1 PROBLEMS WITH THE DEFINITION OF DELUSIONS

Delusions are firmly held despite evidence to the contrary The hallmark of a delusion is that it is held with such conviction that it cannot be altered by presenting evidence to the contrary. For example, a patient who holds the delusion that there are persecutors in the adjoining house will not be convinced by evidence that the house is empty; instead he may suggest that the persecutors left the house shortly before it was searched. The problem of this criterion for delusions is that some of the ideas of normal people are equally impervious to contrary evidence; for example, the beliefs of a convinced spiritualist are not undermined by the counterarguments of a non-believer. Such strongly held non-delusional beliefs are called over-valued ideas (see below).

A further problem about this part of the definition of delusion relates to **partial delusions**. Although delusions are usually held strongly from the start, sometimes they are at first held with a degree of doubt. Also, during recovery, it is not uncommon for patients to pass through a stage of increasing doubt about their delusions before finally rejecting them. The term partial delusion refers to both these situations of doubt. It should be used during recovery only when it is known that the beliefs were preceded by a full delusion, and applied to the development of a delusion only when it is known in retrospect that a full delusion developed later. Partial delusions are not, in isolation, helpful in diagnosis – akin to the status of pseudohallucinations mentioned on p. 8.

Delusions are held on inadequate grounds Delusions are not arrived at by the ordinary processes of observation and logic. Some delusions appear suddenly without any previous thinking about the subject (**primary delusions** – see below). Other delusions appear to be attempts to explain another abnormal experience, for example, the delusion that hallucinated voices are those of people who are spying on the patient.

Delusions are not beliefs shared by others in the same culture This criterion is important when the patient is a member of a culture or subculture (including a religious faith) because healthy people in such a group may hold beliefs that are not accepted outside it. Like delusions, such cultural beliefs are generally impervious to contrary evidence and reasoned argument, for example, beliefs in evil spirits. Therefore, before deciding that an idea is delusional, it is important to determine whether other members of the same culture share the belief.

Delusions as false beliefs Some definitions of delusion indicate that they are false beliefs but this criterion was not included in the definition given above. This omission is because in exceptional circumstances a delusional belief can be true or subsequently become true. A well-recognized example relates to pathological jealousy (p. 314). It is not falsity that determines whether the belief is delusional, but the nature of the mental processes that led up to it. (The difficulty of this statement is that we cannot define these mental processes precisely.) There is a further practical problem about the use of falsity as a criterion for delusion. It is that if the criterion is used, it may be assumed that because a belief is highly improbable, it is false. This is certainly not a sound assumption because improbable stories of, for example, persecution by neighbours, sometimes turn out to be true and arrived at through sound observations and logical thought. Ideas should be investigated thoroughly before they are accepted as delusions.

These issues are discussed further in Spitzer (1990) and Butler and Braff (1991).

way that strongly held normal beliefs do. Since the behavioural response to the delusion may itself be out of keeping or even bizarre, it is often this which first brings the person to psychiatric attention, and leads to the delusion being elicited. For example, a man with the delusion that he was being irradiated by sonic waves covered his windows in silver foil and barricaded his door. Occasionally, however, a delusion has little influence on feelings and actions. For example, a patient may believe he is a member of the royal family while living contentedly in a group home. This separation is called **double orientation** and usually occurs in chronic schizophrenia.

Types of delusions

Several types of delusions are recognized, and categorized either by the characteristics or the theme of the delusion (Table 1.2). Many of the terms are simply useful descriptors, but a few carry particular diagnostic implications. For further descriptions, see also Sims (2003).

TABLE 1.2 Descriptions of delusions

According to fixity (see Box 1.1)
◆ complete
◆ partial
According to onset
◆ primary
◆ secondary
Other delusional experiences
◆ delusional mood
◆ delusional perception
◆ delusional memory
According to theme
◆ persecutory (paranoid)
◆ delusions of reference
◆ grandiose (expansive)
◆ delusions of guilt
◆ nihilistic
◆ hypochondriacal
◆ religious
◆ jealous
◆ sexual or amorous
◆ delusions of control
◆ delusions concerning possession of thought
◆ thought insertion
◆ thought withdrawal
◆ thought broadcasting
According to other features
◆ shared delusions

Primary and secondary delusions

A **primary** or **autochthonous** delusion is one that appears suddenly and with full conviction but without any mental events leading up to it. For example, a schizophrenic patient may be suddenly and completely convinced, for no reason and with no prior thoughts of this kind, that he is changing sex. Not all primary delusional experiences start with an idea. Sometimes the first experience is a delusional mood (see below) or a delusional perception (see below). Because patients do not find it easy to remember the exact sequence of such unusual and distressing mental events, it is often difficult to be certain which experience came first. Primary delusions are given considerable weight in the diagnosis of schizophrenia, and they should be recorded only when it is certain that they are present.

Secondary delusions are delusions apparently derived from a preceding morbid experience. The latter may be of several kinds, including hallucinations (e.g. someone who hears voices may believe that he is being followed), low mood (e.g. a profoundly depressed woman may believe people think she is worthless), or an existing delusion (e.g. a person convinced he is being framed may come to believe he will be imprisoned). Some secondary delusions seem to have an integrative function, making the original experiences more comprehensible to the patient, as in the first example above. Others seem to do the opposite, increasing the sense of persecution or failure, as in the third example. Secondary delusions may accumulate until there is a complicated and stable delusional system. When this happens the delusions are said to be **systematized**.

Delusional mood

When a patient first experiences a delusion, he responds emotionally. For example, a person who believes that a group of people intend to kill him is likely to feel afraid. Occasionally, the change of mood precedes the delusion. This preceding mood is often a feeling of foreboding that some as yet unidentified sinister event is about to take place. When the delusion follows, it appears to explain this feeling. In German this antecedent mood is called *Wahnstimmung*. This term is usually translated as **delusional mood** although it is really the mood from which a delusion arises.

Delusional perception

Sometimes the first abnormal experience is the attaching of a new significance to a familiar percept without any reason to do so. For example, the position of a letter left on the patient's desk may be interpreted as a signal that she is to die. This experience is called **delusional perception**. Note, however, that the perception is normal, it is the delusional interpretation which is abnormal.

Delusional misidentification

This is the delusional misidentification of oneself or of specific other people. Several eponymous forms are described, and have been considered to be both symptoms and syndromes. In line with the latter view, 'delusional misidentification disorder' is described in Chapter 13.

Delusional memory

In **delusional memory**, a delusional interpretation is attached to a past event. In the commoner form of delusional memory, the past event was genuine, and the 'delusional' refers to the significance which has now become attached to it. For example, a patient who believes that there is a current plot to poison her may remember (correctly) that she vomited after a meal, eaten long before her psychosis began, and now concludes (incorrectly) that she had been intentionally poisoned. Alternatively, a sudden (autochthonous) delusion arises which is wrongly dated to a past event. This latter form might be viewed as a true delusional memory (i.e. the memory itself is the delusion), whereas in the first kind described, the memory is normal but a delusional interpretation is placed upon it.

Shared delusions

As a rule, other people recognize delusions as false and argue with the patient in an attempt to correct them. Occasionally, a person who lives with a deluded patient comes to share his delusional beliefs. This condition is known as shared delusions or **folie à deux** (p. 318). Although the second person's delusional conviction is as strong as the partner's while the couple remain together, it often recedes quickly when they are separated.

Delusional themes

For the purposes of clinical work, it is useful to group delusions according to their main themes, since the themes have some diagnostic significance. However, it is first worth considering the word paranoid, which is used widely but not always clearly in this context (Box 1.2).

BOX 1.2 THE TERM PARANOID

The term paranoid is often used as if it were equivalent to persecutory. Strictly interpreted, however, paranoid has a broader meaning (Lewis, 1970). The word was used in ancient Greek writings to mean the equivalent of 'out of his mind'; for example, Hippocrates used it to describe patients with febrile delirium. Many later writers applied the term to grandiose, erotic, jealous, and religious delusions as well as to persecutory delusions. Although, for historical reasons, it is preferable to retain the broader meaning of paranoid, the narrower usage is now commoner, as sanctioned in the diagnostic category of paranoid personality disorder. Because the term paranoid has two possible meanings, the term persecutory is preferable when the narrow sense of paranoid is required. The issue also affects the use of the word to describe syndromes in which such symptoms predominate; the older term 'paranoid psychoses' (or 'paranoid states') is now replaced by 'delusional disorders', in part to avoid the ambiguities (see also Chapter 13).

Persecutory delusions

These are most commonly concerned with persons or organizations that are thought to be trying to inflict harm on the patient, damage his reputation, or make him insane. Such delusions are common but of little help in diagnosis, because they can also occur in organic states, schizophrenia, and severe affective disorders. However, the patient's attitude to the delusion may point to the diagnosis. In a severe depressive disorder, a patient with persecutory delusions characteristically accepts the supposed activities of the persecutors as justified by his own wickedness. In schizophrenia, however, he resents these activities as unwarranted. In assessing persecutory ideas, it is essential to remember the warning, given above, that improbable accounts of persecution are occasionally true, and that it is normal in some cultures to ascribe misfortunes to the malign activities of other people, for example through witchcraft.

Delusions of reference

These are concerned with the idea that objects, events, or people, unconnected with the patient, have a personal significance for him. For example, the patient may believe that an article in a newspaper or a remark on television is directed specifically to himself, either as a message to him or to inform others about him. Delusions of reference may also relate to actions or gestures made by other people which are thought to convey a message about the patient; for example, a person who touches his hair may be thought by the patient to be signalling that he, the patient, is turning into a woman. Although most delusions of reference have persecutory associations, some relate to grandiose or reassuring themes.

Grandiose delusions

These are beliefs of exaggerated self-importance. The patient may think herself wealthy, endowed with unusual abilities, or a special person. Such expansive ideas occur particularly in mania, and in schizophrenia.

Delusions of guilt

These are found most often in depressive illness, and for this reason are sometimes called **depressive delusions**. Typical themes are that a minor infringement of the law in the past will be discovered and bring shame upon the patient, or that her sinfulness will lead to retribution on her family.

Nihilistic delusions

These are beliefs that some person or thing has ceased, or is about to cease, to exist. Examples include a patient's delusion that he has no money, that his career is ruined or that the world is about to end. Nihilistic delusions are seen in severe depression. Occasionally, nihilistic delusions concern failures of bodily function, often that the bowels are blocked, and often called **Cotard's syndrome** (see p. 221).

Hypochondriacal delusions

These are concerned with illness. The patient believes, wrongly and in the face of all medical evidence to the contrary, that he is suffering from a disease. Such delusions are more common in the elderly, reflecting the increasing concern with health among the people of this age group. Other hypochondriacal delusions are concerned with cancer or venereal disease, or with the appearance of parts of the body, especially the nose. They must be distinguished from the health worries of hypochondriasis (p. 209), which are not delusional.

Delusions of jealousy

These are more common among men than women. Not all jealous ideas are delusions; less intense jealous preoccupations and obsessions are common. Jealous delusions are important because they may lead to aggressive behaviour towards the person(s) thought to be unfaithful. A patient with delusional jealousy is not satisfied if he fails to find evidence supporting his beliefs; his search will continue. These important and potentially dangerous problems are discussed further in Chapter 13.

Sexual or amorous delusions

These are rare, and more frequent in women. Sexual delusions are occasionally secondary to somatic hallucinations felt in the genitalia. A person with amorous delusions believes that she is loved by a man who is usually inaccessible to her, and often of higher social status. In many cases she has never spoken to the person. Erotic delusions are the most prominent feature of **De Clérambault's syndrome** (p. 316).

Delusions of control

A patient who has a delusion of control believes that his actions, impulses, or thoughts are controlled by an outside agency. These are also called **passivity phenomena**. Because the symptom strongly suggests schizophrenia, and has forensic implications, it is important not to record it unless it is definitely present. The symptom may be confused with voluntary obedience to commands from hallucinatory voices, with religious beliefs that God controls human actions, or with a metaphorical view of one's free will. By contrast, a patient with a delusion of control firmly believes that his movements or actions are brought about by an outside agency (other than the divine), and not willed by himself; moreover, there are usually other symptoms of schizophrenia present as well.

Delusions concerning the possession of thoughts

Healthy people take it for granted that their thoughts are their own. They know also that thoughts are private experiences that become known to other people only if spoken aloud, or revealed in writing or through facial expression, gesture, or action. Patients with delusions concerning the possession of thoughts lose these normal convictions in one or more of three ways. All are strongly associated with schizophrenia:

- **Thought insertion** is the delusion that certain thoughts are not the patient's own but implanted by an outside agency. Often there is an associated explanatory delusion, for example, that persecutors have used radio waves to insert the thoughts. This experience must not be confused with that of the obsessional patient who may be distressed by thoughts that he feels are alien to his nature but who never doubts that these thoughts are his own. The patient with a delusion of thought insertion believes that the thoughts are not his own but have been placed into his mind.
- **Thought withdrawal** is the delusion that thoughts have been taken out of the mind. The delusion usually accompanies thought blocking: the patient experiences a sudden break in the flow of thoughts and believes that the 'missing' thoughts have been taken away by some outside agency. Often there are associated explanatory delusions comparable to those accompanying delusions of thought insertion.
- **Thought broadcasting** is the delusion that unspoken thoughts are known to other people through radio, telepathy, or in some other way. Some patients also believe that their thoughts can be heard out loud by other people, a belief which also accompanies the experience of hearing one's own thoughts spoken (*Gedankenlautwerden*), described above.

Obsessional and compulsive symptoms

Obsessions

Obsessions are recurrent persistent thoughts, impulses, or images that enter the mind despite efforts to exclude them. One characteristic feature is the subjective sense of a struggle – the patient resists the obsession, which nevertheless intrudes into awareness. Another characteristic feature is a conviction that to think something is to make it more likely to happen. Obsessions are recognized by the person as her own and not implanted from elsewhere (in contrast to delusions of thought insertion). Another important distinction from delusions is that obsessions are regarded as untrue or senseless. They are generally about matters that the patient finds distressing or otherwise unpleasant and are often but not always accompanied by compulsions (see below).

The presence of resistance is important because, together with the lack of persistent or complete conviction about the truth of the idea, it distinguishes obsessions from delusions. However, in practice this distinction can, in isolation, be more difficult, since the resistance tends to diminish when obsessions have been long-standing; also, when obsessions are very intense, patients may become less certain that they are false. However, a careful history, not only of the symptom but of other relevant features (e.g. compulsions, other evidence of psychosis) should avoid diagnostic difficulties. It is also necessary to distinguish clinically significant obsessions from similar thoughts occurring in healthy people, especially when tired or under stress; this requires evidence of dysfunction and persistence. Obsessional symptoms are also a trait in anankastic personality disorder (p. 139).

Obsessions can take various forms (Table 1.3).

- **Obsessional thoughts** are repeated and intrusive words or phrases which are upsetting to the patient, for example, repeated obscenities or blasphemous phrases coming into the awareness of a religious person.
- **Obsessional ruminations** are repeated worrying themes of a more complex kind, for example, about the ending of the world.

TABLE 1.3 Obsessional and compulsive symptoms

Obsessions
◆ thoughts
◆ ruminations
◆ doubts
◆ impulses
◆ obsessional phobias
Compulsions (rituals)
Obsessional slowness

- **Obsessional doubts** are repeated themes expressing uncertainty about previous actions, for example, whether or not the person turned off an electrical appliance that might cause a fire. Whatever the nature of the doubt, the person realizes that the degree of uncertainty and consequent distress is unreasonable.
- **Obsessional impulses** are repeated urges to carry out actions, usually actions that are aggressive, dangerous, or socially embarrassing. Examples are the urge to pick up a knife and stab another person, to jump in front of a train, or to shout obscenities in church. Whatever the urge, the person has no wish to carry it out, resists it strongly, and does not act on it.
- **Obsessional phobias**. This term denotes an obsessional symptom associated with avoidance as well as anxiety; for example, the obsessional impulse to injure another person with a knife may lead to consequent avoidance of knives. Sometimes obsessional fears of illness are called **illness phobias**.
- **Obsessional slowness**. Many obsessional patients perform actions slowly because their compulsive rituals or repeated doubts take time and distract them from their main purpose. Occasionally, however, the slowness does not seem to be secondary to these other problems but a primary feature of unknown origin.

Although the content (or themes) of obsessions are various, most can be grouped into one or other of six categories:

1. Dirt and contamination
2. Aggression
3. Orderliness
4. Illness
5. Sex
6. Religion.

Thoughts about **dirt and contamination** are usually associated with the idea of harm to others or self through the spread of disease. **Aggressive thoughts** may be about striking another person or shouting angry or obscene remarks in public. Thoughts about **orderliness** may be about the way objects are to be arranged or work is to be organized. Thoughts about **illness** are usually of a fearful kind, for example, a dread of cancer or venereal disease. Obsessional ideas about **sex** usually concern practices that the individual would find shameful. Obsessions about **religion** often take the form of doubts about the fundamentals of belief (e.g. 'does God exist?') or repeated doubts about whether sins have been adequately confessed ('scruples').

Compulsions

Compulsions are repetitive and seemingly purposeful behaviours, performed in a stereotyped way (hence the alternative name of compulsive rituals), in response to an obsession. They are accompanied by a subjective sense that the behaviour must be carried out and by an urge to resist. Like obsessions, compulsions are recognized as senseless. The compulsion usually makes sense given the content of the obsession. For example, a compulsion to wash the hands repeatedly is usually driven by obsessional thoughts that the hands are contaminated. Sometimes obsessional ideas concern the consequences of failing to carry out the compulsion in the 'correct' way, for example, that another person will suffer an accident. Compulsions may cause problems for several reasons:

- They may cause direct harm (e.g. dermatitis from excessive washing).
- They may interfere with normal life because of the time they require.
- Although the compulsive act transiently reduces the anxiety associated with the obsession, in fact the compulsions help maintain the condition. Strategies to reduce them are central to behavioural treatments of obsessive–compulsive disorder.

Compulsive acts are of many kinds, but four are particularly common:

- *Checking rituals* are often concerned with safety, for example checking over and over again that the fire has been turned off, or the doors locked.
- *Cleaning rituals* often take the form of repeated handwashing, but may involve household cleaning.
- *Counting rituals* involve counting in some special way, for example in threes, and are frequently associated with doubting thoughts such that the count must be repeated to make sure that it was carried out adequately in the first place. The counting is usually silent so that an onlooker may be unaware of the ritual.
- In *dressing rituals* the person lays out clothes, or puts them on, in a particular way or order. The ritual is often accompanied by doubting thoughts that lead to seemingly endless repetition.

Overvalued ideas

Overvalued ideas were first described by Wernicke in 1900. An overvalued idea is an isolated, 'acceptable, comprehensible idea pursued by the patient beyond the bounds of reason' (Sims, 2003, p. 143). It may preoccupy and dominate a person's life for many years, and affect their actions. It therefore shares some characteristics of delusions. However, it is essential to distinguish the two types of belief, since their diagnostic implications are very different. Overvalued ideas differ from delusions in three main ways:

- The content of, and basis for, the overvalued idea is usually understandable when the person's background is known, whereas delusions and the person's explanation of them tend to be bizarre. For example, a person whose mother and sister suffered from cancer one after the other may understandably become convinced that cancer is contagious.
- The theme also tends to be culturally common and acceptable, as in the overvalued ideas about body shape which characterize anorexia nervosa.
- With an overvalued idea, there is a small degree of insight and willingness to at least entertain alternative views, albeit this is not persistent and the patient always returns to and retains their belief.

Overvalued ideas must also be distinguished from obsessions; this is usually easier than the distinction from delusions, since there is no sense of intrusiveness or senselessness of the thought, nor resistance to it. Overvalued ideas differ from normal religious beliefs in that the latter are shared by a wider group, arise from religious instruction, and are subject to periodic doubts.

Despite these differences, it can on occasion be difficult to recognize an overvalued idea and distinguish it unequivocally from a delusion, obsession, or normal belief. However, this should not lead often to practical problems because diagnosis depends on more than the presence or absence of a single symptom.

The beliefs concerning body shape and weight held in anorexia nervosa are perhaps the clearest example of overvalued ideas. According to McKenna (1984), the term also applies to abnormal beliefs in many other conditions, including dysmorphophobia, hypochondriasis, paranoid personality disorder, and morbid jealousy. However, it is important to emphasize that overvalued ideas are defined by their form, not their content, and have no inviolable relationship with, or implication for, any particular diagnostic category. Thus, some cases of morbid jealousy are clearly delusional, whilst in hypochondriasis or dysmorphophobia, the belief often has the character of an obsession or a worry, not of an overvalued idea.

Disturbances of thinking processes

Disturbance of the stream of thought

In disturbances of the stream of thought, the amount and the speed of thinking are changed. In **pressure of thought**, ideas arise in unusual variety and abundance and pass through the mind rapidly. In **poverty of thought**, the patient has few thoughts, and these lack variety and richness and seem to move slowly through the mind. Pressure of thought occurs in mania; poverty occurs in depressive disorders. Either may be experienced in schizophrenia. Given that the phenomena are recognized through the person's use of language, they are also known as **pressure of speech** or **poverty of speech**.

Thought block

Sometimes the stream of thought is interrupted suddenly. The patient feels that his mind has gone blank, and an observer notices a sudden interruption in the patient's speech. In a minor degree this experience is common, particularly when tired, anxious or if distracted. In thought blocking, the interruptions are sudden, striking, and repeated, and experienced by the patient as an abrupt and complete emptying of his mind. Thought blocking is an important symptom since it suggests schizophrenia. The diagnostic association with schizophrenia is stronger when the patient interprets the experience in an unusual way, for example, when he says that another person has removed his thoughts.

Disorders of the form of thought

Disorder of the form of thought (also known as **formal thought disorder**) is usually recognized from speech and writing but is sometimes evident from the patient's behaviour; for example, he may be unable to file papers under appropriate category headings. Disorders of the form of thought can be divided into several kinds, as below. Each kind has an association with a particular mental disorder, but none of the associations is strong enough to be diagnostic.

Perseveration

Perseveration is the persistent and inappropriate repetition of the same thoughts. The disorder is detected by examining the person's words or actions. Thus, in response to a series of simple questions, the person may give the correct answer to the first but continue to give the same answer inappropriately to subsequent questions. Perseveration occurs in, but is not limited to, dementia and frontal lobe injury.

Flight of ideas

In flight of ideas, thoughts and speech move quickly from one topic to another so that one train of thought is not carried to completion before another takes its place. The normal logical sequence of ideas is generally preserved, although ideas may be linked by distracting cues in the surroundings and by distractions arising from the words that have been spoken. These verbal distractions are of three kinds: **clang associations** (a second word with a sound similar to the first), **puns** (a second meaning of the first word), and **rhymes**. In practice, the distinction between flight of ideas and loosening of associations (see below) is difficult, especially when the patient speaks rapidly. When this happens it is often helpful to record a sample of speech. Flight of ideas is characteristic of mania.

Loosening of associations

Loosening of associations denotes a loss of the normal structure of thinking. To the interviewer the patient's discourse seems muddled, illogical, or tangential to the matter in hand. It does not become clearer when the patient is questioned further; indeed, the interviewer has the experience that the more he tries to clarify the patient's thinking (or the longer he allows the patient to speak without interruption), the less he understands it. Several specific features of this muddled thinking have been described (see below), but they are difficult to identify with certainty and the most striking clinical impression is often a general lack of clarity, best described by recording an example of the speech and the impression made on the interviewer. This lack of clarity differs from that of people who are anxious or of low intelligence. Anxious people give a more coherent account when they have been put at ease, and people with low intelligence usually express their ideas more clearly when the interviewer simplifies the questions and allows more time for the reply.

Three characteristic kinds of loosening of associations have been described, all of which are seen most often in schizophrenia:

1. In **talking past the point** (*Vorbeireden*) the patient seems always about to get to the end point of the topic in question, but skirts round it and never in fact reaches it.
2. **Knight's move thinking** or **derailment** refers to a transition from one topic to another, either between sentences or in mid-sentence, with no

logical relationship between the two topics and no evidence of the associations described above under flight of ideas.

3. **Verbigeration** is said to be present when speech is reduced to the senseless repetition of sounds, words, or phrases. This abnormality can occur with severe expressive aphasia and occasionally in schizophrenia. When this abnormality is extreme the disorder is called *word salad*.

Other disorders of thinking

Overinclusion refers to a widening of the boundaries of concepts, such that things are grouped together that are not normally regarded as closely connected.

Neologisms are words or phrases, invented by the patient, often to describe a morbid experience. Neologisms must be distinguished from incorrect pronunciation, the wrong use of words by people with limited education, dialect words, obscure technical terms, and the 'private words' that some families invent to amuse themselves. Before deciding that a word is a neologism, the interviewer should ask the patient what he means by it. Neologisms occur most often in chronic schizophrenia.

Depersonalization and derealization

Depersonalization is a change of self-awareness such that the person feels unreal, detached from his own experience and unable to feel emotion. **Derealization** is a similar change in relation to the environment, such that objects appear unreal and people appear as lifeless, two-dimensional 'cardboard' figures. Despite the complaint of inability to feel emotion, both depersonalization and derealization are described as highly unpleasant experiences. These central features are often accompanied by other morbid experiences, including changes in the experience of time, changes in the body image such as a feeling that a limb has altered in size or shape, and occasionally a feeling of being outside one's own body and observing one's own actions, often from above.

Because patients find it difficult to describe the feelings of depersonalization and derealization, they often resort to metaphor and this can lead to confusion between depersonalization and delusional ideas. For example, a patient may say that he feels 'as if part of my brain had stopped working', or 'as if the people I meet are lifeless creatures'. Sometimes careful questioning is required to make the distinction; the 'as if' quality is a useful discriminator.

Depersonalization and derealization are experienced quite commonly by healthy people, especially when tired, as transient phenomena of abrupt onset (Sedman, 1970). The symptoms have been reported after sleep deprivation and sensory deprivation, and as an effect of hallucinogenic drugs. They occur in generalized and phobic anxiety disorders, depressive disorders, schizophrenia, and temporal lobe epilepsy. There is also a rarely used diagnostic category of depersonalization–derealization syndrome.

Motor symptoms and signs

Abnormalities of social behaviour, facial expression, and posture occur frequently in mental disorders of all kinds; motor symptoms and signs can also be side-effects of medication. They are considered in Chapter 3 where the examination of the patient is described. Motor slowing and agitation, which are important features of depressive disorder, are discussed in Chapter 11. With the exception of tics, the specific symptoms listed here are mainly observed in schizophrenia, particularly catatonic schizophrenia (p. 270):

- **Tics** are irregular repeated movements involving a group of muscles, for example, sideways movement of the head or the raising of one shoulder.
- **Mannerisms** are repeated movements that appear to have some functional significance, for example, saluting.
- **Stereotypies** are repeated movements that are regular (unlike tics) and without obvious significance (unlike mannerisms), for example, rocking to and fro.
- **Catatonia** is a state of increased muscle tone affecting extension and flexion and abolished by voluntary movement.
- **Catalepsy (waxy flexibility; flexibiltias cereas)** is a term to describe the tonus in catatonia. It is detected when a patient's limbs can be placed in a position in which they then remain for long periods whilst at the same time muscle tone is uniformly increased. Patients with this abnormality sometimes maintain the head a little way above the pillow in a position that a healthy person could not maintain without extreme discomfort ('psychological pillow'). Catalepsy should not be confused with **cataplexy** (p. 373).
- **Posturing** is the adoption of unusual bodily postures continuously for a long time. The posture may appear to have a symbolic meaning, for example, standing with both arms outstretched as if being crucified, or may have no apparent significance, for example, standing on one leg.

- **Grimacing** has the same meaning as in everyday speech.
- The term **Schauzkrampf** (snout cramp or spasm) denotes pouting of the lips to bring them closer to the nose.
- **Negativism**. Patients are said to show negativism when they do the opposite of what is asked and actively resist efforts to persuade them to comply.
- **Echopraxia** is the imitation of the interviewer's movement automatically even when asked not to do so.
- **Mitgehen** (going along with) describes another kind of excessive compliance in which the patient's limbs can be moved into any position with the slightest pressure.
- **Ambitendence**. Patients are said to exhibit ambitendence when they alternate between opposite movements, for example, putting out the arm to shake hands, then withdrawing it, extending it again, and so on repeatedly.

Disturbances of the body image

The body image or body schema is a person's subjective representation against which the integrity of his body is judged and the movement and positioning of its parts assessed. Specific abnormalities of the body image arise in neurological disorders. These abnormalities include the awareness of a phantom limb after amputation, unilateral lack of awareness or neglect (usually following stroke), **hemisomatognosia** (the person feels, incorrectly, that a limb is missing), and **anosognosia** (lack of awareness of loss of function often of hemiplegia). These abnormalities are described in textbooks of neurology and in Lishman (1998).

Distorted awareness of size and shape of the body occurs occasionally in healthy people when they are tired or falling asleep. The experience, which includes feelings that a limb is enlarging, becoming smaller, or otherwise being distorted, occurs also in migraine, as part of the aura of epilepsy, and after taking LSD. The person is aware that the experience is unreal. However, changes of shape and size of body parts are described by some schizophrenic patients, and in this instance the symptoms are delusional or hallucinatory and there is no insight. **Coenestopathic states** are localized distortions of body awareness, for example, the nose feels as if it is made of cotton wool.

A general distortion of the body image occurs in anorexia nervosa: the patient is convinced that he is fat when in fact he is underweight, sometimes to the point of emaciation.

The **reduplication phenomenon** is the experience that the body has doubled, or that part of the body has done so, for example, that there are two left arms. The experience is reported very occasionally in migraine, temporal lobe epilepsy, and schizophrenia. The related experience of **autoscopic hallucinations** is described on p. 7.

Disturbances of the self

The experience of self has several aspects. It is more than the awareness of the body; we have a feeling of unity between the various aspects of the self; we recognize our activities as our own; we recognize a boundary between the self and the outside world; and we have a feeling of continuity between our past and present selves. The concept of self overlaps with that of the body image. Although the body image is usually experienced as part of the self, it can also be experienced in a more objective way, as when we say 'my leg hurts'. Some of these aspects of the self are changed in certain psychiatric disorders. The experiences are often associated with other abnormal phenomena, so that the account of abnormalities of the self overlaps with several other parts of this chapter.

Disturbances concerned with activities

We take it for granted that, other than in a metaphorical or religious sense, our actions are our own. Patients with delusions of control (see p. 12) lose this awareness. They have the experience that thoughts are not their own and believe instead that they have been inserted from outside. Some patients lose the conviction that their actions are their own and believe instead that they have been imposed by an outside agency.

Disturbed awareness of the unity of the self

Some patients lose the normal experience of existing as a unified being. Patients with **multiple personality disorder** (see p. 213) have the experience of existing as two or more selves, alternating at different times. In the experience of **autoscopy** and the related experience of the *Doppelganger* (see p. 7), the person experiences two selves, present at the same time, but with the conviction that each is a version of the self.

Disturbances of the unity of the self

Although we recognize that we change over time, we retain a conviction of being the same person. Rarely, this feeling of continuity is lost in schizophrenia; a patient may say that he is a different person from the one existing before the disorder began, or that a new self has taken over from the old.

Disturbances of the boundaries of the self

This type of disorder is experienced by some people after taking LSD or other drugs, who may say that they feel as if they were dissolving. Hallucinations can be regarded as involving a loss of awareness of what is within the self and what is located outside. The same inability to determine what is part of the self, and what is not, is seen in passivity phenomena in which actions willed by the patient are experienced as initiated from outside (p. 12).

Disturbances of memory

The features of memory disturbance and its assessment are discussed in detail in Chapters 3 and 14. Here, we introduce some key terms and concepts.

Failure of memory is called **amnesia**. The related term **dysmnesia** is occasionally used. **Paramnesia** is distortion of memory. Several kinds of disturbed memory occur in psychiatric disorders, and it is usual to describe them in terms of the temporal stages which approximate crudely to the scheme of memory derived from psychological research. For discussion, consult a neuropsychology text, or Lishman (1998):

- *Immediate memory* concerns the retention of information over a short period measured in minutes. It is tested clinically by asking the patient to remember a novel name and address and to recall it about five minutes later.
- *Recent memory* concerns events in the last few days. It is tested clinically by asking about events in the patient's daily life which are known also to the interviewer directly or via an informant (for example, what they have eaten) or in the wider environment (for example, well-known news items).
- *Long term (remote) memory* concerns events over longer periods of time. It is tested by asking about events before the presumed onset of memory disorder.

In testing any state of memory, a distinction is made between spontaneous **recall** and **recognition** of information. In some conditions, patients who cannot recall information can recognize it correctly.

Memory loss most commonly occurs in dementia and delirium. It usually affects recall of recent events more than recall of distant ones. In dementia, it usually progresses with time and becomes severe, but rarely total. Some organic conditions give rise to an interesting partial effect known as **amnestic disorder**, in which the person is unable to remember events occurring a few minutes before, but can recall remote events. Total loss of all memory, or selective loss of personal identity, strongly suggests psychogenic causes (see below) or malingering. Some patients with memory disorder recall more when given cues. When this happens, it suggests that the disorder is concerned at least in part with retrieval.

After a period of unconsciousness, memory is impaired for the interval between the ending of complete unconsciousness and the restoration of full consciousness (**anterograde amnesia**). Some causes of unconsciousness (e.g. head injury and electroconvulsive therapy) lead also to inability to recall events before the onset of unconsciousness (**retrograde amnesia**).

Disturbances of recognition

Several **disorders of recognition** occur occasionally in neurological and psychiatric disorders:

- **Jamais vu** is the failure to recognize events that have been encountered before.
- **Déjà vu** is the conviction that an event repeats one that has been experienced in the past when in fact it is novel.
- **Confabulation** is the reporting as memories of events at one time, of events that took place at another time, or never involved the person. It is characteristic of amnestic syndrome.

Recall of events can be biased by the mood at the time of recall. Importantly, in depressive disorders, memories of unhappy events are recalled more readily than other events, a process which adds to the patient's low mood.

Psychogenic amnesia

Psychogenic amnesia is thought to result from an active process of repression which prevents the recall of memories that would otherwise evoke unpleasant emotions. The ideas arose from the study of dissociative amnesia (see p. 213), but the same factors may play a part in some cases of organic amnesia, helping to explain why the return of some memories is delayed longer than others.

False memory syndrome

It is a matter of dispute whether memories can be repressed completely but return many years later. The question arises most often when memories of sexual abuse are reported during psychotherapy by a person who had no recollection of the events before the psychotherapy began, and the events are strongly denied by the alleged abusers. Many clinicians consider that these recollections have been 'implanted' by overzealous questioning; others contend that they are true memories that have previously been completely repressed. Those who hold the latter opinion point to evidence that memories of events other than child abuse can sometimes be completely lost and then regained and also that some recovered memories of child abuse are corroborated subsequently by independent evidence (see Brewin, 2000 for review). Although the quality of the evidence has been questioned, the possibility of complete and sustained repression of memories has not been ruled out. However, it seems likely that only a small minority of cases of 'recovered memory syndrome' can be explained in this way.

Disturbances of consciousness

Consciousness is awareness of the self and the environment. The level of consciousness can vary between the extremes of alertness and coma. The quality of consciousness can also vary: sleep differs from unconsciousness, as does stupor (see below).

- **Coma** is the most extreme form of impaired consciousness. The patient shows no external evidence of mental activity and little motor activity other than breathing. He does not respond even to strong stimuli. Coma can be graded by the extent of the remaining reflex responses and by the type of electroencephologram (EEG) activity.
- **Clouding of consciousness** refers to a state which ranges from barely perceptible impairment to definite drowsiness in which the person reacts incompletely to stimuli. Attention, concentration, and memory are impaired to varying degrees and orientation is disturbed. Thinking seems muddled, and events may be interpreted inaccurately. It is a defining feature of delirium.
- **Stupor**, in the sense used in psychiatry, refers to a condition in which the patient is immobile, mute, and unresponsive but appears to be fully conscious in that the eyes are usually open and follow external objects. If the eyes are closed, the patient resists attempts to open them. Reflexes are normal and resting posture is maintained. It may occur in catatonia. Note that in neurology the term stupor is used differently and generally implies an impairment of consciousness.
- **Confusion** means an inability to think clearly. It occurs characteristically in states of impaired consciousness but it can occur when consciousness is normal. In delirium, confusion occurs together with partial impairment (clouding) of consciousness and other features (p. 329). In the past, delirium was called a confusional state, with the result that the term confusion was also used to mean impairment of consciousness as well as muddled thinking.

Other terms used to describe states of impaired consciousness include:

- **Oneiroid states**, in which there is dream-like imagery although the person is not asleep; if prolonged this may be called a *twilight state*.
- **Torpor**, in which the patient appears drowsy, readily falls asleep, and shows evidence of slow thinking and narrowed range of perception.

In addition, there are sleep–wake disorders that can present with impaired consciousness, such as narcolepsy, in which there are often recurrent, sudden, brief collapses due to loss of muscle tone (**cataplexy**).

Disturbances of attention and concentration

Attention is the ability to focus on the matter in hand. **Concentration** is the ability to maintain that focus. The ability to focus on a selected part of the information reaching the brain is important in many everyday situations, for example, when conversing in a noisy place. It is also important to be able to attend to more than one source of information at the same time, for example, when conversing while driving a car.

Attention and concentration may be impaired in a wide variety of psychiatric disorders including depressive disorders, mania, anxiety disorders, schizophrenia, and organic disorders. Therefore, the finding of abnormalities of attention and concentration does not assist in diagnosis. Nevertheless, these abnormalities are important in management; for example, they affect patients' ability to give or receive information when interviewed, and can interfere with a patient's ability to work, drive a car, or take part in leisure activities.

Insight

In psychopathology, the term insight refers to awareness of morbid change in oneself and a correct attitude to this change including, in appropriate cases, a realization that it signifies a mental disorder. This awareness is difficult for a patient to achieve, since it involves some knowledge of what are the limits of normal mental functioning and mental experience. Also, insight has to be assessed against the background of knowledge and beliefs about psychiatric disorder; it is not the same as complete agreement with the views of the doctor. Insight is also influenced by cultural factors (Saravanan *et al.* 2004).

Although in the past lack of insight was said to be a distinguishing feature between psychosis (where it was said to be absent) and neurosis (where it is present), this distinction is no longer thought to be reliable or useful. The 'lack of insight' in psychosis is better conceptualized in terms of 'impaired reality testing' or 'reality distortion' (see Chapter 12).

Insight is not simply present or absent. It has several facets, each being a matter of degree:

- Is the patient aware of phenomena that others have observed (e.g. that he is unusually active and elated)?
- If so, does he recognize the phenomena as abnormal (rather than, for example, maintaining that his unusual activity and cheerfulness are normal high spirits)?
- If so, does he consider that they are caused by mental illness (as opposed to, say, a physical illness or poison administered by enemies)?
- If so, does he think that he needs treatment?

The answers to these questions are more informative and more reliable than those of the single question, Is insight present or not? (David, 1990). The value of determining the degree of insight is that it helps to predict whether a patient is likely to comply with treatment.

In discussions of psychotherapy, insight has a meaning different from the one considered so far which is used in general psychiatry. In psychotherapy, insight is the capacity to understand one's own motives and to be aware of previously unconscious aspects of mental activity. The term **intellectual insight** is sometimes used to denote the capacity to formulate this understanding, whereas **emotional insight** is the term for the capacity to feel and respond to the understanding.

Further reading

Berrios, GE (1996) *The history of mental symptoms*. Cambridge, Cambridge University Press. (A fascinating history of descriptive psychopathology.)

Jamison, KR (1996) *An unquiet mind*. Knopf, New York. (A valuable insight into the subjective experience of manic-depressive disorder.)

Jaspers, K (1963) *General psychopathology* (trans. from the 7th German edition by J. Hoenig and M. W. Hamilton), Manchester, Manchester University Press. (The classic work on the subject. Chapter 1 is particularly valuable, read in whole or in part.)

Sims, A (2003) *Symptoms in the mind; an introduction to descriptive psychopathology*, 3rd edn, Elsevier Science, London. (A comprehensive modern text.)

CHAPTER 2

Classification and diagnosis

Chapter contents

Chapter 1 outlined the symptoms and signs of psychiatric disorder. In Chapter 3 we describe the psychiatric assessment, by which these symptoms and signs are elicited, interpreted, and used as the basis upon which psychiatric diagnoses are made. However, before doing so, in this chapter we discuss the principles of psychiatric diagnosis and classification, since this provides the framework within which this clinical process happens.

Classification is needed in psychiatry for several purposes:

- To enable clinicians to communicate with one another about the diagnoses given to their patients.
- To understand the implications of these diagnoses, in terms of their symptoms, prognosis, treatment, and sometimes aetiology.
- To relate findings of clinical research to patients seen in everyday practice.
- To facilitate epidemiological studies and the collection of reliable statistics.
- To ensure that research can be conducted with comparable groups of subjects.

Of these, the first three are the most relevant to clinical practice. Indeed, it is difficult to imagine how psychiatry could be practised in any reasonable or evidence-based manner without the order which classification provides. In this respect, the position of classification as one of the fundamental building blocks of psychiatry is no different from that in the rest of medicine. However, in other respects, psychiatric classification does raise particular challenges and controversies, largely as a consequence of the uncertain aetiology of many disorders. These difficulties are of two kinds. The first is conceptual, relating to the nature of mental illness and what, if anything, should be classified. The second is practical, relating to how categories are defined and organized into a classificatory scheme. In this chapter, the conceptual issues and criticisms are covered first, followed by a historical perspective to classification. We then describe and compare the two schemes in widespread use at present – Chapter V of the ICD-10, and DSM-IV—and the organizing principles on which they are based.

Concepts of mental illness

In everyday speech the word 'illness' is used loosely. Similarly, in psychiatric practice, the term 'mental illness' is used with little precision, and often synonymously with 'mental disorder'. In this context, 'mental' and 'psychiatric' are also used interchangeably.

A good definition of mental illness is difficult to achieve, for both practical and philosophical reasons, as outlined here. In routine clinical work the difficulty is important mainly in relation to ethical and legal issues such as compulsory admission to hospital. In forensic psychiatry the definition of mental illness (by the law) is particularly important in the assessment of issues such as criminal responsibility.

Diverse discussion of the concepts of mental illness can be found in Lazare (1973), Kendell (1975), Häfner (1987), and Clare (1997).

Definitions of mental illness

Many attempts have been made to define mental illness. None is satisfactory nor uniformly accepted. A common approach is to examine the concept of illness in general medicine and to identify any analogies with mental illness. In general medicine there are five types of definition:

- **Absence of health.** This approach changes the emphasis of the problem but does not solve it, because health is even more difficult to define. The World Health Organization, for example, defined health as 'a state of complete physical, mental and social well-being, and not merely the absence of disease or infirmity'. As Lewis (1953) rightly commented, 'a definition could hardly be more comprehensive than that, or more meaningless'. Many other definitions of health have been proposed, all equally unsatisfactory.
- **Disease is what doctors treat.** This definition has the attraction of simplicity, but does not really address the issue. The notion that disease is what doctors *can* treat has somewhat more merit, since there is evidence that as a medical treatment for a condition becomes available, for example for alcoholism or obesity, it becomes more likely that the condition will be considered as a disease (Campbell *et al.*, 1979).
- **Biological disadvantage.** Defining disease in terms of biological disadvantage was proposed by Scadding (1967) and is the most extreme biomedical view of disease. Scadding never defined biological disadvantage, but it has been used in psychiatry to include decreased fertility (reproductive fitness) and increased mortality. Viewing disease in terms of 'evolutionary disadvantage' is a similar concept (Wakefield, 1992).
- **Pathological process.** Some extreme theorists, such as Szasz (1960), take the view that illness can be defined only in terms of **physical** pathology. Since most mental disorders do not have demonstrable physical pathology, this view they are not illnesses. Szasz takes the further step of asserting that most mental disorders are therefore not the province of doctors. This kind of argument can be sustained only by taking an extremely narrow view of pathology. It is also arbitrary, based on current knowledge, and is increasingly incompatible with the evidence of a genetic and neurobiological basis to the major psychiatric disorders, and their associated morbidity and mortality.
- **Presence of suffering.** This approach has some practical value because it defines a group of people likely to consult doctors. A disadvantage is that the term cannot be applied to everyone who would usually be regarded as ill in everyday terms. For example, patients with mania may feel unusually well and may not experience suffering, though most people would regard them as mentally ill.

Biomedical versus social concepts

The above concepts may be divided into those that view mental illnesses in purely biomedical terms, and those that consider them to be social constructs or value judgements. This debate is still ongoing, and depends in part on one's opinion about their aetiology, but it is now generally accepted that value judgements play a part in all diagnoses, even if the disorders themselves are considered from a biomedical perspective (Fulford, 1989). For example, beliefs and emotions are central to most psychiatric disorders, yet it is a value judgement as to whether a given belief or emotion is 'good or bad', and therefore what, if any, diagnostic significance it has.

Impairment, disability, and handicap

It is useful in medicine, and particularly in psychiatry, to describe and classify the consequences of a disorder; this approach is related to the concept of disease as involving dysfunction (Wakefield, 1992), as incorporated into the definitions of mental disorder used in ICD10 and DSM-IV (see below). Three related terms, derived from medical sociology and social psychology, are used to describe the harmful consequences of a disorder:

1. **Impairment**, referring to a pathological defect. For example, hemiparesis after a stroke.
2. **Disability** is the limitation of physical or psychological function arising from an impairment; for example, difficulties in self-care caused by the hemiparesis.
3. **Handicap** refers to the resulting social dysfunction. For example, being unable to work because of the hemiparesis.

Incapacity may be seen as another harmful consequence of illness, though the term usually refers in a legal sense to the effect which illness has on one's competence to make treatment decisions (see Chapter 4).

Diagnoses, diseases, and disorders

The term 'diagnosis' has two somewhat different meanings. It has a general meaning of 'telling one thing apart from another', but in medicine it has also acquired a more specific meaning of 'knowing the underlying cause' of the symptoms and signs about which the patient is complaining. Underlying causes are expressed in quite different terms from the symptoms. Thus, the symptoms of acute appendicitis are quite different from the idea that will form in the mind of the doctor that the appendix is inflamed and producing peritoneal irritation. To be able to make a diagnosis of this type is, of course, satisfying for the doctor and very useful for the patient, since it immediately suggests what investigations and treatment are needed. Its clear utility also makes redundant most theoretical or philosophical concerns about classification. Unfortunately, it is rarely possible to arrive at this type of diagnosis with most psychiatric patients. The only exception is, by definition, 'organic' psychiatric disorders (see below).

The lack of clear disease categories, in a medical sense, has led to the use of the more general term 'disorder' in psychiatry. The definition of a disorder in ICD-10 is:

> 'a clinically recognizable set of symptoms or behavior associated in most cases with distress and with interference with personal functions. Social deviance or conflict alone, without personal dysfunction, should not be included in mental disorder as defined here.'

The DSM-IV definition is longer but similar:

> 'a clinically significant behavioral or psychological syndrome or pattern that occurs in an individual and that is associated with present distress (a painful symptom) or disability (impairment of one or more important areas of functioning) or with a significantly increased risk of suffering death, pain, disability, or an important loss of freedom. In addition, this syndrome or pattern must not be merely an expectable response to a particular event, e.g. the death of a loved one. Whatever its original cause, it must currently be considered a manifestation of a behavioral, psychological, or biological dysfunction in the individual. Neither deviant behavior (e.g. political, religious, or sexual) nor conflicts that are primarily between the individual and society are mental disorders unless the deviance or conflict is a symptom of a dysfunction in the individual, as described above.'

Despite the similarity there is one important and easily overlooked difference between the two definitions. 'Interference with personal functions' in ICD-10 refers only to such things as personal care and one's immediate environment; it does not extend to interference with work and other social roles. In DSM-IV 'impairment of one or more important areas of functioning' refers to *all* types of functioning.

Both definitions illustrate that most psychiatric disorders are not based upon theoretical concepts or presumptions about aetiology, but upon recognizable clusters of symptoms and behaviours (Kendler, 1990). This reliance also explains much of the debate about the reliability and validity of the categories being classified, as discussed later in this chapter.

Criticisms of classification

Despite its advantages, the use of psychiatric classification is on occasion criticized as being inappropriate or even harmful. In part, such criticisms stem from the various controversies outlined above: if the concept of mental disorder is itself disputed, then so will any classifications thereof. These criticisms were most prevalent and trenchant at the height of the 'anti-psychiatry' movement in the 1950s and 1960s. Three main criticisms were made:

- Allocating patients to a diagnostic category distracts from the understanding of their unique personal difficulties. The use of classification can certainly be combined with consideration of a patient's unique qualities; indeed, it is important to combine the two because these qualities can modify prognosis and should be taken into account in treatment. The critics of standard classifications have themselves used idiosyncratic classifications with their own technical terms as a means of summarizing information.

BOX 2.1 STIGMA

People stigmatize others when they judge them not on their personal qualities but on the basis of a mark or label which assigns them to a feared or unfavoured group. The tendency to stigmatize seems to be deeply rooted in human nature as a way of responding to people who appear or behave differently. Stigmatization is based on fear that those who seem different may behave in threatening or unpredictable ways, and it is reduced when it becomes clear that the stigmatized person is unlikely to behave in the ways that were expected.

Stigma in psychiatry People fear mental illness and they stigmatize those who are affected by it. The reasons, which are complex, include the notion that people with mental illness cannot control their own behaviour, and that they may act in odd, unpredictable and possibly violent ways. Thus they are seen as directly threatening and perhaps also as indirectly threatening because their lack of self control threatens our belief in our ability to control our actions. Whatever the underlying psychological mechanisms, fear of mental illness makes people react to all mentally ill persons in the same cautious and unfavourable way, that is to stigmatize them.

Diagnoses, as labels, have the potential to be stigmatizing; for example leprosy and AIDS. It has been suggested that the stigma of mental illness would be reduced if diagnoses such as schizophrenia were abandoned, but this proposal misses the point that the basis of stigma is fear and simply removing the label does not reduce the fear. The mentally ill were stigmatized long before modern diagnostic terms were in use, and people who fear mental illness invent their own labels, such as 'nutter', which are far more stigmatizing than a diagnosis. To reduce stigma it is necessary to reduce fear, and this requires accurate information about mental illness and better understanding of mentally ill people.

Concern about dangerousness is a major component of psychiatric stigma. Other important components (Crisp *et al.*, 2000) are the ideas that:

- people with mental illness feel different from the rest of us
- it is hard to talk to them
- mental illness cannot be cured
- it does not recover.

These beliefs make people draw back from those with mental illness and discourage people from talking to the mentally ill. Hence they do not learn that their original assumptions about such people were wrong. Fear of being stigmatized adds greatly to the problems of people with mental illness. It discourages them from seeking help at an early stage, and from sharing their distress with relatives and friends. Stigma also has wider social effects: for example, it makes it harder for mentally ill people to obtain work, or to marry and have children. For some, efforts to conceal their condition, in order to avoid stigma, may create almost as great a burden as is created by the illness. Stigmatization may also affect the allocation of resources for the care of people with mental illness, with a reluctance to fund care in the community or to give appropriate priority to services generally.

Reducing stigma The misperceptions and prejudices underlying stigma are susceptible to public education. Campaigns to reduce stigma generally include:

- information about the true nature of mental illness, and about the low frequency of dangerous behaviour,
- encouragement to persuade public figures who have had a mental illness to speak publically about their experiences, and
- a focus on young people whose attitudes may be less fixed than those of their elders.

While stigma can be reduced, it cannot be done easily or quickly. In the past, epileptic people were stigmatized but as knowledge of the condition spread and as treatment improved, attitudes gradually changed. Changes are now beginning to be seen in the stigma attached to depressive disorders and Alzheimer's disease, though not yet with schizophrenia to any extent. Thus there is an ongoing need for public education campaigns to reduce the fear and misunderstanding that perpetuates stigma. For a comprehensive review of stigma, see Crisp (2004).

- Some sociologists have argued that to allocate a person to a diagnostic category is simply to label deviant behaviour as illness. They argue that such labelling serves only to increase the person's difficulties. There can be no doubt that terms such as epilepsy or schizophrenia attract stigma (see Box 2.1), but this does not lessen the reality of disorders that cause suffering and require treatment. It does, however, emphasize that mental illness should not be defined solely in terms of socially deviant behaviour. For example, the argument is often made that someone must have been mentally ill or 'sick' to commit a cruel murder. Although such behaviour is highly unusual, there is no justification for equating it with mental illness; the presence of the latter must be separately established based on the psychiatric history and mental state examination. Moreover, if mental illness is inferred from socially deviant behaviour alone, political abuse may result (see below). A further reason for excluding social criteria from the definition of mental illness, and from diagnostic criteria, is that many behaviours are appraised differently in different countries and at different times. For example, homosexuality was considered as a mental disorder until the 1970s.

- Individuals do not fit neatly into the available categories. Whilst it is not feasible to classify a minority of disorders (or patients), this is not a reason for abandoning classification for the majority.

It is certainly true that at times classification has been inappropriately used as part of a broader abuse of psychiatry, whether for political, financial or other reasons. A serious example occurred in the Soviet Union, where some psychiatrists colluded with the government in being willing to classify political dissent as evidence of mental illness. Widespread condemnation led the World Psychiatric Association to take a lead in setting out ethical rules that would reduce the risk of further abuses.

Whilst such abuses are fortunately rare, they are an extreme illustration of the fact that making diagnoses and classifying patients are not neutral acts, but carry significant ethical and other implications (Chapter 4). One of these concerns **stigma**, which remains a serious problem for patients with mental health problems, even if one does not accept the rest of the sociological thesis outlined above (Byrne, 2000). The issue of stigma in psychiatry is discussed in Box 2.1. It is incumbent on psychiatrists, and all others using psychiatric diagnostic terms, that they do so appropriately, paying due attention to their correct usage, the purpose, and the context in which they are being applied. Doing so can help reduce the problem of stigmatization, but cannot solve it because stigma results from many other factors too, as noted.

Although these criticisms are important, they are arguments only against the improper use of classification. Disorders such as epilepsy and schizophrenia, and their harmful consequences, cannot be made to disappear by ceasing to give names to them. The ICD-10 and DSM-IV, discussed later, emphasize that classification is a means of communication and a guide to decision-making, but acknowledge that they are provisional and imperfect schemes. Clinicians and researchers must use their experience and common sense, as well as being guided by the descriptions of the disorders that make up the classifications. In addition to the clinical advantages of classification, it is useful in understanding the management of mental problems in relation to crime, decisions about health care rationing or other planning, in deciding grounds for insurance claims, and for informed discussion of the abuse of psychiatry for political purposes.

Other criticisms of classification in psychiatry are mostly concerned with the specifics, not the principles – for example, whether diagnostic categories are reliable and valid. These issues are introduced later in this chapter, and at various points throughout the book.

The history of classification

Efforts to classify abnormal mental states have occurred since antiquity. One reason for including a chronological perspective here is that contemporary psychiatric classifications are, in part, a hybrid of various historical themes and opinions.

The early Greek medical writings contained descriptions of different manifestations of mental disorder, for example, excitement, depression, confusion, and memory loss. This simple classification was adopted by Roman medicine and developed by the Greek physician Galen, whose system of classification remained in use until the eighteenth century.

Interest in the classification of natural phenomena developed in the eighteenth century, partly stimulated by the publication of a classification of plants by Linnaeus, a medically qualified professor of botany who also devised a less well-known classification of diseases in which one major class was mental disorders. Many classifications were proposed, notably one published in 1772 by William Cullen, a Scottish physician. He grouped mental disorders together, apart from delirium which he classified with febrile conditions. In his scheme, mental disorders were part of a broad class of 'neuroses', a term he used to denote diseases affecting the nervous system (Hunter and McAlpine, 1963). Cullen's classification contained an aetiological principle – that mental illnesses were disorders of the nervous system – as well as a descriptive principle for distinguishing individual clinical syndromes within the neuroses. In Cullen's usage, the term neurosis covered the whole range of mental disorders as well as many neurological conditions; the modern narrower usage developed later (see below).

In the early years of the nineteenth century, several French writers published influential classifications. Phillipe Pinel's *Treatise on insanity*, which appeared in an English edition in 1806, divided mental disorders into mania with delirium, mania without delirium, melancholia, dementia, and idiocy. One of Pinel's compatriots, Esquirol, wrote another widely read textbook, published in English in 1845. Esquirol added a new category, 'monomania', which was characterized by 'partial insanity', in which there were fixed false ideas that could not be changed by logical reasoning. Esquirol divided monomania into subgroups including reasoning monomania, erotic monomania, incendiary monomania, homicidal monomania, and monomania resulting from drunkenness. Like other psychiatrists of the time, Pinel and Esquirol did not discuss neuroses (in the modern sense) or behaviour disorders because physicians generally treated these conditions.

Meanwhile, in Germany, Kahlbaum formulated two requirements for research on classification: that the entire course of a mental illness was fundamental to the definition of that illness, and that the total clinical picture must be used in formulating definitions in a system of classification. These ideas were adopted by Kraepelin, who thereby made the important distinction between manic depressive psychosis (bipolar disorder) and schizophrenia (see Box 12.3, p. 274). The successive editions of Kraepelin's textbook led to further refinements in the classification of mental illness that are the basis of today's systems.

At the same time, separate developments in the emerging specialty of neurology led to decreasing medical interest in the 'nervous patient', a term used throughout the nineteenth century in Britain and North America (Bynum, 1985) to refer to a large group of patients with varied complaints. These were gradually seen as a part of the new specialty of psychiatry alongside the major mental illnesses. The writings of Freud and his contemporaries led to greater recognition of the psychological causes of nervous symptoms and 'neurotic' disorders, and to the modern concepts of hysteria and anxiety disorder. See Pichot (1994) for a review of nosological models in psychiatry.

Organizing principles of contemporary classifications

As well as these historical roots, it is worth considering the major issues that contemporary classifications have faced regarding their organizing principles.

Organic and functional

The first issue concerns the distinction conventionally drawn between organic and functional disorders. **Organic disorders** are those which arise from a demonstrable cerebral or systemic pathological process; the core disorders are dementia, delirium, and the various neuropsychiatric syndromes (Lishman, 1998). '**Functional**' is thereby an umbrella or default term for all other psychiatric disorders. The organic–functional dichotomy has two main implications for classification.

1. It has a philosophical dimension, being inextricably linked to dualism and concepts of mind and body. At its extreme, the implication is that functional disorders have no biological basis, whilst psychological and social factors are irrelevant for organic disorders. This polarization may encourage psychiatrists who are either 'mindless' or 'brainless', rather than seeing that both aspects of aetiology always make a contribution (Eisenberg, 1986a; Anonymous, 1994).
2. It has practical implications, since 'organic' defines disorders aetiologically, whereas all other psychiatric disorders are purely descriptive and based on clusters of symptoms and signs. This leads to inconsistencies and difficulties at the intersection.

There is general agreement that for these and other reasons, the organic–functional dichotomy is neither valid nor helpful and should be abandoned (Spitzer *et al.*, 1992). However, it has proved more difficult to come up with an alternative. The ways in which ICD-10 and DSM-IV have dealt with the issue is discussed below and in Chapter 14.

Neurosis and psychosis

In the past, the concepts of psychosis and neurosis were important in most systems of classification. Though neither is used as an organizing principle in ICD-10 or DSM-IV, in everyday clinical practice these terms are still useful as general descriptors, so it is of relevance to understand their history.

Psychosis

The term **psychosis** was suggested by Feuchterleben who, in 1845, published a book entitled *Principles of medical psychology*. This author proposed psychosis as a term for severe mental disorders. He also accepted the term neurosis for mental disorders as a whole; thus he wrote, 'every psychosis is at the same time a neurosis but not every neurosis is a psychosis' (Hunter and MacAlpine, 1963, p. 950). As the concept of neurosis was narrowed, psychoses ceased to be subgroups of neuroses and were regarded as independent conditions. Many of the difficulties encountered today in defining the terms neurosis and psychosis are related to these origins.

In modern usage, the term psychosis refers broadly to severe psychiatric disorders, including schizophrenia, and some organic and affective disorders. Numerous criteria have been proposed to achieve a more precise definition, but there are problems with all of them. Greater severity of illness is a common suggestion, but some cases are relatively mild (and some neuroses are severe and at least as disabling). Lack of insight is often suggested as a criterion, but insight itself is very difficult to define (see pp. 19–20). A somewhat more straightforward criterion is the inability to distinguish between subjective experience and external reality, as shown by the presence of delusions and hallucinations. However, as well as the problems fully defining these terms (ICD-10 even avoids defining 'delusion'), the label 'psychosis' is unsatisfactory because the conditions embraced by the term have little in common and it is usually more informative to classify the particular disorder concerned. For these reasons, the neurosis–psychosis distinction, which was a fundamental organizing principle (until ICD-9), has been abandoned in the current ICD and DSM classifications.

Nevertheless, although psychosis has lost its classificatory eminence, it is still a convenient term for disorders that are usually severe, and which feature delusions, hallucinations, or unusual or bizarre behaviour, especially when a more precise diagnosis cannot yet be made. The adjectival form is also useful, and survives in ICD-10 and DSM-IV in categories such as 'psychotic disorders not otherwise specified'. Other examples are the use of the descriptive terms 'psychotic symptom' and 'antipsychotic drugs'.

Neurosis

As noted, the term **neurosis** was introduced by Cullen to denote diseases of the nervous system. Gradually the category of neurosis narrowed, first as neurological disorders with a distinct neuropathology (such as epilepsy and stroke) were removed, and later with the development of a separate category of psychosis.

The objections to the term neurosis are similar to the objections to the term psychosis, and explain its removal as an organizing principle in current classification. That is, the concept is difficult to define (Gelder, 1986); second, the conditions that neurosis embraces have little in common, and third, more information can be conveyed by using a more specific and descriptive diagnosis, such as anxiety disorder. A further objection is that neurosis has been widely used with the assumption of an aetiological meaning in the psychodynamic literature, but lacking scientific evidence for these assumptions the term is unsuitable for a classification that is to be useful internationally in general psychiatry.

In the same way as for psychosis, the terms 'neurosis' and neurotic remain useful as simple descriptors, to indicate disorders that are often comparatively mild, and usually associated with some form of anxiety or marked tension, especially if the specific disorder cannot yet be determined. Reflecting its familiarity and utility, ICD-10 retains the adjective in the heading of one group of disorders: 'Neurotic, stress-related, and somatoform disorders'. In DSM-IV, even the adjective is not used.

Categories, dimensions, and multiple axes

Categorical classification

Traditionally, psychiatric disorders have been classified by dividing them into categories which are supposed to represent discrete clinical entities. As already noted, in the absence of knowledge of underlying pathology, these categories can only be defined in terms of symptom patterns and course. Such categorization facilitates the decisions that have to be made in clinical work about treatment and management, but has two problems:

1. Although definitions and descriptions can be agreed upon (to improve **reliability**, see below), the criteria are often arbitrary. There is uncertainty about the extent to which these categories represent distinct entities or 'carve Nature at her joints' (**validity**, see below).
2. A significant proportion of patients do not closely match the descriptions of any disorder, or meet criteria for two or more categories (**comorbidity**, see below).

These are all significant points, and addressed further in the following sections. However, a more satisfactory practical alternative system has not yet been devised.

Dimensional classification

Dimensional classification does not use separate categories, but characterizes the subject by means of scores on two or more dimensions. In the past, Kretschmer and several other psychiatrists advocated it, and more recently it was strongly promoted by the psychologist Eysenck, on the grounds that there is no systematic, objective evidence to support the existence of discrete categories. Eysenck (1970b) proposed a system of three dimensions: psychoticism, neuroticism, and introversion–extroversion. By means of answers to questionnaires, patients are scored on each of these three axes. For example, in the case of a person with a disorder that would be assigned to dissociative disorder in a categorical system, in Eysenck's system the person would be likely to have high scores on the axes of neuroticism and extroversion, and a low psychoticism score. Eysenck's three dimensions were established by various procedures of multivariate analysis, using data from large numbers of normal individuals rather than psychiatric patients. The dimensions are attractive in theory, but it should be remembered that they depend considerably on a number of initial assumptions and the choice of subjects and methods. There is a major problem with the dimension of 'psychoticism', which bears little relation to the concept of psychosis as generally used. For example, artists and prisoners score highly on this dimension.

The concept of dimensionality has most recently been revived by epidemiological surveys that have emphasized that there is a continuum between the healthy population and those with diagnosed psychiatric disorders. This applies, for example, to psychotic symptoms and argues that even a severe disorder such as schizophrenia is in fact a dimensional construct (Stefanis *et al.*, 2002). The dimensional view of psychiatric disorder is comparable to that of hypertension and other medical diagnoses that are really extremes of a normal distribution, and it reflects the nature of the underlying genetic predisposition (as a **quantitative trait**, see Chapter 5) much better than a categorical view of disease. However, the problem with dimensions is that they are not of great value in clinical practice. For every patient, yes/no decisions need to be made, the most critical being whether the person requires treatment; this decision is in turn based on whether they have a disorder meriting treatment, and if so which one. These clinical imperatives strongly favour categorical approaches to classification (see van Os *et al.*, 1999 for an alternative view).

The multi-axial approach

The term **multi-axial** is applied to schemes of classifications in which two or more separate sets of information (such as symptoms, aetiology, and personality type) are coded. Essen-Møller was probably the first to propose such a system for use in psychiatry, using one axis for the clinical syndrome and another for aetiology (Essen-Møller, 1971). Multi-axial classification is now integral to DSM-IV and available within ICD-10 (see below). However, though attractive for several reasons, there is a danger that multi-axial schemes are too complicated and time-consuming to be suitable for everyday use, especially if the clinical utility of each axis (e.g. in terms of affecting management or outcome) has not been demonstrated.

Hierarchies of diagnosis

Categorical systems often include an implicit hierarchy of categories. If two or more disorders are present it has been conventional (though not always made explicit) to assume that one takes precedence and is regarded as the main disorder for the purposes of treatment and recording. For example, organic disorders 'trump' schizophrenia, and schizophrenia takes precedence over mood disorders. This type of assumption is justified because there is some clinical evidence for an inbuilt hierarchy of significance between the disorders. For instance, anxiety symptoms occur commonly with depressive disorders and are sometimes the presenting feature. If the anxiety is treated, there is little response, but if the depressive disorder is treated, there may be improvement in anxiety as well as in the depressive symptoms. These points may be important in making decisions about the order of treatment to be used and in deciding which disorder to record in service statistics if only one is required. Nevertheless, they must not obscure the importance of noting in the case-record all disorders and symptoms that are present, and how they change with time and treatment.

Comorbidity

Recently, less emphasis has been placed on hierarchies of diagnosis, with greater weight being placed on comorbidity (also called **dual diagnosis**). This has occurred for three reasons. First, because research has shown that comorbidity is very common (Kessler 2004); for example, about 50 per cent of patients with major depressive disorder also meet criteria for an anxiety disorder. Second, because it encourages the clinician to focus on all the various disorders which may be present, and not assume that the disorder highest in the hierarchy is necessarily the only, or even the most important, target for treatment. The advent of multi-axial systems of classification, mentioned above, in part reflects this perspective. Third, the diagnostic 'rules' used in current classificatory systems (especially DSM-IV) encourage multiple diagnoses to be made, and it has been argued that at least some psychiatric comorbidity is in fact an artefact of this (Maj, 2005).

The term comorbidity covers two different circumstances:

- **Disorders that are currently considered distinct but are probably causally related.** In other words, there is one disease process, but two or more clinical manifestations, which are currently diagnosed separately due to lack of knowledge or because of clinical convention. For example, a patient with a depressive disorder and an anxiety disorder. Research suggests that this is the commonest form of comorbidity (Krueger 1999).
- **Disorders that are causally unrelated.** That is, the chance co-occurrence of two disorders. For example, the onset of presenile dementia in a person with long-standing panic disorder.

Note that comorbidity applies only when criteria for two or more diagnoses are met. It should not be used for patients who fall between diagnostic categories but who do not meet the criteria for any one.

Reliability and validity

Reliability of psychiatric diagnoses

A prerequisite for any satisfactory classification scheme, whatever its organizing principle, is that the items (diagnoses) being classified can be recognized reliably (Kendell, 1975). However, although reliability is now known and is reasonable for most categories, this was not the case until relatively recently, for reasons described below. Studies done in the 1950s and 1960s demonstrated substantial diagnostic disagreement between psychiatrists, arising for two main reasons (Kreitman, 1961):

- **The interviewing technique and characteristics of the psychiatrist.** This included the way in which symptoms and signs were elicited and interpreted and the weight attached to them. These elements in turn reflected many influences, including training, professional culture, etc. For example, when shown filmed interviews, American psychiatrists reported many more symptoms than did British psychiatrists (Sandifer *et al.*, 1968).
- **The differing use of diagnostic terms and criteria.** Until relatively recently, there were no widely accepted glossaries or definitions of key terms. Therefore, it was impossible to ensure that psychiatrists were using the same criteria for symptoms and syndromes. A key study was by Stengel (1959), who illustrated 'the chaotic state of the classifications in current use' by collecting 28 classifications in a variety of languages, of which 11 were 'official, semi-official or national classifications', and 17 had been produced on a more individual basis but were considered worthy of note. None of the 28 was accompanied by any indication of the meaning of the constituent terms.

Illustrating the importance of these factors, a study in Philadelphia concluded that 62 per cent of diagnostic disagreement arose from inadequate use of diagnostic labels, 32 per cent from inadequate interview technique, and only 5 per cent was due to inconsistency in the patient (Ward *et al.*, 1962).

International studies of psychiatric diagnostic criteria

The work of Stengel (1959), and increasing concern in the 1960s about the level of diagnostic disagreement between countries, heralded international studies intended to identify the source of the variation in diagnostic practice, and then to improve the reliability. This work adopted the suggestion of the philosopher Hempel that **operational definitions** should be developed; that is, the specification of a category (e.g. a symptom) by a series of precise inclusion and exclusion statements.

A key study was the US–UK Diagnostic Study (Cooper *et al.*, 1972), which followed on from the demonstration that both diagnostic and admission rates for manic depression and schizophrenia differed considerably between the two countries. For example, the rate for manic-depressive illness in the UK was more than ten times that in equivalent mental hospitals in the USA, whereas the rate for schizophrenia was about twice as high in the USA compared to the UK (Kramer *et al.* 1969). Further investigation suggested that New York was atypical, with diagnostic practice at other places in North America being more similar to that in Britain.

Another seminal study was the International Pilot Study of Schizophrenia (IPSS), a large international collaborative study organized by the World Health Organization. Centres in nine countries took part: Colombia (Cali), Czechoslovakia (Prague), Denmark (Aarhus), England (London), India (Agra), Nigeria (Ibadan), Taiwan (Taipei), the USA (Washington) and the

Russia (Moscow). The IPSS was the first study to demonstrate clearly that structured interviews could be translated and used in different cultures, enabling it to show that patients with typical schizophrenic symptoms could be found in all nine countries (World Health Organization, 1973). The IPSS findings are discussed further in Chapter 12.

Standardized interview schedules

A major step towards improving diagnostic reliability came with the development of standardized interview schedules that minimize the variations in interviewing technique and rating levels between psychiatrists (discussed in Chapter 3). This is achieved by specifying the content and sequence of the interview, and by providing scoring rules by which the presence and severity of symptoms are rated. The development of standardized interview schedules was closely linked with the international studies mentioned above. Thus, the US-UK Diagnostic Study used the Present State Examination (PSE), one of the first structured psychiatric interviews (Wing *et al.*, 1974).

Standardized interview schedules are now widely used. Both specialist and lay forms are available, for use in different settings and with different populations. Further examples are given in Chapter 3.

Diagnosis by computer

The IPSS also revealed that although a great deal of the differences between psychiatrists in the rating of symptoms could be removed by the use of structured interviews, some variation remained in the resulting diagnoses. This was because of different diagnostic interpretations of the symptoms and behaviours. This led to the development of computer programmes such DIAGNO (Spitzer and Endicott, 1968) and CATEGO (Wing *et al.*, 1974), that generate a diagnosis using the symptom ratings, eliminating both the personal bias of the diagnosticians and any chance errors made for other reasons. Though computer-generated diagnoses inevitably reflect the diagnostic preferences of whoever wrote the program, they have proved valuable for epidemiological studies and are widely used in research.

Validity of psychiatric diagnoses

The above discussion has centred upon the reliability of diagnoses, because without a reasonable level of inter-observer reliability, it is not possible to test whether or not a concept is valid. Validity is a much more difficult topic; in a general sense, validity refers to the extent to which a concept means what it is supposed to mean; it is also closely connected with usefulness (utility).

Three forms of validity are usually recognized.

1. **Face validity:** the correspondence with the clinical concepts and descriptions currently accepted in clinical practice; this is fairly easy to achieve by the careful use of glossaries and lists of criteria (illustrating that reliability and validity are not wholly separate).
2. **Predictive validity:** the extent to which disorders predict response to treatment and outcome; this has high utility.
3. **Construct validity:** the third and most fundamental form of validity, in which there is a demonstrable relationship between a disorder and its underlying aetiology and pathophysiology. Unfortunately, most psychiatric disorders have an unknown and probably low construct validity, reflecting the descriptive criteria upon which most are currently based.

To date, little progress has actually been made towards establishing the validity of the existing schemes of classification. For further discussions of reliability and validity in psychiatry, see Kendell (1975), Spitzer and Williams (1985), and Jablensky and Kendell (2003).

Current psychiatric classifications

The International Classification of Diseases (ICD), Chapter V

The International Classification of Diseases (ICD) is produced by the World Health Organization (WHO) as an aid to the collection of international statistics about disease. The system is revised every few years and the present edition is the tenth (ICD10). Of the twenty-one chapters, Chapter V is devoted to psychiatry.

The history of ICD

Mental disorders were included for the first time in 1948, in the sixth revision (ICD-6), but neither ICD-6 nor ICD-7 were widely used, because they consisted merely of a list of names and code numbers by which national statistics of hospital admissions could be tabulated, with no glossary to indicate suggested meanings of the constituent terms. As already noted, the survey of Stengel in 1959 was an important first step in much-needed improvements, setting the stage for an extensive WHO programme towards achieving 'a common language' that has now stretched over thirty years.

ICD-8 was published in 1968. It made some progress towards solving the earlier problems, and was improved by publication of a British-based glossary in 1974. However, ICD-8 was still unsatisfactory, containing too many categories and allowing alternative codings for some syndromes. In 1978, Chapter V of ICD-9 was published. Overall it was very similar to ICD-8 because the WHO believed that national governments would be unwilling to accept many changes, although it was accompanied by a slightly more elaborate and internationally influenced glossary.

ICD-10

By the time ICD-10 was due, it had become evident that a major process of international collaboration was needed. The objectives of this process were that ICD-10 Chapter V should be:

- Suitable for international communication about statistics of morbidity and mortality.
- A reference standard for national and other psychiatric classifications.
- Acceptable and useful to a wide range of users in different cultures.
- An aid to education.

The process started in 1982. Drafts were produced by experts from many countries, and field trials undertaken at 112 centres in 39 countries, using six languages (Sartorius *et al.*, 1993). The field trials established the inter-rater reliability of the categories and ensured that the experts' descriptions fitted the patients seen by the participating psychiatrists. The final version, entitled *Clinical Descriptions and Diagnostic Guidelines*, was published as ICD-10 by WHO in 1992 (World Health Organization, 1992b). It contains descriptions of each of the disorders in the classification in mainly narrative form. The diagnostic instructions for users make it clear that these allow some latitude for clinical judgement.

All the diagnostic codes start with the letter F and, like the other chapters, it has ten major divisions (Table 2.1) each of which can be divided into ten, and so on. For example, F20 schizophrenia, can be followed by a further number for the category within the group (for example, F20.1, hebephrenic schizophrenia). Further characters can be used if necessary. Though ICD-10 is basically a descriptive classification, available knowledge and ingrained clinical practice mean that aetiology is a defining criterion in some of the main categories, notably organic (F0x), substance use-related (F1x), and stress-related (F4x).

Because ICD-10 is used for several purposes, it exists in several forms (Table 2.2), each derived from, and compatible with, the core version. The primary health care version has only 27 categories, each with reminders about likely management and treatment, and this version may eventually be one of the most widely used versions. The research version (DCR-10) contains more specific criteria for diagnosis similar to those in DSM-IV (see below) and also a list and glossary of 'culture-specific' disorders. To date, however, DSM-IV remains much more widely used for research.

TABLE 2.1 The main categories of ICD-10 Chapter V (F)

F00–F09	Organic, including symptomatic, mental disorders
F10–F19	Mental and behavioral disorders due to psychoactive substance use.
F20–F29	Schizophrenia, schizotypal, and delusional disorders
F30–F39	Mood (affective) disorders
F40–F49	Neurotic, stress-related, and somatoform disorders
F50–F59	Behavioural syndromes associated with physiological disturbances and physical factors
F60–F69	Disorders of adult personality and behaviour
F70–F79	Mental retardation
F80–F89	Disorders of psychological development
F90–F99	Behavioural and emotional disorders with onset usually occurring in childhood or adolescence

TABLE 2.2 ICD-10 Chapter V documents.

Document
The 'standard' ICD-10: Clinical descriptions and research guidelines (World Health Organization, 1992b)
Versions for specialist users
Primary health care
Multi-axial systems for adult general psychiatry
Muti-axial system for child psychiatry
Mental retardation
Diagnostic criteria for research
Documents providing additional explanations, descriptions and definitions
Lexicon of mental health terms
Lexicon of cross-cultural terms in mental health
Lexicon of alcohol and drug terms
ICD-10 symptom checklist
Pocket-sized quick-reference guides

The Diagnostic and Statistical Manual (DSM)

The history of DSM

In 1952 the American Psychiatric Association (APA) published the first edition of the Diagnostic and Statistical Manual (DSM-I) as an alternative to the widely criticized ICD-6. DSM-I was strongly influenced by the views of Adolf Meyer and Karl Menninger, and its simple glossary reflected the prevailing acceptance of psychoanalytic ideas in the USA. DSM-II was published in 1968 as the American National Glossary to ICD-8. It combined psychoanalytic ideas with those of Kraepelin.

DSM-III was published in 1980, and was an important step forward (M. Wilson 1993). It contained five main innovations:

- Precise operational criteria were provided for each diagnosis, with rules for inclusion and exclusion (Feighner *et al.*, 1972; Endicott and Spitzer, 1978). This was the first complete classification to do so, and the first to be based on criteria that had been field-tested.
- A multi-axial classification was adopted with five axes (Table 2.3).
- The nomenclature was revised and some syndromes were regrouped; for example, the terms neurosis and hysteria were discarded, and all mood disorders were grouped together.
- Psychodynamic concepts were largely eliminated.
- For some conditions, duration of illness was introduced as one of the criteria for diagnosis.

DSM-III was important not only because it introduced advances in the method of classification and the preparation of diagnostic criteria, but also because it catered for the needs of modern descriptive research. Its approach was empirical in contrast to the previous mainly clinical and psychodynamic thinking in American psychiatry. In 1987, an interim revision (DSM-III-R) was produced, pending the production of DSM-IV.

TABLE 2.3 The five axes of DSM-III and DSM-IV

Axis I	Clinical syndromes and 'conditions not attributable to mental disorder that are the focus of attention and treatment'
Axis II	Personality disorders
Axis III	Physical disorders and conditions
Axis IV	Severity of psychosocial stressors
Axis V	Highest level of adaptive functioning in the last year

DSM-IV

The next revision, DSM-IV, was prepared by thirteen work groups, who carried out a three-stage procedure:

- Comprehensive reviews of published literature.
- Analysis of data already collected.
- Field trials to evaluate proposed changes.

Drafts were circulated for discussion and comments before publication of DSM-IV in 1994 (American Psychiatric Association, 1994). DSM-IV Textual Revision (DSM-IV-TR) was published in 2000; it contains a small number of textual changes and updates the classification as an educational tool, but contains no significant alterations to the diagnostic criteria (American Psychiatric Association, 2000).

DSM-IV retains the multi-axial nature of DSM-III (Table 2.3). The categories of DSM-IV are not shown here, but are provided in the relevant chapters.

Comparing ICD-10 and DSM-IV

ICD-10 and DSM-IV were developed in parallel, and to avoid unnecessary differences there was close consultation between the working parties preparing the two documents. The efforts were largely successful, with the systems sharing most fundamental concepts and categories, but there are some differences (Table 2.4). Most are minor and discussed as appropriate in later chapters. A few are worthy of mention here.

TABLE 2.4 Differences between ICD-10 and DSM-IV

	ICD-10	DSM-IV
Origin	International (WHO)	American Psychiatric Association
Presentation	Different versions for clinical work, research, and use in primary care	A single document
Languages	Available in all widely spoken languages	English version only
Structure	Part of overall ICD framework Single axis in Chapter V; separate multi-axial systems available	Multi-axial
Content	Guidelines and criteria do not include social consequences of disorders	Diagnostic criteria usually include significant impairment in social functions

- The duration of the symptoms required for a diagnosis of schizophrenia. Though the symptoms are very similar, ICD-10 specifies that they should have been present for most of one month, but DSM-IV requires six months including a prodromal period (Chapter 12).
- The terms 'neurotic' and 'neurasthenia' are not used in DSM-IV. Neurasthenia is a very common diagnosis in China (see below), and neurosis is a term of convenience in many countries, so these are included in ICD albeit with some clearly stated reservations (Chapters 8–10).
- The social effects of the disorders are included as an option in the lists of criteria for most disorders in DSM-IV, whereas in ICD-10 these are not regarded as legitimate identifying criteria. Apart from the logical problem of including consequences of a disorder among its identifiers, the varying attitudes towards the same behaviour in different settings make it essential to keep culturally influenced judgements to a minimum in a classification intended for global use.

It is important to realize that the two classifications are complementary rather than competitors. ICD-10 results from an international effort, and was designed for use in all countries with their varied cultures, professional needs and clinical traditions (Sartorius *et al.*, 1995). DSM-IV is a US national classification, reflecting the professional, educational and financial priorities of its parent organization, the APA. For differing views on the relationships between ICD-10 and DSM-IV, see Andrews *et al.* (1999) and First and Pincus (1999).

Current and future issues in psychiatric classification

Many of the issues about classification discussed in this chapter continue to be topical and under active debate. This section raises some additional issues, especially those that may influence future developments.

Cultural issues

Though ICD-10 and DSM-IV make national approaches to classification less important (see Box 2.2), local and cultural factors remain important in classification in several respects (Mezzich *et al.*, 1999).

Psychiatrists and physicians in countries that have their own long-standing and comprehensive systems of ideas about heath and illness such as India, Pakistan and China sometimes complain that classifications developed in Europe and North America give too much emphasis to separation of mind and body. For example, the concept of somatoform disorders depends on seeing mind and body as alternatives; this approach causes problems in Western medicine and is not understood at all elsewhere. Investigation of these issues is difficult, since outsiders may not appreciate important cultural and local factors, or the varying ways in which

BOX 2.2 OTHER NATIONAL SYSTEMS OF CLASSIFICATION

The widespread international acceptance of ICD-10 and DSM-IV has diminished the importance of pre-existing national diagnostic traditions. However, they are of historical interest and, at times, still have some influence upon educational programmes (see Mezzich *et al.*, 2000).

The descriptive concepts introduced by Kraepelin and Bleuler have been very influential in most European countries, particularly in Germany, the UK, and the Scandinavian countries. In Scandinavia, emphasis has also been placed on the concept of psychogenic or reactive psychoses (Strömgren, 1985; Cooper, 1986). Scandinavia was also notable for its early concepts of multidimensional diagnoses.

In France, Kraepelinian views of schizophrenia were less widely accepted, and two other diagnostic categories of psychosis not commonly used elsewhere have persisted: **bouffée délirante** and **délires chroniques**. **Bouffée délirante** is the sudden onset of a delusional state with trance-like feelings, of short duration and good prognosis. This disorder has been included in ICD-10 within the category of 'acute transient psychotic disorder' (F23) which also incorporates features of the Scandinavian concept of reactive psychosis. **Délires chroniques** are conditions that would be classified in ICD-10 as 'persistent delusional disorders', and are subdivided into the 'non-focused', in which several areas of mental activity are affected, and the 'focused' with a single delusional theme, such as erotomania. These disorders are covered in Chapter 13.

Another example of international variation is the latest Chinese national classification (*Chinese classification of mental disorders*, second edn revised – CCMD-2-R). Although largely based upon ICD-10, it excludes almost all the somatoform disorders, so that particular prominence can be given to the category of neurasthenia, still one of the most frequent diagnoses in Chinese psychiatry (Kleinman, 1982).

emotions and behaviour are described in different languages.

The list of so-called 'culture-specific' disorders provided as appendices to ICD-10 and DSM-IV offer an opportunity for field-testing of the usefulness of these syndromes. The limited and largely anecdotal information available at present suggests that most of these conditions are culturally influenced varieties of anxiety, depression, and violent behaviour, rather than distinct disorders of different types.

Problem categories and atypical disorders

Several areas within the current classifications are recognized to be of uncertain status and value. These include stress-related disorders and somatoform disorders (see Widiger and Clark, 2000; Mayou and Sharpe, 2004).

Within several categories, a unsatisfactorily large proportion of disorders are coded as being 'atypical' or 'not otherwise specified'. A striking example is 'atypical eating disorder', which is more common than the combined prevalence of the typical eating disorders (Chapter 15).

Subthreshold disorders and clinical significance

Conditions that resemble the disorders in the classification but do not meet full diagnostic criteria are frequent, especially in primary care and in community samples. A recent study emphasizes that there are several-fold differences in the population prevalence of psychiatric disorders depending on whether 'mild' cases are included or not (WHO World Mental Health Consortium, 2004). There is continuing debate as to where the significance threshold should be set, and upon what grounds (Pincus *et al.*, 1999; Spitzer and Wakefield, 1999; Regier, 2000; Kessler *et al.*, 2003).

The needs of researchers

Although both clinicians and researchers need a reliable classification, their emphasis is slightly different. Research requires rigorous criteria, to select subjects whose symptoms and other characteristics are similar in clearly stated ways. This aim has been facilitated by the development of various ratings scales, interview schedules, and computer programs, as outlined above and in Chapter 3. This approach makes it easy to know the characteristics of the patients in the research but it limits the generalizations that can be made, since borderline or atypical subjects are excluded and such patients are common in practice.

Towards ICD-11 and DSM-V

At the time of writing, the first discussions regarding ICD-11 and DSM-V are underway. The WHO has abandoned its programme of ten-yearly revisions of all of the chapters of the ICD, so future developments will no longer be driven by this obligation. The APA has published a research agenda for DSM-V, with a view to publication after 2010.

DSM-IV mentions several 'new' diagnoses for consideration in DSM-V, such as post-concussional disorder and premenstrual dysphoric disorder. However, the policy for both the WHO and the APA is to make alterations and additions only where justified by new evidence; all that can be said at this very early stage is that changes in the sections on personality disorders are likely (Cooper, 2003). Epidemiological considerations may also be used to improve the validity of diagnostic categories (Robins, 2004).

Classification in this book

In this book, both ICD-10 and DSM-IV classifications are discussed. As in other textbooks, disorders are grouped in chapters for convenience and ease of understanding. The headings of the chapters do not always correspond exactly to the terms used in DSM-IV and ICD-10; any difference means that the heading more appropriately summarizes the scope of the chapter.

Further reading

American Psychiatric Association (2000) *Diagnostic and statistical manual of mental disorders – text revision*, 4th edn. American Psychiatric Association, Washington, DC.

Kendell, RE (1975) *The role of diagnosis in psychiatry*. Blackwell Scientific Publications, Oxford.

World Health Organization (1992) *The ICD-10 classification of mental and behavioural disorders. Clinical descriptions and diagnostic guidelines*. World Health Organization, Geneva.

CHAPTER 3

Assessment

Chapter contents

Psychiatric assessment has three goals:

1. **To make a diagnosis.** Despite its limitations (Chapter 2), diagnosis is central to the practice of psychiatry, since it provides the basis for rational, evidence-based approaches to treatment and prognosis. A major goal of most assessments, especially those of new patients, is therefore to allow a diagnosis or differential diagnosis to be made. This, in turn, requires that the symptoms and signs of psychiatric disorder (Chapter 1) can be elicited, and their diagnostic significance appreciated.
2. **To understand the context of the diagnosis.** That is, to have sufficient information about the patient's life history, current circumstances, and personality in order to understand why the disorder has occurred. This contextual information also affects decisions about treatment and prognosis. This aspect of assessment is covered in this Chapter, but the significance of particular aetiological factors is discussed in Chapter 5.
3. **To establish a therapeutic relationship.** The psychiatrist must ensure that the patient feels able and willing to give an accurate and full history if she is to obtain the necessary diagnostic information. Establishment of a therapeutic relationship is also likely to be essential if the patient is to accept the treatment plan which the psychiatrist later recommends.

The *process* of psychiatric assessment can be broken down into several stages:

- **Preparation.** This includes having the interviewing skills necessary in order to achieve the above goals; deciding who else needs to be interviewed (e.g. a relative), and whether there are factors which require the assessment to be modified (e.g. language difficulties, shortage of time).
- **The collection of information.** This is usually organized under a series of headings covering the psychiatric history and mental state examination.
- **The evaluation of the information** in order to arrive at a diagnosis or differential diagnosis. This is the hardest part of the process to describe to readers new to psychiatry, since it requires knowledge of the diagnostic significance of particular symptoms and symptom combinations.
- **Using the information** to make treatment decisions and prognostic opinions.
- **Recording and communicating the information** and the conclusions drawn. This must be shared with other health professionals involved with the patient both now and in the future, and with the patient and his family.

This chapter covers these areas in turn, concentrating on the full, initial assessment of a patient by a general adult psychiatrist. It also discusses how this process is adapted in other circumstances. First, however, the basic process of psychiatric interviewing is outlined. At the outset, it is worth emphasizing that the description of assessment in textbooks, including this one, tend to make the process seem to be a passive, even predetermined, one of extensive data collection. In practice, however, assessment is an active, selective process, in which diagnostic clues are pursued, and hypotheses tested, and the focus of questioning adapted to the particular circumstances and needs of the patient. This dynamic aspect of assessment can only be learned from practical experience. It also requires a working knowledge of the main psychiatric syndromes, in order for the significance of specific symptoms or history items which emerge during the assessment to be appreciated; it was for this reason that the preceding chapter covered psychiatric classification.

This chapter assumes that readers are already competent in physical examination, and this matter is considered only briefly. Readers who need more information should consult a textbook of medicine.

Psychiatric interviewing

Preparing for the interview

Psychiatric assessments (interviews) have to be carried out in many settings. The following recommendations should be followed as far as is practicable, but they cannot always be achieved completely. In some locations, such as an accident and emergency department, the setting may be far from ideal. It is important, nevertheless, to do what is possible to:

- put the patient at ease,
- ensure privacy,
- ensure the safety of the interviewer.

The interview should be carried out free from interruptions and where it cannot be overheard. The patient should be comfortable and the interviewer should not face the patient directly but arrange their chair at an angle; nor, if possible, should the interviewer sit at a much higher level.

Whenever possible the interviewer should make notes during the interview; writing notes afterwards is time-consuming and not always wholly accurate.

However, it is usually better to delay note taking for some minutes until the patient feels that they have the interviewer's undivided attention. The patient should sit to the left side of a right-handed interviewer. With this arrangement, the interviewer can attend to the patient and maintain an informal atmosphere while writing. Occasionally, when a patient is very anxious or agitated, note-taking may be deferred until after the interview.

Only a small minority of patients are potentially dangerous, but the need for precautions should be considered before every interview. Whenever there is a possibility of violence, the interviewer should:

- make sure that another person knows where and when the interview is taking place and how long it is expected to last. This is especially relevant to interviews in the community, but applies also to certain hospital situations such as interviews at the end of clinic when other staff have left.
- ensure that help can be called if it is needed. In hospital, check for an emergency call button and its position, and otherwise try to arrange for another person to be within earshot.
- ensure that neither the patient nor any obstruction is between the interviewer and the exit.
- remove from sight any objects that could be used as weapons.

If the risk is thought to be high, or if these requirements cannot be met, it may be necessary to defer the interview.

Starting the interview

The interviewer should welcome the patient by name, give their own name and status, and explain in a few words the reason for, and purpose of, the assessment. If the patient is being seen at the request of another doctor, the interviewer should indicate this. If the patient is accompanied, the interviewer should greet the companions and explain how long they should expect to wait and whether they will be interviewed. It is usually better to see the patient alone first, assuming they are able to provide an adequate history. The interviewer should explain that notes will be taken, and that they will be confidential. If the interview is for the purposes of a report to an outside agency (e.g. a legal report) this should be made clear. The general structure of the interview should be explained (e.g. present problems will be considered first, before past events are reviewed) and the time available.

The interview should begin with an open question (one that cannot be answered yes or no) such as: 'Tell me about your problems'. The patient should be allowed to talk freely for several minutes before further questions are asked. As the patient describes their problems, the interviewer should observe their responses and manner, for example, are they reticent or unduly circumstantial.

The following techniques have been shown to improve the results of the interview (Goldberg *et al.*, 1980). The interviewer should:

- adopt a relaxed posture and appear unhurried – even when time is short
- maintain appropriate eye contact with the patient and not appear engrossed in note-taking
- be alert to verbal and non-verbal cues of distress as well as to the factual content of the interview
- control an over-talkative or discursive patient.

Continuing and completing the interview

The first step is to obtain a clear account of the patient's problems. It is important to separate symptoms from their consequences, and from other life problems which the patient may want to discuss. For example, a patient may have low mood, sexual difficulties, or financial worries as their presenting complaint; in each case the common denominator is depression, but it will require your assessment to discover this. Your priority is to focus first upon the symptoms and signs of psychiatric disorder, leaving the other kinds of problem until later.

From the start, consider the possible diagnoses and, as the interview progresses, select questions to confirm or reject these diagnoses. For example, if a patient mentions hearing voices, this immediately raises the possibility of schizophrenia and requires that, at some stage in the assessment, the other cardinal features of the disorder are sought, and their presence or absence noted. The interviewer considers also what information is relevant to prognosis and treatment. Thus interviewing is not simply the asking of a routine set of questions. Interviewing is an active and iterative process in which the focus of attention is directed by hypotheses formed from the information already elicited, and modified repeatedly as more information is collected. This active process of interviewing is particularly necessary when time is short and when immediate treatment decisions must be made. Obviously, as the interviewer gains in confidence and psychiatric knowledge, he becomes better at thinking of possible diagnoses, and proceeding in a way which rules them in or out more rapidly and convincingly.

It is generally better to establish clearly the nature of the symptoms before asking how and when they developed. If there is any doubt about the nature of the symptoms, the patient should be asked to describe specific examples. When all presenting symptoms have been explored sufficiently, direct questions are asked about others that have not come to light but may be relevant. In doing this, the interviewer uses his knowledge of psychiatric syndromes to decide what further questions to ask. For example, a person who complains of feeling depressed would be asked about ideas concerning the future, and about suicidal ideas; if suicidal thoughts are acknowledged, further specific questions should be asked. Also ask about the impact which the symptoms have had on the patient's life, looking for evidence of functional impairment.

The onset and course of the symptoms is clarified next, together with their relationship to any stressful events or physical illness. Considerable persistence may be needed to date the onset or an exacerbation of symptoms accurately. It sometimes helps to ask how the onset related to an event that the patient is likely to remember, such as a birthday. The patient's attempts to cope with the symptoms are noted, for example, increased drinking of alcohol to relieve distress. If treatment has already been given, its nature, timing and effects are noted, together with the patient's concordance with it.

The interviewer completes the relevant parts of the full interview schedule described below. If time is short it may be better to examine the mental state after the present complaints have been clarified. This can make it easier to select the key points to be asked about in the rest of the history. When time is adequate, the mental state is usually examined at the end of the interview, together with any relevant physical examination.

Throughout the interview, allow the patient, as far as possible, to describe their problems spontaneously. In this way, unexpected material may be revealed that might not be come to light in the answers to questions. However, questions may be needed to bring the patient back to the point after a digression, and to elicit specific information, for example, about the relationship between symptoms and stressful events. Whenever possible, the interviewer should use open rather than leading or closed questions (a leading question suggests the answer; a closed question allows only the answers yes or no). Thus instead of the closed question: 'Are you happily married?' the interviewer might ask: 'How do you and your wife get on?' When there is no alternative to a closed question, the answer should be followed by a request for an example. Before ending the interview, it is good practice to ask a general question such as: 'Is there anything that I have not asked you about, that you think I should know?'

Box 3.1 summarizes some techniques promoting effective interviewing.

BOX 3.1 SOME TECHNIQUES FOR EFFECTIVE PSYCHIATRIC ASSESSMENTS

- Help the patient to talk freely. This can be done using open questions, and by cues such as nodding or saying 'go on' or 'tell me more about that'.
- Keep the patient to relevant topics. Non-verbal cues are again useful, also use specific interventions, such as 'At this point I'd like to ask you more about how you've been feeling. We can return to your money worries later.'
- Make systematic enquiries but without asking so many questions that other, unanticipated, issues are not volunteered.
- Check your understanding, and that you have enquired about all the areas the patient thinks are important, by summarizing the key points of the history back to him. This step also helps you begin to formulate your views on the diagnosis and causes.
- Be flexible in assessments, both regarding their length and sequence. Select questions according to the emerging possibilities regarding diagnoses, causes and plans of action.

Interviewing informants

Whenever possible, the patient's history should be supplemented by information from a close relative or another person who knows them well. This is much more important in psychiatry than in the rest of medicine, because some psychiatric patients are unaware of the extent of their symptoms. Other patients are aware of their problems but do not wish to reveal them; for example, people who misuse alcohol often conceal the extent of their drinking. Patients and relatives may also give quite different accounts of personality characteristics. Interviews with a partner or relative are not only used to obtain additional information about the patient's condition, but to assess their attitudes to the patient and the illness, and to involve them in the treatment plan. It is also an opportunity to learn what burdens the illness has placed on them, and how they have tried to cope. A history from an informant is essential when the patient is unable to give an accurate account of his condition, for example, because of impaired memory. Finally, when it is important to know about a patient's childhood, an interview with a parent or older sibling may reveal important information.

Informants can either be seen separately from the patient, or invited to join the interview. The choice depends on both the assessor's and the patient's preference, but in both instances the patient must give their consent. If the patient refuses to allow an informant to be interviewed, explore the reasons for this and explain the difficulties it will pose for the assessment. There are a few situations in which the patient's permission is not necessary before interviewing a relative or other informant; e.g., if the patient is a child, and when adult patients are mute or confused. In other cases, the doctor should explain to the patient the reasons for interviewing the informant, while emphasizing that confidential information given by the patient will not be passed on. If any information needs to be given to a relative, for example, about treatment, the patient's permission should be obtained. Questions from relatives should be dealt with in the same way.

The interviewer begins by explaining the purpose of the interview and may need to reassure the informant. A relative may fear that the interviewer will view them as responsible in some way for the patient's problems, or make demands on them. The interviewer should be sensitive to such ideas and, when appropriate, discuss them in a reassuring way, but without colluding with them or becoming involved in ways that might conflict with her primary duty to her patient. If the informant has been interviewed separately from the patient, the psychiatrist should not tell the patient what has been said unless the informant has given permission. This is important even when the informant has revealed something that should be discussed with the patient, for example, an account of excessive drinking.

Sometimes it is necessary to speak to employers, friends, police or others in order to collect further information about the patient and his illness. This should be done only with the patient's permission, unless there are legal or safety issues which override this principle; for example, if the patient is in custody, or if there are grounds for concern that he may harm a third party.

Patient characteristics that may affect the interview

Interviews can prove difficult for a variety of reasons. Many of these reflect the situation (e.g. noisy surroundings, lack of time) or interviewer characteristics (e.g. inexperience, tiredness). However, other problems arise from the characteristics of the patient, and these are outlined here. Remember that such problems can be diagnostically useful. For example, a patient may be monosyllabic because of depression; a disturbed patient may have delirium.

Anxious patients

Although anxiety may be part of the patient's disorder, it may also relate to the interview. If the person seems unduly anxious, the interviewer can say that many people feel anxious when they first take part in a psychiatric interview, and go on to explore the patient's concerns.

Taciturn patients

Taciturn patients can be encouraged to speak more freely if the interviewer shows non-verbal expressions of concern (e.g. leaning forward a little in the chair with an expression of interest) additional to those that are part of any good interview.

Garrulous patients

It is not easy to curb an over-talkative patient. If efforts to focus the interview are unsuccessful, the interviewer should wait for a natural break in the flow of speech and then explain that, because time is limited, they propose to interrupt from time to time to help the patient keep focused on issues that are important for planning treatment. If this proposal is made tactfully, most garrulous patients will accept it.

Overactive patients

Some patients are so active and restless that systematic questioning about mental state is difficult. The interviewer then has to limit questions to a few that seem particularly important, and concentrates on observing the patient's behaviour. However, if the patient is being seen in an emergency, some of their overactivity may be a reaction to other people's attempts to restrain them. In such a case, a quiet but confident approach by the interviewer may calm the patient enough to allow more adequate examination.

Confused patients

When the patient gives a history in a muddled way, or appears perplexed, the interviewer should test cognitive functions early in the interview. If there is evidence of impaired cognition or consciousness, the interviewer should try to orientate and reassure the patient, before starting the interview again in a simplified form. In such cases every effort should be made to interview another informant.

Uncooperative patients

Some patients are reluctant to be interviewed and have come at the insistence of a third party, e.g. spouse. When the patient seems unwilling to collaborate, the interviewer should talk over the circumstances of the referral, and try to persuade them that the interview will be in their own interests. Remember that lack of cooperation may occur because the patient does not realize that they are ill; for example, some patients with depression, delirium, or psychosis. In such cases it may be necessary to interview an informant before returning to the patient.

Unresponsive patients

If a patient is mute or stuporose, it is essential to interview an informant who can describe the onset and course of the condition. When it comes to the mental state, the interviewer can only observe behaviour, but this can be informative. Because some stuporose patients change rapidly from inactivity to violent overactivity, it is wise to have help at hand when seeing such a patient.

Before deciding that a patient is mute, the interviewer should allow adequate time for reply, and try several topics. If the patient still fails to respond, attempt to persuade him to communicate in writing. Apart from observations of behaviour, the interviewer should note whether the patient's eyes are open or closed. If open, note whether they follow objects, move apparently without purpose, or are fixed. If the eyes are closed, find out whether the patient opens them on request, and, if not, whether attempts at opening them are resisted. A physical examination including neurological assessment is essential in all such cases. Also, certain signs found in catatonic schizophrenia should be sought (p. 16).

Other problems

Some patients try to dominate the interview, especially when the interviewer is younger than themselves. Others adopt an unduly friendly approach that threatens to convert the interview into a social conversation. In either case, the interviewer should explain why she needs to guide the patient to relevant issues. In the longer term, developing a manner which is confident and assertive, but not domineering, helps avoids such problems.

The psychiatric history

The main parts of a psychiatric assessment are the **psychiatric history** and the **mental state examination**. The latter covers the symptoms and signs present during the interview; the former deals with everything else. The assessment is then completed by the **physical examination**, and sometimes by **further investigations**. This section covers the psychiatric history followed by the mental state examination, and then the other aspects of the assessment.

A commonly used scheme for history taking is given below. For ease of reference, the scheme is presented as a list of headings and items. More detail is provided in the subsequent notes. As noted above, much of the interview is designed to elicit diagnostic symptoms, but other questions are intended to obtain information about the patient's life and circumstances, whilst the interview as a whole must try and establish the rapport needed to achieve these goals and form the basis for a subsequent therapeutic relationship.

The following scheme is comprehensive and systematic, since an ability to conduct this form of assessment is essential before briefer interviews are attempted. Moreover, although it is not possible nor necessary to take a full history on every occasion, the information that has been elicited should always be recorded systematically and in a standard order. This practice helps the interviewer to remember all potentially important topics and to add further information later. The practice also makes it easier for colleagues who need to refer to the notes in the future. This order can be followed in the written record, even when it was not possible to elicit the information in the desired sequence. This and all other entries in the notes should be dated and signed.

A scheme for history taking

Information is grouped under the headings shown in Table 3.1. For brevity, this section is written in the style

TABLE 3.1 Outline of the psychiatric history

Name, age, and address of the patient
Name of informants and their relationship to the patient
History of present condition
Family history
Personal history (expanded in Table 3.2)
Past psychiatric and medical history
Personality (expanded in Table 3.3)

of short notes and illustrative questions. The next section explains why these topics are relevant, and some of the problems which may occur when covering them.

Informant(s)

- Usually the principal informant is the patient. If not, state the reason.
- The name(s), relation to patient, and length of acquaintance of any other person interviewed.
- The name of the referrer and reasons for referral.

History of present condition

- List symptoms, with onset, duration, and fluctuation of each.
- Ask about and record symptoms which might have been expected but which were not present (e.g. no suicidal ideation in a person with low mood; no first rank symptoms of schizophrenia in a patient with delusions).
- The temporal relationship between symptoms and any physical disorder, or psychological or social problems.
- The nature and duration of any functional impairment caused by the symptoms.
- Any treatment received, its effects and side-effects.

Family history

- Parents and siblings – age now or at death (if dead, the cause), occupation, personality, quality of relationship with patient, psychiatric and medical history.
- Social position of family.
- When the family history is complex and relevant, summarize it as a family tree.

Personal history (see Table 3.2)

- Pregnancy and birth abnormalities, e.g. infections, prematurity, problems with labour.
- Early developmental milestones: walking, talking, sphincter control, etc.
- Childhood: any prolonged separation from parents and the patient's reaction to it. Any emotional problems – age of onset, course, and treatment. Any serious illness in childhood.
- Schooling and higher education: age of starting and finishing each stage; character of the school, college or university. Academic record; sporting and other extracurricular achievements; relationships with teachers and other students; bullying.

TABLE 3.2 Outline of the personal history

Mother's pregnancy and the birth
Early development
Childhood: separations, emotional problems, illnesses, education
Occupations
Relationships
Children
Social circumstances
Substance use
Past medical history
Past psychiatric history
Forensic history

- Occupations: present job – dates, duties, performance, satisfaction. List earlier jobs, with reasons for changes.
- Current relationship: identity and gender of partner, duration, nature (e.g. married?). Partner's health, attitude to the patient's illness, and the quality of the relationship.
- Sexual history: attitude to sex; heterosexual and homosexual experience; current sexual practices, contraception. Knowing how and how far to enquire about sexual matters is discussed further on p. 43.
- Children: identities; date of any abortions or stillbirths; temperament, emotional development, mental and physical health.
- Social circumstances: accommodation, household composition and any financial problems.
- Use of alcohol, tobacco, illicit drugs.

Past psychiatric and medical history

- Past medical history: illnesses, operations, accidents, drug treatments.
- Past psychiatric history: nature and duration of each illness. Include any episodes of self-harm. Date, duration, nature, location and outcome of any treatment.
- Current medication, including contraceptive pill, over-the-counter medicines, and alternative remedies. Any allergic or other adverse reactions.
- Forensic history: arrests, convictions, imprisonment. Nature of the offences, especially regarding dangerousness.

TABLE 3.3 Assessment of personality

Relationships
Leisure activities
Prevailing mood and emotional tone
Character
Attitudes and standards
Habits

Personality

- By this stage in the interview, the patient's manner and description of their history will have provided some indication of their personality. However, specific focus on the topic is also essential (Table 3.3). See Chapter 7 for discussion of personality and personality disorder.
- Relationships: friendships, few or many, superficial or close, with own or opposite sex; relations with workmates and superiors.
- Use of leisure: hobbies and interests.
- Predominant mood and emotions: e.g. anxious, despondent, optimistic, pessimistic, self-deprecating, overconfident; stable or fluctuating; controlled or demonstrative.
- Other character traits. For example, perfectionist, obsessional, isolated, impulsive, sensitive, controlling.
- Attitudes and standards: moral and religious; attitude towards health and the body.

Notes on history taking

The scheme just outlined lists the items to be considered when a full history is taken, but gives no indication as to why these items are important or what sort of difficulties may arise in eliciting them. These issues are discussed in this section, which is written in the form of notes approximating to the headings used above.

The reason for referral

Only a brief statement need be given, for example, 'severe depression, failing to respond to drug treatment'. The reason for referral usually, but not always, proves to be the main focus of the interview. Check that the patient has the same understanding as to why he has been referred. If not, this in itself is useful information. For example, the patient may disagree that they are depressed, believing that they have cancer; this may be diagnostically significant (e.g. suggestive of hypochondriasis), and it may also affect their willingness to engage fully in the assessment or subsequent treatment.

History of present condition

This part of the history is relatively long, as there will often be several symptoms, and each may require time to characterize fully. Record the severity and duration of each symptom, how it began, and what course it has taken (increasing gradually or stepwise, staying the same, intermittent). Indicate which symptoms co-vary and which take an independent course. Note any treatment, the response, and any adverse effects. When a drug was ineffective, ask whether the patient took it regularly and in the required dosage.

Family history

A family history of psychiatric disorder may indicate genetic or environmental influences. A genetic explanation is more likely for some disorders than others, and increases as more relatives are affected. Though shared environment has proved, as a rule, less important than genes in explaining family history (Chapter 5), knowledge about the family's circumstances remains part of the basic information for understanding the origin and presentation of the patient's problems. Hence ask about factors such as the personality of the parents and siblings, their interrelationships, and the financial and social standing of the family.

Recent events in the family may have been stressful to the patient, for example, the serious illness or divorce of a family member. Events in the family may throw light on the patient's concerns. For example, the death of an older sibling from a brain tumour may partly explain a patient's extreme concern about headaches.

Personal history

Pregnancy and birth

Events in pregnancy and delivery are most likely to be relevant when the patient is learning disabled, though they are also risk factors for several psychiatric disorders. An unwanted pregnancy may be followed by a poor relationship between mother and child.

Child development

Few patients know whether they have passed through developmental stages normally. However, this information is usually more important if the patient is a child or adolescent, in which case the parents are likely to be available for interview. This information is important also in cases of learning disability. The effects of separation from the mother vary considerably, and depend in part on the age of the child, the duration, and the reason. Questioning about the child's emotional development provides information about early temperament and emerging personality, and abnormalities or delays may serve as risk factors for, or early signs of, later problems. However, childhood characteristics as a rule are weak predictors of adult disorders, and only require detailed consideration when assessing children and adolescents. Assessment in child psychiatry is covered in Chapter 24.

Education

The school record gives an indication of intelligence, achievements, and social development. Ask whether the patient made friends and got on well with teachers, and about success at games and other activities. Similar questions are relevant to higher education.

Occupational history

Information about the present job helps the interviewer to understand the patient's current financial and social circumstances and one potential source of stress. A list of previous jobs and reasons for leaving is relevant to the assessment of personality. If the status of jobs has declined, this may reflect chronic illness or alcohol misuse. Repeated changes of job or dismissals may reflect personality difficulties.

Sexual history

The interviewer should use common sense in deciding how much to ask the individual patient, depending on the response to initial questions, demographic factors, and the nature of the presenting complaint. For example, a detailed account may be essential when the patient is seeking help for sexual dysfunction, but more often the interviewer is concerned to establish generally whether the patient's sexual life is involved in their current difficulties, whether as a cause, a correlate, or a consequence.

Judgement must also be used about the optimal timing and amount of detail of questioning about childhood sexual abuse. Unfortunately such past experiences are sufficiently common, especially in women, to merit questioning. However, it may often not be appropriate to bring the matter up in a first interview, unless prompted by the patient. The decision to do so depends on the clinical suspicion, and the time and expertise available to the interviewer. If the matter is not raised, this fact should be recorded. Questions relevant to sexual disorders are considered further in Chapter 19.

Marital history

This heading includes all enduring intimate relationships. Ask about the current and any previous lasting relationships, preferably phrased in a way which does not assume the gender of the partner(s). Frequent broken relationships may reflect abnormalities of personality. The spouse's occupation, personality, and state of health are relevant to the patient's circumstances.

Children

Pregnancy, childbirth, miscarriages, and terminations are important events that are sometimes associated with adverse psychological reactions. Information about the patient's children is relevant to present worries and the pattern of family life. Since children may be affected by the parent's illness, it is important to know, for example, whether a seriously depressed woman has the care of a baby, or whether a violent man who misuses alcohol has children in the home. If admission is being considered for a patient who has the care of children, it is important to find out their needs and, if necessary, arrange for their care.

Past psychiatric and medical history

Previous medical or surgical treatment should always be asked about, and particularly careful inquiries made about previous psychiatric disorders. Patients or relatives may be able to recall the general nature of the illness and treatment but it is nearly always appropriate to request information from others who have treated the patient.

Social circumstances

Questions about housing, finances, and the composition of the household help the interviewer to understand the patient's circumstances. Assets and resources (including potential carers) are assessed as well as problems and sources of stress. There can be no general rule about the amount of detail to elicit, and this must be left to common sense.

Substance use and misuse

This includes past as well as present consumption of alcohol and other substances. Misuse of prescribed drugs should also be considered. Answers may be evasive or misleading and may need to be checked with other informants and sources of information (e.g. urine screens, blood tests). See Chapter 18 for further information about interviewing in this area.

Assessing personality

Aspects of personality can be judged by asking for a self-assessment, by asking others who know the patient well, and by observing behaviour. Mistakes can arise from paying too much attention to the patient's own assessment of their personality. Some people give an unduly favourable account of themselves; for example, antisocial people may conceal the extent of their aggressive behaviour or dishonesty. Conversely, depressed patients often judge themselves negatively and critically. Therefore it is essential to interview other informants whenever possible.

Good indications of personality can often be obtained by asking how the patient has behaved in particular circumstances, especially at times when social roles are changing, such as starting work, marrying, or becoming a parent.

When assessing personality from behaviour at interview, it is essential to take into account the anxiety which the situation often provokes, and to allow for the possible effects of psychiatric disorder. Thus, when depressed, a person who is normally self-possessed and sociable may appear reserved and lacking in self-confidence.

Common sense and experience will indicate the depth and focus of character assessment needed for each patient. If the patient (or informant) has difficulty describing their character with an open question, offer options. For example, 'Would you call yourself an optimist or a pessimist? A loner or a socialite?' Do not focus entirely on negative attributes, but ask about positive ones, including resilience to adversity. This is important not just to gain a balanced impression, but because strengths are usually better targets for intervention if personality proves to be therapeutically relevant.

Relationships

Is the person shy or does he make friends easily? Are his friendships close and are they lasting? Relationships at work, as well as those with friend and relatives, are significant. Leisure activities can throw light on personality, by reflecting a person's interests and preferences for company or solitude, as well as levels of energy and resourcefulness.

Mood

Ask whether the patient is generally cheerful or gloomy and whether she has marked changes of mood, and if so, how quickly they appear, how long they last, and if they follow life events. Information about prevailing mood and mood swings may reveal evidence suggestive of mood disorder, which can be enquired about further.

The mental state examination

The history records symptoms up to the time of the interview. The mental state examination is concerned with symptoms, signs and behaviour during the interview; it is usually conducted after the history. Although the distinction is traditional, and conceptually useful, in practice the boundary between history and mental state examination is somewhat blurred. In particular, very recent symptoms and signs (e.g. hearing hallucinations within the past few hours) are often recorded in the mental state examination, even if the phenomena are not experienced during the interview. The mental state examination is also sometimes used to elicit and record symptoms and signs that, for whatever reason, have not been covered previously (e.g. whether the patient is suicidal). The important point is that the assessor clearly notes the timing of all symptoms and signs, and whether they are currently present.

If the patient is being seen by nurses and other professional staff in hospital or in the community, their observations of mental state are important and sometimes more revealing than the small sample of behaviour observed during the mental state examination.

Mental state examination uses a standard series of headings under which the relevant phenomena, or their absence, are recorded (Table 3.4). The symptoms and signs referred to in the following account are described in Chapter 1 and, with a few exceptions, are not repeated. Mental state examination is a skill that should be learned by watching experienced interviewers and by practising repeatedly under supervision, as well as by reading. The mental state provides much of the key diagnostic information, and the ability to carry out an accurate and comprehensive mental state examination is therefore a core skill needed by all psychiatrists and other mental health professionals.

Appearance and behaviour

General appearance

Much diagnostically useful information can be learned from the patient's appearance and behaviour; indeed, as discussed later, experienced clinicians often make provi-

TABLE 3.4 Outline of the mental state examination
Appearance and behaviour
Speech
Mood
Thoughts
Perceptions
Cognitive function
Insight

sional diagnoses within minutes of meeting a patient, relying heavily on this information. The process of observation starts from the first moment you see the patient. For example, what is their manner and behaviour in the waiting room. Are they sitting quietly, pacing around, or laughing to themselves? When greeted, what is their response? As they walk towards the interview room, is there evidence of parkinsonism, ataxia, or unsteadiness? Note the general attire. A dirty, unkempt look may indicate self-neglect. Manic patients may wear bright colours, or dress incongruously. Occasionally an oddity of dress may provide the clue to diagnosis; for example, a rain-hood worn on a dry day may be the first evidence of a patient's belief that rays are being shone on their head by persecutors. An appearance suggesting recent weight loss should alert the observer to the possibility of depressive disorder, anorexia nervosa, or physical illness.

Facial appearance and emotional expression

The facial appearance provides information about mood. In depression, the corners of the mouth are turned down, and there are vertical furrows on the brow. Anxious patients have horizontal creases on the forehead, widened palpebral fissures, and dilated pupils. Facial expression may reflect elation, irritability, and anger, or the fixed 'wooden' expression due to drugs with parkinsonian side-effects. The facial appearance may also suggest physical disorders, e.g. thyrotoxicosis.

Posture and movement

Posture and movement also reflect mood. A depressed patient characteristically sits with hunched shoulders, the head and gaze inclined downwards. An anxious patient may sit on the edge of the chair with hands gripping its sides. Anxious people and patients with agitated depression may be tremulous and restless, touching jewellery, or picking at the fingernails. Manic patients are overactive and restless. Other abnormalities of movement include tardive dyskinesia (p. 534), and the motor signs seen mainly in catatonic schizophrenia (p. 12).

Social behaviour

A patient's social behaviour and interactions are influenced by their personality, and their attitude to the interview, as outlined above. However, such behaviour can also be influenced by psychiatric disorder, and so it provides another potential source of diagnostic information. Manic patients tend to be unduly familiar or disinhibited, whilst those with dementia may behave as if they were elsewhere than in a medical interview. Patients with schizophrenia may be withdrawn and preoccupied. Patients with antisocial personality disorders may behave aggressively. If social behaviour is highly unusual, note what exactly is unusual, rather than using imprecise terms such as 'bizarre'.

Speech

Speech and thoughts are recorded in different parts of the mental state examination, even though it is only through speech that thoughts become known to the interviewer. By convention, the 'speech' section covers rate, quantity, difficulties speaking, and flow of speech; its content (e.g. preoccupations about death, grandiose delusions) is deferred until the 'Thoughts' section.

Rate and quantity

Speech may be unusually fast and increased in amount, as in mania, or slow, sparse and monotonous, in depression. Depressed or demented patients may pause for a long time before replying to questions and then give short answers, producing little spontaneous speech. The same may be observed among shy people or those of low intelligence.

Difficulties speaking

If the patient is having problems finding or articulating words, consider the possibility of dysphasia or dysarthria. For further details, see Box 3.2 (p. 50) and consult a neurology textbook.

Neologisms

Neologisms are private words invented by the patient, often to describe morbid experiences (p. 16).

The flow of speech

Abnormalities in the flow of speech may simply reflect an anxious, distracted patient, or one of low intelligence. More significantly, such abnormalities may be evidence of disturbances in the stream or form of thoughts (p. 15). For example, sudden interruptions may indicate thought blocking; rapid shifts from one topic to another suggest flight of ideas. It can be difficult to be certain about these abnormalities, and it is often helpful to record a sample of speech and listen to it several times. Write down a representative example in the notes.

Mood

Conventionally, the mood section includes recording of other emotions and related phenomena as well, including suicidal thoughts.

Depression and mania

The assessment of mood begins with the observations of behaviour described already, and continues with direct questions such as 'What is your mood like?' or 'How are you in your spirits?' To assess depression, questions should be asked about a feeling of being about to cry (actual tearfulness is often denied), pessimistic thoughts about the present, hopelessness about the future, and guilt about the past. Suitable questions are 'What do you think will happen to you in the future?' or 'Have you been blaming yourself for anything?' Questions about elevated mood correspond to those about depression; for example, 'How are you in your spirits?' followed, if necessary, by direct questions such as: 'Do you feel in unusually good spirits?' Note that the mood in mania can be irritable as well as cheerful.

Both depressed and elevated mood, if clinically significant, are accompanied by other features of depression and mania respectively. For example, anhedonia, tiredness or poor concentration in depression. In practice, therefore, it is common to extend this part of the mental state examination to include questioning about other diagnostic features of mood disorder, if not asked about already. Whether the interviewer chooses to record them in the notes under this heading, or insert them into the relevant part of the history, is a matter of convenience.

Fluctuating and incongruous mood

As well as assessing the prevailing mood, the interviewer should find out how mood varies. When mood varies excessively, it is said to be **labile**; for example, the patient appears dejected at one point in the interview but quickly changes to a normal or unduly cheerful mood. Any lack of emotional response, sometimes called blunting or flattening of affect (p. 5), should also be noted.

Normally, mood varies during an interview in parallel with the topics discussed. The patient appears sad while talking of unhappy events, angry while describing things that have irritated them, and so on. When the mood is not suited to the context, it is recorded as **incongruent** or inappropriate (p. 5).

Suicidal ideation

Some inexperienced interviewers are wary of asking about suicide in case they should suggest it to the patient. There is no evidence to warrant this caution although questions should be in stages, starting with the question such as 'Have you thought life is not worth living?' and, if appropriate, going on to ask 'Have you wished you could die?' or 'Have you considered any way in which you might end your life?' The interviewer may also be concerned that they will not be able to cope if the patient does admit to suicidal ideation or intent. A basic training in this topic, and knowledge of self-harm and suicide, should preclude these worries. Questions about suicide are considered further on p. 414.

Anxiety

Anxiety is assessed both by asking about subjective feelings, and by enquiring about the physical symptoms and cognitions associated with anxiety. For example, the interviewer should start with a general question such as 'Have you noticed any changes in your body when you feel upset?', and then go on to specific enquiries about palpitations, dry mouth, sweating, trembling, and the various other symptoms of autonomic activity and muscle tension. To detect anxious thoughts, one can ask: 'What goes through your mind when you are feeling anxious?' Possible replies include thoughts of fainting or losing control. Many of these questions overlap with enquiries about the history of the disorder.

Depersonalization and derealization

Depersonalization and derealization are usually symptoms of anxiety disorders. Their importance in the mental state examination is largely because they are easily mistaken for psychotic symptoms and must be distinguished from them. Patients who have experienced depersonalization and derealization find them difficult to describe, and patients who have not experienced them may say that they have because they have misunderstood the questions. Try and obtain specific examples of the patient's experiences. It is useful to begin by asking 'Do you ever feel that things around you are unreal?' and 'Do you ever feel unreal or that part of your body is unreal?' Patients with derealization often describe things in the environment as seeming artificial and lifeless. Patients with depersonalization may say that they feel detached, unable to feel emotion, or as if acting a part.

Thoughts

In this section, any predominant *content* of the person's thoughts can first be noted. For example, a preoccupation with persecutory themes, negative or self-deprecating responses to questions, or a repeated return of the conversation to diet and body shape. This information may signify, respectively, a delusional disorder, depression, and an eating disorder, and indicate areas for further questioning. However, the main purpose of this section is to determine the *nature* of the patient's thoughts, and particularly to identify obsessions and delusions.

Obsessions

Obsessions were described on pp. 12–13. An appropriate question is: 'Do any thoughts keep coming into your mind, even though you try hard to stop them?' If the patient says 'yes', they should be asked for an example. Patients may be ashamed of obsessional thoughts, especially those about violence or sexual themes, so that persistent but sympathetic questioning may be required. Before recording thoughts as obsessional, the interviewer should be certain that the patient accepts them as their own (and not implanted by an outside agency).

Compulsions

Many obsessional thoughts are accompanied by compulsive acts (p. 13). Some can be observed directly (though rarely during the interview), but others are private events (such as repeating phrases silently), detected only because they interrupt the patient's conversation. Appropriate questions are: 'Do you have to keep checking activities that you know you have completed?' 'Do you have to do things over and over again when most people would have done them only once?' 'Do you have to repeat exactly the same action many times?' If the patient answers 'yes' to any of these questions, the interviewer should ask for specific examples.

Delusions

A delusion cannot be asked about directly, because the patient does not recognize it as differing from other beliefs. Because of the difficulty this produces for the interviewer, and because of their diagnostic significance, delusions were described at length in Chapter 1 (pp. 8–12).

The interviewer may be alerted to the possibility of delusions by information from other people or by events in the history. In searching for delusional ideas, it is useful to begin by asking what might be the reason for other symptoms or unpleasant experiences that the patient has described. For example, a patient who says that life is no longer worth living may be convinced that he is thoroughly evil and that his internal organs are already rotting away. Some patients hide delusions skillfully, and the interviewer needs to be alert to evasions, changes of topic, or other hints of information being withheld. However, once the delusion has been uncovered, patients often elaborate on it without much prompting.

When ideas are revealed that could be delusional, the interviewer needs to determine whether they meet the criteria for a delusion (pp. 8–12). First, find out how strongly they are held. To do this without antagonizing the patient requires patience and tact. The patient should feel that they are having a fair hearing. If the interviewer expresses contrary opinions to test the strength of the patient's beliefs, the manner should be enquiring rather than argumentative. The next step is to decide whether the beliefs are culturally determined convictions rather than delusions. This judgment may be difficult if the patient comes from a culture or religious group whose attitudes and beliefs are not known to the interviewer. In such cases any doubt can usually be resolved by finding an informant from the same country or religion, and by asking this person whether others from the same background share his beliefs.

Some types of delusion, characteristic of schizophrenia, present particular problems of recognition:

- **Delusions of thought broadcasting** must be distinguished from the belief that other people can infer a person's thoughts from his expression or behaviour. In eliciting such delusions an appropriate question is: 'Do you ever feel that other people know what you are thinking, even though you have not spoken your thoughts aloud?' If the patient says 'yes', the interviewer should ask how other people know this. (Some patients answer 'yes' when they mean that others can infer their thoughts from their facial expression.)
- **Delusions of thought insertion.** A suitable question is: 'Have you ever felt that some of the thoughts in your mind were not your own but were put there from outside?' A corresponding question about **delusions of thought withdrawal** is: 'Do you ever feel that thoughts are being taken out of your head?' In each case, if the patient answers 'yes', detailed examples should be sought.
- **Delusions of control** (passivity of thought) present similar difficulties. It is appropriate to ask 'Do you ever feel that some outside force is trying to take control of you?' or 'Do you ever feel that your actions are controlled by some person or thing outside you?' Some patients misunderstand the question and answer 'yes' when they mean that they have a religious or philosophical conviction that man is controlled by God or other agency. Others think that the questions refer to the experience of being 'out of control' during extreme anxiety; some patients say 'yes' when in fact they have experienced auditory hallucinations commanding them to do things. Therefore positive answers should be followed by further questions to eliminate these possibilities.

Finally, the reader is reminded of the various categories of delusion described in Chapter 1 (pp. 9–12). The interviewer should also distinguish between primary and secondary delusions, and look out for the experiences of delusional perception and delusional mood. These issues only need to be addressed when there is already clear evidence of a psychosis, when they are useful in distinguishing schizophrenia from other psychotic disorders.

Perceptions

As with delusions, when asking about hallucinations enquiries should be made tactfully, to avoid distressing the patient, and in order to encourage them to elaborate on their experiences without being ridiculed. Questions can be introduced by saying 'Some people find that, when their nerves are upset, they have unusual experiences.' This can be followed by enquiries about hearing sounds or voices when no one else is within earshot. Whenever the history makes it relevant, corresponding questions should be asked about visual hallucinations and those in other modalities. Conversely, in assessments where there has been no prior evidence of psychosis at all, it may be appropriate to omit assessment of them altogether.

Auditory hallucinations

If the patient describes auditory hallucinations, certain further questions are required depending on the type of experience because of their diagnostic significance (pp. 7–8). Has the patient heard a single voice or several and, if the latter, did the voices appear to talk to the patient, or to each other about the patient in the third person? The latter experience must be distinguished from that of hearing actual people talking and believing that they are discussing the patient (an idea or delusion of reference). If the patient says that the voices are speaking to them, the interviewer should find out what the voices say and, if the words are experienced as commands, whether the patient feels that they must be obeyed. Note examples of the words spoken by hallucinatory voices.

Visual hallucinations

Visual hallucinations must be distinguished from visual illusions. Unless the hallucination is experienced at the time of the interview, this distinction may be difficult because it depends on the presence or absence of a visual stimulus which has been misinterpreted. Ascertaining if there is an 'as if' quality to the image, or asking if it is seen 'out there, or in your mind's eye' may help in the distinction. The interviewer should also distinguish hallucinations from dissociative experiences. The latter are described by the patient as the feeling of being in the presence of another person or a spirit with whom he can converse. Such experiences are reported by people with histrionic personality, though not confined to them, and are encouraged by some religious groups. They have little diagnostic significance.

Cognitive function

Early on in the interview, any significant cognitive difficulties will have already become apparent from the patient's interactions with the interviewer and their responses to questions. If so, the assessment of cognitive function should be brought forward, since the result may lead the interviewer to curtail the rest of the interview or postpone it until an informant is available. The Mini-Mental State Examination (see the Appendix at the end of this chapter) is a widely used cognitive screen.

In the evaluation of possible dementia and other organic disorders, cognitive testing is a central part of the assessment and often supplemented by more formal testing (see below and Chapter 14). Conversely, if the interview is nearing completion and no evidence or suspicion of such difficulties has arisen, cognition can be assessed very briefly. For a review of cognitive assessment, see Kipps and Hodges (2005).

Orientation

This is assessed by asking about the patient's awareness of time, place, and person. Specific questions begin with the day, month and year. In assessing the replies, remember that many healthy people do not know the exact date and that, understandably, patients in hospital may be uncertain about the day of the week or their precise location. If the patient cannot answer these basic questions correctly, they should be asked about their own identity; this is preserved except in severe dementia, dissociative disorders, or malingering.

Attention and concentration

Whilst taking the history, the interviewer should look out for evidence of attention and concentration. In this way an opinion will already have been formed about these abilities before reaching the mental state examination. Formal tests add to this information, and can provide a semi-quantitative indication of changes between occasions. It is usual to begin with the serial sevens test. The patient is asked to subtract seven from 100 and then subtract seven from the remainder repeatedly until this is less than seven. The time taken is recorded, together with the number of errors. If poor performance seems to be due to lack of skill in arithmetic, the patient should be asked to do a simpler subtraction or to say the months of the year in reverse order.

Memory

Whilst taking the history, the interviewer should compare the patient's account of past events with that of any other informant, and be alert to gaps or inconsistencies. If memory is impaired, any evidence of confabulation (p. 18) should be noted. During the mental state examination, tests are given of short-term, recent, and remote memory. Since none is wholly satisfactory, the results should be assessed alongside other information about memory and, if there is doubt, supplemented by standardized psychological tests. Objective evidence of memory impairment and its impact on normal activities (e.g. shopping, dressing) is also essential.

Short-term memory can be assessed by asking the patient to memorize a name and a simple address, to repeat it immediately (to make sure it has been registered correctly), and to retain it. The interview continues on other topics for 5 minutes before recall is tested. A healthy person of average intelligence should make only minor errors. If recall is imperfect, memory can be prompted, e.g. by saying '35, Juniper ... ' and the patient may then recall 'Street'.

Memory for recent events can be assessed by asking about news items from the last few days.

Remote memory can be assessed by asking the patient to recall personal events or well-known items of news from former years. Personal items could be the birth dates of children or the names of grandchildren (provided these facts are known to the interviewer); news items could be the names of well-known former political leaders. Awareness of the sequence of events is as important as the recall of individual items.

The reader is again referred to Chapter 14 for detailed assessment of cognitive functioning.

Insight

A note that merely records 'insight present' or 'no insight' is of little value. Instead the interviewer should enquire about the different aspects of insight discussed on p. 19. This includes the patient's appraisal of his difficulties and prospects, and whether he ascribes them to illness or to some other cause (such as persecution). If the patient recognizes that he is ill, does he think that the illness is physical or mental, and does he think that he needs any treatment? If so, what are his views on the options, such as medication, admission, or psychotherapy? The interviewer should also find out whether the patient thinks that stressful life experiences or his actions have played a part in causing his illness. The patient's views on these matters are a guide to her likely collaboration with treatment.

Other components of psychiatric assessment

Although the psychiatric history and mental state examination are the main parts of the psychiatric assessment, several other elements may also be necessary as part of the 'work up' of a patient. This section does not cover more specialized aspects of assessment (e.g. use of rating scales; see p. 62), or those not directly linked to diagnosis or initial management (e.g. assessment for psychotherapy).

Physical examination

Physical examination provides three kinds of information in the assessment:

1. It may reveal diagnostically useful signs, for example, a goitre or absent reflexes, and it is therefore particularly important in the diagnosis, or exclusion, of organic disorders. Neurological (including cerebrovascular) and endocrine systems most commonly require detailed examination, although other systems should not be neglected. The reader should consult a relevant textbook (e.g. Kaufman, 2002) if instruction is required in these aspects of clinical practice.
2. Psychotropic drugs may produce physical side-effects which need to be identified or measured, for example, hypertension, parkinsonism, or a rash.
3. The patient's general health, nutritional status and self-care may all be affected by psychiatric disorders.

For these reasons, a physical examination is an integral part of the psychiatric assessment. In practice, however, the extent of the physical examination, and the medical responsibility for it, varies. For example, many outpatients have been referred by, or are also cared for by, another doctor who may have recently carried out an appropriate physical examination. With day- or inpatients, the psychiatrist is generally responsible for their physical as well as their mental health; certainly, every newly admitted patient should have a full physical examination. Whatever the circumstances, the psychiatrist should decide what physical examination is relevant, and either carry it out themselves or ensure that this is done by another doctor. Discussion

BOX 3.2 THE NEUROPSYCHIATRIC EXAMINATION

Language abilities

Dysarthria is difficulty in the production of speech by the speech organs. **Dysphasia** is partial failure of language function of cortical origin; it can be receptive or expressive. Testing for dysarthria can be done by giving difficult phrases such as 'West Register Street' or a tongue twister.

Receptive dysphasia can be detected by asking the patient to read a passage of appropriate difficulty or, if he fails in this, individual words or letters. If he can read the passage, he is asked to explain it. Comprehension of spoken language is tested by asking a patient to listen to a spoken passage and explain it (first checking that memory is intact), or to respond to simple commands, for example, to point at named objects.

Expressive dysphasia is detected by asking patients to name common objects such as a watch, key, and pen, and some of their parts (for example, the face of a watch), and parts of the body. They are asked also to talk spontaneously (for example, about hobbies) and to write a brief passage, first to dictation, and then spontaneously on a familiar topic (for example, the members of the family). A patient who cannot do these tests should be asked to copy a short passage.

Language disorders point to the left hemisphere in right-handed people. In left-handed patients localization is less certain, but in many it is still the left hemisphere. The type of language disorder gives some further guide to localization: expressive dysphasia suggests an anterior lesion, receptive dysphasia suggests a posterior lesion, mainly auditory dysphasia suggests a lesion in the temporal region, and mainly visual dysphasia a more posterior lesion.

Construction abilities

Apraxia is inability to perform a volitional act even though the motor system and sensorium are sufficiently intact for the person to do so. Apraxia can be tested in several ways.

- **Constructional apraxia** is tested by asking the patient to draw simple figures, e.g. a bicycle, house, or clock face.
- **Dressing apraxia** is tested by asking the person to put on some of his clothes.
- **Ideomotor apraxia** is tested by asking her to perform increasingly complicated tasks to command, usually ending with a three-stage sequence such as: (i) touch the right ear with (ii) the left middle finger while (iii) placing the right thumb on the table.

Apraxias, especially if the patient fails to complete the left side of figures or dressing on the left side, suggests a right-sided lesion in the posterior parietal region. It may be associated with other disorders related to this region, namely sensory inattention and anosognosia.

Agnosia is the inability to understand the significance of sensory stimuli even though the sensory pathways and sensorium are sufficiently intact for the patient to be able to do so. Agnosia cannot be diagnosed until there is good evidence that the sensory pathways are intact and consciousness is not impaired.

- **Astereognosia** is failure to identify three-dimensional form; it is tested by asking the patient to identify objects placed in his hand while his eyes are closed. Suitable items are keys, coins of different sizes, and paper clips.
- **Atopognosia** is failure to know the position of an object on the skin.
- In **finger agnosia** the patient cannot identify which of his fingers has been touched when he has his eyes shut. Right-left confusion is tested by touching one hand or ear and asking the patient which side of the body has been touched.
- **Agraphognosia** is failure to identify letters or numbers 'written' on the skin. It is tested by tracing numbers on the palms with a closed fountain pen or similar object.
- **Anosognosia** is failure to identify functional deficits caused by disease. It is seen most often as unawareness of left-sided weakness and sensory inattention after a right parietal lesion.

Agnosias point to lesions of the association areas around the primary sensory receptive areas. Lesions of either parietal lobe can cause contralateral astereognosia, agraphognosia, and atopognosia. Sensory inattention and anosognosia are more common with right parietal lesions. Finger agnosia and right–left disorientation are said to be more common with lesions of the dominant parietal region.

with a neurologist or other physician is appropriate if the initial examination reveals equivocal or complex findings, or if a second opinion is sought. In some cases, more detailed assessment of higher neurological functions is required, as in the neuropsychiatric examination, summarized in Box 3.2. This may be a prelude to formal neuropsychological assessment or neurological investigations, notably for neuropsychiatric disorders.

Laboratory investigations

These vary according to the nature of the differential diagnosis, the patient's general health, and the resources available. At one extreme, no investigations may be necessary; at the other, brain imaging, genetic testing, and biochemical screening may be needed, especially if there is a strong suspicion of a treatable or heritable organic disorder. There is no one set of routine investigations applicable to every case, although by convention, routine blood tests (full blood count, electrolytes, liver and thyroid function) are usually carried out on admission to hospital. Investigations are discussed further in the chapters on individual syndromes.

Psychological assessment

Clinical psychologists and psychological testing can contribute to psychiatric assessment in several ways. They are not, however, required in most cases, and their availability is limited. We therefore only introduce the topic briefly here. The following are illustrations of the main forms and roles of psychological assessment.

Neuropsychological assessment

There are many psychometric tests, which measure different aspects of neuropsychological performance, ranging from overall intelligence to specific domains of memory, speed of processing, or tests which putatively assess functioning of a particular part of the brain (Lezak *et al.*, 2004). Neuropsychological testing in psychiatry is primarily used in the following areas (Grant and Adams, 1996; Powell, 2000):

- In learning disability, where IQ defines the severity of the condition.
- In dementia, where tests measure the severity and domains of cognitive impairment.
- If a decline in performance from premorbid abilities is suspected. In this instance, a discrepancy may be seen between verbal and performance IQ.
- To monitor the progress of neuropsychological deficits during the course of illness, by repeated administration of tests.
- To reveal deficits which may be subtle and neglected clinically, but which may be functionally important. For example, in schizophrenia, there are persistent impairments in specific domains of memory and attention, and these predict poor outcome. Although this use of neuropsychological testing is primarily a research tool, it may become part of routine clinical assessment as the findings become robust and their implications clear.
- If an organic cause for a patient's psychiatric disorder is suspected, the profile of test results may suggest the location of the lesion. However, this use of neuropsychological testing to localize brain lesions has largely been replaced by neuroimaging.

Cognitive assessment

The term 'cognitive' is sometimes used interchangeably with neuropsychological. In the present context however, cognitive assessment refers to the assessment of a patient's cognitions (thoughts), assumptions, and patterns of thinking. It is used to determine the suitability for, and focus of, cognitive therapy (Chapter 22).

Behavioural assessment

Observations and ratings of behaviour are useful in everyday clinical practice, especially for inpatients (Hall, 2000). When no ready-made rating scale is available, ad hoc ratings can be devised. For example, a scale could be devised for the nurses to show how much of the time a patient with depression was active and occupied. This could be a five-point scale, in which the criteria for each rating refer to behaviour (such as playing cards or talking to other people) relevant to the individual patient. As well as providing baseline information, the scale could also help monitor progress and response to treatment, complementing the information provided by repeated mental state examinations and qualitative observations.

Behavioural assessment is also used to evaluate the components of a patient's disorder (for example, in a phobia, the elements of anticipatory anxiety, avoidance, and coping strategies) and their relationship to stimuli in the environment (for example, heights), or more general circumstances (for example, crowded places), or internal cues (for example, awareness of heart action). Behavioural assessment is a necessary preliminary to behaviour therapy (see p. 590).

Personality assessment

In the past, detailed personality testing, including the use of 'projective' tests such as the Rorschach test, was often part of psychiatric assessment. These are no longer widely used, as they do not measure aspects of personality that are most relevant to psychiatric disorder, and they have not been shown to be valid predictors of diagnosis or outcome. Instead, personality is assessed descriptively as part of the history, described above, supplemented for research purposes with schedules for diagnosing personality disorders, such as the International Personality Disorder Examination, and the Personality Assessment Schedule (Reich and de Girolamo, 2000, and see Chapter 7).

TABLE 3.5 Risk factors for harm to others

Personal factors
Previous violence to others*
Antisocial, impulsive, or irritable personality traits
Male and young
Recent life crisis
Poor social network
Divorced or separated
Unemployed
Social instability
Illness-related factors
Psychotic symptoms*
Substance abuse*
Treatment resistant
Poor compliance with treatment
Stopped medication recently
Factors in the mental state
Irritability, hostility, anger
Suspiciousness
Thoughts of violence towards others
Threats to people to whom patient has access*
Planning of violence*
Persecutory delusions
Delusions of jealousy
Delusions of control
Hallucinations commanding violence to others
Suicidal ideas with severe depression
Clouding of consciousness
Lack of insight about illness
Situational factors
Confrontation and provocation by others
Situations associated with previous violence
Ready availability of weapons*

Risk assessment

Risk assessment is an essential part of psychiatric assessment. Risk in this context refers to risk of harm to others (violence) and risk to self (through suicide, deliberate self harm, or neglect). A failure to carry out and clearly document a risk assessment – and the resulting risk management plan – is a common criticism of enquiries that follow homicides and suicides involving psychiatric patients. Risk to self is covered in Chapter 17. Here we consider assessment of risk to others. Four kinds of information are used to assess such risks: personal factors, factors related to illness, factors in the mental state, and situational factors. These factors are summarized in Table 3.5, with the most important ones in each category starred.

A history of violence is the best predictor of future violence. Therefore seek full information on this not only by questioning the patient but, in appropriate cases, from additional sources including relatives and close acquaintances, previous medical and social services records, and in certain cases the police. Antisocial, impulsive, or irritable features in the personality are a further risk factor. Social circumstances at times of any previous episodes of violence may reveal provoking factors, and should be compared with the patient's current situation (see below). Social isolation and a recent life crisis also increase the risk. Among the illness factors, psychotic disorder and drug or alcohol misuse are important, much more so when present together. The combination of psychosis, substance misuse and personality disorder carries the highest risk of violence.

The mental state factors in Table 3.5 require careful consideration. Thoughts of violence to others are very important, especially if concerned with a specific person to whom the patient has access. The entry concerning suicidal ideas refers to the occasional killing, usually of family members, by a patient with severe (usually psychotic) depression. Features of morbid jealousy and other delusional disorders may pose specific risks of harm against a perceived aggressor or rival (p. 315).

Situational factors are highly important. Actual or perceived confrontational behaviour towards the patient by others may trigger violence, as may a return to situations in which violence has been expressed in the past. Enquiries should always be made about the availability of weapons.

Clinical experience and common-sense judgement have to be used to combine the risk factors into an overall assessment. Risk assessment schedules have been developed but do not replace thorough, and repeated, clinical assessment. The assessment of risk should be shared among the members of the team treating the patient, or if the patient is in individual treatment, may need to be discussed with a colleague. In certain circumstances the assessment may need to be made known to an individual at risk (see p. 71). Risk assessments should be reviewed regularly, combining information from the members of the clinical team. See Maden (1996) and Mullen (2000) for further information.

Although risk assessment is essential, it is important also to put it in context. First, the vast majority of psychiatric patients pose no risk to others, and are more likely to be the victims and not the perpetrators of violence. The assumption that all patients with severe mental illness, especially schizophrenia, are potentially violent is unwarranted and contributes to the stigma of all psychiatric patients. Second, even a complete risk assessment provides only a weak guide to future harm to others; many such acts are carried out by people with no past history of violence, and many of those who have multiple risk factors will never commit further violence. The inability to predict accurately those who will harm others is a strong argument against any legislation intended to preventatively detain those judged at high risk (Szmukler, 2001).

Assessment of needs

For patients with severe or enduring mental illness, particularly psychosis, there is an increasing focus on their needs in the broadest sense, for example, physical health, hygeine, social isolation, domestic skills, etc. The concern arises from findings that such needs are often not well recognized or met. The first step in this process is to assess the needs. Much of the information should already have been collected as part of the history, but further investigation of the patient's circumstances may be required. Scales to formally assess need are also available (e.g. Marshall *et al.*, 1995).

Special kinds of psychiatric assessment

Until now, this chapter has been concerned with the complete psychiatric assessment as carried out by psychiatrists on patients being seen in a psychiatric setting, for whom sufficient time is available. However, the majority of assessments do not meet all these criteria. Many are conducted by non-specialists, in non-psychiatric settings, with limited time and imperfect surroundings. This section considers how psychiatric assessment and interviewing are modified in these circumstances.

Interviews in an emergency

In an emergency, the interview has to be brief, focused on the key issues, and effective in leading to a provisional diagnosis and a plan of action. These assessments generally involve acutely distressed or disturbed patients, and often take place in difficult settings, such as a police station or medical ward. The diagnoses which are usually in question are the psychoses (schizophrenia, mania, drug-induced), and delirium and other organic brain disorders. Throughout, the interviewer should think which questions need to be answered at the time and which can be deferred. The most important issues are those which impact on immediate management decisions. The latter are likely to include whether the patient should be detained, whether laboratory investgiations are indicated, and whether medication should be given.

Because the assessment may be limited by the patient's ability or willingess to participate fully, seek out all available information before commencing the interview. For example, ask whoever is accompanying the person what they know about the patient and the recent events. The patient's belongings may reveal evidence of prior illness or medication. If the patient has a past psychiatric history, strenuous efforts should be made to obtain their case notes or to contact a professional involved in their care. The safety of the patient and those around them must also be actively considered when planning the nature and location of the interview.

An emergency assessment should, wherever possible, include the following core information:

- The presenting problem in terms of symptoms or behaviours, together with their onset, course, and present severity.
- Other relevant symptoms, with their onset, course, and severity.
- History of psychiatric or medical disorder.
- Current medication.
- Use of alcohol and drugs.
- Stressful circumstances around the time of onset and at the present time.

- Family and personal history covered with a few salient questions.
- Social circumstances, and the possibilities of support.
- Risk assessment, including risk of self-harm and the safety of others.

Interviews in general practice and the general hospital

In general practice, many presentations are with psychiatric disorders, notably depression and anxiety disorders, as well as substance misuse and somatoform disorders. Such cases commonly present with physical complaints (e.g. chronic pain, fatigue), and the doctor needs to be aware of the possibility that the symptoms reflect an underlying psychiatric disorder. The interplay of physical and psychological factors is emphasized by the finding that general practitioners who diagnose psychiatric disorder accurately, as compared with a standard assessment, have a good knowledge of general medicine (Goldberg and Huxley, 1980). Other patients present in primary care with an explicit psychological complaint, for example of low mood or panic attacks.

Whether the presentation is physical or psychological, it is a challenge to do an effective psychiatric assessment given the very limited time available. There are two components to achieving this goal. First, to increase the chances of detecting psychiatric disorder by the way the interview is conducted; for example, by being alert to cues in the patient's history, appearance and behaviour. Second, screening questions can be used that detect the common disorders, and identify areas which may require more detailed assessment (Table 3.6).

Goldberg and Huxley (1980) reported the first substantive work in this field, and described how the assessment of a patient in general practice whose complaint may have a psychological cause should cover four areas:

1. *General psychological adjustment:* fatigue, irritability, poor concentration, and the feeling of being under stress;
2. *Anxiety and worries:* physical symptoms of anxiety and tension, phobias, and persistent worrying thoughts;
3. *Symptoms of depression:* persistent depressive mood, tearfulness, crying, hopelessness, self-blame, thoughts that life is unbearable, ideas about suicide, early morning waking, diurnal variation of mood, weight loss, and loss of libido;
4. *The psychological context:* (i.e. the patient's personality and circumstances), although often known to the general practitioner from previous contacts, this should be reviewed and brought up to date.

Subsequently, more formalized sets of screening questions for psychiatric disorders suitable for brief interviews in primary care, and focusing on the disorders common in that setting, have been developed. The questions in Table 3.6 are adapted from Spitzer *et al.* (1994).

If the interview is conducted with psychological issues in mind, and screening questions are used appropriately, then it should be possible to identify many psychiatric disorders in the ten to fifteen minutes available in primary care. A preliminary plan can be made, and a further appointment arranged in order to evaluate the diagnosis and discuss management in more detail.

Similar considerations apply to interviews in a general medical setting, for example an accident and emergency department or medical ward. In these situations, particular attention may again need to be given to physical symptoms and the possibility of somatoform disorder, and to the assessment of suicidal risk. Delirium is also a common reason for a psychiatric consultation amongst medical and surgical inpatients.

TABLE 3.6 Brief screening questions for psychiatric disorders

During the past month:	Screening for:
1. Have you felt low in spirits?	Depression
2. Do you enjoy things less than you usually do?	Depression
3. Have you been feeling generally anxious?	Neurosis (anxiety)
4. Are you worried about your health or other specific things?	Neurosis (health anxiety)
5. Has your eating felt out of control?	Eating disorder
6. Do you drink alcohol? If so, ask CAGE questions (p. 442)	Alcohol problem
7. Present three items and ask patient to recall them after 2 minutes	Dementia/delirium

Interviews in a patient's home

It is often appropriate to add to the information about a patient's circumstances by visiting the home, or arranging for another member of the psychiatric team to do so. Such a visit often throws new light on the patient's home life and gives a more realistic evaluation of the relationship between family members. Home visits are especially important in the assessment of elderly patients (p. 504).

Before arranging a visit the psychiatrist should, if possible, talk to the general practitioner, who often has first-hand knowledge of the family over many years. The safety of the interviewer should always be considered before embarking on a domiciliary visit. The interviewer should ensure that another member of the team is aware of the location and time of the visit; if there is any concern about potential risk, a joint assessment should be made.

Interviews with the family

Sometimes an interview is carried out with several family members together to find out their attitudes to the patient and the illness and the nature of any conflicts within the family. This is usually done in child and adolescent psychiatry. The interviewer should remember that the family has usually tried to help the patient but failed and may feel demoralized, frustrated, or guilty, and should be careful not to add to these feelings.

The interviewer should then ask:

- How has the illness affected family life, and how have the family tried to cope?
- What are the relationships and alliances within the family? Are there important differences of opinion between the members of the family?
- Are the members willing to try new ways of helping the patient?

For further information about family interviews, see Goldberg (1997). Family interviewing in the context of family therapy is covered in Chapter 22.

Interviewing a patient from another culture

If the patient and interviewer do not speak the same language, an interpreter will obviously be needed. However, accurate interpretation is not the only requirement, and the interviewer may not know the patient's culture as well as they know the language. Also, female patients from another culture may be reluctant to describe personal matters to a male interviewer. Even when these problems are absent, the presence of a third person, and the process of translation, affects the interview and lengthens it considerably. If possible the interpreter should be a health professional, as they can then assist in the assessment itself.

Certain events may be more stressful to a patient from another culture than they would be in the interviewer's culture. The stigma of mental illness may be greater. Priorities within the family may be different, with the well-being of the family outweighing that of its individual members. Emotional disorder may be experienced more in terms of physical than mental symptoms. Expectations and fears about treatment may be based on knowledge of less developed services in the country of origin. Behaviours that suggest illness in one culture may be socially sanctioned ways of expressing distress in others, for example, extreme displays of emotion. Ideas about causation may differ; for example, distress may be ascribed to the actions of evil spirits. Also it may be difficult to decide whether strongly held ideas are delusional or normal within the culture or subculture. The influence of cultural differences on diagnosis and classification was discussed in Chapter 2.

Interviewing a patient with limited intelligence

The procedures for interviewing people with low intelligence (learning disability) are similar to those for people with normal intelligence but certain points should receive particular attention. Questions should be brief and worded in a simple way, and avoiding figures of speech. It may be difficult to avoid closed questions, but if they are used, the answers should be checked; for example, if the question 'Are you sad?' is answered 'yes', the question 'Are you happy?' should not be answered in the same way. Some people repeat the interviewer's last word, and such a response should not be accepted as agreement unless checked.

People with learning disability may have difficulty in timing the onset of symptoms or describing their sequence, and to obtain this and other information it is important to interview an informant. Nevertheless, an attempt should always be made to obtain from patients an account of their symptoms and their concerns. See also Chapter 25 for discussion of assessment in learning disability.

Interviewing children and the elderly

Assessment of children and adolescents are considered on pp. 657–60, and the elderly on pp. 503–4.

Integrating and evaluating the information

Thus far, the account of assessment has been largely about data gathering, though with indications that questioning should be aimed at testing hypotheses and following up potential clues about the diagnosis and aetiology. The following section explains further how facts are evaluated and integrated with knowledge of psychiatry. The conclusions should lead directly on to decisions about treatment. We emphasize again that, in practice, information is evaluated as it is collected.

Drawing conclusions and making decisions

The areas in which an opinion must be formed, or a decision made, are listed in Table 3.7. It may also be useful to think in terms of a set of rhetorical questions needing to be answered:

- What is the diagnosis?
- What are the effects on the patient's life?
- Are there immediate risks that need to be managed?
- What are the patient's current circumstances?
- Why has the disorder occurred?
- What treatment is indicated?
- What is the prognosis?
- What other information is needed to answer these questions?
- What does the patient need and want to know?

TABLE 3.7 Topics to be evaluated in a psychiatric assessment

The patient's problem and its consequences
◆ Diagnosis
◆ Impact on self and others (dysfunction)
◆ Risk to self and others
The patient's circumstances
◆ Personal history
◆ Current circumstances
◆ Personality
Aetiology
Treatment
Prognosis
The patient's understanding of the above

What is the diagnosis?

The first step is to make a diagnosis using information about the symptoms and signs gained from the history and mental state examination and, in relevant cases, from the physical examination. This information is then used to make a diagnosis based upon knowledge of psychiatric classification and the criteria for each diagnostic category. Sometimes a diagnosis has to be provisional until further information becomes available. The diagnosis of particular psychiatric disorders is discussed in subsequent chapters; here we are concerned with the general approach to assessment. Diagnosis is accompanied by an assessment of the severity of the disorder into categories of mild, moderate, and severe.

What are the effects on the patient's life?

When patients describe their problems, they will include both symptoms and other matters. A key purpose of the assessment is to identify and characterize the psychopathology, since it is these that determine which disorder will be diagnosed. However, it is also necessary to enquire about the effects that their symptoms have on their life, in part since evidence of impaired functioning is relevant to most diagnoses. It is therefore helpful to reach a view about the patient's usual level of functioning and how far the current state differs from it.

Are there immediate risks which need to be managed?

As we have discussed, risk assessment is a core part of the psychiatric assessment. Having identified any risks, they need to be managed. For example, if the patient is at risk of self-neglect or self-harm, this will influence whether compulsory admission is necessary; if a risk of harm to another party has been identified, that person may need to be warned.

What are the patient's current circumstances?

Knowing about the person's accommodation, finances, interests and relationships may all influence management and prognosis. For example, a homeless person will require a different care package than a patient with the same disorder who has a stable home and a carer. The current circumstances may also act as maintaining factors for the disorder, and be a target for intervention. For example, accommodation worries may be a stressor perpetuating a depressive illness.

Why has the disorder occurred?

Aetiology is discussed in Chapter 5. Here we are concerned with how aetiological factors are applied to the individual patient. A useful approach is chronological: causes are divided into **predisposing, precipitating**, and **perpetuating**. Predisposing factors may be genetic or related to temperament, or to damage to the brain in early life. Precipitating factors are often stressful events. Perpetuating (maintaining) factors may be continuing stressors, or related to the way that the patient attempts to cope with stressors (for example, avoiding anxiety-provoking situations or misusing alcohol). Perpetuating factors are highly relevant to treatment.

A **life chart** is a tool for evaluating the role of life events in aetiology (Sharpe, 1990). It helps to reveal the temporal relationship between episodes of physical and mental disorder and potentially stressful events in the patient's life. It is often useful when the history is long and complicated. The chart has three columns – one for life events, and one each for physical and mental disorder. Its rows represent the years in the patient's life. Completion of a life chart requires detailed enquiry into the timing of events, but is worthwhile as it may clarify the relationships between stressors and the onset of illness, and also between physical and mental disorders.

A word on personality is appropriate here. Clear appreciation of a patient's personality is part of the full understanding of their life history and their psychiatric disorder. Hence we have emphasized the collection of sufficient and reliable personality information during the assessment. As well as helping in the aetiological formulation, this knowledge will be of use when planning management and predicting outcome. For example, comorbid personality disorder worsens prognosis of many conditions, and may also influence decisions about psychological treatment.

What treatment is indicated?

A key decision to be made is what, if any, treatment does the patient require? If treatment is indicated, then the options should be discussed with the patient, and the evidence for each possible treatment presented in terms of efficacy, side-effects, etc. These issues are discussed in later chapters.

What is the prognosis?

Prognosis depends primarily on the disorder concerned. It also depends on individual characteristics of the patient; for example, their age, severity of symptoms, comorbid conditions etc. Not all this information may be available after an initial assessment. However, it is usually possible to make a cautious prediction about short-term outcome at this stage, and most patients will expect and appreciate this. The patient can be told that more accurate and longer-term prognostic judgements will be possible as further information is obtained, and the course of the disorder is followed over subsequent weeks and months.

What other information is needed to answer these questions?

For most patients, assessment is not complete after one interview. Many of the questions posed here cannot be answered with any certainty, and assessment should be viewed as an iterative process in which opinions and conclusions undergo continuing review, as further information about the patient and their illness is obtained. For descriptive purposes, this chapter focuses on the diagnostic purpose of assessment, but in practice there is no firm distinction between this and the other goals of assessment (e.g. to assess risk, or response to treatment). Instead, each interaction between psychiatrist and patient is a mixture of assessment, evaluation, and decision-making. In this sense, assessment is a process which continues throughout treatment and follow-up.

What does the patient need and want to know?

This issue is introduced on p. 62, and in later chapters with regard to specific disorders and treatments.

Other issues affecting how the information is evaluated

Disease and illness

These concepts were introduced in Chapter 2, but brief mention is required here. **Illness** refers to a patient's experience and **disease** to the pathological cause for this experience. Patients can be diseased without feeling ill, or feel ill without having an identifiable disease. In general medicine, patients tell doctors about their experience of illness and doctors seek to discover the disease that is causing the illness since this will guide treatment. Patients and their relatives also want to find a cause and a treatment for their illness but they do not always understand how a medical diagnosis helps in finding them. Psychiatrists also search for disease as a cause of illness, but should always look for other causes too; sometimes the patient's experience can be understood as an extreme variation from the norm, sometimes a reaction to circumstance, and sometimes as a combination of all three. Other mental health professionals may emphasize one or other of these factors depending on their background; for example, psychologists focus on variation from the norm, and a social worker focuses on the role of reaction to circumstances. These differences of emphasis can lead to apparent disagreements during multidisciplinary assessment. It is important that psychiatrists are aware of this possibility, so that they can help to resolve them.

Evaluations by experienced psychiatrists

Throughout this chapter, a systematic and logical approach to assessment has been advocated, in which information is collected carefully, and eliciting of symptoms and signs forms the basis of diagnosis. Anyone new to psychiatry should always follow this approach closely. However, studies show that experienced psychiatrists actually carry out assessments rather differently. They make rapid diagnoses, often within the first few minutes of the interview, presumably reflecting the predictive power of the patient's initial appearance, behaviour and utterances (Gauron and Dickinson, 1966; Kendell, 1975). The psychiatrist may not realize the cues and clues which they are using to form these diagnostic judgements. Schwartz and Wiggins (1987) called this process **typification**. The rest of the interview then functions primarily to confirm and refine this diagnostic opinion.

As experience is gained, a clinician is likely to use this kind of strategy increasingly in assessment. If one has a firm grasp of psychopathology and diagnostic classification, typification can be used effectively. However, we emphasize that this approach should not be attempted until the 'textbook' approach to psychiatric assessment has been mastered and further experience accumulated. The interviewer should always ensure they have not come to premature conclusions about a case, causing them to fail to gather necessary information or to disregard contrary evidence that emerges.

Recording and communicating information

Having completed the assessment, it is necessary to record and communicate your understanding of the case and its management. These records and communications take a variety of forms, according to their intended purpose and recipients, but all should follow certain basic principles:

- Information should be presented clearly and concisely. Include important negatives (e.g. 'He is not suicidal'). In letters, avoid repetition of information already known to the recipient. Use headings and subheadings to highlight key points (e.g. 'Diagnosis: ... '; 'Current Medication ...').
- In many countries, patients are entitled to read what is written about them. This information may also be used for legal purposes. In some countries, including the United Kingdom, it is now expected that patients are copied into correspondence between doctors which concerns them, unless there is a compelling reason not to do so. Ensure that all information is accurate, that any opinions or inferences you make are reasonable, and avoid unwarranted or unnecessarily personal comments. It is sometimes better to communicate verbally with the doctor or other health professional to expand on some details of the case. The patient should be told that they will receive a copy of the letter, and invited to contact you if it is unclear or mistaken in fact.
- All communications should be kept confidential.

Here we consider a range of ways in which assessment information is recorded and shared, within the psychiatric team, between psychiatrist and other doctors, and between psychiatrist and patient.

The importance of case notes

Good case records are important in every branch of medicine. In psychiatry they are vital because a large amount of information has to be collected from a variety of sources. It is important to summarize the information in a way that allows essential points to be grasped readily by someone new to the case, especially a colleague called to deal with an emergency. Case notes are not just an aide memoire for the writer, they are important for others concerned with the patient. Case notes are also of medico-legal importance. If a psychiatrist is called upon to justify his actions in the coroner's court, at a trial, or after a complaint has been made by a patient, he will be greatly assisted by case notes which are comprehensive but concise, well organized, and legible.

Admission notes

When a patient is admitted to hospital urgently, the doctor often has limited time so that it is then particularly important to record the right topics. The admission note should contain at least:

- the reasons for admission
- any information required for a decision about immediate treatment
- any other relevant information that will not be available later such as details of the mental state on admission (and prior to medication), and information from any informant who may not be available again.

If there is time, a systematic history can be added. However, inexperienced interviewers sometimes spend too much time on details that are not essential to the immediate decisions, while failing to record details of mental state that may be transitory and yet of great importance in diagnosis. The rest of the assessment can always be carried out over the next few days. The admission note should end with a brief plan of immediate management, agreed with the senior nurses caring for the patient at the time.

Progress notes

Progress notes need to contain specific information if they are to be of value. Instead of recording merely that the patient feels better or is behaving more normally, record in what ways he feels better (for example, less preoccupied with thoughts of suicide) or is less disturbed (for example, no longer so restless as to be unable to sit at table throughout a meal).

Progress notes should record treatment. Although details of drug treatment appear on the prescription sheet, it is convenient to have this information, together with any non-drug treatments, alongside the record of changes in mental state and behaviour. Sessions of counselling or psychotherapy need not be recorded in full, but notes should be made of the main themes, together with any relevant observations of the patient's response. It is often useful to add an occasional note summarizing progress over several sessions. Also a note should be made of the conclusions of team meetings. If the patient is being seen in an outpatient clinic, major life events and stressors since the last visit should be recorded.

A careful note should be made of any information or advice given by the doctor to the patient or his relatives. This should be sufficient to make it clear whether the patient was appropriately informed when consenting to any new treatment. Also it should enable anyone giving advice later to know whether or not it differs from what was said before, so that any necessary explanation can be given.

Observations of progress are made not only by psychiatrists but also by nurses, occupational therapists, clinical psychologists, and social workers. Often, these other professionals keep separate notes, but it is desirable that important items of information are written in the medical record. A note should also be kept of formal discussions between members of the team. It is particularly important to set out clearly the plans made for the patient's further care on discharge from hospital, including the identity of the key worker. These arrangements are formalized in the United Kingdom in the care programme approach (p. 637).

The case summary

Case summaries are usually used for inpatients. Ideally, they are written in two parts; the first part written soon after admission to record the initial presentation, and the second part at discharge, filling in the subsequent progress. In practice, however, a single summary covering all salient aspects of the case is often produced.

Summaries should be brief but comprehensive, written in telegraphic style, using a standard format, to help others people to find particular items of information. A completed summary should seldom need to be any more than between one and one-and-a-half typewritten pages. An example is given in Box 3.3. The completed summary is a valuable record should the patient become ill again, especially if they are under the care of a different team.

Some of the items in the summary call for comment. The reason for referral should state the problem rather than anticipate the diagnosis, for example: 'found wandering at night in an agitated state, shouting about God and the devil', rather than 'for treatment of schizophrenia'. The description of personality is important, and the writer should strive to find words and phrases which characterize the person. Unless an abnormality has been found, results of physical examination can be summarized briefly. However, when the mental state is recorded, a comment should be made under each heading whether or not any abnormality has been found. Diagnosis should be recorded using terms from ICD-10 or DSM-IV. If the diagnosis is uncertain, alternatives can be listed, with an indication of which is judged more likely. More than one diagnosis may be required in some cases.

The summary of treatment should include the dosage and duration of any medication. The prognosis should be stated briefly but as definitely as possible. Statements such as 'prognosis guarded' are of little help to anyone. Unless the assessor commits herself more firmly she will not learn from comparing her predictions with the actual outcome. The writer should note how certain the prognosis is and the reasons for any uncertainty, such as doubt about the patient's future compliance with treatment. The summary of future treatment should specify not only what is to be done but also who is to do it. The roles of the specialist team and the general practitioner should be made clear.

Formulations

A formulation is an exercise in clinical reasoning that helps the writer think clearly about diagnosis, aetiolo-

BOX 3.3 EXAMPLE OF A CASE SUMMARY

Patient Mrs AB. Date of birth 7.2.71. Age 34.

Consultant Dr C. Summary compiled by Dr D., 25.7.05.

Admitted 27.6.05

Discharged 22.7.05

Reason for referral Severe depression and suicidal ideation.

Family history Father 66, retired gardener, good physical health, mood swings, poor relationship with patient. Mother 57, housewife, healthy, spiritualist, distant relationship. Sibling Joan, 38, divorced, healthy. Home materially adequate, little affection. Mental illness: father's brother in hospital four times – 'manic depression'.

Personal history Birth and early development normal. Childhood health good. School 6–16 uneventful; made friends. Worked 16–22 shop assistant. Several boyfriends; married at 22, husband 2 years older, lorry driver. Unhappy in last year following husband's infidelity. Children Jane, 7, well; Paul, 4, epileptic. Sex life satisfactory until last year. Circumstances: council house, financial problems.

Previous illness Aged 27, (postnatal) depressive illness lasting 8 weeks, saw counsellor.

Previous personality Few friends, variable mood, worries easily, lacks self-confidence. No obsessional traits. Shares mother's interest in the supernatural. Drinks occasionally, non-smoker, denies drugs.

History of present illness For 6 weeks, since learning of husband's infidelity, increasingly low-spirited and tearful, waking early, neglecting children. Loss of appetite and libido. Strong suicidal ideation, culminating in abortive attempt to hang herself on night of admission. Getting worse despite fluoxetine 20 mg daily for 4 weeks, taken regularly.

On examination Physical: n.a.d. Mental state exam: dishevelled and distraught. Speech: slow, halting, normal form. Thoughts: Preoccupied with her unhappy state and with worries that her husband and his mistress are conspiring against her. Wishing she were dead. Prominent ideas of suicide, finding them hard to resist. No delusions or obsessions. Mood: depressed, with self-blame, hopelessness. Perceptions: imagines she hears her dead grandmother talking to her in derogatory tones; however, this is not a hallucination. Cognition: attention and concentration poor. Memory not formally tested. Insight: thinks she is ill but believes she cannot recover.

Special investigations Haemoglobin and electrolytes n.a.d.

Treatment and progress Initially on close observations. Medication changed to amitriptyline, progressively increased to 175 mg per day, graded activities, joint interviews with husband to improve marital relationship. Advice to husband about financial management. Gradual improvement in mood and loss of suicidal ideation. Successful weekend at home before final discharge.

Condition on discharge Mild residual depressive symptoms. Hopeful but worried about future of marriage.

Diagnosis Depressive disorder.

Prognosis Depends on outcome of marital problems. If these improve, the short-term prognosis is good but will be at risk of further depressive illness in the long term.

Further management

- Continue amitriptyline 175mg per day for 9 months before review. Prescriptions from GP.
- Jo Smith, community psychiatric nurse, is her key worker and will visit on 27.7.05.
- Patient has a copy of her care plan and she and her husband know who to contact in an emergency.
- Out patient review with psychiatrist on 4.8.05.

gy, treatment, and prognosis. A formulation should not contain speculation, but it may contain hypotheses that can be tested by obtaining further information. By writing formulations of a wide variety of cases, the trainee can learn to analyse the problems of a case. For an experienced psychiatrist, a written formulation remains a valuable aid to the understanding complex cases.

The headings for a formulation are listed in Table 3.8, and an example given in Box 3.4. After a short opening statement, the differential diagnosis comes next with a

BOX 3.4 EXAMPLE OF A FORMULATION

(Note: This formulation refers to the hypothetical case summarized in Box 3.3. By comparing the two ways of condensing information, the reader can appreciate the difference between the two approaches.)

Mrs AB is a 34-year-old married woman who for 6 weeks has been feeling increasingly depressed and unable to cope at home, despite outpatient treatment with antidepressant drugs.

Diagnosis

Depressive disorder As well as feeling low-spirited, Mrs AB has woken unusually early, felt worse in the morning, and lost her appetite and libido. She has little energy or initiative. She blames herself for being a bad mother (which she is not) and believes that she cannot recover. She is suicidal. No feature is against the diagnosis.

Schizophrenia or other psychosis Mrs AB believes that her husband is conspiring against her, and that her dead grandmother talks to her. However, the belief is not a delusion, and the grandmother's voice is not a hallucination. Both symptoms are mood congruent and consistent with a severe depression. She has no first-rank symptoms of schizophrenia, and retains insight.

Personality disorder Although Mrs AB has had mood variations for many years, these do not meet the criteria for a cyclothymic personality disorder.

Conclusions Depressive disorder.

Aetiology

Symptoms appear to have been precipitated by news of her husband's infidelity. Mrs AB was predisposed to react severely to this news by the insecure and jealous traits in her personality. She may be predisposed to develop a depressive disorder in relation to stressful events in that (a) she became depressed after the birth of her first child, (b) she is subject to mood variations, and (c) her family history of mood disorder which may reflect a genetic predisposition. The disorder has been maintained by continuing marital arguments and by worry about debts. Mrs AB's knowledge of her sister's divorce and subsequent unhappiness has added to her own concerns.

Treatment

The symptoms of the depressive disorder suggests that it is likely to respond to an antidepressant drug given in adequate dosage. Although she has not responded to an SSRI, amitriptyline may be more effective for severe depressive disorder. Joint interviews with the patient and her husband may resolve or reduce the marital problems. The husband should be advised how to get advice about dealing with his debts.

Prognosis

If the marital problems improve, the immediate prognosis is good. However, the predisposing factors noted above indicate that she may develop further depressive disorder, particularly at future times of stress.

TABLE 3.8 The formulation

Statement of the problem
Differential diagnosis
Aetiology
Further investigations
Plan of treatment
Prognosis

list of reasonable possibilities in the order of their probability. A note is made of the evidence for and against each alternative, followed by the writer's conclusion about the most probable diagnosis. Under aetiology, identify predisposing, precipitating, and perpetuating causes. The reasons for any predisposition are then considered, usually in chronological order to show how each factor may have added to those that went before. There follows a list of outstanding problems and any further information needed. Next a concise plan of management is outlined, and finally a statement about prognosis.

Problem lists

A problem list is useful in cases with complicated social problems. Such a list makes it easier to identify clearly what can be done to help the patient, and to monitor progress in achieving agreed objectives of treatment. It is often appropriate to draw up the list with the patient, as a way of helping them to understand which problems can be changed and what they can do to bring this about.

TABLE 3.9 A problem list

Problem	Action	Agent	Review
1 Frequent quarrels with husband	Joint interviews	Dr A	3 weeks
2 3-year old son slow to speak	Speech assessment	Via GP	1 week
3 Housing unsatisfactory	Visit housing department	Patient	2 weeks
4 Sexual dysfunction (?due to 1)	Defer		
5 Panic attacks	Assess for cognitive therapy	Psychologist	6 weeks

Table 3.9 shows a problem list that might be drawn up following the initial assessment of a woman who had taken an overdose and was found to have anxiety symptoms and many social problems. As progress is made in dealing with problems in this list, new ones may be added or existing ones modified or removed. For example, it might transpire that her sexual difficulties are a cause of the marital problem rather than a result, and that counselling should be offered. Item 4 in Table 3.9 would then be amended.

Letters to the general practitioner

When a letter is written to a general practitioner, the first step is to think what they already know about the patient, and what questions were asked when they referred the patient. If the referral letter outlined the salient features of the case, there is no need to repeat them in the reply. When the patient is less well known to the general practitioner, more detailed information should be given. Similarly, if the diagnosis given in the referral letter is correct, it is only necessary to confirm it; otherwise the reasons behind your diagnosis should be outlined.

Treatment and prognosis are dealt with next. When discussing treatment, the dosage, timing, and duration of any drug treatment should be stated. Responsibility for future prescribing should be stated. Name any key worker, therapists or other agencies involved, and the nature of their involvement. State the date of the patient's next appointment, and whether you have advised the patient to see the general practitioner. These details should, if possible, be agreed with the general practitioner by phone before the letter is written to confirm them. The letter should emphasize a collaborative approach, and encourage the general practitioner to get in touch should they be unclear about the arrangements, or concerned about the patient.

Explaining the diagnosis and management plan to the patient

When discussing the conclusions from your assessment with the patient, and with relatives, it may be useful to begin by briefly summarizing the key points back to them. This helps ensure you have understood the history correctly and have not omitted anything which in their opinion is significant. This process is also helpful in that it demonstrates your engagement and empathy with the patient, and sets the scene for discussion about the diagnosis and how you propose to proceed.

When introducing the diagnosis, do not use medical terms without explanation. The patient may misunderstand their meaning or make incorrect assumptions about the implications. Explain the significance of the diagnosis in terms of cause, prognosis, and possibilities for treatment.

When discussing the proposed plan of management, it is useful to begin by asking what treatment the patient has been expecting, and whether they have strong feelings about this, for example regarding the use of medication. The plan should be explained in an unhurried way, checking from time to time that the patient has understood. Whether drugs or psychological treatment are planned, there are several relevant issues to raise and discuss (p. 522 and Chapter 22). It is important to set aside enough time for this explanation during the interview, since it is likely to improve concordance with the treatment plan. If, after full explanation, the patient refuses to accept part of the plan, the interviewer should try to negotiate an acceptable alternative.

Box 3.5 summarizes the points that should be considered when communicating with patients and relatives.

Standardized assessment methods

In research, and sometimes in clinical practice, it is helpful to use standardized methods to assess symptoms and syndromes, as well as disabilities and other consequences of psychiatric disorders. Such methods improve reliability and facilitate comparison of findings across time and between psychiatrists.

Standardized methods of assessment are of three main types, considered in turn below.

BOX 3.5 COMMUNICATING WITH PATIENTS AND RELATIVES

Relevant questions from the following list can be helpful when deciding what information should be given to patients and their relatives:

The diagnosis

- What is the psychiatric diagnosis– if it is uncertain, what are the possibilities?
- Is there a physical diagnosis?
- Is any further information or special investigation required?
- What are the implications of the diagnosis for this patient?
- What may have caused the condition?

The care plan

- What is the plan, and how will it help the patient and the family?
- Are there any legal powers to be used: if so why, and what is their effect?
- What do they need to know about medication?
- What do they need to know about psychological treatments?

Who does what?

- Who is the key worker and what will he or she do?
- What is the role of the psychiatrist, and how often will they see the patient?
- What is the role of the other members of the psychiatric team?
- What is the role of the general practitioner?
- What can the family do to help the patient?

Emergencies

- Are they likely and how might they be avoided?
- Are there possible early warning signs of a crisis?
- Who should be approached in an emergency, and how can they be found quickly?

1. Those which rate symptoms in order to make a diagnosis; these have been important in the development of contemporary psychiatric classifications and were introduced in Chapter 2. The mini-mental state examination (in the Appendix to this chapter) is another example of this type.
2. Those which rate the severity of a symptom or group of symptoms.
3. Those which assess the overall evidence for and effects of psychiatric disorder. These are called global rating scales and include quality of life measures.

For reviews of methods and approaches to standardized ratings, see Task Force for Psychiatric Measures (2000) and Farmer *et al.* (2002).

Standardized diagnostic assessments

A range of diagnostic assessment schedules have been developed. The leading ones in current use are mentioned here. Further examples which relate to specific diagnoses are considered in the chapters on individual syndromes.

An important distinction is between those schedules designed for use by interviewers with training in psychiatry, and those without. The former can simply give the general rules by which symptoms are to be assessed. The **Present State Examination** is an example of this kind of interview and the extract in the upper part of Box 3.6 illustrates its format. Schedules designed for use by interviewers without formal training in psychiatry (as is usually the case in large-scale epidemiological research) use more precise rules for detecting symptoms, and for diagnosing syndromes. An example of this format is shown in the second part of Box 3.6.

Present State Examination

The development of the Present State Examination (PSE) began in the late 1950s. Early versions were used solely in the authors' own research: the ninth edition (PSE 9) was the first to be published for use by others (Wing *et al.*, 1974). It is available in at least 35 languages and has been widely used in many countries. The main principle is that the interview, although clearly structured, retains the features of a clinical examination. A trained interviewer seeks to identify abnormal phenomena that have been present during a defined period of time and to rate their severity. Each of the 140 items is defined in detail in a glossary. Computer programs generate a symptom score, a diagnosis (CATEGO), and a clinically derived measure of the severity of non-psychotic symptoms (the Index of Definition).

BOX 3.6 EXAMPLES OF STANDARDIZED ASSESSMENT QUESTIONS

Example 1: PSE definition of 'delusion of thought being read' (see Wing *et al.*, 1974)

This is usually an explanatory delusion. Often it goes with delusions of reference or misinterpretation which require some explanation of how other people know so much about the subject's future movements. It may be an elaboration of thought broadcast, thought insertion, auditory hallucinations, delusions of control, delusions of persecution, or delusions of influence. It can even occur with expansive delusions (the subject wishing to explain how Einstein, for example, stole his original ideas). Therefore the symptom is in no way diagnostic. It is most important that it should not be mistaken for diagnostically more important symptoms such as thought insertion or broadcast.

If the subject merely entertains the possibility that his thought might be read but is not certain about it, rate '1'; rate delusional conviction '2'. Exclude those who think that people can read their thoughts as a result of belonging to a group that practices 'thought reading' - this would be rated 1 or 2 on symptom no. 83.

The section on hallucinations in the PSE continues with questions about third-person hallucinations and non-verbal hallucinations.

Example 2: SCID questions about delusions (see Spitzer *et al.*, 1987)

Psychotic and associated symptoms This module is for coding psychotic and associated symptoms that have been present at any point in the person's lifetime.

For all psychotic and associated symptoms coded '3', determine whether the symptom is 'not organic', or whether there is a possible or definite organic cause. The following questions may be useful if the overview has not already provided the information: 'When you were experiencing the psychotic symptoms were you taking any drugs or medicine? Drinking a lot? Physically ill?' If the patient has not acknowledged psychotic symptoms: 'Now I am going to ask you about unusual experiences that people sometimes have.'

If the patient has acknowledged psychotic symptoms: 'You have told me about (psychotic experiences). Now I am going to ask you more about those kinds of things.'

Delusions These are false personal belief(s) based on incorrect inference about external reality and firmly sustained in spite of what almost everyone else believes, and in spite of what constitutes incontrovertible and obvious proof or evidence to the contrary. Code overvalued ideas (unreasonable and sustained belief(s) that is/are maintained with less than delusional intensity) as '2'. Note: a single delusion may be coded '3' on more than one of the following items: 'Did it ever seem that people were talking about you or taking special notice of you?'…

Delusions of reference, i.e. personal significance is falsely attributed to objects or events in environment: 'What about receiving special messages from the TV, radio, or newspaper, or from the way things were arranged around you?'

(Describe: as ?:1:2:3 where 1 = Poss/def organic; and 3 = Not organic.)

Persecutory delusions, i.e. the individual (or his or her group) is being attacked, harassed, cheated, persecuted, or conspired against:'What about anyone going out of the way to give you a hard time, or trying to hurt you?' (Describe: as ?:1:2:3 where 1 = Poss/def organic; and 3 = Not organic.)

Grandiose delusions, i.e. content involves exaggerated power, knowledge, or importance: 'Did you ever feel that you were especially important in some way, or that you had powers to do things that other people could not do?'

(Describe: as ?:1:2:3 where 1 = Poss/def organic; and 3 = Not organic.)

The section on delusions in SCID continues with questions about other kinds of delusions (somatic, nihilistic, etc.).

Schedules for Clinical Assessment in Neuropsychiatry

The tenth edition of the PSE was incorporated into the Schedules for Clinical Assessment in Neuropsychiatry (SCAN), a more extensive schedule which can be used to diagnose a broader range of disorders, including eating, somatoform, substance abuse, and cognitive disorders (World Health Organization, 1992a). The system is compatible with PSE 9, and it allows ICD-10, DSM-IIIR, and DSM-IV diagnoses (Janca *et al.*, 1994). A computer-assisted version is available.

Structured Clinical Interview for Diagnosis

The Structured Clinical Interview for Diagnosis (SCID) is a diagnostic assessment procedure designed to make DSM diagnoses, first issued with DSM-IIIR. It can be used by the clinician as part of a normal assessment procedure to confirm a particular diagnosis or in research or screening as a systematic evaluation of a whole range of medical states (Spitzer *et al.*, 1987). SCID is available in a patient edition for use with subjects who have been identified as psychiatric patients and in a non-patient edition suitable for use in epidemiological studies. In addition the SCID-II is available for making 12 Axis II, i.e. personality disorder, diagnoses.

Diagnostic Interview Schedule

This Diagnostic Interview Schedule (DIS) was developed in the United States as part of the Epidemiological Catchment Area (ECA) project (Robins *et al.*, 1981). The fully structured interview schedule was developed for use by non-clinicians but employs diagnostic criteria used by clinicians. The DIS covers the most common adult diagnoses that can be evaluated by assessing the content of the interview alone (for example, it omits bulimia nervosa). Diagnoses are first made on a lifetime basis. Then the interviewer asks how recently the last symptom was experienced. On the basis of the answer, the disorder is recorded as occurring within the last 2 weeks, or within the last 1, 2, 6, or 12 months.

Composite International Diagnostic Interview (CIDI)

The Composite International Diagnostic Interview (CIDI) was produced for the WHO and the US Alcohol Drug Abuse and Mental Health Administration. It is a comprehensive and standardized interview derived from the DIS. It is used for the assessment of mental disorders and to provide diagnoses according to ICD and DSM-IV. It is available in 16 languages and designed to be used by clinicians and non-clinicians in different cultures. The CIDI package includes a core interview in a researcher's version and an interviewer's version (the latter has a diagnostic index that allows linkage of specific CIDI questions to specific diagnostic criteria of ICD-10 and DSM-IV), additional modules (concerned, for example, with antisocial personality and post-traumatic stress disorders), as well as training manuals and computer programs. The interview includes questions about symptoms and problems experienced at any time in life, as well as questions about current state (World Health Organization, 1989; Essau and Wittchen, 1993; Janca *et al.*, 1994).

Instruments for measuring symptoms

In research, and sometimes clinically, it is necessary not only to record whether symptoms are present or absent but also to measure their severity, and how they vary with time or in response to treatment. Some instruments rate a single symptom or a narrow group of symptoms, others rate a broad group of symptoms as an overall measure of the severity of a disorder.

Ratings of anxiety symptoms

Hamilton Anxiety Scale

The Hamilton Anxiety Scale (HAS; Hamilton, 1959) is widely used. Thirteen items are rated by an interviewer on five-point scales, each on the basis of a brief description. The interviewing method is for the rater to decide. Some depressive symptoms are included so that the scale is in fact a measure of the severity of the anxiety syndrome and not of the symptom of anxiety.

Clinical Anxiety Scale

The Clinical Anxiety Scale (CAS; Snaith *et al.*, 1982) was developed from the HAS, to focus more clearly on the symptom of anxiety, and its use is not restricted to patients with a diagnosis of anxiety disorder.

The State–Trait Anxiety Inventory

The State–Trait Anxiety Inventory (STAI; Spielberger *et al.*, 1983) is a self-rating scale with 20 statements, which is completed in two ways: as the person feels when he completed the scale (trait) and how he feels generally (state).

Ratings of depressive symptoms

Hamilton Rating Scale for Depression

The Hamilton Rating Scale for Depression (HRSD; Hamilton, 1967) is filled in by an interviewer who uses an unstructured interview. It measures the severity of the depressive syndrome rather than the symptom of depression.

Beck Depression Inventory

The Beck Depression Inventory (BDI; Beck *et al.*, 1961) is a 21-item inventory and is usually completed by the patient. Each item has four statements, and the patient chooses that which applies best to their feelings over the previous week.

Montgomery-Asberg Depression Rating Scale

The Montgomery-Asberg Depression Rating Scale (MADRS; Montgomery and Asberg, 1979) is an inventory with 10 items rated on a four-point scale by an interviewer using definitions for each point. Only psychological symptoms of depression are rated.

Ratings of other symptoms

Yale–Brown Obsessive Compulsive Scale

The Yale–Brown Obsessive Compulsive Scale (YBOCS) (Goodman *et al.*, 1989a) is clinician-rated and assesses 10 symptoms on a four-point scale in patients diagnosed as having obsessive–compulsive disorder. Depressive and anxiety symptoms and obsessional personality traits are not rated.

Young mania rating scale

Symptoms of mania are rated using the Young mania rating scale (Young *et al.*, 1978), both by the patient and the clinician, on an 11 item scale, with each item rated from 0 to 5.

Ratings of motor symptoms

A range of scales are available, especially related to side-effects of antipsychotic medication. They include the *Extrapyramidal Symptoms Rating Scale* (ESRS; Chouinard *et al.*, 1980) and the *Barnes Akathisia Scale* (Barnes, 1989).

Ratings used in assessment of cognitive impairment and dementia

The Mini-Mental State Examination (MMSE; Folstein *et al.*, 1975), shown in the Appendix to this chapter, has already been introduced. Other scales used to assess cognitive impairment and the behavioural symptoms of dementia are discussed in Chapter 14.

Ratings of symptoms of schizophrenia

The PSE has been mentioned. Other scales are discussed in Chapter 12.

Ratings of broad groups of symptoms

General Health Questionnaire

The original General Health Questionnaire (GHQ; Goldberg, 1972) contained 60 items, but shorter versions have also been developed. The GHQ is designed for use as a screening instrument in primary care, general medical practice, or community surveys. Even the full version can be completed within 10 minutes. The symptom ratings are added to a score that indicates overall severity, which is expressed by the judgement of whether a psychiatrist would judge the patient to be a 'case' or a 'non-case'. There is also a version with subscales for somatic symptoms, anxiety and insomnia, depression, and social dysfunction (Goldberg and Hillier, 1979).

Brief Psychiatric Rating Scale

The Brief Psychiatric Rating Scale (BPRS; Overall and Gorham, 1962) has 16 items, each scored on a seven-point scale. There are criteria to define the symptom items but not for the severity ratings. The time period is not defined and must be decided by the rater. It is suitable for rating severe psychiatric illness but not minor disorders.

Global rating scales

Global Assessment of Functioning

Global Assessment Functioning (GAF) was introduced in DSM-IV, and is a revised version of the Global Assessment Scale (Endicott *et al.*, 1976). The GAF is a 100-point scale on which the clinician rates the overall functioning of the patient. Each decile has a brief description of psychological, social and occupational performance.

Clinical Global Impression

The Clinical Global Impression (CGI; Guy, 1976) has two items. The main one, 'global severity' requires the clinician to rate the overall severity of the patient's illness at the time of interview, relative to other patients with the same diagnosis. The 'global change' index rates change relative to a baseline assessment. The CGI is often used as a measure of efficacy in drug trials.

Quality of life scales

There is increasing interest in quality of life as a key measure of outcomes throughout medicine. Over 100 scales are now available. Commonly used ones in psychiatry include EuroQoL, the SF-36, and the Lancashire scale. Some scales are completed by the patient, and others by a relative or carer.

Health of the Nation Outcome Scale

The Health of the Nation Outcome Scale (HoNOS; Wing *et al.*, 1998) is a 12-item scale which rates clinical problems and social functioning. It was developed as an instrument to measure progress towards a British National Health Service target to improve the health and social functioning of mentally ill people, with a view to its use becoming routine with all psychiatric patients. The HoNOS is also being tested in other countries, and has been adapted for the elderly and those with learning disability.

Further reading

Blumenthal, S and Lavender, T (2000) *Violence and mental disorder: a critical aid to the assessment and management of risk*. Zito Trust, London.

Cooper, JE and Oates, M (2000) The principles of assessment in general psychiatry. In MG Gelder, JJ López Ibor Jr, and NC Andreason (eds) *The new Oxford textbook of psychiatry*, Chapter 1.10.1. Oxford University Press, Oxford.

Maguire, P and Pitceathly, C (2002) Key communication skills and how to acquire them. *BMJ* 325: 697–700.

Task Force for Psychiatric Measures (2000) *Handbook of psychiatric measures*. American Psychiatric Association Press, Washington, DC. (A reference book containing comprehensive information about instruments for the detection and measurement of psychiatric symptoms and syndromes.)

Taylor, MA (1999) *Fundamentals of clinical neuropsychiatry*. Oxford University Press, New York and Oxford. (See especially Chapter 2, Neuropsychiatric evaluation, and Chapter 4, The cognitive and behavioural neurologic examination.)

Appendix The Mini-Mental State Examination

(Add points for each correct response)

			Score	Points
Orientation				
1	What is the	Year?	____	1
		Season?	____	1
		Date?	____	1
		Day?	____	1
		Month?	____	1
2	Where are we?	State?	____	1
		County?	____	1
		Town or city?	____	1
		Hospital?	____	1
		Floor?	____	1
Registration				
3	Name three objects, taking 1 second to say each. Then ask the patient all three after you have said them. Give one point for each correct answer. Repeat the answers until patient learns all three.		____	3
Attention and calculation				
4	Serial sevens. Give one point for each correct answer. Stop after five answers. Alternative: Spell WORLD backwards		____	5
Recall				
5	Ask for name of three objects learned in Q.3. Give one point for each correct answer.		____	3
Language				
6	Point to a pencil and a watch. Have the patient name them as you point.		____	2
7	Have the patient repeat 'No ifs, ands, or buts'.		____	1
8	Have the patient follow a three-stage command: 'Take a paper in your right hand. Fold the paper in half. Put the paper on the floor'.		____	3
9	Have the patient read and obey the following: 'CLOSE YOUR EYES'. (Write it in large letters.)		____	1
10	Have the patient write a sentence of his choice. (The sentence should contain a subject and an object, and should make sense. Ignore spelling errors when scoring.)		____	1
11	Enlarge the design printed below to 1.5 cm per side and have the patient copy it. (Give one point if all sides and angles are preserved and if the intersecting sides form a quadrangle.)		____	1
			____	**Total** = 30

Reprinted with permission from J. C. Anthony, L. Le Resche, U. Niaz, M. R. Von Korff, and M. F. Folstein (1982). Limits of the 'Mini-Mental State' as a screening test for dementia and delirium among hospital patients. *Psychological Medicine* **12**, 397–408.

CHAPTER 4

Ethics and civil law

Chapter contents

This chapter is concerned with the ways in which general ethical principles, relating to matters such as confidentiality, consent, and autonomy, are applied to the care of people with mental disorders. We assume that readers have already studied ethical aspects of general medicine: any who have not should consult Hope, Savalescu and Hendrick (2003) or a comparable textbook of medical ethics.

Ethical considerations are highly important in all branches of medicine: in psychiatry they have an additional importance because some patients lack the capacity to make judgements about their own need for care. Questions about capacity to consent to treatment of psychiatric illness arise commonly, and psychiatrists are sometimes asked, by colleagues in other specialties, for advice about capacity to consent to treatment for physical illness.

In this chapter we consider also some aspects of the law relevant to psychiatry. These aspects are necessarily general ones because the specific provisions of the law differ in different countries. For this reason, readers should find out the relevant legal provisions in the country in which they are working and whenever necessary seek expert advice about details of the law and its application.

The chapter is divided into three parts:

1. General issues
2. Ethical problems in psychiatry
3. Some aspects of civil law relevant to the practice of psychiatry

Readers should note that this not the only chapter in which we consider ethical problems: some that relate specifically to issues discussed in other chapters, are considered in those chapters (see Box 4.1).

General issues

The conclusion that it is ethically right to act in one way rather than another should be:

- based on agreed ethical approaches and principles
- logically sound
- consistent across decisions.

Ethical approaches

In psychiatry, as in ethics generally, two broad approaches to ethical problems are employed: the duty based approach and the utilitarian approach.

The duty-based approach sets out clinicians' obligations in a series of rules, for example the rule that doctors must not have sexual relationships with their patients. These rules may be brought together in a code of practice. Because there are rules, clinicians are readily aware of their duties. However, the approach is inflexible and is difficult to apply to some complex problems.

The utilitarian approach is concerned with balancing judgements about benefit and harm. Instead of applying general rules, each case is assessed individually with the assumption that the ethically correct action is the one that has the best foreseeable overall consequences. The approach can take into account the complexities of some clinical problems, but it does not always result in an agreed conclusion because different people may give different weight to the benefits and harms in a particular case.

In practice the two approaches overlap. A duty-based approach may include a duty to do that which will result in the best outcome; and in a utilitarian approach the best outcome may result from the application of a rule

Ethical principles

Three ethical principles are widely adopted in medical ethics (Beauchamp and Childress, 2001).

1. **Respect for autonomy:** involving patients in healthcare decisions; informing them so that they can make the decisions; and respecting their views
2. **Beneficence (and non-malevolence)** doing what is best for patients (and not doing harm). In practice this usually means doing what the body of professional opinion judges best. Beneficence is sometimes in conflict with respect of autonomy, for example when a patient refuses treatment that professional opinion judges essential (see below).
3. **Justice:** acting fairly and balancing the interests of different people.

Codes of practice

Codes of practice and guidelines are prepared and overseen by professional organizations such as the American Psychiatric Association (1995) and, in the UK, the General Medical Council (2004) and the Royal College of Psychiatrists (2000). In some countries ethical codes are enforced not by the professions but by government: loss of confidence in the professions has led to some demands for this arrangement in the UK.

The other professions involved in psychiatric care, such as nursing and psychology, have their own codes of practice and these are not identical in every respect with those of the medical profession. Such differences may sometimes complicate decisions concerned with ethical aspects of care provided by a multidisciplinary team.

Ethical problems in psychiatric practice

In the following sections of this chapter we discuss ethical problems relating to:

- the doctor/patient relationship
- confidentiality
- consent
- compulsory treatment
- research.

Ethical problems arising in particular aspects of practice are discussed in other chapters (see Box 4.1).

The doctor-patient relationship

A relationship of trust between doctor and patient is the basis of ethical medical practice. This relationship should be in the patient's interests and based on the principles, outlined above, of respect for autonomy, beneficence, non-maleficence, and justice.

Abuse of the relationship

The more intense the doctor-patient relationship, and the more vulnerable the patient, the more readily can it be abused. For these reasons, particular care has to be taken not to abuse the relationship during psychother-

BOX 4.1 ETHICAL PROBLEMS DISCUSSED IN OTHER CHAPTERS

Classification (Chapter 2)

Diagnosis on the basis of moral or political judgements (p. 25)

Evidence-based psychiatry (Chapter 6)

Placebo-controlled trials and randomization (p. 117)

Personality disorder (Chapter 7)

Stigma and patient involvement (p. 149)

Eating disorder (Chapter 15)

Compulsory treatment in anorexia nervosa (p. 365)

Psychiatry and medicine (Chapter 16)

Patients who refuse treatment (p. 393)

Genetic counselling (p. 394)

HIV (p. 399)

Suicide and deliberate self-harm (Chapter 17)

Patients who harm themselves and refuse treatment (p. 427)

Drugs and other physical treatment (Chapter 21)

Drug treatment (p. 523)

ECT and psychosurgery (p. 572 and 575)

Psychiatric services (Chapter 23)

Ethical problems in the provision of psychiatric services (p. 643)

Child psychiatry (Chapter 24)

Conflict of interest, confidentiality and consent (p. 701)

Learning disability (Chapter 25)

Normalization, autonomy and conflict of interests (p. 727)

Consent to treatment, and consent to research (p. 727)

apy. Therapists abuse the doctor patient relationship when they:

- **impose their own values and beliefs** on their patients, for example, when counselling about termination of pregnancy. This influence may be overt, for example, when a doctor refuses termination of pregnancy saying that it is is morally wrong. Or it may be covert, for example, when the doctor expresses no opinion but nevertheless gives more attention to the arguments against termination than to those for it. Similar problems may arise, for example, in marital therapy when therapists' values may intrude on their approach to the question of whether a couple should separate.
- **put the interests of third parties before those of patients**, for example the interests of employers. Nevertheless, the interests of individual patients cannot be considered in isolation. For example, when allocating resources to a community, or when deciding about the treatment of potentially dangerous patients, the interests of the patient have to be balanced against those of other people. These difficult decisions are discussed further on p. 643 and p. 644.
- **exploit patients sexually.** Medical codes of practice contain an absolute prohibition against a sexual relationships with a patient. Particular care is needed when sexual problems are the main topic of the interviews, as in sex therapy.
- **exploit patients for financial gain**, for example by prolonging treatment in private practice for longer than is necessary to achieve the patient's goals.

Confidentiality

Confidentiality is central to the trust between patients and doctors. It is particularly important in psychiatry because information is so often collected about private and highly sensitive matters As a general rule information should not be disclosed without the patient's consent though, as discussed later, there are defined exceptions to this rule. The rule is an ancient one, stated in the Hippocratic Oath:

> Whatever, in connection with my professional practice or not in connection with it, I see or hear in the life of men, which ought not to be spoken abroad, I will not divulge as reckoning that all such should be kept secret.

The rule was restated in 1948 in the Declaration of Geneva which added the important point that the obligation of confidentiality continues after a patient's death:

I will respect the secrets which are confided in me, even after the patient has died.

In many countries, national professional organizations publish guidelines dealing with common clinical situations such as protecting records, sharing information with relatives, and disclosing information to third parties (see for example General Medical Council, 2004, and the updated website www.gmc-uk.org). Confidentiality is also enforced by law and by contract of employment, and although professional guidelines do not have the force of law, they are taken seriously by the courts as evidence of generally accepted standards.

Many countries have laws of privacy, and laws that govern the ways in which written and electronic records can be held and that set out patients' rights to see their personal information. Psychiatrists should be aware of the ethical and legal requirements in the place in which they are working. In the UK, the relevant legislation includes the Data Protection Act (1998).

From the perspective of English law, it is in the **public** interest, as well as that of the individual, that patients should be able to trust their doctors to maintain confidentiality. Therefore the issue of when it is lawful and when it is unlawful for a doctor to breach confidentiality is generally answered by balancing two conflicting public interests rather than balancing a private interest against a public interest.

Ethical principles relating to confidentiality

Safeguarding information

Personal information must be safeguarded and records kept securely and thought must be given to the security of mobile phones or email. Unintentional disclosure should be avoided by carrying out consultations where they cannot be overheard (sometimes difficult when patients are seen at home or in a medical ward) and by avoiding discussions between professional staff in places where they might be overheard.

Consent to disclosure of information

Confidentiality is not breached when a patient has given informed consent to disclosure. In this context, informed consent means consent based on full understanding of the reasons for disclosure, what will be disclosed, and the likely consequences of disclosure. In principle, confidentiality is not breached when the patient cannot be identified, for example in a disguised case report. It is usual, nevertheless, for journals and books to require that patients give informed, signed consent to publication, even when their identities have been disguised.

Confidentiality in the care of children

These and other ethical problems in the care of children are discussed in Chapter 24. Here it is sufficient to note here children over a stated age (usually 16) have the same rights of confidentiality as adults. For younger children, clinical information is usually shared with parents who have a legal duty to act in their children's best interests and therefore need to be properly informed.

Situations in which there may be problems about confidentiality

Seeking information from others As a rule, patients' permission should be obtained before information is sought from other persons. When a patient is mentally disordered and unable to give an account of himself, and the information is essential for good care, the psychiatrist must decide whether to seek it without the patient's consent. The guiding principles are to act in the patient's best interests, and as far as possible to obtain the information from close relatives.

Disclosing information to others Information should be disclosed only with the patient's consent except in the special circumstances discussed below. Disclosure should be limited to the information necessary for the purpose of the disclosure and, whenever possible, unidentifiable data should be used. Relatives often ask for information but this should be given only with the patient's consent. However, when the patient is unable to consent to disclosure (for example, as a result of dementia), information may be shared provided disclosure is in the patient's best interests.

Assessment of behalf of a third party When patients are assessed on behalf of a third party, for example an assessment of fitness to work carried out for an employer, it is essential to ensure at the outset that the patient is aware of the purpose of the assessment and of the obligations of the doctor towards the third party. Written consent should be obtained. Otherwise disclosure can be made only in the public interest (see below) usually to prevent death or serious harm.

Care in the community Patients should know from the start that information will be shared as necessary with other members of the care team and these team members must follow the principles of confidentiality. Some of the team, for example social workers, may be required to discuss information with their supervisors, or pass on information to other agencies, for example when helping patients with housing. It is important to keep such matters in mind as treatment plans develop, and discuss them with the patient when this becomes necessary. When visits are made to patients, neighbours may become aware of the visits; moreover outreach programmes may require enquiries about high risk patients who have not kept appointments. These and similar potential problems should be anticipated as far as possible and discussed with patients so that the necessary permissions are obtained in advance. In an emergency, the right to privacy has to be balanced against the risks of harm to the patient or to others, should necessary enquiries not be made.

If patients refuse the disclosure of information despite clear information about the likely consequences of non-disclosure, their wishes must be respected unless this would put others at risk of serious harm.

Group therapy Group therapy presents special problems of confidentiality because patients reveal personal information not only to the therapist but also to other members of the group. Before treatment begins, the therapist should explain the requirement to treat as confidential the revelations of the others, and the necessary agreement should be obtained from everyone who will take part in the group.

Therapy with couples Usually, the treatment of a couple is preceded by an interview with each person separately. Information obtained in this way from one person should not be revealed to the other without the agreement of the first. If possible, all relevant information should be revealed by the person concerned, during the joint sessions. If, after therapy has started, it becomes necessary to see one of the couple alone, for example, to assess symptoms of depression, it may be better for the therapist to ask a colleague to do this. Similar problems may arise in **family therapy**.

Exceptions to the rule of confidentiality

Exceptions in the patient's interest In exceptional circumstances, doctors may disclose information to a third party without the patient's consent, when this disclosure is in the patient's best interest: for example when information is requested urgently by another doctor dealing with the patient in an emergency, and the patient's permission cannot be obtained, or when a patient is incapable of giving informed consent because of severe mental or physical illness, and the disclosure is essential for his care.

Exceptions in the public interest Although there is a general legal obligation for doctors to keep confidential what patients tell them, there are special circumstances in which doctors are obliged to disclose information to a third party because this is in the interest of the community as a whole or of a group or individual within it. There are **statutory obligations** to do this in relation, for example, to communicable disease, the use of certain controlled drugs, unfitness to drive, and suspicion of child abuse. There is also an obligation to disclose relevant information in response to a Court Order, and when there is evidence of serious crime, usually a crime that will put some person at risk of death or serious harm, for example the abuse of a child. In such a case, every effort should be made to persuade patients to agree to disclosure; if they refuse, the reasons for the disclosure should be explained and written down.

Exceptions for legal representatives A patient's legal representative, like the patient, may read clinical notes and letters that have been written about that patient, although there may be restrictions in relation to the possibility of harm to others (for example from the reading of certain information given in confidence by informants).

For further information about problems related to confidentiality see Hope *et al.* (2004, Chapter 7).

Consent to treatment

Consent is relevant to the whole of medical practice and in the account which follows we assume that readers are familiar with the relevant concepts and procedures from their general medical training. Any readers who are not should consult the latest GMC guidelines if they are working in the UK (see www.gmc-uk.org) or a corresponding document if they are working elsewhere, and read a textbook of ethics such as Hope *et al.* (2004).

Obtaining consent

The patient should:

1. have a **clear and full understanding** of the nature of the condition to be treated, the procedures available and their probable side-effects;
2. **agree freely** to receive the treatment;
3. be **competent** to take decisions, i.e. **to have legal capacity** – see below. (Note that in the US, the word capacity is generally used in the clinical rather than the legal sense adopted in the UK).

Maintaining consent

Some patients consent to treatment of chronic illness but later fail to collaborate with it. When this happens, the clinician should seek to re-establish consent and collaboration. To achieve these, offers of additional help are justified, but threats that help will be reduced are not.

When explicit consent is not required

There are special **situations in which explicit consent is not needed** (their precise nature depends on local law and precedent):

- **implied consent**, for example when a patient holds out his arm to have his blood pressure measured.
- **necessity;** that is a circumstance in which grave harm or death are likely to occur without intervention and there is doubt about the patient's competence (see below).
- **emergency,** in order to prevent immediate serious harm to the patient or to others, or to prevent a crime.

When consent to medical treatment is refused

In the UK, the law distinguishes between consent to medical treatment and consent to psychiatric treatment. This section is concerned with refusal of **medical** treatment; refusal of psychiatric treatment is discussed on p. 75. Competent adults have a right to refuse medical treatment, even if this refusal results in death or permanent disablement.

If a patient refuses medical treatment, the doctor needs to make two judgements before accepting that the patient has the right to refuse: (i) does the patient lack competence (i.e. does he lack the legal capacity, see below) to consent to or refuse treatment, by reason of mental illness? (ii) Has the patient been influenced by others to the extent that a refusal has been coerced or is not voluntary?

Refusal by competent patients Their refusal may be the result of misunderstanding or fear about the illness and its treatment. Clinicians should set aside the time needed to understand the patient's concerns about, and their current understanding of, their condition before explaining the medical issues once more. When this approach is taken, agreement can usually be reached about a treatment plan that is both medically appropriate and acceptable to the patient. Nevertheless, some competent adult patients continue to refuse treatment even after a full discussion, and it is their right to do so.

Refusal by incompetent patients In the UK and various other countries the doctor treating the patient has right to act in the patient's best interests and give immediate treatment in **life-threatening emergencies** when the patient lacks capacity to consent. Whenever possible, other health workers should be consulted and a careful record should be kept of the reasons for the decision. Doctors should know the relevant law in the country in which they are working. For further discussion see Hope *et al.* (2004).

Refusal by mentally disordered patients If a patient who refuses medical treatment has an accompanying mental disorder that appears to impair his ability to give informed consent, the mental disorder should be treated, if necessary and appropriate, under compulsory legal powers. In English law, such powers do not allow treatment of the physical illness against the patient's wishes, they do, however, allow the treatment of the mental disorder. After successful treatment of the mental disorder, the patient may then give informed consent for the treatment of the physical illness which was previously refused.

Legal aspects of consent

The legal concept of **capacity** to consent relates to a patient's ability to: (i) comprehend and retain information about the treatment; (ii) believe this information; and (iii) use it to make an informed choice.

Patients may lack the capacity to give informed consent by reason of:

1. young age – parents give consent for children and and adolescents below the age at which, in law, they are able to consent. Consent to treatment for children and adolescents is considered in Chapter 24;
2. learning disability;
3. mental disorder. Psychiatrists may be asked to assess patients thought to be in this third group; they should do so by making the enquiries listed in Box 4.2.

Judgements of legal capacity to consent **are specific to the particular decision**. Thus a patient with a severe mental disorder may be incompetent in other respects, but nonetheless competent to decide whether to consent to a particular treatment. For example, a patient with schizophrenia and paranoid delusions may be capable of deciding about medical treatment of a heart attack. (See Katz *et al.* 1995 for an account of psychiatric consultation with those refusing medical treatment.)

Consent by a proxy

In English law, at the time of writing, if the adult patient does not have the capacity to consent to treatment for a medical condition, no-one can give proxy consent on behalf of that patient. In some other jurisdictions, there is provision for a form of proxy consent such as, in Scottish law, the appointment of a guardian. When there is no legal provision for proxy consent and the patient has not made an advance directive (see below), and a decision whether to give treatment must be made, this is done on the basis of the patient's best interests as judged by the responsible clinician in accordance with general medical opinion. It is wise to consult relatives (even though, at the time of writing, in English law they cannot give or withhold consent) and to discuss the case with other professional staff. Detailed notes should be kept of the reasons for the decision and of the consultations that took place.

Consent in advance

Advance directives, sometimes called 'living wills', are accepted in many countries (though not, at the time of writing, in England and Wales). They are designed to ensure that those who previously had the capacity to take decisions but have lost it, e.g. because of dementia, are treated as they would have wished. To make an advanced directive, the person must be competent and well informed at the time. Advance directives respect the principle of autonomy and are generally thought by doctors and patients as being helpful. Nevertheless it is sometimes difficult to apply general wishes views made in a state of good health to a subsequent specific decision. In some jurisditions (though not currently in English law) relatives or other proxies may be empowered to decide for the incompetent patient, though this is not an entirely satisfactory way of judging what the person would have wanted. The person making the directive should understand that changing circumstances and the need to consider the interests of others may mean that the directive will have to be interpreted flexibly rather than as a strict instruction to be followed in every detail and every circumstance.

BOX 4.2 ASSESSMENT OF COMPETENCE OF ADULT PATIENTS

Step 1 Identify the decision required and the information relevant to it

- The decision to be made.
- The alternative, reasonable, decisions.
- The pros and cons of each reasonable decision.

Step 2 Assess cognitive ability
Assess whether the person has the cognitive ability to:

- understand the information;
- retain the information;
- evaluate the information and reach a decision.

Step 3 Consider possible causes of impaired cognitive ability

- delirium;
- dementia;
- other neurological disorders which may impair cognition;
- learning disability.

Step 4 Assess other factors which may interfere with capacity
Mental illness:

- delusions
- hallucinations
- mood disorder.

Lack of maturity:

- assess emotional and cognitive maturity.

Compulsory treatment for mental disorder

Special legal provision is made for people who are a danger to themselves or others because of mental disorder, and who refuse to accept necessary treatment usually because they do not accept that they have a mental disorder. Such people present an ethical dilemma: they have a right to liberty but they also have a need for care and treatment, and society has a right to be protected.

Most countries have laws to protect mentally disordered persons and to protect society from the consequences of their mental disorder, although the definition of mental disorder and the procedures vary in different countries. In some Scandinavian countries, procedures for compulsory treatment are simple, whilst in some states of the USA, a court hearing may be required. In England and Wales, provisions for compulsory admission and treatment are embodied, at the time of writing, in the Mental Health Act 1983 although new legislation is planned.

Compulsory powers should be used only when there is no safe alternative. An experienced psychiatrist can often avoid the use of such powers by patient and tactful discussion, with the patient and relatives, of the reasons why admission to hospital is necessary. If this fails to persuade the patient and compulsory treatment is justified, further discussion should take place with family members to seek their support for compulsory admission. When talking to the family, the doctor should bear in mind that they are likely to feel anxious and perhaps guilty.

Once detained, restrictions on the patient should be the minimum required for safety and for adequate treatment. If the staff are sympathetic, patient, and firm but adaptable, detained patients and their relatives soon realize that the treatment differs little from that of voluntary patients, and they collaborate. If they do not, and treatment has to proceed without consent, the reasons should be explained to the patient and relatives and recorded in the notes.

In England and Wales, there are additional legal requirements when a detained patient is judged to need electroconvulsive therapy (ECT) and does not or cannot give valid consent. The problem has to be discussed fully with relatives, and an independent psychiatric opinion must be obtained. The psychiatrist who gives this opinion is required to consult with others who have been professionally concerned with the patient's treatment.

Conflict of interests relating to compulsory treatment

Conflicts of interest arise, for example, when a patient refuses admission and his care outside hospital places substantial burdens upon relatives or other informal carers. Such conflict of interests may be resolved by discussion between the psychiatrist who is reponsible for the patient's care and the general practitioner or another professional whose primary responsibility is to the carers.

Safeguards

An important safeguard in any legal framework for compulsory detention and treatment is a provision for appeal against the original decision. The way in which the appeals are considered differs between the various jurisdictions and readers should find out what the arrangements are in the jurisdiction in which they are working.

Ethics of research

Psychiatric research is bound by the ethical principles that apply to all medical research. These derive from the first internationally agreed guidelines on research involving people. These principles were stimulated by knowledge of the appalling abuse of medical research in Nazi Germany and were set out in the Declaration of Helsinki, first published by the World Medical Association in 1964 (see World Medical Association, 2000). Since then there have been other national and international guidelines, generally enforced national and local research ethics committees. The ethical

BOX 4.3 ASSESSMENT OF SOME ETHICAL ISSUES RELATING TO RESEARCH

Note: Ethical problems related to recruitment for and the conduct of clinical trials are considered on p. 117.

Scientific merits

- Will the findings be of value?
- Are the methods and the size of the groups likely to achieve the aims?
- What are the sources of financial and other support, and is there any potential conflict of interest?
- Are there any potential conflicts of interest for any of the investigators?
- Could the aims be achieved in an ethically better way?

Safety

- Are the procedures safe? If there is a risk, are all necessary precautions being taken?
- Is the assessed level of risk acceptable to investigators, subjects and relatives?

Consent

- Will the subjects be competent to give consent?
- Will subjects receive clear and sufficient information?
- Will they have adequate time to consider and, should they wish, to withdraw consent?
- Will it be clear that refusal will not affect the quality or quantity of care provided?
- Is the relationship beween subject and investigator potentially coersive (e.g. a supervisor and a pupil)?
- Is any payment to subjects for expenses likely to exceed these and act, therefore, as an incentive to consent?
- Is the researcher under any pressure to recruit subjects (e.g. payments from a sponsoring company?)

Confidentiality

- Have subjects consented for the use of confidential information in the research?
- Will the data from the research be kept securely?

Adapted from Hope *et al.* (2004, p. 196), and Weingarten and Leibovici (2004, p. 1013).

problems of psychiatric research are those of other medical research as set out, for example, in the UK General Medical Council guidelines (see www.gmc-uk.org), or the website of the UK Central Office of Research Committees (www.corec.org.uk), with particular emphasis on those related to consent by competent but vulnerable adults who may feel under pressure to consent, and by those who lack capacity.

Informed consent to research

Informed consent is crucial to the ethical conduct of research. Miller (2000) has outlined a number of important considerations:

- Patients must be made specifically aware that the research is not being conducted for their individual benefit.
- Patients must be free from any coercion or inducement.
- Patients have right to withdraw from the study at any time without any kind of penalty.
- In addition to the investigator, a family member or other suitable person should be encouraged to monitor the patient's condition and report to the investigator if there are concerns.
- In placebo controlled trials patients must understand clearly the probability of receiving placebo, the lack of improvement that might result, and the possibility of symptomatic worsening (see also Lavori, 2000).

Research with people who cannot give informed consent

Most psychiatric patients can give informed consent but a few have a disorder which impairs judgement and decision-making. To exclude these patients from all research could deprive future similar patients of the benefits of research. The decision whether to include such patients is made after considering:

- any potential benefit of the research to the person who is being asked to consent
- any possible discomfort or risk to this person
- the potential benefit to others with a similar problem and incapacity
- any signs or other indications suggesting unspoken objection.

It is advisable to consult with relatives or others who may be able to take an informed view of the patient's situation. Juristictions vary in the extent to which this is a legal requirement and investigators should take great care to follow local ethical and legal procedures.

Some aspects of civil law

Civil law deals with the rights and obligations of individuals to one another, including family law which is a particular concern of child psychiatrists. In this respect civil law differs from criminal law, which is concerned with offences against the state (though some are directed against an individual, for example, homicide). As well as the issues discussed earlier in this chapter, civil law is concerned with property, inheritance, and contracts. Proceedings in civil law are undertaken by individuals or groups who believe that they have suffered a breach of the civil law, in contrast to criminal law procedings which are undertaken on behalf of the state.

Psychiatrists are sometimes asked to submit written reports on a patient's mental state in relation to a civil case. Such reports should be prepared only after full discussion with the patient and only with the patient's informed consent, and should be concise and factual. The structure should follow the plan set out on pp. 754–5. Regarding the contents, it is advisable to seek legal advice about the relevant aspects of law relating to the case. The following sections are based on the law in England and Wales although the principles apply more widely.

Testamentary capacity

This term refers to the capacity to make a valid will. If someone is suffering from mental disorder at the time of making a will, its validity may be in doubt and other people may challenge it. The will may still be legally valid if the testator was of 'sound disposing mind' (see below) at the time of making it. Psychiatrists may be asked to report in relation to two issues:

1. testamentary capacity;
2. the possibility that the testator was subjected to undue influence.

In order to decide whether or not a testator is of sound disposing mind, the doctor should decide whether the person making the will:

- understands what a will is and its consequences;
- knows the nature and extent of his property (though not in detail);
- knows the names of close relatives and can assess their claims to his property;
- **is free from an abnormal state of mind that might distort** feelings or judgements relevant to making the will (a deluded person may legitimately make a will, provided that the delusions are unlikely to influence it).

To decide these matters, the doctor should first interview the testator alone, and then see relatives or friends to check the accuracy of factual statements.

Assessment of undue influence is more complex and requires an assessment of the relationship between testator and beneficiary, the mental state of the testator, and what is known of the person's earlier intentions.

Power of attorney and receivership

If a patient is incapable of managing his possessions by reason of mental disorder, alternative arrangements need to be made, particularly if the incapacity is likely to last a long time. Such arrangements may be required for patients living in the community as well as those in hospital. In English law two methods are available – power of attorney and receivership.

Power of attorney is the simpler method, requiring only that the patient give written authorization for someone else to act for him during his illness. In signing such authorization, the patient must be able to understand what he is doing. He may revoke it at any time.

Receivership is the more formal procedure and is likely to be more in the patient's interests. In England and Wales an application is made to the Court of Protection, which may decide to appoint a receiver. The procedure is most commonly required for the elderly. The question of receivership places special responsibility on the psychiatrist. If a patient is capable of managing his affairs on admission to hospital, but later becomes incapable by reason of intellectual deterioration, then it is the doctor's duty to advise the patient's relatives about the risks to property. If the relatives are unwilling to take action, then it is the doctor's duty to make an application to the Court of Protection. The doctor may feel reluctant to act in this way, but any actions taken subsequently are the Court's responsibility and not the doctor's.

Aspects of family law

A **marriage contract** is not valid if at the time of marriage either party was so mentally disordered as not to understand its nature. If mental disorder of this degree can be proved, a marriage may be decreed null and void by a divorce court. If a marriage partner becomes of 'incurably unsound mind' later in a marriage, this may be grounds for divorce and a psychiatrist may be asked to make a prognosis. A doctor may also be asked for an opinion about the **capacity of parents or a guardian** to care adequately for a child.

Torts and contracts

Torts are wrongs for which a person is liable in civil law as opposed to criminal law. They include negligence, libel, slander, trespass, and nuisance. If such a wrong is committed by a person of unsound mind, then any damages awarded in a court of law are usually only nominal. In this context the legal definition of unsound mind is restrictive, and it is advisable for a psychiatrist to take advice about it from a lawyer.

If the person makes a contract and subsequently develops a mental disorder, then the contract is binding. If a person is of unsound mind when the contract is made, then in English law a distinction is made between the 'necessaries' and 'non-necessaries' of life. **Necessaries** are goods (or services) 'suitable to the condition of life of such person and to his actual requirements at the time' (Sale of Goods Act 1893). In a particular case the court decides whether any goods or services are necessaries within this definition. A contract made for necessaries is always binding.

When a contract for **non-necessaries** made by a person of unsound mind, the contract is binding unless it can be shown both that he did not understand what he was doing and that the other person was aware of the incapacity.

Personal injury

Psychiatrists may be asked to write reports in relation to claims for compensation by patients with post-traumatic stress disorder or one of the other psychological sequelae of accidents (see p. 400). Reports should be set out to accord with the relevant local legal procedures and should state clearly (i) the sources of information, (ii) the history of the trauma, (iii) the psychiatric and social history, and (iv) the post-accident course. Reports should include a detailed assessment of function and of the relationship between the trauma and any subsequent symptoms and disability.

Fitness to drive

Questions of fitness to drive may arise in relation to many psychiatric disorders. Dangerous driving may result from suicidal inclinations or manic disinhibition; panicky or aggressive driving may result from persecutory delusions; and indecisive or inaccurate driving may be due to dementia. Concentration on driving may be impaired in severe anxiety or depressive disorders. The question of fitness to drive arises also in relation to the sedative and other side-effects of some psychiatric drugs, such as some anxiolytic or antipsychotic drugs in high dosage.

Doctors should be aware of and follow the legal criteria for fitness to drive in the places in which they are working; these criteria may differ somewhat from those for drivers of cars and drivers of heavy goods vehicles, which are more strict. UK holders of driving licences have a duty to inform the Driving and Vehicle Licensing Agency (DVLA) if they have a condition that may affect their safety as a driver. Doctors should inform patients if they have such a condition, and make sure that they understand their duty to report it. In deciding fitness to drive, doctors should consider whether the patient's condition or its treatment is liable to cause loss of control, impair perception or comprehension, impair judgement, reduce concentration, or affect motor functions involved in handling the vehicle. If after full discussion, a patient with such a condition continues to drive, a doctor working in the UK should disclose the relevant medical information to the medical advisor of the DVLA.

Further reading

General references are listed below. In many countries, National Medical and Psychiatric Organisations also publish guidelines about the ethical and legal aspects of practice.

American Psychiatric Association (2001) *Psychiatric ethics primer*. American Psychiatric Publishing Inc., Washington DC.

Bloch, S, Chodoff, P and Green S (eds) (1999) *Psychiatric ethics*, 3rd edn. Oxford University Press, Oxford. (A series of reviews by leading writers covering the principal theoretical issues.)

Dickenson, D and Fulford, KWM (2000) *In two minds: a case book of psychiatric ethics*. Oxford University Press, Oxford. (A readable, practical account based on discussions of common clinical problems.)

Hope, T, Savelescu, J and Hendrick, J (2003) *Medical ethics and law: the core curriculum*. Churchill Livingstone, London. (A comprehensive introductory text.)

Montgomery, J (2002) *Health care law*, 2nd edn. Oxford University Press, Oxford. (A useful work of reference.)

And a useful website:

National Reference Center for Bioethics Literature: www.georgetown.edu/research/nrcbl

CHAPTER 5

Aetiology

Chapter contents

Approaches to aetiology in psychiatry

Psychiatrists are concerned with aetiology in two ways. First, in everyday clinical work they try to discover the causes of the mental disorders presented by individual patients. Second, in seeking a wider understanding of psychiatry they are interested in aetiological evidence obtained from **clinical studies, community surveys**, or **laboratory investigations**. Correspondingly, the first part of this chapter deals with some general issues about aetiology in the assessment of the individual patient, whilst the second part deals with the various scientific disciplines that have been applied to the study of aetiology.

General issues about aetiology

Aetiology and intuitive understanding

When the clinician assesses an individual patient, he draws on a common fund of aetiological knowledge that has been derived from the study of groups of similar patients, but he cannot understand the patient in these terms alone. He also has to use everyday insights into human nature. For example, in assessing a depressed patient, the psychiatrist should certainly know what has been discovered about the psychological and neurochemical changes accompanying depressive disorders, and what evidence there is about the aetiological role of stressful events and about genetic predisposition to depressive disorder. At the same time he will need intuitive understanding to recognize, for example, that this particular patient feels depressed because he has been informed that his wife has cancer.

Common-sense ideas of this kind are an important part of aetiological formulation in psychiatry, but they must be used carefully if superficial explanation is to be avoided. Aetiological formulation can be done properly only if certain conceptual problems are clearly understood. These problems can be illustrated by a case history.

For 4 weeks a 38-year-old married woman became increasingly depressed. Her symptoms started soon after her husband left her saying he wanted to live by himself. In the past the patient's mother had received psychiatric treatment on two occasions, once for a severe depressive disorder and once for mania; on neither occasion was there any apparent environmental cause for the illness. When the patient was 14 years old, her father went away to live with another woman, leaving his children with their mother. For several years afterwards the patient felt rejected and unhappy but eventually settled down. She married and had two children aged 13 and 10 at the time of her illness. Two weeks after leaving home, the patient's husband returned, saying that he had made a mistake and really loved his wife. Despite his return the patient's symptoms persisted and worsened. She began to wake early, gave up her usual activities, and spoke at times of suicide.

In thinking about the causes of this woman's symptoms, the clinician would first draw on knowledge of aetiology derived from scientific enquiries. Genetic investigations have shown that, if a parent suffers from mania as well as depressive disorder, a predisposition to depressive disorder is particularly likely to be transmitted to the children. Therefore it is possible that this patient received this predisposition from her mother.

Clinical investigation has also provided some information about the effects of separating children from their parents. In the present case, the information is not helpful because it refers to people who were separated from their parents at a younger age than the patient. On scientific grounds there is no particular reason to focus on the departure of the patient's father, but intuitively it seems likely that this was an important event. From everyday experience it is understandable that a woman should feel upset if her husband leaves her; it is also understandable that she is likely to feel even more distressed if this event recapitulates a related distressing experience in her own childhood. Therefore, the clinician would recognize intuitively that the patient's depression is likely to be a reaction to the husband's departure. The same sort of intuition might suggest that the patient would feel start to feel better when her husband came back. In the event she did not recover. Although her symptoms seemed understandable when her husband was away, they seem less so after his return.

This simple case history illustrates some important aetiological issues in psychiatry:

- complexity of causes
- classification of causes
- the concept of stress
- the concept of psychological reaction
- the relative roles of intuition and scientific knowledge in aetiological formulations.

The complexity of causes in psychiatry

In psychiatry the study of causation is complicated by three problems. These problems are met in other branches of medicine, but to a lesser degree.

Lack of temporal association

The first problem is that causes are often **remote in time** from the effects that they produce. For example, it is widely believed that childhood experiences partly determine the occurrence of emotional difficulties in adult life. It is difficult to test this idea because the necessary information can only be gathered either by studying children and tracing them many years later, which is difficult, or by asking adults about their childhood experiences, which is unreliable.

Cause and effect

The second problem is that a single cause may lead to **several effects**. For example, deprivation of parental affection in childhood has been reported to predispose to antisocial behaviour, suicide, depressive disorder, and several other disorders. Conversely, a single effect may arise from several causes. The latter can be illustrated either by different causes in different individuals or by multiple causes in a single individual. For example, learning disability (single effect) may occur in several children, but the cause may be a different genetic abnormality in each child. On the other hand, depressive disorder (single effect) may occur in one individual through a combination of causes, such as genetic factors, adverse childhood experiences, and stressful events in adult life.

Indirect mechanisms

The third problem is that aetiological factors in psychiatry rarely exert their effects directly. For example, the genetic predisposition to depression may be mediated in part through psychological factors which make it more likely that the individual concerned will experience adverse life events. Thus aetiological effects are usually mediated through complex intervening mechanisms which also need to be investigated and understood.

The classification of causes

A single psychiatric disorder, as just explained, may result from several causes. For this reason a scheme for **classifying** causes is required. A useful approach is to divide causes chronologically into **predisposing, precipitating**, and **maintaining**.

Predisposing factors

There are factors, many of them operating from early life, that determine a person's vulnerability to causes acting close to the time of the illness. They include **genetic endowment** and the **environment *in utero***, as well as **physical, psychological, and social factors in infancy and early childhood**. The term constitution is often used to describe the mental and physical make-up of a person at any point in his life. This make-up changes as life goes on under the influence of further physical, psychological, and social influences. Some writers restrict the term constitution to the make-up at the beginning of life, whilst others also include characteristics acquired later (this second usage is adopted in this book). The concept of constitution includes the idea that a person may have a predisposition to develop a disorder (such as schizophrenia) even though the latter never manifests itself. From the standpoint of psychiatric aetiology, one of the important parts of the constitution is the **personality**.

When the aetiology of an individual case is formulated, the personality is always an essential element. For this reason, the clinician should be prepared to spend sufficient time in talking to the patient and to people who know them in order to build up a clear picture of their personality. This assessment often helps to explain why the patient responded to certain stressful events, and why they reacted in a particular way. The obvious importance of personality in the individual patient contrasts with the small amount of relevant scientific information so far available. Therefore, in the evaluation of personality it is particularly important to acquire sound clinical skills through supervised practice.

Precipitating factors

These are events that occur shortly before the onset of a disorder and **appear to have induced it**. They may be physical, psychological, or social. Whether they produce a disorder at all, and what kind of disorder, depends partly on constitutional factors in the patient (as mentioned above). Physical precipitants include cerebral tumours or drugs, for example. Psychological and social precipitants include personal misfortunes such as the loss of a job, and changes in the routine of life such as moving home. Sometimes the same factor can act in more than one way; for example, a head injury can induce psychological disorder either through physical changes in the brain or through its stressful implications to the patient.

Maintaining factors

These factors **prolong the course of a disorder** after it has been provoked. When planning treatment, it is particularly important to pay attention to these factors. The original predisposing and precipitating factors may have ceased to act by the time that the patient is seen, but the perpetuating factors may well be treatable. For example, in their early stages many psychiatric disorders lead to secondary demoralization and withdrawal from social activities, which in turn help to prolong the original disorder. It is often appropriate to treat these secondary factors, whether or not any other specific measures are carried out. Maintaining factors are also called **perpetuating factors**.

The concept of stress

Discussions about **stress** are often confusing because the term is used in two ways. First, it is applied to events or situations, such as working for an examination, which may have an adverse effect on someone. Second, it is applied to the adverse effects that are induced, which may be psychological or physiological change. In considering aetiology it is advisable to separate these components.

The first set of factors can usefully be called **stressors**. They include a large number of physical, psychological, and social factors that can produce adverse effects. The term is sometimes extended to include events that are not experienced as adverse at the time, but may still have adverse long-term effects. For example, intense competition may produce an immediate feeling of pleasant tension, though it may sometimes lead to unfavourable long-term effects.

The effect on the person can usually be called the **stress reaction** to distinguish it from the provoking events. This reaction includes **autonomic responses** (such as a rise in blood pressure), **endocrine changes** (such as the secretion of adrenaline and noradrenaline), and **psychological responses** (such as a feeling of being keyed up). Much current neurobiology research is involved in studying the effects of stress on the brain, particularly in how stress impacts on the mechanisms involved in the regulation of mood and processing of emotional information.

The concept of a psychological reaction

As already mentioned, it is widely recognized that psychological distress can arise as a reaction to unpleasant events. Sometimes the association between event and distress is evident, for example, when a woman becomes depressed after the death of her husband. In other cases, it is far from clear whether the psychological disorder is really a reaction to an event or whether the two have coincided fortuitously, for example, when a person becomes depressed after the death of a distant relative.

Jaspers (1963, p. 392) suggested three criteria for deciding whether a psychological state is a reaction to a particular set of events:

- The events must be adequate in severity and closely related in time to the onset of the psychological state.
- There must be a clear connection between the nature of the events and the content of the psychological disorder (in the example just given, the person should be preoccupied with ideas concerning their distant relative).
- The psychological state should begin to disappear when the events have ceased (unless, of course, it can be shown that perpetuating factors are acting to maintain it).

These three criteria are useful in clinical practice, though they can be difficult to apply (particularly the second criterion).

Understanding and explanation

As already mentioned, aetiological statements about individual patients must combine knowledge derived from research on groups of patients with intuitive understanding derived from everyday experience. Jaspers (1963, p. 302) has called these two ways of making sense of psychiatric disorders '*Erklaren*' and '*Verstehen*', respectively.

In German, these terms mean 'explanation' and 'understanding', respectively, and they are usually translated as such in English translations of Jaspers' writing. However, Jaspers used them in a special sense. He used *Erklaren* to refer to the sort of causative statement that is sought in the natural sciences. It is exemplified by the statement that a patient's aggressive behaviour has occurred because he has a brain tumour. He used *Verstehen* to refer to psychological understanding, or the intuitive grasp of a natural connection between events in a person's life and his psychological state. In colloquial English, this could be called 'putting oneself in another person's shoes'. It is exemplified by the statement, 'I can understand why the patient became angry when her children were shouted at by a neighbour.'

These distinctions are reasonably clear when we consider an individual patient but confusion sometimes arises when attempts are made to generalize from insights obtained in a single case to widely applicable principles. Understanding may then be mistaken for explanation. Jaspers suggested that some psychoanalytical ideas are special kinds of intuitive understanding that are derived from the detailed study of individuals and then applied generally. They are not explanations that can be tested scientifically. They are more akin to insights into human nature that can be gained from reading great works of literature. Such insights are of great value in conducting human affairs. It would be wrong to neglect them in psychiatry, but equally wrong to see them as statements of a scientific kind.

The aetiology of a single case

How to make an aetiological formulation was discussed in Chapter 3. An example was given of a woman in her thirties who had become increasingly depressed. The formulation showed how aetiological factors could be grouped under headings of predisposing, precipitating, and perpetuating factors. It also showed how information from scientific investigations (in this case genetics) could be combined with an intuitive understanding of personality and the likely effects of family problems on the patient. The reader may find it helpful to re-read the formulation on p. 61 before continuing with this chapter.

Aetiological models

Before considering the contribution that different scientific disciplines can make to psychiatric aetiology, attention needs to be given to the kinds of aetiological model that have been employed in psychiatry. A model is a device for ordering information. Like a theory, it seeks to explain certain phenomena, but it does so in a broad and comprehensive way that cannot readily be proved false.

Reductionist and non-reductionist models

Two broad categories of explanatory model can be recognized. **Reductionist models** seek to understand causation by tracing back to simpler and simpler early stages. Examples are the 'narrow' medical model, described below, and the psychoanalytic model. This type of model can be exemplified by the statement that the cause of schizophrenia lies in disordered neurotransmission in a specific area of the brain.

Non-reductionist models try to relate problems to wider rather than narrower issues. The explanatory models used in sociology are generally of this kind. In psychiatry, this type of model can be exemplified by the statement that the cause of a patient's schizophrenia lies in his family; the patient is the most conspicuous element in a disordered group of people. In the same way it can be asserted that certain depressive states are associated with indices of social deprivation and isolation and can be best understood as being caused by these factors.

The neuroscience approach

The technical and conceptual advances in brain sciences has led to what is often called the **neuroscience approach**. Kandel (1998) outlined the key assumptions underlying this approach to aetiology:

- All mental processes derive from operations of the brain. Thus all behavioural disorders are ultimately disturbances of brain function even where the original 'cause' is clearly environmental.
- Genes, through their protein products, have important effects on brain function and therefore exert a significant control over behaviour.
- Social and behavioural effects exert their effects on the brain in part through changes in gene expression. Changes in gene expression and the consequent patterns of synaptic connectivity underlie the ability of experiences such as learning and psychotherapy to change behaviour.

The latter concept derives from the ability of a wide range of environmental stimuli to modulate gene expression by via alterations in **gene transcription factors**. Thus while genes coding for particular proteins are inherited, environmental and developmental influences are involved in determining whether and to what extent a particular gene is expressed. This provides a plausible mechanism by which nature and nurture interact in the production of a behavioural phenotype.

The neuroscience approach therefore seeks to comprehend the role of social, family, and personal factors in behaviour by relating them to changes in brain function. For example, in understanding the effect of childhood neglect on the liability to adult depression, it is important to find out how adverse childhood experiences might alter relevant brain mechanisms (such as the endocrine response to stress) and how this abnormality might predispose to depression when the individual is exposed to difficulties in adulthood. Thus, although a neuroscience approach encompasses the importance of social and personal factors it seeks to understand their consequences in a **reductionist** way.

Medical models

Several models are used in psychiatric aetiology, but the so-called **medical model** is the most prominent. It represents a general strategy of research that has proved useful in medicine, particularly in studying infectious diseases. A disease entity is identified in terms of a consistent pattern of symptoms, a characteristic clinical course, and specific biochemical and pathological findings (see Chapter 2 regarding models of disease). When an entity has been identified in this way, a set of necessary and sufficient causes is sought. In the case of tuberculosis, for example, the tubercle bacillus is the necessary cause, but it is not by itself sufficient: the tubercle bacillus in conjunction with either poor nutrition or low resistance is sufficient cause.

This narrow kind of medical model has been useful in psychiatry, though not for all conditions. It is clearly relevant to syndromes with a well-defined organic aetiology, for example, psychiatric conditions related to obvious cerebral disorder or a general medical condition. It is also applicable to severe psychiatric disorders such as schizophrenia and bipolar disorder. Until recently such disorders were called 'functional' in contrast to 'organic' because the assumption was that brain dysfunction was present but the pathology (with current methods) could not be observed. Recent studies on the aetiology of schizophrenia have shown that this view was essentially correct (see Chapter 12). However, **social and cultural factors** also play a role in the presentation and course of the illness.

The importance of social and cultural factors is now well recognized in general medicine and modern medical models are therefore considerably broader than that based on the elucidation of the mechanism of infectious disease. Modern medical models also recognize that much illness is characterized by quantitative rather than qualitative deviations from normal, for example, high blood pressure. This applies to certain disorders in psychiatry, particularly anxiety and milder depressive disorders which can therefore be accommodated in a broad medical model.

Difficulties with the medical model arise particularly with disorders characterized mainly by **abnormalities of conduct and social behaviour**, for example, antisocial behaviour and substance misuse. As mentioned above, current neuroscience approaches would seek to understand these disorders through changes in relevant brain systems. This is because causal factors in abnormal social behaviour, such as environmental hardship and personal deprivation, must ultimately express their effects on behaviour through changes in brain mechanisms.

While the latter view appears theoretically valid and increases the aetiological power of the medical model, the key decision for clinician and policy-maker is at what level the disorder is best understood and managed. For example, it is possible to understand problems in substance misuse as arising from a defect in brain reward systems which, in a vulnerable individual, results in 'normal' experimentation with illicit substances leading to substance misuse with adverse personal and social consequences. Equally, one can see excessive drug misuse in society as a 'symptom' of social deprivation and family disruption (see Chapter 18). Both kinds of aetiology can be comprehended in a broad medical model, but different forms of intervention would result.

The behavioural model

As explained above, certain disorders psychiatrists treat, particularly those defined in terms of **abnormal behaviour**, do not fit readily into the medical model. The latter include deliberate self-harm, the misuse of drugs and alcohol, and repeated acts of delinquency. The behavioural model is an alternative way of comprehending these disorders. In this model the disorders are explained in terms of factors that determine normal behaviour: drives, reinforcements, social and cultural influences, and internal psychological processes such as attitudes, beliefs, and expectations. The behavioural model predicts that there will not be a sharp distinction between the normal and the abnormal but a continuous gradation. This model can therefore be a useful way of considering many conditions seen by psychiatrists.

Although the behavioural model is mainly concerned with psychological and social causes, it does not exclude genetic, physiological, or biochemical causes. This is because normal patterns of behaviour are partly determined by genetic factors, and because psychological factors such as reinforcement have a basis in physiological and biochemical mechanisms. Also, the behavioural model employs both **reductionist** and **non-reductionist** explanations. For example, abnormalities of behaviour can be explained in terms of abnormal conditioning (a reductionist model), or in terms of a network of social influences.

Developmental models

Medical and behavioural models incorporate the idea of predisposing as well as precipitating causes, i.e. the idea that past events may determine whether or not a current cause gives rise to a disorder. Some models place even more emphasis on past events in the form of a sequence of experiences leading to the present disorder. This approach has been called the 'life story' approach to aetiology. One example is Freud's psychoanalysis; another is Meyer's psychobiology. These ideas are considered further below.

Political models ('anti-psychiatry')

The models outlined above rely on a scientific approach to psychiatric aetiology; this implies that psychiatric disorders can be studied and understood in an objective and empirical way using the methods of natural sciences. In the history of psychiatry this view has often been regarded as far from self-evident and other conceptual frameworks have sometimes been advocated. For example, it was customary in the Middle Ages to explain mental illness in terms of demonic possession and witchcraft (see below). Over the last 50 years, however, criticisms of scientific approaches to aetiology have most often taken the view that psychiatric illness is defined by **social and political imperatives** and represents at best a cultural value judgement and at worst an abusive means of social control.

Arguments of this nature were put forward strongly by the French philosopher, Michel Focault (1926–1984), and further developed by psychiatrists such as RD Laing (1927–1989), who employed a phenomenological approach to argue that schizophrenia is an understandable response of an individual to a culture of exploitation and alienation. Lack of faith in a scientific approach to mental experience was exemplified by the psychiatrist, Thomas Szasz, who commented, 'There is no psychology; there is only biography and autobiography.' These ideas are sometimes called 'anti-psychiatry' to emphasize their fundamental contrast with the medical models employed by conventional psychiatry.

Most psychiatrists have believed that these formulations do not advance the understanding of mental illness, and in fact, provide rather poor explanations of the range of clinical psychopathology. They seem unable, for example, to account for the existence of schizophrenia in all human societies (see Chapter 12). However, political perceptions of psychiatry are important because they have powerful effects on how mentally ill people are treated and on what services are provided (see Chapter 23). Further, there is no doubt that political abuse of psychiatric patients has occurred, as demonstrated by the cooperation of many German psychiatrists with the euthanasia programmes of the Nazi regime (Dudley and Gale, 2002).

While this is an extreme and abhorrent example, political analyses of psychiatric practice underline the need for the **rights of patients to be respected** and their experiences understood in a personal and social context as outlined above. (For a discussion of views of the limits of scientific approaches to psychiatric illness see Thomas and Bracken, 2004).

The historical development of ideas of aetiology

From the earliest times, theories of the causation of mental disorder have recognized both **somatic** and **psychological influences**. Greek medical literature referred to the causes of mental disorders, mainly in the Hippocratic writings (fourth century BC). Serious mental illness was ascribed mainly to physical causes, which were represented in the theory that health depended on a correct balance of the **four body 'humours'** (blood, phlegm, yellow bile, and black bile). Melancholia was ascribed to an excess of black bile. Most of the less severe psychiatric disorders were thought to have supernatural causes and to require religious healing. An exception was hysteria, which was thought to be caused by the displacement of the uterus from its normal position. Nowadays hysteria is attributed mainly to psychological causes.

Roman physicians generally accepted the causal theories of Greek medicine and developed them in some respects. Galen accepted that melancholia was caused by an excess of black bile, but suggested that this excess could result either from cooling of the blood or from overheating of yellow bile. Phrenitis, the name given to an acute febrile condition with delirium, was thought to result from an excess of yellow bile.

Throughout the Middle Ages these early ideas about the causes of mental illness were largely neglected, though maintained by some scholars such as Bartholomeus Anglicus. The causes of mental illness were now formulated in theological terms of sin and evil, with the consequence that many mentally ill people were persecuted as witches. It was not until the middle of the sixteenth century that beliefs in the supernatural and witchcraft were strongly rejected as causes of mental disorder, notably by the Flemish writer Johan Weyer (1515–1588) in his book *De praestigiis demonum*, published in 1563. Earlier, Paracelsus (1491–1541), the renowned physician, had emphasized the natural causes of mental illness.

In the seventeenth and eighteenth centuries, a more scientific approach to the causation of mental illness developed as physicians became interested in mental disorders, mainly hysteria and melancholia. The English physician Thomas Willis attributed melancholia to 'passions of the heart', but considered that madness (illness with thought disorder, delusions, and hallucinations) was due to a 'fault of the brain'. Willis realized that this fault was not a recognizable gross structural lesion, but a functional abnormality. In the terminology of the time, he referred to a disorder of the 'vital spirits' that were thought to account for nervous action. Willis also pointed out that hysteria could not be caused by a displacement of the womb because the organ is firmly secured in the pelvis.

Another seventeenth century English physician, Thomas Sydenham, rejected the alternative theory that hysteria was caused by a functional disorder of the womb ('uterine suffocation') because he had observed it in men. Despite this renewed medical interest in the causes of mental disorder, the most influential seventeenth century treatise was written by a clergyman, Robert Burton. This work, *The anatomy of melancholy* (1621), described in detail the psychological and social causes (such as poverty, fear, and solitude) that were associated with melancholia and seemed to cause it.

Aetiology depends on **nosology**. Unless it is clear how the various types of mental disorder relate to one another, little progress can be made in understanding causation. From his observations of patients with psychiatric disorders, the Italian physician, Morgagni, became convinced that there was not one single kind of madness but many (Morgagni, 1769). Further attempts at classification followed. One of the best known was proposed by William Cullen, who included a category of neurosis for disorders not caused by localized disease of the nervous system.

The idea that individual mental disorders are caused by lesions of particular brain areas can be traced back to the theory of phrenology proposed by Gall (1758–1828) and his pupil Spurzheim (1776–1832). Gall proposed that the brain was the organ of the mind, that the mind was made up of specific faculties, and that these faculties originated in specific brain areas. He also proposed that the size of a brain area determined the strength of the faculty that resided in it, and that the size of brain areas was reflected in the contours of the overlying skull. Hence the shape of the head reflected a person's psychological make-up. Although the last steps in Gall's argument were false, the ideas of cerebral localization were to develop further. An increased interest in brain pathology led to theories that different forms of mental disorder were associated with lesions in different parts of the brain.

It had long been observed that serious mental illness ran in families, but in the nineteenth century this idea took a new form. In 1809, Morel, a French psychiatrist, put forward ideas that became known as the 'theory of degeneration'. He proposed not only that some mental illnesses were inherited, but also that environmental influences (such as poor living conditions and the misuse of alcohol) could lead to physical changes that could be transmitted to the next generation. Morel also proposed that, as a result of the successive effect of environmental agents in each generation, illnesses appeared in increasingly severe forms in successive generations. It was inherent in these ideas that mental disorders did not differ in kind but only in **severity** - neuroses, psychoses, and mental handicap were increasingly severe manifestations of the same inherited process.

These ideas were consistent with the accepted theories of the inheritance of acquired characteristics, and they were accepted widely. They had the unfortunate effect of encouraging a pessimistic approach to treatment. They also supported the Eugenics Movement, which held that the mentally ill should be removed from society in order to prevent them from reproducing. These developments are an important reminder that **aetiological theories may determine undesirable attitudes to the care of patients**.

Mid-nineteenth century views of the causation of mental illness can be judged from the widely acclaimed textbooks of Esquirol, a French psychiatrist, and of Griesinger, a German psychiatrist. Esquirol (1845) focused on the causes of illness in the individual patient and was less concerned with general theories of aetiology. He recorded psychological and physical factors, which he believed to be significant in individual cases, and he distinguished between predisposing and precipitating causes. He regarded heredity as the most important of the predisposing causes, but he also stressed that predisposition was acted on by psychological causes and by social (at that time called 'moral') causes such as domestic troubles, 'disappointed love', and reverses of fortune. Important physical causes of mental disorder included epilepsy, alcohol misuse, excessive masturbation, childbirth and lactation, and suppression of menstruation. Esquirol also observed that age influenced the type of illness; thus dementia was not observed among the young, but mania was uncommon in old age. He recognized that personality was often a predisposing factor.

In 'Pathology and therapy of mental disorders', which was first published in 1845, Wilhelm Griesinger maintained that mental illness was a **physical disorder of the brain**, and he considered at length the neuropathology of mental illness. He paid equal attention to other causes, including heredity, habitual drunkenness, 'domestic unquiet', disappointed love, and childbirth. He emphasized the multiplicity of causes when he wrote:

> A closer examination of the aetiology of insanity soon shows that in the great majority of cases it was not a single specific cause under the influence of which the disease was finally established but a complication of several, sometimes numerous causes, both predisposing and exciting. Very often the germs of the disease are laid in those early periods of life from which the commencement of the formation of character dates. It grows by education and external influences.
>
> (Griesinger 1867, p. 130)

British views on aetiology in the late nineteenth century can be judged from *A manual of psychological medicine* by Bucknill and Tuke (1858), and from *The pathology of mind* by Henry Maudsley (1879). Maudsley described the causes of mental disorder in terms similar to those of Griesinger; thus causes were multiple, whilst **predisposing causes** (including heredity and early upbringing) were as important as the more **obvious proximal causes**. Maudsley held that mistakes in determining causes were often due to 'some single prominent event, which was perhaps one in a chain of events, being selected as fitted by itself to explain the catastrophe. The truth is that in the great majority of cases there has been a concurrence of steadily operating conditions within and without, not a single effective cause' (Maudsley 1879, p. 83).

Although these nineteenth-century writers and teachers of psychiatry emphasized the **multiplicity of causes**, many practitioners focused narrowly on the findings of genetic and pathological investigations, and adopted a pessimistic approach to treatment. However, Adolf Meyer (1866–1950), a Swiss psychiatrist who worked mainly in the United States, emphasized the role of psychological and social factors in the aetiology of psychiatric disorder. Meyer applied the term **psychobiology** to this approach, in which a wide range of previous experiences were considered and then common-sense judgements used to decide which experiences might have led to the present disorder. Meyer acknowledged the importance of heredity and brain disorder but emphasized that these factors were modified by life experiences which often determined whether or not a particular disorder would be clinically expressed. Meyer's approach remains the basis of the evaluation of aetiology for the individual patient.

The aetiological theories considered so far were mainly concerned with the major mental illnesses. Less severe disorders, particularly those that came to be called neurosis, hysteria, and hypochondriasis, and milder states of depression, were treated mainly by physicians. Pierre Janet, a French neurologist, carried out extensive studies of patients with hysteria and of their response to hypnosis. He believed that hysteria resulted from a functional disorder of the brain and could be treated by hypnosis. In the USA, Weir Mitchell proposed that conditions akin to mild chronic depression were due to exhaustion of the nervous system - a condition he called **neurasthenia**.

In Austria another neurologist, Sigmund Freud, tried to develop a more comprehensive explanation of nervous diseases, first of hysteria and then of other conditions. After an initial interest in physiological causes, Freud proposed that the causes were psychological, but hidden from the patient because they were in the unconscious part of the mind. Freud took a developmental approach to aetiology, believing that the seeds of adult disorder lay in the process of child development (see below). In France, Pierre Janet developed an alternative psychological explanation which was based on variations in the strength of nervous activity and on narrowing of the field of consciousness.

Interest in psychological explanations of the whole range of mental disorders grew as neuropathological and genetic studies failed to yield new insights. Freud and his followers attempted to extend their theory of the neuroses to explain the psychoses. Although the psychological theory was elaborated, no new objective data were obtained about the causes of severe mental illness. Nevertheless, the theories provided explanations which some psychiatrists found more acceptable than an admission of ignorance. Psychoanalysis became increasingly influential, particularly in American psychiatry where it predominated until the 1970s. Since then, renewed interest in genetic, biochemical, and neuropathological causes of mental disorder has followed - an approach that has become known as **biological psychiatry** (Guze, 1989).

Perhaps the most important lesson to learn from this brief overview of the history of ideas on the causation of mental disorder is that each generation bases its theories of aetiology on the scientific approaches most active and plausible at the time. Sometimes psychological ideas prevail, sometimes neuropathological, and sometimes genetic. Throughout the centuries, however, observant clinicians have been aware of the **complexity of the causes of psychiatric disorders**, and have recognized that neither aetiology nor treatment should focus narrowly on the scientific ideas of the day. Instead, the approach should be broader, encompassing whatever psychological, social, and biological factors seem most important in the individual case. Modern psychiatrists are working at a time of rapid development of the neurosciences, but they need to keep the same broad clinical perspective of aetiology whilst assimilating any real scientific advances.

Psychoanalysis

In psychoanalysis the method of investigation differs from the scientific methods reviewed later in this chapter in that it was developed specifically for the study of psychiatric disorders. It arose from clinical experience and not from work in the basic sciences. Psychoanalysis is characterized by a particularly elaborate and comprehensive theory of both normal and abnormal mental functioning. Compared with experimental psychology, it is much more concerned with the **irrational** parts of mental activity. Psychoanalytic theory provides a comprehensive range of explanations for clinical phenomena, and therefore has a wide appeal. However, the features that make it all-embracing also make it difficult to test in a scientific way.

Freud originated psychoanalytical theory, but many other workers contributed to it or developed alternative theories. This section refers only to Freud's theory and not to the other theories, some of which are mentioned elsewhere in the book. This section focuses on the basic ideas of psychoanalysis; hypotheses about particular syndromes are discussed in other chapters.

Psychoanalytic theories are mainly derived from data obtained in the course of psychoanalytical treatment. These data relate to the patient's thoughts, fantasies, and dreams, together with their memories of childhood experiences. By adopting a passive role, Freud tried to ensure that the material consisted of the patient's free associations and not of Freud's own preconceptions.

However, Freud also made interpretations of the patient's reports, and in some of Freud's writings it is difficult to distinguish clearly between the patient's statements and Freud's interpretations. This had lead to controversy about, for example, whether reports of childhood sexual experiences related by his adult patients were based on real events or unconscious fantasies. A major reason for this uncertainty is the particular way in which Freud worked and the different techniques he used over the years to elicit unconscious material (see Esterson, 1998).

Psychoanalysis is an example of a broad theory of a kind found in other branches of knowledge. Such theories can be useful in science by providing a framework within which other ideas can be developed. These theories should not be judged solely on their ability to generate testable hypotheses; however, to be useful, such theories must be able to incorporate new observations as they arise. Darwin's theory of evolution is an example of a useful theory; it survives because it has proved compatible with later observations from genetics and from the fossil record. Freud envisaged that his ideas would one day be explained on the basis of brain mechanisms but until recently the brain sciences have lacked the necessary conceptual and technical power. It is, however, now possible to begin to understand and test the neurobiological basis of some important psychoanalytic concepts (see below).

As pointed out earlier in this chapter, an important distinction between understanding and explanation can be made in psychiatry. In the sense of this distinction, psychoanalysis is a highly elaborate form of understanding that seeks to make both normal mental processes and psychiatric disorders more intelligible. Psychoanalysis does not lead to explanatory hypotheses that can be tested experimentally, although attempts have been made to test some of the simpler hypotheses. The value of psychological understanding has been discussed earlier, and is repeated here before psychoanalytic ideas are reviewed. These ideas can deepen our understanding of patients, but they are not the only way of doing so.

At this point a summary of the main features of Freud's theory will be presented. It is too short to do full justice to Freud's ideas, and interested readers are encouraged to consult some of Freud's original writings, for example, the *Introductory Lectures on Psychoanalysis*, which are models of clarity of exposition.

The structure of the healthy mind

Many of the ideas in the theory were current before Freud began his psychological studies, for example, the idea of an **unconscious part of the mind**. However, Freud developed and combined these ideas in an ingenious way. A central feature was his elaborate concept of the unconscious mind. He supposed that all mental processes originated there. Some of these processes were allowed to enter the conscious mind freely (for example, sensations), some not at all (the unconscious proper), and some occasionally (most memories, which made up the 'preconscious'). According to Freud, the unconscious mind had three characteristics that were important in the genesis of neurosis:

1. it was divorced from reality;
2. it was dynamic in that it contained powerful forces;
3. it was in conflict with the conscious mind.

These three characteristics will be discussed in turn.

The **unconscious mind** was held to be divorced from reality in several ways. It contained flagrant contradictions and paradoxes, and it tended to telescope situations and fantasies that were widely separated in time. In Freud's view, these features were well illustrated by dream analysis. Freud believed that the manifest content of a dream (what the dreamer remembered) could be traced back through analysis to a 'latent' content, which was an infantile wish. The sleeper was thought to perform 'dream work' to translate the latent to the manifest content. This translation was effected by a series of mechanisms, such as condensation (several images fused into one), displacement (of feelings from an essential feature to non-essential features of an object), and secondary elaboration (rearrangement of the assembled elements). Freud attached importance to this dream theory because he supposed the composition of neurotic symptoms to be like that of dreams, though with greater secondary elaboration.

Second, the unconscious mind was **dynamic**, i.e. it contained impulses that were kept in equilibrium by a series of checks and balances. In Freud's early writings, these impulses were regarded as entirely sexual. Later, he placed more emphasis on aggressive impulses. Sexual impulses were supposed to be active even in infancy, receding by about the age of 4 years and then remaining latent until re-emergence at puberty. In Freud's view, psychosexual development not only began early, but was long and complicated. The first stage of organization was oral, i.e. the sexual drive was activated by stimulation of the mouth by sucking and touching with the lips. The second stage was anal, i.e. the drive was activated by expelling or retaining faeces. Only in the third stage did the genital organs become the primary source of sexual energy. Sometimes these stages were not passed through smoothly. The libido (the energy of the sexual instincts) could become fixated (partially arrested) at one of the early stages. When this happened, the person would engage in infantile patterns of behaviour or regress to such patterns under stress. In this way the point of fixation determined the nature of any neurosis that developed later in life.

As libido developed, not only was it activated in these three successive ways, but its object was supposed to change. Self-love came first, to be followed in both boys and girls by love of the mother. Next, still in infancy, boys focused their sexual wishes more intensely upon the mother while developing hostile feelings towards the father (the Oedipus complex). Girls developed the reverse attachments. These attachments came to an end through repression of sexual impulses. As a result, the capacity to feel shame and disgust developed, and the child passed into the latency period. Finally, the sexual impulses emerged again at puberty and were directed into relationships with other adults.

The third aspect of the unconscious mind was its **struggle against the conscious mind**. This conflict was regarded as giving rise to anxiety that could persist throughout life and generate neurotic symptoms. One of Freud's lasting contributions was his idea that anxiety could be reduced by a variety of defence mechanisms, which could be discerned at times in the behaviour of healthy people. These mechanisms are considered on p. 153.

Psychoanalysis and psychiatry

Freud's ideas have been of considerable influence in psychiatry and his proposal that developmental processes play an important role in the aetiology of adult psychopathology is widely accepted. However, many of the details of Freud's theories, for example, the importance of unconscious homosexuality in the causation of paranoid states have been not been found helpful, either as an aetiological explanation of clinical syndromes or as a guide to practice. However, psychoanalytically informed approaches to interpersonal relationships continue to be important in many different kinds of psychotherapy as well as day to day psychiatric practice (Chapter 22). In addition, psychoanalytic concepts can provide possible aetiological insights that can now explored using the neuroscience approach outlined above. A number of current points of convergence can be identified (Tutte, 2004):

- The importance of infant attachment to a caregiver for development has been consistently supported by animal experimental and human studies. Disruptions of attachment result in irreversible changes in hypothalamo-pituitary-adrenal (HPA) axis function and impaired physiological and behavioural adaptation to stress in adult life.
- The delineation of a procedural (implicit, unconscious) memory system working together with a declarative (explicit, conscious) memory system has important implications for the way in which traumatic experiences can influence behaviour through non-conscious mechanisms.
- The prefrontal cortex has the task of selecting preconscious material from explicit memory stores and holding it in working memory for conscious evaluation, planning, and action. The prefrontal cortex therefore can be regarded as the brain region that coordinates the activities associated with the 'executive function' of the ego.

The contribution of scientific disciplines to psychiatric aetiology

The main groups of disciplines that have contributed to the knowledge of psychiatric aetiology are shown in Table 5.1. In this section each group is discussed in turn, and the following questions are asked:

- What sort of problem in psychiatric aetiology can be answered by each discipline?
- How, in general, does each discipline attempt to answer the questions?
- Are any particular difficulties encountered in applying its methods to psychiatric disorders?

Clinical descriptive studies

Before reviewing more elaborate scientific approaches to aetiology, attention is drawn to the continuing value of simple **clinical investigations**. Psychiatry was built on such studies. For example, the view that schizophrenia and the mood disorders are likely to have separate causes depends ultimately on the careful descriptive studies and follow-up enquiries carried out by earlier generations of psychiatrists.

Anyone who doubts the value of clinical descriptive studies should read the paper by Aubrey Lewis on

TABLE 5.1 Scientific disciplines contributing to psychiatric aetiology
Clinical descriptive studies
Epidemiology
Social sciences
Experimental and clinical psychology
Genetics
Biochemical studies
Pharmacology
Endocrinology
Physiology
Neuropathology

'melancholia' (Lewis, 1934). The paper describes a detailed investigation of the symptoms and signs of 61 cases of severe depressive disorder. It provided the most complete account in the English language and it remains unsurpassed. It is an invaluable source of information about the clinical features of depressive disorders untreated by modern methods. Lewis's careful observations drew attention to unsolved problems, including the nature of retardation, the relation of depersonalization to affective changes, the presence of manic symptoms, and the validity of the classification of depressive disorders into reactive and endogenous groups. None of these problems has yet been solved completely, but the analysis by Lewis was important in focusing attention on them.

Although many opportunities for this kind of research have been taken already, it does not follow that clinical investigation is no longer worthwhile. For example, the study of Judd *et al.* (2002) described in Chapter 6 is a recent example of how a clinical follow-up study can provide important insight into the aetiology of milder mood disorders in relation to bipolar disorder. Well-conducted clinical enquiries are likely to retain an important place in psychiatric research for many years to come.

Epidemiology

Epidemiology is the study of the distribution of a disease in space and time within a population, and of the factors that influence this distribution. Its concern is with disease in groups of people, not in the individual person.

Concepts and methods of epidemiology

The basic concept of epidemiology is that of **rate**, or the ratio of the number of instances to the numbers of people in a defined population. Instances can be episodes of illness, or people who are or have been ill. Rates may be computed on a particular occasion (**point prevalence**) or over a defined interval (**period prevalence**).

Other concepts include **inception rate**, which is based on the number of people who were healthy at the beginning of a defined period but became ill during that period, and **lifetime expectation or risk**, which is based on an estimate of the number of people who could be expected to develop a particular illness in the course of their whole life. In **cohort studies**, a group of people are followed for a defined period of time to determine the onset or change in some characteristic with or without previous exposure to a potentially important agent (for example, lung cancer and smoking).

Three aspects of method are particularly important in epidemiology:

1. defining the population at risk;
2. defining a case;
3. finding cases.

It is essential to define the **population at risk** accurately. Such a population can be all the people living in a limited area (for example, a country, an island, or a catchment area), or a subgroup chosen by age, gender, or some other potentially important defining characteristic.

Defining a case is the central problem of psychiatric epidemiology. It is relatively easy to define a condition such as Down syndrome, but until recently the reliability of psychiatric diagnosis has not been satisfactory. The development of standardized techniques for defining, identifying, rating, and classifying mental disorders has greatly improved the reliability and validity of epidemiological studies.

Two methods are used for **case finding**. The first is to enumerate all cases known to medical or other agencies (**declared cases**). Hospital admission rates may give a fair indication of rates of major mental illnesses, but not, for example, of most mood or anxiety disorders. Moreover, hospital admission rates are influenced by many variables, such as the geographical accessibility of hospitals, attitudes of doctors, admission policies, and the law relating to compulsory admissions.

The second method is to search for both declared and undeclared cases in the community. In community surveys, the best technique is often to use two stages: preliminary screening to detect potential cases with a self-rated questionnaire such as the General Health Questionnaire (Goldberg, 1972), followed by detailed clinical examination of potential cases with a standardized psychiatric interview.

Aims of epidemiological enquiries

In psychiatry, **epidemiology** attempts to answer three main kinds of question:

1. What is the prevalence of psychiatric disorder in a given population at risk?
2. What are the clinical and social correlates of psychiatric disorder?
3. What factors may be important in aetiology?

Prevalence can be estimated in community samples or among people attending general practitioners or hospital cases. Studies of prevalence in different locations, social groups, or social classes can contribute to aetiology. Studies of associations between a disorder and **clinical and social** variables can do the same and may be useful for clinical practice; for example, epidemiological studies have shown that the risk of suicide is increased in elderly males with certain characteristics, such as living alone, misusing drugs or alcohol, suffering from physical or mental illness, and having a family history of suicide.

Causes in the environment

Epidemiological studies of aetiology have been concerned with predisposing and precipitating factors, and with the analysis of the personal and social correlates of mental illness. Amongst **predisposing factors**, the influence of **heredity** has been examined in studies of families, twins, and adopted people, as described in the later section on genetics. Other examples are the influence of maternal age on the risk of Down syndrome, and the psychological effects of parental loss during childhood. Studies of **precipitating factors** include life-events research, which is described in the following section on the social sciences.

Epidemiological approaches to aetiology can be illustrated by the results of studies of environmental correlates of mental disorders. For example, it has been apparent for many years that schizophrenia is more common in urban environments, particularly in disadvantaged inner-city areas. This finding could be of aetiological importance or it could be a consequence of the experience of schizophrenia with, for example, people in the early stages of illness seeking isolation. In a recent study of this question, van Os *et al.* (2003), confirmed that the prevalence of psychosis increased linearly with the degree of urbanicity (overall odds ratio 1.57, 95 per cent CI 1.30–1.89). This significant effect remained after adjustment for factors such as age, gender, education level, parental psychiatric history and country of birth.

As expected there was, in addition, an independent and highly significant influence of a family history of psychosis on the risk of an individual developing psychosis (odds ratio 4.59, 95 per cent CI 2.41–8.74). Further analysis showed that the effect of urbanicity to increase the risk of psychosis was much greater in individuals with a family history of psychosis than in those without. These findings suggest an important interaction between gene and environment such that the adverse environmental effects of urbanicity are expressed particularly on individuals with a genetic predisposition to psychosis.

Social sciences

Many of the concepts used by sociologists are relevant to psychiatry (see Table 5.2). Unfortunately, some of these potentially fruitful ideas have been used uncritically, for example, in the suggestion that mental illness is no more than a label for socially deviant people, the 'myth of mental illness'. This development points to the obvious need for sociological theories to be tested in the same way as other theories by collecting appropriate data.

TABLE 5.2 Some applications of social theory to psychiatry

Concept	Application
Social class and subculture	Epidemiology of substance misuse
Stigma and labelling	Analysis of handicaps of seriously mentally ill in community
Institutionalization	Negative behavioural effects of hospitalization
Social deviance	Delinquent behaviour
Abnormal illness behaviour	Psychological consequences of physical illness

Some of the concepts of sociology overlap with those of social psychology, for example, attribution theory (which deals with the way in which people interpret the causes of events in their lives) and ideas about self-esteem. An important part of research in sociology, the study of life events, uses epidemiological methods (see below).

Transcultural studies

Studies in different societies help in making an important aetiological distinction. Biologically determined features of mental disorder are likely to be similar in different cultures, whilst psychologically and socially determined features are likely to be dissimilar. Thus the 'core' symptoms of schizophrenia have a similar incidence in people from widely different societies, suggesting that a common neurobiological abnormality is likely to be important in aetiology.

By contrast, depressive disorders have a wider range of prevalence. The Cross-National Collaborative Group (Weissman *et al.*, 1996) found life-time rates of depression ranging from 1.5 per cent in Taiwan to 19 per cent in Lebanon. In addition there are variations in the clinical presentation of depressive states with prominent somatic symptoms being more common in non-Western cultures. In all societies, however, sadness, joylessness, anxiety and lack of energy are common symptoms (see Bhugra and Mastrogianni, 2004).

The study of life events

Epidemiological methods have been used in social studies to examine associations between illness and certain kinds of events in a person's life. In an early study, Wolff (1962) studied the morbidity of several hundred people over many years and found that episodes of illness clustered at times of change in the person's life. Holmes and Rahe (1967) attempted to improve on the highly subjective measures used by Wolff. They used a list of 41 kinds of life event (e.g. work, residence, finance, and family relationships) and weighted each according to its apparent severity, for example, 100 for the death of a spouse and 13 for a spell of leave for a serviceman.

In latter developments the study of the psychological impact of life events has been further improved in a number of ways:

- to reduce memory distortion, limits are set to the period over which events are to be recalled;
- efforts are made to date the onset of the illness accurately;
- attempts are made to exclude events that are not clearly independent of the illness, for example, losing a job because of poor performance;
- events are characterized in terms of their nature (for example, losses or threats) as well as their severity;
- data are collected with a semi-structured interview and rated reliably.

Although significant, life events taken in isolation may be less important than at first appears. For example, in one study events involving the loss or departure of a person from the immediate social field of the respondent ('exit events') were reported in 25 per cent of patients with depressive disorders but in only 5 per cent of controls. This difference was significant at the 1 per cent level and appears impressive, but Paykel (1978) questioned its real significance through the following calculation.

The incidence of depressive disorder is not accurately known, but if it is taken to be 2 per cent for new cases over a 6-month period, then a hypothetical population of 10,000 people would yield 200 new cases. If exit events occurred to 5 per cent of people who did not become cases of depressive disorder, in the hypothetical population, exit events would occur to 490 of the 9800 people who were not new cases. Amongst the 200 new cases, exit events would occur to 25 per cent, i.e. 50 people. Thus the total number of people experiencing exit events would be 490 plus 50, or 540, of whom only 50 (less than 1 in 10) would develop depressive disorders. Hence the greater part of the variance in determining depressive disorder must be attributed to something else. That is, life events trigger depression largely in **predisposed individuals**.

This idea leads us on to the consideration of **vulnerability and protective** factors (see below). However, at this point it is also worth noting that studies of genetic epidemiology have taken life events research a stage further by showing that the tendency to experience adverse life events is itself partly genetically determined. For example, individuals differ genetically in their liability to 'select' those environments which put them at relatively higher risk of experiencing adverse life events. Presumably this is one way in which the genetic vulnerability to depression may be expressed (see Kendler *et al.*, 2004).

Vulnerability and protective factors

People may differ in their response to life events for three reasons. First, the same event may have different meanings for different people, according to their **previous experience**. For example, a family separation may be more stressful to an adult who has suffered separation in childhood. In this way adverse experiences remote in time from the adverse life event itself may predispose to the later development of psychiatric disorder.

The other reasons are that certain contemporary factors may **increase vulnerability** to life events or **protect** against them. Ideas about these last two factors derive largely from the work of Brown and Harris (1978) who found evidence that, among women, vulnerability factors include having the care of small children and being unemployed while protection is conferred by having a confidant who can share problems. The idea of protective factors has been used to explain the observation that some people do not become ill even when exposed to severe adversities. Recent studies suggest that similar protective and vulnerability factors may also modify the response to life stress in other cultures. For example, in women living in an urban setting in Zimbabwe, the risk of depression following a severe adverse life event was substantially reduced by the presence of a supportive family network (Broadhead *et al.*, 2001).

Causes in the family

It has been suggested that some mental disorders are an expression of emotional disorder within a whole family, not just a disorder in the person seeking treatment (the 'identified patient'). Although family problems are common among people with psychiatric disorder, their general importance in aetiology is almost certainly overstated in this formulation since emotional difficulties in other family members may be the result of the patient's problems rather than its cause. In addition, emotional difficulties in close relatives may result from shared genetic inheritance. For example, the parents of children with schizophrenia have an increased risk of schizotypal personality disorder (see p. 282). It seems more likely that family difficulties may modify the course of an established disorder. For example, high levels of 'expressed emotion' from family members increases the risk of relapse in patients with schizophrenia (see p. 295). In terms of aetiology, however, twin studies show that shared (family) environment is less important than shared genes in explaining familial clustering in most psychiatric phenotypes.

Migration

Moving to another country, or even to an unfamiliar part of the same country, is a life change that has been suggested as a cause of various kinds of mental disorder. A number of possible mechanisms have been identified:

- **Selective migration** People in the early stages of an illness such as schizophrenia may migrate because of failing relationships in their country of origin.
- **Process of migration** Events around the process of migration itself for example, physical and emotional trauma, prolonged waiting periods, exhaustion, and social deprivation and isolation may cause several different kinds of stress-related disorder.
- **Post-migration factors** Many factors come into play post-migration which could influence the risk of developing mental illness. These include **social adversity**, caused, for example, by **racial discrimination** and **acculturation** in which the breakdown of traditional cultural structures results in loss of self-esteem and social support. Disparities between aspiration and achievement may also cause stress and depression. Finally, immigrants may be exposed to unfamiliar viruses, which could conceivably affect intrauterine development and predispose to psychiatric disorder in the next generation.

It is fairly well established that immigration is associated higher rates of psychosis in several ethnic groups but the mechanisms are unclear (see Chapter 12). Effects of immigration on other psychiatric disorders are less consistent and some groups experience a relative improvement in mental health compared with their native populations. Clearly refugees who have fled persecution are likely to have elevated rates of stress-related symptomatology and many will meet formal diagnostic criteria for post-traumatic stress disorder. However, it is important that such symptoms are interpreted sensitively in the context of the relevant cultural ways of dealing with trauma (for a review see Bhugra, 2004).

Experimental and clinical psychology

There are a number of characteristic features of the psychological approach to psychiatric aetiology:

- the idea of a **continuity between the normal and abnormal**. This idea leads to investigations that attempt to explain psychiatric abnormalities in terms of processes determining normal behaviour.
- concern with the **interaction between the person and his environment**. The psychological approach differs from the social approach in being concerned less with environmental variables and more with the person's ways of processing information coming from the external environment and from his own body.
- an emphasis on factors **maintaining abnormal behaviour**. Psychologists are less likely to regard behaviour disorders as resulting from internal disease processes, and more likely to assume that persisting behaviour is maintained by abnormal coping mechanisms, for example, by anxiety-reducing avoidance strategies.

Neuropsychology

Neuropsychological approaches share common ground with biological psychiatry in attempting to identify the neurobiological substrates for psychological phenomena. Various methodologies are employed but the aim is to understand psychopathology in the context of brain science. Investigations may therefore involve animal experimental work or a range of human studies including neurological patients with defined brain lesions and patients with psychiatric disorders.

For example, animal experimental models have shown that there is a crucial role for the **amygdala** in fear conditioning. Furthermore, because of its connections to the thalamus, the amygdala is activated by threatening stimuli and can produce autonomic fear responses before any conscious awareness of threat. LeDoux (1998) has related this circuitry to traumatic anxiety by proposing an imbalance in the **implicit (unconscious) emotional memory system** involving the thalamus and amygdala and the **explicit**

(conscious) declarative memory system in the temporal lobe and hippocampus (see below).

As well as animal experimental studies, neuropsychological investigations also involve different groups of human subjects. Valuable information may be gained from subjects who have suffered **well-defined brain lesions**. For example patients with bilateral **amygdala lesions** can recognize the personal identity of faces but not the facial expression of fear. This supports the notion that the amygdala is important in the processing of fear-related stimuli.

Current neuropsychological approaches also make extensive use of **functional brain imaging techniques**. This allows localization of the brain regions and circuits involved in specific psychological processes and facilitates comparisons between healthy subjects and patients who experience abnormalities in the processes concerned. For example, in a magnetic resonance imaging investigation it was found that when patients with depression were shown pictures of fearful facial expressions they showed greater activation than controls in brain circuitry related to the processing of anxiety, including the amygdala. The increased activation was attenuated by treatment with antidepressant medication (Fu *et al.*, 2004). This suggests that increased activity of the amygdala may play a role in the anxious preoccupations characteristic of depression and that antidepressants may act by decreasing amygdala function.

Information processing

The **information theory approach** to psychology proposes that the brain can be regarded as an information channel, which receives, filters, processes, and stores information from sense organs, and retrieves information from memory stores. This approach, which compares the brain to a computer, suggests useful ways of thinking about some of the abnormalities in psychiatric disorders. There are various mechanisms involved at different stages of information processing and therefore different points at which dysfunctional processing could give rise to psychiatric disorder. Two of these mechanisms are **attention** and **memory**, changes in which have been linked to psychiatric symptomatology.

Attention

Attention is viewed as an active process of selecting, from the mass of sensory input, the elements that are relevant to the processing that is being carried out at the time. There is evidence that attentional processes are disturbed in some psychiatric disorders. For example, anxious patients attend more than non-anxious controls to stimuli that contain elements of threat. This can be shown experimentally as a disruption of psychological performance where the task involves ignoring threat-related words. One example is the use of a modified Stroop test where subjects have to name the colour of a background on which a word is written. When the word is a threatening one (such as 'kill') the latency taken to name the background colour is increased and this increase is exaggerated in anxious subjects (see Monk and Pine, 2004).

Subsequent studies have made two additional observations that are clinically important. First, the attentional bias in anxiety disorders is probably due a failure to disengage attention from threat-related stimuli rather than excessive initial orientation towards them. Second, anxious subjects still produce greater responses to threat-related stimuli than controls even when the stimuli are 'masked' so they are received outside conscious awareness. Masking is achieved by presenting the stimulus for a very short time (< 40 milliseconds), immediately followed by the longer presentation of another stimulus (the mask). The fact that masked stimuli elicit greater behavioural responses in anxious subjects suggests that the abnormal attentional mechanisms in anxiety involve the non-conscious threat processing pathways associated with the amygdala (see above and Monk and Pine, 2004). While these findings are of interest it is important to remember that they may, in fact, be a **consequence** of the anxiety disorder rather than a **causal** mechanism. Even in the former case, however, they could still play a maintaining role in symptomatology.

Memory

The **information-processing model** has been applied fruitfully to the study of memory. It suggests that there are different kinds of memory store: sensory stores in which sensory information is held for short periods while awaiting further processing, a short-term store in which information is held for only 20 seconds unless it is continually rehearsed, and a long-term store in which information is retained for long periods. There is a mechanism for retrieving information from this long-term store when required, and this mechanism could break down while memory traces are intact. This model has led to useful experiments. For example, patients with the amnestic syndrome (see p. 327) score better on memory tests requiring recognition of previously encountered material than on tasks requiring unprompted recall; this finding suggests a breakdown of information retrieval rather than of information storage.

It is well established that low mood facilitates recall of unhappy events. This can be demonstrated in healthy subjects undergoing a negative mood induction as well as depressed patients (Clark and Teasdale, 1982). Once again, it is not clear whether in depressed patients this phenomenon is a manifestation of depressed mood rather than one of its causes. However, it is possible that it could play a role in maintaining the depressive state. More recent research has focused on the way that patients with mood disorders recall personal memories. For example when asked to think of a **specific event** associated with the word 'happy', a depressed patient may respond with, 'when I used to go for long walks by myself', a rather general reply. In contrast a non-depressed person is more likely to respond quite specifically 'when I went for a walk in Leighton forest, last Sunday with my family'. This over-generalized style of memory recall is associated with a history of negative life events and also might be linked to impaired problem-solving ability. This could act to perpetuate the depressive state (see Williams, 2000 and van Vreeswijk and De Wilde, 2004).

As noted above, there is increasing interest in how **explicit declarative** and **implicit emotional** memories might be involved in the processing of traumatic events. It has been suggested that during highly traumatic experiences explicit memory of the event is relatively poor while implicit (unconscious emotional memory) is vivid. This could give rise to the automatic intrusions and poor explicit memory seen in post-traumatic stress disorder (Halligan *et al.*, 2003).

Beliefs and expectations

The information processing model also predicts that responses to information, including the emotional response, are determined by **beliefs and expectations**. This idea proposes that behaviour of all individuals is guided by their beliefs and that psychopathology is associated with altered **content of beliefs** about the self and the world. Cognitive psychology assumes that such beliefs are organized into **schemas**. Schemas have important properties in relation to different kinds of psychopathology:

- they influence information processing, conscious thinking, emotion, and behaviour;
- though not necessarily accessible to direct introspection, their content can usually be reconstructed in verbal terms (known as **assumptions or beliefs**);
- in patients with psychiatric disorders, these beliefs are dysfunctional, resistant to refutation, and play a part in the aetiology and maintenance of the disorder.

These ideas have been used in the development of **cognitive therapy** where researchers aim to identify the dysfunctional beliefs associated with particular disorders and apply techniques which help the patient reevaluate and change them. For example, experimental work has shown that patients with panic disorder (p. 192) have inaccurate expectations that sensory information about rapid heart action predicts an imminent heart attack. This expectation results in anxiety when the information is received, with the result that the heart rate accelerates further and a vicious circle of mounting anxiety is set up. Changing these expectations can alleviate panic attacks.

Ethology and evolutionary psychology

Many psychological studies involve quantitative observations of behaviour. In some of these investigations use is made of methods developed originally in the related discipline of ethology. Complex behaviour is divided into simpler components and counted systematically. Regular sequences are noted as well as interactions between individuals, for example, between a mother and her infant. Such methods have been used, for example, to study the effects of separating infant primates from their mothers, and to compare this primate behaviour with that of human infants separated in the same way.

More recent applications of ethology have used insights from the field of **evolutionary psychology** to understand both normal and abnormal behaviour in an evolutionary context. This approach attempts to explain why various behaviours might have arisen in terms of evolutionary **adaptation**.

For example, because depressive states are ubiquitous in human societies, it is reasonable to ask what their adaptive value may be. One suggestion is that depression may reflect a form of subordination in animals who have lost rank in a social hierarchy. Rather than fighting a losing battle, the depressed individual withdraws and conserves emotional resources for another day.

Such ideas are not readily testable experimentally but can give rise to hypotheses concerning possible brain mechanisms. One theoretical difficulty is that psychiatric disorders often appear to represent **maladaptive** rather than adaptive behaviours. Wolpert (1999), for example, has drawn an analogy with cancer in which the consequences of abnormal cell growth are clearly maladaptive and injurious to the individual. As cancer can be regarded as normal cell division 'gone wrong', so depression might be normal emotion 'gone wrong'. From this viewpoint the question is not what is the adaptive value of the abnormal behaviour but rather the adaptive value of the normal behaviour to which the abnormal state is related. For a review of this debate see Nettle (2004).

Genetics

Genetic investigations are concerned with three issues:

1. the relative contributions of genetic and environmental factors to aetiology;
2. the mode of inheritance of disorders that have a hereditary basis;
3. identification of relevant genes and their mutations and polymorphisms.

In psychiatry, important advances have been made with the first issue, but less progress has been made with the other two. Methods in genetics are of three broad kinds: **population and family studies (genetic epidemiology), cytogenetics**, and **molecular genetics**. Population and family studies are mainly concerned with estimating the contribution of genetic factors and the mode of inheritance, whilst cytogenetics and molecular genetics provide information about mechanisms of inheritance. The concepts, methods and terminology of psychiatric genetics are complex and only briefly introduced here. For more detailed coverage, see the textbook by Owen *et al.* (2003).

Extent of genetic contribution

Methods of population genetics (**genetic epidemiology**) are used to assess risk in three groups of people: families, twins, and people who have been adopted. In **family risk studies**, the investigator determines the risk of a psychiatric condition among the relatives of affected persons and compares it with the expected risk in the general population. (The affected persons are usually referred to as **index cases** or **probands**.)

Such studies require a sample selected in a strictly defined way. Moreover, it is not sufficient to ascertain the current prevalence of a psychiatric condition among the relatives because some of the population may go on to develop the condition later in life. For this reason, investigators use corrected figures known as expectancy rates (or morbid risks). However, caution is needed in interpretation of results from studies of this nature for a number of reasons, as will now be discussed.

Family studies

Family risk studies have been used extensively in psychiatry. These studies by themselves cannot distinguish clearly between inheritance and the effects of family environment. However, by demonstrating that the disorder of interest shows familial clustering, they are a valuable first step, pointing to the need for other kinds of investigation.

Twin studies

Twin studies are the most important method for measuring the genetic contribution to a **phenotype** (an observable characteristic, such as a personality trait or a disorder). In twin studies the investigator seeks to separate genetic and environmental influences by comparing **concordance rates** (i.e. where both co-twins have the same disorder) in uniovular (monozygous, MZ) and binovular (dizygous, DZ) twins. If concordance for a psychiatric disorder is higher in MZ twins than in DZ twins, a genetic component is presumed; the greater the difference in concordance, the greater the **heritability**.

Heritability is the proportion of the liability to a disorder in a population that is accounted for by genetic effects; it is usually expressed as a percentage. Recent estimates for common psychiatric disorders, based on population-based twin studies, are shown in Table 5.3. Estimates of heritability apply to the particular population studied, and may vary in different populations under different environmental conditions. Also, a heritability figure cannot be applied to an individual. Most psychiatric disorders, and behavioural traits, are heritable to a degree, and many show a substantial heritability. However, except for some rare autosomal dominant dementias, heritability is always significantly less than 100 per cent, emphasizing that genes are not the sole cause; the environment is important too (Bouchard and McGue, 2003).

Heritability should not be confused with concordance or **penetrance**. A phenotype can show high con-

TABLE 5.3 Heritability estimates for selected psychiatric disorders

Disorder	Heritability estimate (%)
Schizophrenia	80
Bipolar disorder	80
Major depression	40
Generalized anxiety disorder	30
Panic disorder	40
Phobia	35
Alcohol problem or dependence	60

From Owen *et al.* (2000).

BOX 5.1 CONSIDERATIONS IN THE ASSESSMENT OF TWIN STUDIES IN GENETIC EPIDEMIOLOGY

- Has zygosity has been accurately determined? It is assumed that MZ co-twins are genetically identical but this may not be the case because of factors such as mitochondrial inheritance.
- It is assumed that when twins are raised together (as is usually the case), MZ and DZ twin pairs both experience the same degree of environmental sharing. However, this may not necessarily be true, especially if the prenatal (intrauterine) environment is included. (Counterintuitively, this is more *dissimilar* for MZ than DZ co-twins).
- Despite these caveats the '**equal environments assumption**' for twins appears to hold for most disorders. It should also be noted that gene and environment effects often **interact** with each other and so their effects are not simply additive. For example, parents with antisocial personality disorder may pass on genes increasing the risk that children will inherit a liability to conduct disorder but may also produce a family environment that itself increases the risk of behavioural disturbance.
- Most twin studies are now population-based, rather than derived from psychiatric case registers. This reduces the biases of the latter, but does mean that relatively few cases are detected even in large samples, resulting in estimates that sometimes have wide confidence intervals; also, the reliability of diagnoses may be less certain. Finally, being a twin might in itself affect the risk of developing a psychiatric disorder; however, there is little evidence of this.

cordance in MZ twins without being genetic (for example, religious faith, or football team supported); equally, relatively low concordance rates between MZ twins may still denote high heritability: it is the **difference** in concordance rates between MZ and DZ twins which denotes heritability. **Penetrance**, in the present context, refers to the likelihood that a person who has a genotype known to cause a phenotype manifests that characteristic. This does not always happen, probably reflecting protective genetic or environmental factors in that individual; indeed, only a few conditions are fully penetrant.

As well as showing the size of the genetic contribution, modern twin studies allow the environmental contribution to be divided into that which is unique to the individual ('non-shared') and that which reflects the common ('shared') environment experienced by the twins. This is usually done using a sophisticated statistical approach called **structural equation modelling**. With the important exception of schizophrenia, shared environment usually contributes much less than individual specific factors (or than heritability) to psychiatric phenotypes; this calls into question the aetiological importance often attached to the family environment in psychiatry.

Despite their critical role in genetic epidemiology the results of twin studies should not be accepted uncritically, since they make several assumptions which are outlined in Box 5.1.

Adoption studies

Adoption studies provide another useful method of separating genetic and environmental influences. The basic method is to compare rates of a disorder in biological relatives versus adoptive relatives. Three main designs are used:

- Adoptee study: the rate of disorder in the adopted-away children of an affected parent is compared with that in adopted-away children of healthy parents.
- Study of the adoptee's family: the rate of disorder in the biological relatives of affected adoptees is compared with the rate in adopted relatives.
- In a cross-fostering study, the rate of disorder is measured in adoptees who have affected biological parents but unaffected adoptive parents, and compared with the rate in adoptees who have healthy biological parents but affected adoptive parents.

Adoption studies are affected by a number of biases, such as the reasons why the child was adopted, non-random assignment of the children on socioeconomic status, and the effects on adoptive parents of raising a difficult child. They may also be limited by small sample sizes, especially as adoption becomes a rarer event in many countries. A more fundamental limitation is that adoption studies do not control for the prenatal environment, which may be important for disorders associated with intrauterine factors or birth complications.

Boundaries of the phenotype

The studies of genetic epidemiology described above can lead to clearer identifications of the limits of the **clinical phenotype** associated with inheritance of particular genes. For example, such studies have established that that the genetic predisposition to schizophrenia is part of a broader vulnerability, leading to the concept of **schizophrenia spectrum disorders** (p. 283). Similarly, major depression and generalized anxiety disorder appear to share many of the same genes (Kendler *et al.*, 1992a).

As well as trying to clarify the validity and boundaries of diagnostic categories, research has increasingly focused on **endophenotypes** (or **intermediate phenotypes**). These are features thought to be more closely related to a disorder's underlying biology and genes than is the clinical syndrome itself; for example, eye tracking dysfunction and impaired working memory are endophenotypes in schizophrenia. Endophenotypes are thus considered to be more powerful and biologically meaningful constructs than are conventional phenotypes (i.e. syndromes) (Gottesman and Gould, 2003).

The mode of inheritance

A useful intermediate step between finding that a disorder or other phentoype clusters in families and is heritable, and applying molecular methods to find the gene(s) responsible, is to determine the mode of inheritance. In essence, the question is whether the disorder has the characteristics of a Mendelian trait, i.e. the family history shows a classic Mendelian pattern of dominant, recessive, or X-linked inheritance. If so, the disorder can be assumed to be caused by a single major gene, which is then best sought using linkage genetics (see below).

In psychiatry, as in the rest of medicine, such disorders are well known – e.g. familial dementias, and some causes of learning disability – but they cause only a very small fraction of the burden of disease. Most psychiatric disorders do not show classic Mendelian patterns of inheritance; instead, like most common medical disorders such as asthma and diabetes mellitus, psychiatric disorders involve the combined action of several (or many) genes each of moderate (or small) effect. They are called **non-Mendelian, complex,** or **multifactorial genetic disorders**. No gene is either necessary or sufficient to cause the disorder; they are best considered as risk factors, and are termed **susceptibility genes**, which together set the genetic threshold of vulnerability. This kind of 'genetic architecture' explains why it has proven difficult to identify the genes and the variants within them (Owen *et al.*, 2000). Two issues complicate matters further. First, there are additive and interactive effects between the genes (**epistasis**), and between genes and environmental influences; second, the regulation of genes is itself heritable, independent of any change in DNA sequence (**epigenetics**).

Methods for locating and identifying genes

Cytogenetic studies

Cytogenetics is concerned with identifying structural abnormalities in chromosomes and associating them with disease. They are often suspected based on a characteristic physical appearance, are usually associated with learning disability, and can often be diagnosed relatively easily by clinical geneticists using **karyotyping** in which the chromosomes are visualized. A good example in psychiatry is **Down syndrome**. In this condition two kinds of abnormality have been detected: in the commonest kind, there is an additional copy of chromosome 21 (trisomy 21; an example of **aneuploidy** – an incorrect number of chromosomes). Other cases are caused when a segment of chromosome 21 is swapped with a portion of another chromosome, a process called **translocation**. Other examples involve the X and Y chromosomes, such as **Turner's syndrome** (XO) and **Klinefelter's syndrome** (XXY). More subtle cytogenetic disorders affecting small parts of a chromosome are now being recognized, including fragile X syndrome (p. 718) and velocardiofacial syndrome (VCFS), in which part of one copy of the long arm of chromosome 22 is deleted (p. 284).

Although cytogenetic abnormalities are extremely rare causes of disease, their occurrence provides important clues as to where susceptibility genes may be located. For example, it was the observation that Alzheimer's disease is common in Down syndrome which encouraged investigators to search chromosome 21 for genes which might cause the disease even in non-trisomic subjects; in this way, the amyloid precursor gene (APP; Chapter 14) was identified – the first discovery of a causative gene for a psychiatric disorder. Similarly, the increased frequency of psychosis in VCFS has helped identification of three genes within that region that may predispose to psychosis in general (Chapter 12).

Molecular genetics

The aim of molecular genetic studies is to identify the genes explaining the inheritance of a phenotype, in this case a psychiatric disorder. There are two main approaches to finding genes: **linkage studies (positional cloning)** and **association studies**. The reader is referred to Owen *et al.* (2003) for more detailed review, whilst Box 5.2 introduces some concepts and terms pertaining to genetic variability, which is the key to understanding the genetic basis of disease and how this can be investigated.

BOX 5.2 THE TERMINOLOGY OF GENETIC VARIATION: POLYMORPHISMS, ALLELES AND MUTATIONS

- No two people share precisely the same **genome**. That is, each person has a unique DNA sequence (with the exception of MZ twins). DNA sequence variants are called **polymorphisms** or **allelic variants**. They occur on average every 1000 nucleotides across the whole genome, both within genes and between them. A given polymorphism can be very rare, or the variants (**alleles**) can occur at equal frequency in the population.
- Most polymorphisms involve a change in a single nucleotide, hence the term **single nucleotide polymorphism** (SNP), though others involve insertions, deletions or repeats of short stretches of DNA. Most polymorphisms have no known significance, especially those which are silent or conservative substitutions (i.e. where they do not change the aminoacid encoded in the protein, either because they are in non-coding parts of DNA, or because of the degeneracy of the genetic code). However, some polymorphisms do prove to have functional correlates, as discussed below. Because we have two copies of every autosomal gene (**autosomes** = chromosomes other than X or Y), at any point in the genome the two alleles may be identical (**homozygosity**), or they may differ (**heterozygosity**).
- The term **mutation** can be used synonymously with polymorphism to mean any variation in DNA sequence. However, it is often used in a more restricted way to denote a change which is detrimental – usually because it causes a disease. This differs from polymorphisms in general, which, as noted above may have no consequences at all; if they do, they can be beneficial, neutral or harmful, and any effects are not deterministic but merely change the probability of a particular phenotype. The term mutation is therefore used largely with with reference to Mendelian disorders.

Genetic linkage studies

The standard way to identify a causative gene is through study of how segments of DNA are inherited within families affected by a disease. If a particular region or **locus** (plural, **loci**), of a chromosome consistently **segregates** with the disease, then that locus is likely to contain the gene. There is therefore said to be **linkage** between the region and the disease. The likelihood that the locus is linked to the disease is generally expressed as the logarithm of the odds of detection of linkage, or **LOD score**. A LOD score of more than 3 is conventionally taken as reasonable evidence for linkage. Originally, researchers had to study a single chromosome at a time, but it is now usual to do **genome-wide linkage scans**, in which all the chromosomes are studied. A locus can be large, stretching over millions of bases of DNA, and contain many genes. Thus, once a locus has been identified, higher resolution methods are used until the causative gene is identified and sequenced, to reveal the mutation which distinguishes the DNA of affected from unaffected members of the family or families studied. Major successes of the linkage strategy in psychiatry include identification of the APP gene on chromosome 21 in familial Alzheimer's disease, and the huntingtin gene on chromosome 4 in Huntington's disease (Chapter 14).

However, as mentioned, linkage genetics has had very limited success in psychiatry beyond rare, familial dementias and some causes of learning disability. There are several reasons for this (Owen *et al.* 2000), the most important being that linkage works best for Mendelian disorders; that is, when there is a single gene causing the disorder, inherited in classic dominant or recessive fashion, and with high penetrance. The method is poor at detecting multiple genes of small effect, which, as noted, appears to be the case for most psychiatric disorders. Nor does linkage genetics work well if the disorder in the families under study is in fact an admixture of several different single gene disorders (**genetic heterogeneity**) and non-genetic forms of the syndrome (**phenocopies**). There are various ways to try and minimize the limitations of linkage genetics in this situation, e.g. testing different models of inheritance, or using different definitions of the phenotype, and seeing which produces the highest LOD score. Inevitably, however, such manipulations lead to false-positive findings.

A better approach, introduced recently, is to use meta-analysis. Methods have been developed to allow the results from multiple genome-wide scans of a given disorder to be meta-analysed, to identify loci which meet significance when data are pooled, even if they were not significant in individual studies (because of the lack of power and other reasons mentioned above). Meta-analyses have proved particularly useful in schizophrenia, showing beyond reasonable doubt the occurrence of several disease loci (p. 284). Ultimately, proof that a true disease locus has been found comes from identifying the gene, and then the polymorphism(s) or mutation(s) within it, which explains the linkage signal.

Genetic association studies

The existence of polymorphisms (Box 5.2) forms the basis for **association studies**. These are now the most commonly used method in psychiatric genetics. For review of their rationale and design, see Sullivan *et al.* (2001).

In its simplest form, an association study measures the frequency of a genetic polymorphism in a group of people who have the phenotype of interest and compares it with a group of healthy control subjects. The gene to be studied is usually chosen because the researchers consider it to be a **candidate gene** - a plausible gene to contribute to the phenotype under study, and the polymorphism is chosen either because it is common, easy to measure, or has been the subject of a previous positive report. If the frequency of the polymorphism is significantly different between the groups, usually determined with a chi-square test, then the polymorphism or allele is said to be associated with the disorder and, by implication, is a risk factor for it. Odds ratios and confidence intervals can be estimated in the usual fashion.

There have been a huge number of case control association studies in psychiatry, because they are relatively easy to do: groups of unrelated subjects are much easier to collect than the informative families needed for linkage genetics, and genotpying of a polymorphism from DNA extracted from blood or a cheek swab is rapid and straightforward, using techniques based on the **polymerase chain reaction** (PCR), which allows exponential amplification of the DNA. Some findings have proven robust, notably the apoE4 association with Alzheimer's disease (see Box 5.3). However, many others have not, reflecting major limitations to association studies of this kind:

- Sample sizes are often too small (e.g. 50 in each group), leading to many false-negative and false-positive findings - the latter is particularly a problem due to publication bias.
- The groups must have closely similar ethnic backgrounds, since the frequency of polymorphisms can vary markedly. For example, the COMT Met158 allele (see Box 5.3) varies from 1-60 per cent in populations across the world. This can lead to artefactual group differences due to **ethnic stratification**. This can be difficult to detect and avoid.
- There are about 30,000 genes in the genome, and hundreds of thousands of polymorphisms. The prior probability that any one gene, let alone any one polymorphism, is truly associated with the phenotype you are measuring is therefore very small, unless there is already compelling evidence implicating the gene (which is rarely the case in psychiatry).

Recent association studies have tried to overcome these difficulties in various ways (see Page *et al.*, 2003).

- Improving their robustness, by using larger samples, requiring greater statistical stringency, several independent replications, and evidence of biological plausibility (see below). Association studies are also amenable to meta-analysis.
- By using each subject's parents as controls, to see if the subject has inherited the polymorphism more often than expected by chance. The **transmission disequilibrirum test** is often used for this purpose. The family design overcomes the problem of ethnic stratification.
- By measuring several polymorphisms within the gene. A related development is the realisation that polymorphisms within a few thousand nucleotides of each other co-occur (because they will rarely be separated by recombination during meioisis). This is called **linkage disequilibrium**. Once a block of such linked polymorphisms (a **haplotype**) has been identified, it can be 'tagged' by measuring only one of its constituent polymorphisms.
- By coupling association studies to linkage studies. This combination of approaches was used, for example, to identify neuregulin-1 as a susceptibility gene for schizophrenia.
- By genome-wide analysis of polymorphisms. Technical developments are making it possible to simultaneously measure hundreds of thousands of polymorphisms at once (**SNP mapping** or **haplotype mapping**). This will overcome the problem of the paucity of convincing candidate genes on which to focus, and will allow an unbiased search for susceptibility genes.

How genes affect disease risk

A genetic variant can lead to disease for one of two main reasons. If the variant is coding (i.e. it changes the amino-acid sequence of the protein encoded by the gene), the protein may function differently as a direct consequence (as in the first two examples in Box 5.3, or the APP mutations in familial Alzheimer's disease). The effect may either be a failure to function normally (a **loss of function** mutation), or the protein may become toxic in some way (a **gain of function** mutation). However, most genetic variants currently associated with psychiatric disorders are non-coding. In these

BOX 5.3 EXAMPLES OF POLYMORPHISMS IN PSYCHIATRY

Apolipoprotein E4 in Alzheimer's disease The apoE gene on chromosome 19 exists in three common forms (alleles): apoE2, apoE3 and apoE4. Since 1993, dozens of studies in thousands of people have shown an association between apoE4 and Alzheimer's disease; that is, a higher proportion of patients have the apoE4 variant of the gene than do age-matched subjects without the disease. ApoE4 is thus said to be associated with Alzheimer's disease, and is a genetic risk factor for it. Individuals with one copy of apoE4 (heterozygotes) are about threefold more likely to get Alzheimer's disease; the risk is nearer tenfold in homozygotes (where both copies of the gene are apoE4). However, about half of all Alzheimer's disease occurs in people without an apoE4 allele, and apoE4 homozygotes may never develop it, emphasizing that apoE4, like most genes for psychiatric disorders, are polymorphisms which act as risk factors. See Chapter 14 for further discussion of apoE4 in Alzheimer's disease and how it is thought to increase disease risk.

COMT Val158Met, prefrontal performance, and schizophrenia The enzyme catechol-O-methyltransferase (COMT) metabolizes monoamines, especially dopamine. It occurs as a high-activity form and a low-activity form. The difference is due to a coding polymorphism within the gene, which changes a single amino acid: the high-activity allele encodes valine (Val-COMT) and the low-activity allele encodes methionine (Met-COMT). Egan and colleagues (2001) showed that subjects with Val-COMT had a less efficient prefrontal cortex (when doing working memory tasks) than people with Met-COMT; heterozygotes were intermediate. The assumption, supported by other findings, is that the Val form of COMT results in lower levels of dopamine activity than the Met form. The data suggested that this polymorphism explains 4 per cent of the individual variability in prefrontal cortex performance. Egan *et al.* (2001) and some other studies also found a higher frequency of the Val allele in patients with schizophrenia than in healthy subjects, consistent with the evidence linking the disease with dopamine and the prefrontal cortex. Other studies suggest the same polymorphism may predict response to antipsychotic drugs. COMT Val158Met thus illustrates that genetic polymorphisms may influence normal behavioural traits, disease vulnerability, and medication response (*pharmacogenetics*).

5-HT transporter (5-HTT) gene and anxiety The 5-HTT is the target of SSRIs and regulates synaptic 5-HT activity. Its gene contains a polymorphism in the promoter (control) region of the gene. The polymorphism is unlike the examples above, in two ways. First, it is non-coding (i.e. does not change the amino acid sequence of the protein). Second, it is not a SNP but a length polymorphism, the two alleles being called short (S) and long (L). In European populations, the frequency of the L allele is about 55 per cent. Lesch *et al.* (1996) showed that the S allele was associated with neuroticism (trait anxiety), and Caspi *et al.* (2004) found that it predisposes to depression following adverse early life events. The polymorphism may also contribute to individual differences in the therapeutic response to, and side-effects of, SSRIs.

instances, the mechanism most likely involves a change in the expression of the gene and thus the synthesis of the protein. The change may affect the quantity, timing, or specific features of the protein. For example, a polymorphism in a regulatory region may increase transcription of the gene, causing more mRNA and then more protein to be synthesized (as in the final example in Box 5.3, whereby the S allele of the 5-HTT is associated with reduced synthesis of the 5-HT transporter, and less 5-HT reuptake). Other non-coding polymorphisms affect the processing of the mRNA, called **alternative splicing**, by which a single gene can give rise to two or more protein variants (**isoforms**). The isoforms of a protein can have different properties, and a change in their proportion can have physiological and pathophysiological consequences. An increasing number of susceptibility genes are now suspected to exert their effects by modulating gene expression and alternative splicing; schizophrenia may be one of them (Harrison and Weinberger, 2005).

A final point to note is that the regulation of gene expression is itself partly inherited, separate from DNA sequence variation. This is called **epigenetics**. It is important both because it complicates the interpretation of genetic studies, and because it may be relevant for several psychiatric disorders (Petronis, 2004). An example is where only the copy of a gene that was inherited from the father (or mother) is expressed, with the copy on the other chromosome being inactivated. This is called **genomic imprinting**, and the syndromes of Prader–Willi and Angelman provide classic illustrations (Chapter 25).

Genes and gene expression

Molecular genetic techniques can be readily adapted to study gene expression. It is possible to detect and quantitate mRNAs in the brain, and compare cases and controls, using methods such as ***in situ* hybridization** and **reverse-transcriptase polymerase chain reaction** (RT-PCR). The encoded proteins can be studied similarly using specific antibodies for **immunocytochemistry** or **western blotting**. It is now also possible to study thousands of mRNAs simultaneously using **microarrays** (gene chips), a field called **transcriptomics**, and analogous approaches for proteins are also emerging (**proteomics**). All these techniques can also be used to study changes in gene expression caused by injury, drugs, hormones, etc, and can be applied to mRNA or protein extracted from peripheral blood, or in cell culture or other experimental paradigms (see Bunney *et al.*, 2003; Rohlff and Hollis, 2003).

Finally, **transgenic mice** provide a complementary way to investigate the roles of genes and gene expression in psychiatric disorders. It is now relatively easy to delete a gene ('a knock out'), introduce one ('knock-in'), or regulate its level of expression using **RNA interference**. Transgenic animals have been valuable in the study of diseases due to single gene mutations (e.g. mice containing a mutated form of the human APP gene develop Alzheimer's disease; Chapter 14). Genetic manipulations are now the main form of animal model used in psychiatry (Seong *et al.*, 2002).

Biochemical studies

Biochemical studies can be directed either to the causes of diseases or to the mechanisms by which disease produces its effects. The methods of biochemical investigation are too numerous to consider here, and it is assumed that the reader has some knowledge of them. The main aim here is to consider some of the problems of using biochemical methods to investigate psychiatric disorder.

It will be clear from the above account that the scope for molecular genetic studies is greatly enhanced by the presence of a **biochemical abnormality** that reliably distinguishes patients with a particular psychiatric disorder. The value of such an abnormality would be greater still if the biochemical abnormality concerned played a significant role in the cause of the illness or its pathophysiology. However, the nature of the biochemical changes associated with most psychiatric disorders remains unknown. This is due both to our lack of knowledge about the biochemical complexities of the normal brain and to the difficulty of investigating the biochemistry of the living human brain directly. Moreover, because most psychiatric disorders do not lead to death (other than by suicide), post-mortem material is not widely available except among the elderly.

Because of these problems, workers have adopted a variety of **indirect methods** involving sampling of peripheral tissues and fluids such as cerebrospinal fluid, blood cells, and urine. These studies, whilst more feasible to carry out, are not always easy to interpret. For example, concentrations of neurotransmitters and their metabolites in lumbar cerebrospinal fluid have an uncertain relationship to the corresponding functionally active neurotransmitter in the brain. Equally, neurotransmitter receptors and their second messengers in blood platelets and lymphocytes often appear to be regulated in a different way to their brain counterparts. Finally, measures in plasma and urine are very susceptible to confounding dietary and behavioural changes (see below).

The reader will find accounts of the results of biochemical research in subsequent chapters, especially those on mood disorders and schizophrenia. At this point a few examples will be given of the different kinds of investigation.

Post-mortem studies

Post-mortem studies of the brain can provide direct evidence of chemical changes within it. Unfortunately, interpretation of the findings is difficult because it must be established that any changes in the concentrations of neurotransmitters or enzymes did not occur after death. Moreover, because psychiatric disorders do not lead directly to death, the ultimate cause of death is another condition (often bronchopneumonia or the effects of a drug overdose) that could have caused the observed changes in the brain.

Even if this possibility can be ruled out, it is still possible that the chemical findings are the results of treatment rather than of disease. For example, the increases in density of dopamine receptors in the nucleus accumbens and caudate nucleus in patients with schizophrenia might be interpreted as supporting the hypothesis that schizophrenia is caused by changes in dopamine function in these areas of the brain. On the other hand, the finding could equally be the result of long-term treatment with antipsychotic drugs which block dopamine receptors and might lead to a compensatory increase of receptors.

As mentioned above, **molecular genetic techniques** can be used to complement biochemical investigations in post-mortem brain. For example, *in situ* hybridization provides information about the gene expression (mRNA production) of neurotransmitter receptors of interest. Using this technique it was shown that the mRNA for glutamate receptors is decreased in the hippocampus of patients with schizophrenia, a finding that complements ligand-binding studies of the glutamate receptors in this area of the brain (see Harrison, 2004). An important development in post-mortem studies is the combined use of gene expression, neurochemical and neuropathological techniques to investigate abnormalities in neural function in carefully defined brain regions.

Brain biochemistry and brain imaging

Over the last few years effective methods of studying biochemical events in the living brain have become available and have been used in some studies of psychiatric disorders. These methods include:

- magnetic resonance imaging (MRI)
- single-photon emission tomography (SPET)
- positron emission tomography (PET).

The use of these techniques to measure cerebral structure and blood flow is discussed below under the relevant headings. However, brain imaging can also be employed to measure aspects of brain biochemistry. For example, it is possible to carry out *in vivo* receptor binding in different groups of psychiatric patients using positron-labelled ligands and PET or SPET imaging (see Seibyl *et al.*, 2004).

Receptor binding with PET and SPET

The 5-HT_{1A} receptor plays an important role in the regulation of 5-HT neurotransmission and is an important target for antidepressant medications. Using PET imaging in conjunction with a positron-labelled 5-HT_{1A} receptor antagonist, a number of groups have found that the binding of 5-HT_{1A} receptors in the brain is decreased in patients with major depression. Moreover this abnormality appears to persist in patients who have recovered from depression and are no longer taking medication. This suggests that low 5-HT_{1A} receptor binding might represent a trait marker for vulnerability to depression. Alternatively the diminished receptor availability could be a consequence of having been depressed (see Bhagwagar *et al.*, 2004).

For reasons of cost, studies employing PET are likely to remain restricted to a small number of specialist research centres. However, SPET imaging is more widely available and increasing numbers of specific receptor ligands suitable for SPET studies are being developed. For example, there are already several studies using SPET in conjunction with specific dopamine receptor ligands examining dopamine receptor binding in mood disorders and schizophrenia.

Neurotransmitter release in vivo

Studies using PET and SPET in conjunction with specific dopamine receptor ligands have enabled estimation of **dopamine release** *in vivo*. The principle is to scan subjects on two occasions, one after administering a drug that modulates endogenous dopamine release, such as amphetamine, and once after placebo. Amphetamine increases dopamine release pre-synaptically and the increased levels of endogenous dopamine compete with the tracer ligand for access to post-synaptic receptors. Therefore, the specific binding of the tracer is reduced and the difference in tracer signal between the amphetamine and placebo scans provides a measure of how much dopamine was released by the amphetamine.

A similar approach can be taken with drugs that lower endogenous dopamine release, such as the tyrosine hydroxylase inhibitor, α-methyl-para-tyrosine (AMPT). Use of these models has led to the conclusion that dopamine release is increased in patients with acute schizophrenia (see p. 288). Current studies are investigating how these techniques can be applied to the release of other neurotransmitters.

Magnetic resonance imaging

MRI has the advantage over SPET and PET that subjects are not exposed to radiation. Whilst MRI has proved an excellent tool for structural brain imaging and more recently for the examination of cerebral blood flow, its application to the study of brain biochemistry (magnetic resonance spectroscopy, MRS) has been somewhat limited by lack of sensitivity. However, there are a growing number of applications of MRS to the study of psychiatric disorders and their treatment (Lyoo and Renshaw, 2002).

- Proton (^1H) MRS can be used to detect a number of compounds of neurobiological interest, including the important amino acid neurotransmitters, GABA and glutamate (Table 5.4).
- MRS can also be used to identify the spectrum of phosphorus-containing compounds and thereby can provide information about **energy metabolism and intracellular pH**.
- A number of psychotropic drugs, for example, fluoxetine, possess fluorine atoms, which can be imaged by MRS; this provides a means of imaging the distribution of such drugs at their specific receptor sites in the brain.
- MRS has also been used to image **lithium** in the human brain where it appears that brain levels of lithium are about half those seen in plasma.

TABLE 5.4 Neuronal metabolites and transmitters measured by MRS

^{1}H-NMR	^{31}P-NMR
N-Acetyl-aspartate (NAA)	ATP
Creatine	Phosphocreatine
Myoinositol	Inorganic phosphate
GABA	Phosphodiesters
Glutamate	Phosphomonoesters

One reasonably consistent finding from proton MRS is that the patients with depression have decreased levels of cortical GABA. This has shed some new light on a condition where aetiological hypotheses have been dominated for decades by the monoamine theory.

Peripheral measures

There have been long-standing doubts as to whether changes in the composition of neurotransmitters in the cerebrospinal fluid (CSF) reflect functionally significant changes in the brain. However, there are reasonably reproducible links between lowered CSF levels of 5-hydroxindoleacetic acid (5-HIAA) and impulsive aggressive behaviour in both human and non-human primates (Gerald *et al.*, 2002). This suggests that CSF 5-HIAA does correlate with certain defined aspects of behaviour. The major limitation of CSF studies is that it is often ethically and practically difficult to obtain CSF samples from psychiatric patients. In addition, it is not feasible to monitor time-dependent changes in neurotransmitter metabolism through repeated sampling.

Ingenious attempts have been made to infer biochemical changes in the brain from measurements of substances in the blood. For example, it is known that the rate of synthesis of 5-HT depends on the concentration of the 5-HT precursor tryptophan in the brain. Several studies have shown that **plasma tryptophan is decreased in patients with major depression**, a finding which supports the hypothesis that brain 5-HT function may be impaired in depressive disorders. However, it cannot be assumed that a modest reduction in concentrations of plasma tryptophan will necessarily be associated with impaired brain 5-HT neurotransmission. Furthermore, the same reduction in plasma tryptophan concentrations is found when healthy people lose weight through dieting. Therefore, it is quite possible that the decrease in plasma tryptophan found in depressed patients is a consequence of concomitant weight loss.

In general, investigations of biochemical abnormalities in blood and urine have not proved particularly fruitful in understanding the aetiology of psychiatric disorders. The real advances from such studies are in the field of learning disability, where measurement of metabolites in blood and urine have sometimes provided a useful picture of the abnormalities present in the brain as well as valuable diagnostic tests. A good example is phenylketonuria (see p. 715).

Peripheral blood cells such as platelets and lymphocytes possess receptors for neurotransmitters that often resemble the analogous receptor binding sites in the brain. There have been many studies of monoamine receptors in platelets of depressed patients, but the findings tend to be inconsistent and easily confounded by factors such as drug treatment. In addition, it is far from clear that abnormalities found in these peripheral binding sites will necessarily also be present in the brain. Indeed, those studies that have looked simultaneously at peripheral receptor binding and *in vivo* receptor imaging have not found correlations (see, for example, Yatham *et al.* 2000). Similar comments apply to the use of blood cells to investigate neurotransmitter-linked second messengers and ion flux processes such as calcium entry.

Pharmacology

The study of effective treatment of disease can often throw light on aetiology. In psychiatry, because of the great problems of studying the brain directly, research workers have examined the **actions of effective psychotropic drugs** in the hope that the latter might indicate the biochemical abnormalities in disease. Of course, such an approach must be used cautiously. If an effective drug blocks a particular transmitter system, it cannot be concluded that the disease is caused by an excess of that transmitter. The example of Parkinsonism makes this clear; anticholinergic drugs modify the symptoms, but the disease is due to a deficiency in dopaminergic transmission and not an excess of cholinergic transmission.

It is assumed here that the general methods of neuropharmacology are familiar to the reader, and attention is focused on the particular difficulties of using these methods in psychiatry. There are two main problems. First, most psychotropic drugs have more than one action and it is often difficult to decide which is relevant to the therapeutic effects. For example, although lithium carbonate has a large number of known pharmacological effects, it has so far been impossible to explain its remarkable effect of stabilizing the mood of patients with bipolar disorder.

The second difficulty arises because the therapeutic effects of many psychotropic drugs are slow to develop, whereas most pharmacological effects identified in the laboratory are quick to appear. For example, it has been suggested that the beneficial effect of antidepressant drugs depends on alterations in the re-uptake of transmitter at pre-synaptic neurons. However, changes in re-uptake occur quickly, whereas the therapeutic effects are usually delayed for about 2 weeks, suggesting that 'adaptive' responses of the brain to medication are important in clinical antidepressant action. Over the years several different adaptive responses to antidepressant drugs have been identified but none has yet led to new kinds of antidepressant medication. Current ideas in this area focus on the effects of antidepressants to modify synaptic growth and plasticity via actions on gene transcription factors and neurotropins such as brain-derived neurotropic factor (BDNF) (see Duman, 2004).

The introduction of new drugs with different pharmacological actions from conventional compounds can often be used to generate hypotheses about the mode of action of beneficial treatments and the pathophysiology of the disorder concerned. For example, with the introduction of **selective serotonin re-uptake inhibitors** (SSRIs), it became clear that only antidepressant drugs with potent 5-HT re-uptake inhibitor properties are effective in the pharmacological treatment of obsessive–compulsive disorder. Conventional tricyclic antidepressants (with the exception of clomipramine) are not useful. This suggests that the pathophysiology of obsessive–compulsive disorder is likely to differ from that of major depression, for which both classes of compounds are equally effective.

Another drug that has stimulated research in this way is **clozapine**, an antipsychotic drug which is effective in a significant proportion of patients who are unresponsive to traditional antipsychotic agents. Most antipsychotic drugs are believed to produce their therapeutic effects through blockade of dopamine D_2 receptors, but clozapine has a weak affinity for this binding site. In fact, clozapine binds potently to certain 5-HT receptor subtypes, particularly the 5-HT_{2A} receptor.

This has led to development of numerous 'atypical' antipsychotic agents that have combined 5-HT_2 and dopamine D_2 receptor antagonist properties. Whilst these agents have some advantages over conventional antipsychotic drugs, they do not seem to be as effective as clozapine in patients with treatment-resistance illness.

Endocrinology

Changes in circulating concentrations of hormones can have profound effects on mood and behaviour, whilst abnormalities in endocrine function are responsible for a number of well-defined clinical syndromes, some of which have characteristic neuropsychiatric presentations, for example, depression in **Cushing's disease**.

Despite these intriguing associations measurement of **basal plasma hormone levels** in psychiatric disorders has not, in general, shown consistent abnormalities in psychiatric patients or thrown much light on aetiology. The exception is major depression, in which a significant proportion of patients **hypersecrete cortisol**. There is increasing evidence that in some depressed patients elevated cortisol levels may play a role in the pathophysiology of depression (see p. 241).

Hormones and gene expression

Recently, knowledge of how hormones may alter brain function has increased, which makes it possible to see pathophysiological links between altered hormone secretion and changes in relevant brain mechanisms. Hormones can alter both intracellular and extracellular signalling, usually by altering **gene expression**.

For example, corticosteroids act on the cell nucleus to alter the expression of receptors for various neurotransmitters. In animal experimental studies, the density of 5-HT_{1A} receptors is modulated by circulating corticosterone levels, and it has been proposed that excessive cortisol secretion may predispose to a depressive disorder through an attenuation of 5-HT_{1A} receptor function in limbic brain regions. Animal studies have also indicated that corticosteroid administration can cause cell loss in the hippocampus. This finding has led to the hypothesis that the cognitive impairment seen in elderly depressed patients may be a consequence of neuronal damage produced by excessive cortisol secretion (see Holsboer and Kunzel, 2004, and p. 241).

Peptide-releasing factors

Hormones such as thyroid stimulating hormone (TSH) and adenocorticotropic hormone (ACTH) are regulated by peptide-releasing factors that have additional signalling roles in other brain regions, often those involved in the regulation of emotion. These peptides often coexist with classical neurotransmitters; for example, thyrotropin releasing hormone (TRH) is co-localized with 5-HT in 5-HT neurons. There is growing interest in the development of drugs that act on peptide receptors. An example is the possible use of corticotropic releasing hormone (CRH) antagonists in depression (see p. 241).

Neuroendocrine tests

Another use of plasma hormone measurement is to monitor the functional activity of brain neurotransmitters. The secretion of pituitary hormones is controlled by a variety of neurotransmitters. Under certain circumstances, changes in the concentration of a plasma hormone can be used to assess the function of the neurotransmitters involved in its release. For example, stimulating brain 5-HT function with a specific drug gives rise to an increase in plasma prolactin levels; accordingly, the rise in prolactin concentration that accompanies administration of a standard dose of the drug gives a measure of the functional state of brain 5-HT pathways.

These **neuroendocrine challenge tests** provide dynamic functional measures of brain neurotransmitter pathways, and in certain psychiatric disorders they have yielded consistent evidence of impairments in neurotransmitter function. For example, in depressed patients there is good evidence that the prolactin response to 5-HT stimulation is blunted and remains blunted on clinical recovery.

This suggests that depressive disorders are associated with a deficit in brain 5-HT neurotransmission. However, as with other biological measures, great care must be taken to control for possible confounding effects such as weight loss and impaired sleep (for a review of this field, see Cowen, 2005).

Neuroendocrine challenge tests can also be used to assess the effect of psychotropic drugs on brain neurotransmitter function. For example, the cortisol response to the 5-HT_{2c} receptor agonist, *m*-chlorophenylpiperazine, is blocked in patients receiving treatment with the atypical antipsychotic drug clozapine, but not in patients receiving a conventional antipsychotic agent such as fluphenazine. This suggests that clozapine treatment attenuates neurotransmission at a specific subpopulation of 5-HT receptors (in this case the 5-HT_{2c} receptor), and this action may relate to its unusual therapeutic efficacy or perhaps to aspects of its side-effect profile such as excessive weight gain.

Physiology

Physiological methods can be used to investigate the cerebral and peripheral disorders associated with disease states. Several methods have been used:

- psychophysiological methods including measurements of pulse rate, blood pressure, blood flow, skin conductance, and muscle activity;
- studies of cerebral blood flow;
- electroencephalographic (EEG studies).

Psychophysiological measures

Psychophysiological measures can be interpreted in at least two ways. The first interpretation is straightforward. The data are used as information about the activity of peripheral organs in disease, for example, to determine whether electromyographic (EMG) activity is increased in the scalp muscles of patients who complain of tension headaches. The second interpretation depends on the assumption that peripheral measurements can be used to infer changes in the state of **arousal of the central nervous system**. Thus increases in skin conductance, pulse rate, and blood pressure are taken to indicate greater arousal.

Measurement of cerebral blood flow and metabolism

Advances in brain imaging methods have led to increasing sophistication in the measurement of cerebral blood flow in psychiatric disorders. Studies using PET and SPET have replaced older techniques using xenon inhalation because the addition of tomographic techniques allows a three-dimensional measurement of regional cerebral blood flow to be achieved.

Functional MRI

Another important recent development is the demonstration that **MRI techniques using the water proton signal** are sufficiently sensitive to define regional increases in cerebral blood flow following neuronal activation. This technique is usually referred to as **functional MRI** (fMRI). The principal method of fMRI is **blood oxygenation-level-dependent (BOLD) imaging**. The use of BOLD depends on the fact that **deoxyhaemoglobin** is paramagnetic; it therefore aligns with an applied magnetic field, making the local magnetic field stronger. By contrast, oxygenated haemoglobin is only slightly diamagnetic and creates weak local field disturbances.

Increases in neuronal activity are associated with increases local cerebral blood flow, which causes **decreases in deoxyhaemoglobin**. This is because under normal conditions of activation there is a relatively greater increase in blood flow than neuronal oxygen consumption. The change in local deoxyhaemoglobin levels can be imaged and measured. It will be seen from this that fMRI can measure changes in activation but not baseline local cerebral blood flow. Accordingly, it has to be used with an 'activation' paradigm. Such paradigms are usually those that can be readily repeated in an 'off–on' manner over time, for example, a simple test of cognitive function. The advantages of fMRI is that it **has greater spatial and temporal resolution** than other imaging techniques and does not require the use of radioactivity.

fMRI has been used widely to map the neuronal representation of psychological functions in healthy subjects and many interesting findings have emerged. For example, Pantev *et al.* (1998) were able to show that in trained musicians, musical tones activated a greater area of sensory cortex than in non-musical subjects. This study is a good demonstration of how the cortex is able to reorganize itself during learning, presumably via alterations in gene expression. Conceivably, aberrant effects of this nature could be important in the development of certain psychiatric disorders. More recently, Anderson *et al.* (2004) used fMRI to demonstrate that the active forgetting of unwanted material was associated with increased activation of dorsolateral prefrontal cortex and decreased activation of hippocampus. These finding indicate a possible biological substrate for repression, one of the key defence mechanisms described by Freud (p. 153). For a discussion of the use of fMRI in psychiatric disorders see Seibyl *et al.* (2004).

PET

PET imaging can be used to measure either **cerebral metabolism or cerebral blood flow**. Usually the two measures are closely correlated. In the adult brain, functional activity is almost entirely dependent on oxidative metabolism, which requires glucose and oxygen as substrates. Hence rates of metabolism can be determined by measuring the utilization of oxygen or accumulation of **deoxyglucose**. Measurement of regional cerebral blood flow can be made by assessing the accumulation of radioactivity in the brain during inhalation of suitably labelled CO_2 (Seibyl *et al.* 2004).

SPET

Measurement of blood flow with SPET employs lipophilic radiotracers such as technetium-labelled hexamethyl propyleneamine oxime (^{99m}Tc-HMPAO). Following intravenous administration, these compounds are retained in the brain in a stable form for several hours. This enables high resolution images to be obtained with the use of a conventional detector such as a rotating gamma camera. The uptake of ^{99m}Tc-HMPAO is linearly related to cerebral blood flow. However, unlike PET, SPET cannot provide an absolute measure of regional cerebral blood flow; therefore, the results of SPET studies are often expressed by comparing the radioactive counts in each brain region of interest with a reference area, usually either whole brain or cerebellum.

Baseline blood flow in psychiatric disorders

There have been many studies of **basal blood flow** in various psychiatric disorders, but the results of different investigations have often been contradictory. To a large extent the conflicting data may result from the considerable methodological difficulties in standardizing the imaging conditions and the patient population. It is possible that resting conditions are not ideal for the detection of differences between patients and controls because the resting state is inherently physiologically and psychologically variable.

Despite these difficulties, more recent, carefully controlled investigations in rigorously assessed drug-free patients are reaching a greater level of consensus. For example, both PET and SPET studies of patients with obsessive–compulsive disorder have revealed increased metabolic activity and blood flow in the frontal cortex, notably in orbitofrontal regions (Saxena and Rausch, 2000). In addition, further information can be gained by correlating basal regional cerebral blood flow with the psychopathology of the patients at the time of scanning. This approach has been successful in mapping symptom clusters in patients with schizophrenia to specific brain regions (see p. 271).

Activation paradigms

As with fMRI, **psychological activation paradigms** have been widely used in PET studies of healthy volunteers to map the brain regions and distributed neuronal circuits involved in fundamental processes such as memory and language. Activation paradigms can also be applied to patients with psychiatric disorders with perhaps more consistent results emerging than with baseline blood flow studies.

For example, when normal control subjects undertake the Wisconsin Card Sort Test, there is an increase in blood flow in the prefrontal cortex. On this test, patients with schizophrenia perform less well than controls, and produce a different pattern of blood flow in the corresponding cortical area. This suggests that some patients with schizophrenia may have a dysfunction of the **prefrontal cortex**, which is associated with poor performance on tasks that depend on increased neuronal activity in this brain region. More recent studies have linked this altered performance and blood flow change with polymorphisms of the gene for catechol-*O*-methyltransferase (COMT) an enzyme involved in the metabolism of dopamine and a candidate gene for schizophrenia (see Box 5.3). Investigations, which integrate genetic polymorphisms with variance in cognitive performance and changes in cerebral perfusion, hold great promise for improving the understanding of schizophrenia (see Berman and Myer-Lindenberg, 2004).

Electroencephalography

Methods

The electroencephalograph (EEG) provides a measure of **cortical neuronal activity** through detection of potential differences across the scalp. A number of different techniques are relevant to studies of aetiology in psychiatry:

- standard (analogue) EEG
- quantified (digital) EEG
- sleep EEG (polysomnogram)
- magnetoencephalography (MEG)
- evoked potentials.

Standard EEG

The standard clinical EEG is a qualitative assessment of a paper trace by a trained observer using visual inspection. These kind of recordings have been most helpful in studying the relationships between **epilepsy** and psychiatric disorders but otherwise have not been particularly informative about aetiology. About 30 per cent of psychiatric patients referred for an EEG are reported as having an abnormal recording but the relevance of this has proved elusive. Artefacts from drug treatment are probably common. The standard EEG has good temporal but relatively poor spatial resolution.

Quantified EEG

The EEG signal can also be examined **quantitatively** using a number of different mathematical approaches. The most commonly used method employs power spectral analysis with Fourier transformation. Characteristic spectral patterns have been reported for certain disorders, although relating these to underlying brain mechanisms is not straightforward. Statistical removal of EEG artefact is also problematic. Thus far the main clinical research application has been in the analysis and detection of the effects of different drugs with the hope of developing an objective method of screening for novel psychotropic compounds (see Saletu *et al.*, 2002).

Sleep EEG (polysomnogram)

During sleep the EEG shows a characteristic recurrent pattern of waves which can be divided into stages. The fundamental distinction is between **rapid eye movement** (REM or dream sleep) and **non-REM** (or quiet) sleep. The sleep EEG or polysomnogram shows fairly consistent abnormalities in depressed patients, notably a decrease in the **latency to the onset of REM sleep**. Some of these abnormalities may persist into clinical remission and may indicate vulnerability to mood disorder.

The main disadvantage of polysomnography has been the need for a specialized facility (a 'sleep laboratory'). However, the development of home-based monitoring with ambulatory equipment has been helpful in this respect (Sharpley *et al.*, 2000). The polysomnogram has also been useful in measuring the effects of drugs on sleep quality and architecture (for a review of the use of the polysomnogram in psychiatric research see Nishino *et al.*, 2004).

Magnetoencephalography

Magnetoencephalography (MEG) is able to measure changes in extracranial magnetic fields to detect ion fluxes in cortical neurons. Like EEG, MEG has the ability to detect changes in physiological signals over millisecond time intervals. MEG can provide better localization of signals than EEG, but the most useful information may come from using the techniques in combination or by combining MEG with functional imaging. In this way superior temporal and spatial resolution of cortical processing can be obtained. Neither MEG nor EEG is generally helpful in identifying changes in subcortical neuronal activity. In some studies of psychiatric patients, MEG has been used to measure evoked potentials (for a review of the use of the MEG in psychiatry see Stern and Silbersweig, 2001).

Evoked potentials

EEG techniques can also be used to detect changes in brain electrical activity in response to environmental stimuli. These evoked (or event-related) potentials can be detected by computerized averaging methods, and can be identified as waveforms occurring at particular times after the stimulus. For example, the P300 response is a positive deflection that occurs 300 ms after a subject identifies a target stimulus embedded in a series of irrelevant stimuli.

The P300 wave probably corresponds to the cognitive processes required for the recognition, retrieval from memory, and evaluation of a specific stimulus. In patients with schizophrenia, the amplitude of the P300 wave is reduced. It is notable that the same abnormality can be found in first-degree relatives of schizophrenic patients and those with schizotypal personalities.

In these subjects, the change in the P300 response is likely to stem from an abnormality in information processing, and may represent a vulnerability trait marker factor for the development of schizophrenia. However, these changes are not specific in that they can also be found in patients with other disorders such as alcohol misuse (see Blackwood, 2000). In addition, interpretation of evoked potentials in terms of brain mechanism is not easy because the potential recorded from the scalp is far from its generational source and reflects the activity of many different neural systems operating in parallel (Grillon and Ameli, 2004).

Neuropathology

Neuropathological studies attempt to answer the question as to whether a **structural change** in the brain accompanies a particular kind of mental disorder. Brain structure can now be studied in life, usually with MRI scans, as well as by the traditional direct examination of the brain post-mortem.

Neuropathology has been central to the understanding of dementia and a few other psychiatric disorders in which lesions can readily and reliably be found, and if necessary quantified. It has not shown equivalent diagnostic kinds of lesion in other psychiatric disorders, a factor which contributed to the conventional view that most psychiatric conditions were functional as opposed to organic disorders. However, the advent of MRI and improved neuropathological methods has shown that there are structural correlates of many psychiatric disorders. For example, the brain is smaller and lighter in schizophrenia, associated with changes in its cellular and synaptic composition (Chapter 12). Similarly, alterations in volumes of parts of the limbic system and its cytoarchitecture have also been reported in depression (Chapter 12). Whilst none of these changes can yet be used for diagnostic purposes (because of overlap in each parameter with comparison subjects, and across diagnostic boundaries), they do argue strongly against the functional versus organic dichotomy.

These research advances are also a useful reminder that methods of investigation available at a particular time may fail to detect relevant biological abnormalities even when the latter are present. (For example, Alois Alzheimer spent a decade searching for the neuropathology of schizophrenia before he came across the case of presenile dementia and identified the lesions which now define the disease named after him.) In addition, as neuropathological investigations embrace the molecular level, drawing distinctions between 'functional' and 'structural' disorders becomes somewhat arbitrary anyway. Finally, it is worth noting that progress in determining aetiology is most likely to be made through the combination of genetic, pathological and biochemical investigations, and combining these with epidemiological ascertainment and careful clinical, psychological and social characterization of subjects. In this way, the various approaches can be used to inform and guide each other, and a more integrated view of psychiatric aetiology can ultimately emerge.

Relationship of this chapter to those on psychiatric syndromes

This chapter has reviewed several diverse approaches to aetiology. It may be easier for the reader to put these approaches into perspective when reading the sections on aetiology in the chapters on the different psychiatric syndromes, especially those on mood disorders (p. 231) and schizophrenia (p. 280).

Further reading

Charney, DS, Nestler, EJ (2004) *Neurobiology of mental illness,* 2nd edn. Oxford University Press, Oxford. (Comprehensive overview of the developing methods and concepts in biological psychiatry.)

Freud, S (1916–17) *Introductory lectures on psychoanalysis.* Reprinted in Penguin Freud Library, Vol. 1. Penguin, Harmondsworth. (A lucid account of psychoanalytic theory by its original proponent.)

Jaspers, K (1963) *General psychopathology* (trans. J Hoenig and MW Hamilton), pp. 301–11, 355–64, 383–99. Manchester University Press, Manchester. (The classical text: these pages explain the concepts of meaningful connections and psychological reactions.)

Owen MJ, O'Donovan M, Gottesman II. (2003) *Psychiatric genetics and genomics.* Oxford, Oxford University Press. (a clear exposition of the principles of psychiatric genetics and their application.)

CHAPTER 6

Evidence-based approaches to psychiatry

Chapter contents

What is evidence-based medicine?

Evidence-based medicine (EBM) is a systematic way of obtaining clinically important information about aetiology, diagnosis, prognosis, and treatment. The evidence-based approach is a *process* in which the following steps are applied:

- formulation of an answerable clinical question;
- identification of the best evidence;
- critical appraisal of the evidence for validity and utility;
- implementation of the findings;
- evaluation of performance.

The principles of EBM can be applied to a variety of medical procedures. For psychiatry, the main use of EBM at present is assessing the value of **therapeutic interventions**. For this reason, in the following sections the application of EBM will be linked to studies of treatment. Applications to other areas such as diagnosis and prognosis are discussed later.

History of evidence-based approaches

Examples of what we now might call 'evidence-based approaches' to the investigation of treatments have a long if sporadic history in medicine. For example, in 1747 James Lind, a naval surgeon, studied six pairs of sailors 'as similar as I could have them' who were suffering from scurvy. The sailors who received oranges and lemons recovered within a few weeks in contrast to those who simply received the same housing and general diet. Lind's study was not carried out 'blind' but in 1784 Benjamin Franklin applied blindfolds to the participants of a mesmerism study who were therefore unaware whether or not the treatment was being applied. The 'blinding' abolished the treatment effect of mesmerism, strong evidence that its effects were mediated by suggestion (Devereaux *et al.*, 2002).

The application of modern randomized trial methodology to medicine is attributed to Sir Austin Bradford Hill (1897–1991) who designed the MRC trial of streptomycin treatment of tuberculosis in 1948. Subsequently, Bradford-Hill lent his influence to the application of randomized trials in the evaluation of psychiatric treatments, often in the face of vociferous opposition from the profession. The first psychiatric trial to use this methodology was carried out at the Maudsley Hospital in 1955 by David Davies and Michael Shepherd, who demonstrated that, relative to placebo, reserpine had beneficial effects in anxiety and depression. A few years later Ackner and Oldham (1962) used double-blind randomized methods to debunk insulin coma therapy. Subsequently, in 1965, an MRC group reported the first large scale, multicentre, randomized controlled trial in psychiatry, in which imipramine and ECT were shown to be therapeutically superior to placebo in the treatment of hospitalized depressed patients (see Tansella, 2002).

More recent developments in evidence-based approaches owe much to Archibald Cochrane (1909–1988) an epidemiologist and author of an influential book, *Effectiveness and efficiency: random reflections on health services*, published in 1972. Cochrane emphasized the need, when planning treatment provision, to use evidence from randomized controlled trials because it is more reliable than any other kind. In a frequently cited quotation (1979), he wrote, 'It is surely a great criticism of our profession that we have not organized a critical summary, by specialty or subspecialty, adapted periodically, of all relevant randomized controlled trials.'

Cochrane's views were widely accepted and two further developments enabled his vision to be realized. First, the availability of electronic databases and computerized searching made it feasible to find all (or nearly all) of the relevant randomized trials when gathering evidence on particular therapeutic questions. Second, the statistical techniques of meta-analysis enabled randomized trials to be combined providing greater power and allowing a reliable quantification of treatment effects. Results from studies using these methodologies are called 'systematic reviews' to distinguish them from the more traditional, less reliable, 'narrative reviews' where the judgement of the authors plays a major role in deciding what evidence to include and what weight to give it. The Cochrane Collaboration, which was formed in 1993, is now the largest organisation in the world engaged in the production and maintenance of systematic reviews (http://www.cochrane.org). In the UK, the Centre For Reviews and Dissemination, based at the University of York, maintain an up-to-date database of systematic reviews of health care interventions (http://www.york.ac.uk/inst/crd/index.htm).

Why do we need evidence-based medicine?

There are two main related problems in clinical practice which can be helped by the application of EBM:

- the difficulty in keeping up to date with clinical and scientific advances;
- the tendency of practitioners to work in idiosyncratic ways that are not justified by available evidence.

With the burgeoning number of clinical and scientific journals, the most assiduous clinician is unable to keep up to date with all relevant articles, even in their own field. In fact, it has been estimated that to accomplish this task would require scrutiny of 20 publications a day! Clinicians therefore have to rely on information gathered from other sources which might include, for example, unsystematic expert reviews, opinions of colleagues, information from pharmaceutical representatives, and their own clinical experiences and beliefs. This can lead to wide variations in practice, for example, those described for the use of electroconvulsive therapy (see UK ECT Review Group, 2003).

Kinds of evidence

The fundamental assumption of EBM is that some kinds of evidence are *better* (that is, more valid and of greater clinical applicability) than others. This view is most easily elaborated for questions about therapy. A commonly used 'hierarchy' is shown in Table 6.1.

TABLE 6.1 Hierarchy of research for treatment studies

Ia	Evidence from a systematic review of randomized controlled trials
Ib	Evidence from at least one randomized controlled trial
IIa	Evidence from at least one controlled study without randomization
IIb	Evidence from at least one other type of quasi-experimental study
III	Evidence from non-experimental descriptive studies, such as comparative studies, correlation studies, and case control studies
IV	Evidence from expert committee reports or opinions and/or clinical experience of respected authorities

In this hierarchy, evidence from **randomized trials** is regarded as more **valid** than evidence from non-randomized trials, while **systematic reviews of randomized trials** are seen as the gold standard for answering clinical questions (see Geddes and Harrison, 1997). This assumption has itself yet to be tested systematically and some argue that large trials with simple clinically relevant endpoints may be more valid than meta-analyses (see Furukawa, 2004). It is certainly important that clinicians are trained in critical evaluation of systematic reviews before applying their results to clinical practice (see below and Collins *et al.*, 2003).

Individual treatment studies

Validity

The key criterion for validity in treatment studies is **randomization**. In addition, clinicians entering patients into a therapeutic trial should be unaware of the treatment group to which their patients are being allocated. This is usually referred to as **concealment of the randomization list**. Without concealed randomization, the validity of a study is questionable and its results may be misleading.

Other important points when assessing the validity of a study are:

- Were all the patients who entered the trial accounted for at its conclusion?
- Were patients analysed in the groups to which they were allocated (so-called 'intention to treat' analysis)?
- Were patients and clinicians blind to the treatment received (a different question to that of blind **allocation**)?
- Apart from the experimental treatment, were the groups treated equally?
- Did the randomization process result in the groups being similar at baseline?

Presentation of results

Odds ratios

When the outcome of a clinical trial is an event (for example, admission to hospital), a commonly used measure of effectiveness is the **odds ratio**. The odds ratio is the odds of an event occurring in the experimental group divided by the odds of it occurring in the control group. The odds ratio is given with 95 per cent confidence intervals (which indicate the range of values within which we have a 95 per cent certainty that the **true** value falls). The narrower the confidence intervals the greater the precision of the study.

If the odds ratio of an event such as admission to hospital is 1.0, this means the rates of readmission do not differ between control and experimental groups. Therefore if the confidence interval of the odds ratio of an individual study includes the value of 1.0, the study has failed to show that the experimental and control treatments differ from each other.

Effect sizes

In many studies the outcome measure of interest is a continuous variable, such as a mean score on the Hamilton Rating Scale for Depression. It is possible to use the original measure in the meta-analysis although more often an estimate of **effect size** is made because it is more statistically robust.

Effect sizes are obtained by dividing the difference in effect between the experimental group and the control group by the standard deviation of their difference. The clinical interpretation of the effect size is discussed below.

Clinical utility of interventions

Risk reduction and number needed to treat

An important part of EBM is using the results of randomized trials of groups of patients to derive the impact of an intervention at the level of the individual patient. A useful concept when assessing the value of a treatment is that of **absolute risk reduction**. This compares the proportion of patients receiving the experimental treatment who experienced a clinically significant adverse outcome (for example, clinical relapse) compared to the rate in patients receiving the comparison treatment. These are known as the **experimental event rate (EER)** and **control event rate (CER)**, respectively, and are calculated as percentages. The difference between these two outcome rates is **the absolute risk reduction (ARR)**.

The ARR can be converted into a more clinically useful number, the **number needed to treat (NNT)**. The NNT is the reciprocal of the ARR and tells us how many patients would need to be treated to experience one more positive outcome event compared to a comparator treatment (or no treatment) (Box 6.1). Like odds ratios, NNTs are usually given with 95 per cent confidence intervals (see Geddes and Harrison, 1997).

Example

Paykel *et al.* (1999) randomized 158 patients with residual depressive symptoms following an episode of major depression to either clinical management or clinical

BOX 6.1 INDICES FOR TRANSLATING RESEARCH RESULTS INTO CLINICAL PRACTICE

Experimental control

	Treatment X	Treatment Y
Positive outcome	a	b
Negative outcome	c	d

Control Event Rate (CER) = b/(b + d)
Experimental Event Rate (EER) = a/(a + c)
Absolute Risk Reduction (ARR)
The difference in the proportions with a positive outcome on treatments X and Y = (CER - EER)

Odds ratio (OR)

The ratio of the odds of a positive outcome on treatments X and Y = (a/c)/(b/d) = ad/bc
Number Needed to Treat (NNT) - how many patients need to be treated with treatment X to get one more positive outcome than would be expected on treatment Y (= 1/AAR)

From Geddes and Harrison (1997)

management with 18 sessions of cognitive behaviour therapy (CBT). Over the following 68 weeks the relapse rate in CBT-treated group (29 per cent) was significantly less than that of the clinical management group (47 per cent; $P = 0.02$).

The absolute risk reduction (ARR) in relapse with CBT is 47 - 29 = 18%. The number needed to treat (NNT) is the reciprocal of this number, which is approximately 6 (usually the NNT is rounded up to the next highest integer). This means that six patients with residual depressive symptoms have to be treated with CBT to avoid one relapse. In general, an NNT of less than 10 denotes a useful treatment effect. However, interpretation of the NNT will also depend on the nature of the treatment together with the extent of its therapeutic and adverse effects. The NNT for some common psychiatric treatments are shown in Table 6.2.

If the outcome measure of an intervention is a beneficial event (such as recovery) rather than avoidance of an adverse one, the effect of the intervention is calculated as the **absolute benefit increase (ABI)** in the same way as the ARR (see above) with the NNT being similarly computed. A related concept to NNT is the **number needed to harm (NNH)** which describes the adverse risks of particular therapies, for example, extrapyramidal symptoms with antipsychotic drugs.

TABLE 6.2 Examples of number needed to treat (NNT) for interventions in psychiatry

Intervention	Outcome	NNT
Cognitive therapy in bulimia nervosa	Remission	2
Light treatment in winter depression	Clinical response (50% decrease in symptom score)	2
Lithium augmentation in resistant depression	Clinical response (50% decrease in symptom score)	4
Chlorpromazine in schizophrenia	Relapse prevention	4
Family therapy in schizophrenia	Relapse at 1 year	7
SSRIs compared with TCAs in acute depression	Remain in treatment at 6 weeks	33

SSRIs, selective serotonin re-uptake inhibitors; TCAs, tricyclic antidepressants.

Computing the NNT from odds ratios

If a study or meta-analysis provides an odds ratio it is possible to compute an NNT that may be more relevant to the clinical circumstances of the practitioner and their patient. For example, in the example given above (Paykel *et al.*, 1999), relapses occurred in 35 of 78 subjects in the clinical management group compared with 23 of 80 in the CBT group. This gives an odds ratio in the risk of relapse between the two treatments of 0.49. To obtain an NNT from the odds ratio it is necessary to know, or estimate, the expected relapse rate in the control group. This is known as the **patient expected event rate (PEER)**. The PEER is combined with the odds ratio (OR) in the following formula:

$$\text{NNT} = \frac{1 - \text{PEER}(1 - \text{OR})}{(1 - \text{PEER})\,\text{PEER}(1 - \text{OR})}$$

If we take the relapse rate in the patients given clinical management in the above study (45%) we have:

$$\text{NNT} = \frac{1 - [0.45 \times (1 - 0.49)]}{(1 - 0.45) \times 0.45 \times (1 - 0.49)}$$

This gives an NNT of about 6, which we also derived from the other method of calculation involving the ARR. If however, from a local audit, we know that the relapse rate in our own service of patients with residual depressive symptoms is about 20 per cent (rather than the 45 per cent of Paykel *et al.*), using the formula above, the NNT becomes about 11. This means in our own service we would need to treat 11 patients with CBT to obtain one less relapse. In this way odds ratios can be used to adjust NNTs to local clinical conditions, thereby helping decisions over the applicability of interventions.

Clinical relevance of effect size

Like the odds ratio, the **effect size** is not easy to interpret clinically. A useful approach is to use the effect size to estimate the degree of overlap between the control and experimental populations. In this way we obtain the proportion of control group scores that are lower than those in the experimental group. (A negative effect size simply means that scores in the control group are **higher** than those in the experimental group.)

For example, in a review of the effects of benzodiazepines and zolpidem on total sleep time relative to placebo, Nowell *et al.* (1997) found an overall effect size of 0.71. From normal distribution tables this means that 76 per cent of controls had less total sleep time than the average sleep time in the hypnotic-treated patients. Effect sizes have been classified in the following way:

- 0.2 = small
- 0.5 = moderate
- 0.8 or more = large.

The effect size of antidepressant medication relative to placebo is about 0.4–0.5. Furukawa (1999) has devised a tabular method of converting effect sizes to NNT values. At the sort of response levels seen in antidepressant-treated patients (about 30 per cent response rate in the placebo group and 60 per cent in the experimental group) an effect size of 0.2 is equivalent to an NNT of about 10. With an effect size of 0.5, the NNT falls to 5.

Ethical aspects of therapeutic trials

Randomization

As we have seen, randomization is a key process in the conduct of an evidence-based clinical trial because it is best way of avoiding bias due to chance and random error. However, a clinician may feel uncomfortable about randomization when, for example, he has a strong belief in the efficacy of one of the treatments being assessed. Randomization is ethical where there is genuine **uncertainty** about the best treatment for the individual concerned. In fact, EBM suggests that this situation is more common than clinicians may realize, in that many strongly held beliefs about efficacy of therapeutic interventions are based on anecdotal experience rather than systematic evidence.

Use of placebo

The use of drug placebo in trials of psychotropic agents is controversial. However, such studies are required by many drug-licensing authorities before, for example, a new antidepressant drug is licensed. The arguments for the use of placebo in antidepressant drug trials have been summarized (see Miller, 2000):

- The placebo response in major depression is variable and unpredictable, and is not infrequently equivalent in therapeutic effect to active treatment.
- Placebo is required to establish efficacy of new antidepressants. Comparison against an active treatment is not methodologically sufficient because while a finding of 'no difference' in antidepressant activity might mean that the new and established treatments have equivalent efficacy, it might also mean that neither treatment was actually effective under the particular trial conditions employed.
- The lack of placebo-controlled design in antidepressant drug development might lead to the marketing of a drug that is ineffective, thereby harming public health.

These arguments have to be weighed against the knowledge that antidepressants are generally somewhat more effective than placebo in the treatment of depression. Therefore, a patient treated with placebo in a randomized trial is not receiving the best available therapy. One way of trying to deal with this is to ensure that patients in such trials receive particularly close clinical monitoring which will result in their being withdrawn from the study if they are not doing well.

Informed consent

The role of informed consent is crucial to the ethical conduct of randomized and placebo controlled trials. This raises difficulties with some psychiatric disorders where the judgement and decision-making abilities of patients may be impaired. Miller (2000) has outlined a number of important factors:

- Patients must be made specifically aware that the trial is not being conducted for their individual benefit.
- With placebo treatment there must be clear specification of the probability of receiving placebo, the lack of improvement that might result, and the possibility of symptomatic worsening.
- Patients must be free from any coercion or inducement.

- Patients have right to withdraw from the study at any time without any kind of penalty.
- In addition to the investigator, a family member or other suitable person should be encouraged to monitor the patient's condition and report to the investigator if there are concerns.

The key issues therefore are **open and explicit** information sharing with patient and family, and all necessary measures to avoid placebo treatment leading to **harm to the subject**. The issue, however, remains controversial.

Systematic reviews

Validity

The aim of a systematic review is to obtain all available *valid* evidence about a specific procedure or intervention and from this to provide a more precise quantitative assessment of its efficacy. Two advances have greatly increased the feasibility of systematic reviews: first, the availability of electronic databases such as Medline and Embase, and second, new statistical techniques through which results from different studies can be combined in a quantitative manner. Because a meta-analysis uses all available valid data, its **statistical power** is greater than that of an individual study; it may therefore demonstrate moderate but clinically important effects of treatment that were not apparent in individual randomized studies.

Systematic reviews of treatment, like single therapeutic studies, have to be tested for **validity** and **quality**. The following questions should be posed.

- **Is it a systematic review of relevant and randomized studies?** We have already seen that the first task in the EBM process is to ask a clearly formulated question. It is therefore necessary to determine whether the subject of the systematic review is truly relevant to the therapeutic question that needs to be answered. The next step is to make sure that only randomized studies have been included. Systematic reviews that contain a mixture of randomized and non-randomized studies may give misleading results.
- **Do the authors describe the methods by which relevant trials were located?** Whilst electronic searching greatly facilitates identification of clinical trials, up to half the relevant studies may be missed because of miscoding. It is therefore important for authors to make clear whether they supplemented electronic searching with hand-searching of appropriate journals. They may also, for example, have contacted authors of trials, as well as relevant groups in the pharmaceutical industry. In general, negative studies are less likely to be published than positive ones, which can lead to falsely optimistic conclusions about the efficacy and tolerability of particular treatments. For example, analysis of all completed studies of new antidepressants in adolescents indicated that some SSRIs and venlafaxine might increase the risk of suicidal behaviour. This potentially important finding was not apparent from analyses of the published data alone (Whittington *et al.*, 2004).
- **How did the authors decide which studies should be included in the systematic review?** In a systematic review, authors have to decide which of the various studies they identify should be included in the overall analysis. This means defining **explicit measures of quality**, which will be based on the factors outlined above. Because these judgements are in part subjective, it is desirable for them to be made independently by at least two of the investigators.
- **Were the results of the therapeutic intervention consistent from study to study?** It is common to see differences in the size of the effect of a therapeutic intervention from study to study. However, if the effects are mixed, with some studies showing a large clinical effect while others find none at all, the trials are said to show **heterogeneity**. Sometimes heterogeneity can be accounted for by factors such as lower doses of a drug treatment or differences in patient characteristics. If there is no likely explanation for it, the results of the review must be considered tentative.

Presentation of results

Combining odds ratios

Results of meta-analyses are often presented as a 'forest plot' in which the findings of the various studies are shown in diagrammatic form (Figure 6.1). As noted above, studies in which the outcome is an event are presented as odds ratios with 95 per cent confidence intervals.

The aim of meta-analysis is to obtain a **pooled estimate** of the treatment effect by combining the odds ratios or effect sizes of all the studies. This is not simply an average of all the odds ratios but is **weighted** so that studies with more statistical information and greater precision (with narrower confidence intervals) contribute relatively more to the final result. The pooled odds ratio also has a 95 per cent confidence interval. Once again, if this interval overlaps with value of 1.0, the experimental intervention does not differ from the control.

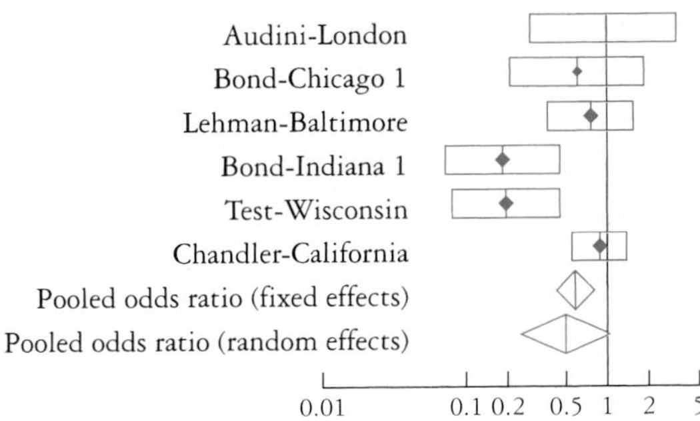

Fig. 6.1 Effect of active community treatment on the odds of admission to hospital. From Freemantle and Geddes (1998).

In Figure 6.1 some of the studies show a significant effect of assertive community treatment (ACT) to decrease readmission, whilst others do not. The two pooled analyses are difficult to interpret because the confidence intervals of one of them (**the fixed effects model**) do not overlap with 1.0, making ACT significantly different from control, whereas the other (**the random effects model**) just overlaps with 1.0 and is therefore of marginal statistical significance.

We have already seen that the studies in a meta-analysis may indicate **heterogeneity**. This can be tested statistically with a modification of the chi-squared test. If significant heterogeneity is present the most appropriate meta-analytic technique is a **pooled random effects model**. This model assumes that different treatment effects will occur in different studies and takes this into account in the pooled estimate. This usually results in wider confidence intervals as in the pooled random effect odds ratio in the ACT studies. If the studies suggest a single underlying population treatment effect (that is, lack of heterogeneity) then the pooled treatment analysis should use a **fixed effects model**. This estimate has narrower confidence intervals that may, however, be misleading in the presence of significant heterogeneity.

In Figure 6.1 there is statistically significant heterogeneity between the studies, and inspection of the data shows that the majority of the benefit is contributed by two of the studies, which are not the largest. The random and fixed effects models find a similar mean benefit of ACT in preventing readmission but the random effects model has a wider confidence interval and, as noted above, just overlaps with 1.0. Because of the heterogeneity of the studies, the random effects model is the more appropriate way of analysing the data. Overall therefore we would be cautious about accepting the efficacy of ACT in lowering readmission rates, unless we were able to find a convincing reason for the variation in study results (see Freemantle and Geddes, 1998).

Effect sizes

As noted above, where the outcome measure is a continuous variable, the usual method of calculating results is to use effect sizes. As with odds ratios, the effect sizes can be combined to give a pooled estimate of greater precision.

Clinical utility

The clinical utility of meta-analyses is assessed as described for individual studies above. Meta-analyses will often provide figures for the NNT. As shown above, however, it is also possible to calculate NNT values from meta-analysis data using ARR or odds ratios.

Problems with meta-analysis

Biased conclusions

Apart from a systematic location of evidence, the aim of meta-analysis is to combine data from multiple studies into a single estimate of treatment effect. There are a number of ways in which results of such an exercise can be misleading:

- **Publication bias** Evidence indicates that studies showing positive treatment effects are more likely to be published than negative studies. If negative studies are not included in the meta-analysis the effect of treatment will be inflated.
- **Duplication of publication** Just as negative treatment studies may go unpublished, positive studies may be published several times in different forms, sometimes with different authors! This, again, will falsely elevate treatment effects if the same study is included more than once.
- **Heterogeneity of studies** As noted above, individual studies may vary widely in the results obtained because of quite subtle differences in study design, quality, and patient population. If such heterogeneity is not recognized and accounted for in the meta-analysis, misleading conclusions will be drawn.

How accurate is meta-analysis?

There are some well-known examples where results of meta-analyses have been contradicted subsequently by single, large randomized trials. For example, a meta-analysis which showed that intravenous magnesium improved outcome in patients with myocardial infarction was later decisively refuted by a single, large randomized trial of 58,000 patients. The misleading result of the meta-analysis was later explained on the basis of publication bias, poor methodological quality in the smaller trials, and clinical heterogeneity (Collins *et al.*, 2003).

Reviews of this area have generally found that about 80 per cent of meta-analyses agree with single large trials in terms of direction of effect of treatment, but the size and statistical significance of the effect often differs between the two methods. Also, separate meta-analyses of the same therapeutic intervention may come to quite different conclusions (see Furukawa, 2004).

Funnel plots

One way of improving the reliability of meta-analyses is by the use of 'funnel plots'. The funnel plot is based on the assumption that the precision (confidence interval) of the estimated treatment effect will be greater in studies with a larger sample size. Therefore, the effect sizes of larger studies should cluster around the overall mean difference between experimental and control groups. By contrast, results from smaller studies should be more dispersed around the mean. This means that when the precision of individual studies is plotted against their odds ratios or effect sizes, the resulting graphical plot should resemble a symmetrical inverted funnel (the funnel plot). Statistically significant deviations from this plot suggest that that the meta-analysis may be biased and should be received with caution (see Egger *et al.*, 1997).

Large-scale randomized trials

As noted above, the advantage of meta-analysis is that by combining individual studies it can assemble sufficient patient numbers to allow detection of moderate-sized, but clinically important, therapeutic effects. Another way of detecting moderate-sized treatment effects is to randomize very large numbers of patients to a single study. These large-scale randomized (simple) trials (or **mega-trials**) have advantages over meta-analysis in that all patients can be allocated to a single study design. Such studies need numerous collaborators and therefore require a **simple study design** and a **clear endpoint**.

This metholodology has been most successfully applied to areas of medicine, such as cardiovascular disorders, where interventions can sometimes be simple (for example, one dose of aspirin daily) and end points (cardiac infarction, or death) clearly identified. The challenge for psychiatric trials is to adapt such methodology to conditions where interventions are more complex and end points more subtle (Rendell *et al.*, 2004).

Applicability

A general problem of applying evidence from randomized trials and meta-analysis to routine clinical work is that clinical trials are often carried out in rather 'ideal' conditions which in a number of respects may not match routine clinical work:

- **Patient population** Patients in controlled trials may differ systematically from those in routine clinical care in being less severely ill and having fewer comorbid difficulties. Thus trials may be carried out on patients who are, in fact, rather unrepresentative of a usual patient population.
- **Level of supervision** In drug trials concordance is regularly monitored by frequent review and supervision. Thus patients are less likely to drop out of treatment even where drugs are not particularly well-tolerated.
- **Therapist variables** Particularly in psychotherapy trials, treatment may be administered by skilled and experienced therapists. In routine practice treatments may be given by people with less experience. Also in trials the performance of therapists is often monitored closely to ensure that it conforms to the treatment protocol. Everyday practice may match the protocol less well.

Pragmatic trials

To overcome these limitations, it has been suggested that **pragmatic trials** might be a more appropriate way study the effect of certain psychiatric interventions. Such studies aim to carry out randomized trials in 'real-life' situations. Methodologically they have much in common with the mega-trials described earlier in that they are designed to answer simple and important clinical questions. As far as possible, pragmatic trials are carried out in a **routine clinical setting**. Other important features are:

- Randomization of very large numbers of subjects to take account of the fact that most advances in treatment will yield effect sizes of only moderate effect. Blinding is seen as less important than randomization, particularly where active treatments are compared;
- Simplification of process of recruitment by avoiding restrictive entry criteria. The principle criterion is that both doctor and patient should feel substantial uncertainty as to which of the trial treatments is best;
- Streamlining of assessments so they fit in with routine clinical practice. 'Many trials would be of much

greater scientific value if they collected 10 times less data … on 10 times more patients' (Collins *et al.*, 2003);

- Use of clinically relevant outcome measures. For example, in a trial of a therapeutic intervention in schizophrenia, a rating by patient and family member on a simple scale of well-being may carry more clinical relevance than a score on a standardized rating scale.

Implementation of EBM

Implementing EBM for the individual patient

Having obtained the best evidence on a therapeutic intervention and decided that it is valid and therapeutically useful, it is necessary to decide how applicable it is to the individual patient you are considering. In large measure this depends on the answers to the questions on 'applicability' listed above. The key issues are:

- How similar is the patient to those in the randomized trials?
- Can the local service deliver the intervention successfully? (For example, it is no use recommending interpersonal therapy if there are no trained therapists available to carry it out.)

In making the decision about implementation it may be useful to adjust the NNT for local clinical conditions if the relevant information is available (see above). A further way of taking more information into account in clinical decision making is provided by the concept of 'likelihood of being helped or harmed (LHH)'. Straus and McAlister (2001) give an example where a patient and clinician are considering the use of the anticholinesterase, donepezil, to decrease the risk of cognitive decline. The NNT of donepezil for this indication is 6 while the NNH to experience an adverse event with donepezil is 11. The LLH is calculated as the ratio of (1/NNT) to (1/NNH) or (1/6):(1/11) which is about 2 to 1 in favour of donepezil. It is also possible to weight the NNT and NNH with factors that incorporate the patient's attitude to the value of avoiding cognitive decline relative to that of experiencing adverse effects. Whether such efforts at quantification add significantly to a careful clinical assessment and discussion with the patient is questionable. The important point is that results from randomized trials need to be adapted to the differing needs of individuals.

Implementing EBM at a service level

Haynes (1999) suggested that the following stages are important in the implementation of a new treatment:

- *Efficacy* Does the intervention work under carefully controlled ('ideal') conditions?
- *Effectiveness* Does the intervention work when provided under the usual circumstances of health care practice?
- *Efficiency* What is the effectiveness of the intervention in relation to the resources it consumes (cost-effectiveness or cost-benefit?

Ideally, the full implementation of EBM would involve successful negotiation all these stages, and only interventions that have satisfied the three criteria of efficacy, effectiveness, and efficiency would be used. In practice many therapeutic interventions in psychiatry (particularly drug treatment and cognitive–behaviour therapy) are of proven **efficacy** but there is often uncertainty about **effectiveness** and **efficiency**. For example, lithium treatment is **efficacious** in the prophylaxis of bipolar disorder but appears to have disappointing **effectiveness**, mainly because under standard clinical conditions relatively few patients take lithium reliably (see Goodwin, 1999).

Clinical practice guidelines

In some medical fields there is a substantial amount of evidence of different kinds but still considerable clinical uncertainty about the best therapeutic management. In this situation it may be worth developing **clinical practice guidelines**, which are explicitly evidence-based.

Such guidelines are best developed in the following way:

- A guideline development group, composed of a multidisciplinary group and patient representatives, decide the precise clinical questions to be answered.
- The available evidence is systematically reviewed and classified according to the hierarchy shown in Table 6.1.
- The guideline development group make recommendations, explicitly demonstrating how their recommendations are linked to the available evidence.

Clinical guidelines are best developed at national level by appropriate professional organizations but usually require modification to take local clinical conditions into account. Guidelines will only be effective if they are actively disseminated and implemented.

In the United Kingdom, the National Institute for Clinical Excellence has taken a prominent role in analysing and promulgating evidence about therapeutic interventions in the form of national guidelines (http://www.nice.org.uk/). The success of this process in changing clinical practice is thus far uncertain and may depend on other factors such as strength and stability of evidence and cost issues (Freemantle, 2004). A further problem is that sometimes the evidence used in guideline development is based on a few trials whose relevance to the real world may be questionable. Nevertheless workable guidelines need relatively definitive advice which can lead to the issuing of rather arbitrary guidance together with a diminished probability that more informative studies will be carried out.

Evaluation of EBM

EBM needs to evaluated through randomized trials of effectiveness as described above for the guidelines on treating depression. Individual practitioners can also evaluate their EBM performance by:

- auditing what proportion of their clinical decisions are evidence-based;
- recognizing gaps in practice that require a search and appraisal of relevant evidence;
- auditing the effectiveness of evidence-based practice changes.

In this way the process of EBM can become an integral part of continuing professional development and the audit cycle.

Other applications of EBM

The foregoing account has focused on the use of EBM in the assessment of therapeutic interventions in psychiatry. Other applications of EBM include assessment of evidence relating to diagnosis, prognosis, and aetiology. These applications require rather different methodologies from the randomized trials previously considered, and diagnosis and prognosis will be discussed in the remainder of the chapter. Approaches to aetiology have been discussed in Chapter 5. All these applications start with a focused question which, as with treatment related questions, must:

- be directly relevant to the identified problem;
- be constructed in a way that facilitates searching for a precise answer (see Geddes 1999, Table 6.3).

Diagnosis

If we are trying to assess the value of a particular study assessing a diagnostic test, the practitioner needs to consider a number of questions (see Sackett *et al.* 1997):

- Was there an independent, blind comparison of the test with a diagnostic gold standard?
- Did the sample include the range of patients to whom the test is likely to be applied in clinical practice?
- What is the sensitivity and specificity of the test?
- Will it help the management of my patients?

Example

Question: How useful is the CAGE questionnaire in detecting problem drinking in medical and surgical inpatients?

The CAGE questionnaire is a simple four-item questionnaire designed to detect patients with alcohol misuse (see Chapter 18, p. 442). Sackett (1996) describes a study in a community-based teaching hospital in Boston where the CAGE questionnaire was administered to

TABLE 6.3 Common types of clinical question

Form of the question	Most reliable study architecture
How likely is a patient who has a particular symptom, sign, or diagnostic result to have a specific disorder?	A cross-sectional study of patients suspected of having the disorder comparing the proportion of the patients who really have the disorder and have a positive test with the proportion of patients who do not have the disorder and have a positive test result
Is the treatment of interest more effective in producing a desired outcome than an alternative treatment (including no treatment)?	Randomized evidence in which the patients are randomly allocated to receive either the treatment of interest or the alternative (Table 6.1)
What is the probability of a specific outcome in this patient?	A study in which an inception cohort patients at a common stage in the development of the illness – especially first onset) are followed up for an adequate length of time
What has caused the disorder (or, how likely is a particular intervention to cause a specific adverse effect)?	A study comparing the frequency of an exposure in a group of people with the disease (cases) of interest with a group of people without the disease (controls) – this may be a randomized controlled trial, a case control study, or a cohort study

From Geddes (1999).

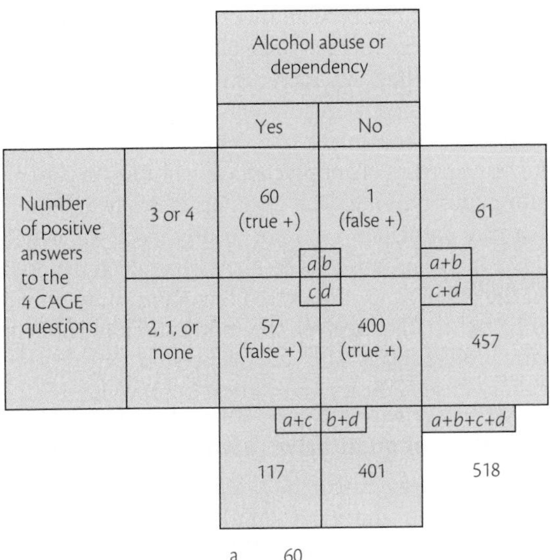

$$\text{sensitivity} = \frac{a}{(a+c)} = \frac{60}{117} = 0.51 \text{ or } 51\%$$

$$\text{specificity} = \frac{d}{(b+d)} = \frac{400}{401} = 0.998 \text{ or } 99.8\%$$

Fig. 6.2 The CAGE questions for alcohol abuse/dependency. From Sackett (1996).

518 patients. The gold standard to which the CAGE questionnaire was compared was an extensive social history and clinical examination supplemented by liver biopsy where indicated. We can be reasonably confident therefore that cases of alcohol misuse were reliably identified.

On clinical ('gold standard') grounds, 117 patients met criteria for alcohol misuse or dependence. Of the 61 patients who scored positively on the CAGE questionnaire (scores of 3 or 4), 60 were found to have gold standard evidence of alcohol misuse. The CAGE is therefore highly specific (Figure 6.2). However the remaining 57 patients with alcohol misuse were not identified by the CAGE. The CAGE therefore has only a modest sensitivity.

These results show that the CAGE is a useful screening instrument for problem drinking in a general hospital setting, in that a positive response is highly predictive of alcohol problems. However, the test would have to be applied in the knowledge that a negative CAGE response does not rule out alcohol misuse, particularly if there is other evidence of problem drinking.

Prognosis

Studies relating to prognosis should be assessed in the following way (see Sackett *et al.*, 1997):

- Was a defined, representative sample of patients identified at a common point, early in the course of the disorder?
- Was the follow-up sufficiently long and was it complete?
- Were objective outcome criteria applied in a blind fashion?
- Are these follow-up data likely to apply my own patients?

A common problem with prognostic studies is lack of complete follow-up. As a rule of thumb, less than 5 per cent drop-out is ideal and more than 20 per cent makes the study of questionable validity. As with treatment trials, the applicability of the study will depend critically on the how far the patients in it resemble those whom the practitioner is considering.

Example

Question: How much of the time during long-term follow-up do patients with bipolar disorder experience affective symptomatology and what is the pattern of symptoms?

Judd *et al.* (2002) recruited 146 patients with diagnosis of bipolar disorder and a current episode of major mood disturbance from five tertiary care centres in the USA. They were followed up with interviews every 6 months for the first 5 years and annually thereafter. At interview, affective symptoms were elicited using Psychiatric Status Rating Scales linked to the Research Diagnostic criteria. Affective symptoms that did not meet criteria for RDC diagnosis were assigned to sub-syndromal categories of depression or mania.

The mean follow-up period was 14.2 years and 93 per cent of subjects were followed up for more than 2 years. Patients were symptomatically ill about half the time. Overall about 90 per cent of patients spent one or more weeks during follow-up with depressive symptoms and almost the same number (86 per cent) experienced at least one week of manic or hypomanic symptoms. However, depressive symptoms during follow-up (32 per cent of follow-up weeks) were about three times as common as manic or hypomanic symptoms (9.3 per cent). Most of these depressive states were classified as sub-syndromal depression or minor mood disorder rather than major depression. At least one week of mood cycling or mixed affective states were noted in about 48 per cent of patients.

This study suggests that patients with bipolar disorder who are referred to a tertiary centre with an episode of major mood disturbance will have some symptoms of mood disturbance about half the time over the next few years. Overall depressive symptoms predominate, particularly minor and sub-syndromal depressive states; however, over time patients can experience considerable fluctuation in symptoms both manic and depressive or mixed. This study also has some aetiological implications because it suggests that bipolar disorder and other milder depressive and hypomanic states are different expressions of the same underlying disorder. In terms of applicability, we would note that the patients in the study are tertiary referrals, so the findings might not apply, for example, to patients in primary care.

Qualitative research

Qualitative research methods are used to collect and analyse data that cannot be easily represented by numbers (see Brown and Lloyd, 2001). While current evidence-based approaches in psychiatry have focused on the use of randomized controlled trials with quantitative endpoints, the use of qualitative approaches has a long history and encompasses, for example, the classificatory work of Kraepelin and the case studies of Freud. More modern case series, such as that of Russell (1979) describing bulimia nervosa, also rely on a qualitative approach.

Key differences between qualitative and quantitative research are summarized in Table 6.4.

When should qualitative methods be used?

There are a number of circumstances in which the application of qualitative methods is appropriate in psychiatric research and service development (Brown and Lloyd, 2001):

- In the initial stages of research, to conceptualize and clarify the relevant questions and to generate hypotheses.
- To gather and collate attitudes, beliefs and experiences of service users, carers and professionals.
- Development of assessment tools and rating scales.
- Examining the use of evidence-based interventions in practice and to understand problems in implementation.

From this it can be seen that qualitative and quantitative approaches are not antagonistic but have particular uses in defined situations. For example, Rogers *et al.* (2004) combined a qualitative methodology with a quantitative randomized trial, which aimed to improve the management of antipsychotic medication in patients with schizophrenia. The qualitative study indicated that trial participants did not readily recall the details of the interventions to which they had been exposed. On the other hand they valued the opportunity provided by the trial for greater communication and contact with professionals. This was associated with greater feelings of self-efficacy and clinical improvement.

Evaluation of qualitative research

Like quantitative research, qualitative research needs to be relevant and valid. Similar general principles apply to processes of participant selection, which should be clear and justified. It is important to be explicit about the reasons for choosing a qualitative approach and to give clear description of methods of data collection and analysis. **The concept of permeability**, or the extent to which observations have influenced understanding, is important in qualitative research. Stiles (1999) outlined factors which influence study permeability:

- **The degree of engagement** with the material. How far were theories generated by direct contact, for example, through interviews, naturalistic observation, and familiarity with textual sources?
- **Iteration.** Did the investigators continually reformulate and re-examine their interpretations in the light of continuing observations?
- **Grounding.** Were the procedures for linking interpretations with observations clearly presented and were illustrative examples given?
- **Context.** Were the values and expectations of the investigator disclosed? Was the cultural context of

TABLE 6.4 Key differences between qualitative and quantitative research

	Quantitative research	Qualitative research
Fundamental aim	Objectivity, reliability, scientific truth	Understanding through personal encounter and observation. 'Permeability.'
Sampling	Random selection; designed to represent general population of subjects and avoid bias	'Purposive'. Subjects chosen deliberately to possess characteristics relevant to study question
Data collection	Standardized, 'objective'; validated rating scales, biochemical end points etc	Observation and interview, often interactive and open-ended. Systematic study of written material
Analysis of data	Quantitative, statistical, hypothesis testing	Narrative, generation of categories and themes. Analysis occurs iteratively with data collection

the research and its meaning to the participants made explicit?

Validity

The concept of validity in qualitative research refers to the soundness and reasoning of interpretation rather than comparison to an objective external criterion. Validity also differs according to role. For example, readers of a study will look for coherence and internal consistency of material while participants must feel that their experiences are accurately described by the interpretations. Finally the authors of the research need to take into account the effect the research process itself might have on the data they have collected ('**reflexivity**').

Assessing qualitative research is not always straightforward and the specialist terminology may defeat general readers. Brown and Lloyd (2001) have pointed out the lack of utility of evaluative checklists whose terminology is not readily understood by health service researchers.

Further reading

Sackett, DL, Richardson, WS, Rosenberg, W and Haynes, RB (1997) *Evidence-based medicine*. Churchill Livingstone, New York. (Concise handbook with clear exposition of principles of EBM.)

CHAPTER 7

Personality and personality disorder

Chapter contents

Personality

The term personality refers to enduring qualities of an individual that are shown in his ways of behaving in a wide variety of circumstances. Personality therefore differs from mental disorder in that the behaviours which define it have been present throughout adult life, whereas the behaviours that define mental disorder differ from the person's previous behaviour. The distinction is easy to make when behaviour changes markedly over a short period of time (as in a manic disorder), but difficult when behaviour changes slowly over a longer time (as in some early cases of schizophrenia).

The importance of personality

Variations in personality are important because they may predispose to psychiatric disorder, they may account for unusual features in a psychiatric disorder (they are 'pathoplastic' factors) – and they may affect the way that patients approach psychiatric treatment.

Personality as predisposition

Personality can predispose to psychiatric disorder by modifying the response to stressful events. For example, adverse circumstances are more likely to induce an anxiety disorder in a person who has always worried about minor problems.

Personality as a pathoplastic factor

Personality can account for unusual features of a disorder. This usually occurs when features of personality have become exaggerated in response to stressful events associated with illness. For example, histrionic features suggesting a diagnosis of dissociative disorder may arise from histrionic personality traits. When such unusual features are marked, diagnosis is difficult if the psychiatrist has not made an accurate assessment of personality.

Personality in relation to treatment

Personality is an important determinant of a person's approach to treatment. For example, people with obsessional traits may become angry if treatment does not follow their expectations exactly; anxiety-prone people may be overcautious when asked to do more during rehabilitation; and people with antisocial traits may be uncooperative with treatment or aggressive towards staff who are caring for them. Some people with a severe disorder of personality have difficulty in accessing services because clinicians are reluctant are reluctant to accept them (see Lewis and Appleby, 1988).

Personality types

A first step in understanding personality is to identify basic types. Clinicians have generally derived these types from their collective experience, which suggests several generally recognizable categories such as a sociable and outgoing type and a solitary and self-conscious type. Psychologists have attempted to produce a more scientific set of categories by using personality tests to measure certain aspects of personality ('traits'), and then employing statistical methods to discover which traits cluster together as 'factors'. Examples of personality traits include: anxiety, energy, flexibility, hostility, impulsiveness, moodiness, orderliness, and self-reliance. The various investigators have derived rather different personality factors from such traits: Cattell (1963) identified five factors, while Eysenck (1970a) proposed a scheme that originally had only two 'dimensions' (high-level factors) labelled extraversion–introversion and neuroticism. Subsequently Eysenck added a third dimension, psychoticism (Eysenck and Eysenck, 1976). He used the term in a special way to denote a constellation of traits of coldness, aggressivity, cruelty, and a propensity to antisocial behaviour.

It is now generally agreed that personality can be described by five factors. These have been variously named but can be referred to usefully as openness to experience (or novelty seeking), conscientiousness, extraversion–introversion, agreeableness (or affiliation), neuroticism. (The initial letters of these factors form the mnemonic OCEAN.) Widiger and Costa (1994) have proposed a scheme in which each of these five factors is made up from scores on six traits. Assessment inventories for these factors have been developed based on self-report and report from informants (Costa and McCrae, 1992), as well as a semi-structured interview (Trull and Widiger, 1997).

Cloninger (1986) and Cloninger *et al.* (1993) developed an alternative scheme with three 'basic behavioural dispositions' which are expressed as four basic temperaments (the seven-factor model). The behavioural dispositions are behavioural activation, behavioural inhibition, and behavioural maintenance. According to Cloninger, behavioural activation is associated with the basic temperament of **novelty seeking**; behavioural inhibition is associated with **harm avoidance**; and behavioural maintenance is associated with **reward dependence**. The fourth basic temperament is **persistence**. It has been suggested that novelty seeking is related to dopaminergic function, and harm avoidance to serotonergic function. Cloninger's scheme also includes three character traits of **self-directedness**, **cooperativeness**, and **transcendence**. These character traits are thought to originate in experiences during childhood and adolescence rather than from the biologically determined behavioural dispositions.

The various types of personality and personality disorder are constructed from these four basic temperaments and three character traits. For example, novelty seeking may be expressed as curiosity, readiness to boredom, enthusiasm, and unconventional behaviour. Cloninger's scheme is noteworthy for its attempt to identify basic behavioural dispositions which can account for the observable behaviours that characterize personality, and for its inclusion of both inherited differences in brain function and the effects of experience. The Temperament and Character Inventory has been developed to assess the seven factors (see Brandstrom *et al.*, 2003) and attempts are being made to relate scores on the inventory to measures of brain function though so far without conclusive results (see for example, Turner *et al.* 2003).

Despite these scientific findings, clinicians continue to use everyday words to describe the positive and negative features of normal personality. Positive attributes include outgoing, self-confident, stable, and adaptable. Negative attributes include shy, reserved, lacking in confidence, sensitive, jealous, irritable, impulsive, self-centred, rigid, and aggressive. In addition, two terms are in general use to describe sets of attributes which are often found together. These terms are as follows.

Obsessional traits These traits include the positive qualities of being dependable, persistent, and precise. People who have them set high standards, observe social conventions, and keep to the law. When these traits are more marked, they are expressed in a negative way as obstinacy, preoccupation with unimportant detail, bigotry, and lack of a sense of fun.

Histrionic traits In a minor form, these traits are socially advantageous. People who possess them are lively and engaging company, popular as hosts and guests, successful in amateur dramatics, and entertaining as public speakers. When the traits are more pronounced they carry disadvantages. Such people are easily moved to tears and dramatize situations. They react to illness in the same demonstrative way, in the past called 'hysterical overlay', which makes it difficult to assess the severity of their suffering. As patients they may be demanding or flirtatious.

The origins of personality

The biological basis of personality types

Genetic influences

Everyday observation suggests that children often resemble their parents in personality. Such similarities could be inherited, or acquired through social learning. Three kinds of scientific study have been used to study the inheritance of personality.

Studies of body build and personality It is sometimes thought that personality is linked to body build and if this is true, a possible link between the two could be genetic. Kretschmer (1936) described three types of body build: pyknic (stocky and rounded), athletic, and asthenic (lean and narrow). He suggested that the pyknic body build was linked to the cyclothymic personality type (sociable, with variable moods), whereas the asthenic build was related to the 'schizotypal' personality type (cold, aloof, and self-sufficient). Kretschmer's ideas were based on subjective judgements. Sheldon *et al.* (1940) repeated the studies using quantitative methods for assessing physique and more objective ratings of personality. The results did not support any simple relationship between body build and personality type (Sheldon *et al.*, 1940).

Studies of twins More direct evidence of a genetic basis of personality has been obtained by studying the degree of similarity between the scores on personality tests of identical twins reared together or reared apart. The general conclusion from these and other studies is that the hereditability for traits of extraversion and neuroticism is 35–50 per cent (McGuffin and Thapar, 1992). The hereditability of other traits is broadly similar, non-shared environmental factors, with shared environment having little effect. These results may hold only for normal populations: a twin study based on DSM-III-R personality disorder categories found little heritability (Torgesen *et al.* 1993).

Linkage studies Methods of molecular genetics have been used to seek for linkages with measures of novelty seeking and of neuroticism. Several quantitative trait loci have been identified that influence variations in neuroticism (Fullerton *et al.*, 2003). These and other findings await confirmation though linkage between harm avoidance and a region on 8p21 has been reported and confirmed in one study (Zohar *et al.*, 2003). Such studies are difficult but important because they may eventually show the biological basis of aspects of personality.

Childhood temperament and adult personality

Young infants differ in patterns of sleeping and waking, approach or withdrawal from new situations, intensity of emotional responses, and span of attention. These differences, which are described further in Chapter 24, could be a basis from which differences in personality develop. However, whilst the differences persist into the later years of childhood, they have not been shown to be related to specific features of adult personality (Berger, 1985).

Childhood experience and personality development

Everyday experience suggests that experiences in childhood shape personality. It is not easy, however, to produce objective evidence to test this impression. Experiences that seem relevant are difficult to quantify or even to record reliably, and it is difficult to arrange prospective studies that span the long interval between childhood events and adult personality. Retrospective studies are easier to arrange but recall by adults of childhood experiences is unreliable. Nevertheless some information is available (see the aetiology of personality disorder, below). Meanwhile the psychodynamic theories of Freud and others continue to be quoted.

Freudian theory Freud's scheme of personality development emphases events in the first five years of life. It is proposed that crucial stages of development of the libido (oral, anal, and genital) must be passed through successfully if personality development is to proceed normally. Failure at particular stages is thought to account for certain features of adult personality, for example, difficulties at the anal stage are said to lead to obsessional personality traits. The scheme allows for some modification of personality at later stages of development through identification with people other than the parents, but this influence is thought to be less important than the earlier ones. The scheme is comprehensive and flexible so that it is possible to explain many features of personality in terms of earlier experience. However, the same features of the theory make it difficult to test it scientifically.

Jung's theory This theory of personality development resembles Freud's in recognizing the importance of psychic events in early life. Unlike Freud, however, Jung thought of personality development as a lifelong process. He referred to events in the first part of life as merely 'fulfilling one's obligations' and applied this term to events such as severing ties with parents, finding a spouse, and starting a family. Jung's account is useful in drawing attention to the adjustments in personality that occur throughout life, but in other ways it has not been as influential as Freud's theory and it is equally difficult to test.

Adler and the neo-Freudians Adler rejected Freud's ideas of libido development, proposing instead that personality develops through efforts to compensate for basic feelings of inferiority. The 'neo-Freudians' (Fromm, Horney, and Sullivan) emphasized social factors in development rather than the biologically determined stages of Freud's scheme, though they differed amongst themselves in the details of these social factors. The details of these theories have not been widely accepted but their general emphasis of social factors has been influential.

Erikson The theory proposed by Erikson is essentially similar to Freud's though the nomenclature is different. Erikson referred to the oral stage as the stage of **trust versus mistrust**, to indicate that this is the period in which feelings of security develop. He referred to the anal stage as the stage of **autonomy versus doubt**, to indicate that it is the period in which the child learns self-control, social rules, and self-confidence. Erikson referred to the genital stage as the stage of **initiative versus guilt**, to indicate that it is the stage at which children develop an image of themselves as people. If this stage goes well, the child emerges with confidence and initiative; otherwise, the child emerges insecure and inhibited. Erikson adopted Freud's idea of a latency period but extended it into adolescence. He called this last stage the period of **industry versus inferiority**. In it the child learns the value of achievements in work and at school, and in social relationships outside the family. Erikson's scheme has been influential in the study of adolescents, largely because it recognizes the importance of this period of life while Freud gave it little attention.

The assessment of personality

The assessment of personality is discussed in Chapter 2, but two points need to be mentioned again. The first is that the means of assessment of personality used in everyday life cannot be applied reliably in clinical practice. In everyday life, we assume that current behaviour reflects the person's habitual ways of behaving (the personality) and generally this assumption is correct. The same assumption is often misleading when patients are assessed because the current behaviour of an ill person reflects the effects of the illness as well as the personality. The personality of an ill person can be judged effectively only from reliable accounts of past behaviour, obtained wherever possible from informants as well as from the patient.

Some assessment instruments for personality were mentioned in the section on personality types (p. 128). It might be supposed that these and similar standardized tests would give better information about personality than the clinician could obtain. However, although personality tests are more reliable in healthy people, their results can be affected by the presence of mental disorder. Also, they do not measure the traits that are most relevant to clinical practice. For this reason, tests of personality, although useful in research, are seldom used in clinical practice.

For a review of methods of assessment of personality see Westen (1997) and Clark and Harrison (2001).

The importance of personality assessment

As explained in the introduction to this chapter, the assessment of personality is important in decisions about aetiology, diagnosis, and treatment. In aetiology, knowledge of personality helps to explain why certain events are stressful to the patient. In diagnosis, an understanding of personality may explain the presence of unusual features in a disorder, which would otherwise cause uncertainty. In treatment, an assessment of personality helps understanding of the way that patients react to illness and to its treatment, and affects prognosis. Personality should be assessed in every case and not just in those where there is a disorder of personality (i.e. an extreme deviation from the normal – see below).

The assessment is recorded best with a series of descriptive terms, chosen with the features of abnormal personality in mind. This is because the personality factors described above are too general to convey the information that is important to the clinician. Examples of such descriptions are sensitive, lacking in self-confidence, and prone to worry unreasonably; or abnormally aggressive with little remorse or concern for others. Descriptions of this kind are useful in constructing a picture of the unique features of each patient, and this is one of the bases of good clinical practice.

Personality disorder

The concept of abnormal personality

Some personalities are obviously abnormal, for example, paranoid personalities characterized by extreme suspiciousness, sensitivity, and mistrust. It is, however, impossible to draw a sharp dividing line between normal and abnormal personalities. Indeed, it is even difficult to decide what criterion should be used to make this distinction. Two kinds of criteria have been suggested, the first statistical and the second social.

On the **statistical criterion**, abnormal personalities are quantitative variations from the normal and the dividing line is decided by a cut-off score on an appropriate measure. In principle, this scheme is attractive as it parallels the approach used successfully in defining abnormalities of intelligence, and it has obvious value in research. However, its usefulness in clinical work has yet to be established.

Using a **social criterion**, abnormal personalities are those that cause the individual to suffer, or cause suffering to other people. For example, an abnormally sensitive and gloomy personality causes suffering for the individual, and an emotionally cold and aggressive personality causes suffering for others. Although such criteria are subjective and lack the precision of the first approach, they correspond well to the realities of clinical practice and they have been adopted widely.

Given the conceptual problems, it is not surprising that it is difficult to frame a satisfactory definition of abnormal personality. In ICD-9, personality disorders were described as follows:

> Severe disturbances in the personality and behavioural tendencies of the individual, not directly resulting from disease, damage or other insult to the brain, or from another psychiatric disorder. They usually involve several areas of the personality and are nearly always associated with considerable personal distress and social disruption. They are usually manifest since childhood or adolescence and continue throughout adulthood.

ICD-10 has a somewhat different definition in terms of enduring patterns of behaviour, but the ICD-9 definition is more concise, and still valuable.

It can be added that the personal distress referred to in the ICD-9 definition may become apparent only late in the course of the condition (for example, when a long-standing supportive relationship is lost), and that there are usually, though not always, significant problems in occupational and social performance.

Whilst definitions naturally focus on abnormal features, it is important to recognize that people with abnormal personalities generally have favourable as well as unfavourable traits. The clinician should always assess positive as well as unfavourable features, since it may be possible to build on the former in a plan of management.

Personality change

In some circumstances during adult life, there may be a profound and enduring change in personality, distinct from the temporary changes in behaviour that may accompany stressful events or illness. These lasting changes may result from:

- injury to or organic disease of the brain;
- severe mental disorder, especially schizophrenia;
- exceptionally severe stressful experiences, for example, those experienced by hostages or prisoners undergoing torture.

ICD-10 has categories for each type of change. **Change in personality due to organic disease of the brain** is classified with the organic mental disorders in section F00, which contains a category for personality and behavioural disorders due to brain disease, damage, and dysfunction. Examples include the changes in personality following encephalitis and head injury. In DSM-IV this condition is diagnosed as personality change due to a general medical condition.

In ICD-10 the other two forms of personality change listed above are classified in section F60, disorders of adult personality and behaviour. To diagnose **enduring personality change after psychiatric illness**, the change of personality must have lasted for at least 2 years, be clearly related to the experience of the illness, and not present before it. The person with this condition may, for example, be dependent, passive, and demanding, or socially withdrawn and isolated because of the (non-delusional) conviction of being changed or stigmatized. The authors of ICD noted that the change must be understandable in terms of the person's experiences during the illness, and their previous attitudes, adjustment, and life situation. However, it is generally thought that schizophrenic illness can change personality directly as well as in these indirect ways.

In ICD-10, **enduring personality change after a catastrophic experience** must also have lasted for at least

2 years. The stressful experience must have been extreme, for example, a disaster, prolonged captivity with the imminent possibility of being killed, being the victim of terrorism, torture, or confinement in a concentration camp. The person with this condition is hostile, irritable, distrustful, and socially withdrawn, and feels empty, hopeless, estranged, and on edge. These features were not present before the experience and, although the condition may follow post-traumatic stress disorder, it is separate from it.

How ideas about abnormal personality developed

In psychiatry the concept of abnormal personality can be traced to the beginning of the nineteenth century, when the French psychiatrist Pinel described *manie sans délire*. Pinel applied this term to patients who were prone to outbursts of rage and violence but were not deluded (at that time delusions were regarded as the hallmark of mental illness, and *délire* is the French term for delusion). Presumably this group of patients included not only those who would now be regarded as having an antisocial personality, but also some who were mentally ill but not deluded, for example some manic patients. (See Kavka, 1949 for a translation of the relevant section of the second edition of Pinel's book, first published in 1801.)

Although other writers, such as the American Benjamin Rush, were interested in similar clinical problems, it was an English physician who took the next important step forward. In 1835, J. C. Prichard, senior physician to the Bristol Infirmary, published his *A treatise on insanity and other disorders of the mind*. After referring to Pinel's *manie sans délire*, he suggested a new term, *moral insanity*, which he defined as a

> morbid perversion of the natural feelings, affections, inclinations, temper, habits, moral dispositions and natural impulses without any remarkable disorder or defect of the intellect or knowing or reasoning faculties and in particular without any insane delusion or hallucination.
>
> (Prichard 1835, p. 6)

Although this description included the violent patients described by Pinel, Prichard clearly had a wider group in mind, since he added: 'a propensity to theft is sometimes a feature of moral insanity and sometimes it is its leading if not sole characteristic' (p. 27).

Prichard's category of moral insanity, like Pinel's *manie sans délire*, seems to have included some affective disorders, for he wrote: 'a considerable proportion among the most striking instances of moral insanity are those in which a tendency to gloom or sorrow is the predominant feature' (p. 18); and added: 'a state of gloom and melancholy depression occasionally gives way to the opposite condition of preternatural excitement' (p. 19).

Prichard's moral insanity included conditions we would now diagnose as personality disorder. However, he did not confine the term to people who had always behaved in these ways:

> When however such phenomena are observed in connection with a wayward and intractable temper, with a decay of social affections, an aversion to the nearest relatives and friends formerly beloved – in short, with a change in the moral character of the individual, the case becomes tolerably well marked.

In this passage the reference to change in character indicates that Prichard had in mind not only conditions we would classify as personality disorder but also some that we would classify as mental disorder.

Later in the nineteenth century, it was recognized that mental illness could occur without delusions and the concept of moral insanity took on a more restricted meaning. Thus, Henry Maudsley applied the term to someone whom he described as having

> no capacity for true moral feeling – all his impulses and desires, to which he yields without check, are egoistic, his conduct appears to be governed by immoral motives, which are cherished and obeyed without any evident desire to resist them.
>
> (Maudsley 1885, p. 171)

Maudsley commented on the current dissatisfaction with the term moral insanity, which he referred to as ' a form of mental alienation which has so much the look of vice or crime that many people regard it is an unfounded medical invention' (p. 170).

The next step towards modern ideas was the introduction by Koch (1891) of the term psychopathic inferiority to denote this same group of people who have marked abnormalities of behaviour in the absence of mental illness or intellectual impairment. (Later, the word inferiority was replaced by personality to avoid judgemental overtones.) Kraepelin was, at first, uncertain how to classify these people, and it was not until the eighth edition of his textbook that he finally adopted the term psychopathic personality and devoted a long chapter to it. He included not only the antisocial type but also six others: the excitable, unstable, quarrelsome, and eccentric, together with liars and swindlers.

Kurt Schneider broadened the concept of psychopathic personality. Whereas Kraepelin's seven types of psychopathic personality applied to people causing inconvenience, annoyance, or suffering to other people, Schneider included as well people who suffered themselves. For example, he included people with markedly depressive or insecure characters. Thus, in Schneider's usage, psychopathic personality covered the whole range of abnormal personality, not just antisocial personality. In this way the term came to have two meanings: the wider meaning of abnormal personality of all kinds, and the narrower meaning of antisocial personality.

Confusion about the term psychopathic personality does not end with Schneider's broader definition. Two other usages call for attention. The first originated in the work of the Scottish psychiatrist, Sir David Henderson, who in 1939 published the influential book *Psychopathic states*. He defined psychopaths as people who, although not mentally subnormal,

> throughout their lives or from a comparatively early age, have exhibited disorders of conduct of an antisocial or asocial nature, usually of a recurrent or episodic type which in many instances have proved difficult to influence by methods of social, penal and medical care or for whom we have no adequate provision of a preventative or curative nature.

So far this definition corresponds to the previous narrow concept of psychopathic personality. However, Henderson extended his definition by referring to three groups of psychopaths:

1. **predominantly aggressive** personalities, including not only those who are repeatedly aggressive, but also those prone to suicide, drug addiction, and alcohol abuse;
2. **passive and inadequate** personalities, including unstable, hypochondriacal, and sensitive people, pathological liars, and those with a schizoid nature;
3. **creative psychopaths**, a group so wide that it is of little value.

Henderson gave as examples of the third group, T. E. Lawrence and Joan of Arc who, though both creative, had little else in common. Henderson's main contribution was to draw attention to the group of inadequate personalities.

Yet another variation in the meaning of the term psychopathic was introduced in the 1959 Mental Health Act for England and Wales and repeated in the 1983 Act where psychopathic disorder is as defined in Section 41(42) as

> a persistent disorder or disability of mind (whether or not including significant impairment of intelligence) which results in abnormally aggressive or seriously irresponsible conduct on the part of the person concerned.

This definition is a return to the narrow concept of aggressive or irresponsible behaviour causing suffering to other people and adds the possibility that the suffereing may be only to the person concerned so that it covers a wide range of personality diagnoses. The Act adds the proviso for admission for treatment (section 3(2b)) that: 'in the case of psychopathic disorder ... treatment is likely to alleviate or prevent a deterioration of his condition'.

Not surprisingly, many difficulties have attended the use of this definition and the rider. (In Britain new mental health legislation is under discussion at the time of writing). The most recent development is the use of the term **dangerous and severe personality disorder** (DSPD), mainly to refer to men with antisocial disorder and a history of violence, and in the context of initiatives to reduce the risk they pose (Home Office, 1999). The term has a political rather than clinical or scientific provenance.

The two meanings of psychopathic personality – the wider meaning of all abnormal personality, and the narrower meaning of antisocial personality – persist to the present day. Because the term psychopathic personality is ambiguous, the preferred terms are personality disorder and antisocial personality disorder to denote the wide and narrow senses, respectively.

The classification of abnormal personalities

General issues

The use of categories

Personality is a continuous variable but systems for the classification of psychiatric disorders use categories that require cut-off points. Categories are useful when cases have to be counted in epidemiological studies and clinical audit. However, the chosen criterion – distress to the person or to others – is both arbitrary and imprecise, and cases that just fall short of it (subthreshold cases) are frequent and often present clinical problems similar to those of definite cases.

Comorbidity

It is not only the boundary between normal and abnormal personality that is imprecise and arbitrary; the boundaries between different types of personality are also ill defined. In addition, many patients have features contained among the criteria for more than one personality disorder (see Fyer *et al.* 1988). When more than one personality diagnosis can be made in a single patient, the term comorbidity is used. The same term is used when a patient meets the criteria for both a mental disorder and a personality disorder. In the latter case, it can be argued that two separate conditions are present but when two personality disorders can be diagnosed, the same cannot be maintained convincingly. It seems more likely that the patient has a single personality disorder which has features which overlap two of the arbitrary sets of criteria used in the current systems of diagnosis.

Conditions related to personality disorder and classified elsewhere

Cyclothymia and schizotypal disorder were previously classified as personality disorders on the grounds that they are long-lasting patterns of behaviour that can cause distress. In ICD-10 both have been removed from the personality disorders and classified instead with the mental disorders: cyclothymia with affective disorders, schizotypal disorder with schizophrenia. This arrangement takes account of the fact that these two conditions may begin in adult life, after the time when personality has developed fully and in the case of schizotypal disorder evidence from family studies that link it genetically to schizophrenia (see p. 282). In DSM-IV, cyclothymic disorder is classified with mood disorders, but schizotypal disorder is retained as a personality disorder. In both classifications, multiple personality disorder is classified with dissociative disorders (see p. 213).

Classification of personality disorders in ICD-10 and DSM-IV

In Table 7.1, the classification of personality disorders in ICD-10 is compared with that in DSM-IV. The two schemes are broadly similar but the following differences should be noted.

The use of Axis II

In DSM-IV, personality disorders are classified on a different 'axis' (Axis II) from mental disorders (classified on Axis I). This arrangement recognizes the different nature of the two diagnoses and it encourages a search for personality disorder in every case. This convention is not adopted in ICD-10. (If no personality disorder is present, the normal personality should still be assessed for the reasons given above, and recorded in the formulation even though it cannot be included among the diagnoses).

Grouping into clusters

In DSM-IV, but not in ICD-10, personality disorders are grouped into three 'clusters':

TABLE 7.1 Classification of personality disorders

ICD-10	DSM-IV
Paranoid	Paranoid
Schizoid	Schizoid
(Schizotypal, see text)	Schizotypal
Dissocial	Antisocial
Emotionally unstable	Borderline
Impulsive type	
Borderline type	
Histrionic	Histrionic
–	Narcissistic
Anankastic (obsessive–compulsive)	Obsessive–compulsive
Anxious (avoidant)	Avoidant
Dependent	Dependent
–	Passive–aggressive

1. *Cluster A* paranoid, schizoid, schizotypal;
2. *Cluster B* antisocial, borderline, histrionic, narcissistic;
3. *Cluster C* avoidant, dependent, obsessive-compulsive.

This useful convention is adopted later in this chapter.

Different names for the same personality disorder:

- In ICD-10 the term dissocial is used for the personality disorder referred to as antisocial in DSM-IV (the term antisocial is used in this book).
- In ICD-10 anankastic is the preferred term for the personality disorder called obsessive- compulsive in DSM-IV.
- In ICD-10 anxious is the preferred term for the personality disorder called avoidant in DSM-IV.

Categories included in one system only:

Present in ICD-10 but not in DSM-IV

- Emotionally unstable impulsive personality disorder.
- Enduring personality change, not attributable to brain damage or disease (see above).

Present in DSM-IV but not in ICD-10

- Narcissistic personality disorder.
- Passive-aggressive personality disorder (listed as a category for further study).

Conditions classified differently in DSM-IV and ICD-10

As noted above, schizotypal personality disorder is classified with schizophrenia in ICD-10 (and named schizotypal disorder). In DSM-IV it is classified as a personality disorder.

Descriptions and diagnostic criteria

This section contains an account of the abnormal personalities listed in the ICD-10 and DSM-IV (see Table 7.1). The criteria for diagnosis are lengthy and differ somewhat in wording and emphasis in the two systems. The following description refers to the main common features of the two sets of definitions and, where appropriate, has simplified or paraphrased the criteria to present a more general description of the personality disorder.

In each case the condition must meet the general criteria for personality disorder for which the ICD10 criteria for research can be summarized as follows:

- the person's characteristic and enduring patterns of behaviour deviate markedly from the cultural norm, with deviation in more than one of the areas of cognition (i.e. attitudes and ways of perceiving and interpreting), affectivity, control of impulses and gratification, and ways of relating to others;
- the deviation is pervasive, and the behaviour is inflexible, and maladaptive or dysfunctional in a broad range of situations;
- there is personal distress or an adverse impact on others;
- the deviation is stable and long-lasting, beginning usually in late childhood or adolescence;
- the deviant behaviour is not caused by another mental disorder;
- the deviant behaviour is not caused by brain injury, disease, or dysfunction.

There are several diagnostic instruments (see the Appendix to this chapter, p. 150). They are of value in research, but less useful in clinical practice

Cluster A personality disorders

Paranoid personality disorder

People with this kind of abnormal personality are suspicious and sensitive (Table 7.2). They have a marked sense of self-importance, but easily feel shame and humiliation. They are suspicious and constantly on the lookout for attempts by others to deceive them or play tricks on them. As a result, other people find them difficult and unreasonable. These people are mistrustful and jealous. They doubt the loyalty of other people and do not trust them. Sexual jealousy is common. They do not make friends easily and avoid involvement in groups. They appear secretive, devious, and self-sufficient to a fault. They take offence easily and see rebuffs where none is intended. Presented with a new proposal, they look for ways in which it might be designed to harm their interests.

TABLE 7.2 Features of a paranoid personality disorder

Suspicious
Mistrustful
Jealous
Sensitive
Resentful
Bears grudges
Self-important

These people are **sensitive** to rebuff, prickly, and argumentative. They read demeaning or threatening meanings into innocent remarks. Kretschmer described how such people's sensitivity leads to feelings of humiliation and to suspicious ideas so intense that they can be mistaken for persecutory delusions. These '**sensitive ideas of reference**' are considered further in Chapter 13. These people are also **resentful and bear grudges**, and they do not forgive real or perceived insults. They have a strong sense of their rights and may engage in litigation, with which they may persist long after others would have abandoned the case.

Paranoid personalities have a strong sense of **self-importance**. They believe that they are unusually talented and capable of great achievements. This unrealistic idea is maintained, despite modest accomplishments, by beliefs that others have prevented them from fulfilling their potential.

Schizoid personality disorder

The name schizoid was suggested by Kretschmer (1936), who believed that this type of personality is related to schizophrenia, but the idea has not been confirmed (see Chapter 12). People with this disorder are emotionally cold, detached, aloof, humourless, introspective, and prone to engage in fantasy (Table 7.3).

These people are emotionally cold and incapable of expressing either tender feelings or anger. They show little interest in sexual relationships. When the disorder is extreme, they appear cold and callous. They are **detached and aloof** and show little concern for the opinions of other people. They are ill at ease in company, do not make intimate relationships, and show little satisfaction in membership of a family group. They are seclusive, following a solitary course through life, and

TABLE 7.3 Features of schizoid personality disorder

Emotionally cold
Detached
Aloof
Lacking enjoyment
Introspective

often remain unmarried. These people also **lack a sense of enjoyment**, have little sense of humour, and take little pleasure in activities that most people enjoy. These qualities contribute to their separation from other people.

These people are **introspective and prone to fantasy**. They are more interested in intellectual matters than in people. They have a complex inner world of fantasy, although this lacks emotional content.

Schizotypal personality disorder

People with schizotypal personality disorder are socially anxious, experience cognitive and perceptual distortions, show oddities of speech and inappropriate affective responses, and behave eccentrically. This personality disorder appears to be related to schizophrenia, and in ICD-10 (but not DSM-IV) it is not classified as a personality disorder but placed with schizophrenia and called schizotypal disorder.

These people have **social anxiety**. They feel anxious in company so that they have difficulty in making relationships and lack friends and confidants. They feel different from other people and do not fit in. **Cognitive and perceptual distortions** include ideas (but not delusions) of reference, suspicious ideas, odd beliefs, and magical thinking (for example, belief in clairvoyance, mind reading, and telepathy), and unusual perceptual experiences (for example, awareness of a presence, or experiences bordering on hallucinations). They also show **oddities of speech** such as unusual constructions, words and phrasing, as well as vagueness, and a tendency to digression.

Their **affective responses are unusual** and they appear stiff, odd, and constricted in their emotions. Their **behaviour is eccentric** with odd mannerisms, unusual choices of clothing, disregard of conventions, and awkward social behaviour.

Cluster B personality disorder

Antisocial (dissocial) personality disorder

The term antisocial is used in DSM-IV; dissocial is the term in ICD-10. In this book, the term antisocial is preferred. People with this disorder show a callous lack of concern for the feelings of others. They disregard the rights of others, act impulsively, lack guilt, and fail to learn from adverse experiences (Table 7.4). Often their abnormal behaviour is made worse by the abuse of alcohol or drugs. An influential description of this type of personality disorder was written in 1941 by Cleckley in his book *The mask of sanity* (1964).

TABLE 7.4 Features of antisocial personality disorder

Callous
Transient relationships
Irresponsible
Impulsive and irritable
Lack guilt and remorse
Fail to accept responsibility

The criteria for diagnosis differ slightly in the two classifications; the following are taken from ICD-10. The DSM-IV criteria include the requirement of conduct disorder before the age of 15 years.

These people have a **callous lack of concern for others**. Their sexual activity is without tender feelings. They may inflict cruel or degrading acts on other people, including the sexual partner and any children, who may be physically or sexually abused. Their **relationships are shallow and short-lived** despite their superficial charm. They are **irresponsible and depart from social norms**. They do not obey rules and may repeatedly break the law, often committing violent offences. Their offending typically begins in adolescence.

These people are **impulsive**. They lack goals, do not plan ahead, and typically have an unstable work record marked by frequent dismissals. They take risks, disregarding their own safety and that of other people. They are **irritable** and when angry sometimes assault others in a violent way. These features of personality are accompanied by a striking **lack of guilt or remorse** and a failure to change their behaviour in response to punishment or other adverse outcomes. They **avoid responsibility**, transferring blame onto other people, and rationalizing their own failures. They are also deceitful and irresponsible about finances.

Borderline personality disorder

The term borderline personality was used originally to describe people who show marked 'instability'. This instability was originally described in psychodynamic terms, notably by Kernberg (1975), as involving (a) ego weakness, with poor control of impulses, (b) 'primary process' (i.e. irrational) thinking despite intact reality testing, (c) use of less 'mature' defence mechanisms such as projection and denial, and (d) diffuse personal identity.

When this type of personality disorder was recognized in the classification systems, more objective criteria were developed, but it proved difficult to isolate a few core features. Also, different names have been adopted in the two systems of classification: in DSM-IV the term is borderline personality disorder, whereas in ICD-10 the term is emotionally unstable personality disorder. The latter is divided into a borderline type and an impulsive type. In DSM-IV borderline personality disorder is characterized by nine features, of which five are required to make a DSM-IV diagnosis. In ICD-10 there are five criteria for each subtype and four are required for diagnosis. The criteria are shown in summary form in Table 7.5 using terms that summarize those in the published criteria but do not repeat the exact wording. Table 7.5 shows that several features of the ICD-10 impulsive type are among the criteria for borderline personality disorder in DSM-IV.

TABLE 7.5 Abbreviated criteria for emotionally unstable and for borderline personality disorders

ICD-10	DSM-IV
Emotionally unstable personality disorder, borderline type	Borderline personality disorder
Disturbed or uncertain self-image	Identity disturbance
Intense and unstable relationships	Intense and unstable relationships
Efforts to avoid abandonment	Efforts to avoid abandonment
Recurrent threats or acts of self-harm	Recurrent suicidal behaviour
Chronic feelings of emptiness	Chronic feelings of emptiness
–	Transient stress-related paranoid ideation
Impulsive type	
Impulsive	Impulsive
Liability to anger and violence	Difficulty controlling anger
Unstable, capricious mood	Affective instability
Quarrelsome	–
Difficulty maintaining a course of action	–

Despite these attempts to define a borderline personality disorder, it is uncertain whether it exists as a separate entity. Many people who meet the criteria for borderline personality disorder in DSM-IV also meet the criteria for histrionic, narcissistic, and antisocial personality disorder (Skodal, 2002a).

Impulsive personality disorder

As explained above, this disorder is recognized in ICD-10 as a subtype of emotionally labile personality disorder. It is not included separately in DSM-IV though several of its features are listed as criteria for borderline personality disorder. Diagnostic criteria are shown in Table 7.5; three are required to make the diagnosis. People with impulsive personality disorder cannot control their emotions adequately. They are liable to sudden unrestrained anger, which they regret subsequently. These outbursts are not always confined to words, but may include physical violence, which may at times cause serious harm. Unlike people with antisocial personality disorder, who also exhibit explosions of anger, the impulsive group does not have other difficulties in relationships.

Histrionic personality disorder

Although histrionic personality disorder is included in both ICD-10 and DSM-IV, the criteria adopted are somewhat different. Table 7.6 shows the features that are diagnostic criteria in ICD-10 and notes also the criteria which differ between the two systems.

Self-dramatization is a striking feature of this personality disorder. It may extend to emotional 'blackmail', angry scenes, and demonstrative suicide attempts. These people are **suggestible** and easily influenced by others, especially by figures of authority. They follow the tastes and opinions of others, and adopt the latest

TABLE 7.6 Features of histrionic personality disorder

Self-dramatization
Suggestibility
Shallow, labile affect
Seeks attention and excitement
Inappropriately seductive
Over-concern with physical attractiveness
Note DSM-IV has two additional criteria: • speech excessively impressionistic; and • considers relationships more intimate than they are

fads and fashions. These people **seek attention and excitement**. They crave new experiences, are easily bored, and have short-lived enthusiasms.

These people have a **shallow labile affect**. They display their emotions in a dramatic manner, and may exhaust others with tantrums of rage or unrestrained expressions of despair. There is little depth to these emotional outpourings and they recover quickly, and seem surprised that other people have not forgotten the scenes as quickly as they have done. They are flirtatious and **inappropriately seductive**, but their sexual feelings, like their other emotions, are shallow and they may fail to reach orgasm despite elaborate displays of passion.

These people are **overconcerned with physical attractiveness**. In an attempt to impress others they spend excessive amounts of time and money on clothes, and personal grooming, and they are unreasonably upset by even minor criticism of their appearance.

As well as the above features, which are used as diagnostic criteria, two other aspects of the histrionic personality disorder deserve mention. These people are **self-centred**. They lack consideration for others, and put their own interests and enjoyment first. They appear vain, inconsiderate, and demanding, and may go to extreme lengths to force other people to fall in with their wishes. They also have a marked capacity for **self-deception**. They believe their own lies, however elaborate and improbable, even when other people have seen through the deceit. This pattern of behaviour is observed in its most extreme form in 'pathological liars' and swindlers.

Since some of the above qualities are normal in children (for example, transient enthusiasms, and make-believe), some psychiatrists have applied the term 'immature' to this type of personality disorder. However, the term should be avoided because it is imprecise and pejorative.

Narcissistic personality disorder

This personality disorder is listed in DSM-IV but not in ICD-10 where it is one of the disorders coded in the residual category 'other specific personality disorder'. The DSM-IV criteria are summarized and paraphrased in Table 7.7.

People with this disorder have a grandiose sense of self-importance and are boastful and pretentious. They are preoccupied with fantasies of unlimited success, power, beauty, or intellectual brilliance. They think themselves special and expect others to admire them and offer special services and favours. They feel entitled to the best and seek to associate with people of high status. They exploit people and do not empathize with, or show concern for, their feelings. They envy the possessions and achievements of others, and expect that others will envy them in the same way. They appear arrogant, disdainful, and haughty, and behave in a patronizing or condescending way.

TABLE 7.7 Features of narcissistic personality disorder

Grandiose self-importance
Fantasizes unlimited success, power, etc.
Believes himself special
Requires excessive admiration
Sense of entitlement to favours and compliance
Exploits others
Lacks empathy
Envious; believes others envy him
Arrogant and haughty

Cluster C personality disorders

Avoidant (anxious) personality disorder

In DSM-IV the term avoidant is used to denote this kind of personality disorder, whilst in ICD-10 the term anxious personality is preferred, with 'avoidant' as an accepted alternative. Slightly different features are used as diagnostic criteria in the two classifications, as shown in Table 7.8 in which the features are summarized. Liability to tension is a criterion only in ICD-10.

People with this disorder are **persistently tense**. They feel insecure and lack self-esteem. They feel **socially inferior**, unappealing, and socially inept. They

TABLE 7.8 Features of avoidant (anxious) personality disorder

Feelings of tension*
Feels socially inferior
Preoccupied with rejection
Avoids involvement
Avoids risk
Avoids social activity

Note DSM-IV has two additional criteria:
- restraint in intimate relationships because of fear of being shamed or ridiculed; and
- inhibited in new personal situations because of feelings of inadequacy.

* Not a DSM-IV criterion.

are **preoccupied with the possibility of rejection**, disapproval, or criticism, and worry that they will be embarrassed or ridiculed. They are cautious about new experiences and **avoid involvement** with unfamiliar people. They are timid in the face of everyday hazards and **avoid risk**. They are ill at ease in company and **avoid social activity**. They have few close friends, are inhibited in new personal situations, and their intimate relationships are constrained by fears of being shamed or ridiculed. Unlike people with schizoid personalities, they are not emotionally cold; indeed, they crave the social relationships that they cannot attain.

Dependent personality disorder

Table 7.9 shows that the features used as diagnostic criteria differ slightly in ICD-10 and DSM-IV. People with this disorder **allow others to take responsibility** for important decisions in their lives. They appear weak-willed and **unduly compliant** with the wishes of others. Nevertheless, they are **unwilling to make direct demands** on other people, but do this indirectly by appearing unable to help themselves. They lack vigour and **feel unable to care for themselves** and fear that they may have to do so. They lack self-reliance, avoid responsibility, and need **excessive help to make decisions**, asking repeatedly for advice and reassurance.

If married, such people may be protected from the full effects of their personality by support from a more energetic and determined spouse who is willing to make decisions and arrange activities. Their difficulties come to medical attention only when the spouse leaves or dies. Left to themselves, some drift down the social scale and are found among the long-term unemployed and the homeless. In the past this type of personality was called asthenic, inadequate, or passive.

TABLE 7.9 Features of dependent personality disorder

Allows others to take responsibility
Unduly compliant
Unwilling to make reasonable demands*
Feels unable to care for himself
Fear of being left to care for himself
Needs excessive help to make decisions

Note Three additional criteria are used in DSM-IV. They can be summarized as:
- difficulty in initiating projects;
- goes to excessive lengths to obtain support; and
- urgently seeks a supportive relationship.

*Not a criterion in DSM-IV.

TABLE 7.10 Features of obsessive–compulsive (anankastic) personality disorder

Preoccupied with details, rules, etc.
Inhibited by perfectionism
Overconscientious and scrupulous
Excessively concerned with productivity
Rigid and stubborn
Expects others to submit to his ways
Excessively pedantic and bound by convention*
Excessively doubting and cautious*

Note DSM-IV has two additional criteria:
- cannot discard worthless or worn out objects; and
- miserly; hoards money.

*These are not included in the DSM-IV criteria.

Obsessive–compulsive personality disorder

The term obsessive–compulsive personality disorder is used in DSM-IV. In ICD-10 the term anankastic (originated by Kahn, 1928), is used to avoid the false implication that this type of personality is directly linked to obsessional-compulsive disorder (see p. 197). Table 7.10 shows that slightly different features are used as diagnostic criteria in ICD-10 and DSM-IV.

These people are **preoccupied with details and rules**, order and schedules. They have an **inhibiting perfectionism** that makes ordinary work a burden and leaves the person immersed in trivial detail. They lack imagination and fail to take advantage of opportunities. They have high moral standards evident as **excessive conscientiousness and scruples**, and a judgemental approach. These characteristics stifle enjoyment so that these people seem humourless and are ill at ease when others are enjoying themselves. They are **unduly concerned with productivity at work** to the exclusion of relationships.

These people lack adaptability to new situations. They are **rigid and inflexible**; they dislike change and prefer a safe and familiar routine. They are **stubborn and controlling**, expecting others to submit to their ways. They are mean, sometimes to the point of being miserly, and they do not enjoy giving or receiving gifts. They do not like throwing things away and may hoard objects and money.

They are **pedantic and unduly concerned with social conventions**. Such people display **excessive doubt and caution** and they are indecisive. They find it hard to weigh up the advantages and disadvantages of new situations; they delay decisions, and often ask for more and more advice. They fear making mistakes, and after coming to a decision, they worry lest the choice was wrong.

Two other features are important, though they are not used as diagnostic criteria. **Sensitivity to criticism** is shown in an undue concern about other people's opinions, and an expectation of being judged harshly. These people show little emotion. They are, however, given to smouldering and unexpressed **feelings of anger and resentment**, often directed to people who have interfered with their routine of life. Such angry feelings may be accompanied by obsessional thoughts and images of an aggressive kind.

Passive–aggressive personality disorder

This term is applied to a person who, when demands are made upon him for adequate performance, responds with some form of passive resistance, such as procrastination, dawdling, stubbornness, deliberate inefficiency, pretended forgetfulness, and unreasonable criticism of people in authority. The category does not appear among the personality disorders in ICD-10 or DSM-IV.

Affective personality disorders

Some people have lifelong disorders of mood regulation. They may be persistently gloomy (depressive personality disorder) or habitually in a state of inappropriate elation (hyperthymic personality disorder). A third group alternates between these two extremes (cycloid or cyclothymic personality disorder). These types of personality disorder have been described for many years and are readily recognized in clinical practice. However, they do not appear in either the ICD-10 or DSM-IV systems of classification. The reason is that in both systems these disorders are classified under disorders of mood and not under disorders of personality. Thus they are classified under 'persistent mood (affective) states' (cyclothymia or dysthymia) in ICD-10, and under cyclothymia or dysthymia in DSM-IV. Nevertheless, it is convenient to describe them briefly here.

People with **depressive personality disorder** always seem to be in low spirits. They take a persistently gloomy view of life, anticipating the worst outcome of every event. They brood about their misfortunes and worry unduly. They often have a strong sense of duty. They show little capacity for enjoyment and they express dissatisfaction with their lives. Some are irritable and bad-tempered.

People with **hyperthymic personality disorder** are habitually cheerful and optimistic, and show a striking zest for living. If they have these traits to a moderate degree, they are often effective and successful. If they have these traits to an extreme degree, they show poor judgement and may be uncritical and hasty in coming to conclusions. Their habitual cheerfulness is often interrupted by periods of irritability, especially when their aims are frustrated. In the past, exceptionally contentious people in this group were called pseudoquerulant.

People with **cycloid personality disorder** alternate between the extremes of depressive and hyperthymic states described above. This instability of mood is much more disruptive than either of the persisting conditions. People with this disorder are periodically extremely cheerful, active, and productive. At such times they take on additional commitments in their work and social lives. Eventually their mood changes. Instead of confident optimism, they have a gloomy defeatist approach to life. Their energy is reduced. Whereas in the elated phase they took up activities with much relish, now they find them a burden. They make different but equally unwise decisions, and they refuse opportunities that could be managed. Eventually they return to a normal mood or to further elation.

Terms to avoid

It has been explained above that the term psychopathic personality is unsatisfactory (see pp. 132–3). Two other commonly used terms are also unsatisfactory and should be avoided. Both tend to be used when the interviewer has not thought clearly enough about the precise nature of his patient's difficulties. The first, **inadequate personality**, is often used pejoratively. In place of this term, it is better to specify precisely the ways in which the person is inadequate to the demands of life. Such a specification will lead to more constructive ideas about helping the person to cope better.

The second term, **immature personality**, is often used vaguely to denote a non-specific discrepancy between the patient's behaviour and his chronological age, such that the behaviour is more appropriate to a younger person than to a person of the patient's age. To avoid the vagueness of the term immature, it is better to specify the exact nature of the problem, whether it is in social relationships, the control of emotions, willingness to take responsibility, or elsewhere. Such specification of the patient's problems is more likely to lead to a constructive approach than is the mere labelling of the personality as immature. It also avoids the implication of an unsubstantiated cause, namely a failure of maturation.

Epidemiology

Epidemiological research into personality disorders (PD) in the general population began after the development of standardized instruments using DSM-III criteria. The studies require large samples because the prevalence rates of some personality disorders are low. Also, it is difficult to identify personality disorder reliably in community surveys in which interviewers seldom have access to information from informants. Data come mainly from eight studies in the USA, the UK, and Germany (reviewed by de Girolamo and Gotto, 2000).

Estimates of the **total prevalence** (i.e. the sum of all types) of personality disorder vary from about 6–15 per cent in the eight studies. Rates are generally higher in urban than in rural populations (see, for example, Casey and Tyrer, 1986). The latest and probably most reliable figure for the UK is lower, at 4.4 per cent (Singleton *et al.*, 2000). The rates of personality disorder are about the same in men and women and decrease with age.

Higher overall rates of personality disorder have been reported in patients with psychiatric symptoms including those attending primary care. Among the latter the rate is as high as 30 per cent (Moran *et al.*, 2000). Among psychiatric outpatients and inpatients, overall rates of personality disorders of up to 50 per cent have been reported (see de Girolamo and Gotto, 2000).

Estimates of the **prevalence of the various types** of personality disorder are shown in Table 7.11. In these studies sample sizes ranged from 200 to 1600. Some of these estimates have a substantial range, reflecting, among other sources of variation, the use of different assessment instruments. Rates of some disorders vary between men and women: antisocial personality disorder is more common among men (estimated ratios vary between 2.1 and 7.1). Although borderline and histrionic personality disorders are often described as more frequent among women, this was not a consistent finding in these studies.

Some curious apparent variations in the prevalence of specific PD categories has been found between countries, such as a low prevalence of antisocial PD in Taiwan. No convincing explanations have been offered for the large variations in prevalence figures, even from well-designed surveys using large numbers. The prevalence of some PDs may vary with cultural environment and practice, perhaps through the mediator of childhood environment (see below), local genetic variations, or the effect of the inclusion of reference to cultural norms in current definitions of personality disorder.

Aetiology

General issues

The causes of personality disorder are uncertain. Genetic factors have been proposed, together with various kinds of early life experience. Some personality disorders have been linked aetiologically with the psychiatric disorders which they resemble.

Genetic causes are considered below, where the aetiology of particular kinds of personality disorder is outlined. The study of the influence of **early life experiences** is made difficult by the long interval between these experiences and diagnosis of personality disorder in adult life. Psychodynamic theories linking childhood experience and personality are mentioned in the account that follows where they have been influential.

Whether or not they accept psychodyamic theories of personality, most clinicians agree that there are causal links between childhood experience, personality and personality disorder. It is agreed good practice to assess childhood experiences and to use common-sense judgement to decide whether any of these experiences could have influenced the development of personality. For example, extreme and repeated rejection by the parents may be linked to low self-esteem in adult life. Retrospective studies present obvious problems, but prospective studies are becoming available. In one such study independently documented gross physical neglect or abuse or sexual abuse in childhood was found to be associated with an increased risk of cluster B personality disorders in later life (Johnson *et al.*, 1999).

TABLE 7.11 Median prevalence rates of personality disorders in epidemiological surveys

Personality cluster	Personality disorder	Number of studies	Rate (per cent)
Cluster A	Paranoid	8	0.6
	Schizoid	9	0.4
	Schizotypal	8	0.6
Cluster B	Antisocial	18	1.9
	Borderline	9	1.6
	Histrionic	8	2.0
Cluster C	Obsessive–compulsive	8	1.7
	Avoidant	7	0.7
	Dependent	8	0.7
	Passive–aggressive	7	1.7

Data from de Girolamo and Dotto (2000).

The relationship between some **personality disorders and mental disorders** has already been considered. The similarity between cyclothymic personality and manic-depressive disorder led to the suggestion that they are causally related and this view is reflected in the classification system (see above p. 140). Similarly it has been suggested that schizoid personality disorder is a partial expression of schizophrenia but this is not supported by evidence (see p. 291) – though schizotypal personality disorder is so related. Likewise, the suggested relationship between obsessional personality disorder and obsessive–compulsive disorder has not been confirmed (Pfohl and Blum, 1991).

Since rather different causes have been suggested for the various types of personality disorder, they are considered separately below. Antisocial personality disorder is considered first because more research has been reported on this than on the other disorders. The rest are considered in the order in which they were described earlier in the chapter.

Antisocial personality disorder

Genetic causes

Twin studies The much quoted early twin studies by Lange (1931) and Rosanoff *et al.* (1934) were concerned with probands with repeated conviction for criminal offences, rather than antisocial personality disorder, so that their relevance to the latter is uncertain. More recent twin studies have confirmed the hereditability of antisocial behaviour in adults and shown that genetic factors are more important in adults than in antisocial children or adolescents where shared environmental factors are more important (Lyons *et al.*, 1995).

Adoption studies In an important study Cadoret (1978) found that adoptees separated at birth from a parent who had persistent antisocial behaviour, had higher rates of antisocial personality disorder than did adoptees whose parents were not antisocial. This finding held whether the biological father or biological mother had shown antisocial behaviour. Among the offspring, however, antisocial personality disorder was diagnosed more often in men than women, although the women had an increased rate of what was then diagnosed hysteria. Cadoret suggested that hysteria is an expression in women of the genetic endowment that causes antisocial personality disorder in men. Although this study had the shortcoming of a refusal rate of almost 30 per cent among those approached for interview, it confirmed the findings of a previous study (Crowe, 1974). A small study of the biological parents of adoptees with antisocial behaviour found an excess of antisocial behaviour compared with the biological parents of children who were not antisocial (Schulsinger, 1982).

Cadoret *et al.* (1995) studied the family environment as well as the parentage of adoptees. Again antisocial personality disorder in the biological parents predicted antisocial disorder in the adopted-away children. However, adverse factors in the adoptive environment (for example, marital problems or substance abuse) independently predicted adult antisocial behaviours.

Linkage studies These have proved difficult and at the time of writing no confirmed linkage has been reported.

Cerebral pathology and cerebral maturation

The observation that some brain-injured patients show aggressive behaviour suggested that minor degrees of brain injury might be a cause of antisocial personality. However, there is no convincing evidence to support of this idea. A report of evidence from MRI of reduced pre-frontal grey matter in the absence of gross brain lesions in people with antisocial personality disorder (Raine *et al.*, 2000) could indicate some kind of prefontal dysfunction. However, the findings need confirmation before their significance can be assessed. More recent brain imaging studies have revealed deficits in the amygdala response to emotional stimuli. In addition, amygdala volume may be decreased in sociopathic individuals. These findings have been linked to the lack of empathy which sociopathic people display towards the suffering of others (see Blair, 2003).

5-Hydroxytryptamine and aggression

Abnormalities in brain 5-hydroxytryptamine (5-HT) neurotransmission have been reported in patients with impulsive and aggressive behaviour, though not specifically in relation to antisocial personality disorder. Low levels of the 5-HT metabolite, 5-hydroxyindoleacetic acid (5-HIAA), have been found in the cerebrospinal fluid of subjects who have committed acts of unpremeditated violence (Linnoila and Virkkunen, 1992); and 5-HT-mediated prolactin release is lower in subjects with histories of impulsive aggressiveness (Coccaro *et al.*, 1989). It has been suggested that the same abnormalities may be relevant to personality disorders characterized by impulsive behaviour, particularly in the presence of pre-frontal deficits (Dolan *et al.*, 2002; New *et al.*, 2004).

Developmental theories

Separation In a much-quoted early study, Bowlby (1944, 1946) studied 44 'juvenile thieves' and concluded that separation of a young child from its mother could lead to antisocial behaviour and failure to form close relationships. This work stimulated much research into the effects of separating children from their mothers (see p. 654) and this research showed that the effects of separation are more varied than Bowlby had originally supposed. Not all separated children are affected adversely and the effects of separation depend on many factors, including the child's age, the previous relationship with the mother and father, and the reasons for separation.

Parental causes Separation from a parent usually follows a long period of tension and arguments between parents that could itself affect the child's development. Thus in an important study, Rutter (1972) showed that marital disharmony partly accounts for the association between separation and antisocial disorder in sons. As antisocial behaviour in childhood is linked to antisocial behaviour disorder in adult life (see below), these findings suggest a relationship between parental factors and antisocial personality disorder.

Social learning in childhood Many years ago, Scott (1960) proposed four ways in which antisocial behaviour could develop through social learning:

1. through growing up in an antisocial family;
2. through lack of consistent rules in the family;
3. learnt as a way of overcoming another problem (for example, aggressive behaviour to hide feelings of inferiority);
4. from poor ability to sustain attention and other impediments to learning.

There is evidence for some of these factors. For example, antisocial personality disorder is associated with physical abuse and with violent parenting without consistently applied rules (Pollock *et al.*, 1990), and with low IQ and large family of origin (Farrington *et al.*, 1988). However the main value of the scheme is that it provides the clinician with a useful framework for the assessment of possible causes of antisocial personality.

Childhood behaviour problems and antisocial personality An important 30-year follow-up study of children attending a child guidance clinic found an association between behaviour problems in childhood and antisocial personality disorder in adult life (Robins, 1966). Although only a minority of those even with the more serious antisocial behaviour in childhood went on to persistent antisocial behaviour in adult life, most of the adults with antisocial personality disorder had behaviour problems in childhood. This outcome was particularly likely if, in childhood, there was more than one kind of antisocial behaviour and if antisocial acts were repeated. Stealing among boys and sexual delinquency among girls were especially likely to be followed by antisocial behaviour in adult life. These early findings have been confirmed and early conduct problems have been shown to predict antioscial personality independently of associated adverse family and social factors (Hill, 2003).

Paranoid personality disorder

Little is known about the causes of this disorder. Some investigators have reported that paranoid personality disorder is more frequent among first degree relatives of probands with schizophrenia than among the general population (Kendler *et al.*, 1985a), but others have not confirmed this finding (Coryell and Zimmerman, 1989).

Schizoid personality disorder

The cause of this disorder is unknown. As noted above, schizoid personality does not appear to be closely related genetically to schizophrenia (Fulton and Winokur, 1993). Psychoanalytic ideas focus on the inability to give or receive love. This inability is thought to be a defence that developed early in life in response to inadequate mother–child relationships. Klein (1952) suggested that all infants pass through a stage of development, which she called 'schizoid position', in which oral and sadistic impulses are experienced as dangerous and are projected on to the parent. According to this theory, most children pass through this stage, but a few retain some of the projective defences. These ideas were not, however, applied to schizoid personality disorders as defined in current diagnostic manuals.

Schizotypal personality disorder

Increased rates of schizotypal personality disorder are found amongst relatives of probands with this disorder compared with relatives of co-twins (Torgersen, 1984) and with other family members (Baron *et al.*, 1985), suggesting a genetic aetiology. Schizotypal personality disorder is also more frequent among biological relatives of probands with schizophrenia than among adopted relatives or controls (Kendler *et al.*, 1981). A review of 17 structural imaging studies of people with this personality disorder found brain abonormalities similar in most ways to those in people with schizophrenia except for the temporal lobe and lateral ventrical abnormalities found in schizophrenia (Dickey *et al.*, 2002). These findings suggest that this personality disorder may be a milder form of schizophrenia, or that the two are related in some other way.

Borderline personality disorder

There is no convincing evidence of important genetic causes. Studies of the prevalence of borderline personality disorder among the relatives of probands with this disorder, have produced conflicting results. However, there may be an increased rate of affective disorder (Stone, 1987) and of other personality disorders (Pope *et al.*, 1983). It may be more fruitful to study the genetics of some of the traits that contribute to the overall clinical picture: for example dysregulation of affect, and poor impulse control (see Siever *et al.*, 2002). Psychoanalytic theories propose a disturbed relationship with the mother at the stage of individuation of the child (Kernberg, 1975). In keeping with this idea, people with the borderline personality are more likely than controls to report physical and sexual abuse in childhood (Berelowicz and Tarnopolsky, 1993). In a 28-year follow-up study Helgeland *et al.* found an association between abuse and neglect in childhood and later development of borderline disorder. Artistic and other talents and intellectual ability were found to be protective.

Histrionic personality disorder

There have been few objective studies of the causes of this personality disorder. The genetics of histrionic personality disorder has not been studied with standardized methods of assessment, and the few reported investigations have yielded inconsistent findings (McGuffin and Thapar, 1992). Psychoanalytic explanations relate this disorder either to failure to resolve Oedipal conflicts (Fenichel, 1945) or to oral conflicts (Marmor, 1953).

Obsessional personality disorder

Obsessional personality appears to have a substantial genetic aetiology (Murray and Reveley, 1981), although its nature is unknown. Psychoanalytic theory explains obsessional personality disorder as originating in problems at the anal stage of development. The clinical features of the disorder are explained as the result of the defence mechanisms of regression, reaction formation, and isolation (see p. 153). Neither explanation is supported by scientific evidence.

Anxious (avoidant) personality disorder

The genetics of anxious–avoidant personality disorder has not been studied separately from those of anxiety disorder. A cognitive model has been proposed by Beck and Freeman (1990) in which the central features are fear of rejection, self-criticism, and inaccurate evaluations of the reactions of other people, and the other features of the personality derive from them. The theory has not been supported by evidence.

Dependent and passive–aggressive personality disorders

The cause of these personality disorders is unknown. No genetic causes have been identified. Psychoanalytic ideas suggest that both disorders originate in problems at the oral stage of development. People with dependent personality disorder report intrusive parenting (Head *et al.*, 1991) but the limitations of such reports were noted above.

The prognosis of personality disorder

Personality disorders are defined as lifelong conditions, so little change would be expected with time. There is little reliable evidence about their outcome. A review of nine follow-up studies showed that only two were over periods of more that 4 years. The studies varied widely in methods of sampling and assessment, and most were concerned with rather small groups. A large-scale ongoing study by the US National Institute of Mental Health should provide better information.

Aggressive and antisocial personality disorders Clinical impressions indicate that minor improvement may take place, slowly and especially in aggressive and antisocial behaviour. In the study by Robins mentioned above, about a third of people with persistent antisocial behaviour in early adult life improved later, as judged by arrests and contacts with social agencies. However, they still had problems in relationships, as shown by hostility to wives and neighbours, as well as an increased rate of suicide.

Borderline personality disorder The outcome is very varied, suggesting that it may not be a single entity (Skodal *et al.*, 2002b). For example, Stone *et al.* (1987) found that only about one in four of those from the higher social classes who received this diagnosis in their twenties still met criteria for the same diagnosis in middle age. However, most met the criteria for another personality disorder, including histrionic, avoidant, and obsessive types. People who continued to meet the criteria for the original diagnosis more often had comorbid substance abuse or a criminal record. A high rate of suicide has been found in some studies (8.5 per cent in the study by Stone *et al.* 1987) but not in others.

Schizotypal personality disorder Mehlum *et al.* (1991) reported a 3–5-year follow-up in which the outcome of this personality disorder was worse than that of borderline personality disorder.

'Cluster C' personality disorders (see p. 138) seem to have a better outcome than the other groups.

Treatment

There is little evidence to guide the clinician in the choice of treatment for personality disorders. Few studies have met the basic requirements of randomization, blind assessment, and an appropriate control treatment. Tyrer and Davidson (2000) have identified other reasons for the lack of clinically relevant research, as follows.

Comorbidity

Comorbidity is common between personality disorders and other disorders, especially mood disorders and substance abuse. Few trials have ruled out the possibility that changes following treatment are due to improvement in a comorbid condition rather than in the personality disorder. This is particulary the case with borderline personality disorder in which mood disorder is common.

Ideally, two kinds of trial are required: trials with pure personality disorder to show whether treatment has an effect independent of any comorbid condition; and pragmatic trials, each with one of the comorbid disorders, to show the treatment effect that can be expected in clinical practice where comorbidity is common.

Duration of treatment and follow-up

Most clinical trials report changes over periods that are too short when judged against the natural course of personality disorders. Tyrer and Davidson suggest 2 years as the necessary minimum.

Collaboration and drop out

Personality disorder is often associated with poor collaboration with treatment but clinical trials necessarily involve patients who will collaborate. Even with the more collaborative patient, the size of the drop-out rates makes it difficult to generalize from the results. The problem is made worse by the long follow-up period required - see above.

Outcome measures

Assessments of personality disorder reflect change in mental state as well as change in personality (and change in mental state may be due to change in a comorbid disorder - see above). Also, personality disorder is defined by suffering to the self or others but it is difficult to measure change in these variables. In trials of treatment of antisocial personality, easily counted events such as reoffending have been used as an outcome measure but changes in these measures may be due to factors other than change in personality.

Drug treatments

Apart form their effect on comorbid mood disorder, drug treatment could affect the biological basis of a personality disorder (see aetiology above), or it might have a non-specific effect on anxiety, aggression, or other symptoms.

Antipsychotic drugs

Typical antipsychotics have been used to treat borderline and schizotypal personality disorders but the clinical trials have had mixed results (see Tyrer and Bateman, 2004). The atypical antipsychotics olanzepine and risperidone have been reported to reduce the hostility and chronic dysphoria of borderline personality disorder (Bogenschutz *et al.*, 2004; Zanarini *et al.*, 2001). These drugs are also reported to be of benefit in schizotypal personality disorder (Keshaven *et al.*, 2004; Koenigsberg *et al.*, 2003).

Antidepressant drugs

Amitriptyline has been tested against placebo as a treatment for borderline personality disorder (Soloff *et al.*, 1986; Soloff, 1994). Some patients responded well, others not at all, a finding that could be due to an effect on associated depressive disorder. Fluoxetine has also been reported to be more effective than placebo in reducing anger in people with borderline personality disorder (Salzmann *et al.*, 1995; Coccaro and Kavoussi, 1997). An open trial Venlafaxine was found to reduce self-injury in borderline disorder (Markovitz and Wagner, 1995). Safety in overdose is a crucial factor in prescribing antidepressants to people with a history of overdosing.

Mood stabilizers

Valproate has been investigated in borderline disorder in a small randomized trial and reported to produce improvements in aggression, depression and general symptomatology (Hollander *et al.*, 2003). Reports that lithium reduces anger and impulsiveness in antisocial personalities have not been convincingly replicated (see Nilsson, 1993 for a review). In any case, there is a practical difficulty that people with aggressive behaviour may not comply with the strict regimen required for the safe use of lithium. Carbamazepine has been used in the management of personality disorders but findings have not been consistent.

For a review of drug treatment for personality disorder, see Tyrer and Bateman (2004).

Psychological treatments

Supportive therapy

Psychological support is the mainstay of treatment of people with personality disorder. For some, modest but useful progress can be achieved over a period of months, but for antisocial personality disorders support may be required for years. Support may be provided by a member of the psychiatric team, or if the person has broken the law, by a probation officer. A probation order can be a useful external control for people with antisocial behaviour whose initial motivation to change was poor.

Counselling

Problem-solving counselling (see p. 585) can help patients deal with stressful circumstances that provoke abnormal behaviour or painful feelings. The approach is less likely than other forms of counselling to lead to dependency and transference problems in patients with cluster C disorders. Its practical step-by-step aspects are also valuable for patients with cluster B disorders.

Psychodynamic counselling which links past experiences to present difficulties should be used selectively for personality disorders. It is most likely to help young people who lack confidence, have difficulty in making relationships, and are uncertain about the direction that their lives should take. Also they should be highly motivated to examine and reconsider their attitudes and emotions. For borderline and antisocial personalities, psychodynamic approaches are generally less helpful than problem solving counselling.

Dynamic psychotherapy

This treatment requires that the person wishes to change and is able to collaborate. Even when these requirements are met, the technique has had to be modified with less emphasis on the reconstruction of past events and more on ways of relating to others, coping with external difficulties, and dealing with feelings. The analysis of transference and counter-transference is important as a way of identifying problems in relationships. A more recent modification has been called mentalization. It aims to help patients understand in terms of feelings, beliefs and desires, their own reactions to others and other people's reactions to the patient's behaviour (see Bateman and Fonagy, 2004).

There have been too few controlled studies of this kind of treatment for personality disorder to reach a conclusion about its effectiveness (see Bateman and Tyrer, 2004a). One often quoted study compared short-term dynamic psychotherapy and a short-term therapy directed to better adaptation. Both were superior to a waiting list condition, but they did not differ from one another (Winston *et al.*, 1991).

Cognitive therapy

Cognitive therapy was adapted for use with personality disorders by Beck and Freeman (1990). Therapists focus on modes of thinking and beliefs that characterize the personality disorder and underlie the problematic emotions and behaviour. They attempt to change these cognitions with the usual cognitive therapy techniques (see p. 594). Good results have been claimed but the methods have not been proved effective; for example manual assisted cognitive therapy failed to reduce the repetition of self harm in borderine personality disorder (Tyrer *et al.*, 2004).

Cognitive–analytic therapy

This approach (see p. 601) has been applied to borderline personality disorder (Ryle, 1997), but its value has not been established in clinical trials. Young's schema focused approach is also used (Young, 1999), but this too awaits evaluation in controlled trials.

A meta-analysis of trials of 14 studies of psychodynamic and 11 studies of cognitive therapies for personality disorders found an effect size of 1.46 for psychodynamic therapy and of only 1.00 for cognitive therapy (Leichsenring and Leibing, 2003). However, the effect sizes cannot be compared directly because of differences in patient populations and other variables.

For a review of psychological treatments for personality disorder see Bateman and Tyrer (2004a).

The management of personality disorders

Assessment

As well as deciding the diagnosis, the **strengths and weaknesses** of the individual should be assessed. Strengths are important because treatment should build on favourable features as well as to attempt to modify unfavourable ones. The patient's **circumstances** should be assessed next. Detailed observations over several weeks should be made to discover any circumstances that provoke undesirable behaviour, such as aggression. Patients generally appreciate the value of this practical approach and collaborate in the assessment. If such enquiries reveal factors that worsen the abnormal behaviour, attempts should be made to change or avoid them. Sometimes the enquiries suggest a new approach to treatment. For example, a man who is aggressive to women may become angry when he is rejected, and this rejection may be provoked by his clumsy approach to women. He might be helped by counselling and social skills training directed to this clumsiness.

General aims of management

Although there has been some progress in finding ways of effecting change in personality disorders, management still consists largely of helping people find a way of life that conflicts less with their character. Whatever treatment is used, aims should be modest and considerable time should be allowed to achieve them. A trusting and confiding relationship is the basis of treatment. However, the relationship should not be allowed to become one of dependency, as it may do when the personality disorder includes traits of dependency. To avoid this, people should not be seen too frequently, and the therapist should be alert to the early signs of dependency (see p. 584). Group treatment can sometimes be a way of lessening this problem. Often, more than one professional is involved in the care of these patients, helping with pharmacological, psychological and social aspects of care, and close collaboration is needed to avoid inconsistencies of approach. Many of these patients react badly to changes in staff which may re-enact painful losses, rejections, or separations in their earlier life.

The overall plan should include attempts to help the patient have less contact with situations that provoke difficulties, and more opportunity to develop assets in the personality. Patients should be encouraged to take an active part in planning their care and the reasons for decisions should be explained clearly and discussed fully. Patients should be helped to avoid adding to their problems by misusing drugs or alcohol, or by entering into unsatisfactory relationships. They should be encouraged to develop leisure interests, pursue further education, and increase their social network. Even if no improvement is achieved, these basic steps may stabilize the situation until some fortuitous change in the patient's life brings about improvement.

Choice of psychotherapy Psychodynamic or cognitive psychotherapy may be added to these basic procedures when the patient is well motivated and enough stability has been achieved to enable him to focus on the treatment. The choice of approach will depend on the type of personality disorder (see below) and on the person's preferences.

Choice of medication Medication has only a small part in the treatment of personality disorders. Medication should not be the first choice and, when it is prescribed, it should be part of a wider plan embracing psychological and social care. Anxiolytic medication should be used with special caution because of the risk of dependency. Antidepressants are used mainly for associated mood disorder – which is a common reason for the worsening of the emotional and behavioural problems associated with the personality disorder (for the use of antidepressants in borderline personality disorder, see below). Antipsychotics are occasionally useful in reduce aggressive behaviour. These and other special uses were considered above (in the section on treatment) and are referred to again in the section on the management of specific personality disorders, below.

Organization of services People with personality disorder can be cared for by a single practitioner who integrates the psychological, pharmacological, and social aspects of treatment, calling on specialist help when needed. The arrangement makes it easier for the practitioner to understand and help with relationship problems and it emphasizes the essential unity of the person's diverse problems. Howvere, it can be difficult to sustain when the personality disorder is severe. Alternatively, care can be provided by a community team, with a key worker who coordinates the contributions of other team members. In some places, there are specialist teams whose members develop additional expertise in helping people with personality disorder. See Bateman and Tyrer (2004b) for a review of services for personality disorder.

Progress

Progress is often achieved as a series of small steps by which the person gradually moves nearer to a satisfactory adjustment. Setbacks are common but they can be used constructively since it is at these times that people are most likely to be willing to confront their problems. Although therapists should try hard and long to help people with personality disorder, they should recognize that some people may not benefit.

The management of specific personality disorders

The type of personality disorder is not always a good guide to the choice of effective treatment. Nevertheless, some associations have been described, mainly on the basis of clinical experience, and these will be considered next.

Paranoid personality disorder

Patients with this disorder do not engage well in treatment because they are touchy and suspicious. If this problem can be overcome, supportive treatment may prevent the accumulation of problems caused by the patient's suspicious or angry responses to other people.

Schizoid personality disorder

Patients with schizoid personality avoid close personal contact and often drop out after a few sessions of treatment. If they can be persuaded to continue, they tend to intellectualize their problems and question the value of their treatment. The therapist should try to help these people become more aware of their problems, and respond to them in ways that cause fewer difficulties. At best, the process is slow and the results are limited. Exploratory psychotherapy is unlikely to succeed, and medication is generally unhelpful.

Antisocial (dissocial) personality disorder

Treatment usually consists of the general measures discussed above. Medication has little value except that an antipsychotic drug may have a temporary effect of calming aggressive behaviour arising in response to increased stress, and antidepressant medication may be needed for a comorbid depressive disorder. Lithium has been claimed to reduce aggressive behaviour in some patients (see p. 145). It should not be prescribed unless it is reasonably certain that the patient will collaborate closely with the dosage regimen and the other requirements for safety (see p. 560). Anxiolytic drugs should be avoided because they may cause for disinhibition and dependency.

If resources are available, individual or group psychotherapy can be considered but the results are uncertain. The following points should be considered.

Individual psychotherapy

Good results have been reported with a modified form of dynamic psychotherapy in which people are confronted repeatedly and directly with evidence of their own abnormal behaviour. The method, derived from the work of Schmideberg (1947), requires a therapist with a particularly forceful and robust personality. The claims for good results are so far unproved.

Small-group therapy

People with antisocial personality disorder seldom benefit from the usual kind of small-group therapy, and often disrupt the treatment of the others in the group. Groups composed entirely of antisocial patients can sometimes be more constructive but they are difficult to conduct. The therapist needs considerable general skills in psychotherapy, and special training with this group of patients.

Therapeutic communities

Some of the earliest therapeutic communities such as the Henderson Hospital in England specialized in the treatment of antisocial personality disorder. (For the principles of this form of treatment see p. 607). No controlled evaluation of this treatment has been carried out, and there is no consensus about its value.

Other group regimens

Group methods have been applied in a more authoritarian setting to prisoners with personality disorder. At Grendon Prison in England this approach has been applied to the care and rehabilitation of prisoners who have not responded well in other prison environments. Good results have been reported, although a well controlled trial has not yet been conducted.

Histrionic personality disorder

These patients make many demands on their carers. Frequent problems include attempts to impose impractical conditions on treatment, requests for inappropriate medication, and demands for help at unreasonable times. Other problems include seductive behaviour, threats of self-harm, and attempts to prolong interviews unreasonably. It is important to identify these problems early because, once established, they cannot easily be controlled. The behaviours should be discussed with the patient, and clear limits set by offering appropriate help while explaining which behaviours cannot be accepted. One to one exploratory psychotherapy should be avoided, and treatment should focus on developing more adaptive ways of responding to stressful situations. Medication has little value unless there is a comorbid depressive disorder.

Borderline personality disorder

The general problems in managing borderline personality disorders are similar to that encountered with histrionic personality disorder (described above). However, there are more therapeutic options. Problem-solving counselling (see p. 585) is sometimes helpful. Small doses of an antipsychotic drug may reduce aggressive behaviour in the short term. A selective serotonin re-uptake inhibitor (SSRI) can be tried since some at least of these drugs appear to reduce impulsive behaviour in some patients (see p. 145). Anxiolytic medication should be avoided because of its potential for disinhibition and dependence. If prescribed, mediaction should be part of a wider plan of treatment.

Several kinds of psychological treatment can be tried when resources are available, though none has been proved to have a substantial and reliable effect. The following points should be considered.

Dynamic psychotherapy

People with borderline personality disorder do not respond well to the usual forms of dynamic psychotherapy, and unskilled treatment may result in reduced emotional control and increased impulsiveness. Kernberg (1993) described an alternative approach for these patients, which is less likely to have these adverse effects but still deals with what is thought to be the core psychopathology. This approach, called **expressive psychotherapy**, is claimed to give good results (see, for example, Stone *et al.*, 1987), but to date no randomized controlled trials have been reported. For a review of dynamic psychotherapy for borderline personality disorder see Higgitt and Fonagy (1993).

Group psychotherapy

This treatment has the advantages that transference relationships are spread over the group instead of focused on the therapist, and that the group's comments on acting out behaviour may be accepted more readily than those of the therapist. The therapist needs considerable skill if the borderline patient is to be helped without disrupting the treatment of the other group members. It is seldom practicable to treat more than one borderline patient in a group. For a review of group treatment see Clarkin *et al.* (1991).

Dialectical behaviour therapy

This type of therapy is described on p. 599. As noted above, this treatment is one of the few that have been evaluated in a controlled trial – with females with borderline personaly disorder who had made repeated suicide attempts. Dialectic behaviour therapy was more effective than the control treatment in reducing self-harm but the effect on the personality disorder was not assessed directly and most of the benefits were lost on longer follow-up (Linehan *et al.*, 1991).

Psychoanalytically oriented day treatment

The treatment combines analytic groups and psychoanalytic individual treatment and is designed to increase the patient's ability to better understand the mental states of others. The treatment is supported by the results of a small randomized controlled trial with borderline patients showing improvemen in all tested domains after 18 months treatment (Bateman and Fonagy, 1999). The gains were maintained or improved at 18 month follow-up (Bateman and Fonagy, 2001).

Obsessional personality disorder

People with this personality disorder do not respond well to psychotherapy. Unskilled treatment can lead to excessive morbid introspection, which leaves the person worse rather than better. Treatment should be directed to avoiding situations that increase the patient's difficulties, and to developing better ways of coping with stressful situations. Patients often seek help during an associated depressive disorder, and it is important to identify and treat this comorbid condition.

Avoidant (anxious) personality disorders

These patients generally have low self-esteem and fear disapproval and criticism. They can be helped by a therapeutic relationship in which they feel valued and able to reconsider their perception of themselves. Some leave treatment, fearing criticism or rejection, and such feelings should be anticipated and discussed constructively as soon as they appear. The therapist should be alert to the possibility of a comorbid depressive disorder, requiring treatment.

Dependent personality disorder

Dynamic psychotherapy may increase these patients' dependence. They are usually helped more by problem-solving counselling, in which they are encouraged to take increasingly more responsibility for themselves. Medication should be avoided unless there is an associated depressive disorder.

Ethical problems

Stigma and patient involvement

From early ideas of moral insanity to the present time, the concept of personality disorder has been linked to a moral judgement; people told they have a disordered personality believe there is something inadequate in who they are. This problem finds its echoes in some professionals attitudes and in the difficulty people with personality disorder have in accessing psychiatric and other services. Once made, the diagnosis tends to stick and to affect the person's subsequent care as well as the way other people think of them over the longer term. For this reason many clinicians are reluctant to make the diagnosis. The increasing involvement of patients in planning of service delivery and research, stemming partly from the ideas of therapeutic community movement, may help to reduce these disadvantages. The emphasis on encouraging patients' involvement in decisions about their care, which is a central part of the modern management of all psychiatric disorders, is especially important in the management of personality disorder.

Further reading

Gelder, MG, López-Ibor, JJ Jr and Andreasen, NC (eds) (2000) *The new Oxford textbook of psychiatry*, Section 4.12: Personality disorder. Oxford University Press, Oxford. (The seven chapters in this section provide a comprehensive review of personality disorder.)

Gunderson, JG and Hoffman, PD (eds) (2005) *Understanding and treating borderline personality disorder; a guide for professionala and families*. American Psychiatric Publishing, Washington D.C.

Schneider, K (1950) *Psychopathic personalities* (trans. MW Hamilton). Cassell, London. (A classic text of great importance in the development of ideas about personality disorder.)

Tyrer, P (ed.) (2000) *Personality disorders: diagnosis, management and course*, 2nd edn.Butterworth-Heinemann, Oxford. (Contains systematic reviews of the subject, and an account of the editor's Personality Assessment Schedule.)

Appendix

BOX 7.1 SOME INSTRUMENTS FOR DIAGNOSING PERSONALITY DISORDERS

International Personality Disorders Examination (Loranger *et al.*, 1994)

- Assesses DSM-IV and/or ICD-10 personality disorders categorically and/or dimensionally;
- Semi-structured clinical interview in two versions: a DSM-IV version with 99 sets of questions and an ICD-10 version with 67 sets of questions. There is a screening questionnaire for each version which can be used to identify people who are unlikely to have a personality disorder.

Structured Clinical Interview for DSM-IV Axis II Personality Disorders (SCID-II) (First *et al.*, 1995)

- Assesses DSM-IV personality disorders either categorically or dimensionally;
- Semi-structured clinical interview with 119 sets of questions. There is a screening interview to identify people unlikely to have a personality disorder.

Structured Interview for DSM-IV Personality (SIDP-IV) (Pfohl *et al.*, 1997)

- Assess DSM-IV and ICD-10 personality disorders either categorically or dimensionally;
- A semi-structured clinical interview with 101 questions in a thematic version and 107 questions in a disorder-by-disorder version.

For further information on these and other instruments for personality assessment see Task Force for Psychiatric Measures (2000), Chapter 32.

CHAPTER 8

Reactions to stressful experiences

Chapter contents

Stressful events frequently provoke psychiatric disorders. Such events can also provoke emotional reactions that are distressing but not of the nature or severity required for the diagnosis of an anxiety disorder or a mood disorder. These less severe reactions are discussed in this chapter together with post-traumatic stress disorder, which is an intense and prolonged reaction to a severe stressor. With the exception of normal grief reactions, the conditions described in this chapter are listed as disorders in ICD-10 and DSM-IV.

The chapter begins with a description of the several components of the response to stressful events, including coping strategies and mechanisms of defence. The classification of reactions to stressful experience is discussed next. The various syndromes are then described, including acute stress reactions, post-traumatic stress disorder, special forms of response to severe stress, and adjustment disorders. The chapter ends with an account of special forms of adjustment reaction, including adjustment to bereavement (grief) and to terminal illness, and the problems of adults who experienced sexual abuse in childhood.

The response to stressful events

The response to stressful events has three components:

1. An emotional response, with somatic accompaniments;
2. A coping strategy;
3. A defence mechanism.

Coping strategies and defence mechanisms are overlapping concepts but they originated from different schools of thought and for this reason they are described separately in the following account.

Emotional and somatic responses

These responses are of two kinds: **anxiety** responses with autonomic arousal leading to apprehension, irritability, tachycardia, increased muscle tension, and dry mouth, and **depressive** responses with pessimistic thinking and reduced physical activity. Anxiety responses are generally associated with events that pose a **threat**, whilst depressive responses are usually associated with events that involve separation or **loss**. These features of these responses are similar to, but less intense than, the symptoms of anxiety and depressive disorders (described in Chapters 9 and 11, respectively).

Coping strategies

Coping strategies serve to reduce the impact of stressful events, thus attenuating the emotional and somatic responses and making it more possible to maintain normal performance at the time (though not always in the longer term, see below). The term coping strategy is derived from research in social psychology; it is applied to activities of which the person is aware, for example, deliberately avoiding further stressors. (Responses of which the person is unaware are called defence mechanisms, and are described below.)

Coping strategies are of two kinds: problem-solving strategies, which can be used to make adverse circumstances less stressful, and emotion-reducing strategies, which alleviate the emotional response to the stressors.

Problem-solving strategies include:

- **seeking help** from another person;
- **obtaining information or advice** that would help to solve the problem;
- **solving problems** – making and implementing plans to deal with the problem;
- **confrontation** – defending one's rights, and persuading other people to change their behaviour.

Emotion-reducing strategies include:

- **ventilation of emotion** – talking to another person and expressing emotion;
- **evaluation of the problem** – to assess what can be changed and try to change it (by problem-solving), and what cannot be changed and to accept it;
- **positive reappraisal of the problem** – recognizing that it has led to some good, for example, that the loss of a job is an opportunity to find a more satisfying occupation;
- **avoidance of the problem** – by refusing to think about it, avoiding people who are causing it, or avoiding reminders of it.

Coping strategies are generally useful in reducing the problem or in lessening the emotional reaction. However, they are not always adaptive. For example, avoidance may not be adaptive in the early stages of physical illness because it can lead to delay in seeking appropriate treatment. Hence a person needs not only the ability to use coping strategies but also the ability to judge which strategy should be used in particular circumstances.

Maladaptive coping strategies

These strategies reduce the emotional response to stressful circumstances in the short term, but lead to greater difficulties in the long term. Maladaptive coping strategies include the following:

- **use of alcohol or unprescribed drugs** to reduce the emotional response or to reduce awareness of stressful circumstances.
- **deliberate self-harm** either by drug overdose or self-injury. Some people gain relief from tension by cutting the skin with a sharp instrument to induce pain and draw blood. Others take overdoses to withdraw from the situation or to show their need for help.
- **unrestrained display of feelings** can reduce tension, and in some societies such behaviour is sanctioned in particular circumstances, for example, grieving. In other circumstances, such behaviour can damage relationships with people who would otherwise have been supportive.
- **aggressive behaviour** aggression provides immediate release of feelings of anger. In the longer term, it may increase the person's difficulties by damaging relationships.

Coping styles

When particular coping mechanisms are used repeatedly by the same person in different situations, they are said to constitute a coping style. Some people change their coping strategies according to the circumstances;

BOX 8.1 DEFENCE MECHANISMS

Repression This is the exclusion from consciousness of impulses, emotions, or memories that would otherwise cause distress. For example, especially painful aspects of the memory of distressing events such as sexual abuse in childhood may be kept out of awareness for many years.

Denial This is a related concept: it is inferred when a person behaves as if unaware of something that he may reasonably be expected to know. For example, on learning that he is dying of cancer, a patient may continue to live normally as if unaware of the diagnosis. In this example, denial is adaptive since it can help to reduce depression. However, in the early stage of illness denial may delay seeking help or lead to refusal of necessary investigations and treatment. In this second example, denial is maladaptive.

Displacement This is the transfer of emotion from a person, object, or situation with which it is properly associated, to another source. For example, after the recent death of his wife, a man may blame the doctor for failure to give adequate care, and may thus avoid blaming himself for putting his work before her needs in the last months of her life.

Projection This is the attribution to another person of thoughts or feelings similar to one's own, thereby rendering one's own thoughts or feelings more acceptable. For example, a person who dislikes a colleague may attribute reciprocal feelings of dislike to him; it is then easier to justify his own feelings of dislike for the colleague.

Regression This is the adoption of behaviour appropriate to an earlier stage of development, for example, dependence on others. Regression often occurs among physically ill people. In the acute stages of illness it can be adaptive, enabling the person to acquiesce passively to intensive medical and nursing care. If regression persists into the stage of recovery and rehabilitation, it can be maladaptive because it reduces the patient's ability to make efforts to help themself.

Reaction formation This is the unconscious adoption of behaviour opposite to behaviour that would reflect true feelings and intentions. For example, excessively prudish attitudes to sex are sometimes (but not always) a reaction to the person's own sexual urges that they cannot accept.

Rationalization This is the unconscious provision of a false but acceptable explanation for behaviour that has a less acceptable origin. For example, a husband may leave his wife at home because he does not enjoy her company, but he may reassure himself falsely that she is shy and would not enjoy going out.

Sublimation This is the unconscious diversion of unacceptable impulses into more acceptable outlets, for example, turning the need to dominate others into the organization of good works for charity. (There are, of course, many other motives for charitable work.)

Identification This is the unconscious adoption of the characteristics or activities of another person, often to reduce the pain of separation or loss. For example, a widow may undertake the same voluntary work that her husband used to do.

for example, they use problem-solving strategies at work but employ avoidance when unwell. Some people habitually use maladaptive strategies; for example, they repeatedly abuse alcohol or take overdoses of drugs when under stress. For a review of coping strategies see Lazarus (1993). Later work has distinguished between 'coping style', which is seen as a relatively enduring behavioural trait, and 'coping response' which is much more specific to particular stressful environments (see Beutler *et al.*, 2003).

Defence mechanisms

Defence mechanisms (Box 8.1) are unconscious responses to external stressors as well as to anxiety arising from internal conflict. They were described originally by Sigmund Freud and later elaborated by his daughter Anna Freud (1936). In response to stressful circumstances, the most frequent mechanisms are repression, denial, displacement, projection, and regression. Defence mechanisms are unconscious processes, i.e. people do not use them deliberately and are unaware of their own real motives, although they may become aware later through introspection or through another person's comments. Freud identified defence mechanisms in his study of the 'psychopathology of everyday life', a term that he applied to slips of the tongue and lapses of memory. The concept of defence mechanisms has proved useful in understanding many aspects of the day-to-day behaviour of people under stress, notably those with physical or psychiatric illness. Freud also used the concept of mechanisms of defence to explain the aetiology of mental disorders, but this extension of his original observations has not proved useful.

The main mechanisms of defence are illustrated in Box 8.1.

Present circumstances, previous experience, and response to stressful events

Brown and Harris (1978) showed that the response to a stressful life event is modified by present circumstances and by past experience. Some current circumstances make a person more vulnerable to stressful life events, for example, the lack of a confidant with whom to share problems. Such circumstances are called **vulnerability factors**. Previous experience can also increase vulnerability; for example, the experience of losing a parent in childhood may make a person more vulnerable in adult life to stressful events involving loss. It is difficult to examine these more remote associations scientifically. (Life events and vulnerability factors are considered further on p. 94.)

Classification of reactions to stressful events

Although included within the classifications of diseases, not all reactions to stressful events are abnormal. Grief is a normal reaction to the stressful experience of bereavement, and only a minority of people have a very severe or abnormally prolonged reaction. There is also a normal pattern of reaction to a dangerous or traumatic event such as a car accident. Most people have an immediate feeling of great anxiety, are dazed and restless for a few hours afterwards, and then recover; a few people have more severe and prolonged symptoms – an abnormal reaction. It is difficult to decide where to make a separation between normal and abnormal reactions to stressful events in terms of severity or of duration, and in practice the division is arbitrary. Similarly, amongst patients in hospital for medical or surgical treatment, most are anxious but a few are severely anxious and show extreme denial or other defence mechanisms that impair cooperation with treatment.

ICD-10 and DSM-IV reactions to stressful experiences are classified into three groups (Table 8.1).

Acute reactions to stress

This category is for immediate and brief responses to sudden intense stressors in a person who does not have another psychiatric disorder at the time. The ICD-10

TABLE 8.1 Classification of reactions to stressful experience

ICD-10	DSM-IV
Acute stress reaction	Acute stress disorder
Post-traumatic stress disorder	Post-traumatic stress disorder
Adjustment disorder	Adjustment disorder
◆ Brief depressive reaction	◆ With depressed mood
◆ Mixed anxiety and depressive reaction	◆ With mixed anxiety and depressed mood
◆ Predominant disturbance of other emotions	◆ With anxiety
◆ Predominant disturbance of conduct	◆ With disturbance of conduct
◆ Mixed disturbance of emotions and conduct	◆ With mixed disturbance of emotions and conduct
◆ Other specified symptoms	◆ Unspecified

The order of the subgroups has been changed to show similarities and differences between the two systems.

definition of acute stress reaction requires that the response should start within an hour of exposure to the stressor and begins to diminish after not more than 48 hours. The DSM-IV definition of acute stress disorder states that the onset should be while or after experiencing the distressing event and requires that the condition lasts for at least 2 days and for no more than 4 weeks. These two definitions capture different phases of the anxiety response as the different terms, reaction and disorder, suggest. ICD refers to the short-lived normal response. DSM-IV refers to the more prolonged response, which is less common. Both diagnostic systems require that the stressor must be of an exceptional nature and, in the case of DSM-IV, that actual or threatened injury to self or others has occurred.

Post-traumatic stress disorder

This is a prolonged and abnormal response to exceptionally intense stressful circumstances such as a natural disaster or a sexual or other physical assault.

Adjustment disorder

This is a more gradual and prolonged response to stressful changes in a person's life. In both ICD-10 and DSM-IV, adjustment disorders are subdivided, according to the predominant symptoms, into depressive, mixed anxiety, and depressive, with disturbance of conduct, and with mixed disturbance of emotions and conduct. DSM-IV has an additional category of adjustment disorder with anxiety. ICD-10 has an additional category of 'predominant disturbance of other emotion', which includes not only adjustment disorder with anxiety but also adjustment disorder with anger.

In ICD-10 the three types of reaction to stressful experience are classified together under 'reactions to stress and adjustment disorders', which is a subdivision of section F4, 'neurotic, stress-related and somatoform disorders'. The defining characteristics of this group of reactions to stress and of adjustment disorders are:

- they arise as a **direct consequence** of either acute stress or continued unpleasant circumstances;
- it is judged that the disorder would not have arisen without these factors.

A different organizing principle is used in DSM-IV: acute stress disorder and post-traumatic stress disorder are classified as anxiety disorders, whilst adjustment disorders have their own place in the classification, separate from the anxiety disorders.

Additional codes in ICD-10

If any of these reactions is accompanied by an act of deliberate self-harm, another code can be added to record this fact (codes X60–X82 list 23 methods of self-harm). It is also possible to specify certain kinds of stressful event by adding a code from Chapter Z; for example, Z58 problems related to employment and unemployment, and Z63 problems related to family circumstances.

Coding grief reactions

In ICD-10, abnormal grief reactions are coded as adjustment disorders. Reactions to bereavement that are appropriate to the person's culture are not included. If it is appropriate to code them as part of the description of the patient's condition, code Z63.4 (death of a family member) can be used.

Acute stress reaction and acute stress disorder

Clinical picture

The **core symptoms** of an acute psychological response to stress are anxiety or depression. Anxiety is the response to threatening experiences; depression is the response to loss. Anxiety and depression often occur together, because stressful events often combine danger and loss; an extreme example is a road accident in which a companion is killed. Other symptoms include feelings of being numb or dazed, difficulty in remembering the whole sequence of the traumatic event, insomnia, restlessness, poor concentration, and physical symptoms of autonomic arousal, especially sweating, palpitations, and tremor. Anger or histrionic behaviour may be part of the response. Occasionally there is a flight reaction, for example, when a driver runs away from the scene of a road accident.

Coping strategies and defence mechanisms are also part of the acute response to stressful events. Avoidance is the most frequent coping strategy; the person avoids talking or thinking about the stressful events, and avoids reminders of them. The most frequent defence mechanism is denial.

Usually avoidance and denial recede as anxiety diminishes: memories of the events can be more readily accessed and the person is able to think or talk about them with less distress. This sequence allows working through and coming to terms with the stressful experience, though there may be continuing difficulty in recalling details of highly stressful events.

Variations in the clinical picture

Not all responses to acute stress follow this orderly sequence, in which coping strategies and defences are maintained long enough to allow the person to function until anxiety and depression subside and are then abandoned so that working through can occur. Not all coping strategies are adaptive; an example is excessive use of alcohol or drugs to reduce distress. Defence mechanisms may also be of the less adaptive types such as regression or displacement. Sometimes defence mechanisms persist longer than is adaptive; for example, denial may persist so long that 'working through' is delayed. Sometimes vivid memories of the stressful events intrude into awareness as images and flashbacks or disturbing dreams. When this state persists, the condition is called a post-traumatic stress disorder (PTSD).

Diagnostic conventions

As noted above, 'acute stress reaction' in ICD-10 and 'acute stress disorder' in DSM-IV capture different phases of the psychological response to stress (p. 157). The DSM definition refers to cases of more clinical importance and it is widely used. People who develop acute stress disorder are more likely to experience subsequent post-traumatic stress disorder (Brewin *et al.*, 2003). Indeed the symptomatology of PTSD is similar to acute stress disorder; the main difference is in the timing and duration of symptoms. However, around 50 per cent of those who eventually develop PTSD after a trauma do not meet criteria for acute stress disorder soon after it (McNally *et al.*, 2003).

Both systems of classification describe typical symptoms of the disorder. In DSM-IV the diagnosis of acute stress disorder requires marked symptoms of anxiety or increased arousal; re-experiencing of the event; and three from a list of five 'dissociative' symptoms, namely:

1. a sense of numbing or detachment;
2. reduced awareness of the surroundings ('being in a daze');
3. derealization;
4. depersonalization;
5. dissociative amnesia.

There must also be avoidance of stimuli that arouse recollections of the trauma, and significant distress or impaired social functioning. ICD-10 also requires that the symptom criteria for generalized anxiety disorder are met.

In ICD 10 dissociative and other symptoms are not required to diagnose the disorder in its mild form (F43.00) but two are required for the moderate form (F43.01) and four for the severe form (F43.02) from a list of seven, namely:

- withdrawal from expected social interaction;
- narrowing of attention;
- apparent disorientation;
- anger and verbal aggression;
- despair and hopelessness;
- inappropriate or purposeless activity; and
- uncontrollable and excessive grief.

The terms acute stress reaction and acute stress disorder are used only when the person was free from these symptoms immediately before the impact of the stressful event; otherwise the response is classified as an exacerbation of pre-existing psychiatric disorder.

Epidemiology

Rates in the population are unknown. The rate of acute stress disorder reported among survivors of motor vehicle accidents is 13 per cent among survivors (Harvey and Bryant, 1998), among victims of violent crime 19 per cent (Brewin *et al.*, 1999), and among the witnesses of a mass shooting 33 per cent (Classen *et al.*, 1998).

Aetiology

Many kinds of event can provoke an acute response to stress. Examples are involvement in a significant but brief event such as a motor accident or a fire, an event that involves actual or threatened injury such as a physical assault or rape, or the sudden discovery of serious illness. Some of these stressful events involve life changes to which further adjustment is required, for example, the serious injury of a close friend involved in the same accident. Not all people exposed to the same stressful situation develop the same degree of response (see epidemiology, above); this variation suggests that differences in constitution, previous experience, and coping styles may play a part in aetiology. However, there is little factual information since research has focused on the more severe and lasting PTSD.

Treatment

Planning for disaster

Planning is needed to ensure an immediate and appropriate response to the psychological effects of a major disaster. Such a response can be achieved by enrolling and training helpers who can support victims and are

BOX 8.2 THE PRINCIPAL COMPONENTS OF PSYCHOLOGICAL FIRST AID

- Comfort and consolation
- Protection from further threat and distress
- Immediate physical care
- Helping reunion with loved ones
- Sharing the experience (but not forced)
- Linking survivors with sources of support
- Facilitating a sense of being in control
- Identifying those who need further help (triage)

willing to be called on at short notice, and by agreeing procedures for contacting these helpers promptly. At the time of the disaster, priorities have to be decided between the needs of the victims of the disaster, those of relatives (including children), and those of members of the emergency services who may be severely affected by their experiences. The essential elements of psychological assistance for victims of disaster have been described by Alexander (2005) (Box 8.2).

Debriefing

After a major incident, counselling has often taken the form known as debriefing, or Critical Incident Stress Debriefing (CISD), provided individually or in a group. In debriefing the victim goes through the following stages after the counsellor has first explained the procedure:

- facts - the victims relate what happened;
- thoughts - they describe their thoughts immediately after the incident;
- feelings - they recall the emotions associated with the incident;
- assessment - they take stock of their responses;
- education - the counsellor offers information about stress responses and how to manage them.

Debriefing has been used widely but current evidence suggests that single session 'stand alone' debriefing is not helpful in lowering subsequent psychological distress and might even be harmful (for a meta-analysis see Rose *et al.*, 2003). It remains unclear whether debriefing might be useful as part of a coordinated treatment programme or whether delivery in a group setting might be more helpful.

Management

After a traumatic event, many people talk informally to a sympathetic relative or friends, or to a member of the professional staff dealing with any physical injuries originating during the incident. Since in most cases stress reactions will resolve with time, a policy of watchful waiting is appropriate, though it is good practice to offer a follow up appointment in about a month to identify subjects whose stressful symptoms are not settling and who might therefore be at high risk of developing PTSD.

More formal psychotherapy may be needed if there is no friend or professional who can assist, or if the stressful circumstances cannot easily be discussed with a relative or friend (for example, in some cases of rape), or if the response is prolonged or severe. The victim can be reassured that the condition is frequent, and often short lived. Advice may be needed about ways of dealing with the consequences of the traumatic events. If anxiety is severe, an anxiolytic drug may be prescribed for a day or two, and when sleep is severely disrupted a hypnotic drug may be given for one or two nights. If more formal psychotherapy is needed, there is evidence that brief trauma-focused cognitive behaviour therapy is more effective than supportive counselling and may help prevent the subsequent development of post-traumatic stress disorder (Bryant *et al.*, 1998; McNally *et al.*, 2003).

Post-traumatic stress disorder

This term denotes an intense, prolonged, and sometimes delayed reaction to an intensely stressful event. The essential features of a post-traumatic stress reaction are:

1. Hyperarousal,
2. Re-experiencing of aspects of the stressful events,
3. Avoidance of reminders.

Examples of extreme stressors that may cause this disorder are natural disasters such as floods and earthquakes, man-made calamities such as major fires, serious transport accidents, or the circumstances of war, and rape or serious physical assault on the person. The original concept of post-traumatic stress disorder (PTSD) was of a reaction to such an extreme stressor that any person would be affected. Epidemiological studies have shown that not everyone exposed to the same extreme stressor develops PTSD; hence personal predisposition plays a part. In many disasters the victims suffer not only psychological distress but also physical injury, which may increase the likelihood of a PTSD. Other predisposing factors are reviewed below under aetiology.

The condition now known as PTSD has been recognized for many years, though under other names. The term PTSD originated in the study of American servicemen returning from the Vietnam War. The diagnosis meant that affected servicemen could be given medical and social help without being diagnosed as suffering from another psychiatric disorder. Similar psychological effects have been reported (under other names) among servicemen in both world wars, and amongst survivors of peacetime disasters such as the serious fire at the Coconut Grove nightclub in America (Adler, 1943). For a historical review of the concept of PTSD see Jones *et al.* (2003).

Other reactions to severe stress

PTSD occurs only after exceptionally stressful events, but not every response to such events is represents PTSD. Combat veterans have high rates of depression, somatization disorder, and alcohol and drug misuse as well as PTSD. After road accidents, various other kinds of anxiety disorders are actually more frequent than PTSD. Survivors of concentration camps may develop PTSD, but also persistent irritability and poor memory. ICD-10 has a category of 'Enduring personality changes after catastrophic experience' (Box 8.3). This and other conditions may occur instead of, but also as well as, PTSD. For example, of Vietnam war veterans meeting diagnostic criteria for PTSD, 43 per cent had at least one other diagnosis. The most frequent were atypical depression, alcohol dependence, anxiety disorder, substance misuse, and somatization disorder (MacFarlane, 1985).

BOX 8.3 ICD-10 CRITERIA FOR 'ENDURING PERSONALITY CHANGES AFTER CATASTROPHIC EXPERIENCE'

(A) At least two of the following

- a permanent hostile or distrustful attitude toward the world
- social withdrawal
- a constant feeling of emptiness or hopelessness
- an enduring feeling of being on edge or being threatened without external cause
- a permanent feeling of being changed or being different from others

(B) The change causes significant interference with personal or social functioning or significant distress

(C) The personality change developed after the catastrophic event, and the person did not have a personality disorder prior to the event that explains the current traits.

(D) The personality change must have been present for at least two years, and is not related to episodes of any other mental disorder (other than PTSD) or brain damage or disease.

Clinical picture of PTSD

The clinical features of PTSD can be divided into three groups (Table 8.2). The first group of symptoms are related to **hyperarousal** and include persistent anxiety, irritability, insomnia, and poor concentration. The second group of symptoms centres round **intrusion**; there is intense intrusive imagery of the events, sudden flashbacks, and recurrent distressing dreams. The third group of symptoms is concerned with **avoidance**: difficulty in recalling stressful events at will, avoidance of reminders of the events, a feeling of detachment,

TABLE 8.2 The principal symptoms of post-traumatic stress disorder

Hyperarousal
◆ Persistent anxiety
◆ Irritability
◆ Insomnia
◆ Poor concentration
Intrusions
◆ Intense intrusive imagery
◆ 'Flashbacks'
◆ Recurrent distressing dreams
Avoidance
◆ Difficulty in recalling stressful events at will
◆ Avoidance of reminders of the events
◆ Detachment
◆ Inability to feel emotion ('numbness')
◆ Diminished interest in activities

inability to feel emotion ('numbing'), and diminished interest in activities. The most characteristic symptoms are flashbacks, nightmares, and intrusive images, sometimes known collectively as **re-experiencing symptoms**. Maladaptive coping responses may occur, including persistent aggressive behaviour, the excessive use of alcohol or drugs, and deliberate self-harm and suicide (Hendin and Haas, 1991).

Other features

Depressive symptoms are common, and guilt is often experienced by the survivors of a disaster. After some traumatic events, survivors feel forced into a painful reconsideration of their beliefs about the meaning and purpose of life (Janoff-Bulman, 1985). It has been suggested that dissociative symptoms and depersonalization are important symptoms of the disorder (Foa *et al.*, 1995).

Onset and course

Symptoms of PTSD may begin very soon after the stressful event or after an interval usually of days, but occasionally of months, though rarely more than 6 months (McFarlane, 1988). In DSM-IV, PTSD cannot be diagnosed until at least a month of symptomatology has elapsed; until then the condition is regarded an acute stress disorder. However, in these circumstances it is doubtful that the diagnosis of stress-related disorder and PTSD represent two separate conditions (Brewin *et al.*, 2003). If the person experiences a new traumatic event, symptoms may return even if the second event is less severe than the original. Many cases are persistent; about half recover within a year but up to a third do not recover even after many years (Kessler *et al.*, 1995).

Diagnosis

The diagnostic criteria in ICD-10 and DSM-IV are similar, though the latter assigns rather more importance to numbing. DSM-IV has two criteria not present in ICD-10: symptoms must have been present for at least a month and must cause significant distress or impaired social functioning. As a result of these differences, the concordance between the diagnosis of PTSD using the two sets of criteria is only 35 per cent (Andrews *et al.*, 1999). By convention, PTSD can be diagnosed in people who have a history of psychiatric disorder before the stressful events.

Differential diagnoses include:

- stress-induced exacerbations of previous anxiety or mood disorders;
- acute stress disorders (distinguished by the time course);
- adjustment disorders (distinguished by the different pattern of symptoms).
- enduring personality changes after catastrophic experience.

PTSD may present as deliberate self-harm or substance abuse which have developed as maladaptive coping strategies (see above).

Epidemiology

Estimates of the PTSD in the general population are mainly from the USA. Rates in other countries are likely to differ somewhat in relation to the frequency of natural and man-made disasters in these places. In a large representative USA sample, Kessler et al. (1995) estimated a lifetime prevalence of PTSD of 7.8 per cent (women: 10.4 per cent; men: 5.0 per cent), using DSM-IIIR criteria. Estimates for the 12-month prevalence range between 1.3 per cent in Australia (Creamer et al., 2001) and 3.6 per cent in the USA (Narrow et al., 2002).

Aetiology

The stressor

The necessary cause of PTSD is an exceptionally stressful event. It is not necessary that the person should have been harmed physically or threatened personally; those involved in other ways may develop the disorder, for example, the driver of a train in whose path someone has thrown himself for suicide, and the bystanders at a major accident. The authors of DSM-IV describe such events as involving actual or threatened death or serious injury or a threat to the physical integrity of the person or others. In a study of people affected by a volcanic eruption, the highest rate of PTSD was amongst those who experienced the greatest exposure to the stressful events (Shore *et al.*, 1989). Even so, not all those most affected by the stressor developed PTSD, a finding that indicates that some form of personal vulnerability plays a part. Such vulnerability might be genetic or acquired. Epidemiological research (Kessler *et al.*, 1995; Stein *et al.*, 1997 and Creamer *et al.*, 1992) has shown the following:

- The majority of people will experience at least one traumatic event in their lifetime.
- Intentional acts of interpersonal violence, in particular sexual assault, and combat are more likely to lead to PTSD than accidents or disasters.

- Men tend to experience more traumatic events in general than women, but women experience more events that are likely to lead to PTSD, for example, childhood sexual abuse, rape and domestic violence.
- Women are also more likely to develop PTSD in response to a traumatic event than men. This enhanced risk is not explained by differences in the type of traumatic event.

Genetic factors

Studies of twins suggest that differences in susceptibility are in part genetic. True *et al.* (1993) studied 2224 monozygotic and 1818 dizygotic male twin pairs who had served in the US armed forces during the Vietnam war. After allowance had been made for the amount of exposure to combat, genetic variation accounted for about one-third of the variance in susceptibility to self-reported PTSD. Self-reported childhood and adolescent environment did not contribute substantially to this variance. The risk of PTSD is increased by a family history of psychiatric disorder which may reflect genetic factors (Koenen *et al.*, 2002).

Other predisposing factors

The individual factors that increase vulnerability to the development of PTSD have been summarized by Ozer *et al.* (2003). They include:

- Personal history of mood and anxiety disorder
- Previous history of trauma
- Female gender
- Neuroticism
- Lower intelligence
- Lack of social support.

Neurobiological factors

Work to date on the neurobiology of PTSD has focused on monoamine neurotransmitters and the HPA axis, both of which are involved in mediating defensive responses to stressful events. In addition brain imaging studies have implicated changes in the **hippocampus**, a brain region important in memory formation, and the **amygdala** which plays a role in non-conscious emotional processing (Box 8.4). These findings suggest that hippocampal dysfunction prevents adequate memory processing while increased activity in noradrenergic innervation of the amygdala increases arousal and facilitates the automatic encoding and recall of traumatic memories (O'Donnell *et al.*, 2004).

BOX 8.4 BOX 8.4 NEUROBIOLOGICAL ABNORMALITIES IN PTSD

HPA axis Evidence for low plasma cortisol levels and increased sensitivity to dexamethasone suppresion. Increased levels of CRH in CSF. Longitudinal sampling suggests dysregulation of HPA axis with general increase in lability following environmental stress (Mason *et al.*, 2002).

Noradrenaline Increased sympathetic tone. Increased startle response. Increased levels of MHPG in CSF. Increased anxiety response to noradrenaline challenge (O'Donnell *et al.*, 2004).

Brain imaging Smaller volume of the hippocampus (which may be a vulnerability factor), overactivity of the amygdala to traumatic psychological stimuli (Nutt and Malizia, 2004).

Psychological factors

Fear conditioning

Some patients with PTSD experience vivid memories of the traumatic events in response to sensory cues such as smells and sounds related to the stressful situation. This finding suggests that classical conditioning may be involved.

Cognitive theories

These suggest that PTSD arises when the normal processing of emotionally charged information is overwhelmed, so that memories persist in an unprocessed form in which they can intrude into conscious awareness. In support of this idea, patients with PTSD tend to have incomplete and disorganized recall of the traumatic events (Van Kolk and Fisler, 1995). Individual differences in response to the same traumatic events are explained as due to differences in the appraisal of the trauma and of its effects. Similarly, difference in the appraisal of the early symptoms may explain why these symptoms persist longer in some people. Negative interpretations of intrusive thoughts (for example, I am going mad) after road accidents predict the continuing presence of PTSD after one year (Ehlers *et al.*, 1998). The cognitive model of PTSD has been reviewed by Ehlers and Clark (2000).

Psychodynamic theories

These emphasize the role of emotional development in determining individual variations in the response to severely stressful events (see, for example, Horowitz,

1986). The general approach is plausible, but it is not supported by scientific evidence.

Maintaining factors

As noted above, symptoms of PTSD may be maintained in part by negative appraisals of the early symptoms. Other suggested maintaining factors include avoidance of reminders of the traumatic situation (which prevents deconditioning and cognitive reappraisal); suppression of intrusive memories which is known to make them more likely to recur and rumination (Murray *et al.*, 2002).

Assessment

This should include enquiries about the nature and duration of symptoms, previous personality, and psychiatric history. When the traumatic events have included head injury (for example, in an assault or transport accident), a neurological examination should be performed. Feelings of anger and thoughts of self-harm are common in PTSD and an appropriate risk assessment needs to be carried out. Secondary complications such as substance misuse may require treatment in their own right (see Chapter 18).

Treatment

Counselling

The treatment of PTSD can be difficult, particularly once symptoms have been established for more than a year. The general approach to more short-lived cases is to provide emotional support, to encourage recall of the traumatic events to integrate them into the patient's experience, and to facilitate working through the associated emotions. Treatment may also need to deal with the person's feelings of guilt about perceived shortcomings in responding during the events, grief, and guilt about surviving when others have died. There may be existential concerns about the meaning and purpose of life and death (Horowitz, 1986). Victims of personal assault or rape have additional concerns.

Cognitive–behavioural treatment

Where symptoms are severe or long-standing, cognitive behaviour therapy is the most appropriate treatment. This treatment has several components:

- information about the normal response to severe stress, and the importance of confronting situations and memories related to the traumatic events;
- self-monitoring of symptoms;
- exposure to situations that are being avoided;
- recall of images of the traumatic events, to integrate these with the rest of the patient's experience. When first recalled these images are often fragmentary and are not related clearly in time to the other contents of memory;
- cognitive restructuring through the discussion of evidence for and against the appraisals and assumptions;
- anger management for people who still feel angry about the traumatic events and their causes.

A meta-analysis of psychotherapy studies of PTSD suggests that cognitive behavioural treatments have a therapeutic effect size of 1.65 compared to an inactive control, and 1.01 when compared to relaxation and supportive therapies. An effect size of 1 corresponds to an improvement of one standard deviation on the relevant symptomatic measure, and effect sizes of >1 indicate a large treatment effect (see p. 117). At the end of psychological treatment about 55 per cent of patients no longer meet criteria for PTSD, though many are still symptomatic. While these results are encouraging, further work is required to show that similar benefit can be obtained in everyday clinical settings (Bradley *et al.*, 2005).

Eye movement and desensitization reprocessing was designed for the treatment of PTSD. Treatment trials using this technique in subjects with PTSD have shown similar effect sizes as those obtained with cognitive behaviour therapy, but the evidence base is not as large (Bradley *et al.*, 2005). Some have questioned whether the eye movements associated with this treatment add any specific therapeutic value to element of exposure (Davidson and Parker, 2001).

There is little evidence for effectiveness of other psychotherapies such psychodynamic therapy and hypnotherapy. For a review see the National Institute of Clinical Excellence (2005).

Medication

Anxiolytic drugs should be avoided for established PTSD because prolonged use may lead to dependence. A number of antidepressant drugs have shown efficacy in clinical trials including SSRIs, TCAs and MAOIs. There are also more preliminary data supporting the efficacy of mirtazapine (see Davidson, 2003). However a meta-analysis carried out by the National Institute of Clinical Excellence (2005) indicated that in PTSD drug treatment has a lower effect size than structured psychotherapy and medication should not therefore be a first-line treatment unless the patient expresses a preference for it, or if psychotherapy is not available.

BOX 8.5 NICE GUIDANCE FOR THE MANAGEMENT OF PTSD AND RELATED TRAUMATIC SYNDROMES

1. The routine use of a brief screening instrument for PTSD at one-month post incident should be considered for all people who have been involved in a major disaster.
2. Where symptoms are mild and have been present for less than four weeks after the trauma, watchful waiting, as a way of managing the difficulties presented by individual suffers, should be considered by healthcare professionals. A follow up contact should be arranged within one month.
3. Trauma-focused cognitive behavioural therapy should be considered for those with severe post-traumatic symptoms during the first month after the traumatic event. All PTSD sufferers should be offered a course of trauma-focused psychological treatment These treatments are usually given individually on an outpatient basis.
4. Drug treatments for PTSD should not be used as a routine first line treatment in preference to a trauma-focused psychological therapy.
5. Drug treatments (paroxetine, tricyclic antidepressants or mirtazapine) should be considered for the treatment of PTSD where a sufferer expresses a preference not to engage in a trauma-focused psychological treatment.

Adapted from the National Institute of Critical Excellence (2005)

However where patients with PTSD have a significant comorbid depressive disorder, then antidepressant treatment should be considered as an adjunct to psychotherapy. For a review of the treatment of PTSD see Ehlers (2000), the National Institute of Clinical Excellence (2005) (Box 8.5) and Bradley *et al.* (2005).

Response to special kinds of severe stress

Rape and physical assault

Victims of rape or physical assault experience acute reactions to stress, PTSD, anxiety and depressive disorders, and psychosexual dysfunction. PTSD is the most frequent of these consequences. In one study of women victims of rape, 94 per cent had acute stress disorder after the assault, and 47 per cent had the symptoms 3 months later (Rothbaum *et al.*, 1992). In another study of rape victims, two-thirds of women reported reduced sexual activity, whilst 40 per cent gave up intercourse or had impaired orgasm for 6 months after the rape (Burgess and Holmstrom, 1979).

As well as experiencing symptoms of PTSD, victims of rape and assault feel humiliated, ashamed, and vulnerable to further attack. They lose confidence and self-esteem, question why they were chosen as victims, and blame themselves for putting themselves in unnecessary danger (Janoff-Bulman and Frieze, 1983). To these problems are added issues of betrayal and secrecy when the rapist is a family member or a friend. The victims may have problems in trusting, persistent anger and irritability, and excessive dependence. These problems were described first among women victims of rape but similar difficulties have been described among male victims of sexual assault (Mezey and King, 1989).

Problems are more likely to persist when there has been an actual or perceived threat to life, previous psychological and social problems, past victimization, particularly abuse in childhood, past psychiatric illness or substance abuse, or a lack of social support (see Mezey and Robbins, 2000).

Treatment

Social support is important in providing opportunities for the victim to talk over the problem and to regain self-esteem. Specific treatment is similar to that of other kinds of PTSD, including prolonged exposure by reliving the events in imagination, with additional emphasis on overcoming feelings of vulnerability and self-blame (see Jaycox *et al.*, 2002). A different form of psychotherapy which emphasizes the role of cognitive processing has shown efficacy equal to that of exposure therapy (Resick *et al.*, 2002).

War and other armed conflict

Shell shock, battle fatigue, or war neurosis were terms used during the First World War to describe psychological reactions to battle in British and American servicemen. Most of the reactions appear to resemble cases now diagnosed as PTSD; others seem to have resembled panic disorder or depressive disorders. Cases with panic attacks and concerns about the heart, now diagnosed as panic disorder (see p. 192), were known then as Da Costa's syndrome or disorderly action of the heart. Army psychiatrists were few in number, and were unable to deal with the many cases. In any case, their experience of mental hospital work with severely ill patients did not equip them to treat these reactions to battle. Therefore, patients with shell shock were treated mainly by neurologists or psychologists. W. H. Rivers, William Brown, and William McDougall were British psychologists who treated shell shock during the war, and used this experience to write influential books on medical psychology in the years after the war (Rivers, 1920; McDougall, 1926; Brown, 1934).

Treatment

At first, shell shock was treated with the methods in use at the time for neurasthenia (see p. 386), namely rest, isolation, massage, and diet, but these methods had a low success rate. Hypnosis achieved some dramatic cures but was not generally effective. Medical psychologists tried psychotherapeutic methods advocated by Freud, including the recall of stressful events to remove repression and the expression of associated emotion. There was an increasing emphasis on early treatment, and it became evident that psychotherapy had to be combined with military drill to maintain general fitness and morale. This combined treatment led to improved results.

These general principles of early treatment, abreaction, and maintenance of fitness and morale were adopted in the Second World War and in subsequent conflicts. Abreaction with anxiolytic drugs was used widely in the Second World War (see Sargant and Slater, 1940). In subsequent conflicts it has been reported that, with immediate counselling (without drug-induced abreaction), about 70 per cent of 'battle shock' personnel can be returned to their units within 5 days (Brandon, 1991). The treatment of shell shock in the British army in the First World War has been described by Stone (1985).

Problems of refugees and victims of torture

Refugees may have experienced a wide range of traumatic events, including:

- the conditions of war
- loss by death or separation of relatives and friends
- loss of home and possessions
- physical injury (including brain injury) either from the actions of war or from assault, rape or torture, and the witnessing of violence to others.

Those involved may develop any of the reactions to stressful events, especially PTSD and depressive disorders (Turner *et al.*, 2003). These conditions have been identified in refugees from many cultures, though the presenting complaints may differ somewhat in people from different cultures, with more emphasis on physical than on psychological symptoms among people from non-Western countries. Victims of torture often experience PTSD as well as the physical consequences of the experience. It is important to remember, however, that stressors related to a refugee's current situation can be just as difficult to deal with as those that led to flight in the first place (Box 8.6). In a systematic review, Fazel *et al.* (2005) estimated that of refugees re-settled in Western countries, about 10 per cent met diagnostic criteria for PTSD, 5 per cent had major depression and 4 per cent had generalized anxiety disorder. In many individuals these disorders overlapped.

Treatment

Treatment should combine physical and psychiatric care. The latter should be introduced carefully since it may be resisted as stigmatizing, not only by the refugee but also by aid workers. Special care is needed to establish a trusting relationship. Practical help is often an

BOX 8.6 SOME STRESSFUL ISSUES FACED BY REFUGEES

Causes

War
Human rights abuses
Persecution on grounds of politics, religion, gender or ethnicity

Resultant losses

Country
Culture
Family
Profession
Language
Friends
Possessions
Plans for the future

Issues in country of asylum

Psychological and practical adjustment
Uncertain future
Traumatic life events
Social exclusion and poverty
Racism
Stereotyping by host country
Unknown cultural traditions

From Tribe (2002)

essential preliminary to engagement. Many refugees have problems related to separation, bereavement, and loss of material possessions, so that it is important not to focus narrowly on PTSD. Victims of torture may need additional help to cope with feelings of personal humiliation and of remorse for the suffering of others. Health beliefs and understanding of the 'normal' psychological response to stress may well differ between a health worker from one culture and a refugee from another. Therefore it is necessary to consider in each individual how far formal psychological therapies may be indicated and whether or not they should be presented in the language of mental illness and trauma (Tribe, 2002).

Care is needed in working through interpreters. If possible, they should not be family members, community elders, or others to whom the refugee is unlikely to speak of shameful experiences. This point is especially important in situations in which women may have experienced sexual assaults, for these may bring shame to the whole family. Ideally, such problems should be dealt with by a female mental health professional who understands the patient's language and culture, but this may be difficult to arrange.

For further information about the psychiatric problems of refugees see Mollica (2000) and Lustig *et al.* (2004).

Adjustment disorders

This term refers to the psychological reactions arising in relation to adapting to new circumstances. Such circumstances include divorce and separation, a major change of work and abode, such as transition from school to university or migration, and the birth of a handicapped child. Bereavement, the onset of a terminal illness, and sexual abuse involve special kinds of adjustment which are discussed below.

Clinical features

The symptoms of an adjustment disorder include anxiety, worry, poor concentration, depression, and irritability, together with physical symptoms caused by autonomic arousal such as palpitations and tremor. There may be outbursts of dramatic or aggressive behaviour, single or repeated episodes of deliberate self-harm, or the misuse of alcohol or drugs. The onset is more gradual than that of an acute reaction to stress, and the course is more prolonged. Usually social functioning is impaired. The impairment in social function as well as the intensity of distress is what distinguishes adjustment disorder from normal adaptive reactions (Casey *et al.*, 2001).

Stressful life events may precipitate depression, anxiety, schizophrenia, and other psychiatric disorders; for this reason the diagnosis of adjustment disorder is not made when diagnostic criteria for another psychiatric disorder are met. In practice, therefore, the diagnosis is usually made by excluding an anxiety or depressive disorder. A further requirement for diagnosis is that the disorder starts soon after the change of circumstances. Both ICD-10 and DSM-IV require that the disorder starts within 3 months, and ICD-10 indicates that it usually starts within 1 month. An essential point is that the reaction is understandably related to, and in proportion to, the stressful experience when account is taken of the patient's previous experiences and personality.

Diagnostic conventions

As explained on p. 155, in ICD-10 adjustment disorders are divided into depressive reactions, mixed anxiety and depressive reactions, reactions with disturbance of other emotions, and reactions with disturbed conduct with or without emotional disturbance. DSM-IV lists six types of adjustment disorder (see Table 8.2).

Epidemiology

The prevalence of adjustment disorder in the community is unknown. It is presumed that in certain settings, for example, the general hospital and primary care, prevalence rates are increased. For example in a large study of medical patients referred for psychiatric assessment, 12 per cent met criteria for adjustment disorder and in patients attending a stroke unit the prevalence of adjustment disorder was 27 per cent (see Strain *et al.*, 1998).

Aetiology

Stressful circumstances are the necessary cause of an adjustment disorder, but individual vulnerability is also important because not all people exposed to the same stressful circumstances develop an adjustment disorder. The nature of this vulnerability is unknown; it seems to vary from person to person, and may relate in part to previous life experiences.

Prognosis

Clinical experience suggests that most adjustment disorders last for several months and a few persist for years. There is little systematic follow-up information though Andreasen and Hoenck (1982) reported that while the prognosis is good for adults, some adolescents with adjustment disorder develop psychiatric disorders in adult life.

Treatment

Treatment is designed to help the patient resolve the stressful problems if this is possible, and to aid the natural processes of adjustment. The latter is done by reducing denial and avoidance of the stressful events, encouraging problem-solving, and discouraging maladaptive coping responses. Anxiety can usually be reduced by encouraging the patient to talk about the problems and to express feelings. Occasionally, an anxiolytic or hypnotic drug is needed for a few days.

Problem-solving counselling (see p. 585) encourages the patient to seek solutions to stressful problems, and to consider the advantages and disadvantages of various kinds of action. The patient is then helped to select and implement a course of action to solve the problem. If this action succeeds, another problem is considered. If the first attempt fails, another approach to the original problem is tried. If problems cannot be resolved, the patient is encouraged to come to terms with them. Maina *et al.* (2005) reported that in patients with adjustment disorder, both brief dynamic and supportive psychotherapy were more effective than waiting list control.

Special kinds of adjustment

Adjustment to physical illness and handicap

Appraisal of illness

Adjustment to illness cannot be understood simply in terms of the facts about the disease and its objective consequences. Adjustment depends on patients' beliefs about their disorder and its effects on their lives - on their appraisal of their illness. This appraisal may be similar to that of the professionals who are treating them, or it may be very different because it is based on false information or on emotions rather than facts or influenced by cultural beliefs. The appraisal may be reinforced by members of the family who share the patient's views, or it may be contradicted by them, thus adding to the patient's distress. Two terms are much used in the discussions of adjustment to illness and handicap: illness behaviour and the sick role. These terms are considered next.

Illness behaviour

Mechanic (1978) suggested the term illness behaviour for behaviour associated with adjustment to physical or mental disorder, whether adaptive or not. Illness behaviour includes consulting doctors, taking medicines, seeking help from relatives and friends, and giving up inappropriate activities. These behaviours are adaptive in the early stages of illness, but may become maladaptive if they persist into the stage of convalescence when the patient should be becoming independent. Illness behaviour results from the person's conviction that he is ill rather than from the objective presence of disease, and it may develop when no disease is present. Illness behaviour without disease is an important problem in general practice, and once firmly established it is difficult to treat. The concept of illness behaviour overlaps with that of the sick role (described next) but the two are described separately because they have different origins.

The sick role

Society bestows a special role for people who are ill. Parsons (1951) called this the sick role, which is made up of two privileges and two duties:

- exemption from certain social responsibilities;
- the right to expect help and care from others;
- the obligation to seek and cooperate with treatment
- the expectation of a desire to recover.

While the person is ill, the sick role is adaptive. If people continue in the sick role after the illness is over, recovery is delayed since they continue to avoid responsibilities and depend on others instead of becoming independent.

Adjustment to the onset of physical illness

When people become physically ill, they may feel anxious, depressed, or angry. Usually this emotional reaction is transient, subsiding as the patient comes to terms with the new situation. As in other adjustment reactions, denial or minimization can protect the patient against overwhelming anxiety when the diagnosis is first known. Although helpful in this way, denial can be maladaptive: in the early stage of illness it may lead to delay in seeking help; at a later stage it may lead to poor compliance with treatment. Other coping strategies can be divided into emotion-reducing and problem-solving groups (see p. 152). Coping strategies that reduce emotion are often appropriate in the early stages of illness but should give way to problem-solving coping. Coping may fail when demands are very great, or when coping resources are limited either in the long term, or as a temporary result of disease of, or trauma to, the brain.

Physical illness as a direct cause of psychiatric symptoms

As well as acting as a stressor, physical illness may induce psychiatric symptoms directly. Anxiety, depression, fatigue, weakness, weight loss, or abnormal behaviour may all be caused directly by physical disorders; common examples are listed in Chapter 16 (Table 16.5). Similarly, sexual dysfunction may be impaired by physical illness or its treatment (see p. 477). Any of these symptoms may be the reason for referral, and psychiatrists should always be alert to the possibility of undetected physical illness in their patients.

Psychiatric symptoms due to treatments for physical illness

Some drugs used in the treatment of physical illness may affect mood, behaviour, and consciousness. The drugs most likely to have these effects are listed in Chapter 16 (Table 16.6).

Help for people adjusting to physical illness

Most people adjust well to physical illness, but when adjustment is slow and incomplete, psychological treatment may be needed. This treatment need not be complicated and can usually be provided effectively by the general practitioner or the hospital doctors or nurses dealing with the physical illness. Generally, the psychiatrist has a role in treating only the most severe problems or in supporting the medical and nursing staff.

The first step is to identify patients who are adjusting badly (failing to cope). This is generally done by the professional staff who are caring for the physical illness. They can do this most easily by looking out for patients who are progressing less well than would be expected from the severity of the disease. Mood disorders are a common cause of slow progress, but some are dismissed as normal responses to the problems of the illness. Screening questionnaires can be used to detect mood disorders among this group, but the results should be checked at least by a brief interview, carried out, if possible, in surroundings in which the replies will not be overheard. Generally, one or more members of the family should be interviewed to obtain information about the patient's previous adjustment to problems and illness, and to discover how the family views the illness.

Some patients require medication but for many counselling (p. 584) is more appropriate. Counselling requires a trusting relationship with the patient and this in turn requires adequate time for the interviews. Counselling begins with an explanation of the nature of the illness and its treatment; the patient is then helped to accept the implication of the diagnosis, to adjust to illness, and to give up any maladaptive behaviours such as excessive dependence on others or denial of the need for treatment. Graded activities, motivational interviewing, and anger management may be useful in some cases.

If the reaction to physical illness is an anxiety or a depressive disorder, treatment appropriate to the disorder should be given (see Chapters 9 and 11).

Adjustment to terminal illness

Amongst patients dying in hospital, about half have emotional symptoms of anxiety, depression, anger, or guilt (Meyer *et al.*, 2003). Determinants of emotional reactions include the patient's personality, and the amount and quality of support from family, friends, and carers. Understandably, emotional reactions are more common among young dying patients than among the elderly. They are less common among patients who believe in an after-life.

Anxiety

Anxiety may be provoked by the prospect of severe pain, disfigurement, or incontinence, by fear of death, and by concerns about the future of the family. Families and carers sometimes try to spare the patient anxiety by concealing the truth about the condition. Since most patients become aware of the diagnosis, attempts at concealment only increase their fear of possible consequences of the disease such as pain or incontinence.

Depression

Depression may be provoked by the prospect of separation from family and friends and the loss of valued activities. Changes in physical appearance caused by the illness, the effects of surgery, and the debilitating effects of radiotherapy are other causes of low mood.

Guilt and anger

Some patients experience guilt because they believe that they are making excessive demands on relatives or friends. Patients with religious beliefs may believe that illness is a punishment for previous wrongdoing. Anger may be felt about the unjustness of impending death; this anger may be displaced onto doctors, nurses, and relatives, making care more difficult (see below).

Defence mechanisms

Defence mechanisms observed in dying patients are most often denial, dependency, and displacement:

- **Denial** is usually the first reaction to the news of fatal illness. It may be experienced as a feeling of disbelief and may lead to an initial period of calm. Denial diminishes as the patient becomes reconciled to the illness but may return as the disease progresses, and the patient may again behave as if unaware of the nature of the illness.

- **Dependency** is adaptive in the early stages of severe physical illness when the patient needs to comply passively with treatment. Excessive or prolonged dependency makes subsequent treatment more difficult, and increases the burden on the family. A further stage of dependency may be appropriate as the patient nears death.
- **Displacement** is often of anger, which may be directed to staff and relatives, who may not understand this reaction so that they find it difficult to tolerate. As a result they may spend less time with the patient, thereby increasing their feelings of despair.

Denial, dependency, and displacement are usually followed by **acceptance**. The doctor's aim should be to help the patient to reach this acceptance before the final stage of the illness. This aim is more likely to be achieved when there is good communication between patients, the staff caring for them, and relatives.

Psychological symptoms

Psychological symptoms induced by the disease or its treatment may add to the patient's distress. The more frequent associations between disease and psychological symptoms are summarized in Table 16.5. There is a particularly strong association between dyspnoea and anxiety. The associations between drug treatment and psychological symptoms are summarized in Table 16.6.

Treatment

Usually dying patients are helped to adjust by the staff who are caring for the physical illness. Psychiatrists are called upon only when there are special problems (see below), or to assist with staff support and training.

The aims of treatment

According to Hackett and Weissman (1962), the aim of treating the dying patient should be to achieve an 'appropriate death'. By this they meant that

> the person should be relatively free from pain, should operate on as effective a level as possible, should recognize and resolve remaining conflicts, should satisfy as far as possible remaining wishes, and should be able to yield control to others in whom he has confidence.

Kubler-Ross (1969) formulated the aims in different terms and described five phases of psychological adjustment to death. The phases do not necessarily occur in the same sequence, and some may not occur at all, but they are a useful guide for professionals helping dying patients. The phases are:

- denial and isolation,
- anger,
- partial acceptance ('bargaining for time'), depression, and
- acceptance.

Reducing symptoms

Adequate control of pain and breathlessness and the reduction of confusion due to delirium are particularly important. Anxiety and depression may diminish as pain and breathlessness are controlled. The causes of delirium are listed on p. 329. Among dying patients, important remediable causes are dehydration, the side-effects of drugs, secondary infection, cardiac or respiratory failure, and hypercalcaemia.

Helping the patient to adjust

It is essential to establish a good relationship with the patient so that they can talk about their problems and ask questions. The nature of the illness should be explained honestly and in simple language. Sometimes doctors are apprehensive that such an explanation will increase patients' distress. Although excessive detail given unsympathetically can have this effect, it is seldom difficult to decide how much to say about diagnosis and prognosis provided that patients are allowed to lead the discussion, express their worries, and say what they want to know. If patients ask about the prognosis, they should be told the truth; evasive answers undermine trust in the carers. If patients do not seem to wish to know the full extent of their problems, it is usually better to save this information until later. At an appropriate stage patients should be told what can be done to make their remaining time as comfortable as possible. Whilst the whole account should be truthful, the amount disclosed on a single occasion should be judged by patients' reactions and by their questions. If necessary, the doctor should be prepared to return for further discussion when patients are ready to continue. It is important to bear in mind that most dying patients become aware of their prognosis whether or not they are told directly, because they infer the truth from the behaviour of those who are caring for them. They notice when answers to questions are evasive and when people avoid talking to them. Patients who are anxious, angry, or despairing need to be able to express these feelings and to discuss the ideas that induce them.

Informing the staff

The information given to the patient should be known to all the staff, otherwise conflicting advice and opinions may be given. If all those involved know what has been said, they will feel more at ease in talking to the patient. Otherwise they will draw back from the patient, isolating them, and increasing their difficulty in adjusting.

Informing and supporting relatives

Relatives need to know what has been said to the patient so that they will feel less ill at ease when talking to them. Relatives may need as much help as the patient. They may become anxious and depressed, and they may respond with guilt, anger, or denial. Such reactions make it difficult for them to communicate helpfully with the patient or the staff. Relatives need information, and opportunities to talk about their feelings, and to prepare for the impending bereavement. Without these the patient and the family may become increasingly distant and alienated.

Special services

In many hospitals, **specialist nurses** work with the family doctor and with the hospital staff caring for dying patients. These nurses are trained in the psychological as well as the physical care of the dying. Sometimes care is provided in **hospices** where it is possible to provide close attention to the details of care that improve quality of life for the dying person. These hospices care for patients when home care is impractical, and provide periods of respite care to relieve those who are caring for the patient at home.

Referral to a psychiatrist

Referral to a psychiatrist is appropriate when psychiatric symptoms or behaviour disturbance are severe (Lyness, 2004). The referrals are concerned with the assessment and management of:

- **depressed patients**, to decide the cause and whether they require medication or more structured psychotherapy;
- **uncommunicative patients** who will not talk about the illness;
- **uncooperative patients** who do not accept the social restrictions imposed by the illness, will not make appropriate plans, or take necessary decisions;
- long-standing problems made worse by the illness and related to personality or family conflicts;
- **other symptoms**. Although anxiety and delirium are common, these problems are more often dealt with appropriately by medical staff, than referred to a psychiatrist. The exception is delirium with paranoid symptoms.

Management of depressive disorders

Depressive disorders may be caused by symptoms such as pain or breathlessness, all of which should be treated appropriately. Any drugs that can cause depression (see Table 16.6) should be reviewed and, if possible, given in lower dose or replaced. Some symptoms of depressive disorder are difficult to evaluate in patients with advanced cancer; thus weight loss, anorexia, insomnia, loss of interest, and fatigue may be caused by the physical illness. Early morning wakening, extreme hopelessness, and self-blame are surer guides to diagnosis. Suicidal ideation should be assessed carefully. If counselling and improved medical management do not improve the low mood, antidepressant drugs should be prescribed with careful supervision. The starting dose should be small, and medication should be changed if necessary to find a compound that is well tolerated (see Dein, 2003).

Liaison with medical and nursing staff

Liaison with medical and nursing staff is important. Often these staff can provide treatment when the psychiatrist has formulated a plan. For further information about the care of the dying, see Billings (2000).

Grief and adjustment to bereavement

Terminology

Although the words bereavement, mourning, and grief are sometimes used interchangeably, they have separate meanings which incorporate distinctions that are useful in psychiatry:

- **Bereavement** is the loss through death of a loved person.
- **Grief** is the involuntary emotional and behavioural response to bereavement.
- **Mourning** is the voluntary expression of behaviours and rituals that are socially sanctioned responses to bereavement. These behaviours and rituals differ between societies and between religious groups both in their form and in their duration.

The systems of classification do not make these distinctions in consistent ways. In ICD-10, bereavement is coded appropriately as Z63.4, that is as one of the 'factors influencing health status and contact with health services'. In DSM-IV, however, bereavement is coded as a 'condition that may be the focus of clinical attention'; thus, the term is used to denote the response to bereavement rather than the event itself. ICD-10 codes grief under adjustment disorders, but uses the term grief reaction. Mourning – a form of social behaviour – is not a disorder and, appropriately, is not listed in the index to either classification. In this chapter the term bereavement reaction is used to denote all responses to bereavement, normal and abnormal. Normal reactions are called grief, abnormal reactions include abnormal (or pathological) grief, and depressive disorders.

Grief

Grief is a continuous process, but for clarity can be described as having three stages (Table 8.3).

The first stage lasts from a few hours to several days. There is denial, which is manifested as a lack of emotional response ('numbness'), often with a feeling of unreality, and incomplete acceptance that the death has taken place. The bereaved person may be restless, as if searching for the dead person.

The second stage usually lasts from a few weeks to about 6 months but may be much longer. There may be extreme sadness, weeping, loneliness, and often overwhelming waves of yearning for the dead person. Anxiety is common; the bereaved person is anxious and restless, sleeps poorly, lacks appetite, and may experience panic attacks. Many bereaved people feel guilt that they failed to do enough for the deceased. Some feel anger and project their feelings of guilt, blaming doctors or others for failing to provide optimal care for the dead person. Many bereaved people have a vivid experience of being in the presence of the dead person, and about one in ten experience brief hallucinations (Clayton, 1979). The bereaved person is preoccupied with memories of the dead person, sometimes in the form of intrusive images. Withdrawal from social relationships is frequent. Complaints of physical symptoms are common (Parkes and Brown, 1972), and widows seek medical care more often than comparable people who are not bereaved (Stein and Susser, 1969).

In the third stage, these symptoms subside and everyday activities are resumed. The bereaved person gradually comes to terms with the loss and recalls the good times shared with the deceased in the past. Often there is a temporary return of symptoms on the anniversary of the death.

Although these stages are a useful guideline, individual responses are not all the same and no one feature is universal (Schuchter and Zisook, 1993).

TABLE 8.3 Normal grief reaction

Stage I: hours to days
Denial, disbelief
'Numbness'
Stage II: weeks to 6 months
Sadness, weeping, waves of grief
Somatic symptoms of anxiety
Restlessness
Poor sleep
Diminished appetite
Guilt, blame of others
Experience of a presence
Illusions, vivid imagery
Hallucinations of the dead person's voice
Preoccupation with memories of deceased
Social withdrawal
Stage III: weeks to months
Symptoms resolve
Social activities resumed
Memories of good times
(Symptoms may recur at anniversaries.)

Abnormal or pathological grief

Grief is considered abnormal if it is unusually intense, unusually prolonged, delayed, or inhibited or distorted. The criterion for abnormal intensity is that the symptoms meet the criteria for a depressive disorder. The criterion for abnormal duration is that the response lasts more than 6 months. The usual criterion for delay is that the first stage of grief has not occurred by 2 weeks after the death of the loved person. In all these forms of grief, persistent avoidance of situations and of other reminders of death are common.

Abnormally intense grief Depressive symptoms are a frequent component of normal grief and up to 35 per cent of bereaved people meet the criteria for a depressive disorder at some time during their grieving (Schuchter and Zisook, 1993). Most of these depressive disorders resolve within 6 months but about 20 per cent persist for longer. It might be argued that if about a third of bereaved people meet the criterion for depressive disorder at some time, the threshold has been set too low. However, people who meet the criteria for a depressive disorder are more likely to have poor social adjustment, to visit doctors frequently), and to use alcohol (Shuchter and Zisook, 1993). Therefore, it is of practical value to use the criterion and to record the additional diagnosis of a depressive disorder in these cases. When there is doubt whether depressive disorder should be recorded, particular attention should be paid to symptoms of retardation and global loss of self-esteem (clearly greater than regret about omissions of care during the terminal illness), because these features are seldom present in uncomplicated grief (Jacobs *et al.*, 1989).

Suicidal thoughts may occur when grief is intense. The rate of suicide is increased most in the year after bereavement, but continues to be high for 5 years after the death of a spouse or parent. Young widows and elderly widowers are at higher risk than other bereaved people (Bunch, 1972). The presence of suicidal ideas should prompt appropriate assessment of suicide risk (see p. 414).

Prolonged grief As explained above, prolonged (or chronic) grief is often defined as grief lasting for more than 6 months. Instead of the normal progression, symptoms of the first and second stages persist. However, it is difficult to set a precise limit to normal grief, and complete resolution may take much longer. One study found that only a minority of widows had ceased to grieve a year after the death (Parkes 1971). Prolonged grief may be associated with a depressive disorder but can occur without it. Prolonged grief has also been described as 'traumatic grief' in which subjects show persistent searching, yearning, disbelief regarding the death and preoccupation with thoughts of the deceased (Boelen et al., 2003).

Delayed grief By convention, delayed grief is said to occur when the first stage of grief does not appear until more than 2 weeks after the death. It is said to be more frequent after sudden, traumatic, or unexpected deaths (Jacobs 1993, p. 175).

Inhibited and distorted grief The term inhibited grief refers to a reaction which lacks some normal features. Distorted grief refers to features (other than depressive symptoms) that are either unusual in degree, for example, marked hostility, overactivity, and extreme social withdrawal, or else unusual in kind, for example, physical symptoms that were part of the last illness of the deceased. These distorted presentations were described by Lindemann (1944) in a study of survivors of a fire in a nightclub.

In all these forms of grief, persistent avoidance of situations and of other reminders of death are common.

Causes of abnormal grief

Abnormal grief is generally thought to be more likely when:

- the death was sudden and unexpected
- the bereaved person had a very close, or dependent, or ambivalent relationship with the deceased
- the survivor is insecure, or has difficulty in expressing feelings, or has suffered a previous psychiatric disorder
- the survivor has to care for dependent children and so cannot show grief easily.

Morbidity after bereavement

Several studies (reviewed by Stroebe and Stroebe, 1993) have shown an increased rate of mortality among bereaved spouses and other close relatives, with the greatest increase being in the first 6 months after bereavement. Most studies report increased rates of death from heart disease, and some have reported increased rates of death from cancer, liver cirrhosis, suicide, and accidents. The reasons for these associations are uncertain, and are likely to be different for different conditions. Increased rates of suicide have been reported (Bunch, 1972). There also increased rates of psychological morbidity and economic disadvantage (Valdimarsdottir *et al.*, 2003).

Management of grief

Grief is a normal response and most people pass through it with the help of family, friends, spiritual advisors, and the rituals of mourning. In some Western societies, many people may not have links with a religion, the rituals of mourning may be attenuated, and family may not be close at hand. For these and other reasons, family doctors have an important part to play in helping the bereaved. Psychiatrists may be asked to help people with abnormal grief.

Although bereaved people have some problems in common, they also have problems that are individual. For example, a young widow with small children has many difficulties that are not shared by an elderly widow whose adult children can support her. A mother grieving for a stillborn child will have special problems (discussed below). In planning management it is important to take into account the individual circumstances of the patient as well as the general guidelines outlined below.

Counselling

When counselling is appropriate, it is similar to counselling for other kinds of adjustment reaction. The bereaved person needs to talk about the loss, to express feelings of sadness, guilt, or anger, and to understand the normal course of grieving. It is helpful to forewarn a bereaved person about unusual experiences such as feeling as if the dead person were present, illusions, and hallucinations; otherwise these experiences may be alarming. Help may be needed to:

- Accept that the loss is real.
- Work through the stages of grief.
- Adjust to life without the deceased.

The bereaved person may need help to progress from the first stage of denial of loss to the acceptance of reality. Viewing the dead body and putting away the dead person's belongings help this transition, and a bereaved person should be encouraged to perform these actions. Practical problems may need to be discussed, including funeral arrangements and financial difficulties. A young widow may need help in maintaining and caring for young children, and in supporting them without inhibiting her own grief excessively. As time passes, the bereaved person should be encouraged to resume social contacts, to talk to other people about the loss, to remember happy and fulfilling experiences that were shared with the deceased, and to consider positive activities that the latter would have wanted survivors to undertake. (For further information about grief counselling see Clark, 2004.)

Parents grieving for a stillborn child need special help. They should be encouraged to name the dead baby and to view the body. If they do not feel able to take these steps, it is often helpful to obtain a photograph of the body, which the parents can see later if they wish. If these steps are combined with counselling, the mothers of stillborn children experience less distress than those not given this help (Forrest and Standish, 1984).

Medication

Drug treatment cannot remove the distress of normal grief, but it may be needed in specific circumstances. In the first stage of grief, a hypnotic or anxiolytic drug may be needed for a few days to restore sleep or to relieve any severe anxiety. In the second stage, antidepressant drugs may be beneficial if the criteria for depressive disorder are met, though such usage has not been much evaluated in this special group. Medication may be needed for a short period in the second stage to relieve severe anxiety.

Support groups

Support groups have been developed to help recently bereaved people, particularly young widows. One such organization in the UK is known as CRUSE. By sharing their experience with others who have dealt successfully with bereavement, recently bereaved people can share grief, obtain practical advice, and discuss ways of coping (Clark, 2004).

Psychotherapy

It is not practical, nor is there evidence that it is helpful, to provide psychotherapy for all bereaved persons. There is some evidence that crisis intervention may be helpful for people who are at high risk of an abnormal grief reaction (Raphael, 1977), though not for unselected grieving people Marmar *et al.* (1988) studied brief dynamic psychotherapy and they found it no more effective than a mutual support group. Similarly, Lieberman and Yalom (1992) found no significant difference in outcome between bereaved spouses treated with group psychotherapy and a control group who were not treated. For abnormal grief, dynamic psychotherapy has a clear rationale and approach but its effectiveness has not been formally evaluated (Clark, 2004).

Guided mourning

Guided mourning is the name given to a procedure which reduces avoidant behaviours that are thought to prolong grief. The bereaved person is helped to confront memories of the dead person and to enter situations that provoke these memories (it is a form of exposure treatment, see p. 591). In a controlled evaluation, this approach produced modest benefit (Foa *et al.*, 1991). For a review of the psychological treatment of abnormal grief, see Clark (2004).

Long-term adjustment to sexual abuse in childhood

When sexually abused, children may experience anxiety, depression, and post-traumatic stress disorder (see p. 157). These effects usually subside during childhood, but people who have been abused in childhood are more vulnerable than others to psychiatric disorder in adult life. Also, sexual abuse in childhood may be followed by persistent low self-esteem and psychosexual difficulties whether or not a psychiatric disorder develops.

Some adults who were previously unaware that they had been sexually abused in childhood suddenly recall the abuse in a vivid and disturbing way. Sometimes this recall occurs spontaneously, often when the person has encountered a reminder of the events. It may occur also during counselling or psychotherapy, at a time when childhood experiences are being discussed. Some of these recollections are confirmed by other evidence, but many are vigorously denied by the alleged abuser, who is often one of the parents. It has been suggested that some, perhaps most, of these unconfirmed reports of abuse are not accurate memories and that some have been induced by questions, suggestions, or interpretations from the therapists. This phenomenon has been called the false memory syndrome (see McNally, 2003).

Recovered memory and false memory

Many victims of sexual abuse, and of other severe stressful events, have partial amnesia for the most stressful parts of the experience, even though they have suffered no head injury that could lead to post-traumatic amnesia. Indeed, partial amnesia is part of the clinical picture of PTSD. However, complete amnesia is less frequent and, to many psychiatrists, complete amnesia for repeated stressful events followed by their recall, is improbable, especially when there is no supporting evidence for the events from another source. This doubt is increased by evidence that 'memories' of single non-abusive childhood events can be implanted by suggestion in about a quarter of subjects (Brewin, 2000; McNally, 2003).

Evidence for the proposition that true memories can be inaccessible for many years and then recovered, comes mainly from clinical reports (see Brewin, 2000). These reports suggest that between about a quarter and a half of people reporting childhood sexual abuse describe long periods in which they did not remember the abuse. Also, clinicians have reported that up to 40 per cent of memories recovered in therapy are confirmed by other evidence.

In the absence of conclusive evidence about the status of memories recovered in counselling or psychotherapy, the clinician who is carrying out these procedures should:

- take special care not to suggest memories of sexual abuse; and
- consider most carefully apparent recovered memories arising for the first time in therapy, before concluding that they are true memories of actual events.

It seems reasonable to conclude that many of the 'recovered memories' elicited without these precautions are likely to be false, and that true recovered memories of repeated sexual abuse are uncommon.

Epidemiology

Adults who report sexual abuse in childhood have higher rates of psychiatric disorder in adult life (Mullen *et al.*, 1993; Kendler *et al.*, 2000). Most studies have been retrospective and have involved women. Female psychiatric patients are more likely than healthy controls to report sexual abuse in childhood; such reporting is particularly frequent in those with somatization disorder, disassociative states and borderline personality disorder (see Sar *et al.*, 2004). It is not clear what proportion of women who were sexually abused in childhood develop these disorders in adult life, but some make a good adjustment. In a prospective study of over 1600 abused children, Spataro *et al.* (2004) found that that 12.4 per cent of the abused group subsequently received psychiatric treatment compared to 3.6 per cent of controls. Male children were significantly more likely to have received treatment than females. Abused subjects had higher rates of several psychiatric disorders including a range of childhood mental disorders as well as adult mood disorders, somatoform disorders, stress disorders, personality disorder and substance use disorders. In general, psychiatric consequences are particularly likely when the abusing person is a parent, when there are multiple abusers and when abuse is prolonged (Steel *et al.*, 2004).

Aetiology

There could be three explanations for an association between the reporting of childhood sexual abuse and the symptoms of psychiatric disorder in adult life:

1. People with psychiatric disorder may be more likely than controls to report childhood sexual abuse, perhaps because they have been asked questions about their childhood in the course of psychiatric assessment.
2. Childhood sexual abuse may be a direct cause of vulnerability to adult psychiatric disorder.
3. Sexual abuse may be a marker of some other factor, such as disturbed relationships within the family, which is the real cause of the excess psychiatric disorder in adult life.

These three possible causes will now be considered in turn.

It seems unlikely that the association can be explained solely by the greater recall of sexual abuse by women who have psychiatric disorder because community studies have also found an association between the reporting of childhood sexual abuse and the reporting of psychiatric symptoms (Bushnell *et al.*, 1993). In addition, as noted above there are also prospective data indicating that sexual abuse in childhood is indeed associated with adult psychiatric disorder (Spataro *et al.*, 2004).

How far sexual abuse itself directly causes adult psychiatric disorder is uncertain. For example, an association between childhood abuse and adult psychiatric disorder may be explained in part by disturbed relationships in the family of the abused child (Neumann *et al.*, 1996). Thus people who have been abused as children are more likely to report to others that their parents were uncaring or emotionally distant (Alexander and Lupfer, 1987). Mullen *et al.* (1993) found that, with less severe forms of abuse, the relationship between abuse and subsequent disorder could be accounted for by the family factors alone, but when abuse was severe, it had an independent and direct effect.

Treatment

The late effects of childhood sexual abuse have been treated with counselling, dynamic psychotherapy, cognitive therapy, and group treatments. The various methods have several common features:

- the general aim is to help the patient understand the earlier experiences and their effects on her life, in order to improve present adjustment;
- the therapeutic relationship is used to help the patient feel trusted, understood, and respected, and to increase self-esteem;
- the patient is allowed to set the pace at which she talks about the experience of being abused. (Otherwise they may be overwhelmed by an extreme emotional response to the memories of abuse, and withdraw from treatment);
- present problems of adjustment are identified, especially any avoidance of problems and difficulties in expressing anger. Help is given to overcome these difficulties;
- some patients need help with psychosexual problems.

The main difference between the dynamic and cognitive behavioural approaches is the greater emphasis given in the former to understanding the effects of the trauma on self-esteem and emotional expression, and the greater emphasis given in the latter to more precise specification of ways in which current patterns of thinking affect present behaviour.

For a review of psychological treatment of the long-term effects of sexual abuse see Kessler *et al.* (2003) and Callahan *et al.* (2004).

Further reading

Gelder, MG, López-Ibor, JJ Jr, and Andreasen, NC (eds) (2000) *The new Oxford textbook of psychiatry*, Section 4.6: Stress-related and adjustment disorders. Oxford University Press, Oxford. (The four chapters in this section contain systematic reviews of acute stress reactions, post-traumatic stress disorder, recovered and false memories, and adjustment disorders.)

Parkes, CM (1996) *Bereavement: studies of grief in adult life*, 3rd edn. Penguin Books, Harmondsworth. (A brief but comprehensive review, written for the layman but containing useful information for the professional, including a scientific appendix.)

McNally, RJ (2003) *Remembering trauma*. Harvard University Press, Cambridge, MA. (Thorough and critical account of how trauma can influence memory.)

CHAPTER 9

Anxiety and obsessive–compulsive disorders

Chapter contents

Terminology and classification

The symptom of anxiety is found in many disorders. In the anxiety disorders, it is the most severe and prominent symptom, and it is also prominent in the obsessional disorders though these are characterized by their striking obsessional symptoms. In DSM-IV, obsessional disorders are classified as a type of anxiety disorder, but in ICD10 they are classified separately. We have followed the DSM convention and included obsessional disorders in this chapter.

Anxiety disorders

Anxiety disorders are abnormal states in which the most striking features are mental and physical symptoms of anxiety, occurring in the absence of organic brain disease or another psychiatric disorder. The symptoms of anxiety are described on p. 5 and are listed for convenience in Table 9.1. Although all the symptoms can occur in any of the anxiety disorders, there is a characteristic pattern in each disorder which will be described later. The disorders share many features of their clinical picture and aetiology but there are also differences:

- In generalized anxiety disorders, anxiety is continuous – though it may fluctuate in intensity.
- In phobic anxiety disorders, anxiety is intermittent, arising in particular circumstances.
- In panic disorder, anxiety is intermittent but its occurrence is unrelated to any particular circumstances.

These differences (and some exceptions to these initial generalizations) will be explained further when the various types of anxiety disorders are described.

The development of ideas about anxiety disorders

Anxiety has long been recognized as a prominent symptom of many psychiatric disorders. Anxiety and depression often occur together and, until the last part of the nineteenth century, anxiety disorders were not classified separately from other mood disorders. It was Freud (1895b) who first suggested that cases with mainly anxiety symptoms should be recognized as a separate entity under the name of anxiety neurosis.

Freud's original anxiety neurosis included patients with phobias and panic attacks, but subsequently he divided it into two groups. The first, which retained the name anxiety neurosis, was of cases with mainly psychological symptoms of anxiety; the second group, which he called anxiety hysteria, was for cases with mainly physical symptoms of anxiety and with phobias. Thus anxiety hysteria included the cases we now diagnose as agoraphobia. Freud originally proposed that the causes of anxiety neurosis and anxiety hysteria were related to sexual conflicts, though he later accepted a rather wider range of causes. By the 1930s most psychiatrists considered that a very wide range of stressful problems could cause anxiety neurosis (see, for example, Henderson and Gillespie, 1930, pp. 416–17).

Phobic disorders have been recognized since antiquity, but the first systematic medical study of these conditions was probably that of Le Camus in the eighteenth century (Errera, 1962). The early nineteenth century classifications assigned phobias to the group of monomanias, which were disorders of thinking rather than emotion. However, when Westphal (1872) first described agoraphobia, he emphasized the importance of anxiety in the condition. Later, in 1895, Freud divided phobias into two groups: common phobias, in which there was an exaggerated fear of something that is commonly feared (for example, darkness or high places), and specific phobias, that is, fears of situations not feared by healthy people, such as open spaces (Freud 1895a, pp. 135–6). As explained later, the term specific phobia now has a rather different meaning.

In the 1960s, the different responses of certain phobias to behavioural methods suggested a grouping into simple phobias, social phobia, and agoraphobia, and these groups were found to differ also in their age of onset. (Simple phobias generally begin in childhood, social phobia in adolescence, and agoraphobia in early adult life.) At about the same time, it was observed that when phobias were accompanied by marked panic attacks, they responded poorly to behaviour therapy

TABLE 9.1 Symptoms of anxiety

Symptoms of anxiety
Psychological arousal
Fearful anticipation
Irritability
Sensitivity to noise
Restlessness
Poor concentration
Worrying thoughts
Autonomic arousal
Gastrointestinal
Dry mouth
Difficulty in swallowing
Epigastric discomfort
Excessive wind
Frequent or loose motions
Respiratory
Constriction in the chest
Difficulty inhaling
Cardiovascular
Palpitations
Discomfort in the chest
Awareness of missed heartbeats
Genitourinary
Frequent or urgent micturition
Failure of erection
Menstrual discomfort
Amenorrhoea
Muscle tension
Tremor
Headache
Aching muscles
Hyperventilation
Dizziness
Tingling in the extremities
Feeling of breathlessness
Sleep disturbance
Insomnia
Night terror

and better to imipramine (Klein, 1964). These cases were subsequently classified separately as panic disorder. This advance led to the present scheme of classification into generalized anxiety disorder, phobic anxiety disorder (simple, social, and agoraphobic), and panic disorder.

The relationship between obsessive-compulsive disorders and anxiety disorders has been and remains uncertain. Freud thought at first that phobias and obsessions were closely related (see Freud, 1895a). He proposed later that anxiety is the central problem in both conditions and that their characteristic symptoms - phobias and obsessions- resulted from different kinds of defence mechanisms against anxiety. Others considered that obsessional disorders were a separate group of neuroses of uncertain aetiology. As explained above, this division of opinion is reflected today in the two major classification systems: in DSM-IV obsessive-compulsive disorders are classified as a subgroup of the anxiety disorders; in ICD-10, anxiety disorders and obsessive-compulsive disorders have separate places in the classification.

The classification of anxiety disorders

The classification of anxiety disorders in DSM-IV and ICD-10 is shown shown in Table 9.2. Although the two are broadly similar, there are four important differences:

- in ICD-10, anxiety disorders are divided into two named subgroups: (a) phobic anxiety disorder (F40) and (b) other anxiety disorder (F41), which includes panic disorder and generalized anxiety disorder;
- panic disorder is classified differently in the two schemes (the reasons are explained on p. 192);
- in DSM-IV, obsessive-compulsive disorder is classified as one of the anxiety disorders, but in ICD-10 it has a separate place in the classification;
- ICD-10 contains a category of mixed anxietydepressive disorder, but DSM-IV does not.

TABLE 9.2 Classification of anxiety disorders

	ICD–10	DSM-IV
F4	Anxiety disorders	Anxiety disorders*
F40	Phobic anxiety disorder	
	Agoraphobia	Agoraphobia
	Without panic disorder	Without a history of panic disorder
	With panic disorder	Panic disorder with agoraphobia
	Social phobia	Social phobia
	Specific phobia	Specific phobia
F41	Other anxiety disorders	
	Panic disorder	Panic disorder without agoraphobia
	Generalized anxiety disorder	Generalized anxiety disorder
	Mixed anxiety and depressive disorder	–

* The order of presentation has been altered to facilitate comparison of the schemes.

Generalized anxiety disorders

Clinical picture

The symptoms of generalized anxiety disorder (GAD) (Table 9.3) are persistent and are not restricted to, or markedly increased in, any particular set of circumstances (in contrast to phobic anxiety disorders). All the symptoms of anxiety (see Table 9.1) can occur in GAD but there a characteristic pattern comprised of the following features:

- **worry and apprehension** that are more prolonged than those of healthy people. The worries are widespread and not focused on a specific issue as they are in panic disorder (on having a panic attack) or social phobia (on being embarrassed) or obsessive-compulsive disorder (on contamination). The person feels that these widespread worries are difficult to control.
- **psychological arousal**, which may be evident as irritability, poor concentration, and sensitivity to noise.

TABLE 9.3 Symptoms of generalized anxiety disorder

Symptoms
Worry and apprehension
Muscle tension*
Autonomic overactivity*
Psychological arousal*
Sleep disturbance*
Other features
Depression
Obsessions
Depersonalization

*See Table 9.1.

Some patients complain of poor memory but this is due to poor concentration. If true memory impairment is found, a careful search should be made for a cause other than anxiety.

- **autonomic overactivity**, which is experienced most often as sweating, palpitations, dry mouth, epigastric discomfort, and dizziness. However, patients may complain of any of the symptoms listed in Table 9.1. Some patients ask for help with any of these symptoms without mentioning spontaneously the psychological symptoms of anxiety.
- **muscle tension**, which may be experienced as restlessness, trembling, inability to relax, headache (usually bilateral and frontal or occipital) and aching in the shoulders and back.
- **hyperventilation**, which may lead to dizziness, tingling in the extremities and, paradoxically, a feeling of shortness of breath.
- **sleep disturbances**, which include difficulty in falling asleep and persistent worrying thoughts. Sleep is often intermittent, unrefreshing, and accompanied by unpleasant dreams. Some patients have night terrors in which they wake suddenly feeling intensely anxious. Early morning waking is not a feature of generalized anxiety disorder and its presence strongly suggests a depressive disorder.
- **other features** include tiredness, depressive symptoms, obsessional symptoms, and depersonalization. These symptoms are never the most prominent feature of a generalized anxiety disorder. If they are prominent, another diagnosis should be considered (see differential diagnosis below).

Clinical signs

The face appears strained, the brow is furrowed, and the posture is tense. The person is restless and may tremble. The skin is pale and sweating is common, especially from the hands, feet, and axillae. Readiness to tears, which may at first suggest depression, reflects the generally apprehensive state.

Diagnostic conventions

There is no clear dividing line between generalized anxiety disorder and normal anxiety. They differ both in the extent of the symptoms and in their duration. The diagnostic criteria for both extent and duration are arbitrary, and they differ in several ways between DSM-IV and ICD-10. Regarding **extent**, both DSM-IV and the research version of ICD-10 require the presence of a minimum number of symptoms from a list. However, the ICD-10 list contains 22 physical symptoms of anxiety, whilst there are only 6 in the DSM-IV list. Also in DSM but not in ICD, worry is a key symptom

Regarding duration, in DSM-IV and the research version of ICD-10 symptoms must have been present for 6 months. However, the ICD-10 criterion for clinical practice is more flexible; symptoms should have been present on 'most days for at least several weeks at a time, and usually several months'.

Comorbidity

Anxiety and depression

The two classifications differ in their approach to cases which fulfil the diagnostic criteria for both depressive disorder and generalized anxiety disorder. ICD-10 has a separate category for these cases, namely mixed anxiety and depressive disorder. This category is not included in DSM-IV (though it is included among 'criteria sets for further study') therefore both diagnoses are made. These conditions are discussed further below (p. 195) and in Chapter 11.

Generalized anxiety disorder and other anxiety disorders.

The guidance differs in ICD-10 and DSM-IV about the circumstances in which two diagnoses should be made:

- **in ICD-10**, generalized anxiety disorder is not diagnosed when the symptoms fulfill the diagnostic criteria for phobic anxiety disorder (F40), panic disorder (F41), or obsessive compulsive disorder (F42).
- **in DSM-IV** the emphasis placed on the worrying ideas in general anxiety disorder makes it possible to diagnose generalized anxiety disorder when these are present even in the presence of symptoms of one of the other three anxiety diagnoses When this convention is followed, comorbidity between generalized anxiety disorder and other anxiety disorders is frequent: social phobia in 23 per cent of cases of GAD, simple phobia in 21%, and panic disorder in 11 per cent (Brawman-Mintzer *et al.*, 1993).

Differential diagnosis

General anxiety disorder has to be distinguished not only from other psychiatric disorders but also from certain physical conditions. Anxiety symptoms can occur in nearly all the psychiatric disorders, but there are some in which particular diagnostic difficulties arise.

Depressive disorder

Anxiety is a common symptom in depressive disorder, and generalized anxiety disorder often includes some depressive symptoms. The usual convention is that the diagnosis is decided on the basis of the severity of two kinds of symptom and the order in which they appeared. Information on these two points should be obtained, if possible, from a relative or other informant as well as from the patient. Whichever type of symptoms appeared first and is more severe is considered primary. An important diagnostic error is to misdiagnose the agitated type of severe depressive disorder for generalized anxiety disorder. This mistake will seldom be made if anxious patients are asked routinely about symptoms of a depressive disorder including depressive thinking and, when appropriate, suicidal ideas. Depressive disorders are often worst in the morning, and anxiety that is worst at this time suggests a depressive disorder.

Schizophrenia

People with schizophrenia sometimes complain of anxiety before other symptoms are recognized. The chance of misdiagnosis can be reduced by asking anxious patients routinely what they think caused their symptoms. Schizophrenic patients may give an unusual reply, which leads to the discovery of previously unexpressed delusional ideas.

Dementia

Anxiety may be the first abnormality complained of by a person with presenile or senile dementia. When this happens, the clinician may not detect an associated impairment of memory or may dismiss it as the result of poor concentration. Therefore, memory should be assessed in middle-aged or older patients presenting with anxiety.

Substance misuse

Some people take drugs or alcohol to relieve anxiety. Patients who are dependent on drugs or alcohol sometimes believe that the symptoms of drug withdrawal are those of anxiety and take anxiolytic or other drugs to control them. The clinician should be alert to this possibility, particularly when anxiety is severe on waking in the morning, the time when alcohol and drug withdrawal symptoms tend to occur. (Anxiety that is worst in the morning also suggests depressive disorder – see above.)

Physical illness

Some physical illnesses have symptoms that can be mistaken for those of an anxiety disorder. This possibility should be considered in all cases but especially when there is no obvious psychological cause for anxiety or no history of past anxiety. The following conditions are particularly important:

- **thyrotoxicosis** in which the patient may be irritable and restless with tremor and tachycardia. Physical examination may reveal characteristic signs of thyrotoxicosis, such as enlarged thyroid, atrial fibrillation, and exophthalmos. If there is doubt, thyroid function tests should be arranged.
- **phaeochromocytoma and hypoglycaemia** usually cause episodic symptoms and are therefore more likely to mimic a phobic disorder or panic disorder. However, they should also be considered as a differential diagnosis of generalized anxiety disorder. When there is doubt, appropriate physical examination and laboratory tests should be carried out.

Anxiety secondary to the symptoms of physical illness

Sometimes the first complaint of a physically ill person is anxiety caused by worry that certain physical symptoms portend a serious illness. If the physical symptoms are non-specific, they may be mistakenly attributed to anxiety. Also some patients do not mention all the physical symptoms unless questioned. This is particularly likely when the patient has a special reason to fear serious illness, for example, if a relative or friend died of cancer after developing similar symptoms. It is good practice to ask anxious patients with physical symptoms whether they know anyone who has had similar symptoms.

Generalized anxiety disorder mistaken for physical illness

When this happens, extensive investigations may be carried out which increase the patient's anxiety. While physical illness should be considered in every case, it is also important to remember the diversity of the anxiety symptoms. Palpitations, headache, frequency of micturition, and abdominal discomfort can all be the primary complaint of an anxious patient. Correct diagnosis requires systematic enquiries about other symptoms of generalized anxiety disorder, and about the order in which the various symptoms began.

Epidemiology

Estimates of incidence and prevalence vary according to the diagnostic criteria used in the survey and whether a clinical significance criterion is used. Estimates for one year rates are around 3 per cent and lifetime rates around 4–5 per cent, with women affected more often than men. Thus, in the US Epidemiological Catchment Area Study, the one year prevalence of generalized anxiety disorder, using DSM-IIIR criteria was 3.8 per cent (Blazer *et al.*, 1991). In the US National Comorbidity Survey, the one-year prevalence rates was 2.8 per cent when a clinical significance criterion was applied (Narrow *et al.*, 2002). A survey in Africa using DSM-IV criteria found a weighted prevalence of 3.7 per cent (Bhagwanjee *et al.*, 1998). For a review of the epidemiology of generalized anxiety disorder see Kessler *et al.* (2001).

Aetiology

In general terms, generalized anxiety disorder appears to be caused by stressors acting on a personality predisposed by a combination of genetic factors and environmental influences in childhood. However, evidence for the nature and importance of these causes is incomplete.

Stressful events

Clinical observations indicate that generalized anxiety disorders often begin in relation to stressful events, and some become chronic when stressful problems persist. Stressful events involving threat are particularly related to anxiety disorder - loss events are associated more with depression (Finlay-Jones and Brown, 1981). In the Epidemiological Catchment Area Study, men who reported four or more stressful life events in the preceding year were eight times more likely to meet DSM-IIIR criteria for generalized anxiety disorder than were men reporting three or fewer such events in that period (Blazer *et al.*, 1991).

Genetic causes

Family studies Generalized anxiety disorders are more frequent among the first-degree relatives of probands with generalized anxiety disorder than among first-degree relatives of controls.

Twin studies Early twin studies (for example, Slater and Shields [1969] showed a higher concordance for anxiety disorder between monozygotic than dizygotic pairs, suggesting that the familial association has a genetic cause. However, the study did not distinguish between different kinds of anxiety disorder. A meta-analysis showed that the familial aggregation is largely explained by genes, with an important role for non-shared environmental factors while the role of family environment is uncertian Hettema *et al.* (2001). The hereditability appears to be shared with mood disorders, suggesting that environmental factors somehow determine how the inherited vulnerability is expressed (Roy *et al.*, 1995).

Early experience

Accounts given by anxious patients of their experience in childhood suggest that early adverse experiences is a cause of generalized anxiety disorder. These accounts have given rise to objective studies and to psychoanalytic theories.

Objective studies Brown and Harris (1993) studied the relation between adverse experience in childhood and anxiety disorder in adult life in 404 working-class women living in an inner city. Adverse early experience was assessed from patients' accounts of parental indifference and of physical or sexual abuse. Women reporting early adversity had increased rates of generalized anxiety disorder (and also agoraphobia, and depressive disorder, but not simple phobia). Also Kendler *et al.* (1992b) found that the rate of anxiety disorder (and several other psychiatric disorders) was greater in women separated from the mother before the age of 17 years.

Psychoanalytic theories Psychoanalytical theory proposes that anxiety arises from intrapsychic conflict. It arises when the ego is overwhelmed by excitation from any of three sources:

1. the outside world (realistic anxiety);
2. the instinctual level of the id, including love, anger, and sex (neurotic anxiety);
3. the superego (moral anxiety).

According to this theory, in generalized anxiety disorder, anxiety is experienced directly unmodified by the defence mechanisms that are thought to be the basis of phobias or obsessions (see pp. 184 and 199). The theory proposes that in generalized anxiety disorders, the ego is readily overwhelmed because it has been weakened by a developmental failure in childhood. Separation and loss are thought to be particularly important causes of this failure (Bowlby, 1969). Normally, children overcome anxiety through secure relationships with loving parents. If they do not achieve this security, they will be liable, as adults, to anxiety when experiencing separation. Freud suggested that, at a later stage of childhood, anxiety is linked to rivalry with the father. He used the term castration anxiety, and described the rivalry as the Oedipal conflict (see p. 91). He believed that failure to surmount this stage of development successfully was another cause of vulnerability to anxiety in adult life. These theories have not been confirmed by scientific study.

Cognitive–behavioural theories

Conditioning theories propose that generalized anxiety disorders arise when there is an inherited predisposition to excessive responsiveness of the autonomic nervous system, together with generalization of the responses through conditioning of anxiety to previously neutral stimuli. This theory has not been supported by a body of objective data.

Cognitive theory proposes that generalized anxiety disorder arises from a tendency to worry unproductively about problems and to focus attention on potentially threatening circumstances. This theory is supported directly by studies of thinking in anxious patients and controls, and indirectly by the efficacy of cognitive-behavioural treatments (see p. 182). (For a review of research on the cognitive aspects of generalized anxiety disorder see Wells and Butler, 1997.)

Personality

Personality traits: The symptom of anxiety is associated with neuroticism, and twin studies have shown an overlap between the genetic factors related to neuroticism and those related to generalized anxiety disorder (Hettema *et al.*, 2004).

Personality disorder: Generalized anxiety disorder occurs in people with anxious-avoidant personality disorders, but also in people with other personality disorders.

Neurobiological mechanisms

The neurobiological mechanisms involved in general anxiety disorders are presumably those which mediate normal anxiety. The mechanisms are complex, involving several brain systems and several neurotransmitters. Studies in animals have indicated a key role for the amygdala, which receives sensory information both directly from the thalamus and from a longer pathway involving somatosensory cortex and anterior cingulate cortex. Cortical involvement in anxiety is important because it indicates a role for cognitive processes in its expression (see le Doux, 2000). The hippocampus is also believed to have an important role in the regulation of anxiety because it relates fearful memories to relevant present contexts. Breakdown of this mechanism could lead to an overgeneralization of fear in response to non-threatening stimuli.

Animal studies have also led to an understanding of the regulation of anxiety in the brain by neurotransmitters and neuromodulators. Noradrenergic neurons originating in the locus ceruleus increase arousal and anxiety. Serotonergic eurons originating in the raphe nuclei appear to have complex effects, some inhibitory, others anxiogenic. Gamma-aminobutyric acid (GABA) receptors, which are widely distributed in the brain, are inhibitory, as are the associated benzodiazepine binding sites. There is probably an important role also for corticotrophin releasing hormone which increases anxiety-related behaviours and is found in high concentration in the amygdala (see Charney and Bremner, 2004).

These mechanisms are likely to be involved also in generalized anxiety disorder but there is little relevant research in humans. Functional scanning of the brain has shown increased cortical activity and decreased basal ganglia activity in patients with generalized anxiety disorder but the functional significance of these changes is uncertain. For a review of these and other neurobiological changes in generalized anxiety disorder see Nutt (2001).

Prognosis

One of the DSM-IV criteria for generalized anxiety disorder is that the symptoms should have been present for 6 months. One of the reasons for this cut-off is that anxiety disorders lasting for longer than 6 months have a poor prognosis: thus in one study, 80 per cent were still present after 3 years (Abelson *et al.*, 1991). The prognosis beyond 3 years is less certain though in a study of medical patients with anxiety disorder, two-thirds improved substantially or recovered within 6 years (Yonkers *et al.*, 1996).

The risk of major depression is increased among patients with generalized anxiety disorders (as it is with other anxiety disorders) (Bittner *et al.*, 2004). However, the rates of schizophrenia and bipolar disorder are not increased (Kerr *et al.*, 1974). The relationship between anxiety and depression is considered further on p. 222.

Treatment

Counselling

In the absence of a sufficient data from well conducted controlled trials, guidance has to be based on clinical experience. In the early stages of a generalized anxiety disorder (before symptoms have been established for the 6 months necessary for a DSM-IV diagnosis), counselling is often effective. Some patients with more persistent generalized anxiety disorders also respond to counselling, but others need either cognitive-behavioural therapy or medication (both are described below). Counselling for generalized anxiety disorder follows the general lines described on p. 584 with particular emphasis on the following:

- **a clear plan** of management agreed with the patient and, when appropriate, a relative or partners.
- an **explanation** of the nature of the disorder and **reassurance** that any physical symptoms of anxiety are not caused by physical disease. (Since anxious people often concentrate poorly, it is useful to provide an information leaflet that contains the same points.)
- **problem-solving** or help in adjusting to problems.
- advice about the use of **caffeine**. Patients with generalized anxiety disorder are more sensitive than

normal subjects to the anxiogenic effects of caffeine (Bruce *et al.*, 1992). Although many patients discover this for themselves and reduce their caffeine intake, those who have not done so may be helped by advice to avoid excessive caffeine.

Relaxation training

Because there have been no satisfactory controlled trials with patients with formally diagnosed generalized anxiety disorder, advice has to be based on clinical experience. If practised regularly, relaxation seems able to reduce anxiety in the less severe cases. However, many patients with such disorders do not practise the relaxation exercises regularly. Motivation may be improved if the training is in a group, and some people engage more with treatment when relaxation is taught as part of a programme of yoga exercises.

Cognitive–behaviour therapy

This treatment combines relaxation with cognitive procedures designed to help patients to control worrying thoughts. The method is described on p. 594. Its produces improvement greater that no treatment or non-specific treatment (Borkovec and Ruscio, 2000) with a decrease in symptom severity of about 50 per cent and a low dropout rate (Barlow *et al.*, 1997). The effects are maintained for at least two years (Borkovec *et al.*, 2002) and possibly much longer (Durham *et al.*, 2003). However it has not been shown that the full procedure is more effective than either relaxation alone or cognitive therapy without relaxation (Borkovec *et al.*, 2002).

Medication

Anxiolytic drugs are described on p. 526. Here we are concerned with some special points about their use in generalized anxiety disorders. Medication can be used to bring symptoms under control quickly, while the effects of psychological treatment are awaited. It can be used also when psychological treatment has failed. However, medication is often prescribed too readily and for too long. Before prescribing, it is appropriate to recall that the placebo response rate with generalized anxiety disorder is about 40 per cent (Fossey and Lydiard, 1990), showing that improvement can often occur without medication.

Short-term treatment One of the longer acting benzodiazepines is appropriate for the short-term treatment of generalized anxiety disorders, for example, diazepam in a dose from 5 mg twice daily in mild cases to 10 mg three times a day in the most severe. Anxiolytic drugs should seldom be prescribed for more than 3 weeks because of the risk of dependence when given for longer. Buspirone (see p. 527) is similarly effective for short-term management of generalized anxiety disorder and less likely to cause dependency has but has a slower onset of action. Beta adrenergic antagonists (see p. 528) are sometimes used to control anxiety associated with severe palpitations that have not responded to other treatment. However,they are used more often for performance anxiety (see p. 188) than for generalized anxiety disorder. If one of these drugs is used, care should be taken to observe the contraindications to treatment and the advice given on p. 528 and in the manufacturer's literature.

Long-term treatment Because generalized anxiety disorders often require lengthy treatment, for which benzodiazepines are unsuitable (see above), and because depressive disorders often develop during follow-up, long-term treatment is usually with one of the anxiolytic antidepressants (see Chapter 21). Both tricyclic and specific serotonin release inhibitors can be used for this purpose. Antipsychotic drugs, given in low doses, can also be employed but their use is usually restricted to anxiety in people with aggressive personalities, or people who have become dependent on other drugs.

Although long-term treatment is often needed, clinical trials of antidepressants for anxiety disorders have seldom lasted for more than two to three months. It is necessary, therefore, to extrapolate from the extensive experience of the use of these drugs in the long-term treatment of depressive disorders. This experience indicates that medication can be continued safely and effectively for many months. Amongst the available drugs, venlafaxine and paroxetine have been tested for longer than most others and have shown to be effective (see Rouillon, 2004). **Monoamine oxidase inhibitors** were the first antidepressants to be used to treat anxiety disorders (Sargant and Dally, 1962) but they are seldom used for this purpose nowadays because of their many interactions with other drugs and foodstuffs (see p. 550).

For a Cochrane review of the use of antidepressants in generalized anxiety disorder see Kapczinski *et al.* (2003).

Management

In primary care, many patients are seen in the early stage of an anxiety disorder before a formal diagnosis of generalized anxiety disorder can be made. As noted above, these patients often respond to counselling. If anxiety is severe, a short course of a benzodiazepine can bring rapid relief. Psychiatrists are more likely to encounter established cases. The steps in the management of such patients are:

- **Check diagnosis and comorbidity** especially depressive disorder, substance abuse, or a physical cause such as thyrotoxicosis. If present treat appropriately.
- **Evaluate psychosocial maintaining factors** such as persistent social problems, marital conflict, and concerns that physical symptoms of anxiety are evidence of serious physical disease.
- **Explain the evaluation and proposed treatment** especially the origins of any physical symptoms of anxiety. Discuss the way in which the patient might describe the condition to employers, friends and family. Self-help books (for example Kennerley, 1997), reinforce the explanation and describe simple cognitive–behavioural techniques that people can use on their own or as part of a wider plan of treatment.
- **Offer psychological or social help** either in the form of counselling as described above, or practical help with social problems, or cognitive behaviour therapy.
- **Consider medication:** a short course of benzodiazepines may be prescribed to reduce high anxiety initially but seldom for more than about 3 weeks. Low dose antidepressant therapy is used for longer term control of anxiety either until psychological treatment can be arranged or after it has been tried and failed. The main and side effects of medication should be discussed as in the use of the same drugs in the treatment of depression (see p. 258).
- **Discuss the plan with the patient, the general practtoner and the community team** to allocate tasks and responsibility appropriately. Plans should recognize that generalized anxiety disorder is often a long term problem.

Phobic anxiety disorders

Phobic anxiety disorders have the same core symptoms as generalized anxiety disorders, but these symptoms occur only in particular circumstances. In some phobic disorders these circumstances are few and the patient is free from anxiety for most of the time. In other phobic disorders many circumstances provoke anxiety, with the result that anxiety is more frequent, but even so there are situations in which no anxiety is experienced. Two other features characterize phobic disorders: the person avoids circumstances that provoke anxiety, and experiences anticipatory anxiety when there is the prospect of encountering these circumstances. The circumstances provoking anxiety can be grouped into **situations** (for example, crowded places), **'objects'** (a term that includes living things such as spiders), and **natural phenomena** (for example, thunder). For clinical purposes, three principal phobic syndromes are recognized: specific phobia, social phobia, and agoraphobia. These syndromes will be described next.

Classification of phobic disorders

In DSM-IV and ICD-10 phobic disorders are divided into specific phobia, social phobia, and agoraphobia. In DSM-IV, but not in ICD-10, agoraphobic patients who have regular panic attacks (more than four in 4 weeks, or one attack followed by a month of persistent fear of having another) are classified as having panic disorder. The reasons for this convention are explained on p. 192.

Specific phobia

Clinical picture

A person with a specific phobia is inappropriately anxious in the presence of a particular object or situation. In the presence of the object or in the situation, the person experiences the symptoms of anxiety listed above in Table 9.1. Anticipatory anxiety is common, and the person ususally seeks to escape from and avoid the feared situation. Specific phobias can be characterized further by adding the name of the stimulus; for example spider phobia. In the past it was common to use terms such as arachnophobia (instead of spider phobia) or acrophobia (instead of phobia of heights), but this practice adds nothing of value to the use of the simpler names.

In DSM-IV, four types of specific phobia are recognized concerned with:

1. animals
2. aspects of the natural environment
3. blood, injection, and injury
4. situations and other provoking agents. This group includes fears of dental and medical situations and fears of choking.

The following specific phobias merit brief separate consideration.

Phobia of dental treatment

About 5 per cent of adults have fears of dental treatment. These fears can become so severe that all dental treatment is avoided and serious caries develops. A meta-analysis of 38 studies of behavioural treatment found a significant reduction in fear with on average 77 per cent attending for dental treatment four years after the treatment (Kvale *et al.*, 2004).

Phobia of flying

Anxiety during aeroplane travel is common. A few people have such intense anxiety that they are unable to travel in an aeroplane and some seek treatment. This fear occurs occasionally among pilots who have had an accident while flying. Desensitization treatment (see p. 591) is provided by some airlines, and self-help books are available. Virtual reality programmes have been used to replace actual and imagined exposure. Good resuts have been reported (Rothbaum *et al.*, 2002) but not confirmed (Maltby *et al.*, 2002).

Blood injury phobia

In this phobia, the sight of blood or of an injury results in anxiety. However, the accompanying autonomic response differs from that in other phobic disorders. The initial tachycardia is followed by a vasovagal response with bradycardia, pallor, dizziness, nausea, and sometimes fainting. It has been reported that people who have this kind of phobia are prone to develop to neurally mediated syncope even without the specific blood injury stimulus (Accurso *et al.*, 2001). Thus tensing the muscles may help prevent syncope. There is a high prevalence of the condition among first-degree relatives of affected people. For further information see Marks (1988).

Phobia of choking

People with this kind of phobia are intensely concerned that they will choke when attempting to swallow. They have an exaggerated gag reflex and feel intensely anxious when they attempt to swallow. The onset is either in childhood, or after choking on food in adult life. Some of these people also fear dental treatment, others avoid eating in public. Treatment is with desensitization. For further information see McNally (1994).

Phobia of illness

People with this phobia experience repeated fearful thoughts that they might have cancer, venereal disease, or some other serious illness. Unlike people with delusions, people with phobias of illness recognize that the thoughts are irrational, at least when the thoughts are not present. Moreover, they do not resist the thoughts as obsessional thoughts are resisted. Such people may avoid hospitals, but are not otherwise specific to situations. If the patient is convinced that he has the disease, the condition is classified as hypochondriasis (see p. 209). When the thoughts are recognized as irrational and are resisted, the condition is classified as obsessive–compulsive disorder.

Epidemiology

Among adults the lifetime **prevalence** of specific phobias has been estimated, using DSM-IIIR criteria, as 4 per cent in men and 13 per cent in women (Kessler *et al.*, 1994). When a clinical significance criterion is applied, the overall one year rate is 4.4 per cent (Narrow *et al.*, 2002). The **age of onset** of most specific phobias is in childhood: phobias of animals at average age 7 years, blood phobia at 9, dental phobia at 12 (Öst, 1987a).

Aetiology

Persistence of childhood fears

Most specific phobias of adult life are a continuation of childhood phobias. Specific phobias are common in childhood (see p. 682). By early teenage years most of these childhood fears have been lost, but a few persist into adult life. Why the few persist is not certain, except that the most severe phobias are likely to last the longest.

Genetic factors

In one study, 31 per cent of first-degree relatives of people with specific phobia also had the condition (Fyer *et al.*, 1995). The results of a study of female twins with specific phobia fitted an aetiological model in which a modest genetic vulnerability combined with phobia-specific stressful events (Kendler *et al.*, 1992a). The genetic vulnerability may involve difference in the strength of fear conditioning which has a hereditability of around 40 per cent Hettema *et al.*, 2003).

Psychoanalytical theories

These theories suggest that phobias are not related to the obvious external stimulus but to an internal source of anxiety. This internal source is excluded from consciousness by repression and attached to the external object by displacement.The theory is not supported by objective evidence.

Conditioning and cognitive theories

Conditioning theory suggests that specific phobias arise through association learning. A minority of specific phobias appear to begin in this way in adult life, in relation to a highly stressful experience; for example, a phobia of horses may start after a dangerous encounter with a bolting horse. Some specific phobias may be acquired by observational learning: the child observes another person's fear responses and learns to fear the same stimuli. Cognitive factors are involved also in the maintenance of the fear, especially fearful anticipation of, and selective attention to the phobic stimuli.

Prepared learning

This term refers to an innate predisposition to develop persistent fear responses to certain stimuli. Some young primates seem to be prepared to develop fears of snakes, but it is not certain whether the same process accounts for some of the specific phobias of human children.

Cerebral localization

Positron emission tomography has been used to study changes in blood-flow when people with a specific phobia are exposed to a feared stimulus. When people with specific phobia are exposed to a stimulus for their phobia they have a startle response and there is an accompanying increase in activity in the anterior cingulate cortex, the amygdala and hippocampal areas (Pissiota *et al.*, 2003; Frederickson and Furmark, 2003).

Differential diagnosis

Diagnosis is seldom difficult. The possibility of an underlying depressive disorder should always be kept in mind, since some patients seek help for long-standing specific phobias when a depressive disorder makes them less able to tolerate their phobic symptoms. Obsessional disorders sometimes present with fear and avoidance of objects such as knives (see p. 197). In such cases a systematic history and mental state examination will reveal the associated obsessional thoughts (for example, thoughts of harming a person with a knife).

Prognosis

The prognosis of specific phobia in adult life has not been studied systematically. Clinical experience suggests that specific phobias originating in childhood continue for many years, whilst those starting after stressful events in adult life have a better prognosis.

Treatment

The main treatment is the exposure form of behaviour therapy (see p. 591). With this treatment, the phobia is usually reduced considerably in intensity and so is the social disability. However it is unusual for the phobia to be lost completely. Outcome depends importantly on repeated and prolonged exposure and drop-out rates of up to 50 per cent have been reported (Schneier *et al.* 1995). Some patients seek help soon before an important engagement that will be made difficult by the phobia. When this happens, a few doses of a benzodiazepine may be prescribed to relieve phobic anxiety until a treatment can be arranged. Exposure is usually over several one-hour sessions, but it can be carried out in a single very long and intensive session lasting several hours (Ost *et al.*, 2001).

TABLE 9.4 Abbreviated diagnostic criteria for social phobia in ICD–10 and DSM-IV*

ICD-10	DSM-IV
Marked fear or avoidance of being the focus of attention or of behaving in an embarrassing or humiliating way – manifested in social situations	Marked fear or avoidance of situations in which the person is exposed to unfamiliar people or to scrutiny with fear of behaving in an embarrassing or humiliating way
Two symptoms of anxiety in the feared situations plus at least one from blushing/shaking, fear of vomiting and fear or urgency of micturition or defecation	–
Significant emotional distress, recognized as excessive or unreasonable	Recognizes that the fear is excessive or unreasonable, interferes with functioning or causes marked distress
Symptoms restricted to or predominate in feared situations or their contemplation	–
Not secondary to another disorder	Not secondary to another disorder Duration at least 6 months if the person is under 18 years of age

* To facilitate comparison between the two sets of criteria, the wordings have been paraphrased and the order of some items has been changed.

Social phobia

Clinical picture

In this disorder, inappropriate anxiety is experienced in social situations in which the person feels observed by others and could be criticized by them. Socially phobic people attempt to avoid such situations. If they cannot avoid them, they try not to engage in them fully; for example, they avoid making conversation, or they sit in the place where they are least conspicuous. Even the prospect of encountering the object or situation may cause considerable anxiety.

The situations include restaurants, canteens, dinner parties, seminars, board meetings, and other places where the person feels observed by other people. Some patients become anxious in a wide range of social situations (**generalized social phobia**), whilst others are anxious only in specific situations such as public speaking, writing in front of others, or playing a musical instrument in public. These discrete social phobias are classified separately in DSM-IV (though not in ICD-10).

The symptoms People with social phobia may experience any of the anxiety symptoms listed in Table 9.3, but complaints of blushing and trembling are particularly frequent. Socially phobic people are often preoccupied with the idea of being observed critically, though they are aware that the idea is groundless.

The cognitions centre round a fear of being evaluated critically by others. These cognitions are described further under aetiology, below.

Other problems Some patients take alcohol to relieve the symptoms of anxiety, and alcohol misuse is more common in social phobia than in other phobias; also social phobia is a predictor of alcohol misuse (Zimmermann *et al.*, 2003). Comorbid depressive disorder is common, and suicide attempts seem to be more frequent than in the general population (Schneier *et al.*, 1992).

Onset and development The condition usually begins in the early teenage years. The first episode occurs in a public place, usually without an apparent reason. Subsequently, anxiety is felt in similar places and the episodes become progressively more severe with increasing avoidance.

Two discrete social phobias require separate consideration:

1. **Phobia of excretion** Patients with these phobias either become anxious and unable to pass urine in public lavatories, or have frequent urges to pass urine with an associated fear of incontinence. Such patients arrange their lives so as never to be far from a lavatory. A few have comparable symptoms centred around defecation.

2. **Phobias of vomiting** Some patients fear that they may vomit in a public place, often a bus or train; in these surroundings they feel nausea and anxiety. A smaller group have repeated fears that other people will vomit in their presence.

Diagnostic conventions

Table 9.4 shows in summary form the criteria for the diagnosis of social phobia in ICD-10 and DSM-IV. The requirements are similar (although the original wordings differ more than the paraphrased versions in the table) though there is greater emphasis in ICD-10 on symptoms of anxiety: two general symptoms of anxiety and one of three symptoms associated with social phobia. DSM-IV has an additional criterion that symptoms must have been present for at least 6 months if the person is under 18 years of age.

Differential diagnosis

Agoraphobia and panic disorder The symptom of social phobia can occur in either of these disorders. When this occurs both diagnoses can be made, though it is generally more useful for the clinician to decide which syndrome should be given priority.

Generalized anxiety disorder and depressive disorder Social phobia has to be distinguished from the former by establishing the situations in which anxiety occurs; and from the latter from the history and mental state.

Schizophrenia Some patients with schizophrenia avoid social situations because they have persecutory delusions. Although when they are in the feared situation, people with social phobia may feel convinced by their ideas of being observed, when they are away from the situation they know that their ideas are false.

Body dysmorphic disorder People with this disorder may avoid social situations but the diagnosis is usually clear from the patient's account of the problem.

Avoidant personality disorder Social phobia has to be distinguished from a personality characterized by life-long shyness and lack of self-confidence. In principle, social phobia has a recognizable onset and a shorter history, but in practice the distinction may be difficult to make since social phobia usually begins in adolescence and the exact onset may be difficult to recall. Many people have disorders that meet criteria for both diagnoses (Schneier *et al.*, 1992).

Inadequate social skills This is a primary lack of social skills with secondary anxiety; it is not a phobic disorder but a type of behaviour that occurs in personality disorders, in schizophrenia, and among people of low intelligence. Its features include hesitant, dull, and inaudible diction, inappropriate use of facial expression and gesture, and failure to look at other people during conversation.

Normal shyness Some people who have none of the above disorders are shy and feel ill at ease in company. The diagnostic criteria for social phobia set a level of severity intended to exclude these people.

Epidemiology

The one-year prevalence of social phobia in the US National Comorbidity Study was 7.4 per cent, falling to 3.7 per cent of 18–54 year olds when a clinical significance criterion was applied. Social phobias are about equally frequent among the men and women who seek treatment, but in the community surveys they are reported rather more frequently by women (Kessler *et al.*, 1994). As noted above, social phobia is associated with depression and alcoholism.

Aetiology

Genetic factors

Genetic factors are suggested by the finding that social phobias (but not other anxiety disorders) are more common among the relatives of social phobics than in the population (Fyer *et al.*, 1993). The rates of social phobia in first-degree relatives is greater when the probands have generalized social phobia than when they have non-generalized social phobia (Stein *et al.*, 1998a). In a population-based sample of over 2000 female twins, the results from probands with social phobia fitted a model in which moderate genetic influences, accounting for less than a third of the variance, interact with nonspecific environmental factors (Kendler *et al.*, 1992a).

Conditioning

Most social phobias begin with a sudden episode of anxiety in circumstances similar to those which become the stimulus for the phobia, and it is possible that the subsequent development of phobic symptoms is partly through conditioning.

Cognitive factors

The principal cognitive factor in the aetiology of social phobia is an undue concern that other people will be critical of the person in social situations (often referred to as a 'fear of negative evaluation'). This concern is accompanied by several other ways of thinking including:

- Excessively high standards for social performance
- Negative beliefs about the self – e.g. I am boring
- Excessive monitoring of their own performance in social situations
- Intrusive negative images of the self as supposedly seen by others.

People with social phobia often adopt *safety behaviours* (see p. 588) such as avoiding eye contact, which makes it harder for the phobic person to interact normally. For a review of the cognitive model of social phobia see Clark (2001).

Neural mechanisms

A PET study of social phobics experiencing anticipatory anxiety found increased blood flow in the right dorsolateral prefrontal cortex, left inferior temporal cortex and left amygdaloid–hippocampal region. This pattern of activation is similar to that during anticipatory anxiety in healthy people except that (i) the amygdala is not activated in the latter and (ii) activation is more widespread in social phobics (Tilfors *et al.*, 2001). The functional significance of these findings could be that the amygdala is a brain region involved in response to threat. Successful treatment with either citalopram or cognitive behaviour therapy results in decreased blood flow in the amygdala and related brain areas (Furmark *et al.*, 2002).

Course and prognosis

People with social phobia identified in community surveys had experienced the symptoms for an average of 20–25 years (Davidson *et al.*, 1993). As noted already, alcoholism and depression occur during follow-up. Although there have been reports of an increased rate of deliberate self-harm in these patients, it seems that this behaviour occurs only when there is a comorbid condition such as depressive disorder and alcohol misuse (Schneier *et al.*, 1992).

Treatment

Psychological treatment

Cognitive–behaviour therapy is the psychological treatment of choice for social phobia (this treatment is described on p. 594). The original cognitive procedures were based on those used successfully for agoraphobia and panic disorder, and when added to exposure, did not greatly increase the benefit (Gould *et al.*, 1997; Taylor, 1996). A modified form of cognitive–behaviour therapy appears to be more effective (See Clark 2001, Clark *et al.*, 2003). This modified treatment is (i) based on the particular cognitive abnormalities found in social phobia (see above under Aetiology); (ii) coupled with measures to reduce safety behaviours (see p. 588); and (iii) using video or audio feedback. Cognitive–behaviour therapy can be given in a group format but this may not be as effective as individual treatment (Stangier *et al.*, 2003).

Relaxation training given alone appears to be ineffective for social phobia (Alström *et al.*, 1984), though it may have greater effect when combined with exposure though it is probably less effective than cognitive therapy (Jerremalm *et al.*, 1986).

Dynamic psychotherapy Clinical experience suggests that this treatment may help some patients, particularly those whose social phobia is associated with pre-existing problems in personal relationships. However, there have been no controlled trials to test this impression.

Drug treatment

Specific serotonin re-uptake inhibitors are often the first choice. Fluvoxamine (van Vliet *et al.*, 1994), paroxetine (Stein *et al.*, 1998b), and sertraline (Katzelnick *et al.*, 1995) have been shown in controlled trials to be effective for social phobia. Fluoxetine may also be effective (Davidson *et al.*, 2004). With any of these drugs, the onset of action may take up to 6 weeks. Medication is usually continued for 9 months to a year, since up to a half of patients relapse if is stopped earlier (see for example Haug *et al.*, 2003). When medication is reduced, it should be done slowly.

Monoamine oxidase inhibitors Phenelzine is more effective in the treatment of social phobia than placebo (Liebowitz *et al.*, 1988) or atenolol (Liebowitz *et al.*, 1992) and comparable to phenelzine (Heimberg *et al.*, 1998). Moclobemide, the reversible inhibitor of monoamine oxidase, can also be prescribed but reported response rates vary. In an industry-sponsored trial, 47 per cent were much improved (International Multicenter Clinical Trial Group on Moclobemide in Social Phobia, 1997); in another smaller trial, only 17.5 per cent were rated as responders (Schneier *et al.*, 1998). If a MAOI is used after failure to respond to an SSRI, there should be at least 2 weeks interval, and when fluoxetine is used, 5 weeks (see p. 551).

Benzodiazepines can be used for short term relief of symptoms but should not be prescribed for long because of the risk of dependency (see p. 527). The main use of benzodiazepines is to help patients cope with essential social commitments while waiting for another treatment to take effect.

Beta-adrenergic blockers Beta-adrenergic blockers such as atenolol may achieve short-term control of tremor and palpitations, which can be the most handicapping symptoms of specific social phobias such as performance anxiety among musicians. However, their effect in social phobia overall seems not to be significantly greater than that of placebo (Turner *et al.*, 1994).

For a review of the treatment of social phobia, see Veale (2003).

Management

What patients need to know Patients need to understand that although constitutional factors may play a part, the extent and severity of their social anxiety has built up as a result of adopting maladaptive ways of thinking and behaving when socially anxious. These patterns of thinking and behaviour can be reversed either with psychological treatment or with medication. Self-help books (for example Butler, 1999) can inform patients and help them to use simple cognitive behavioural approaches while awaiting further help.

The choice of treatment The choice between medication and psychological treatment should be discussed with the patient, after explaining the side-effects of medication and the need to take it for several months; and, with psychological treatment, the requirement for regular attendance and strong involvement. In many services, psychological treatments have a long waiting period, whilst medication is available immediately.

The choice of medication Benzodiazepines should be used only for short-term relief of symptoms while other treatment takes effect. If there is comorbid substance abuse, benzodiazepines should not be used. The next choice is between a monoamine oxidase inhibitor (MAOI) and a selective serotonin re-uptake inhibitor (SSRI). Generally, one of the SSRIs is likely to be the first choice. If psychological treatment is chosen, cognitive–behaviour therapy is supported by the strongest evidence of effectiveness. Psychodynamic treatment may help some patients, but its use is not based on evidence from clinical trials.

Agoraphobia

Clinical features

Agoraphobic patients are anxious when they are away from home, in crowds, or in situations that they cannot leave easily. They avoid these situations, feel anxious when anticipating them, and experience other symptoms. These features will now be onsidered one by one.

Anxiety

The anxiety symptoms experienced by agoraphobic patients in the phobic situations are similar to those of other anxiety disorders (see Table 9.1) although two features are particularly important:

1. Panic attacks, whether in response to environmental stimuli or arising spontaneously.
2. Anxious cognitions about fainting and loss of control.

In DSM-IV, cases with more than four panic attacks in 4 weeks are not classified as agoraphobia but as panic disorder with secondary agoraphobic symptoms; the reasons for this convention are discussed on p. 192.

Situations

Many situations provoke anxiety and avoidance. They seem at first to have little in common but there are three common themes of **distance from home**, **crowding**, and **confinement**. The situations include buses and trains, shops and supermarkets, and places that cannot be left suddenly without attracting attention, such as the hairdresser's chair or a seat in the middle of a row in a place of entertainment. As the condition progresses, patients avoid more and more of these situations until in severe cases they may be more or less confined to their homes (sometimes called the 'housebound housewife syndrome', though not all these people are housewives). Apparent variations in this pattern are usually due to factors that reduce symptoms for a while. For example, most patients are less anxious when accompanied by a trusted companion and some are helped even by the presence of a child or pet dog. The variability in anxiety produced in this way may suggest erroneously that when symptoms are severe they are being exaggerated.

Anticipatory anxiety

This is common. In severe cases this anxiety appears hours before the person enters the feared situation, adding to the patient's distress and sometimes suggesting that the anxiety is generalized rather than phobic.

Other symptoms

Depressive symptoms are common. Sometimes they are a consequence of the limitations to normal life caused by anxiety and avoidance; in other cases they seem to be part of disorder, as in other anxiety disorders. **Depersonalization** can be severe.

Onset and course

The onset and course of agoraphobia differ in several ways from those of other phobic disorders.

Age of onset Most cases begin in the early or middle twenties, with a further period of high onset in the mid-thirties. Both these ages are later than the average ages of onset of simple phobias (childhood) and social phobias (mostly teenage years).

Circumstances of onset Typically, the first episode occurs while the person, more often a woman (see below), is waiting for public transport or shopping in a crowded store. Suddenly she becomes extremely anxious without knowing why, feels faint, and experiences palpitations. She rushes away from the place and goes home or to hospital, where she recovers rapidly. When she enters the same or similar surroundings, she becomes anxious again and makes another hurried escape. However, not all patients describe such an onset starting from an unexplained panic attack. It is unusual to discover any serious immediate stress that could account for the first panic attack, though some patients describe a background of serious problems (e.g. worry about a sick child); in a few cases the symptoms begin soon after a physical illness or childbirth.

Subsequent course The sequence of anxiety and avoidance recurs over the next weeks and months with panic attacks experienced in more and more places, and an increasing habit of avoidance develops.

Effect on the family As the condition progresses, agoraphobic patients become increasingly dependent on their partner relatives for help with activities, such as shopping, that provoke anxiety. The consequent demands on the spouse often lead to arguments, but serious marital problems are no more common among agoraphobics than among other people of similar social background (Buglass *et al.*, 1977).

Diagnostic conventions

Most, but not all, patients with agoraphobia have panic attacks, which may be situational or spontaneous, and many of these patients meet criteria for panic disorder as well as for agoraphobia. In ICD-10, conditions that meet both sets of criteria are diagnosed as agoraphobia but in DSM-IV they are diagnosed as panic disorder with agoraphobia. A consequence of this convention is that DSM-IV contains a category of agoraphobia without panic attacks. Another difference is that the ICD criteria require definitive anxiety symptoms (see Table 9.1). (The criteria for the diagnosis of panic disorder in DSM-IV are considered on p. 193.)

Differential diagnosis

Social phobia

Some patients with agoraphobia feel anxious in social situations, and some social phobics avoid crowded

TABLE 9.5 Abbreviated diagnostic criteria for agoraphobia in ICD–10 and agoraphobia without panic in DSM-IV

ICD–10	DSM-IV
Marked, consistent fear in, or avoidance of at least two situations from: crowds, public places, travelling alone, travel away from home	Anxiety in situations in which escape may be difficult, or help unavailable were there a panic attack, e.g. outside the home, crowds, travel, bridges
Significant distress caused by the avoidance, or the anxiety, recognized as excessive or unreasonable	These situations are avoided, or endured with distress
At least one symptom of autonomic arousal plus one other anxiety symptom in the feared	Criteria for panic disorder never met
Symptoms restricted to, or predominate in, the feared situations or contemplation thereof	
Not the result of another disorder, nor to cultural beliefs	Not accounted for by another disorder

* The criteria have been abbreviated and paraphrased, and the order has been changed to facilitate comparison of the two systems.

buses and shops where they feel under scrutiny. Detailed enquiry into the current pattern of avoidance and into the order in which the two sets of symptoms developed will usually decide the diagnosis.

Generalized anxiety disorder

When the agoraphobia is severe, anxiety may develop in so many situations that the condition resembles generalized anxiety disorder. In these cases, the history of development of the disorder will usually point to the correct diagnosis.

Panic disorder

Agoraphobia often includes panic attacks. The distiction between the two disorders has been discussed above.

Depressive disorder

Agoraphobic symptoms can occur in a depressive disorder, and many agoraphobic patients have depressive symptoms. Enquiry about the order in which the symptoms developed will usually point to the correct diagnosis. Sometimes a depressive disorder develops in a person with long-standing agoraphobia and it is important to identify such cases and treat the depressive disorder (see below).

Paranoid disorders

Occasionally a patient with paranoid delusions (arising in the early stages of schizophrenia or in a delusional disorder) avoids going out and meeting people in shops and other places. The true diagnosis is usually revealed by thorough mental state examination which generally uncovers delusions of persecution or of reference.

Epidemiology

In a study using DSM-IIIR criteria, the 1-year prevalence of agoraphobia without panic disorder was estimated as 1.7 per cent in men and 3.8 per cent in women (Kessler *et al.*, 1994) and the lifetime prevalence about 6–10 per cent (Weissman and Merikangas, 1986).

Aetiology

Theories of the aetiology of agoraphobia have to explain both the initial anxiety attacks and their spread and recurrrence. The two problems will be considered in turn.

Theories of onset

Agoraphobia begins with anxiety in a public place, generally but not always, as a panic attack. There are three explanations for the initial anxiety.

1. The **cognitive hypothesis** proposes that the anxiety attack develops because the person is unreasonably afraid of some aspect of the situation or of certain of the physical symptoms experienced in the situation (see below under panic disorder, p. 194). Although such fears are expressed by people with established agoraphobia, it is not known whether they were present before the onset.
2. The **biological theory** proposes that the initial anxiety attack results from chance environmental stimuli acting on a person who is constitutionally predisposed to over-respond with anxiety. There is some evidence for a genetic component to this predisposition (Kendler *et al.*, 1992a).
3. The **psychoanalytic theory** proposes, essentially, that the initial anxiety is caused by unconscious mental conflicts related to unacceptable sexual or aggressive impulses which are triggered indirectly by the original situation. Although widely held in the past, this theory has not been supported by independent evidence.

Theories of spread and maintenance

Learning theories Conditioning could account for the association of anxiety with more and more situations, and avoidance learning could account for the subsequent avoidance of these situations. Although this explanation is plausible and in keeping with observations of learning in animals, there is no direct evidence to support it.

Personality Agoraphobic patients are often described as dependent, and prone to avoid rather than confront problems. This dependency could have arisen from overprotection in childhood, which is reported more often by agoraphobics than by controls. However, despite such retrospective reports, it is not certain that the dependency was present before the onset of the agoraphobia.

Family influences Agoraphobia could be maintained by family problems. However, in a well-controlled study, Buglass *et al.* (1977) found no evidence that agoraphobics had more family problems than controls. Clinical observation suggests that symptoms are sometimes prolonged by overprotective attitudes of other family members, but this feature is not found in all cases.

Prognosis

Although short-lived cases may be seen in general practice, agoraphobia that has lasted for 1 year generally remains for the next 5 years (Marks, 1969). Brief episodes of depression are common in the course of chronic agoraphobia, and clinical experience suggests that people are more likely to seek help during these episodes.

Treatment

Psychological treatment

Exposure treatment was the first of the behavioural treatments for agoraphobia. It was shown to be effective, but more effective when combined with anxiety management (see p. 594, also Cohen *et al.*, 1984). Prognosis was shown to be better in people with good marital relationships before treatment (Monteiro *et al.*, 1985) and worse in those experiencing chronic life stress (Wade *et al.*, 1993).

Cognitive-behaviour therapy for panic and agoraphobia is described on p. 594. Clinical trials (reviewed under panic disorder on p. 194) indicate that, in the short term, cognitive therapy is about as effective as medication and that in the long term it is probably more effective.

Medication

The drug treatment of agoraphobia resembles that for panic disorder (see p. 194) except that medication is usually combined with repeated practice in re-entering situations that are feared and avoided. This exposure may account for some of the observed change. Most studies of drug treatment contain both agoraphobic and panic disorder patients, and it is difficult to separate the treatment response of the two disorders. The following account should be read in conjunction with the discussion of medication for panic disorder on p. 194.

Anxiolytic drugs These may be used for a specific, short-term purpose such as helping a patient to undertake an important engagement before other treatment has taken effect. Anxiolytic drugs should not be prescribed for more than a few weeks because of the risk of dependence (see p. 527). In some countries, though seldom in the UK, the high potency benzodiazepine, alprazolam, is used to treat agoraphobia with frequent panic attacks (in DSM-IV terms, panic disorder with agoraphobia). This treatment is discussed further under panic disorder (p. 194). Most clinical trials of alprazolam have included patients with panic disorder as well as patients with agoraphobia with panic. An exception is the trial by Marks *et al.* (1993a, b), in which all patients had agoraphobia; these authors found that the short-term benefit with alprazolam was about half that obtained with exposure treatment, and that relapse after treatment was more frequent with alprazolam. However, the methodology of the study has been criticized.

Antidepressant drugs As well as the obvious use to treat a concurrent depressive disorder, these drugs have a therapeutic effect in agoraphobic patients who are not depressed but have frequent panic attacks. Imipramine has been tested most thoroughly, but similar effects have been reported with clomipramine (e.g. Gentil *et al.*, 1993). The treatment regime is the same as that described for panic disorder on p. 194. A high rate of relapse has been reported when imipramine is stopped (Zitrin *et al.*, 1978).

Selective serotonin re-uptake inhibitors (SSRIs) Several SSRIs have been shown to be effective in panic disorder with and without agoraphobia (see p. 194). One meta-analysis suggested that SSRIs are superior to imipramine and alprazolam for these patients (Boyer, 1995).

Monoamine oxidase inhibitors (MAOIs) One of the earliest reports of drug treatment for agoraphobia concerned the MAOIs (Sargant and Dally, 1962), but they are now used infrequently because they interact with some drugs and foodstuffs (see p. 550). Moreover the relapse rate is high when MAOIs are stopped even after many months of treatment.

Management

What patients need to know People with agoraphobia and those around them usually have difficulty in understanding the nature of agoraphobia and may think of it as the result of lack of determination to overcome normal anxiety. A two-stage explanation, starting with the panic attacks is generally helpful. Panic attacks can be likened to false alarms occuring in an over sensitive intruder alarm system. The excessive sensitivity can be explained in terms of constitution or chronic stress, whichever the patient's history suggests. Avoidance can be explained in terms of conditioning with examples such as anxiety persisting after falling from a bicycle or a car accident. Partners, friends and relatives can usually understand the principles of behaviour therapy but may be unsympathetic to drug treatment and puzzled when antidepressants are prescribed for anxiety. Patients can say in explanation that the medication is to reduce the sensitivity of the 'alarm system', and explain that some antidepressant drugs do this.

Patients also need to know that medication is likely to be effective only when accompanied by determined and persistent efforts to overcome avoidance. The therapist should explain how to do this and emphasize that the result will depend on the patients' own efforts. Self-help books (see below) are a useful source of information about the disorder and about the ways in which people can help themselves. When the population includes recent migrants who have a poor understanding of English, information booklets should if possible be provided in appropriate other languages.

Behavioural management In early cases, patients should be strongly encouraged to return to the situations that they are avoiding. The treatment of choice for established cases is probably a combination of exposure to phobic situations with cognitive therapy for panic attacks (see p. 594). If there is a waiting list for cognitive therapy, the referring clinicians should supervise exposure treatment. Several self-help manuals have been published which reduce the time that therapists need to spend in doing this (for example, Andrews *et al.*, 1994).

Medication can be offered as a first treatment especially when panic attacks are frequent and/or severe. However, medication needs to be accompanied by repeated exposure to previously feared and avoided situations. In the UK, the medication is usually an antidepressant - generally imipramine or an SSRI. In other countries alprazolam may be chosen. It is not certain how long medication should be maintained but on the analogy of depressive disorder, antidepressants are often prescribed for 9 months to a year. Any medication should be discontinued gradually, and alprazolam should be reduced particularly slowly.

Patients who have relapsed after drug treatment can be offered behaviour therapy, though no controlled trials have been carried out specifically with such patients.

Most patients improve but few lose the symptoms completely following treatment. Relapse is common, and patients should be encouraged to seek further help at an early stage should relapse occur.

Panic disorder

Although the diagnosis of panic disorder did not appear in the nomenclature until 1980 when it was introduced in DSM-III, similar cases have been described under a variety of names for more than a century. The central feature is the occurrence of panic attacks, i.e. sudden attacks of anxiety in which physical symptoms predominate and are accompanied by fear of a serious medical consequence such as a heart attack. In the past, these symptoms have been variously referred to as irritable heart, Da Costa's syndrome, neurocirculatory asthenia, disorderly action of the heart, and effort syndrome. These early terms assumed that patients were correct in fearing a disorder of cardiac function. Some later authors suggested psychological causes, but it was not until the Second World War (when interest in the condition revived) that Wood (1941) showed convincingly that the condition was a form of anxiety disorder. From then until 1980 patients with panic attacks were classified as having either generalized or phobic anxiety disorders. In 1980, the authors of DSM-III introduced the new diagnostic category, panic disorder, which included patients whose panic attacks occurred with or without generalized anxiety, but excluded those whose panic attacks appeared in the course of agoraphobia. In DSM-IV, all patients with frequent panic attacks are classified as having panic disorder whether or not they have agoraphobia. (Agoraphobia without panic attacks has a separate rubric - see p. 189.) Panic disorder is included in ICD-10; however, unlike DSMIV, the diagnosis is not made when panic attacks are accompanied by agoraphobia.

TABLE 9.6 Symptoms caused by hyperventilation

Dizziness
Tinnitus
Headache
Feeling of weakness
Faintness
Numbness
Tingling in the hands, feet, and face
Carpopedal spasms
Precordial discomfort
Feeling of breathlessness

Clinical features

The symptoms of a panic attack are listed in Table 9.7. Not every patient has all these symptoms in the panic attack and to diagnose panic disorder, DSM-IV requires the presence of only four or more symptoms. Important features of panic attacks are that

- anxiety builds up quickly,
- the symptoms are severe,
- the person fears a catastrophic outcome.

Some people with panic disorder hyperventilate, and this adds to their symptoms.

Hyperventilation is breathing in a rapid and shallow way with a resultant fall in the concentration of carbon dioxide in the blood. The resulting hypocapnia may cause the symptoms listed in Table 9.6. The last symptom in the list, the feeling of breathlessness, is paradoxical since the person is breathing excessively. It is important because it leads to a further increase in breathing which worsens the condition. Hyperventilation should always be borne in mind as a cause of unexplained bodily symptoms. The diagnosis can usually be

TABLE 9.7 Symptoms of a panic attack (from DSM-IV)

Shortness of breath and smothering sensations
Choking
Palpitations and accelerated heart rate
Chest discomfort or pain
Sweating
Dizziness, unsteady feelings or faintness
Nausea or abdominal distress
Depersonalization or derealization
Numbness or tingling sensations
Flushes or chills
Trembling or shaking
Fear of dying
Fears of going crazy or doing something uncontrolled

made by watching the pattern of breathing when the symptoms are present. If there is doubt, blood gas analysis will decide the matter in recent cases but the findings may be normal in chronic ones.

Diagnostic criteria

In DSM-IV the diagnosis of panic disorder is made when (i) panic attacks occur unexpectedly (i.e. not in response to an identified phobic stimulus), and (ii) more than four attacks have occurred in 4 weeks, or one attack has been followed by 4 weeks of persistent fear of another attack and worry about its implications (for example having a heart attack). The research criteria in ICD-10 are similar except that those concerned with course are rather less precise: the attacks must have been recurrent and not consistently associated with a phobic situation or object, or with marked exertion or exposure to dangerous or life-threatening situations.

Differential diagnosis

Panic attacks occur in generalized anxiety disorders, phobic anxiety disorders (most often agoraphobia), depressive disorders, and acute organic disorder. Two of the DSM diagnostic criteria help to distinguish these secondary attacks from panic disorder: the presence in panic disorder of a persistent marked concern about having further attacks, and worry about the implication of the attacks.

Epidemiology

Using DSM-IIIR criteria, the one-year prevalence of panic disorder in the general population is about 14 per 1000 (Narrow *et al.*, 2002). This figure includes panic disorder with agoraphobia which accounts for about half of the cases in the general population. In most studies, the prevalence in women is about twice that in men. As explained above, the diagnostic criteria include a threshold of frequency and severity but research suggests a continuous variation in the number of attacks. Therefore studies have been made of panic attacks that are too infrequent or insufficiently severe to meet criteria for panic disorder. Their 6-month prevalence is about 30 per 1000 (Von Korff *et al.*, 1985) and their lifetime prevalence as about 56 per 1000 (Katerndahl, 1993).

Aetiology

Genetics

Panic disorder is familial (see for example Mendelwicz *et al.*, 1993). Rates in monozygotic twins are higher than in dizygotic twins, indicating that the family aggregation is likely to be at least partly due to genetic factors (Skre *et al.*, 1993) with a hereditability of 30–40 per cent (Kendler *et al.*, 1993e). Numerous linkage studies have been carried out with, among others, reports of linkages to chromosomes 7, 9q and 13q but at the time of writing, none has yielded a convincing confirmed positive result.

There are two main hypotheses about other causes of panic disorder. The first proposes a biochemical abnormality, and the second a cognitive abnormality.

The **biochemical hypothesis** is based on two sets of observations.

- **Induction of panic attacks** Chemical agents, notably sodium lactate (Pitts and McClure, 1967) and yohimbine (Charney *et al.*, 1984), but also flumazenil (a benzodiazepine receptor antagonist), cholecystokinin, and mCCP (a 5-HT receptor agonist) (Nutt and Lawson, 1992) can induce panic attacks more readily in patients with panic disorder than in healthy people. The multitude of chemical agents that provoke panic attacks in panic disorder patients make it difficult to identify a single causal mechanism. Suggestions include abnormalities in the presynaptic adrenoceptors that normally restrain the activity of presynaptic neurons in brain areas concerned with the control of anxiety; and an abnormality of 5-HT or benzodiazepine receptor function. The latter suggestion is supported by brain imaging studies showing a decrease in benzodizapine receptor binding sites in patients with panic disorder (Malizia *et al.*, 1998).
- **Reduction of panic attacks** Panic attacks are reduced by imipramine which affects both 5-HT and nor-

adrenergic systems; by clomipramine and fluvoxamine which mainly affect 5-HT transmission; but not by maprotiline, a selective noradrenergic uptake blocker (Den Boer and Westerberg, 1988). Clomipramine appears to be more potent than imipramine as an antipanic agent and this could be because the latter is a relatively weak 5-HT uptake blocker.

See Ballenger (2000) for a review of the biological theories concerning the aetiology of panic disorder.

The **cognitive hypothesis** is based on the observation that fears about serious physical or mental illness are more frequent among patients with panic attacks than among anxious patients without panic attacks. It is proposed that there is a spiral of anxiety in panic disorder as the physical symptoms of anxiety activate fears of illness and thereby generate more anxiety (Clark, 1986). These observations have led to a cognitive treatment for panic disorder (see below).

Hyperventilation as a cause

A subsidiary hypothesis proposes that hyperventilation is a cause of panic disorder. Whilst there is no doubt that voluntary overbreathing can produce a panic attack, it has not been shown that panic disorder is caused by involuntary hyperventilation.

Course and prognosis

Follow-up studies have generally included patients with panic attacks and agoraphobia as well as patients with panic disorder alone. Earlier studies which used categories such as effort syndrome, found that most patients still had symptoms 20 years later, though most had a good social outcome (e.g. Wheeler *et al.*, 1950). Studies of patients diagnosed as panic disorder also reveal a long course with fluctuating anxiety and depression (Roy-Byrne and Cowley, 1995). Mortality rates from unnatural causes and, among men, from cardiovascular disorders are higher than average (Coryell *et al.*, 1982).

Treatment

Apart from supportive measures and help with any causative life problems, treatment is with medication or cognitive therapy. Three kinds of medication can be used.

Benzodiazepines

When given in high doses, benzodiazepines control panic attacks. In these doses, most benzodiazepines cause sedation but alprazolam, a high-potency compound, is an exception. Hence it has been used to treat panic disorder and its effectiveness over placebo has been shown in many controlled trials (see Ballenger, 2000). At the end of treatment, alprazolam should be reduced very gradually to avoid withdrawal symptoms. Even when reduced over 30 days, about a third of patients report significant withdrawal symptoms (Cross-National Collaborative Panic Study, 1992).This treatment developed in the United States and has not been taken up widely in the UK, where benzodiazepines are not now recommended for the treatment of panic disorder in the NHS (National Institute for Clinical Excellence, 2004a).

Imipramine and clomipramine

Imipramine was the first antidepressant to be shown effective for panic disorder (Klein, 1964). The first effect of the drug is often to produce an unpleasant feeling of apprehension, sleeplessness, and palpitations. For this reason the initial dose should be small, for example 10 mg/day for 3 days, increasing by 10 mg every 3 days to 50 mg/day, and then by 25 mg/week to 150 mg/day. If symptoms are not controlled at this dose, further increments of 25 mg may be given to physically fit patients up to a maximum of 175–225 mg/day. Before high doses are given, an ECG should be obtained if there is any doubt about cardiac function. Full dosage is continued for 3–6 months. A relapse rate of up to 30 per cent has been reported after stopping imipramine (Zitrin *et al.*, 1978), but the rate may be less if a reduced dose is continued forseveral months more (Mavissakalian and Perel, 1992).

Clomipramine has been found to be as effective as imipramine (Cassano *et al.*, 1988).

Specific serotonin re-uptake inhibitors (SSRIs)

Several SSRIs have been reported to be effective in panic disorder and they do not have the cardiac side effects of imipramine. They include fluvoxamine (Bakish *et al.*, 1996), paroxetine (Ochberg *et al.*, 1995), sertraline (see Ballenger, 2000), and fluoxetine (Michelson *et al.*, 2001).

Cognitive therapy

Cognitive therapy reduces the fears of the physical effects of anxiety, which are thought to provoke and maintain the panic attacks. Common fears of this kind are that palpitations indicate an impending heart attack, or that dizziness indicates impending loss of consciousness. In treatment, the physical symptoms that the patient fears are induced by hyperventilation or exercise. The therapist points out the sequence of physical symptoms leading to fear and explains that similar sequence occurs in the early stages of a panic attack. The therapist goes on to question the patient's belief in the feared outcome. The procedure is described further on p. 594.

Controlled studies have shown that cognitive therapy is at least as effective as imipramine for panic disorder (Clark *et al.*, 1994; Barlow *et al.*, 2000). In both trials, patients treated with imipramine were more likely to relapse soon after treatment had ended than were those treated with cognitive-behaviour therapy. The few well conducted studies comparing the long-term effectiveness of cognitive behaviour therapy and medications also suggest a modestly greater effect of cognitive behaviour therapy (Nadiga *et al.*, 2003). In the trial by Barlow, the combination of cognitive therapy and imipramine was no more effective that either singly.

Management

What patients need to know Patients need to be able to explain the disorder to relatives and friends and the explanation outlined in relation to agoraphobia (p. 191) is usually appropriate. Patients also need to understand how ways of thinking and behaviours increase and prolong the disorder (see cognitive therapy above). Books are available to reinforce this (for example Rachman and De Silver, 1998). When the population includes recent migrants with a poor understanding of English, information should be provided, if possible, in appropriate other languages.

Choice of treatment As cognitive therapy and medication have similar effects, and the therapeutic result may be no greater when they are combined, the choice of treatment depends on the patient's preference, the availability of cognitive therapy, and considerations of cost and long- term benefit (cognitive therapy is more costly but may have more lasting effects). If medication is chosen, one of the SSRIs may be preferred to imipramine because they have fewer side-effects. Alprazolam has been used in some countries, but is not recommended in the UK (see above). Information about the main and side effects should that given when the same medication is given for other reasons, including the delayed onset of action, the dangers of overdose, and the need to withdraw medication gradually. If there is no improvement after about 12 weeks, the treatment can be changed to an antideprssant of a different class, or cognitive therapy can be started.

If, as often happens, panic disorder is accompanied by some degree of agoraphobic avoidance, exposure treatment should be added to the medication or cognitive-behavioural treatment (see the treatment of agoraphobia, p. 191).

Mixed anxiety and depressive disorder

As explained on p. 178, anxiety and depressive symptoms often occur together. The overlap is greatest when the symptoms are mild (52 per cent in the study of psychiatric patients by Hiller *et al.*, 1989) and least when they are severe enough for a diagnosis of psychiatric disorder (29 per cent in the same study). Similar findings were obtained in a community epidemiological study of people meeting diagnostic criteria for anxiety disorder: 28 per cent also met criteria for minor depression and a further 21 per cent met criteria for major depression (Angst and Dobler-Mikola, 1985).

Diagnostic conventions

When the anxiety and depressive symptoms are not severe enough to meet diagnostic criteria, the condition is sometimes referred to as a **minor affective disorder** (see Chapter 11) or as **cothymia**. Other diagnostic terms are:

- **mixed anxiety and depressive disorder**. This category is included in ICD10 but not in the main classification of DSM-IV, though it is listed as acondition for further study.
- **adjustment disorder** is diagnosed when minor anxiety and depressive symptoms are related to a change in life circumstances.

Aetiology

There are three reasons why anxiety and depression may occur together:

1. They may have the **same predisposing causes**. Brown and Harris (1993) found that childhood adversity is associated with both anxiety and depressive disorders in adult life.
2. Some **stressful events combine elements of loss and danger**, the former are associated with depression and the latter with anxiety.
3. Persistent **anxiety leading to secondary depression**. Follow-up studies have shown that onsets of depression are more common among people with persistent anxiety than are onsets of anxiety among people with persistent depression.

The **prognosis** of mixed anxiety and depressive disorders is not clearly established.

Treatment

Treatment is generally with one of the antidepressants that have an anxiolytic as well as antidepressant effects (Chapter 11). A tricyclic may be chosen; sometimes a MAOI is the second-line treatment, but care must be taken to avoid side-effects or interactions (see p. 550). SSRIs can be used although they may lead to an initial increase of anxiety in these patients.

For further information see p. 222 and Tyrer *et al.* (2003).

Transcultural variations of anxiety disorder

In several cultures the presenting symptoms of anxiety disorder are more often somatic than psychological. Leff (1981) has pointed out that this difference parallels the different words used to describe anxiety in the corresponding languages. Thus there is no word for anxiety in some African, Oriental, and American Indian languages; instead, a phrase denoting bodily function is used. For example in Yoruba, an African language, the phrase is 'the heart is not at rest'. In addition, several conditions have been described that may be transcultural variants of anxiety disorders, though their exact relation to these disorders is uncertain.

Koro, which occurs amongst men in Asia, more commonly among the Chinese, has similarities with panic disorder. Cantonese people call it *suk-yeong*, which means shrinking of the penis. There are episodes of acute anxiety, lasting from 30 minutes to a day or two, in which the person complains of palpitations, sweating, pericardial discomfort, and trembling. At the same time he is convinced that the penis will retract into the abdomen and that when this process is complete he will die. Most episodes occur at night, sometimes after sexual activity. To prevent the feared outcome, patients may tie the penis to an object, or ask another person to hold the organ. This belief parallels the conviction held by patients during a panic attack that the heart is damaged and they will die. Epidemics of *koro* have been described among people made anxious by social stressors and superstitious ideas (Tseng *et al.*, 1988).

Variants of social phobia have been described in the east, originally among Japanese people where it is known as *taijin-kyofu-sho* or phobia of interpersonal relations. There is an intense anxiety in social situations and an intense conviction bordering on the delusional that the person is being thought of unfavourably by others. Other symptoms include fears of producing body odours, dysmorphophobia, and aversion to eye contact (Tseng *et al.*, 1992).

Obsessive–compulsive disorder

The concise description of obsessive-compulsive disorder, contained in ICD-9, is still valuable:

> The outstanding symptom is a feeling of subjective compulsion - which must be resisted - to carry out some action, to dwell on an idea, to recall an experience, or ruminate on an abstract topic. Unwanted thoughts, which include the insistency of words or ideas, ruminations or trains of thought, are perceived by the patient to be inappropriate or nonsensical. The obsessional urge or idea is recognized as alien to the personality but as coming from within the self. Obsessional actions may be quasi ritual performances designed to relieve anxiety, e.g. washing the hands to deal with contamination. Attempts to dispel the unwelcome thoughts or urges may lead to a severe inner struggle, with intense anxiety.

Clinical picture

Obsessive–compulsive disorders are characterized by obsessional thinking, compulsive behaviour, and varying degrees of anxiety, depression, and depersonalization. Obsessional and compulsive symptoms are listed in Table 9.8. They were described on pp. 13–14 but the reader may find it helpful to be reminded of the main features.

Obsessional thoughts are words, ideas, and beliefs, recognized patients as their own, that intrude forcibly into the mind. They are usually unpleasant, and attempts are made to exclude them. It is the combination of an inner sense of **compulsion** and of efforts at **resistance** that characterize obsessional symptoms, but the effort of resistance is the more variable of the two. Obsessional thoughts may take the form of single words, phrases, or rhymes; they are usually unpleasant or shocking to the person, and may be obscene or blasphemous. Obsessional images are vividly imagined scenes, often of a violent or disgusting kind involving, for example, abnormal sexual practices.

Obsessional ruminations are internal debates in which arguments for and against even the simplest

TABLE 9.8 Principal features of obsessive–compulsive disorder

Obsessional symptoms
Thoughts
Ruminations
Impulses
'Phobias'
Compulsive rituals
Abnormal slowness
Anxiety
Depression
Depersonalization

everyday actions are reviewed endlessly. Some obsessional doubts concern actions that may not have been completed adequately, such as turning off a gas tap or securing a door; other doubts concern actions that might have harmed other people, for example, that driving a car past a cyclist might have caused him to fall off his bicycle. Sometimes doubts are related to religious convictions or observances ('scruples') – a phenomenon well known to those who hear confession.

Obsessional impulses are urges to perform acts, usually of a violent or embarrassing kind, for example leaping in front of a car, injuring a child, or shouting blasphemies in church.

Obsessional rituals include both mental activities, such as counting repeatedly in a special way or repeating a certain form of words, and repeated but senseless behaviours, such as washing the hands 20 or more times a day. Some rituals have an understandable connection with the obsessional thoughts that precede them, for example, repeated handwashing following thoughts about contamination. Other rituals have no such connection, for example, arranging objects in a particular way. The person may feel compelled to repeat such actions a certain number of times; if this sequence is interrupted, it has to be repeated from the beginning. People with rituals are invariably aware that they are illogical and usually try to hide them. Some people fear that their symptoms are a sign of incipient madness and are greatly helped by reassurance that this is not so.

Obsessional slowness Although obsessional thoughts and rituals lead to slow performance, a few obsessional patients are afflicted by extreme slowness that is out of proportion to other symptoms.

Obsessional phobias Obsessional thoughts and compulsive rituals may worsen in certain situations; for example, obsessional thoughts about harming other people may increase in a kitchen or other place where knives are kept. The person may the avoid these such situations because they cause distress, just as people with phobic disorders avoid situations. Because of this resemblance, the condition is called an obsessional phobia.

Anxiety Anxiety is a prominent component of obsessive–compulsive disorders. Some rituals are followed by a lessening of anxiety, whilst others are followed by increased anxiety

Depression Obsessional patients are often depressed. In some patients, depression is an understandable reaction to the obsessional symptoms; in others, depression seem to vary independently.

Depersonalization Some obsessional patients complain of depersonalization. The relationship between this distressing symptom and the other features of the disorder is not clear.

Relation to obsessional personality Obsessional personality is described in Chapter 7. There is no simple, one-to-one relationship between obsessive-compulsive disorder and this kind of personality. Although obsessional personality is over represented among people who develop obsessive–compulsive disorder, about a third of obsessional patients have other types of personality (as noted in a classical paper by Lewis, 1936). Also, people with obsessional personality are more likely to develop depressive disorders than obsessive–compulsive disorders.

Differential diagnosis

Obsessive–compulsive disorders must be distinguished from other disorders in which obsessional symptoms occur.

Anxiety disorders

The distinction from generalized anxiety disorder, panic disorder, or phobic disorder is seldom difficult provided that a careful history is taken and the mental state is examined thoroughly.

Depressive disorder

The course of obsessive–compulsive disorder is often punctuated by periods of depression in which the obsessional symptoms increase; when this happens the depressive disorder may be overlooked. Also, obsessional symptoms sometimes occur in the course of a primary depressive disorder.

Schizophrenia

Occasionally, obsessive–compulsive symptoms disorder may resemble delusions because the content of the obsessional thoughts are peculiar, or the rituals are exceptionally odd, and resistance is weak. The disorder can then be mistaken for schizophrenia. In such cases, the correct diagnosis can be made following thorough history taking and a careful search for other symptoms of schizophrenia.

Organic disorders

Obsessional symptoms are found occasionally in organic cerebral disorders. They were observed most strikingly in chronic cases of encephalitis lethargica following the epidemic in the 1920s.

Epidemiology

The total one-year prevalence of obsessive compulsive disorder is 2.1 per cent; the one-year prevalence of obsessive compulsive disorder not comorbid with another anxiety disorder is 1.2 percent (Narrow *et al.*, 2002).

Estimates of the ratio of lifetime prevalence of women to men in the population varies from 1.2 (in Puerto Rico) to 3.8 (in New Zealand). However in clinic populations, the ratio is usually about 1:1. In community samples, 20–60 per cent of people reported obsessions only, while among clinic attenders more than 70 per cent report both obsessions and compulsions (see Weissman *et al.*, 1994).

Aetiology

Healthy people experience occasional intrusive thoughts, some of which are concerned with sexual, aggressive, and other themes similar to those of obsessional patients (as shown many years ago by Rachman and Hodgson, 1980). It is the frequency, intensity, and, above all, the persistence of obsessional phenomena that have to be explained.

Genetics

In early studies, obsessive-compulsive disorders were found in 5–7 per cent of the parents of patients with obsessive-compulsive disorders (Brown, 1942; Rüdin, 1953) a rate that is higher than in the general population (see above). In the small number of twin studies, the concordance rate was greater in monozygotic than in dizygotic pairs (Rasmussen and Tsuang, 1986), indicating that at least part of the familial loading is genetic. Molecular genetic studies have found a number of associations between OCD and various certain genes coding for 5-HT receptors such as the 5-HT_{1D} receptor. However, these findings have not yet been convincingly replicated (Mundo *et al.*, 2002).

Evidence of a brain disorder

Two kinds of evidence suggest a disorder of brain function in obsessive-compulsive disorder: associations with conditions that have known effects on brain function, and evidence from brain scanning.

Associations with other brain disorders As noted above, obsessional symptoms were recorded frequently among patients affected by encephalitis lethargica after the epidemic of the 1920s. Also, Gilles de la Tourette included obsessional symptoms in his original description of the disorder that now bears his name (Gilles de la Tourette, 1885), and more recent studies have confirmed this observation (for example Cummings and Frankel, 1985; Robertson *et al.*, 1988). In childhood, 70 per cent of cases of Sydenham's chorea, which affects the caudate nucleus, are reported to have obsessive-compulsive symptoms. The development of obsessive-compulsive disorder in some children has been linked to Group A streptococcal infections (see Snider and Swedo, 2004). The condition which is referred to as PANDAS (paediatric autoimmune neuropsychiatric disorder associated with streptococcal infection) is considered further on p. 685.

Brain imaging studies Computerized tomography and magnetic resonance imaging have not revealed any consistent **structural** brain abnormality specific to patients with obsessive-compulsive disorder (Saxena *et al.*, 1998). However, studies with single-photon emission tomography (SPET) and PET have shown **functional** abnormalities. There is increased activity in the orbitofrontal cortex, anterior cingulate, caudate nucleus and parts of the thalamus (see Saxena *et al.*, 2001) suggesting abnormal activity in a neurological circuit involving these structures. Treatment appears to reverse at least some of the abnormalities (Saxena *et al.*, 2002). A different pattern of activity has been reported in patients with compulsive hoarding suggesting the possibility that this rare variant may not have the same pathophysiology as the other obsessive-compulsive disorders (Saxena *et al.*, 2003).

Abnormal serotonergic function

The finding that obsessive-compulsive symptoms respond to drugs that affect 5-HT function suggests that 5-HT function might be abnormal in obsessive-compulsive disorder. The effect of 5-HT uptake inhibitors on obsessive-compulsive symptoms takes several weeks so the late effects are likely to be most relevant. However, these late effects are complex and it is not known which are important. In any case, the response of obsessive-compulsive symptoms to drugs that affect 5-HT function does not prove that 5-HT function is abnormal in obsessive-compulsive disorder. The situation might resemble that of parkinsonism in which anticholinergic drugs control symptoms by acting on the normal cholinergic systems of patients whose disorder is due to abnormal dopaminergic function.

Attempts to assess 5-HT function in obsessive-compulsive disorder have used both neuro-endocrine tests (e.g. Barr *et al.*, 1992; Hollander *et al.*, 1992) and measures of serotonin transport using PET and SPET (Pogarell *et al.*, 2003; Simpson *et al.*, 2003). The results of these studies have been contradictory and no clear conclusion is possible. Other studies have examined the effect on obsessive-compulsive symptoms of challenges with agents with effects specific to particular kinds of 5-HT receptors. Some studies have implicated 5-HT_{1D} and 5-HT_{2C} subtypes but again the results are contradictory (see Zohar *et al.*, 2004).

Early experience

It is uncertain whether early experience plays a part in the aetiology of obsessive–compulsive disorder. Mothers with the disorder might be expected to transmit symptoms to their children by imitative learning. However, an early study found that although the children of patients with obsessive–compulsive disorder have an increased risk of non-specific neurotic symptoms, they do not have more obsessional symptoms (Cowie, 1961).

Psychoanalytical theories

Although not supported by evidence, these theories are summarized here for their historical importance. Freud (1895a) originally suggested that obsessional symptoms result from unconscious impulses of an aggressive or sexual nature. These impulses could potentially cause extreme anxiety, but anxiety is reduced by the action of the defence mechanisms of repression and reaction formation. This idea reflects the aggressive and sexual fantasies of many obsessional patients, and with their restraints on their own aggressive and sexual impulses. Freud also proposed that obsessional symptoms occur when there is a regression to the anal stage of development as a way of avoiding impulses related to the subsequent genital and Oedipal stages. This idea reflects obsessional patients' frequent concerns with excretory functions and dirt.

Learning theory

This theory attempts to explain obsessive–compulsive disorder as the result of abnormal learning, for example that obsessional rituals are a form of avoidance response. While such mechanisms could account for some aspects of obsessional symptoms, they do not convincingly explain the disorder as a whole.

Cognitive theory

Cognitive theory starts with the premise that it is not the occurrence of intrusive thoughts that has to be explained (they are experienced at times by healthy people – see above) but the obsessional patient's inability to control them. Salkovskis (1997) proposed that people with obsessional disorder respond to such thoughts as if they were personally responsible for their possible consequences, for example, for harm to another person. This feeling of responsibility, it is suggested, leads to excessive attempts to ward off the thoughts and their supposed consequences by adopting compulsive behaviours and avoidance, and seeking repeated reassurance. Although the theory is unproven, it directs attention to aspects of the disorder other than the obvious obsessions and compulsions.

Prognosis

About two-thirds of cases improve to some extent by the end of a year. Of the cases lasting for more than a year, some run a fluctuating course, but others are chronic (Ravizza *et al.*, 1997). Prognosis is better when (i) there has been a precipitating event, (ii) social and occupational adjustment is good, and (iii) the symptoms are episodic. Prognosis is worse when there is a personality disorder, and onset is in childhood (see Iancu *et al.*, 2000). Severe cases may be exceedingly persistent; for example, in a study of obsessional patients admitted to hospital, Kringlen (1965) found that three-quarters remained unchanged 13–20 years later, and in another study almost half had obsessive–compulsive disorders lasting for more than 50 years (Skoog and Skoog, 1999).

Treatment

Medication

Clomipramine Clomipramine is a tricyclic antidepressant with potent 5-HT uptake blocking effects. When given in high doses (200–250 mg/day) it is more effective than placebo in reducing the obsessional symptoms of patients with obsessive–compulsive disorder (Clomipramine Collaborative Study Group, 1991). Most patients tolerate the treatment, but at these high doses, anticholinergic side-effects are common and a few patients develop seizures. A clinically useful effect may not be reached until about 6 weeks of treatment; and further improvement may take another 6 weeks. Many patients relapse in the first few weeks after the drug is stopped (Pato *et al.*, 1988) but relapse is reduced when clomipramine is combined with exposure (Simpson *et al.*, 2004). Other tricyclic antidepressants that are less potent 5-HT uptake blockers do not have this therapeutic effect in obsessive–compulsive disorder (Foa *et al.*, 1987).

Specific serotonin uptake inhibitors (SSRIs) SSRIs, including fluoxetine and fluvoxamine, paroxetine and sertraline, are effective in reducing obsessional symptoms (Goodman *et al.*, 1989b; Jenike *et al.*, 1990). A meta-analysis indicates that these drugs may be rather less effective than clomipramine (Ackerman and Greenland, 2002) though this finding has to be balanced with their lack of anticholinergic side effects. Since only about half the treated patients improve substantially, attempts have been made to improve the response rate by adding a second drug to the SSRI. The only approach with a consistent, albeit rather limited, therapeutic effect concerns addition of an antipsychotic agent usually at low dose. Beneficial effects have been seen with both typical and atypical antipsychotic drugs but the latter are usually better tolerated (see Sareen *et al.*, 2004). As with clomipramine, relapse is common in the few weeks after an SSRI has been stopped.

Anxiolytic drugs Anxiolytic drugs give some short term symptomatic relief but should not be prescribed for more than about 3 weeks at a time. If anxiolytic treatment is needed for longer, small doses of a tricyclic antidepressant or an antipsychotic may be used.

Cognitive–behaviour therapy

Response prevention Obsessional rituals usually improve with a combination of response prevention (see p. 591) with exposure to any environmental cues that increase the symptoms. About two-thirds of patients with moderately severe rituals can be expected to improve substantially though not completely (Rachman and Hodgson, 1980). When rituals respond to this treatment, the accompanying obsessional thoughts usually improve as well. The results seem comparable with those of treatment with clomipramine and SSRIs (Cox *et al.*, 1993; van Bolkom *et al.*, 1998).

Behavioural treatment is much less effective for obsessional thoughts occurring without rituals. The technique of thought stopping has been used for many years, but there is no good evidence that it has a specific effect. Indeed, Stern *et al.* (1973) found an effect which did not differ from that of thought-stopping directed to irrelevant thoughts.

Cognitive therapy Cognitive therapy seeks to reduce attempts to suppress and avoid obsessional thoughts, since these attempts have been shown to increase, rather than decrease, their frequency. Patients are helped to record the frequency of obsessional thoughts to compare the effects of suppression and distraction. Since suppression and avoidance seem to be driven by the conviction that to think something is to make it happen, attempts are made to weaken this conviction by reviewing the evidence for and against it. These techniques may be combined with exposure to tape-recorded repetition of the thoughts, and by discussion of any other cognitive distortions along the general lines of cognitive therapy (see p. 594). At the time of writing, there is insufficient evidence to decide the long-term effectiveness of this treatment. (See Salkovskis, 1997 for an account of a cognitive therapy for obsessive–compulsive disorder).

Dynamic psychotherapy

Exploratory and interpretative psychotherapy seldom helps obsessional patients. Indeed, some are made worse because these procedures encourage painful and unproductive rumination about the subjects discussed during treatment.

Neurosurgery

The immediate results of neurosurgery for severe obsessive–compulsive disorder is often a striking reduction in tension and distress. However, the long-term effects are uncertain, since no prospective controlled trial has been carried out Hay *et al.* (1993) reported a 10-year follow-up of 26 obsessive–compulsive patients treated with orbitomedial or cingulate lesions, or both. Of the 18 patients interviewed, eight had a second operation, two died by suicide, and about a third of the survivors improved. The frequency of second operations and the low improvement rates indicate the limitations of this treatment. For a review see Christmas *et al.* (2004).

If neurosurgery is considered for these patients, it should be only for the most chronic cases that have resisted intensive inpatient or day-patient treatment, including drug and behavioural methods, for at least a year. Using these criteria, the authors have not referred patients for surgical treatment.

Management

In treatment, it is important to remember that some cases of obsessive–compulsive disorder run a fluctuating course with long periods of remission. Also, depressive disorder frequently accompanies obsessive–compulsive disorder, and in such cases effective treatment of the depressive disorder often leads to improvement in the obsessional symptoms. For this reason a thorough search for depressive disorder should be made in every patient presenting with obsessive–compulsive disorder.

What patients need to know Treatment should begin with an explanation of the symptoms, and if necessary with reassurance that these symptoms are not an early sign of insanity (a common concern of obsessional patients). If the patient agrees, the partner or another close relative can be involved in educational sessions about the nature and treatment of the disorder. Patients and family members are often helped by reading a book on obsessional compulsive disorder. Obsessional patients may attempt to involve other family members in their rituals. When this happens, the relatives should be helped to find ways of resisting such requests in a way that is appropriately sympathetic but firm.

Choice of treatment As noted above, medication controls symptoms in many cases but when it is stopped, many relapse. Exposure with response prevention seems to produce better long-term results but it is difficult to achieve response prevention when symptoms are severe. For this reason, medication and response prevention should often be combined unless the patient is against medication. When there is a waiting list for behaviour therapy, medication can be started first.

For a review of obsessive-compulsive disorder see Jenicke (2004).

Further reading

Gelder, MG, López-Ibor, JJ Jr and Andreasen, NC (eds) (2000) *The new Oxford textbook of psychiatry*. Oxford University Press, Oxford. See section 4.7: Anxiety disorders (generalized anxiety disorders; social and specific phobias; and panic disorder and agoraphobia), and section 4.8: Obsessional disorders.

Menzies, R and de Silva, P (eds) (2003) *Obsessive compulsive disorders: theory, research and treatment*. John Wiley, Chicester. (A comprehensive review.)

Nathan, PE and Gorman, JM (eds) (2002) *A guide to treatments that work*, 2nd edn. Oxford University Press, New York. (See the chapters concerned with psychosocial and pharmacological treatments for panic disorders, phobia, generalized anxiety disorders, and obsessional compulsive disorders.)

National Institute for Clinical Excellence (2004) Anxiety: management of anxiety (panic disorder, with and without agoraphobia, and generalized anxiety disorder) in adults in primary, secondary and community care. National Institute for Clinical Excellence Guideline 22. (A periodically updated comprehensive review, available at www.nice.org.uk.)

CHAPTER 10

Somatoform and dissociative disorders

Chapter contents

This chapter is concerned mainly with physical symptoms that have no detectable physical cause and appear to have instead a psychological cause. These disorders are called somatoform disorders. It also considers disorders characterized by disturbances of consciousness or identity, such as amnesia and multiple personality (dissociative disorders) which also have no physical cause. The two are considered together in this chapter because they are classified together in DSM-IV. Apart from this, the disorders are not closely linked, so that the subject matter and argument of this chapter cannot be quite as coherent as that of chapters in which the disorders are more closely related aetiologically.

Some of the terms that will used in this chapter are defined in Box 10.1.

Classification

In DSM-IV, the overall term somatoform disor is used to denote a group of conditions (listed in Table 10.1) characterized by physical symptoms occuring without an aqequate physical cause. In ICD-10, these disorders are not allocated a separate category; instead they are classified as members of a wider category of **neurotic**, **stress-related**, and **somatoform** disorders.

A further, potentially confusing difference between the classifications is that in ICD-10 the condition called conversion disorder in DSM is a member of a group called dissociative disorders, while in DSM-IV conversion disorder is classified as a somatoform disorder. In this chapter we follow the DSM-IV convention.

BOX 10.1 SOME DEFINITIONS

Somatoform disorders A generic term used in DSM for a group of disorders characterized by physical symptoms that are not explained by organic factors.

Somatization The (little understood) processes whereby physical symptoms are experienced in the absence of an adequate organic cause.

Somatization disorder a condition with multiple physical symptoms without physical cause and of long duration.

Dissociation A hypothetical mechanism whereby psychological processes relating to consciousness are split or fragmented. Dissociation is discussed further in Chapter 8 under Stress-related disorders.

Dissociative symptoms Symptoms that have been thought to arise through the mechanism of dissociation.

Conversion A term introduced by Freud for a hypothetical mechanism by which psychological stress leads to (is converted into) physical symptoms.

Conversion disorder A term for conditions that may result from conversion; conditions that in the past were called hysteria.

Somatoform disorder

The following section should be read in conjunction with the section on unexplained physical symptoms in Chapter 16. This section is concerned only with the groups of unexplained physical symptoms classified within the somatoform disorder category.

Somatoform disorder was introduced as a provisional diagnostic category many years ago in DSM-III, and many years later its value is still uncertain. The defining feature is the presence of:

> physical symptoms suggesting a physical disorder for which there are no demonstrable organic findings or known physiological mechanisms, and for which there is strong evidence, or a strong presumption, that the symptoms are linked to psychological factors or conflicts.

There is no doubt, of course, that many people experience such symptoms, and that they are associated with significant distress and disability (Bass *et al.*, 2001). There is doubt, however, about the value of grouping together under this one rubric, conditions which are dissimilar in many ways and which overlap (are comorbid) with anxiety disorders and depressive disorders Also two of the conditions - hypochondriasis and somatization disorder - are so enduring that it has been suggested that they should be classified as personality disorders. See Sharpe and Mayou (2004) for a critique of the concept of somatoform disorder.

Classification in DSM-IV and ICD-10

Although there are broad similarities, there are also two important differences between the categories in ICD and DSM (see Table 10.1).

- **Neurasthenia** is not included in DSM because the category is seldom used in the USA. It is included in ICD-10 because it is an international classification and the category is used in some Far Eastern counties.
- **Conversion disorder** is a somatoform disorder in DSM-IV but not in ICD (see above).
- **Body dysmorphic disorder** does not exist as a separate category in ICD-10; instead it is included in the diagnostic criteria for hypochondriacal disorder.

There are also problems which both classifications share:

- **Diagnostic criteria within the group** are based on a mixture of principles - aetiology, symptom count, consultation, and response to **medical** treatment.

TABLE 10.1 Categories of somatoform disorders in ICD-10 and DSM-IV

ICD-10	DSM-IV
Somatization disorder	Somatization disorder
Undifferentiated somatoform disorder	Undifferentiated somatoform disorder
Hypochondriacal disorder	Hypochondriasis
Somatoform autonomic dysfunction	*No category*
Persistent pain disorder	Pain disorder associated with psychological factors (and a general medical condition)
Other somatoform disorders	Somatoform disorders not otherwise specified
No category	Body dysmorphic disorder
No category	Conversion disorder
Neurasthenia	*No category*

- **Diagnostic criteria for hypochondriacal disorder** were derived largely from patients attending hospitals and do not apply readily to many of the people with unexplained symptoms in the community.
- Many cases in the community do not meet the diagnostic criteria for any specific somatoform disorder and have to be placed in one of the two non-specific categories of **undifferentiated somatoform disorder** or **other somatoform disorders**. These residual categories have attracted little research and their diagnostic criteria are so broad that almost all persistent unexplained physical symptoms can be included.
- The seemingly small differences between DSM-IV and ICD-10 criteria have resulted in large differences in estimates of prevalence of somatoform disorder as a whole and of the subcategories (see Simon, 2000).

We lack the information needed for a thorough revision of this part of the classification and there would be little advantage in making minor changes. A useful alternative might be a multidimensional description in terms of clinical syndrome, duration, number of symptoms, cognitions, and associated psychiatric disorder (see Sharpe and Mayou 2004).

BOX 10.2 A BRIEF HISTORY OF HYSTERIA

There are descriptions of hysteria in ancient Greek medical texts. At that time the disorder was thought to result from abnormalities of position or function of the uterus, a view that persisted until the seventeenth century. Gradually, the idea became accepted that hysteria is a disorder of the brain and, by the nineteenth century, the importance of predisposing constitutional and organic causes of this brain disorder were recognized. It was accepted also that the usual provoking cause was strong emotion.

In the later years of the nineteenth century, the studies of hysteria by Charcot, a French neurologist working at the Salpêtrière Hospital in Paris, were particularly influential. Charcot believed at first that the symptoms of hysteria were caused by a functional disorder of the brain, and that this disorder also rendered patients susceptible to hypnosis. As a result of this susceptibility, new symptoms could be induced in these patients by suggestion, and existing ones could be modified. Later, Charcot became interested in the idea of his former pupil, Pierre Janet, that the basic disorder in hysteria is not suggestability but a tendency to dissociation. By this Janet meant that the patients had lost the normal integration between various parts of mental functioning (see also p. 212). Janet believed that this dissociation led to a loss of awareness of certain aspects of psychological functioning that would otherwise be within awareness. Janet's ideas were influential for a while but never had the impact of those of Freud. For a review of Janet's ideas about hysteria see van der Kolk and van der Hart (1989).

Freud visited Charcot in the winter of 1895–96 and was impressed by demonstrations of the susceptibility of patients to hypnosis, and of the power of suggestion (see Sulloway, 1979). On his return to Vienna, Freud and his colleague Breuer studied patients with hysteria and reported their findings first in a seminal paper 'On the psychical mechanisms of hysterical phenomena' (Freud, 1893) and subsequently in a monograph *Studies on hysteria* (1893–5). They proposed that hysteria was caused by emotionally charged ideas, usually sexual, which had become lodged in the patient's unconscious mind as a result of some past experience, and which were excluded from conscious awareness by repression (see p. 153). Freud adopted the word 'conversion' to refer to the hypothetical process whereby this hidden, unexpressed emotion was transformed into physical symptoms. Breuer and Freud summarized this idea in the phrase 'hysterics suffer mainly from reminiscences'.

In the years that followed, Freud came to believe that this original formulation was wrong and had been based on fabricated accounts obtained from suggestible patients, and from then on he wrote no more on hysteria. There was little interest in hysteria on the part of others and no real progress in understanding it. Hysteria was thought to be a declining problem in developed countries and there was concern that many apparent cases were in fact unrecognized organic disease. This view was put vigorously by Slater (1965) who reported a 7-year follow-up study of 85 patients diagnosed as having hysteria. At follow-up 30 had definite organic disease and 34 had a definite psychiatric disorder other than hysteria. Subsequent changes of opinion are considered on p. 207.

For the history of hysteria see Shorter (1992); for the history of the concept of conversion see Mace (2001).

Conversion disorder

Conversion disorder is the term used in DSM to replace the older term hysteria; it is the equivalent of Dissociative (Conversion) Disorder in ICD-10. The term refers to a condition in which there are isolated *neurological* symptoms that cannot be explained in terms of known mechanisms of pathology and in which there has been a significant psychological stressor. The study of such symptoms has a long history. Some understanding of this history is a necessary background to knowledge of the present status of the concept of conversion disorder. The account in Box 10.2 is longer than is strictly needed for this purpose because the history of ideas about hysteria is important also in understanding the development of Freud's ideas which so greatly influenced twentieth-century psychiatry.

BOX 10.3 TREATMENT OF ACUTE CONVERSION DISORDER

- Obtain medical and psychiatric history from patient and informants
- Carry out appropriate medical and psychiatric examination and arrange investigations for physical causes
- Reassure that the condition is temporary, well recognized and, for motor disorders, due to a problem of converting intention into action
- Avoid reinforcing symptoms or disability
- Offer continuing help with any related psychiatric or social problems

Clinical features

In DSM-IV, conversion disorder is divided into four subtypes:

1. **With motor symptom or deficit** This subtype includes such symptoms as impaired coordination or balance, paralysis or localized weakness, difficulty swallowing or 'lump in throat', aphonia, and urinary retention.
2. **With sensory symptom or deficit** This subtype includes such symptoms as loss of touch or pain sensation, double vision, blindness, deafness, and hallucinations.
3. **With seizures or convulsions** This subtype includes seizures or convulsions with voluntary motor or sensory components.
4. **With mixed presentation** This subtype is used if symptoms of more than one category are evident.

Conversion symptoms do not normally reflect the physiological or pathological mechanisms that are involved in other neurological lesions. They are also highly responsive to suggestion and may vary considerably in response to the comments of other people, especially doctors. Symptoms may be 'reinforced' by measures such as providing a wheelchair for the patient who has difficulty walking. In addition, people with conversion disorders may show a relative lack of obvious concern about the nature and implications of the symptoms (a feature sometimes known by a term used by nineteenth century French writers – *la belle indifference*). However this last feature is not invariable.

It is often said that sufferers derive **secondary gain** from their symptoms; that is to say external benefits or avoidance of unwanted responsibilities. (The term 'primary gain' refers to the relief allegedly obtained by the conversion of mental distress into physical symptoms.) It is sometimes impossible to identify such gains and, in any case, benefits of being ill are observed at times in many psychiatric and physical disorders.

Epidemiology

The prevalence of conversion disorder in the general population is difficult to determine. Estimates vary with the criteria used and the population studies. A review of five studies indicated an incidence rate of 5–12 per 100, 000 per annum with the lowest rates in a study of psychiatric practice, in keeping with the view that many of these patients are not referred to psychiatrists. Estimates of prevalence vary even more but with figures around 50 per 100, 000 (see for example Singh and Lee, 1997). The few studies that examined change over time do not support the belief that the condition is disappearing (Akagi and House, 2002).

Aetiology

The aetiology is unknown.There are several theories but few research findings to support any of them:

- **Psychodynamic theories** use the explanatory concept of conversion of emotional distress into physical symptoms which have a symbolic meaning.
- **Social factors** appear to be major determinants of the onset and development of conversion symptoms.
- **Neurophysiological mechanisms:** functional neuroimaging has yielded results which are compatible

with the idea of malfunctioning of the normal interactions between regions of the brain concerned with the intention to move and those involved in the initiation of movement (Athwal *et al.*, 2001).

- **Cognitive explanations** Brown (2002) suggested that the symptoms are caused by the chronic activation of representations of the symptoms stored within memory, the process being driven by attention directed to these representations.
- **Cultural explanations:** some of the phenomena classified as conversion disorder in Western countries may, in some other cultures, be accepted as possession states (see Trance and possession disorders, p. 215).

See Halligan *et al.* (2001) for reviews of theories of aetiology.

Prognosis

Prognosis for subsequent neurological disorder Most of the patients seen in general practice or hospital emergency departments with conversion disorders of recent onset recover quickly. Disorders lasting longer than a year are likely to persist for many years. In a widely cited follow-up study, noted above, Slater (1965) described the development of a physical and psychiatric disorder in a high proportion of patients. This finding is now thought to relate to the highly atypical nature of Slater's sample of neurological patients obtained from attenders at a tertiary referral hospital. A more recent follow-up of patients attending the same hospital, with symptoms that were unexplained after modern methods of investigation, found a very low incidence of physical or psychiatric diagnoses of a kind that could have explained the original symptoms (Crimlisk *et al.*, 1998). When the diagnosis of conversion disorder was made, it remained stable over time.

Prognosis for subsequent psychiatric disorder Although subsequent neurological disorder is uncommon in these patients, psychiatric morbidity is high. Usually the psychiatric symptoms are present when the patients were first seen and it is unusual for psychiatric disorder to develop for the first time, years later.

Predictors of prognosis Predictors of good outcome are short history and young age; predictors of poor outcome are long history, personality disorder, and receipt of disability benefit or involvement in litigation (Ron, 2001).

Treatment

For **acute conversion disorders** seen in primary care or hospital emergency departments, reassurance and suggestion of improvement are usually appropriate, together with immediate efforts to resolve any stressful circumstances that provoked the reaction (Box 10.3). The doctor should be sympathetic and positive, and provide a socially acceptable opportunity for rapid return to normal physical functioning, for example by arranging a brief course of physiotherapy. The patient should feel that the problem is accepted as deserving assessment, that it is common, and that a good outcome can be expected. The therapist should discuss any personal difficulties that have been identified, and suggest that they deserve attention in their own right.

Where symptoms have persisted for more than a few weeks more elaborate treatment is required. The general approach is to focus on removing any factors that are reinforcing the symptoms and disability and on encouraging of normal behaviour. It should be explained that the symptoms and disability (as in remembering, or moving his arm) are not caused by physical disease but by an inability to convert willed intention into action; and that sensory problems are caused by an inability to become aware of sensory information not by a lesion interfering with sensory pathways. This problem is provoked by psychological factors. Patients should be told also that they can regain control of the disturbed function and, if necessary, offered help to do so – usually through physiotherapy.

Attention is then directed away from the symptoms and towards problems that have provoked the disorder. Staff should show concern for the patient, but at the same time should encourage self-help. They should not make undue concessions to patients' disabilities; for example, a patient who cannot walk should be encouraged to walk again, not be provided with a wheelchair. The approach should be supportive and sympathetic: it should not appear in any way uncaring or punitive. To achieve this end, there must be a clear plan so that all members of staff adopt a consistent approach to the patient.

Medication has no direct part to play in the treatment of these disorders. However, when a conversion disorder is secondary to a depressive or anxiety disorder, treatment of the primary condition usually leads to improvement in the secondary symptoms. Cognitive behaviour therapy appear to be of little specific value though it may act as a non-specific aid to recovery.

It is essential that measures to reduce symptoms are accompanied by help with any associated personal and social difficulties. Brief and focused psychological treatments are helpful, but more intensive therapy may result in transference reactions which are difficult to manage.

Those who do not improve should be reviewed thoroughly for undiscovered physical illness. All patients, whether improved or not, should be followed carefully for long enough to exclude any organic disease that might have been missed at the original assessment.

'Epidemic hysteria'

Occasionally, dissociative (or conversion) disorder spreads within a group of people as an 'epidemic'. This spread happens most often in closed groups of young women, for example, in a girls' school, a nurses' home, or a convent. Usually anxiety has been heightened among the members of the group by some threat to the community, such as the possibility of being involved in an epidemic of actual and serious physical disease present in the neighbourhood. Typically, the epidemic starts in one person who is highly suggestible, histrionic, and a focus of attention in the group. This first case may result from a general apprehension about the threat of physical illness, or from a specific concern about an acquaintance who has contracted the illness. Gradually, other cases appear, first in the most suggestible and then, as anxiety mounts, among those with less predisposition. The symptoms are variable, but fainting and dizziness are common. Outbreaks among schoolchildren have been documented. Some writers believe that the 'dancing manias' of the Middle Ages may have been hysterical epidemics in people aroused by religious fervour (see Wessely, 1987).

Somatization disorder

The essential feature of somatization disorder is **multiple** somatic complaints **of long duration**, beginning before the age of 30. In 1962, psychiatrists in St Louis (Perley and Guze, 1962) described a syndrome of chronic multiple somatic complaints without any identified organic cause, which they regarded as a form of hysteria. They named it **Briquet's syndrome** after a nineteenth-century French physician who wrote a monograph on hysteria. In fact, Briquet did not describe the syndrome to which his name was given and the symptoms do not accord with usual concepts of hysteria.

A similar syndrome was introduced in DSM-III The diagnostic criteria were highly restrictive, so that many patients with multiple somatic complaints of long duration were excluded and had to be allocated to the residual category of **undifferentiated somatoform disorder**. In DSM-IV, the criteria for diagnosis were made less restrictive: they require four pain symptoms, two gastrointestinal symptoms, one sexual symptom, and one pseudo-neurological symptom, none of which is fully explained by a medical condition. The ICD-10 criteria require at least six symptoms relating to at least two organ systems from among a list of fourteen predefined symptoms distributed in four groups - gastrointestinal, cardiovascular, neurogenital, and skin or pain symptoms.

Epidemiology

The reported prevalence of somatization disorder depends on the assessment methods used. However estimates from community surveys have reported prevalences of less than 1 per cent while those in primary care have usually been between 1–2 per cent. The disorder is twice as common in women as in men. There is substantial comorbidity with other psychiatric disorders, such as major depression. Diagnosis is considerably less stable over time than was suggested in the original description of the syndrome. See Simon (2000) and Fink (2000) for reviews.

Aetiology

The St Louis group reported a familial association between somatization disorder in females and sociopathy and alcoholism in their male relatives. They also concluded that follow-up studies and family studies showed that somatization disorder was a unitary syndrome, stable over time. These views have not been confirmed. The long course essential for the diagnosis of somatization disorder has led to the suggestion that it may better be considered as a personality disorder. However this suggestion does not increase understanding of the causes of the condition. The causes of unexpalined physical symptoms are discussed further in Chapter 16.

Treatment

Treatment is difficult and patients often consume large amounts of resources. Continuing care by one doctor using only the essential investigations, can reduce the use of health services and may improve patients' functional state (Smith *et al.*, 1986; G. R. Smith, 1995). Psychiatric assessment can help to clarify a complicated history, to negotiate a simplified pattern of care, and to agree the aims of treatment with the patient, the family, and the responsible physician. The aim of treatment is more often to limit further progression than to cure. See Fink (2000) for a review.

Undifferentiated somatoform disorder

This is a residual category for unexplained physical symptoms, lasting at least 6 months, which are below the threshold for a diagnosis of somatization disorder. Its prevalence is much greater than that of somatization disorder. Since data do not show any clear boundary between the two conditions, based on the number or distribution of unexplained symptoms, it has been suggested that the criteria for somatization disorder should be made less restrictive (for example Escobar *et al.*, 1998). The problem would remain, however, that it is unsatisfactory to define a syndrome by an arbitrary number of unexplained symptoms when research suggests a continuum.

Hypochondriasis

The term hypochondriasis is one of the oldest medical terms, originally used to describe disorders believed to be due to disease of the organs situated in the hypochondrium. Since then, the term has been used in many ways. It is now defined by DSM-IV and ICD-10 in terms of conviction and/or fear of disease unsupported by the results of appropriate medical investigation. DSM-IV describes the condition as a

> preoccupation with a fear or belief of having a serious disease based on the individual's interpretation of physical signs of sensations as evidence of physical illness. Appropriate physical evaluation does not support the diagnosis of any physical disorder than can account for the physical signs or sensations or for the individual's unrealistic interpretation of them. The fear of having, or belief that one has a disease, persists despite medical reassurance.

The criteria go on to exclude patients with panic disorder or delusions, and require that symptoms have been present for at least 6 months. There is continuing uncertainty about the status of similar conditions that last for less than 6 months; whether there is a hypochondriacal personality disorder; and whether illness phobias should be included in the category.

Epidemiology

Attempts to estimate prevalence have been hindered by the absence of proven standardized methods of assessment. Whilst some primary care surveys have estimated a prevalence of around 5 per cent, the WHO multicentre primary care survey (Gureje *et al.*, 1997a) found a prevalence of only 0.8 per cent. Using a less restrictive definition, the prevalence was 2.2 per cent. This later definition omitted the criterion 'persistent refusal to accept medical reassurance' but retained the triad of illness worry, associated distress, and medical help-seeking. Comorbidity with depression and anxiety disorders is frequent. See Simon (2000) for a review of epidemiology.

Prognosis

A 4–5 year follow-up by Barsky *et al.* (1998) showed that the condition is often persists for this period.

Aetiology

The cause is unknown. Cognitive formulations suggest that there is faulty appraisal of normal bodily sensations which are interpreted as evidence of disease. This misinterpretation is maintained by behaviours such as continually seeking reassurance and examining or rubbing the supposedly affected part. The aetiology of unexplained symptoms is discussed further in Chapter 16.

Treatment

Since the disorder is chronic or recurrent, management is difficult. Repeated reassurance is unhelpful and may serve to prolong the patient's concerns. Investigations should be limited to those indicated by the medical priorities and not extended to satisfy the patient's other concerns. Misinterpretations of the significance of bodily sensations should be corrected, and encouragement given to constructive ways of coping with symptoms. Trials have shown more benefit for hypochondriacal symptoms from cognitive–behavioural treatment than from behavioural stress management or a waiting list control (Clark *et al.*, 1998) and more effectiveness than usual medical care (Barsky and Aherne, 2004). Poor response is predicted by greater psychopathology and higher social impairement (Hiller *et al.*, 2002).

See Noyes (2000) for a general review of hypochondriasis.

Body dysmorphic disorder

Body dysmorphic disorder is the DSM term for a subgroup of the broader but ill-defined syndrome of **dysmorphophobia**, which was first described by Morselli (1886) as 'a subjective description of ugliness and physical defect which the patient feels is noticeable to others'. In DSM the term body dysmorphic disorder denotes dysmorphophobia that is not better accounted for by another psychiatric disorder. The preoccupation with the imagined defect in appearance is usually an overvalued idea, but individuals 'can receive an additional diagnosis of Delusional Disorder, Somatic type'.

The syndrome overlaps with delusional disorder, hypochondriasis, and obsessive–compulsive disorder. In ICD-10 the condition is a subgroup of the broader category of hypochondriasis.

Patients with dysmorphophobia are convinced that some part of their body is too large, too small, or misshapen. To other people the appearance is normal, or there is a trivial abnormality. In the latter case, it may be difficult to decide whether the preoccupation is disproportionate. The common concerns are about the nose, ears, mouth, breasts, buttocks, or penis, but any part of the body may be involved. Patients may be constantly preoccupied with and tormented by their mistaken beliefs. It seems to them that other people notice and talk about the supposed deformity. They may blame all their other difficulties on it: if only their nose were a better shape, they would be more successful in their work, social life, and sexual relationships. Time-consuming behaviours which aim to re-examine, improve, or hide the perceived defect are frequent. Social impairment is considerable. There is substantial comorbidity, especially with major depression and social phobia.

The condition usually begins in adolescence. It is chronic, though it often fluctuates over time. It is probable that there is some improvement over many years but there have been no long-term prospective studies.

The severe cases described in the psychiatric literature are infrequent, but less severe forms of dysmorphophobia are more common, and especially among those seeking plastic surgery or seeing dermatologists. As with the more severe cases, some of those with this milder syndrome meet diagnostic criteria for other disorders.

Assessment

Assessment should include questions about the nature of the preoccupations with appearance and of the ways in which this has interfered with personal and social life. Diagnosis can be difficult because some sufferers fail to reveal the precise nature of their symptoms because of embarrassment. This failure may result in misdiagnosis as social phobia, panic disorder, or obsessive–compulsive disorder.

Treatment

When body dysmorphic disorder is secondary to a psychiatric disorder such as major depression, the latter should be treated in the usual way. The treatment of primary body dysmorphic disorder is often difficult. It is essential to establish a working relationship in which the patient feels that the psychiatrist is sympathetic, understands the severity of the problems, and is willing to help. Since many patients will be requesting surgery, it is important to explain the lack of success of this approach and suggest that there are other effective treatments. Counselling and practical help should be provided for any occupational, social, or sexual difficulties that accompany the condition. Although some patients are helped by this approach coupled with continued support, many are not.

Cosmetic surgery is often successful for patients with conditions other than dysmorphophobia. Surgery is usually contraindicated, however, for people who have body dysmorphic disorder, many of whom are very dissatisfied after the operation. Selection for surgery therefore requires careful assessment of the patient's expectations: those who do not have realistic views of the possible benefits of surgery generally have a poor prognosis. Assessment is difficult, and collaboration between plastic surgeons, psychiatrists, and psychologists is valuable.

Antidepressants There is evidence of beneficial effects from antidepressant medication (especially with selective serotonin re-uptake inhibitor [SSRI]), especially but not only in patients with prominent depressive symptoms.

Whatever treatment is offered, it is essential that patients feel that their views have been listened to sympathetically. Unintended rebuffs by surgeons or psychiatrists can increase the difficulties of management. See Phillips (2000) for a review of dysmorphophobia.

Somatoform disorder not otherwise specified

This residual diagnostic category is used for a wide range of somatoform symptoms that do not meet the criteria for the specific somatoform categories discussed so far or for adjustment disorder with physical complaints.

Pain disorder

This term denotes patients with chronic pain that is not caused by any physical or specific psychiatric disorder. DSM-IV states that the essential feature of this disorder is pain that is the predominant focus of the clinical presentation and is of sufficient severity to cause distress or impairment of functioning, and that either no organic pathology or pathophysiological mechanism has been found to account for the pain, or, when there is related organic pathology, the pain or resulting social or occupational impairment is grossly in excess of what would be expected from the physical findings.

Epidemiology

Pain is widely reported in surveys of the general population. Most people report pain that is transient, but a minority describe persistent or recurrent pain leading to disability (Gureje *et al.*, 1998). Pain is the most common symptom among people who consult doctors. Acute pain usually has an organic cause, but psychological factors can affect the subjective response to pain whatever the main cause.

In general practice, pain is a common presenting symptom of emotional problems. In psychiatric practice, it has been reported that pain is experienced by about one-fifth of inpatients and over half of outpatients. Pain is particularly associated with depression, anxiety, panic, and somatoform disorders. Patients with multiple pains are especially likely to have associated psychiatric disorder (Gureje *et al.*, 1998).

Aetiology

Chronic pain occurs in many conditions, including neurological or musculoskeletal disorders. It often has both physical and psychological causes. Some patients (with or without physical pathology) have a depressive disorder. In the past, it was suggested that others have a 'pain-prone disorder' which was a variant of depressive disorder. There is little evidence to support this idea (Von Korff and Simon, 1996). It is more likely that in these cases the pain arises from personal and social factors, and that beliefs about pain are important in maintaining it (Linton, 2000). Chronic pain may impose great burdens on the patient's family; also, the attitude of family members and other caregivers can influence the perception of pain, its course, and the response to treatment.

Assessment

The assessment of a patient complaining of pain of unknown cause should include:

- **thorough investigation of possible physical causes.** When the results of this investigation are negative, it should be remembered that pain may be the first symptoms of a physical illness that cannot be detected at an early stage;
- **full description** of the pain and the circumstances in which it occurs;
- **search for symptoms** of a depressive or other psychiatric disorder;
- **description of pain behaviours** – for example the presentation of symptoms, requests for medication, and responses to pain;
- **beliefs** about the causes of pain and of its implications.

Treatment

The management of chronic pain should be individually planned, comprehensive, and involve the patient's family. Skill is required to maintain a working relationship with patients unwilling to accept an approach that uses psychological treatments as part of the treatment of pain. Any associated physical disorder should be treated and adequate analgesics provided. The treatment of pain associated with a psychiatric disorder is the treatment of the primary condition.

Psychological care is directed to assessing:

- **any associated mental disorder.** This assessment should be made on positive findings and not solely because no specific organic cause has been identified. If depressive illness is present it should be treated vigorously. Antidepressant medication is effective in some patients with chronic pain in the absence of evidence of a depressive disorder (O'Malley *et al.*, 1999).
- **Whether psychological techniques are indicated** to modify the pain or any associated behaviours. Cognitive–behavioural treatment aims to encourage the use of distraction, relaxation and other ways of coping with the pain, and to reduce social reinforcement of pain related behaviour. In a meta-analysis comparing them with wait list controls and alternative treatments, these treatments had a significant though modest effect (Morley *et al.*, 1999).

Multidisciplinary pain clinics bring together expertise in somatic and psychological treatments for pain.

See Bass and Jack (2002) for a review of psychological approaches to chronic pain.

Some specific pain syndromes

Many kinds of pain are common in the population. This section is concerned with headache, facial pain, back pain, and pelvic pain. Some other specific pain syndromes are discussed in Chapter 16, including non-cardiac chest pain (p. 397), abdominal pain (p. 388), phantom limb pain (p. 395), and fibromyalgia (p. 388).

Headache

Patients with chronic or recurrent headache are sometimes referred to psychiatrists. There are many physical causes of headache, notably migraine which affects about one in ten of the population at some time of their life. Many patients attending neurological clinics have headaches for which no physical cause can be found. The commonest of these is 'tension' headache, which is usually described as a dull generalized feeling of pressure or tightness extending around the head. It is frequently of short duration and is relieved by analgesia or a good night's sleep, but may occasionally be constant and unremitting. Some patients describe depressive symptoms and others describe anxiety in relation to obvious life stresses. Psychological factors seem to contribute to aetiology, but there is no evidence that the headaches result from increased muscle tension, and vascular mechanisms are more likely.

Most patients with headaches for which no physical cause can be found are reassured by an explanation of the negative results of investigations. Antidepressants and stress management both produce modest improvement (Holroyd *et al.*, 2001).

Facial pain

Facial pain has many physical causes; there are at least two forms in which psychological variables appear to be important. The more common is temporomandibular dysfunction (Costen's syndrome or facial arthralgia). There is a dull ache around the temporomandibular joint, and the condition usually presents to dentists. 'Atypical' facial pain is a deeper aching or throbbing pain which is more likely to present to neurologists. Patients with either of these symptoms are often reluctant to see a psychiatrist, but several trials suggest that some antidepressants can relieve symptoms even when there is no evidence of a depressive disorder. Cognitive-behaviour therapy has been found to enhance the effect of the usual dental care for temporomandibular disorders (Dworkin *et al.*, 2002).

See Feinmann (1999) for a review of psychological aspects of facial pain.

Back pain

Back pain is the second leading cause for visits to primary-care doctors and a major cause of disability. Most acute pain is transient, but in about a fifth of patients it persists for more than 6 months. Psychological and behavioural problems at the onset predict a poor outcome (Linton, 2000). Treatment includes the provision of accurate information about the cause and outcome of the condition, limited use of analgesics, and a graded increase in activity. Von Korff *et al.* (1994) reported that, in primary care, systematic advice about self-care led to a functional outcome as good as that with analgesia and bed rest, cost less, and was more satisfactory to patients. A review using the Cochrane methodology found that behavioural treatment had an effect greater than no treatment or a waiting list control, but did not add significantly to the effect of the usual treatment programmes for chronic low back pain (van Tulder *et al.*, 2002). Another meta-analysis concluded that antidepressants are more effective that placebo in reducing back pain but not in increasing functional status (Salerno *et al.*, 2002).

Chronic pelvic pain

Pelvic pain is one of the most common symptoms reported by women attending gynaecology clinics. The pain often persists despite negative investigations, and psychological factors appear to be significant causes of the pain and the disability. Cognitive-behavioural interventions may be effective in some cases (Glover and Pearce, 1995).

Dissociative disorders

In DSMIV, the essential feature of dissociative disorders is a disruption of the usually integrated functions of consciousness, memory, identity or perception. This disturbance may be sudden or gradual, transient or chronic.

The history of the term dissociation is reviewed briefly in Box 10.4.

Types of dissociative disorder

Dissociative disorder are the conditions listed in table 10.2 with the corresponding terms in ICD-10. The

BOX 10.4 A BRIEF HISTORY OF DISSOCIATION

The term dissociation is associated particularly to the French philosopher and psychiatrist, Pierre Janet (1859–1947) who worked for a time with Charcot at the Salpêtrière in Paris. He studied aspects of sensory perception and mental integration in hysteria and other neuroses, and used the term 'désagregation psychologique' (translated as dissociation) to describe the breakdown of this integration. For a while Janet's ideas were influential (see van der Kolk and van der Hart, 1989) however, his theories were overshadowed by those of Freud.

In the 1970s interest in dissociation revived as a result of studies of the effects of psychological trauma, especially among Vietnam war veterans. These studies documented symptoms occuring in response to traumatic events, and suggested a common origin in the mechanism of dissociation, a new name of dissociative symptoms (see Table 10.2), and a new diagnostic category of dissociative disorders.

TABLE 10.2 Dissociative symptoms

Subjective numbing
Detachment
Reduced awareness of surroundings
Fragmentation or loss of memory
Derealization and depersonalization

TABLE 10.3 DSM-IV classification of dissociative disorder and their ICD–10 equivalents

DSM-IV	ICD–10
Dissociative disorder	**F44 Dissociative (conversion) disorder**
Dissociative amnesia	Dissociative amnesia
Dissociative fugue	Dissociative fugue
Dissociative identity disorder	Multiple personality disorder
Depersonalization disorder	(classified in F. 48.1)
Dissociative disorder not otherwise specified	Dissociative (conversion) disorder not otherwise specified
	Dissociative stupor
	Trance and possession disorders
	Ganser's syndrome

Note: ICD–10 also includes categories of sensory and motor disturbance which DSM-IV classifies within somatoform disorders in a subcategory of conversion disorder.

inclusion in ICD-10 of the bracketed term conversion in the title of the group, reflects the previous convention of classifying these conditions with the conversion disorders.

Some authors consider that these disorders are well established and common (for example Coons, 1998); others doubt the evidence base both for the category and for its constituents.(for example, Merskey, 2000).

Dissociative amnesia

The essential feature is an inability to recall important personal memories, usually of a stressful nature, that is too extensive to be explained by normal forgetfulness. Dissociative amnesia occurs alone and during the course of other dissociative disorders and of post-traumatic stress disorder, acute stress disorder, and somatization disorder. The diagnosis is made only when these other conditions are not present.

Dissociative amnesia must be distinguished from amnesia having a medical cause. It has been described in two forms:

1. circumscribed amnesia for a single recent traumatic event;
2. inability to recall long periods of childhood. Amongst patients who present in this way, some have concurrent organic disease.

See Coons (1998) for a review.

Dissociative fugue

Dissociative fugue is extremely rare. In a dissociative fugue, there is loss of memory coupled with wandering away from the person's usual surroundings. These people usually deny all memory of their whereabouts during the period of wandering, and some deny knowledge of personal identity. Many dramatic case histories have been published (see Hacking, 1998). The disorder must be distinguished from organic disorder, including epilepsy and substance intoxication.

Dissociative identity disorder

In this disorder (widely known by the ICD-10 term **multiple personality disorder**) there are sudden alternations between two patterns of behaviour, each of which is forgotten by the patient when the other is present. One pattern is the person's normal personality, the other 'personality' is an integrated array of emotional responses, attitudes, memories, and social behaviour, which contrasts, often strikingly, with the normal. Sometimes there is more than one additional 'personality'. The criteria for the DSM-IV diagnosis are shown in Box 10.4. The condition is probably rare, but it has been reported more frequently in certain periods, notably around the end of the nineteenth century. These variations over time probably reflect the changing interests of doctors rather than true changes in prevalence. In the course of last 40 years there has been another increase in the number of reported cases, especially in the USA. It is not certain whether this change is real and epidemiological studies do not provide the answer because they report such widely varying prevalence rates.

Patients who meet the criteria in Box 10.5 often meet the criteria for other diagnoses including schizophrenia, personality disorder, and substance abuse. Many also have symptoms of anxiety and depression.The relationship between dissociative identity disorder and these other conditions would be clarified by long-term follow-up studies, but no systematic studies of this kind have been reported.

Two issues have dominated the discussion of **aetiology:**

1. **The role of severe trauma** Clinical experience and research show that many of those with the disorder

BOX 10.5 DSM-IV DIAGNOSTIC CRITERIA FOR DISSOCIATIVE IDENTITY DISORDER

A The presence of two or more distinct identities or personality states (each with its own relatively enduring pattern of perceiving, relating to, and thinking about, the environment and self).

B At least two of these identities or personality states recurrently take control of the person's behaviour.

C Inability to recall important personal information that is too extensive to be explained by ordinary forgetfulness.

D The disturbance is not due to the direct physiological effects of a substance (e.g. blackouts or chaotic behaviour during alcohol intoxication) or a general medical condition (e.g. complex partial seizures).

Note In children, the symptoms are not attributable to imaginary playmates or other fantasy play.

describe severe physical or sexual abuse taking place in childhood. It has been suggested that dissociation began as a psychological defence mechanism that reduced distress at the time of the original trauma but had unfortunate lasting consequences.

2. **Iatrogenic factors** It has been argued that the widespread publicity given to some people with multiple personality, the credulity of some therapists, and the use of hypnosis, have been responsible for at least some instances of the disorder. For a review see Putnam and Loewenstein (2000). For a sceptical opinion see Merskey (2000).

Depersonalization disorder

Depersonalization disorder is characterized by an unpleasant state in which external objects or parts of the body are experienced as changed in their quality and feel unreal or remote. Transient symptoms of depersonalization are quite common as a minor feature of other syndromes, and the symptoms of depersonalization disorder occurs occasionally in association with other psychiatric disorders (see differential diagnosis below), but primary depersonalization disorder is rare. How rare is uncertain because estimates of the prevalence vary so widely that no useful conclusion can be reached (see Hunter et al., 2004).

Although classified as a dissociative disorder in DSM-IV, it is not certain whether dissociation is indeed the causal mechanism of depersonalization disorder (see aetiology below). In ICD this uncertainty is recognized by giving the disorder its own place in the classification, separate from the dissociation disorders.

Clinical picture

The central features are a feeling of being unreal and an unreal quality to perceptions. Emotions seem dulled and actions feel mechanical. Paradoxically, this lack of feeling is experienced as extremely unpleasant. Insight is retained into the subjective nature of their experiences. These symptoms may be intense, and accompanied by *déjà vu* and by changes in the experience of passage of time. Some patients complain also of sensory distortions affecting a single part of the body (usually the head, the nose, or a limb), a feeling which some describe as if made of cotton wool.

Two-thirds of the patients are women. The onset is often in adolescence or early adult life, with the condition starting before the age of 30 in about half the cases. The symptoms usually begin suddenly, sometimes when the person is active but sometimes in the course of relaxation after intense physical exercise (Shorvon *et al.*, 1946). Once established, the disorder often persists for years, though with periods of partial or complete remission.

Differential diagnosis

Before diagnosing depersonalization disorder, any primary disorder must be excluded, especially temporal lobe epilepsy, schizophrenia, depressive disorder, obsessional disorder, conversion disorder, another dissociative disorder, generalized and phobic anxiety disorders, and panic disorder. It is also associated with migraine and epilepsy (Lambert *et al.*, 2002) and the use of illicit drugs (Medford *et al.*, 2003). Severe and persistent depersonalization is experienced by some people with schizoid personality disorder.

Most patients who present with depersonalization will be found to have one of these other disorders. The primary syndrome is rare.

Aetiology

The causes of a primary depersonalization disorder are not known. Apart from the possible association with schizoid personality disorder, no definite constitutional factors have been identified. Sierra *et al.* (2002) reported that the response to a startling noise was earlier in depersonalization disorder than in controls, suggesting a heightened state of alertness. At the same time autonomic responses to unpleasant stimuli were reduced, suggesting a selective inhibition of emotional processing. An fMRI study (Phillips *et al.*, 2001) compared responses to emotionally salient stimuli in people with depersonalization disorder, obsessive–compulsive disorder and healthy controls. Those with depersonalization disorder had a smaller response in the insula and occipito-temporal cortex, and a greater response in the right ventral prefrontal cortex. These findings, if confirmed, could be interpreted as a reduced response in areas concerned with the representation of emotion and an increased response in areas concerned with the regulation of emotion - again suggesting inhibition of emotional responses in depersonalization disorder. None of these findings explain why in most people depersonalization is short lived, while in a small minority it persists as depersonalization disorder.

Prognosis

Secondary cases have the prognosis of the primary condition. The rare primary depersonalization disorder has not been followed systematically; clinical experience indicates that cases lasting longer than a year have a poor long-term outcome.

Treatment

When depersonalization is secondary to another disorder, treatment should be directed to the primary condition. For primary depersonalization disorder, anxiolytic drugs may give short-term relief but they should not be prescribed for long periods because of the risk of dependency. Supportive interviews can help the patient to function more normally despite the symptoms, and any stressors should be addressed. Claims for the value of lamotrigine which reduces glutamate release (Sierra *et al.*, 2003), have not been confirmed, nor have claims for cognitive–behavioural treatments or dynamic psychotherapy (see Simeon *et al.*, 2003). In this, as in other conditions that are difficult to treat, it is important to resist the temptation to give ineffective treatments in order to appear to be doing something for the patient. It is better to give adequate time for supportive care.

See de Pauw (2000) for a review of depersonalization syndrome.

Other dissociative syndromes in ICD-10 (not specifically listed in DSM-IV)

Dissociative stupor

In dissociative stupor, patients show the characteristic features of stupor. They are motionless and mute, and they do not respond to stimulation, but they are aware of their surroundings. Dissociative stupor is rare. It is essential to exclude other possible conditions, namely schizophrenia, depressive disorder, mania, and organic brain diseases.

Ganser's syndrome

Ganser's syndrome is a very rare condition with four features:

1. giving 'approximate answers' (see below) to questions designed to test intellectual functions,
2. psychogenic physical symptoms,
3. hallucinations,
4. apparent clouding of consciousness.

The syndrome was first described among prisoners (Ganser, 1898) but is not confined to them. The term 'approximate answers' denotes answers (to simple questions) that are plainly wrong but are clearly related to the correct answer in a way that suggests that the latter is known. For example, when asked to add two and two a patient might answer five, while to three plus three he might answer seven. The obvious advantage to be gained from the condition, coupled with the approximate answers, suggests malingering. However, the condition is maintained so consistently that unconscious mental mechanisms have been thought to play a part. It is important to exclude an organic brain disease or schizophrenia; the former should be considered particularly carefully when muddled thinking and visual hallucinations are part of the clinical picture.

For a review see Dwyer and Reid (2004).

Trance and possession disorder

Trance and possession disorder is included in dissociative (conversion) disorder in ICD-10. DSM-IV lists it in Appendix B (Criteria Sets and Axes provided for further study) as **Dissociative Trance Disorder**.

Trance and possession states are characterized by a temporary loss of the sense of personal identity and of full awareness of the surroundings. Such states are induced temporarily in willing participants in religious or other ceremonies. When they arise in this way, the states are not recorded as disorders. According to DSM-IV they become disorders when there is:

> an involuntary state of trance not accepted by the person's culture as a normal part of a collective cultural or religious practice and that causes clinically significant distress or functional impairment.

Some cases resemble multiple personality disorder, in that the person behaves as if taken over by another personality for a brief period. When the condition is induced by religious ritual, the person may feel taken over by a deity or spirit. The focus of attention is narrowed to a few aspects of the immediate environment, for example, to the priest carrying out a religious ceremony. The affected person may repeatedly perform the same movements, or adopt postures, or repeat utterances.

Cultural syndromes

Certain patterns of unusual behaviour, resticted to certain cultures, have been thought to reflect psychological mechanisms of dissociation. Some these behaviours can be classified as cultural syndromes. (This term has been criticized because it is applied to syndromes in non-Western cultures but not to syndromes which are found particularly in Western cultures - for example eating disorders, and chronic fatigue syndrome). Examples of cultural syndromes include the following:

- ***Latah***, which is found among women in Malaya, is characterized by echolalia, echopraxia, and other kinds of abnormally compliant behaviour. The condition usually begins after a frightening experience.
- **Amok** has been described among men in Indonesia and Malaya (Van Loon, 1927). It begins with a period of brooding, which is followed by violent behaviour and sometimes dangerous use of weapons. Amnesia is usually reported afterwards. It is unlikely that all patients with this pattern of behaviour are suffering from a dissociative disorder; the others may be suffering from mania, schizophrenia, or a post-epileptic state.
- **Arctic hysteria** is seen among the Eskimo, more often in the women. The affected person tears off her clothing, screams and cries, runs about wildly, and may endanger her life by exposure to cold. Sometimes the behaviour is violent. The relationship of this syndrome to dissociative disorder is not firmly established, and there may be more than one cause.

Recovered memories and false-memory syndrome

These conditions are described on p. 172.

Factitious dissociative identity disorder

There is wide agreement, even among those who believe that dissociative identity disorder is common, that both factitious and malingered presentations are common (see Coons, 1998).

Further reading

Gelder, MG, López-Ibor JJ Jr and Andreasen, NC (eds) (2000) *New Oxford textbook of psychiatry*. Oxford, Oxford University Press. (See sections 4.6.3; 4.9; 5.2.)

Halligan, PW, Bass, C and Marshall, JC (eds) (2001) *Contemporary approaches to the study of hysteria: clinical and theoretical perspectives*. Oxford, Oxford University Press. (A useful source book for all aspects of the conditions considered in this chapter.)

Manu, P (ed.) (1998) *Functional somatic syndromes*. Cambridge, Cambridge University Press. (Reviews the common functional syndromes.)

CHAPTER 11

Mood disorders

Chapter contents

Introduction

The **mood disorders** are so called because one of their main features is abnormality of mood. Nowadays the term is usually restricted to disorders in which this mood is depression or elation, but in the past some authors have included states of anxiety as well. In this book, anxiety disorders are described in Chapter 9. Mood disorders have in the past been referred to as 'affective disorders', a term still used fairly widely.

Depression

It is part of normal experience to feel unhappy at times of adversity. The symptom of depressed mood is a component of many psychiatric syndromes and is also commonly found in certain physical diseases, for example, in infections such as hepatitis and some neurological disorders. In this chapter we are concerned neither with normal feelings of unhappiness nor with depressed mood as a symptom of other disorders, but with the syndromes known as **depressive disorders**.

The central features of these syndromes are:

- depressed mood
- negative thinking
- lack of enjoyment
- reduced energy
- slowness.

Of these, depressed mood is usually, but not invariably, the most prominent symptom.

TABLE 11.1 Symptoms needed to meet criteria for 'depressive episode' in ICD–10

A
◆ Depressed mood
◆ Loss of interest and enjoyment
◆ Reduced energy and decreased activity
B
◆ Reduced concentration
◆ Reduced self-esteem and confidence
◆ Ideas of guilt and unworthiness
◆ Pessimistic thoughts
◆ Ideas of self-harm
◆ Disturbed sleep
◆ Diminished appetite
Mild depressive episode: at least 2 of A and at least 2 of B
Moderate depressive episode: at least 2 of A and at least 3 of B
Severe depressive episode: all 3 of A and at least 4 of B
Severity of symptoms and degree of functional impairment also guide classification

Mania

Similar considerations apply to **states of elation**. A degree of elated mood is part of normal experience at times of good fortune. Elation can also occur as a symptom in several psychiatric syndromes, though it is less widely encountered than depressed mood. In this chapter we are concerned with a syndrome in which the central features are:

- overactivity
- elevated or irritable mood
- self-important ideas.

This syndrome is called **mania**. Some diagnostic classifications distinguish a less severe form of mania, **hypomania** (see below).

Clinical features

Depressive syndromes

The clinical presentations of depressive states are varied and they can be subdivided in a number of different ways. In the following account, disorders are grouped by their **severity**. The account begins with a description of the clinical features of an episode of depression of **moderate severity**. More severe disorders are then described together with certain important clinical variants. Finally, the special features of the **less severe** depressive disorders are outlined. What constitutes an 'episode' of clinical depression is inevitably a somewhat arbitrary concept. The symptoms listed for the diagnosis of 'depressive episode' in the ICD-10 classification and the various levels of severity are shown in Table 11.1. Table 11.2 shows the criteria for 'major depressive episode' in DSM-IV.

Moderate depressive episode

In a moderate episode of depression, the central features are **low mood, lack of enjoyment, negative thinking**, and **reduced energy**, all of which lead to decreased **social and occupational functioning**.

Appearance

The patient's **appearance** is characteristic. **Dress and grooming** may be neglected. The facial features are characterized by a turning downwards of the corners of the mouth and by vertical furrowing of the centre of the brow. The rate of blinking may be reduced. The shoulders are bent and the head is inclined forwards so that the direction of gaze is downwards. Gestural movements are reduced. It is important to note that some patients maintain a smiling exterior despite deep feelings of depression.

TABLE 11.2 Criteria for major depressive episode – DSM-IV

Five (or more) of the following symptoms have been present during the same 2-week period and represent a change from previous functioning; at least one of the symptoms is either (1) depressed mood or (2) loss of interest or pleasure
1. Depressed mood most of the day, nearly every day, as indicated by either subjective report (e.g. feels sad or empty) or observation made by others (e.g. appears tearful)
2. Markedly diminished interest or pleasure in all, or almost all, activities most of the day, nearly every day (as indicated by either subjective account or observation made by others)
3. Significant weight loss when not dieting or weight gain (e.g. a change of more than 5% of body weight in a month), or decrease or increase in appetite nearly every day
4. Insomnia or hypersomnia nearly every day
5. Psychomotor agitation or retardation nearly every day (observable by others, nor merely subjective feelings of restlessness or being slowed down)
6. Fatigue or loss of energy nearly every day
7. Feelings of worthlessness or excessive or inappropriate guilt (which may be delusional) nearly every day (not merely self-reproach or guilt about being sick)
8. Diminished ability to think or concentrate, or indecisiveness, nearly every day (either by subjective account or as observed by others)
9. Recurrent thoughts of death (not just fear of dying), recurrent suicidal ideation without a specific plan, or a suicide attempt or a specific plan for committing suicide

Mood

The **mood** of the patient is one of **misery**. This mood does not improve substantially in circumstances where ordinary feelings of sadness would be alleviated, for example, in pleasant company or after hearing good news. Moreover, the mood is often experienced as different from **ordinary sadness**. Patients sometimes speak of a black cloud pervading all mental activities. Some patients can conceal this mood change from other people, at least for short periods. Some try to hide their low mood during clinical interviews, making it more difficult for the doctor to detect. The mood is often worse first thing in the morning when the patient awakes, improving a little as the day wears on. This is called diurnal variation of mood.

Depressive cognitions

Negative thoughts ('depressive cognitions') are important symptoms which can be divided into three groups:

1. worthlessness
2. pessimism
3. guilt.

In feeling **worthless**, the patient thinks that he is failing in everything that he does and that other people see him as a failure; he no longer feels confident, and discounts any success as a chance happening for which he can take no credit. **Pessimistic thoughts** concern future prospects. The patient expects the worst. He foresees failure in his work, the ruin of his finances, misfortune for his family, and an inevitable deterioration in his health. These ideas of **hopelessness** are often accompanied by the thought that life is no longer worth living and that death would come as a welcome release. These gloomy preoccupations may progress to thoughts of, and plans for, **suicide**. It is important to ask about these ideas in every case (the assessment of suicidal risk is considered further in Chapter 17).

Feelings of **guilt** often take the form of unreasonable self-blame about minor matters; for example, a patient may feel guilty about past trivial acts of dishonesty or letting someone down. Usually these events have not been in the patient's thoughts for years but, when he becomes depressed, they flood back into his memory, accompanied by intense feelings. Preoccupations of this kind strongly suggest depressive disorder. Some patients have similar feelings of guilt but do not attach them to any particular event. Other memories are focused on unhappy events; the patient remembers occasions when he was sad, when he failed, or when his fortunes were at a low ebb. These gloomy memories become increasingly frequent as the depression deepens. The patient blames himself for his misery and incapacity and attributes it to personal failing and moral weakness (a view not uncommonly held by the wider public).

Goal-directed behaviour

Lack of interest and enjoyment (also known as **anhedonia**) is frequent though not always complained of spontaneously. The patient shows no enthusiasm for activities and hobbies that he would normally enjoy. He feels no zest for living and no pleasure in everyday things. He often withdraws from **social encounters**. Reduced energy is characteristic (though sometimes associated with a degree of physical restlessness that can mislead the observer). The patient feels lethargic, finds everything an effort, and leaves tasks unfinished. For example, a normally house-proud person may leave the beds unmade and dirty plates on the table. Work outside the home becomes increasingly difficult.

Understandably, many patients attribute this lack of energy to physical illness.

Psychomotor changes

Psychomotor retardation is frequent (though, as described later, some patients are **agitated** rather than slowed up). The retarded patient walks and acts slowly. Slowing of thought is reflected in the patient's speech; there is a significant delay before questions are answered, and pauses in conversation may unusually prolonged. **Agitation** is a state of restlessness that is experienced by the patient as inability to relax and is seen by an observer as restless activity. When it is mild, the patient is seen to be plucking at his fingers and making restless movements of his legs; when it is severe, he cannot sit for long but paces up and down.

Anxiety is frequent though not invariable in moderate depression. (As described later, it is common in less severe depressive disorders.) Another common symptom is **irritability**, which is the tendency to respond with undue annoyance to minor demands and frustrations.

Biological symptoms

A group of symptoms often called 'biological' (also 'melancholic', 'somatic' and' vegetative') is important. These symptoms include sleep disturbance, diurnal variation of mood, loss of appetite, loss of weight, constipation, loss of libido, and, among women, amenorrhoea. They are frequent but not invariable in depressive disorders of moderate degree. (They are less usual in mild depressive disorders and particularly common in severe ones.) Some of these symptoms require further comment.

Sleep disturbance in depressive disorders is of several kinds. Most characteristic is **early morning waking**, but delay in falling asleep and waking during the night also occur. Early morning waking occurs 2 or 3 hours before the patient's usual time; he does not fall asleep again, but lies awake feeling unrefreshed and often restless and agitated. He thinks about the coming day with pessimism, broods about past failures, and ponders gloomily about the future. It is this combination of **early waking with depressive thinking** that is important in diagnosis. It should be noted that some depressed patients sleep excessively rather than wake early, but they still report waking unrefreshed.

Weight loss in depressive disorders often seems greater than can be accounted for merely by the patient's reported lack of appetite. In some patients the disturbances of eating and weight are towards excess – they eat more and gain weight. Usually eating brings temporary relief to their distressing feelings.

Complaints about **physical symptoms** are common in depressive disorders. They take many forms, but complaints of constipation, fatigue, and aching discomfort anywhere in the body are particularly common. Complaints about any pre-existing physical disorder usually increase and **hypochondriacal preoccupations** are common.

Other features

Several other psychiatric symptoms may occur as part of a depressive disorder, and occasionally one of them dominates the clinical picture. They include **depersonalization, obsessional symptoms, panic attacks**, and **dissociative symptoms** such as fugue or loss of function of a limb. Complaints of **poor memory** are also common; depressed patients commonly show deficits on a wide range of neuropsychological tasks, but impairments in the retrieval and recognition of recently learned material are particularly prominent. Sometimes the impairment of memory in a depressed patient is so severe that the clinical presentation resembles that of dementia. This presentation, which is particularly common in the elderly, is sometimes called depressive **pseudodementia** (see p. 511).

Severe depression and psychotic depression

As depressive disorders become more severe, all the features described above occur with greater intensity. There is complete loss of function in social and occupational spheres. Inattention to basic hygiene and nutrition may give rise to fears for the patient's well-being. Psychomotor retardation may make interview difficult or impossible. In addition, there may be delusions and hallucinations; the disorder is then called **psychotic depression**.

The delusions of severe depressive disorders are concerned with the same themes as the non-delusional thinking of moderate depressive disorders. Therefore they are termed **mood congruent**. These themes are worthlessness, guilt, ill-health, and, more rarely, poverty. Such delusions have been described in Chapter 1, but a few examples may be helpful at this point. The patient with a **delusion of guilt** may believe that some dishonest act, such as a minor concealment in making a tax return, will be discovered and that he will be punished severely and humiliated. He is likely to believe that such punishment is deserved. A patient with **hypochondriacal delusions** may be convinced that he has cancer or venereal disease. A patient with a **delusion of impoverishment** may wrongly believe that he has lost all his money in a business venture.

Persecutory delusions also occur. The patient may believe that other people are discussing him in a derogatory way or are about to take revenge on him. When persecutory delusions are part of a depressive syndrome, typically the patient accepts the supposed persecution as something that he has brought upon himself. In his view, he is ultimately to blame. Some depressed patients experience delusions and hallucinations that are not clearly related to themes of depression ('mood-incongruent'). Their presence appears to worsen the prognosis of the illness.

Particularly severe depressive delusions are found in **Cotard's syndrome**, which was described by a French psychiatrist, Cotard in 1882. The characteristic feature is an extreme kind of nihilistic delusion. For example, some patients may complain that their bowels have been destroyed so that they will never pass faeces again. Others may assert that they are penniless and without any prospect of having money again. Still others may be convinced that their whole family has ceased to exist and that they themselves are dead. Although the extreme nature of these symptoms is striking, such cases do not appear to differ in important ways from other severe depressive disorders.

Other clinical variants of moderate and severe depression

Agitated depression

This term is applied to depressive disorders in which **agitation** is prominent. As already noted, agitation occurs in many severe depressive disorders, but in agitated depression it is particularly severe. Agitated depression is seen more commonly among the middle-aged and elderly than among younger patients.

Retarded depression

This name is sometimes applied to depressive disorders in which psychomotor retardation is especially prominent. There is no evidence that they represent a separate syndrome, though retardation does predict a good response to electroconvulsive therapy (ECT). If the term is used, it should be in a purely descriptive sense. In its most severe form, retarded depression shades into **depressive stupor**.

Depressive stupor

In severe depressive disorder, slowing of movement and poverty of speech may become so extreme that the patient is motionless and mute. Such depressive stupor is rarely seen now that active treatment is available. Therefore the description by Kraepelin (1921, p. 80) is of particular interest:

> The patients lie mute in bed, give no answer of any sort, at most withdraw themselves timidly from approaches, but often do not defend themselves from pinpricks .... They sit helpless before their food, perhaps, however, they let themselves be spoon-fed without making any difficulty....

Kraepelin commented that recall of the events taking place during stupor was sometimes impaired when the patient recovered. Nowadays, the general view is that on recovery patients are able to recall nearly all the events taking place during the period of stupor. It is possible that in some of Kraepelin's cases there was clouding of consciousness (possibly related to inadequate fluid intake, which is common in these patients). Patients in states of depressive stupor may exhibit catatonic motor disturbances (see p. 16).

Atypical depression

The term **atypical depression** is generally applied to disorders of moderate clinical severity. The meaning of the term has varied over the years but currently it is applied to disorders characterized by:

- variably depressed mood with **mood reactivity** to positive events;
- overeating and oversleeping;
- extreme fatigue and heaviness in the limbs (leaden paralysis);
- pronounced **anxiety**.

Many patients with these clinical symptoms have a lifelong tendency to react in an exaggerated way to perceived or real rejection (**rejection sensitivity**), though this character trait can be exacerbated by the presence of a depressive disorder. The importance of recognizing atypical depression is that, because of their interpersonal sensitivity, patients with this disorder can be hard to manage and may be regarded as having 'difficult' personalities rather than depressive disorder. Also, atypical depression seems to be associated with a poor response to tricyclic antidepressant treatment but a better response to monoamine oxidase inhibitors (MAOIs) and selective serotonin reuptake inhibitors (SSRIs) (Quitkin *et al.*, 1993; Joyce *et al.*, 2004).

Mild depressive states

It might be expected that **mild depressive disorders** would present with symptoms similar to those of the depressive disorders described already, but with less intensity. To some extent this is so, but in mild depressive disorder there are frequently **additional symptoms** that are less prominent in severe disorders. These symptoms have been characterized in the past as 'neurotic', and they include **anxiety, phobias, obsessional**

symptoms, and, less often, **dissociative symptoms**. In terms of classification, both DSM-IV and ICD-10 have categories of **mild depression** where criteria for a depressive episode are met but the depressive symptoms are fewer and less severe (see Table 11.1).

Apart from the 'neurotic' symptoms found in some cases, mild depressive disorders are characterized by the expected symptoms of low mood, lack of energy and interest, and irritability. There is sleep disturbance, but not the early morning waking that is so characteristic of more severe depressive disorders. Instead, there is more often difficulty in falling asleep and periods of waking during the night, usually followed by a period of sleep at the end of the night. 'Biological' features (poor appetite, weight loss, and low libido) are not usually found. Although mood may vary during the day, it is usually worse in the evening than in the morning. The patient may not be obviously dejected in his appearance or slowed in his movement. Delusions and hallucinations are not present.

In their mildest forms, these cases shade into the minor affective disorders considered below. As described later, they pose considerable problems of classification. Many of these mild depressive disorders are brief, starting at a time of personal misfortune and subsiding when fortunes have changed or a new adjustment has been achieved. However, some cases persist for months or years, causing considerable suffering, even though the symptoms do not increase. These chronic depressive states are called **dysthymia**. The term **cyclothymic disorder** refers to a persistent instability of mood in which there are numerous periods of mild elation or mild depression. It is seen as a milder variant of bipolar disorder. It is not unusual for episodes of more severe mood disorder to supervene in patients who experience dysthymia or cyclothymia and the converse can also occur (Judd *et al.*, 1998, 2002). This suggests that in some people milder symptoms are a limited expression of an underlying major mood disturbance.

Minor mood disorders

We have already seen that anxiety and depressive symptoms often occur together. Indeed, earlier writers (see Lewis, 1956) considered that anxiety and depressive disorders could not be separated clearly even in patients admitted to hospital with severe disorders. Although most psychiatrists now accept that the distinction can usually be made among the more severe forms presenting in psychiatric practice, the distinction is less easy to make in the milder forms presenting in primary care.

Classification

As psychiatrists work increasingly with general practitioners, the importance of minor anxiety depressive disorders has been recognized but without any agreement about classification.

ICD-10 includes a category of 'mixed anxiety and depressive disorder' which can be applied when neither anxiety symptoms nor depressive symptoms are severe enough to meet criteria for an anxiety disorder or a depressive disorder, and when the symptoms do not have the close association with stressful events or significant life changes required for a diagnosis of acute stress reaction or adjustment disorder.

According to ICD-10, patients with this presentation are seen frequently in primary care and there are many others in the general population who are not seen by doctors. In ICD-10 this diagnosis appears amongst anxiety disorders, although some psychiatrists consider that the condition is more closely related to the mood disorders, a view that is reflected in the alternative term **minor affective disorder**.

In DSM-IV, no comparable diagnosis appears in the classification. The appendix to the classification contains two provisional diagnoses that might be used for these cases: **mixed anxiety and depressive disorder** and **minor depressive disorder**. It is stated that there is insufficient factual information to justify the inclusion of either in the classification. Although little is known about these conditions or about their relationship to other disorders, patients present to doctors with this group of symptoms. A suitable category is needed even if it is not possible to write strict criteria for diagnosis.

Clinical picture

One of the best descriptions of minor affective disorder has been given by Goldberg *et al.*, (1976) who studied 88 patients from a general practice in Philadelphia. The most frequent symptoms were:

- fatigue
- anxiety
- depression
- irritability
- poor concentration
- insomnia
- somatic symptoms and bodily preoccupation.

A very similar range of symptoms was found was found in the National Psychiatric Morbidity Household Survey (Jenkins *et al.*, 1997) which surveyed the frequency of 'neurotic' symptomatology in a community

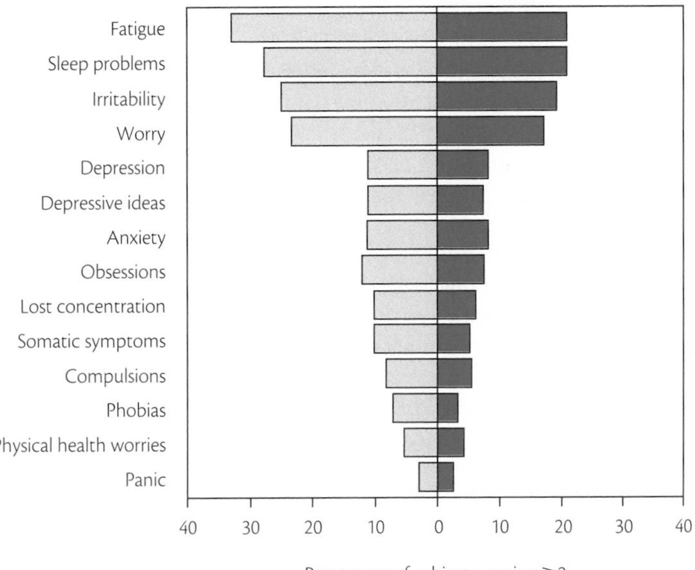

Fig. 11.1 Scores for neurotic symptoms on the revised clinical interview schedule (CIS-R) of a randomly selected sample of 10 000 adults in the National Survey of Psychiatric Morbidity. All symptoms are commoner in women (light hatching) than men (darker hatching). The commonest symptom is 'fatigue', reported by 27% of subjects. (From Jenkins *et al.* 1997.)

sample (Figure 11.1). Patients with minor affective disorders commonly present to medical practitioners with **prominent somatic symptoms**. The reason for this is uncertain; some symptoms are autonomic features of anxiety, and it is possible that patients expect somatic complaints to be received more sympathetically than emotional problems. Another point of clinical relevance is that minor affective disorders can be prolonged and in some cases cause incapacitating difficulties in personal and occupational function. Thus the term 'minor' may not capture the serious consequences of the disorder for an individual. As noted above, in some people minor affective disorders may represent a residual form of a major mood disturbance (Judd *et al.*, 1998, 2002).

Mania

As already mentioned, the central features of the syndrome of mania are **elevation of mood**, **increased activity**, and **self-important ideas**.

Mood

When the mood is elevated, the patient seems cheerful and optimistic, and he may have a quality described by earlier writers as **infectious gaiety**. However, other patients are irritable rather than euphoric, and this irritability can easily turn to anger. The mood often varies during the day, though not with the regular rhythm characteristic of many severe depressive disorders. In patients who are elated, not uncommonly, high spirits are interrupted by brief episodes of **depression**.

Appearance and behaviour

The patient's appearance often reflects their prevailing mood. Clothes may be brightly coloured and ill-assorted. When the condition is more severe, the patient's appearance is often **untidy and dishevelled**. Manic patients are overactive. Sometimes the persistent overactivity leads to **physical exhaustion**. Manic patients start many activities but leave them unfinished as new ones catch their fancy. Appetite is increased and food may be eaten greedily with little attention to conventional manners. Sexual desires are increased and sexual behaviour may be uninhibited and quite out of character. Women may neglect precautions against pregnancy, a point calling for particular attention when a patient is of childbearing age. Sleep is often reduced. Patients wake early, feeling lively and energetic; often they get up and busy themselves noisily, to the surprise of other people.

Speech and thought

Speech of manic patients is often **rapid and copious** as thoughts crowd into their minds in quick succession. When the disorder is more severe, there is **flight of ideas** (see p. 15) with such rapid changes that it is difficult to follow the train of thought. However, the links are usually understandable if the speech can be recorded and reviewed. This is in contrast to thought disorder in schizophrenia where changes in the flow of thought may not be comprehensible even on reflection.

Expansive ideas are common. Patients believe that their ideas are original, their opinions important, and their work of outstanding quality. Many patients become **extravagant**, spending more than they can afford on expensive cars or jewellery. Others make reckless decisions to give up good jobs, or embark on plans for hare-brained and risky business ventures.

Sometimes these expansive themes are accompanied by **grandiose delusions**. Some patients may believe that they are religious prophets or destined to advise statesmen about great issues. At times there are **delusions of persecution**, with patients believing that people are conspiring against them because of their special importance. Delusions of reference and passivity feelings also occur. Schneiderian first-rank symptoms (see Chapter 12, Table 12.4) have been reported in about 10–20 per cent of manic patients. Neither the delusions nor the first-rank symptoms last long - most disappear or change in content within days.

Perceptual disturbances

Hallucinations occur. They are usually consistent with the mood, taking the form of voices speaking to the patient about his special powers or, occasionally, of visions with a religious content.

Other features

Insight is invariably impaired in more severe manic states. Patients see no reason why their grandiose plans should be restrained or their extravagant expenditure curtailed. They seldom think of themselves as ill or in need of treatment.

Most patients can exert some control over their symptoms for a short time, and many do so when the question of treatment is being assessed. For this reason it is important to obtain a history from an **informant** whenever possible. Henry Maudsley (1879, p. 398) expressed the problem well:

> Just as it is with a person who is not too far gone in intoxication, so it is with a person who is not too far gone in acute mania; he may on occasion pull his scattered ideas together by an effort of will, stop his irrational doings and for a short time talk with an appearance of calmness and reasonableness that may well raise false hopes in inexperienced people.

The symptoms needed to fulfill the criteria for Manic Episode in DSM-IV are shown in Table 11.3. The criteria for manic episode in ICD-10 are very similar, though they do not specify so precisely the number of manic symptoms required for diagnosis.

TABLE 11.3 Criteria for manic episode (DSM-IV)

A. A distinct period of abnormally and persistently elevated, expansive, or irritable mood, lasting at least 1 week (or any duration if hospitalization is necessary)
B. During the period of mood disturbance, three (or more) of the following symptoms have persisted (four if the mood is only irritable) and have been present to a certain degree:
1. Inflated self-esteem or grandiosity
2. Decreased need for sleep (e.g., feels rested after only 3 hours of sleep)
3. More talkative than usual or pressure to keep talking
4. Flight of ideas or subjective experience that thoughts are racing
5. Distractibility (i.e., attention too easily drawn to unimportant or irrelevant external stimuli)
6 Increase in goal-directed activity (either socially, at work or school, or sexually) psychomotor agitation
7. Excessive involvement in pleasurable activities that have a high potential for painful consequences (e.g., engaging in unrestrained buying sprees, sexual indiscretions, or foolish business investments)
C. The symptoms do not meet criteria for a mixed episode
D. The mood disturbance is sufficiently severe to cause marked impairment in occupational functioning or in usual social activities or relationships with others, or to necessitate hospitalization to prevent harm to self or others, or there are psychotic features
E. The symptoms are not due to the direct physiological effects of a substance e.g., a drug of abuse, a medication, or other treatment) or a general medical condition (e.g., hyperthyroidism)

Mixed mood (affective) states

Depressive and manic symptoms sometimes occur at the same time. Patients who are overactive and over-talkative may be having profoundly depressive thoughts. In other patients, mania and depression follow each other in a sequence of rapid changes; for example, a manic patient may become intensely depressed for a few hours and then return quickly to his manic state. These changes were mentioned in early descriptions of mania by Griesinger (1867), and have been re-emphasized in recent years because they seem to predict a better response to certain mood stabilizers such as valproate.

Rapid cycling disorders

Some bipolar disorders recur regularly with intervals of only days or weeks between episodes. In the nineteenth century these regularly recurring disorders were designated *folie circulaire* (circular insanity) by the French psychiatrist Falret (1854). At present, the frequent recurrence of mood disturbance in bipolar patients is usually called **rapid cycling disorder**. These recurrent episodes may be depressive, manic, or mixed. The main features are that recurrence is frequent (conventionally, at least four distinct episodes a year) and that episodes are separated by a period of remission or a switch to an episode of opposite polarity. A number of clinical features of rapid cycling disorder are important in management and prevention:

- they occur more frequently in women;
- concomitant hypothyroidism is common;
- they can be triggered by antidepressant drug treatment;
- lithium treatment is relatively ineffective.

For a review of the clinical features and treatment of rapid cycling see Mackin and Young (2004).

Manic stupor

In this unusual disorder, patients are **mute and immobile**. Their facial expression suggests elation and on recovery they describe having experienced a rapid succession of thoughts typical of mania. The condition is rarely seen now that active treatment is available for mania. Hence an earlier description by Kraepelin (1921, p. 106) is of interest:

> The patients are usually quite inaccessible, do not trouble themselves about their surroundings, give no answer, or at most speak in a low voice ... smile without recognizable cause, lie perfectly quiet in bed or tidy about at their clothes and bedclothes, decorate themselves in an extraordinary way, all this without any sign of outward excitement.

On recovery, patients can remember the events that occurred during their period of stupor. The condition may begin from a state of manic excitement, but at times it is a stage in the transition between depressive stupor and mania.

Transcultural factors

Mania appears to be present in all cultures. However, caution in diagnosis is needed because culture-specific means of expressing distress can lead to behaviours which may be misdiagnosed as mania (Kirmayer and Groleau, 2001). There are cultural variations in the clinical presentation of depressive states but in most countries depression appears to be under-diagnosed, particularly in primary care. While somatic features are undoubtedly found in all societies, they are more frequent and prominent in non-Western cultures. However, it is necessary to distinguish between somatization (see Chapter 10) and somatic metaphors for an emotional state. For examples, Punjabi women living London used expressions such 'weight on my heart' and 'feelings of heat' to express emotional suffering, the presence of which they were well aware. It should also be noted that sadness, joylessness, anxiety and lack of energy are common symptoms of depression in all cultures (for a review see Bhugra and Mastrogianni, 2004).

Classification of mood disorders

The fundamental clinical distinction in the classification of mood disorders is between depression and mania. Depressive episodes have been subdivided in various ways which are outlined below, but the results of much of this work have not been particularly useful. However, studies of the longitudinal course of mood disorders have indicated that there are useful clinical distinctions to be made between people who never experience mania or hypomania (recurrent depressive disorder) and those who do (bipolar disorder).

Classification of depression

There is no general agreement about the best method of classifying depressive disorders. A number of approaches have been tried:

- based on presumed aetiology
- based on symptomatic picture
- based on course.

Classification by presumed aetiology

Historically, depressive disorders were sometimes classified into two kinds; in one the symptoms were caused by factors within the individual, and were independent of outside factors (**endogenous depression**), whereas in the other, the symptoms were a response to external stressors (**reactive depression**). This distinction has been recognized to be unsatisfactory for many years. For example, Lewis (1934) wrote:

> every illness is a product of two factors - of the environment working on the organism - whether the constitutional factor is the determining influence or the environmental one ... is never a question to be dealt with as either/or.

As noted in Chapter 5, when considering the aetiology of individual cases of depression, the relative contributions of a variety of aetiological factors must be considered. Neither ICD-10 nor DSM-IV contains categories of reactive or endogenous depression.

Classification by symptomatic picture

Melancholic depression It is well recognized that episodes of depression vary in symptomatic profile both within and between subjects. In the section on clinical description it was noted that some depressive conditions are characterized by 'biological' symptoms such as loss of appetite, psychomotor changes, weight loss, constipation, reduced libido, amenorrhoea, and early morning waking. These symptoms have sometime been called **melancholic** and they have been used to delineate a specific subgroup of depressive disorders, namely major depression with **melancholia** in DSM-IV, or depressive episode with **somatic symptoms** in ICD-10 (Table 11.4). The difficulty with this classification is that most patients have melancholic symptoms of some kind, though it may require a careful search to reveal them. Therefore the number of symptoms needed to fulfill the criterion for depression with melancholia is somewhat arbitrary. Despite this caveat it is generally agreed that clear-cut melancholic depression is associated with a number of clinical correlates (Parker *et al.*, 2001):

- More severe symptomatology
- Poor response to placebo medication
- Good response to ECT
- More evidence of neurobiological abnormalities (decreased latency to rapid eye movement sleep, cortisol hypersecretion).

TABLE 11.4 Clinical features of melancholic and somatic depression

Melancholic features (DSM-IV)
Loss of interest or pleasure in usual activities*
Lack of reactivity to pleasurable stimuli* *plus at least three of the following:*
Distinct quality of mood (unlike normal sadness)
Morning worsening of mood*
Early morning waking*
Psychomotor agitation or retardation*
Significant anorexia or weight loss*
Excessive guilt
Marked loss of libido* (ICD–10 only)

* Somatic symptoms of depression in ICD–10 (at least four required for diagnosis).

It is still not clear whether melancholic depression is a distinct condition or rather represents a point on a continuum of severity, towards the more severe end. Kendler (1997) attempted to answer this question using a population sample of twins. He found evidence that melancholic depression did represent a valid subtype in that it identified a group of individuals with a particularly high familial risk of depression. However, the diagnosis of melancholia indicated the presence of a *quantitatively* more severe form of depression rather than a distinct aetiological subtype.

Psychotic depression As noted above severe depression can also manifest with **psychotic features**, (though in depressive psychosis the features of melancholia are almost invariably present as well). The presence of psychotic features indicates that treatment with antidepressant medication alone is unlikely to be successful and that combination with antipsychotic drugs is usually needed (see Cowen, 2005).

Non-melancholic depression In this classification by symptom profile, the remaining forms of major depression (**'non-melancholic' depression)** include several different kinds of clinical disorder including, for example, mild depressive episodes, atypical depression, and dysthymia. These depressions are more likely to have a relative prominence of features such as **anxiety, hostility, phobias**, and **obsessional symptoms**. In the past, because of these symptoms, non-melancholic depressions were sometimes called 'neurotic depression' but this term does not appear in current diagnostic classifications. As noted above (p. 221), **atypical depression** has a particular clinical characteristics and response to treatment; it is therefore appears to merit a specific category within the non-melancholic depressions.

Classification by course

Unipolar and bipolar disorders Mood disorders are characteristically **recurrent** and Kraepelin was guided by the course of illness when he brought mania and depression together as a single entity. He found that the course was essentially the same whether the original disorder was manic or depressive, and so he put the two together in a single category of **manic-depressive psychosis**.

This view was widely accepted until 1962 when Leonhard *et al.* suggested a division into three groups:

1. patients who had had a depressive disorder only – **unipolar depression**;
2. those who had had mania only – **unipolar mania**;
3. those who had had both depressive disorder and mania – **bipolar**.

Nowadays, it is the usual practice not to use the term unipolar mania, but to include all cases of mania in the bipolar group on the grounds that nearly all patients who have mania eventually experience a depressive disorder.

In support of the distinction between unipolar and bipolar disorders, Leonhard *et al.* (1962) described differences in heredity between the groups, which have been confirmed by later studies (see p. 232). However, it is agreed that the two groups do not generally differ in their symptoms when depressed. There must be some overlap between the two groups, because a patient classified as having unipolar depression at one time may have a manic disorder later. In other words, the unipolar group inevitably contains some bipolar cases that have not yet declared themselves. Despite this limitation, the division into unipolar and bipolar cases is a useful classification because it has implications for treatment (see pp. 246–65).

Seasonal affective disorder Some patients repeatedly develop a depressive disorder at the same time of year, usually the autumn or winter. In some cases the timing reflects extra demands placed on the person at a particular season of the year, either in work or in other aspects of their life. In other cases there is no such cause and it has been suggested that seasonal affective disorder is related in some way to the changes in the seasons, for example, to the length of daylight. Although these seasonal affective disorders are characterized mainly by the time at which they occur, some symptoms are said to occur more often than in other mood disorders. These symptoms are:

- hypersomnia
- increased appetite with craving for carbohydrate
- afternoon slump in energy.

The most common pattern is onset in autumn or winter, and recovery in spring or summer. This is also called 'winter depression'. Some patients show evidence of hypomania or mania in the summer, suggesting that they have a seasonal bipolar illness. This pattern has led to the suggestion that shortening of daylight is important in the pathophysiology of winter depression and treatment methods include exposure to bright artificial light during hours of darkness. For a review, see Eagles (2004). (The use of bright light treatment is reviewed on p. 572).

Brief recurrent depression Some individuals experience recurrent depressive episodes of short duration, typically 2–7 days, that are not of sufficient duration to meet criteria for major depression or depressive episode. These episodes recur with some frequency, about once a month on average. There is no apparent link with the menstrual cycle in female sufferers. Whilst the depressive episodes are short, they are as severe as the more enduring depressive disorders and can be associated with suicidal behaviour. Hence recurrent brief depression is associated with much personal distress and social and occupational impairment. There appears to be little comorbidity with manic illness or dysthymia. Individuals with recurrent brief depression often receive treatment with antidepressant medication but its value is questionable (see Baldwin, 2003).

Classification in ICD and DSM

The main categories in the sections on mood disorders in DSM-IV and the ICD-10 are shown in Tables 11.4 and 11.5. Broad similarities are evident, together with some differences. The first similarity is that both systems contain categories for **single episodes** of mood disorder as well as categories for **recurrent episodes**. The second is that both recognize mild but persistent mood disturbances in which there is either a repeated alternation of high and low mood (**cyclothymia**) or a sustained depression of mood (**dysthymia**). In neither case are the mood disturbances sufficiently severe to meet criteria for a hypomanic or depressive episode. In DSM-IV, mood disorders judged to be secondary to a medical condition are included as a subcategory of mood disorders, whereas in ICD-10 these conditions are classified as mood disorders under 'Organic mental disorders'.

Bipolar disorder

Both classifications delineate hypomania from mania on grounds of duration of symptoms, absence of psychotic features and lesser degree of social and occupational impairment. A manic episode can be further subdivided according to severity and whether or not psychotic symptoms are present. In DSM-IV, the presence of a single episode of hypomania or mania is sufficient to meet criteria for bipolar disorder. In ICD-10, however, at least two episodes of mood disturbance are needed for this diagnosis. DSM-IV also separates bipolar disorder into

- bipolar I (in which **mania** has occurred on least one occasion);
- bipolar II (where **hypomania** has occurred but mania has not).

The diagnosis of bipolar II disorder is intended to indicate the importance of detecting mild hypomanic episodes in patients who might otherwise be diagnosed as having recurrent major depression. The presence of

TABLE 11.5 Classification of bipolar disorder

ICD-10	DSM-IV
Manic episode	Hypomanic episode
Hypomania	Manic episode
Mania	Mild
Mania with psychosis	Moderate
	Severe
	Severe with psychosis
Bipolar affective disorder	Bipolar I and bipolar II
	Disorders
Currently hypomanic	Current (or most recent episode)
Currently manic	Hypomanic
Currently depressed	Manic*
Currently mixed	Depressed
In remission	Mixed*
Cyclothymia	Cyclothymic disorder

* Excludes bipolar II.

TABLE 11.6 Classification of depressive disorders

ICD-10	DSM-IV
Depressive episode	Major depressive episode
Mild	Mild
Moderate	Moderate
Severe	Severe
Severe with psychosis	Severe with psychosis
Other depressive episodes	
Atypical depression	
Recurrent depressive disorders	Major depressive disorder
	Recurrent
Currently mild	
Currently moderate	
Currently severe	
Currently severe with psychosis	
In remission	
Persistent mood disorders	Dysthymic disorder
Cyclothymia	
Dysthymia	
Other mood disorders	Depressive disorders not otherwise specified
Recurrent brief depression	Recurrent brief depression

such episodes may have implications for treatment response. In DSM-IV, if a hypomanic or manic episode appears to have been precipitated by a **somatic treatment**, for example, antidepressant drug therapy, it is not counted towards the diagnosis of bipolar I or bipolar II disorder though there is a growing body of opinion that antidepressant-induced mania or hypomania should be taken as indicating an underlying bipolar disorder (Goodwin, 2003).

Depressive disorders

Both ICD-10 and DSM-IV classify depressive episodes on the basis of **severity** and whether or not **psychotic features** are present. It is also possible to specify whether the depressive episode has melancholic (DSM-IV) or somatic (ICD-10) features. In DSM-IV, an episode of major depression with appropriate clinical symptomatology (see above) can be specified as atypical depression. In ICD-10, atypical depression is classified separately under 'Other depressive episodes'. Both ICD-10 and DSM-IV allow the diagnosis of recurrent brief depression, but under slightly different headings (Table 11.6).

Classification and description in everyday practice

Although neither DSM-IV nor ICD-10 is entirely satisfactory, it seems unlikely that further rearrangement of descriptive categories will be better. The solution will come only when we have a better understanding of aetiology. Meanwhile, either ICD or DSM-IV should be used for statistical returns. For most clinical purposes, it is better to describe disorders systematically than to classify them.

This can be done for every case by referring to the severity, the type of episode, distinguishing symptomatic features, and the course of the disorder, together with an evaluation of the relative importance of known aetiological factors (Table 11.7). It has become conventional to record all cases with a manic episode as bipolar, even if there has been no depressive disorder, on the grounds that most manic patients develop a depressive disorder eventually; and in several important ways manic patients resemble patients who have had both types of episode. This convention is followed in this textbook.

Differential diagnosis

Depressive disorder

Depressive disorders have to be distinguished from:

- normal sadness
- anxiety disorders

TABLE 11.7 A systematic scheme for the clinical description of mood disorders

The episode	
Severity	Mild, moderate, or severe
Type	Depressive, manic, mixed
Special features	With melancholic symptoms
	With atypical symptoms
	With prominent anxiety
	With psychotic symptoms
	With agitation
	With retardation or stupor
The course	Unipolar or bipolar
Aetiological factors	Organic
	Family history of mood disorder
	Personal history of mood disorder
	Childhood experiences
	Personality
	Social support
	Life events

- schizophrenia
- organic brain syndromes.

As already explained on p. 218, the distinction from **normal sadness** is made on the presence of other symptoms of the syndrome of depressive disorder. Depressive disorders also have rates of **comorbidity** with a wide range of other disorders, for example, anxiety disorders, eating disorders, substance misuse, and personality disorder. In all these cases, it is important to recognize and treat the depressive disorder.

Anxiety disorders

Mild depressive disorders are sometimes difficult to distinguish from anxiety disorders. Accurate diagnosis depends on assessment of the relative severity of anxiety and depressive symptoms, and on the order in which they appeared. Similar problems arise when there are prominent phobic or obsessional symptoms, or when there are **dissociative** symptoms with or without histrionic behaviour. In all these cases, the clinician may fail to identify the depressive symptoms and so prescribe the wrong treatment.

Schizophrenia

The differential diagnosis from **schizophrenia** depends on a careful search for the characteristic features of this condition (see Chapter 12). Difficult diagnostic problems may arise when the patient has **depressive psychosis**, but here again the distinction can usually be made on careful examination of the mental state and on the order in which symptoms appeared. Information about the past psychiatric history may also be useful. Particular difficulties also arise when symptoms characteristic of depressive disorder and of schizophrenia are found in equal measure in the same patient; these so-called schizoaffective disorders are discussed on p. 278.

Dementia and other organic conditions

In middle and late life, depressive disorders are sometimes difficult to distinguish from **dementia** because some patients with depressive symptoms complain of considerable difficulty in remembering. In fact, patients with severe depression can perform very badly on tests of cognitive function and distinction between the two conditions purely in terms of the nature of the cognitive impairment may not be possible. Here the presence of depressive symptoms is the key to diagnosis, which should be confirmed with improvement of the memory disorder as normal mood is restored. Numerous other general medication conditions can present with depressive features (see p. 382). The key to diagnosis is a careful history and physical examination, supplemented by special investigations where appropriate.

Mania

Manic disorders have to be distinguished from:

- schizophrenia
- organic brain disease involving the frontal lobes (including brain tumour and HIV infection)
- states of brief excitement induced by amphetamines and other illicit drugs.

Schizophrenia

The diagnosis from schizophrenia can be most difficult. Auditory hallucinations and delusions, including some that are characteristic of schizophrenia such as delusions of reference, can occur in manic disorders. However, these symptoms usually change quickly in content, and seldom outlast the phase of overactivity. When there is a more or less equal mixture of features of the two syndromes, the term schizoaffective is often used. This term is discussed further in Chapter 12. Further clues to diagnosis can often be elicited by a careful personal and family psychiatric history.

Organic brain disorder and drug misuse

An organic brain lesion should always be considered, especially in middle-aged or older patients with expansive behaviour and no past history of mood disorder. In the absence of gross mood disorder, extreme social disinhibition (for example urinating in public) strongly suggests **frontal lobe pathology**. In such cases appropriate neurological investigation is essential. In younger adults infection with HIV or head injury may lead to the manifestation of mania.

The distinction between mania and excited behaviour due to **drug misuse** depends on the history and an examination of the urine for drugs. Drug-induced states usually subside quickly once the patient is in hospital. It should be remembered, however, that a significant proportion of patients with bipolar disorder misuse alcohol and other drugs.

The epidemiology of mood disorders

It is difficult to determine the prevalence of depressive disorder, partly because different investigators have used different diagnostic definitions. More modern investigations have used structured diagnostic interviews linked to standardized diagnostic criteria such as the Diagnostic Interview Schedule (DIS), the Composite International Diagnostic Interview (CIDI) and the Schedule for Clinical assessment in Neuropsychiatry (SCAN) which incorporates the 10th edition of the Present State Examination (PSE) (p. 62). Of all the mood disorders, bipolar cases are probably identified more reliably because mania is somewhat easier to define and diagnose.

Bipolar disorder

More recent community surveys in industrialized countries (Kessler *et al.*, 1997) have suggested that:

- the lifetime risk for bipolar disorder lies between 0.3 and 1.5 per cent;
- the 6-month prevalence of bipolar disorder is not much less than the lifetime prevalence, indicating the chronic nature of the disorder;
- the prevalence in men and women is the same;
- the mean age of onset is about 17 years of age in community studies;
- bipolar disorder is highly comorbid with other disorders, particularly anxiety disorders and substance misuse.

Depression

Defining the boundaries of depressive episodes in community surveys presents difficulties. However, if the DSM-IV criteria for major depression are applied, recent surveys in industrialized countries (Alonso *et al.*, 2004) suggest that:

- the 12-month prevalence of major depression in the community is between 2 and 5 per cent;
- the lifetime rates in different studies vary considerably (4–30 per cent). The true figure probably lies between 10 and 20 per cent;
- the mean age of onset is about 27 years;
- rates of major depression are about twice as great in women as men, across different cultures;
- there may be increased rates of depression in people born since 1945;
- rates of depression are higher in the unemployed and divorced;
- major depression has a high comorbidity with other disorders, particularly anxiety disorders and substance misuse.

The reasons for **higher rates among women** are uncertain. The increase starts to be apparent at puberty and could be due in part to a greater readiness in women to admit depressive symptoms; however, such selective reporting is unlikely to be the whole explanation. It is possible that some depressed men misuse alcohol and are diagnosed as suffering from alcohol-related disorders rather than depression with the consequence that the true number of major depressive disorders is underestimated. Again, misdiagnosis of this kind is unlikely to account for the whole of the difference. Whether gender-related differences in neurobiology (for example, the organization of central 5-HT pathways) might underlie differences in susceptibility to depression requires further investigation. Also in many societies women are subject to various kinds of social disadvantage and, for example, are more likely than men to experience sexual abuse and domestic violence. Factors of this sort are also likely to be involved in their increased risk of depression.

Whilst it used to be thought that the risk of depressive disorders increased with age, recent surveys suggest that major depression is most prevalent in the 18–44 age group. A number of studies have suggested that people born since 1945 in industrialized countries have both a higher lifetime risk of major depression and an earlier age of onset. These studies have mainly been retrospective and it is possible that the apparent increased rate of major depression in young people is because older people forget (or are less willing to reveal) that they have been depressed (see Paykel, 2000). For a review of the epidemiology of mood disorders, see Joyce (2000).

Dysthymia and recurrent brief depression

The lifetime risk for **dysthymia** is about 4 per cent (Alonso *et al.*, 2004). Rates of dysthymia are greater in **women** and the **divorced**. There is less epidemiological information about **recurrent brief depression** but in the Zurich prospective study the 12-month prevalence for recurrent brief depression was about 2.6 per cent, very similar to the rate found for dysthmia (2.3 per cent) (Pezawas *et al.*, 2003).

Minor mood disorders

Estimates of the frequency of **minor mood disorders** show wide variations because the different studies have not defined cases in the same way. However, these disorders are probably the most prevalent psychiatric disorder in the community. For example, in the National Psychiatric Morbidity Household Survey, the overall 1-week prevalence of **neurotic disorder** was 16 per cent (12.3 per cent in males and 19.5 per cent in females). Nearly half this group met ICD-10 criteria for **mixed anxiety depression** (Jenkins *et al.*, 1997). There are also epidemiological studies of minor depression (as defined in DSM-IV). In a systematic review of community studies of people aged over 55, the prevalence of minor depression was 9.8 per cent (Beekman *et al.*, 1999). A remarkably similar rate (9.9 per cent) was identified in a group of adolescents and young adults (Kessler and Walters, 1998).

The aetiology of mood disorders

There have been many different approaches to the aetiology of mood disorders. There is substantial knowledge about the **genetic epidemiology** of depression and how certain **childhood experiences** can lay down a predisposition to mood disorders in adult life. There is also a good understanding of the role of **current life difficulties and stresses** in provoking mood disorders in predisposed individuals. There is much less knowledge about the mechanism involved in the translation of these predisposing and provoking factors into clinical symptomatology.

In trying to elucidate these mechanisms (which, of course, have important implications for treatment), investigators have employed two main conceptual approaches, which can be broadly termed 'psychological' and 'biological'. It is likely, of course, that these approaches represent different levels of enquiry that will eventually inform each other. The main kinds of investigations that will be discussed are listed in Table 11.8. To help guide the reader through the studies in the next section Box 11.1 summarizes how the knowledge gained from them contributes to our current understanding of the pathogenesis of mood disorder. In most research areas there are much more data available concerning the aetiology of depression than of mania.

TABLE 11.8

Area of investigation	Relevant studies
Genetic	Genetic epidemiology
	Molecular genetics
Personality	Temperament
	Cognitive style
Early environment	Parental deprivation
	Childhood adversity and abuse
Social environment	Life events
	Chronic difficulties
Psychological	Psychodynamic
	Cognitive
Biological	Monoamines
	HPA axis
	Neuropsychology and brain imaging
	Neuropathology

Genetic causes

Family and twin studies

Familial aggregation

The risk of mood disorders is increased in first-degree relatives of both bipolar and unipolar probands with the risk being about **twice as great** in relatives of bipolar patients (Table 11.9). Relatives of bipolar probands have increased risks of **unipolar depression** and **schizoaffective disorder** as well as **bipolar disorder**. By contrast, relatives of patients with **unipolar depression** do not have increased rates of bipolar disorder or schizoaffective disorder.

Twin studies

Twin studies suggest that the aggregation of mood disorders in families is due to genetic factors, with the

BOX 11.1 MULTIFACTORIAL ORIGIN OF MOOD DISORDERS

- An important genetic contribution to mood disorder is made by multiple genes of small individual effect. This genetic contribution may be expressed directly through modification of relevant cortical circuitry or indirectly through effects on personality and psychological coping mechanisms.
- Adverse early life experiences also shape personality and limit subsequent attachment behaviour and ability to access social support. Early adverse experience may also affect development of the HPA axis and neurobiological responses to stress in adulthood.
- Mood disorders are often triggered by current life events, particularly in people who lack social support. The impact of life events is modified by early life experience, personality and genetic inheritance. The interaction of these factors determines the resilience or vulnerability of an individual to a life event and subsequent risk of clinical mood disturbance.
- The neurobiology of episodes of mood disorder is associated with changes in the activity of monoamine neurons and the HPA axis which together modify the activity of neural circuitry involved in mood regulation. Some structural brain abnormalities in mood disorder suggest persistent biological vulnerability probably produced by genetic inheritance or early developmental factors.

TABLE 11.9 Genetic epidemiology of bipolar disorder and major depression

	Bipolar disorder	Unipolar disorder
Lifetime risk	About 1%	10–20%
Sex ratio (M:F)	1:1	1:2
First-degree		
Relatives:		
Lifetime risk for		
Bipolar disorder	About 10%	About 2%
Lifetime risk for		
Unipolar disorder	20–30%	20–30%
Average age of onset	21 years	27 years

concordance rate for both bipolar and unipolar disorder being higher in monozygotic than dizygotic twins. For example, the concordance rate for mood disorder in the monozygotic co-twin of a proband with bipolar disorder is between 60–70 per cent, but for dizygotic twins the rate is only about 20 per cent. In unipolar depression the concordance rate is also greater in monozygotic twins (46 per cent) than dizygotic twins (20 per cent). Overall, the genetic influence seems greater in bipolar disorder than in unipolar disorder (see McGuffin *et al.*, 1996).

Genetic evidence on classification of mood disorders

Genetic studies can also throw light on the aetiological relationship between different subtypes of mood disorder. For example, in an epidemiological sample of twins, Karkowski and Kendler (1997) obtained results suggesting that in terms of genetic liability, unipolar and bipolar *depression* lie on a continuum of severity rather than being aetiologically distinct. In contrast, McGuffin *et al.* (2003) found evidence that the genetic liability to *mania* appeared to be inherited more specifically and did not seem to represent simply a more severe form of mood disorder.

Twin studies have also suggested that the liability to major depression and generalized anxiety disorder involves similar genes but different environmental risk factors (Kendler, 1996). In addition, the effect of the environment on liability to depression predominantly involves experiences specific to an individual rather than shared (family) experiences.

Mode of inheritance

The familial segregation of mood disorders does not fit a simple Mendelian pattern. The female preponderance of depression is well established and it is possible that genetic factors play a somewhat greater aetiological role in women, particularly if broad diagnostic criteria are used (Kendler *et al.*, 2001). This raises the possibility that in linkage and association studies the impact of different genetic loci on liability to depression will need to be examined separately in men and women. Overall, it seems likely that the genetic liability to mood disorders result from the combined action of several genes of modest, or small effect, so-called **polygenic** inheritance.

Molecular genetics

Linkage studies

Molecular linkage studies of mood disorders have not thus far been particularly revealing, perhaps because the genes involved are of small effect or because of genetic heterogeneity. Positive findings have emerged but have often proved difficult to replicate. More recent investigations of **bipolar disorder** have revealed a number of significant linkages involving chromosomes 13q and 22q (see Badner and Gershon, 2003). Replication of these findings is required.

Association studies

The monoamine theory of depression suggest that allelic variation in genes coding for monoamine synthesis or metabolism or specific receptors may contribute to the risk of mood disorders. There have been numerous association studies of such **candidate genes**, though thus far results have not been compelling (Fanous and Kendler, 2004). The gene coding for the **serotonin transporter** has a number of allelic variants, one of which, in the promotor region, influences the expression of transporter sites. The evidence implicating this polymorphism in major depression in population studies is inconsistent (Anguelova *et al.*, 2003); however, in a prospective study Caspi *et al.* (2003) found evidence suggesting that subjects carrying a particular allele for the serotonin transporter were more likely experience a subsequent episode of major depression when exposed to an adverse life event. This could represent an interesting example of interaction between environmental adversity and a genetic susceptibility factor.

Personality

Certain kinds of personality development could be associated with predisposition to mood disorder. For example, it is a common clinical observation that patients with depression often seem to have high levels of anxiety pre-morbidly. Aspects of personality could be associated with mood disorder in a number of ways:

1. What is recognized as a personality characteristic may in fact represent a mild form of the illness. For example, Kraepelin (1921) suggested that people with **cyclothymic personality** (i.e. those with repeated and sustained mood swings) were more prone to develop manic-depressive disorder. Nowadays this personality type is classified as a mood disorder (cyclothymic disorder), and is seen as a mild form of bipolar disorder.
2. Some personality features might influence the way that people respond to adverse circumstances and thus make depressive disorders more likely. For example, a cognitive style characterized by 'sociotropy' (a high need for approval) is associated with increased risk of depression after adverse life events (Mazure and Maciejewski, 2003).
3. Certain kinds of personality development and psychiatric disorder may share common genes. For example, ***neuroticism***, as measured by the Eysenck Personality Questionnaire, predisposes to major depression but twin studies suggest that neuroticism and major depression have genes in common (see Fanous and Kendler, 2004).

Overall, current findings suggest that part of the genetic risk of depression takes the form of inheritance of particular character traits and cognitive styles, which may limit ability to cope with specific kinds of life stresses (see Goodyer, 2002).

Early environment

Parental deprivation

Psychoanalysts have suggested that childhood deprivation of maternal affection through separation or loss predisposes to depressive disorders in adult life. Overall, however, epidemiological studies do not suggest that loss of a parent by death in childhood increases the risk of depressive disorder in adult life. By contrast, there is more support for the proposal that depressive disorder in later life is associated with **parental separation**, particularly divorce. The key factor here appears to be less the loss itself than the discord and diminished care that result from it. Indeed family discord and lack of adequate care predispose to depression even in families where separation does not occur (see Harris, 2001).

Relationships with parents

It is clear that gross disruption of parent-child relationships, as occurs, for example, in **physical and sexual abuse**, is a risk factor for several kinds of adult psychiatric disorder, including major depression (Harris, 2001). It is less certain whether more subtle differences in **parental style** may also predispose to depression. One problem is the difficulty of determining retrospectively what kind of relationship a patient may have had with their parents in childhood. The patient's recollection of the relationship may be distorted by many factors, including the depressive disorder itself. However, it appears that both **non-caring** and **overprotective parenting** styles are associated with non-melancholic depression in adult life. The mechanism of this association requires further study (Enns *et al.*, 2000). Mothers with **post-natal depression** may manifest a rearing style characterized by neglect and emotional indifference. This could lead to longer-term deleterious effects on self-esteem and attachment style in the child hence increasing the risk of depression in the subsequent generation.

Precipitating factors

Recent life events

Methodological considerations

It is an everyday clinical observation that depressive disorders often follow **stressful events**. However, several other possibilities must be discounted before it can be concluded that stressful events cause the depressive disorders that succeed them. First, the association might be **coincidental**. Second, the association might be **non-specific**; there might be as many stressful events in the weeks preceding other kinds of illness. Third, it might be **spurious**; the patient might have regarded the events as stressful only in retrospect when seeking an explanation for his illness, or he might have experienced them as stressful only because he was already depressed at the time. Finally the depression itself might have caused the life event.

Research workers have tried to overcome each of these methodological difficulties. The first two problems - whether the events are coincidental or whether any association is non-specific - require the use of control groups suitably chosen from the general population and from people with other illnesses. The third problem - whether the association is spurious - requires two other approaches. The first approach is to separate events that are undoubtedly independent of illness (such as losing a job because a whole factory closes) from events that may have been secondary to the illness (such as losing a job when no one else is dismissed). The second approach is to assign a rating to each event according to the consensus view of healthy people about its stressful qualities.

Findings

Methodologically reliable research has shown that:

- there is a sixfold excess of adverse life events in the months before the onset of depressive disorder.
- an excess of similar events has also been shown to precede suicide attempts, and the onset of anxiety disorders and schizophrenia.
- generally, 'loss' events are associated with depression and 'threat' events with anxiety.
- life events are important antecedents of all forms of depression but appear relatively less important in established melancholic-type disorders and where there is a strong family history of depression.

Recent studies suggest that events that lead to feelings of **entrapment and humiliation** may be particularly relevant to the onset of depression. In contrast, remission from depression is often associated with 'fresh-start' life events (such as establishing a new relationship or starting an educational course) (Harris, 2001). It is also important to note that **genetic factors** may be involved in the liability of an individual to experience life events. Thus certain individuals seem more prone to select **risky environments** and genetic factors also play a role in how life events are **perceived** by a particular individual perhaps through the personality mechanisms discussed above (Kendler *et al.*, 1999).

In general the importance of life events in the onset of a depressive episode decreases as the number of episodes increases. This suggests that once a depressive disorder is clearly established, depressive episodes can occur in the absence of major environmental precipitants. This relationship is much less clear where there is a strong family history of depression raising the possibility that one of the mechanisms by which a family history increases the risk of depression is by diminishing the need for a major environmental stressor during the first episodes of the illness (Kendler *et al.*, 2001).

Mania

It is less certain whether **mania** is provoked by life events. In the past, mania was thought to arise entirely from **endogenous** causes. However, clinical experience suggests that a proportion of cases are precipitated, sometimes by events that might have been expected to induce depression, for example, **bereavement**. As in the case of recurrent depression it is possible that the impact of life events may be more important early in the course of a recurrent manic-depressive illness because once the illness is established environmental precipitants are less pertinent. However, adverse life events increase symptomatology in the course of bipolar illness though the effect seems predominantly on depression. Interestingly, manic symptoms may be triggered when people attain an important goal, suggesting that 'normal' feelings of happiness and well-being can develop into manic illness in predisposed people (see Rush, 2003).

Vulnerability factors and life difficulties

It is a common clinical impression that the events immediately preceding a depressive disorder act as a 'last straw' for a person who has been subjected to a long period of adverse circumstances such as an unhappy marriage, problems at work, or unsatisfactory housing. Brown and Harris (1978) divided predisposing events into two kinds. The first are **prolonged stressful circumstances** which can themselves cause depression as well as adding to the effects of short-term life events. Brown and Harris gave the name **long-term difficulties** to these circumstances.

The second kind of predisposing circumstance does not itself cause depression; instead, it acts only by increasing the effects of short-term life events. This kind of circumstance is known as a **vulnerability factor**. In practice, the distinction between the two kinds of circumstance is not clear cut. Thus, long continued marital problems (a long-term difficulty) are likely to be associated with a lack of a confiding relationship, and the latter has been identified by Brown as a vulnerability factor.

Overall, the studies suggest that the following are social vulnerability factors that increase the risk that life events will trigger a depressive episode:

- having the care of young children;
- not working outside the home;
- having no one to confide in.

Generally, there is good evidence that **poor social support**, measured as lack of intimacy or social integration, is associated with an increased risk of depression. The mechanism of this association is not clear and is open to different interpretations. First, it may be that a lack of opportunities to confide makes people more vulnerable. Second, it may indicate that depressed people have a distorted perception of the degree of intimacy that they achieved before becoming depressed. Third, some other factor, presumably an abnormality in personality, may result in difficulty confiding in others and thereby lead to vulnerability to depression (Harris, 2001). For a further discussion of this work see p. 94.

The effects of physical illness

All medical illnesses and their treatment can act as **non-specific stressors** which may lead to mood disorders in predisposed subjects. Sometimes, however, medical conditions are believed to play a more direct role in causing the mood disorder; examples of such medical conditions are brain disease, certain infections, including HIV, and endocrine disorders. The resulting mood disorders are known as organic mood disorders; they are discussed further in Chapter 16.

Inevitably, the above distinction is arbitrary. For example, major depression occurs in about half of patients with **Cushing's disease**; since not all patients with Cushing's disease suffer from depressive disorder, it follows that variables other than raised plasma cortisol levels are involved. However, organic mood disorders can give clues to aetiology. For example, depressive disorders in Cushing's disease remit after cortisol levels are restored to normal; this finding had led to the proposal that increased cortisol secretion may play a role in the pathophysiology of major depression (see p. 241). It is also worth noting here that the **puerperium** (although not an illness) is associated with an increased risk of mood disorders (see p. 402).

Psychological approaches to aetiology

These theories are concerned with the **psychological mechanisms** by which recent and remote life experiences can lead to depressive disorders. Much of the literature on this subject fails to distinguish adequately between the symptom of depression and the syndrome of depressive disorder. The main approaches to the problem are derived from the ideas of psychoanalysis, and cognitive–behavioural theories.

Psychoanalytical theory

The psychoanalytical theory of depression began with a paper by Abraham in 1911, and was developed by Freud in 1917 in a paper called 'Mourning and melancholia'. Freud drew attention to the resemblance between the **phenomena of mourning and symptoms of depressive disorders**, and suggested that their causes might be similar. Although this and subsequent theories have not been strongly supported by evidence, they are outlined here because of their importance in understanding the historical development of ideas about depressive disorder.

It is important to note that Freud did not suppose that all severe depressive disorders necessarily had the same cause. Thus he commented that some disorders 'suggest somatic rather than psychogenic affections' and indicated that his ideas were to be applied only to those 'whose psychogenic nature was indisputable' (Freud, 1917, p. 243). Freud suggested that, just as mourning results from loss by death, so melancholia results from **loss of other kinds**. Since it was apparent that not every depressed patient had suffered an actual loss, it was necessary to postulate a loss of 'some abstraction' or internal representation, or in Freud's terms the loss of an 'object'.

Freud pointed out that depressed patients often appear critical of themselves, and he proposed that this self-accusation was really a disguised accusation of someone else for whom the patient 'felt affection'. In other words, depression was thought to occur when feelings of love and hostility were present at the same time (**ambivalence**). When a loved 'object' is lost, the patient feels despair; at the same time any hostile feelings attached to this 'object' are redirected against the patient himself as self-reproach.

Freud's ideas were developed subsequently by Melanie Klein (1882–1960) who believed that weaning (absence of the breast) represents a major symbolic loss for the infant who then feels remorse and guilt about the disappearance of this 'good object'. In normal development this 'depressive anxiety' leads to attempts at reparation and concern for others. Failure to negotiate this process can result in depressive reactions in the face of future losses. Klein laid rather little emphasis on what maternal behaviour was actually like during this process, apparently believing that the internal instinctual drive of the infant was the key factor. However, the work of John Bowlby (1907–1990), showed that the rearing abilities of the main caregiver (usually the mother in Western cultures) plays an important role in giving the infant a secure emotional 'attachment' which is of critical importance in the development of satisfactory interpersonal relationships. Insecure attachments can increase the risk of various kinds of adult psychopathology including depression. The mechanism of this effect might involve diminished ability in adult life to access appropriate emotional support when in difficulties (see Gabbard, 2000).

Cognitive theories

Depressed patients characteristically have recurrent and intrusive **negative thoughts ('automatic thoughts')**. Beck (1967) proposed that these depressive cognitions reveal negative views of the **self**, the **world**, and the **future** (the depressed patient usually reviews the past in a similar vein). These automatic thoughts appear to persist because of illogical ways of thinking (which Beck called **cognitive distortions**). These include:

- **arbitrary inference** (drawing a conclusion when there is no evidence for it and even some against it);
- **selective abstraction** (focusing on a detail and ignoring more important features of a situation);
- **overgeneralization** (drawing a general conclusion on the basis of a single incident);
- **personalization** (relating external events to oneself in an unwarranted way).

Whilst most psychiatrists regarded these cognitions as secondary to a primary disturbance of mood, Beck suggested that another set of cognitions precede depression and predispose to it. These cognitions are **dysfunctional beliefs** such as 'If I am not perfectly successful then I am a nobody'. These beliefs are thought to affect the way a person responds to stress and adversity. For example, a failure at work is more likely to provoke depression in a person who holds the belief described above. Others have shown that, when depressed, people are more likely to remember unhappy events (Clark and Teasdale, 1982). This selective recall adds to the person's depression, making it more difficult to reverse.

One of the major problems for the cognitive model is that whilst dysfunctional attitudes and beliefs, as well as negatively biased information processing, are easy to demonstrate when patients are depressed, these phenomena usually remit on clinical recovery. For this reason, more recent cognitive theory has suggested that dysfunctional beliefs may be present but difficult to demonstrate ('latent') until activated by a relevant stressor or by a minor change of mood (within the normal range). In this model a minor (normal) lowering of mood can activate all the concepts and constructs associated with clinical depression. An interactive cycle of low mood and negative thinking will result (Abela and D'Alessandro, 2002 and Figure 11.2).

Other developments of cognitive theories include the idea that mood-related biases in cognitive processing reflect changes in the **mental models** we all use to make sense of our experiences. This has led to the

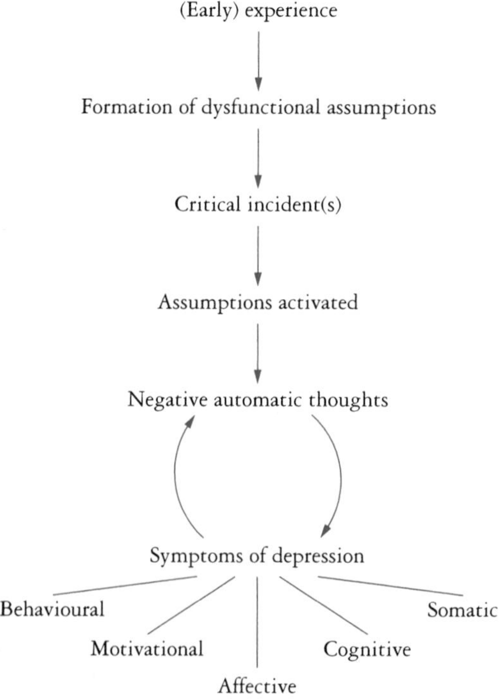

Fig. 11.2 Cognitive model of how latent dysfunctional assumptions (laid down by early experience) are activated by critical incidents leading to vicious cycle of negative thinking and depressed mood. (From Fennell 1993)

development of the concept of loss of 'meta-cognitive awareness' in depression, that is of awareness that negative thoughts and feelings are mental events rather than objective truths about the self. 'Mindfulness-based' cognitive therapy aims to increase meta-cognitive awareness and thereby prevent depressive relapse (see Teasdale *et al.*, 2002).

Neurobiological approaches to aetiology

Whatever their aetiology, the clinical manifestations of depressive disorders must ultimately be mediated through changes in brain neurochemistry and the circuitry involved in emotional regulation. Biochemical investigations in depressed patients have focused on the **monoamine neurotransmitters** because monoamine pathways appear to play an important role in the actions of effective antidepressant drugs (see below). Of course, the actions of antidepressant drugs may not reverse the cause of depression but may merely change the expression of symptoms. However, another reason for studying monoamines is that they play an important role in mediating **adaptive responses to stressful events**, and depressive disorders can be viewed as a failure of these adaptive responses.

Monoamine pathways, particularly noradrenaline and 5-HT, innervate cortical and subcortical brain regions thought to be involved in mood regulation. Recent studies have used structural and functional imaging techniques to elicit changes in the neural circuitry that underpins the expression of clinical affective symptomatology. In hand with this has come the realization that mood disorders, despite their fluctuating and remitting clinical course, are associated with distinct neuropathological changes in relevant brain regions. Some of these changes are likely to be developmental in origin; this could encompass either genetic inheritance or the consequences of adverse childhood experiences. There is currently much research effort in both animal and human studies to assess how traumatic experiences in development might affect the subsequent maturation of the HPA axis and thereby influence responses to environmental stress. A final point worth considering is that the prognosis of mood disorders worsens as the number of episodes increases. While this phenomenon may represent simply an association between severity and poor prognosis, it is also possible that acute episodes of mood disturbance themselves produce neurobiological effects that worsen subsequent prognosis (a phenomenon sometime known as 'scarring').

The monoamine hypothesis

The **monoamine hypothesis** suggests that depressive disorder is due to an abnormality in a monoamine neurotransmitter system at one or more sites in the brain. In its early form, the hypothesis suggested a changed provision of the monoamine; more recent elaborations postulate alterations in receptors as well as in the concentrations or the turnover of the amines. Three monoamine transmitters have been implicated: **serotonin (5-hydroxytryptamine, 5-HT)**, **noradrenaline**, and **dopamine**. The latter two neurotransmitters are called **catecholamines**.

The hypothesis has been tested by observing three kinds of phenomenon:

1. the biochemistry of neurotransmitters in patients with mood disorders;
2. the effects of selective drugs on measurable indices of the function of monoamine systems (usually neuroendocrine indices);
3. the pharmacological properties shared by antidepressant drugs.

The biochemical effects of antidepressant drugs are considered in Chapter 21. The present chapter will

BOX 11.2 ABNORMALITIES IN MONOAMINE NEUROTRANSMISSION IN DEPRESSION

5-HT

Decreased plasma tryptophan

Blunted 5-HT neuroendocrine responses

Decreased brain 5-HT_{1A} receptor binding (PET)

Decreased brain 5-HT re-uptake sites (SPET)

Clinical relapse after tryptophan depletion

Noradrenaline

Blunted noradrenaline-mediated growth hormone release

Clinical relapse after AMPT

Dopamine

Decreased homovanillic acid (HVA) levels in CSF

Increased dopamine D_2 receptor binding (PET/SPET)

Clinical relapse after AMPT

consider the evidence for abnormalities in monoamine neurotransmitters in untreated depressed patients (Box 11.2). Much less work of this kind has been carried out in mania. Therefore the present discussion will be largely restricted to depressive disorders, although the dopamine hypothesis of mania will also be outlined.

5-HT function

Plasma trypytophan The synthesis of 5-HT in the brain depends on the availability of its precursor amino acid, L-tryptophan. Plasma tryptophan levels are decreased in untreated depressed patients, particularly in those with melancholic depression. Studies in healthy subjects have shown that weight loss through dieting can lower plasma tryptophan, and this factor appears to explain some, but not all, of the reduction in plasma tryptophan seen in depression. Decreases in plasma tryptophan may contribute to the impairments seen in brain 5-HT function in depressed patients but are probably not an important causal factor (see Cowen, 2005).

Studies of cerebrospinal fluid Indirect evidence about 5-HT function in the brains of depressed patients has been sought by examining cerebrospinal fluid (CSF). Numerous studies have been carried out, but overall the data do not suggest that drug-free patients with major depression have a consistent reduction in CSF concentrations of **5-hydroxyindoleacetic acid (5-HIAA)**, the main **metabolite** of 5-HT formed in the brain. However, there is more consistent evidence that depressed patients who have made impulsive and more dangerous suicide attempts have **low CSF 5-HIAA level**. This finding is not restricted to patients with depression. It has also been reported in, for example, patients with schizophrenia and personality disorder who have histories of aggressive behaviour directed towards themselves or other people. It has been proposed that low levels of CSF 5-HIAA, whilst not related specifically to depression, may be associated with a tendency of individuals to respond in an impulsive and hostile way to life difficulties (Placidi *et al.*, 2001).

Studies of post-mortem brain Measurements of 5-HT and 5-HIAA have been made in the brains of depressed patients who have died, usually by suicide. Although this is a more direct test of the monoamine hypothesis, the results are difficult to interpret for two reasons. First, the observed changes may have taken place after death. Second, the changes may have been caused before death but by factors other than the depressive disorder, for example, by anoxia or by drugs used in treatment or taken to commit suicide. Overall there is little consistent evidence that depressed patients dying from natural causes or suicide have lowered brain concentrations of 5-HT or 5-HIAA. More recent studies have adopted techniques such as receptor autoradiography and mRNA expression. Such studies have suggested that suicide victims have increased expression of 5-HT$_{2A}$ receptors and decreases in serotonin transporters (5-HT re-uptake sites) in pre-frontal cortex (see Stockmeier, 2003).

Neurochemical brain imaging studies Recent developments in brain imaging with selective labelled ligands has allowed assessment of certain brain 5-HT receptor subtypes *in vivo*. There is evidence of a widespread modest decrease **in 5-HT$_{1A}$ receptor binding** throughout cortical and subcortical regions (Sargent *et al.*, 2000). Also there appear to be reductions **in brainstem 5-HT re-uptake sites** in depressed subjects, consistent with a decrease in the density of 5-HT cell bodies; however, such changes have not been detected in cortical areas (Meyer *et al.*, 2004).

Neuroendocrine tests The functional activity of 5-HT systems in the brain has been assessed by giving a substance that stimulates 5-HT function and by measuring an endocrine response that is controlled by 5-HT pathways – usually the release of **prolactin, growth hormone**, or **cortisol**. Neuroendocrine challenge tests have the advantage that they measure an aspect of brain 5-HT **function**. However, the 5-HT synapses involved presumably reside in the **hypothalamus**, which means that important changes in 5-HT pathways in other brain regions could be missed. A number of drugs have been used to increase brain 5-HT function for the purposes of neuroendocrine challenge.

Studies in unmedicated depressed patients have shown consistent evidence that 5-HT-mediated endocrine responses are blunted in depressed patients. A number of these abnormalities persist into clinical recovery suggesting persistent dysfunction of some aspects of 5-HT function in those at risk of depression (see Cowen, 2005).

Tryptophan depletion While the findings outlined above provide strong evidence that aspects of brain 5-HT neurotransmission are abnormal in depression, they do not reveal whether these changes are central to **pathophysiology** or might instead represent some form of **epiphenomenon**. To assess this, it is necessary to study the psychological consequences of lowering brain 5-HT function in healthy subjects and those at risk of mood disorder.

As mentioned above, the synthesis of brain 5-HT is dependent on the brain availability of its amino acid precursor, L-tryptophan. It is possible to produce a transient lowering of plasma tryptophan and brain 5-HT function over a few hours by administering a mixture of amino acids that lacks tryptophan. This procedure is called **tryptophan depletion**. Tryptophan depletion in subjects with no personal or family history of mood disorder has little measurable effect on mood and certainly does not produce significant clinical depressive symptomatology. By contrast, unmedicated euthymic patients with a personal history of mood disorder undergo a **rapid but temporary depressive relapse** when exposed to tryptophan depletion (K. A. Smith *et al.*, 1997). The following conclusions can be drawn:

- Low brain 5-HT function is not **sufficient** to cause depression because tryptophan depletion fails to alter mood in those not vulnerable to mood disorder.
- In people **vulnerable to mood disorder**, lowering brain 5-HT function results in clinical depressive symptomatology.
- Low brain 5-HT function interacts with **other vulnerability factors** to cause depressive disorders in at-risk individuals.

The nature of these other vulnerability factors remains conjectural. It is possible that the 5-HT pathways of vulnerable individuals react abnormally to precursor deficit. Alternatively, there may be pre-existing deficits in central mood-regulating circuitry which are 'revealed' in the presence of low brain 5-HT states (Smith *et al.*, 1999).

Noradrenaline function

Metabolism and receptors There is no consistent evidence that **brain or CSF concentrations of noradrenaline** or its major metabolite **3-methoxy-4-hydroxy-phenyleth-ylene glycol (MHPG)** are altered in depressed patients (see Anand and Charney, 2000). As with 5-HT receptors, noradrenaline receptors in the brain can be divided into a number of subclasses. There is some evidence that depressed patients dying from suicide have increased expression of **α_2-adrenoceptor binding** in some brain regions (see Escriba *et al.*, 2004).

Neuroendocrine tests Increasing brain noradrenaline function elevates plasma concentrations of **adrenocorticotropic hormone (ACTH)**, **cortisol**, and **growth hormone**. There is fairly consistent evidence that the growth hormone response to both the noradrenaline re-uptake inhibitor **desipramine** and the noradrenaline receptor agonist **clonidine** is blunted in patients with melancholic depression. Clonidine acts directly on postsynaptic α_2-adrenoceptors in the hypothalamus to increase plasma growth hormone, and therefore the blunted response in depressed patients suggests a decreased responsivity of hypothalamic postsynaptic α_2-adrenoceptors (Anand and Charney, 2000). Clearly this finding appears inconsistent with the increased expression of α_2-adrenoceptors in cortical regions noted above.

Catecholamine depletion It is possible to lower the synthesis of catecholamines by inhibiting the enzyme **tyrosine hydroxylase**, which catalyses the conversion of the amino acid, tyrosine to L-DOPA, a precursor of both noradrenaline and dopamine. The drug used to achieve this effect is **α-methyl-para-tyrosine (AMPT)**. In healthy subjects, AMPT produces sedation but not significant depressive symptoms. As with tryptophan depletion, however, when administered to recovered depressed patients off drug treatment, it causes a **striking clinical relapse in depressive symptomatology** (Berman *et al.*, 1999). This could be mediated either by diminished dopamine or noradrenaline function, or by combined inhibition of both these neurotransmitters.

These findings suggest that subjects at risk of mood disorder are **vulnerable to decreases in both 5-HT and catecholamine neurotransmission**. This is consistent with the clinical evidence that drugs acting selectively on noradrenaline or 5-HT pathways are effective antidepressant treatments.

Dopamine function

Depression The function of dopamine in depression has been less studied than that of 5-HT or noradrenaline but there are a number of reasons for thinking that dopamine neurons may be involved in the pathophysiology of the depressed state:

- Dopamine neurons in the mesolimbic system play a key role in incentive behaviour and reward, processes that are disrupted in depression, particularly melancholic states.
- Antidepressant treatments in animals increase the expression of dopamine receptors in part of the mesolimbic system called the **nucleus accumbens**.

There are some pieces of evidence that suggest that dopamine function may be abnormal in depression:

- CSF levels of the dopamine metabolite homovanillic acid (HVA) are consistently low in depressed patients.
- Some brain imaging studies in depressed patients have found increased binding of dopamine D_2/D_3 receptors in striatal regions; this has been attributed to lowered presynaptic release of dopamine (see Verhoeff, 1999).

These findings, taken with the effect of AMPT to cause relapse in recovered depression, suggest that impaired dopamine function may play a role in the manifestation of the depressive syndrome and in the effects of antidepressant drug treatment.

Mania An influential hypothesis links excessive dopamine activity to the pathophysiology of schizophrenia (see p. 288). It has also been proposed that **manic states** may be attributable to dopamine overactivity (Silverstone and Cookson, 1982). Studies of dopamine metabolism and function have provided little direct evidence for this suggestion, but mania can be provoked by dopamine agonists such as bromocriptine, and the euphoriant and arousing effects of psychostimulants such as amphetamine and cocaine are well known. Finally, dopamine receptor antagonist drugs such as haloperidol are useful in the treatment of mania.

A study in recovered bipolar patients showed that they had a greater psychological response to intravenous amphetamine but no greater release of presynaptic dopamine as measured by the technique of raclopride displacement (see p. 288). This suggests that there may be a heightened responsivity to increased dopamine neurotransmission in patients at risk of mania but this is unlikely to be due to increased presynaptic dopamine release (Yatham *et al.*, 2002).

Role of monoamines

There is now good evidence that unmedicated depressed patients have abnormalities in various aspects of monoamine function. However, these abnormalities vary in extent from case to case, and the changes are not large and are not sufficiently sensitive to be diagnostic.

The most convincing studies that show a key role for monoamines in the pathophysiology of depression are the 5-HT and catecholamine depletion paradigms. It is now established that in vulnerable individuals, lowering of 5-HT and noradrenaline and dopamine function is sufficient to cause clinical depression. Two major questions emerge from this work:

1. How does altered monoamine function impact on the cortical circuitry involved in mood regulation?
2. How does altered monoamine function contribute to the clinical symptomatology of depression?

The first question might be addressed by improving our understanding of the actions of monoamines at a cellular level. There is now increasing knowledge of the effects of monoamines on **second messenger production and intracellular signalling**. For example, recent animal experimental studies have shown that stimulating the cyclic AMP system leads to changes in expression of specific target genes including those involved in the elaboration of neurotropins such as **brain-derived neurotropic factor (BDNF)**. These neurotropins are necessary for the function and survival of CNS neurons. Hence altered monoamine function could lead to changes in the function and viability of cortical neurons involved in mood regulation.

BDNF expression in experimental animals is decreased by stress and enhanced by antidepressant medication. This has given rise to the hypothesis that stress-induced precipitation of mood disorders and the therapeutic effect of monoamine potentiating treatments are mediated via changes in intracellular mechanisms responsible for the production of neurotropins (see Duman, 2004). This suggestion could also account for how environmental adversity can give rise to changes in neuronal survival and perhaps thereby in the anatomy on brain structures important in mood regulation (see below).

Information concerning the second question has been obtained by studying the effect of monoamine manipulation on the processing of emotional information. Specifically both serotonergic and noradrenergic antidepressants decrease negative bias and increase positive bias in tasks involving social perception and emotional memory. These changes occur early in treatment in the absence of subjective mood change. This suggests a possible mechanism whereby changes in monoamine activity can modify cognitions known to be important in the onset and maintenance of depressed mood (see Harmer *et al.*, 2004).

Endocrine abnormalities

Abnormalities in endocrine function may be important in aetiology for two reasons:

1. Some disorders of endocrine function are followed by mood disorders more often than would be expected by chance, suggesting a causative relationship.
2. Endocrine abnormalities found in depressive disorder indicate that there may be a disorder of the hypothalamic centres controlling the endocrine system.

Endocrine pathology and depression

About half of patients with **Cushing's syndrome** suffer from major depression, which usually remits when the cortisol hypersecretion is corrected. Depression also occurs in **Addison's disease**, **hypothyroidism**, and **hyperparathyroidism**. Endocrine changes may account for depressive disorders occurring **premenstrually**, during the **menopause**, and after **childbirth**. These clinical associations are discussed further in Chapter 16.

Hypothalamic-pituitary-adrenal (HPA) axis

Much research effort has been concerned with abnormalities in the control of cortisol in depressive disorders. In about half of patients whose depressive disorder is at least moderately severe, *plasma cortisol secretion is increased* throughout the 24-hour cycle. The increase in cortisol secretion is associated with enlargement in the adrenal gland and increased cortisol response to corticotropin (ACTH) challenge.

In studying depressed patients, use has been made of the **dexamethasone suppression test**, which suppresses cortisol levels via inhibition of **ACTH** release at pituitary level. About 50 per cent of depressed inpatients do not show the normal suppression of cortisol secretion induced by giving a 1 mg dose of the synthetic corticosteroid dexamethasone, an agent which suppresses ACTH via interaction with specific **glucocorticoid receptors**.

Dexamethasone non-suppression is more common in depressed patients with **melancholia**, but it has not been reliably linked with any more specific psychopathological feature. However, abnormalities in the dexamethasone suppression test are not confined to mood disorders; they have also been reported in mania, chronic schizophrenia, and dementia. This lack of diagnostic specificity diminished early hopes that dexamethasone non-suppression could be used as a diagnostic marker of melancholic depression.

A further methodological development has involved administration of an evening dose of dexamethasone followed the next day by challenge with corticotrophin-releasing hormone (CRH), the hypothalamic releasing factor which stimulates ACTH release from the pituitary. In healthy subjects dexamethasone pre-treatment abolishes the ACTH and cortisol response to CRH; however in patients with depression a robust ACTH and cortisol response occurs. This again suggests that depressed patients are insensitive to the effects of the dexamethasone to suppress ACTH release. This has led to the '**glucocorticoid receptor hypothesis**' of depression whereby dysfunction of the HPA axis and the resulting depressive syndrome are linked to genetic or acquired defects of glucocorticoid receptors. Together with this have come findings from animal experimental studies that different classes of antidepressant medication increase expression of glucocorticoid receptors. Therefore one therapeutic mechanism of antidepressant drug action may be to normalize excessive HPA axis activity via increased ability of glucocorticoid receptors to provide feedback regulation (see Holsboer and Kunzel, 2004).

In general, HPA axis changes in depressed patients have been regarded as **state abnormalities**, that is, they remit when the patient recovers. There is some evidence, however, that subtle changes in HPA axis function may persist in recovered depressed subjects. This suggests that some vulnerable individuals may have fairly enduring abnormalities is HPA axis regulation. In experimental animals, early adverse experiences produce long-standing changes in HPA axis regulation, indicating a possible neurobiological mechanism whereby childhood trauma could be translated into increased vulnerability to mood disorder. Recent studies confirm that adults who were abused as children have heightened HPA axis responses to stress (Heim and Nemeroff, 2000).

CRH and depression In addition to its effects on cortisol secretion, CRH may play a more direct role in the aetiology of depression. It is well established that **CRH has a neurotransmitter role** in limbic regions of the brain where it is involved in regulating biochemical and behavioural responses to stress. Administration of CRH to animals produces changes in neuroendocrine regulation, sleep, and appetite that parallel those found in depressed patients. Furthermore, CRF levels may be increased in the CSF of depressed patients. Therefore it is possible that **hypersecretion of CRH** could be involved in the pathophysiology of the depressed state and non-peptide antagonists of CRH receptors may have value as antidepressant agents (see Heim and Nemeroff 2000).

Cortisol, monoamine function, and neuronal toxicity Recent work has shown that corticosteroids regulate the genomic expression and function of a number of monoamine receptors in the brain. For example, it has been shown that corticosteroids can decrease the **expression of post-synaptic 5-HT$_{1A}$ receptors in the hippocampus**; this finding has led to the suggestion that excessive cortisol secretion may precipitate depressive states through decreasing 5-HT neurotransmission. Experimental studies of animals have also linked excessive cortisol secretion to **damage to neurons in the hippocampus**. Subsequently, it has been suggested that chronic cortisol hypersecretion could be associated with the cognitive impairment which may be a particular feature of chronic depression (for a review see Holsboer and Kunzel, 2004).

Thyroid function

Circulating plasma levels of free thyroxine appear to be normal in depressed patients, but levels of **free triiodothyronine** may be decreased. About a quarter of depressed patients have a **blunted thyrotropin-stimulating hormone** (TSH) response to intravenous thyrotropin-releasing hormone (TRH); this abnormality is not specific to depression, as it is also found in alcoholism and panic disorder. Like CRH, TRH has a role in brain neurotransmission and is found in brain neurons co-localized with classical monoamine neurotransmitters such as 5-HT. Therefore, it is possible that the abnormalities in thyroid function found in depressed patients may be associated with changes in central TRH regulation (see Holsboer and Kunzel, 2004).

Depression and the immune system

There is growing evidence that patients with depression manifest a variety of disturbances of **immune function**. Older studies found decreases in the cellular immune responses of lymphocytes in depressed patients (Herbert and Cohen, 1993) but more recent work has produced evidence of immune activation with increases particularly in the release of certain **cytokines** (Box 11.3). Cytokines are known to provoke HPA axis activity and therefore changes in immune regulation may play a part in HPA axis dysfunction in depression.

It is also possible that the changes seen in immune activity are secondary to other depressive features, for example, lowered food intake and diminished self-care. However, the fact that medical administration of some cytokines (for example, interferon and tumour necrosis factor) can cause significant depressive symptoms argues that in some situations, changes in immune function may have a more direct role in provoking mood disorders. Current formulations propose that cytokines can induce expression of the tryptophan metabolizing enzyme, tryptophan oxygenase. This lowers circulating tryptophan levels which could put vulnerable individuals at risk of depression (see Capuron and Miller, 2004).

Sleep changes in depression

Disturbed sleep is characteristic of depression. Recordings of the sleep EEG (polysomnogram) have shown a number of abnormalities in **sleep architecture** in patients with major depression:

- impaired sleep continuity and duration;
- decreased deep sleep (stages 3 and 4);
- decreased latency to the onset of rapid eye movement (REM) sleep;
- increase in the proportion of REM sleep in the early part of the night.

Decreased REM sleep latency is of interest in relation to aetiology because there is some evidence that it may persist in recovered depressed patients and indicate a vulnerability to relapse. A further link between REM sleep and depression is that many (but not all) effective antidepressant drugs decrease REM sleep time and increase the latency to its onset. In addition, both total **sleep deprivation** and selective REM sleep deprivation can produce a temporary alleviation of mood in depressed patients (for a review see Nishino *et al.*, 2004).

The neurochemical mechanism that links changes in REM sleep and mood is not known. The abnormalities in REM sleep in depressed patients could be attributable to excessive sensitivity of **muscarinic cholinergic receptors** (Perlis *et al.*, 2002).

BOX 11.3 IMMUNE CHANGES IN DEPRESSION

Lowered proliferative responses of lymphocytes to mitogens

Lowered natural killer cell activity

Increases in positive acute phase proteins

Increases in cytokine levels (e.g. IL–1, IL–6)

Brain imaging in mood disorder

Structural brain imaging

Changes in brain volume Computerized tomography (CT) and magnetic resonance imaging (MRI) have found a number of abnormalities in patients with major depression, particularly in those with more **severe and chronic disorder**. The most consistent findings are:

- enlarged lateral ventricles (predominantly in elderly subjects with late onset depression);
- decreased hippocampal volume (more consistently in unipolar than bipolar subjects);
- decreased volume of basal ganglia structures (in unipolar but not bipolar subjects);
- decreased grey matter volume of subgenual prefrontal cortex (unipolar and bipolar subjects)
- increased amygdala volume (bipolar subjects).

The origin of these structural abnormalities is unclear but might be related to the cellular neuropathological abnormalities that are increasingly described in depression (Box 11.4). The **neurotrophic hypothesis** of depression suggest that stress (perhaps aided by cortisol hypersecretion) can lead to atrophy and death of neurons and down-regulation of adult neurogenesis,

BOX 11.4 SOME CELLULAR PATHOLOGICAL ABNORMALITIES IN PATIENTS WITH MOOD DISORDERS

1. Decreased glial cell numbers (anterior cingulate cortex)
2. Decreased neuronal size and density (anterior cingulate, pre-frontal cortex)
3. Decreased synaptic markers (pre-frontal cortex)

From Harrison, 2002

particularly in hippocampus (see Duman, 2004). Conceivably processes of this kind could lead to the kind of structural deficits listed above.

White matter hyperintensities Hyperintense MRI signals can be detected in a number of regions in both normal ageing and patients with major depression. The usual sites are in the deep white matter and periventricular white matter. In major depression, increased deep white matter hyperintensities are associated with:

- late onset of depressive disorder;
- greater illness severity and poorer treatment response;
- apathy, psychomotor slowness, and retardation;
- presence of vascular risk factors.

It has been proposed that major depression with these clinical and radiological features is likely to be caused by vascular disease which presumably impairs functioning in the pathways involved in mood regulation (see Drevets *et al.*, 2004). There are also reports that white matter hyperintensities can be found in both old and young patients with **bipolar disorder**. However, the significance of these abnormalities is not clear at present.

Cerebral blood flow and metabolism

Cerebral blood flow can be measured in a number of ways with, for example, single-photon emission tomography (SPET), positron emission tomography (PET) or fMRI; the latter can also measure cerebral metabolism. Cerebral blood flow and metabolism are normally highly correlated.

Numerous studies have examined both cerebral metabolism and blood flow in groups of depressed patients. The findings have often been contradictory, and there are many methodological factors such as patient selection, drug status, and imaging techniques that may account for the discrepant findings. Nevertheless, there is some consensus that depressed patients have evidence of altered cerebral blood flow and metabolism in the following regions:

- prefrontal cortex (orbitofrontal, dorsolateral and dorsomedial cortex)
- anterior cingulate cortex
- amygdala and thalamus
- caudate nucleus.

Taken together, the abnormalities in functional brain imaging in depression support a circuitry model in which mood disorders are associated with **abnormal interactions between several brain regions** rather than a major abnormality in a single structure. The circuits implicated involve regions of the frontal and temporal lobe as well as related areas of basal ganglia and thalamus (see Drevets *et al.*, 2004). Some tentative correlations between these brain regions and clinical depressive features are shown in Box 11.5.

BOX 11.5 SOME NEUROPSYCHOLOGICAL CORRELATES OF ALTERED CENTRAL PERFUSION IN DEPRESSED PATIENTS

Dorsolateral and dorsomedial prefrontal cortex

- Cognitive dysfunction (particularly executive dysfunction) and cognitive slowness

Orbital and lateral prefrontal cortex

- Abnormal emotional processing
- Perseverative thinking

Anterior cingulate

- Impaired attentional processes
- Abnormal emotional processing

Amygdala

- Abnormal emotional processing

Basal ganglia

- Impaired incentive behaviour
- Psychomotor disturbances

Neuropsychological changes in mood disorder

Patients with acute depression and mania show poor performance on several measures of neuropsychological function. Impairment is typically seen over a wide range of neuropsychological domains including attention, learning, memory, and executive function. There is disagreement as to whether these defects are best regarded as global and diffuse or whether there may be some selectivity to the changes seen. However, some have suggested that deficits in executive function may be particularly prominent which would be consistent with abnormalities seen in prefrontal perfusion in imaging studies.

Most of the cognitive impairments resolve as the mood disorder remits, but a growing literature attests to the persistence of cognitive defects, albeit less striking, in euythmic patients with recurrent depression and bipolar disorder (Chamberlain and Sahakian, 2004). Such deficits are particularly apparent in elderly patients where they have been found to correlate with decreases in hippocampal volume (O'Brien *et al.*, 2004).

Aetiology—conclusion

The **predisposition** to develop mania and severe depressive disorders has an important genetic contribution. The levels at which genetic factors operate are not fully clear. They could be via effects on the regulation of monoamine neurotransmitters or through more remote factors such as temperament and the psychological response to stressful life events. Adverse early experience such as parental discord or abuse of various kinds may play a part in shaping features of personality which in turn determine whether, in adult life, individuals are able to access emotional support to help buffer the stressful effects of social adversity. In addition, early life experiences could programme the HPA axis to respond to stress in a way that might predispose to the development of mood disorder.

The **precipitating causes** of mood disorders are stressful life events and certain kinds of physical illness. Some progress has been made in discovering the types of event that provoke depression and in quantifying their stressful qualities. Such studies show that **loss** can be an important precipitant, but not the only one. The effects of particular events may be modified by a number of background factors that may make a person more vulnerable, for example, caring for several small children without help and being socially isolated. As noted in the preceding paragraph, the impact of potentially stressful events also depends on early life experience, personality factors and probably on genetic inheritance.

Two kinds of **pathophysiological mechanism** have been proposed to explain how precipitating events lead to the phenomena observed in depressive disorders. The first mechanism is psychological and the second is neurobiological. The two sets of mechanism are not mutually exclusive, for they may represent different levels of organization of the same pathological process. The psychological studies are at an early stage. Abnormalities have been shown in the thinking of depressed patients and they may play a part in perpetuating depressive disorder. However, there is no convincing evidence that they induce it.

Various biochemical theories can be used to explain how life stress and difficulty could be translated into the **neurochemical changes** that characterize depressive disorders. Monoamine neurotransmitters are involved in regulating responses to stress and in modifying behaviours known to be altered in mood disorders. It seems likely that both external events and a genetic predisposition bring about the changes in brain monoamine function that are seen in depressed patients. In predisposed subjects, reduction in monoamine neurotransmission can bring about clinical symptomatology. Depressive states are associated with

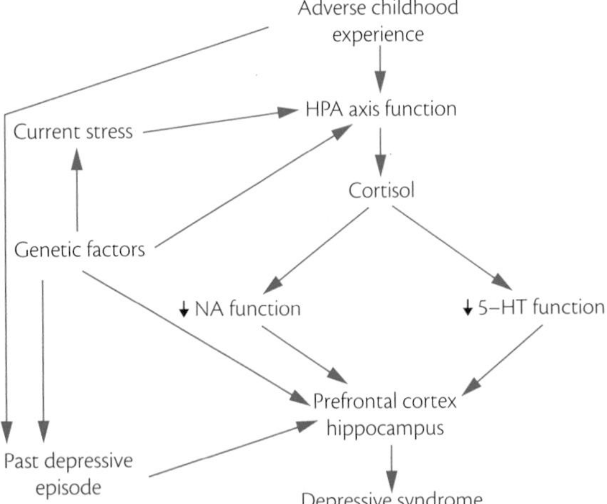

Fig. 11.3 Simplified neurobiological model of the pathophysiology of major depression. Adverse childhood experience has enduring effects on HPA axis function which is further modified by stressful life events (the susceptibility to which is influenced by genetic factors). Abnormalities in cortisol secretion decrease monoamine function which can lead to clinical depression in the setting of developmental and acquired abnormalities in prefrontal cortex and hippocampus circuitry.

altered cerebral activity, particularly in prefrontal cortex. In some patients, particularly those with a poor prognosis, there is evidence for underlying **neuropathological changes**, which probably act as a further predisposing factor (for a simplified model see Figure 11.3).

Recent studies have used sophisticated statistical techniques in an attempt to derive quantitative estimates of the roles of different risk factors in the development of depressive disorders. For example, from a prospective study of 1,942 female twin pairs, Kendler *et al.* (2002) calculated that about half the liability to an episode of major depression in the attributable to the following factors (in order of relative importance):

- Recent stressful life events and difficulties;
- Adolescent risk factors (neuroticism, early onset anxiety and conduct disorder);
- Genetic risk;
- Past history of major depression.

The same study found that adverse childhood experiences also played a significant role in the risk of subsequent depression but this was expressed indirectly through an increased risk of life events and difficulties and diminished social support. Interestingly some of the impact of genetic factors was mediated through an increased risk of early adverse experiences. This suggests that part of the genetic risk associated with depression is expressed though greater likelihood of exposure to an adverse family environment. This in turn could be linked to temperamental factors in both parents and children.

Taken together, recent studies show that major depression is a disorder with important genetic, environmental, and interpersonal determinants. These factors do not interact in a simple additive manner but modify each other in direct and indirect ways. Whilst this formulation precludes the use of simple models to explain the aetiology of major depression, it does correspond more closely to clinical experience. In addition, it suggests that a number of different kinds of intervention could be useful in decreasing the liability of individuals to develop mood disorders.

Course and prognosis

In considering course and prognosis it is necessary to deal with **bipolar and unipolar** disorders separately. It should be remembered, however, that any sample of patients with unipolar depression will contain a proportion of patients whose bipolar illness has not yet declared itself. It has been estimated that about 10 per cent of patients presenting with a depressive disorder will eventually have a manic illness. Such patients are more likely to have a family history of mania or to show brief, mild manic mood swings during antidepressant treatment. From recent hospital and population-based studies, the following general conclusions can be derived (see Angst, 2000).

Bipolar disorders

- The age of onset of bipolar disorder is typically about 21 years in hospital studies but earlier (about 17 years) in community surveys. Late-onset bipolar disorder is rare and may be precipitated by organic brain disease.
- The average length of a manic episode (treated or untreated) is about 6 months.
- At least 90 per cent of patients with mania experience further episodes of mood disturbance.
- Over a 25 year follow-up, on average bipolar patients experience about 10 further episodes of mood disturbance.
- The interval between episodes becomes progressively shorter with both age and the number of episodes.
- Nearly all bipolar patients recover from acute episodes but the long-term prognosis is rather poor. For example, less than 20 per cent of bipolar patients achieve a period of 5 years of clinical stability with good social and occupational performance. Patients with bipolar II disorder have a somewhat better outcome, whilst rapid cycling has a worse prognosis.

Unipolar depressive disorders (recurrent major depression)

- The age of onset of unipolar disorders varies widely; it is generally agreed to be later on average than for bipolar cases. There is a fairly uniform incidence of onset of cases throughout the life span but the relative contribution of different aetiological factors probably differs between early- and late-onset cases.
- The average length of a depressive episode is about 6 months but about 25 per cent of patients have episodes of more than a year and about 10–20 per cent develop a chronic unremitting course.
- About 80 per cent of patients with major depression will experience further episodes (that is, have recurrent major depression).

- Over a 25-year follow-up, on average, patients with recurrent major depression experience about five further episodes.
- As with bipolar patients, the interval between episodes becomes progressively shorter.
- A high proportion (about one-third) of depressed patients do not achieve complete symptom remission between episodes.
- The longer-term prognosis of recurrent major depression may be a little better in some ways than that of bipolar disorder but is still modest. For example, only about 25 per cent of patients with recurrent depression achieve a period of 5 years of clinical stability with good social and occupational performance.

Dysthymia

Dysthymia is by definition a chronic disorder lasting many years and community studies show a low spontaneous recovery rate. Over the life span, some patients with dysthymia develop major depression (so-called **double depression**) whilst some patients originally presenting with major depression subside into dysthymia. The development of mania is rare.

Minor mood disorder

Most information is available for **minor depression** which shows a recurrence rate similar to that of major depression. Patients who meet criteria for minor depression at one point in follow-up may then subsequently be diagnosed as suffering from major depression and vice versa. Thus, similarly to dysthymia, minor depression is likely to be a **risk factor** for major depression and may also be a **residual state** following remission of major depression. Overall, the longitudinal data suggest that major and minor depression and dysthymia are not distinct conditions but are part of a **spectrum of depressive disorders** (see Hermens *et al.*, 2004).

Mortality of mood disorders

Mortality is significantly increased in patients with mood disorders, largely, though not exclusively from **suicide**. The standardized mortality ratio in mood disorders is about twice that found in the general population. Apart from suicide, excess deaths are due to accidents, cardiovascular disease, and comorbid substance misuse. Epidemiological studies suggest that treatment lowers the mortality in mood disorders (see Angst *et al.*, 2002)

Rates of suicide in mood disorders are at least 12 times greater than those of the general population (Harris and Barraclough, 1997). The risk varies with diagnostic subcategory but is greatest for major depression (Box 11.6). Longer-term follow-up of patients with depression have given differing rates of lifetime risk of suicide. In those with severe illnesses who have been treated as inpatients the risk may be as high as 15 per cent. However, in community samples the risk is less. The proportion of patients who die by suicide in mood disorders lessens as the period of follow-up increases, presumably because mortality from natural causes becomes more significant. It is also possible, however, that the risk of suicide is highest in the early stages of the illness.

BOX 11.6 STANDARDIZED MORTALITY RATIOS FOR SOME DEPRESSIVE DISORDERS

- Major depression 20.35
- Bipolar disorder 15.05
- Dysthymia 12.12

Harris and Barraclough (1997)

Prognostic factors

The best predictor of the future course is the history of **previous episodes**. Not surprisingly, the risk of recurrence is much greater in those with **several previous episodes**. Other factors that predict a greater risk of future episodes are:

- incomplete symptomatic remission
- bipolar disorder
- early age of onset
- poor social support
- poor physical health
- comorbid substance misuse
- comorbid personality disorder.

The various risk factors, particularly previous pattern of recurrence, and extent of current remission have important implications for the use of longer-term maintenance treatments (see below). In many patients, mood disorders are best conceptualized as chronic relapsing conditions which require an integrated long-term treatment approach (see Young, 2001).

The acute treatment of depression

This section is concerned with the **efficacy of various forms of treatment** in the acute management of depression. Details of treatment with drugs and ECT are given in Chapter 21, which should be consulted before reading this section. Advice on the selection of treatments and the day-to-day care of patients is given in the section on management.

Antidepressant drugs

Antidepressant drugs are effective in the acute treatment of major depression. The largest effects relative to placebo are seen in patients with major depression whose symptoms are of at least **moderate severity**. Short-term response rates in controlled trials are about 60 per cent for patients on active treatment and about 30 per cent for those on placebo (number needed to treat [NNT] = 4–5) (see Anderson *et al.*, 2003). In terms of efficacy there is little to choose between the various antidepressants, although some are better in certain defined situations (see below).

Similar clinical response rates are seen in **dysthymia** where again several classes of antidepressant drugs including tricyclics and SSRIs have shown therapeutic efficacy. A meta-analysis by de Lima *et al.* (1999) showed a response rate with active of treatment of 55 per cent, compared with 30 per cent on placebo (NNT = 4).

The value of antidepressant drugs in milder depressive disorders such as minor depression and mixed anxiety-depression is not established. It is generally believed that tricyclics are relatively ineffective in these disorders and though SSRI treatment may produce benefit, its clinical relevance is not established (Judd *et al.*, 2004).

Tricyclic antidepressants

Tricyclic antidepressants have been extensively compared with placebo in both inpatients and outpatients with major depression. In all but the most severely depressed patients, tricyclic antidepressants are clearly more effective than placebo (Morris and Beck, 1974). There is little evidence that tricyclic antidepressant drugs differ from one another in clinical efficacy, but they do differ in side-effect profile (see Chapter 21). **Lofepramine** is relatively safe in overdose. Among the other classes of antidepressant drug, none is more effective than the tricyclics, although individual patients may show a preferential response to other compounds (see below).

Response in clinical subgroups

Tricyclics appear to be less effective in patients with:

- depressive psychosis (as a sole treatment);
- milder depressive states with Hamilton Depression Scores less than about 14;
- patients with atypical depression.

Monoamine oxidase inhibitors

The efficacy of **monoamine oxidase inhibitors (MAOIs)** in the treatment of major depression (particularly with melancholic features) has been a matter of controversy. However, placebo-controlled trials have shown that MAOIs are effective antidepressants and equal in therapeutic activity to tricyclic antidepressants for moderate-to-severe depressive disorders.

MAOIs are liable to produce dangerous reactions with other drugs and some foods; therefore, they are not recommended as first-line antidepressant drugs. However, controlled trials have shown that for the following conditions MAOIs carry an advantage over tricyclic antidepressants:

- atypical depression;
- anergic bipolar depression (characterized by fatigue, retardation, increased appetite, and sleep);
- depression resistant to tricyclics and SSRIs.

The reversible type-A MAOI **moclobemide** has the advantage of not requiring adherence to a low-tyramine diet. However, it can still produce hazardous interactions with other drugs (see p. 552). Controlled trials have shown that moclobemide is more effective than placebo in the treatment of uncomplicated major depression. It is doubtful, however, whether moclobemide at standard doses is as effective as conventional MAOIs for atypical and tricyclic-resistant depression (see Cowen, 2005).

Combination of MAOIs and tricyclic antidepressants

It has been reported that, in cases resistant to treatment with a tricyclic or MAOI, a combination of the two drugs is more effective than either drug given alone in corresponding dosage. This claim has not been proved; indeed, two clinical trials have failed to confirm it (see Cowen, 2005). However, it can be argued that neither trial was concerned with patients known to be resistant to single drugs (the patient group to whom combined treatment is most often given).

Selective serotonin re-uptake inhibitors (SSRIs) and serotonin and noradrenaline re-uptake inhibitors

Selective serotonin re-uptake inhibitors (SSRIs) have undergone extensive trials both against placebo and comparator antidepressants. There is good evidence that they are as effective as tricyclics in the broad range of depressed patients, although they may be less effective in hospitalized depressed patients. Venlafaxine, a serotonin and noradrenaline re-uptake inhibitor (SNRI), also appears a little more effective than SSRIs in patients with more severe depressive states (Smith *et al.*, 2002). SSRIs are more effective than tricyclics (with the exception of clomipramine) where depression occurs in association with **obsessive-compulsive disorder** (see Anderson *et al.*, 2000).

Tolerance relative to tricyclics

In short-term clinical trials, compared to tricyclics SSRIs are associated with lower drop-out rates due to side-effects, but the differences are modest (relative risk of drop-out due to side-effects is 0.73, NNT = 33). However, the differences in favour of SSRIs increase in routine clinical situations, particularly when length of treatment exceeds a few weeks (see Anderson *et al.*, 2000). Clearly, relative safety in overdose gives SSRIs an advantage in certain clinical situations, though venlafaxine appears less safe in overdose than SSRIs (Cheeta *et al.*, 2004).

Other antidepressants

A wide variety of other antidepressant drugs is now available (see Chapter 21). All have established efficacy relative to placebo. The main differences between the various preparations are in side-effect profile (Table 11.10). Apart from reboxetine, anti-cholinergic-type side-effects are uncommon. Trazodone and mirtazapine are sedating. The adverse effects of the SNRI, duloxetine, are similar to those of SSRIs. All these agents are safer than tricyclics in overdose.

Lithium

Lithium as a sole treatment

This section is concerned only with lithium as a treatment for depressive disorders. The use of lithium in the **treatment of mania** and in the **maintenance treatment of mood disorders** is considered later. Placebo-controlled trials suggest that lithium has antidepressant efficacy in bipolar depression but its effects in unipolar depression as a sole treatment are modest (Goodwin, 2003).

Lithium in combination with antidepressants

Despite its limited utility as a sole drug treatment for depression, lithium can produce useful therapeutic effects when added to antidepressant medication in treatment-resistant patients (**lithium augmentation**). In a meta-analysis, Bauer and Döpfmer (1999) found about 50 per cent of depressed patients responded to lithium augmentation of their antidepressant regimen, compared with about 20 per cent of patients given placebo (NNT = 3–4).

Whilst some studies have reported a rapid amelioration of the depressed state within as little as 48 hours after the addition of lithium, the more usual pattern of response is a gradual resolution of symptoms over 2–3 weeks. Unipolar depressed patients seem to respond as well as bipolar patients and thus far there are no reliable clinical or biochemical predictors that identify depressed patients likely to respond to lithium augmentation. The effects of lithium augmentation do not seem to be restricted to any specific class of antidepressants.

Anticonvulsants

Anticonvulsants such as carbamazepine, valproate, and lamotrogine are useful in the management of bipolar disorder and in these circumstances can prevent episodes of major depression. There is less evidence that these drugs have acute antidepressant efficacy but lamotrogine has been shown to produce antidepressant

TABLE 11.10 Clinical characteristics of some antidepressant drugs

	Anticholinergic	Sedation	Weight gain	Sexual dysfunction	Toxicity in overdose
Amitriptyline	+++	+++	+++	+	+++
Lofepramine	+	0	0	+	0
SSRIs	0	0	+	+++	0*
Venlafaxine	0	0	+	+++	++
Duloxetine	0	0	+	+++	?
Trazodone	0	+++	+	0	+
Reboxetine	+	0	0	+	0
Mirtazapine	0	+++	+++	0	0

0, none; +, mild; ++, moderate; +++, marked.

* Citalopram may be somewhat more toxic than other SSRIs.

effects in a placebo-controlled trial in bipolar depressed patients (Calabrese *et al.*, 1999).

Electroconvulsive therapy

This treatment is described in Chapter 21, where its unwanted effects are also considered. The present section is concerned with evidence about the therapeutic effects of ECT for depressive disorders.

Comparison with simulated ECT

Six double-blind controlled trials have compared the efficacy of ECT and simulated ECT (anaesthesia with electrode application but no passage of current) in patients with major depression. Five of these studies found ECT to be more effective than the simulation. In the study which did not find the full procedure more effective, unilateral low-dose ECT was used, a procedure which is thought on other grounds to be relatively ineffective. The overall response rate is about 70 per cent for ECT and 40 per cent for simulated treatment (NNT 3–4) (see UK ECT Review Group, 2003 and Chapter 21).

Comparison with other treatments

Several studies have compared depressed inpatients receiving ECT with those receiving antidepressant drugs. In nine comparisons with tricyclic antidepressants, ECT was therapeutically more effective in six studies and equally effective in the remaining three. In five comparisons with MAOIs, ECT was superior in each trial and worked more quickly. These data suggest that in severely depressed inpatients ECT is probably superior to antidepressant drug treatment, at least in the short term (UK ECT Review Group, 2003, Box 21.12).

Indications for ECT

Clinicians generally agree that the therapeutic effects of ECT are greatest in severe depressive disorders, especially those with **marked weight loss, early morning waking, retardation**, and **delusions**. From the trials comparing full ECT with simulated ECT, it appears that delusions and (less strongly) retardation are the features that distinguish patients who respond to full ECT from those who respond to placebo (UK ECT Review Group, 2003).

Other studies have established that patients with **depressive psychosis** respond better to ECT than to tricyclic antidepressants or antipsychotic drugs given alone. However, combined treatment with tricyclic antidepressants and **antipsychotic drugs** may be about as effective as ECT although no direct comparisons have been made (see Cowen, 2005). Another point of practical importance is that ECT may often prove effective in depressed patients who have not responded to full trials of medication, whether or not psychotic features are present; however in such patients relapse rates are high (Sackheim *et al.*, 1990). (For recent NICE guidance on the use of ECT see p. 565.)

Psychological treatment

All depressed patients, whatever other treatment they may be receiving, need psychotherapy in a general sense, which provides education, reassurance, and encouragement. These measures ('clinical management') can provide some symptomatic relief and can also ensure that pessimistic patients comply with specific treatments. Education and reassurance should also be given to the **patient's partner**, other close family members, and other people involved in care.

The psychological treatments used for depressive disorders can be divided as follows:

- supportive psychotherapy
- cognitive behaviour therapy
- interpersonal psychotherapy
- marital therapy
- dynamic psychotherapy.

These psychotherapies can be employed as alternatives to antidepressant medication or as adjuncts. Psychotherapies have been less well evaluated than antidepressant medication in major depression but the most extensive evidence base is for cognitive behaviour therapy. In general psychotherapies are somewhat more effective than treatment as usual in the management of mild to moderate depression, particularly in primary care. In this setting, however, structured treatments such as cognitive behaviour therapy do not appear superior to other therapies such as non-directive counselling (Wampold *et al.*, 2002). This suggests that factors common to all psychological treatments are likely to be important in mediating the therapeutic effect (p. 583). In randomized trials psychotherapies usually perform as well as drug treatment in moderately depressed patients (National Institute for Clinical Excellence, 2004).

Support and problem solving

Supportive psychotherapy goes beyond clinical management in focusing on the identification and resolution of current life difficulties, and in using the patient's strengths and available coping resources. A development of this approach is **problem-solving**, in which the therapist and patient identify the main problems of concern and devise feasible step-by-step ways of tackling them. Randomized trials suggest that problem-solving treatment is better than treatment as usual in moderately depressed patients in primary care. Its efficacy relative to drug treatment and other psychotherapies is unclear (National Institute for Clinical Excellence, 2004d).

Cognitive behaviour therapy

For depressive disorder, the essential aim of **cognitive behaviour therapy** is to help patients to modify their ways of thinking and acting about life situations and depressive symptoms (see p. 588 for further information). There have been numerous studies of cognitive behaviour therapy in acute major depression which have been reviewed (National Institute for Clinical Excellence, 2004d). Current conclusions are:

- There is strong evidence that cognitive behaviour therapy is superior to waiting list control in relieving depressive symptomatology
- There is insufficient evidence to show whether in depressed patients, cognitive behaviour therapy is superior to placebo medication with clinical management or GP treatment as usual
- There is insufficient evidence to show whether in depressed patients cognitive behaviour therapy is superior to other psychotherapies (either structured or unstructured).

When compared to antidepressant medication, however, cognitive behaviour therapy has fared somewhat better. For example, no difference in antidepressant effect was seen when cognitive behaviour therapy was compared to antidepressant medication but the longer-term effect of cognitive treatment on depressive symptoms was somewhat more sustained (Evans *et al.*, 1992). In addition, the combination of cognitive behaviour therapy with antidepressant medication was superior to medication alone in moderately to severely depressed patients (National Institute for Clinical Excellence, 2004d). The opinion of many clinicians is that cognitive behaviour therapy is not effective as a sole treatment for patients with severe depression (Thase and Friedman, 1999) but this view is not supported clearly by trial evidence (National Institute for Clinical Excellence, 2004d). Issues such as what is meant by 'severity' in different settings as well as the problem of generalizing from randomized trials to everyday practice are likely to be involved in this controversy. In addition, therapist expertise may be important (DeRubeis *et al.*, 2005). In milder depressive states there is evidence that cognitive behaviour therapy delivered by computer or through guided self-help may be beneficial (National Institute for Clinical Excellence, 2004d).

Interpersonal psychotherapy

Interpersonal therapy is a systematic and standardized treatment approach to personal relationships and life problems (see p. 587). It has been less studied than cognitive therapy in depression but seems to be effective (Weisman *et al.*, 1979; Elkin *et al.*, 1989). The National Institute for Clinical Excellence (2004d) concluded that in depressed patients, interpersonal therapy:

- Is more effective than placebo with clinical management and GP treatment as usual.
- Is as effective as antidepressant medication.
- Is more effective when combined with antidepressants than when given alone. However, it is not clear whether the combination of interpersonal therapy and antidepressants is better than antidepressants alone for the treatment of acute depression

Couple therapy

Couple therapy can be given to depressed patients for whom **interactions with a partner** appear to have contributed to causing or maintaining the depressive disorder. The aim of the intervention is to understand the nature of these interactions and modify them so that the relationship becomes more mutually supportive. There are few randomized trials available but the evidence suggests that couple therapy is significantly more effective than a waiting list control. However, there is insufficient data to indicate how couple therapy compares to other psychotherapies or antidepressant medication (National Institute for Clinical Excellence, 2004d). In practice, antidepressant treatment and couple therapy are often used together but the combination has not been well evaluated.

Dynamic psychotherapy

Dynamic psychotherapy has a different aim from the treatments described so far, which is to resolve underlying personal conflicts and attendant life difficulties that are believed to cause or maintain the depressive disorder. Opinions differ about its value. There have been few attempts to evaluate treatment, and they have mainly been concerned with brief dynamic psychotherapy in groups. The results for the treatment of depression suggest that dynamic psychotherapy may be less effective than cognitive behaviour therapy or antidepressant medication (National Institute for Clinical Excellence, 2004d).

Other treatments

Sleep deprivation

Several studies suggest that, in some depressive disorders, rapid short-term changes in mood can be brought about by keeping patients **awake overnight**. The alleviation of depressed mood after total sleep deprivation is nearly always **temporary**; it disappears after the next night's sleep or even during a daytime nap after the night of sleep deprivation. Whilst the antidepressant effect of sleep deprivation is of great theoretical interest, its brevity makes it unpractical. However, there are reports that sleep deprivation can be used to quicken the onset of effect of antidepressant drugs and also that some pharmacological manipulations can prolong the effect of sleep deprivation (see Berger *et al.*, 2003).

Bright light treatment

Over 50 per cent of patients with recurrent winter depression respond to **bright light treatment** (about 10,000 lux). Treatment is usually given for an hour or two in the morning but the timing of light treatment is not always critical and evening light or even midday exposure can be effective. The duration of exposure usually needs to be 1–2 hours (p. 572).

Designing placebo-controlled trials of bright light for winter depression presents problems, because most patients are aware before treatment that bright light is believed to be the important therapeutic ingredient. Within this limitation, most studies have found that dim light is less effective than bright light. The usual onset of the antidepressant effect of bright light is within 2–5 days, but longer periods of treatment seem to be needed in some patients. Patients with **'atypical'** depressive features such as **overeating and oversleeping** appear to respond best. To avoid relapse, light treatment usually needs to be maintained until the usual time of natural remission, in the early spring. For reviews of bright light treatment and winter depression see Eagles (2004), Golden *et al.*, (2005), and p. 572.

The acute treatment of mania

The treatment of mania presents a formidable clinical challenge which often tests the management skills of the psychiatric team. Drug treatment plays a pivotal role in the management of mania and has the aim of reducing physical and mental overactivity, improving features of psychosis, and preventing deterioration in health due to exhaustion, sleep deprivation, and poor fluid intake. It is worth noting that before the advent of modern drug treatment the mortality of mania in hospital setting was over 20 per cent; nearly half these patients died from exhaustion (Derby, 1933).

Medication

Antipsychotic drugs

Typical antipsychotic drugs

Several randomized controlled trials have shown efficacy of **chlorpromazine** and **haloperidol** in treating mania, whether or not patients have clear psychotic features (Chou *et al.*, 2000). However, the use of typical antipsychotic drugs has limitations; manic patients often receive high doses and may be particularly susceptible to extrapyramidal side-effects. In addition, conventional antipsychotic drugs do not protect against the depressive downswings that can follow resolution of a manic illness.

Atypical antipsychotic drugs

Because of their improved tolerability profile, atypical antipsychotic agents are being increasingly used in mania. In a systematic review Rendell *et al.* (2003) found that in the management of acute mania, olanzapine had superior efficacy to both placebo and valproate but not haloperidol. Placebo-controlled trials also support the efficacy of quetiapine, aripirazole and risperidone in mania (Schatzberg, 2004). It should be noted, however, that more severely ill patients may not be included in placebo-controlled trials, which could limit the generalizibility of these findings.

Mood stabilizers

Lithium

Five placebo-controlled trials have shown that lithium is effective in the acute treatment of mania. In the only study which compared lithium to both placebo and an active comparator, Bowden *et al.* (1994) found a response rate of 49 per cent for lithium, 48 per cent for valproate and 25 per cent for placebo. A meta-analytic review concluded that lithium approximately doubled the placebo response in mania with an NNT of 5 (Poolsup *et al.*, 2000). Lithium is at least as effective as antipsychotic medication but its onset of action is slower (see Grunze *et al.*, 2003). Prominent depressive symptoms and psychotic features predict a poorer response to lithium alone, as does a rapid cycling disorder (Goodwin, 2003).

Carbamazepine

Assessment of the efficacy of **carbamazepine** in acute mania has been limited by problems in study design. These include small numbers, the use of adjunctive medications, and mixed diagnostic groupings. However, a more recent placebo-controlled study of an extended-release carbamazepine in 200 patients found a significantly higher response rate to carbamazepine (42 per cent) than to placebo (21 per cent). In general, carbamazepine appears equivalent in efficacy to antipsychotic drugs, in the treatment of acute mania, although it may be slightly less effective than lithium and valproate (Grunze *et al.*, 2003). As with lithium, carbamazepine requires careful upward titration to help tolerance giving it a slow onset of action. In addition, carbamazepine induces liver metabolizing enzymes which can lead to lower plasma levels of concomitantly administered drugs.

Valproate

Several randomized controlled trials have shown that **valproate** possesses antimanic activity greater than placebo and equivalent to lithium. Valproate may be more effective than lithium in the subgroup of patients with prominent dysphoric symptoms and rapid-cycling. Current evidence suggests that valproate is somewhat less effective than olanzapine in the treatment of acute mania but causes less sedation and weight gain (see Macritchie *et al.*, 2003).

An advantage possessed by valproate is that the onset of its activity is sooner than other mood stabilizers. For example, with 'valproate loading' (20 mg/kg/day) the onset of manic effect can be as early as within 1–4 days. This is probably because the tolerability of valproate allows rapid dose escalation whilst lithium and carbamazepine must be introduced more gradually (Goodwin, 2003). Studies have suggested that an antimanic response to valproate is more likely to occur with plasma levels above 50 µg/ml (see Hirschfeld *et al.*, 1999).

Benzodiazepines

Benzodiazepines are useful **adjuncts** in the treatment of mania because they can rapidly diminish overactivity, and restore sleep. Benzodiazepines have been used as a sole therapy in the treatment of mania but this carries a risk of disinhibition. Their most useful role is an adjunct to mood stabilizers because the latter drugs can take several days to become effective. Benzodiazepines can also be given in combination with antipsychotic drugs because this lowers the doses of antipsychotic drug needed to calm agitated and overactive patients. The usual benzodiazepines employed are the high-potency agents, lorazepam and clonazepam. Use should be 'as needed' and for as short a time as possible to minimize the risk of tolerance and dependence (Grunze *et al.*, 2004).

Electroconvulsive therapy

ECT has been widely used to treat mania, although there are only two prospective controlled trials in the modern era. In one, bilateral ECT was found to be superior to lithium (Small *et al.*, 1988). In another study, unilateral and bilateral ECT were compared with a combination of lithium and haloperidol in patients who had not responded to antipsychotic drugs alone. The response rate of these patients to ECT (13 of 22) was greater than that to combined drug treatment (none of five). The efficacy of unilateral and bilateral ECT did not differ (Mukherjee *et al.*, 1988).

Retrospective investigations have shown ECT to be effective in acute mania, with the overall response rate being about 80 per cent. Many of the patients had been unresponsive to medication (Mukherjee *et al.*, 1994). In clinical practice, there is a tendency to give ECT to patients unresponsive to drug treatment, or to patients with a manic illness of life-threatening proportions due to extreme overactivity and physical exhaustion. ECT is often given at shorter intervals in the treatment of mania than in the treatment of depression, but there is no evidence that this regimen is necessary or speeds treatment response. It is unclear whether bilateral electrode placement is better than unilateral placement in manic patients (for a review see Mukherjee *et al.*, 1994).

The longer-term treatment of mood disorders

Follow-up studies have shown that mood disorders often recur and, untreated, have a rather poor long-term prognosis. For this reason there is now increasing emphasis on **long-term management**.

Prevention of relapse and recurrence

Strictly, the word **relapse** refers to the worsening of symptoms after an initial improvement during the treatment of a single episode of mood disorder, whilst **recurrence** refers to a new episode after a period of complete recovery. Treatment to prevent relapse should be called **continuation treatment**, and treatment to prevent recurrence should be called **prophylactic or maintenance treatment**. In practice, however, it is not always easy to maintain the distinction between these two kinds of treatment because a therapy may be given at first to prevent relapse and then may be used to prevent recurrence.

Drug treatment of unipolar depression

Continuation treatment

It is now well established that stopping antidepressants soon after treatment response is associated with a high risk of *relapse*. About a third of patients withdrawn from medication relapse over the next year with the majority of the relapses occurring in the first 6 months. Placebo-controlled studies of the role of continuation therapy have reached the following conclusions (see Anderson *et al.*, 2000):

- continuing antidepressant treatment for 6 months past the point of remission halves the relapse rate;
- treatment should be at the originally effective dose of medication if possible;
- in patients at low risk of further episodes, continuation of antidepressant treatment longer than 6 months confers little extra benefit except in the elderly where 12 months continuation therapy is more appropriate.

Maintenance treatment

Controlled studies involving patients with recurrent depression (usually defined as at least three episodes over the last 5 years) have shown that maintenance antidepressant treatment can substantially reduce relapse rates. For example, in a 3-year study of 128 patients, Frank *et al.*, (1990) found a relapse rate of 22 per cent in patients taking imipramine compared with 78 per cent in patients treated with placebo. The effects of longer-term maintenance treatment were confirmed in a systematic review (Geddes *et al.*, 2003) where over one to two years of continued antidepressant treatment the relapse rate was lowered from 41 per cent on placebo to 18 per cent on active medication. During longer-term treatment, it is common practice to lower the dose of medication, especially tricyclic antidepressant, to a 'maintenance' level, but this may lessen prophylactic efficacy unless it carried out carefully with close monitoring. The general rule is 'what gets you well, keeps you well' (Anderson *et al.*, 2000).

Lithium carbonate has also been used in the prevention of recurrent unipolar depression but while some patients show a clear response the overall evidence for its efficacy is less robust than for the prevention of bipolar disorder (see Burgess *et al.*, 2001). Lithium may, however, be a useful treatment for depressed patients who have shown any sign of elevated mood because (unlike antidepressant drugs) it also prevents mania (see below).

Drug treatment of bipolar disorder

Continuation treatment

The role of continuation treatment in bipolar disorder following an episode of mania has been less studied. However, it a common clinical experience that too

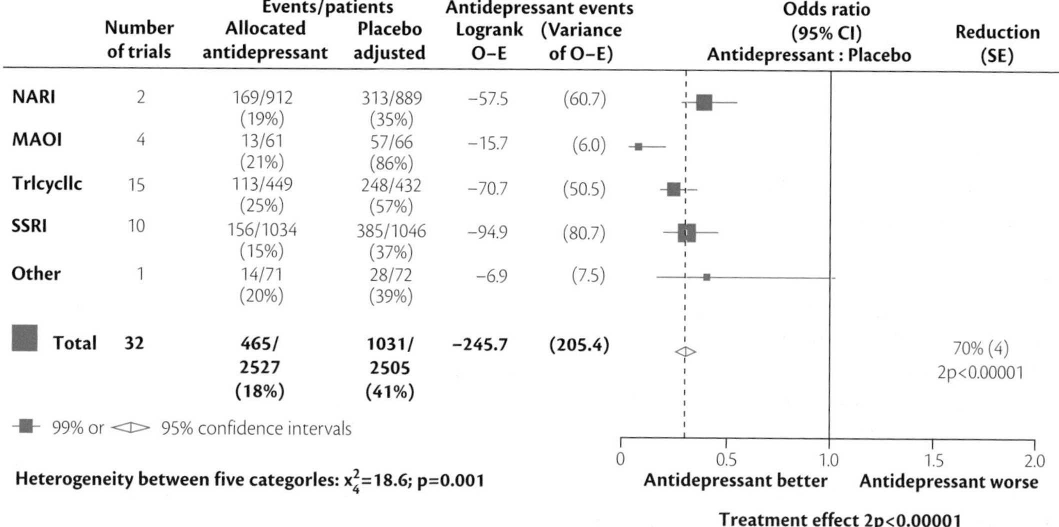

	Number of trials	Events/patients: Allocated antidepressant	Events/patients: Placebo adjusted	Antidepressant events: Logrank O–E	Antidepressant events: (Variance of O–E)	Reduction (SE)
NARI	2	169/912 (19%)	313/889 (35%)	−57.5	(60.7)	
MAOI	4	13/61 (21%)	57/66 (86%)	−15.7	(6.0)	
Trlcycllc	15	113/449 (25%)	248/432 (57%)	−70.7	(50.5)	
SSRI	10	156/1034 (15%)	385/1046 (37%)	−94.9	(80.7)	
Other	1	14/71 (20%)	28/72 (39%)	−6.9	(7.5)	
Total	**32**	**465/ 2527 (18%)**	**1031/ 2505 (41%)**	**−245.7**	**(205.4)**	70% (4) 2p<0.00001

Fig. 11.4 Meta-analysis of rates of depressive relapse in patients randomly allocated to receive continuation treatment for on average about one year with antidepressant medication or placebo. (From Geddes *et al.*, 2003.)

rapid a reduction in doses of drug treatment can lead to the sudden recrudescence of an apparently treated manic disorder. Since the average length of a manic episode is about 6 months, it seems prudent to continue some form of medication for at least this period. Patients who have been severely ill may well be taking both a mood stabilizer and an antipsychotic agent. Because of the adverse effects of antipsychotic drugs, it will often be appropriate slowly to withdraw this form of treatment first.

Maintenance treatment

Lithium There is substantial evidence for the efficacy of lithium in the maintenance treatment of recurrent mood disturbances in patients with bipolar disorders. In a systematic review, Geddes *et al.* (2004) found that lithium was significantly more effective than placebo in preventing relapses of all mood disorder (mean relative risk 0.65, 95 per cent CI = 0.5–0.84). However, while lithium was clearly effective in preventing manic relapse its effect in preventing depressive episodes was more equivocal (mean relative risk 0.72, 95 per cent CI = 0.49–1.07).

In general about half of bipolar patients treated with lithium respond well. The following predict a **relatively poorer** response to lithium maintenance treatment:

- rapid-cycling disorders or chronic depression;
- mixed affective states;
- alcohol and drug misuse;
- mood-incongruent psychotic features.

There is also evidence that use of lithium in patients with recurrent mood disorders is associated with a **significant reduction in mortality from suicide** (Cipriani *et al.*, 2005). This effect is most often seen in dedicated lithium clinics and the mechanism and specificity of the association requires further study. Nevertheless, it is clinically important that the carefully supervised use of lithium is associated with a lowered risk of suicidal behaviour. This effect is not necessarily shared by other mood stabilizers (Muller-Oerlinghausen *et al.*, 2003).

Carbamazepine Although the number of patients studied in randomized controlled studies is relatively few, carbamazepine appears to have efficacy in the prophylaxis of bipolar disorder though it appears to be less effective than lithium in 'classical' bipolar illness (Goodwin, 2003). Therefore, carbamazepine can be considered in patients who respond poorly to lithium, particularly those with rapid-cycling disorders. Carbamazepine can be given alone or in combination with lithium.

Valproate Valproate is increasingly used in the treatment of acute mania and therefore evidence of its longer-term maintenance effects is needed. Bowden *et al.* (2000) randomized 372 patients to one year maintenance treatment with valproate, lithium and placebo. There were no significant differences between the three treatment groups on the primary outcome measure of time to recurrence of any mood disorder. However, the number of patients who left the study because of the occurrence of a mood episode was significantly less in those taking valproate relative to placebo. Patients taking valproate experienced more tremor, alopecia and weight gain than those on placebo. At present, the evidence supporting the use of valproate in longer-term maintenance of bipolar disorder is rather slender and less than that for lithium.

There are numerous case series indicating that valproate may have useful prophylactic effects in patients with refractory bipolar illness, even when there has been a poor response to lithium and carbamazepine. In these studies valproate has often been combined with lithium or other mood stabilizers (Goodwin, 2003).

Lamotrigine Two prospective placebo-controlled trials have shown that lamotrigine has prophylactic effects in patients with bipolar illness. While lamotrigine may have some modest benefit in the prevention of mania it has a clearer prophylactic effect against depression; its profile of activity, therefore, contrasts with lithium and valproate which are more effective in preventing mania (Goodwin *et al.*, 2004). However, lamotrigine is not licensed for the treatment of mood disorder in the UK.

Antipsychotic drugs Patients with bipolar disorder have sometimes been maintained on typical antipsychotic drugs, usually given in addition to mood-stabilizing agents. It is usually wise to minimize this form of treatment where possible because conventional antipsychotic drugs do not protect against depression and may be more liable to cause tardive dyskinesia in bipolar patients.

Atypical antipsychotic drugs are also being employed in the longer-term maintenance treatment of bipolar disorder either as a sole treatment or as an adjunct to mood stabilizers. There is good evidence for the efficacy of olanzapine in this respect which is equivalent overall in efficacy to lithium (McCormack and Wiseman, 2004). While atypical antipsychotic drugs are well-tolerated from the point of view of movement disorders, there is growing concern about their adverse metabolic effects such as weight gain and diabetes. Therefore their long-term use in bipolar disorder requires caution and careful monitoring.

Psychotherapy

Cognitive therapy

Unipolar depression

As noted above, there is some evidence that cognitive therapy given during an acute phase of depression leads to a more sustained improvement in depressive symptomatology and lessens the risk of subsequent relapse (Hollon *et al.*, 2005). There is also growing interest in the use of continuation and maintenance treatment with cognitive therapy, particularly in patients who have **residual depressive symptomatology** and are thereby at increased risk of relapse. For example, Paykel *et al.* (1999) studied 158 patients who experienced significant residual symptoms after treatment of an episode of major depression. All patients received clinical management and continuation treatment with antidepressant medication and half also received 16 sessions of cognitive therapy. Over the next 16 months, the relapse rate in the patients receiving cognitive therapy was 29 per cent, compared with 47 per cent in the group who received clinical management only.

Bipolar disorder

Psychotherapy has been less studied in bipolar patients but cognitive techniques may be valuable in helping patients accept their illness and the need for medical treatment. A randomized study showed that education about early signs of relapse, reduced rates of manic illness in bipolar patients over 18 months by 30 per cent (Perry *et al.*, 1999). More specific cognitive behaviour therapies have also shown benefit in deceasing affective symptomatology and increasing social functioning but control for non-specific effects of treatment are often lacking (Jones, 2004). Better controlled studies that identify more specific therapeutic mechanisms are needed.

TABLE 11.11 Effect of nortriptyline and interpersonal therapy (IPT) on relapse rate over three years in depressed patients aged 60 years and over

Treatment	n	Relapse rate (95% CI)
Nortriptyline + IPT	22	20% (4–36)
Nortriptyline	24	43% (25–61)
IPT and placebo	21	64% (45–83)
Placebo	29	90% (79–100)

Interpersonal therapy

In patients with recurrent depressive episodes, **interpersonal therapy** given once monthly delayed, but did not prevent, depressive relapse compared with standard clinical management. In the same study, interpersonal therapy was less effective than imipramine maintenance treatment and the combination of psychotherapy and imipramine was no better than imipramine alone (Frank *et al.*, 1990). However, a more recent study in elderly depressed patients found that a combination of nortriptyline and interpersonal therapy was superior to nortriptyline and clinical management in preventing depressive relapse over 3 years (Reynolds *et al.*, 1999) (Box 11.7).

The assessment of depressive disorders

The steps in assessment are:

- to decide whether the diagnosis is depressive disorder;
- to judge the severity of the disorder, including the risk of suicide;
- to form an opinion about the causes;
- to assess the patient's social resources;
- to gauge the effect of the disorder on other people.

Diagnosis depends on thorough **history taking** and examination of the **physical and mental state**. It has been discussed earlier in this chapter. Particular care should be taken not to overlook a depressive disorder in the patient who does not complain spontaneously of being depressed ('masked depression'). It is equally important not to diagnose a depressive disorder simply on the grounds of prominent depressive symptoms; the latter could be part of another disorder, for example, a general medical condition. It should also be remembered that certain drugs both licit and illicit can induce depression (see p. 302 and Chapter 18).

The **history of previous mood disturbance** is important in assessment. Some patients will have had recurrent episodes of mood disorder. A history of these episodes often provides clues to the probable course of the current disorder and its response to treatment. It is particularly important to ask about possible previous episodes of **mania and hypomania**, even if mild and short-lived. If there is a history of mania, the mood disorder is bipolar. Interviews with relatives and close friends may help to establish whether such episodes have occurred.

The **severity** of the disorder is judged from the symptoms. Considerable severity is indicated by 'biological' symptoms, hallucinations, and delusions, particularly the latter two. It is also important to assess how the depressive disorder has reduced the patient's capacity to work or to engage in family life and social activities. In this assessment, the duration and course of the condition should be taken into account as well as the severity of the present symptoms. Not only does the length of history affect prognosis, but it also gives an indication of the patient's capacity to tolerate further distress. A long-continued disorder, even if not severe, can bring the patient to the point of desperation. The **risk of suicide** must be judged in every case (the methods of assessment are described on p. 414).

Aetiology is assessed next, with reference to precipitating, predisposing, and maintaining factors. No attempt need be made to allocate the syndrome to an exclusively 'endogenous' or 'reactive' category; instead, the importance of all relevant risk factors should be evaluated in every case.

Provoking causes may be psychological and social (the 'life events' discussed earlier in this chapter), or they may be physical illness and its treatment. In assessing such cases, it is good practice to enquire routinely into the patient's work, finances, family life, social activities, general living conditions, and physical health. Problems in these areas may be recent and acute, or may take the form of chronic background difficulties such as prolonged marital tension, problems with children, and financial hardship.

The patient's **social resources** are considered next. Enquires should cover family, friends, and work. A loving family can help to support a patient through a period of depressive disorder by providing company, encouraging them when they have lost confidence, and guiding him into suitable activities. For some patients, work is a valuable social resource, providing distraction and comradeship. For others it is a source of stress. A careful assessment is needed in each case.

The **effects of the disorder on other people** must be considered carefully. The most obvious problems arise when a severely depressed patient is the mother of young children who depend on her. This clinical observation has been confirmed in objective studies which have demonstrated that depressive disorder in either parent is associated with emotional disorder in the children (Cooper and Murray, 1998). It is important to consider whether the patient could endanger other people by remaining at work, for example, as a bus driver. When there are **depressive delusions**, it is necessary to consider what would happen if the patient were to act on them. For example, severely depressed mothers may occasionally kill their children because they believe them doomed to suffer if they remain alive.

BOX 11.7 WHAT PATIENTS AND FAMILIES WANT TO KNOW

Particularly for patients with a first episode of moderate to severe depression, questions such as the following are important:

1. What is wrong with me?
2. Can I recover?
3. What treatment do I need?
4. What can I do to improve the situation?
5. Can my family be helped?

The answers to these questions require a good knowledge of the patient and their circumstances. Patients will understand and appreciate that a careful practitioner will need to gather information before giving definitive answers to important questions. However, some general advice is given below:

- Depression is regarded as a medical condition and not any fault of the individual concerned. Feelings of guilt are common and are seen as part of the condition.
- The prognosis for individual episodes of depression is good, though people with depression are naturally pessimistic about the future.
- Treatment consists of a comprehensive package with psychological support and medication if indicated. The treatment plan will be developed as a collaborative exercise between patient and clinical team and the patient's rights and choices will be respected.
- Part of the treatment plan will involve a full discussion about the most appropriate level of occupational and social activity for the current circumstances. This will be reviewed frequently to allow adjustment with changing clinical state.
- It is very useful for the family to be fully involved in discussions about the nature of depression and the treatment plan; their support can be invaluable. Conversely critical comments can be demoralizing for depressed people. One of the aims of family involvement is to help improve mutual communication and support.

BOX 11.8 GUIDELINES FOR THE MANAGEMENT OF DEPRESSION

1. Patients with mild depression who may recover quickly without treatment should be offered an early review ('watchful waiting').
2. Antidepressants are not recommended for the treatment of mild depression.
3. Patients with persistent mild depression should be recommended to follow a guided self-help programme based on cognitive behaviour therapy. An exercise programme and sleep hygiene can also be recommended.
4. In both mild and moderate depression psychological treatment specifically focused on depression (such as problem-solving, brief cognitive behaviour therapy and counselling) should be considered.
5. If antidepressant treatment is used in moderate depression it should generally be with an SSRI.
6. Patients presenting with severe depression should be treated with a combination of cognitive behaviour therapy and antidepressant medication.
7. Patients with two or more significant depressive episodes in the recent past should be advised to continue antidepressant treatment for two years.
8. Combination treatment with cognitive behaviour therapy and antidepressant medication should be considered for patients in whom depression is treatment-resistant.
9. Cognitive behaviour therapy should be considered for patients with recurrent depression who have relapsed despite antidepressant treatment or who express a preference for psychological intervention.

National Institute for Clinical Excellence, 2004d

The management of depressive disorders

This section starts with the management of a patient with a depressive disorder of moderate or greater severity. The first question is whether the patient requires **inpatient or day-patient care**. The answer depends on the **severity of the disorder** and the quality of the patient's **social resources**. In judging severity, particular attention should be paid to the **risk of suicide** (or any risk to the life or welfare of family members, particularly dependent children) and to any failure to eat or drink that might endanger the patient's life. Provided that these risks are absent, most patients with a supportive family can be treated at home, even when severely depressed. Patients who live alone, or whose families cannot care for them during the day, may need inpatient or day-patient care, unless intensive community treatment is available. It is important that these important management decisions, as well subsequent treatment plans, are taken together with the patient in a collaborative way. Involvement of the family wherever possible is also likely to improve the outcome (Box 11.7).

If a patient is to remain out of hospital, the next question is whether they should continue to work. If the disorder is mild, work can provide a valuable distraction from depressive thoughts and a source of companionship. When the disorder is more severe, retardation, poor concentration, and lack of drive are likely to impair performance at work, and such failure may add to the patient's feelings of hopelessness. In severe disorders, there may be dangers to other people if the patient remains at his job.

The need for **antidepressant drug treatment** should be considered next. This treatment is indicated for most patients with a **major depressive syndrome** of at least moderate severity, and particularly those with **melancholic symptoms**. Other indications include a family history or personal history of depression, particularly if there has been a clear response to drug treatment. **Dysthymia** is also an indication for antidepressant medication but the role of antidepressants in **minor depressive disorders** is not established. Where, however, a patient with a clear history of major depression develops symptoms of minor depression antidepressant medication can be considered. Guidelines for a stepped care approach to the management of depression have been developed by the National Committee for Clinical Excellence (2004d) (Box 11.8).

Choice and use of antidepressant drug

Several kinds of antidepressant drug treatment are available, and the choice should be made in collaboration with the patient with particular consideration of likely side-effects. These are fully described in Chapter 21.

- **SSRIs** are the usual first choice in moderately depressed patients, unless the patient considers that he has done well previously with a different agent. **Lofepramine**, a tricyclic antidepressant that is relatively safe in overdose, is another non-sedating compound with a different side-effect profile (Table 11.8).

- **Mirtazapine** may be considered if patients need concomitant sedation.
- **Tricyclic antidepressants such as amitriptyline** may be the first choice for patients with severe depression, and particularly for depressed inpatients. For severely ill patients unable to tolerate tricyclics or where there are medical contraindications, **venlafaxine** is an alternative (though practitioners should be aware of recent restrictions on venlafaxine prescription issued by the UK Committee on Safety of Medicines, p. 555). Both amitriptyline and venlafaxine are less safe in overdose than the other compounds listed here.

The dosage of these drugs, the precautions to be observed in using them, and the instructions to be given to patients are described in Chapter 21. Here it is necessary only to emphasize again the importance of explaining to the patient that, although side-effects will appear quickly, the therapeutic effect is likely to be delayed for 2 weeks, with maximum improvement occurring over 6–12 weeks. During this time patients should be seen regularly to provide suitable clinical management (see above); those with more severe disorders may need to be seen every 2 or 3 days, and other patients once a week. It is important to make sure that the drugs are taken in the prescribed dose. Patients should be warned about the effects of **taking alcohol**. They should be advised about **driving**, particularly that they should not drive while experiencing sedative side-effects or any other effects that might impair their performance in an emergency.

The use of ECT

ECT will very rarely be part of the first-line treatment of depression and will usually be considered only for patients already admitted to hospital. The only indication for ECT as a first measure is the need to bring about improvement as rapidly as possible. In practice this applies to two main groups of patients:

- those who refuse to drink enough fluid to maintain an adequate output of urine (including the rare cases of depressive stupor)
- those who present a highly dangerous suicidal risk.

Occasionally, ECT is indicated for a patient who is suffering such extreme distress that the most rapid form of treatment is deemed justifiable. Such cases are rare. It should be remembered that, with the exception of patients who are unresponsive to antidepressant drugs, the effects of ECT differ from those of antidepressant drugs in greater rapidity of action rather than in the final therapeutic result. In patients with **depressive psychosis**, ECT is considerably more effective than an antidepressant given alone, but probably about the same therapeutic effect can be achieved, albeit more slowly, if a combination of an antidepressant drug and an antipsychotic drug is used.

Activity

The need for **suitable activity** should be considered for every patient. Depressed patients give up activities and withdraw from other people. In this way they become deprived of social stimulation and rewarding experiences, and their original feelings of depression are increased. It is important to make sure that the patient is occupied adequately, though they should not be pushed into activities where they are likely to fail because of slowness or poor concentration. Hence there is a fairly narrow range of activity that is appropriate for the individual depressed patient, and the range changes as the illness runs its course. If the patient remains at home, it is important to discuss with relatives how much they should be encouraged to do each day. For inpatients, the question should be decided by the clinical team.

Psychotherapy

The kind of appropriate psychological treatment should also be decided in every case. As noted earlier, all depressed patients require support, encouragement, and a thorough explanation that they are suffering from illness and not moral failure. Similar counselling of partners and other family members is often useful.

The use of one of the more specific psychological treatments discussed earlier should also be considered. These treatments can be used as the sole therapy for patients with mild-to-moderate depression without melancholic features, particularly when the patient prefers not to take drug therapy (National Institute for Clinical Excellence, 2004d). The kind of psychological treatment used depends largely on the availability of a suitably trained therapist and the preference of the patient although the more structured therapies (such as interpersonal therapy and cognitive therapy) have a greater evidence base in the treatment of moderate to severe depression. The therapeutic response to antidepressant drugs is usually quicker than that to psychotherapy.

Current recommendations are that in patients with severe depression it is helpful to add cognitive behaviour therapy to antidepressant medication (National Institute for Clinical Excellence, 2004d). In practice some time is usually needed to arrange cognitive

BOX 11.9 SOME PHARMACOLOGICAL TREATMENTS FOR RESISTANT DEPRESSION

- Increase antidepressant to maximum tolerated dose; measure tricyclic antidepressant levels; if patient has depressive psychosis add an antipsychotic drug; try different class of antidepressant drug, including venlafaxine and tricyclics
- Try antidepressant combination (eg SSRI or venlafaxine with mirtazapine)
- Add lithium to antidepressant drug treatment
- Add atypical antipsychotic drug to SSRI or venlafaxine
- Add tri-iodothyronine to tricyclic antidepressant treatment
- MAOIs (can be usefully combined with lithium)
- ECT

behaviour therapy and, in any event, some initial improvement produced by antidepressant medication may enable patients to make more use of psychological treatment (see Wolpert, 1999). It is also important to tackle psychosocial problems that make an important contribution to the depression. In particular, **couple therapy** can be a helpful addition in depressed patients where problems with a partner play a role in maintaining the disorder.

If the depressive disorder is severe, too much discussion of problems at an early stage is likely to increase the patient's feeling of hopelessness. Therapy directed to self-examination is particularly likely to make the disorder worse. During intervals between acute episodes, such therapy may be given to patients who have recurrent depressive disorders largely caused by their ways of reacting to life events.

Failure to respond to initial treatment

If a depressive disorder does not respond within a reasonable time to a chosen combination of antidepressant drugs, graded activity, and psychological treatment, the plan should be reviewed. The first step is to check again that the patient has been **taking medication** as prescribed. If not, the reasons should be sought. The patient may be convinced that no treatment can help, or may find the side-effects unpleasant. The diagnosis should also be reviewed carefully, and a check made that important stressful life events or continuing difficulties have not been overlooked.

If this enquiry is unrevealing, antidepressants should be continued at increased dose if possible. With certain tricyclic antidepressants, particularly in doses greater than 150 mg daily, it may be worth checking plasma concentrations (see p. 542). In general SSRIs do not have clear dose response relationships though some patients respond to higher doses, particularly if a partial response has been observed at a standard dose. Venlafaxine probably is more effective at higher doses in patients with treatment-resistant depression (see Cowen, 2005). If it becomes clear that the patient is not improving, a number of further steps can be taken (Box 11.9).

Change in antidepressant drug treatment

If a patient does not respond to one antidepressant, the first step is usually to stop the first medication and try another. Most published studies of this approach have studied patients in an open sequential way; clearly this cannot control for the placebo effect or the possibility of spontaneous remission. Overall, however, there is reasonable evidence that switching to a second antidepressant can produce benefit in about 50 per cent of patients unresponsive to an initial medication trial (see Nelson, 2003).

If a patient has not responded to one kind of antidepressant, it would seem sensible to switch to an antidepressant with a different pharmacological profile. However, it must be acknowledged that open studies have shown equally good response rates when patients who failed on one SSRI were switched to another. Switching from a drug with serotonergic properties to another serotonergic compound should be carried out cautiously because of the risk of serotonin toxicity. In practice this means that the first compound should be fully withdrawn if at all possible and the second started at a half-dose or less. In the case of fluoxetine, because of its long duration of action, at least a week should elapse before starting a second serotonergic agent. However, when switching between agents with different pharmacological properties (for example from citalopram to mirtazapine or reboxetine) cross-tapering can be employed. Detailed instructions are provided by the Maudsley Prescribing Guidelines (Taylor *et al.*, 2003).

Both amitriptyline (Barbui and Hotopf, 2001) and venlafaxine (Smith *et al.*, 2002) appear a little more effective than SSRIs; these drugs are therefore worth trying at some point in the management of patients unresponsive to initial medication trials. Similar comments apply to the use of conventional MAOIs, which have a clearly beneficial effect in some patients with resistant depression (Nolen *et al.*, 1988). However, the drug and food restrictions associated with MAOIs means that it is unusual to use them early in drug-resistant depression unless a patient has responded well to them in the past.

Augmentation of antidepressant drug treatment

In switching antidepressant preparations, a problem is that withdrawal of the first compound may not be straightforward. Patients may have gained some small benefit from the treatment, for example, improved sleep or reduced tension, and this benefit may be lost. Also, if the first medication is stopped quickly, withdrawal symptoms may result (see Chapter 21); however, if the dose is reduced gradually, the changeover in medication may be protracted and may not be easily tolerated by a depressed and despairing patient.

For this reason, in patients unresponsive or partly responsive to first-line medication it may be more appropriate to add a second compound to the antidepressant – so-called '**augmentation therapy**'. A disadvantage of augmentation therapy is the increased risk of adverse effects through drug interaction.

Lithium augmentation

We have already seen that data from randomized trials indicates that lithium can be effective in the treatment of resistant depression. Provided that there are no contraindications (see p. 560), the addition of lithium to antidepressant drug treatment is usually safe and well tolerated. About half of depressed patients will show a useful response over 1–3 weeks. Lithium can be added to any primary antidepressant medication with good effect, although combination with SSRIs and venlafaxine should be used with caution because of the risk of **5-HT neurotoxicity** (see p. 551). In the latter case it is appropriate to start lithium at a low dose (200 mg daily) and increase by a maximum of 200 mg weekly. In augmentation treatment, the aim should be to obtain a lithium level within the range used for prophylactic purposes (0.5–0.8 mmol/l); the lower end is appropriate for combination with serotonergic antidepressants. It has been suggested that the combination of lithium with MAOIs or clomipramine (sometimes supplemented with tryptophan) can be effective in depressed patients otherwise refractory to treatment (see Cowen, 2005).

Antipsychotic drugs

As noted above, in patients with psychotic depression it is usually best to prescribe a combination treatment of antidepressant and antipsychotic medication (see above). In non-psychotic resistant depression, conventional antipsychotic drugs are of little value except, at low doses, to ameliorate agitation and distress. There is, however, preliminary evidence that some atypical antipsychotic drugs may have antidepressant effects when used in combination with SSRIs in patients with non-psychotic depression. In a randomized controlled trial Shelton *et al.* (2001) found that in patients resistant to fluoxetine treatment the addition of olanzapine (5–20 mg) produced a significantly greater response rate than placebo addition or olanzapine monotherapy. Open studies also support the usefulness of low-dose risperidone augmentation of SSRI-resistant patients (see Cowen, 2005).

The use of atypical antidepressants to augment SSRIs employs lower doses than would be used to treat schizophrenia, perhaps because the key pharmacological mechanism involves 5-HT_2 receptor rather than dopamine D_2 receptor blockade. Despite this, olanzapine, even at low doses can cause troublesome sedation and weight gain while concomitant use of risperidone also produces a degree of weight gain together with hyperprolactinaemia.

Tri-iodothyronine (T3)

Some open and controlled studies have suggested that the addition of tri-iodothyronine (T3) in doses of 20–40 μg daily to ineffective TCA treatment can bring about a useful clinical response. However, a meta-analysis of four published randomized trials which assessed the efficacy of T3 addition to ineffective TCA treatment was not encouraging (Aronson *et al.*, 1996). It is also worth noting there are no controlled trials that have studied the effect of T3 augmentation of newer antidepressant drugs such as SSRIs. Despite this some depressed patients do seem to be helped by T3 addition which can start in a dose of 10μg daily and increase to 20 μg after a week, if tolerance is good. At this dose side effects are mild but tremor and sweating can occur. It is prudent not to use T3 addition in patients with evidence of cardiovascular disease.

Combination treatment with antidepressants

Combination strategies aim to supplement the antidepressant effect of an ineffective or partially effective medication with another antidepressant agent. This approach can therefore be considered an augmentation strategy though if the patient's condition remits it may be unclear whether the response is due to the combined effect of the two antidepressants or the second agent acting alone.

The pharmacological rationale of combination treatment is the use of two agents to produce a broader spectrum of activity on monoamine pathways than either agent could produce alone. In practice this means that SSRIs or venlafaxine are usually combined with noradrenergic promoting agents such as TCAs, reboxetine or mirtazapine (which increases noradrenaline function through blockade of auto-inhibitory α_2-adrenoceptors).

The evidence for any of these strategies is limited though they are endorsed in case series and expert reviews. The best evidence is probably for the addition of mirtazapine or its predecessor, mianserin, to ineffective SSRI treatment, though a large randomized trial in resistant depression failed to find a benefit of combined sertraline and mianserin over mianserin alone (see Cowen, 2005). Combination of tricyclic with SSRIs must be approached with caution because of the risk of elevation of tricyclic levels (see p. 547).

The use of ECT in resistant depression

If severe depression persists, ECT should be considered. ECT is often beneficial to patients who have not responded to antidepressant drugs, and it is probably more effective than drugs in the most severe depressions, particularly when psychotic features are present. Nevertheless, naturalistic studies suggest that the response rate in depressed patients **resistant to medication** (about 50 per cent) is lower than that expected in patients who are not medication resistant (about 80 per cent) (Prudic *et al.*, 1990).

It is important to note that, among patients who have not responded to full-dose antidepressant medication, the relapse rate in the year after ECT may be as high as 50 per cent. This may be because patients are often continued on the same antidepressant medication to which they previously failed to respond (Sackheim *et al.*, 1990). In these circumstances it seems reasonable to use an antidepressant of a different class or lithium for continuation treatment after ECT, but there is currently no evidence that this procedure lowers the relapse rate.

Other important measures

Continuing support is essential or patients who do not respond to treatment. Lack of improvement increases the pessimism experienced by the depressed patient. Hence it is important to give reassurance that depressive disorders have a good chance of recovering eventually, whether or not treatment speeds recovery. Meanwhile, if the patient is not too depressed, any problems that have contributed to their depressed state should be discussed further. Techniques derived from cognitive therapy can be used to help the patient to limit distorted thinking and judgement. In resistant cases, it is particularly important to watch carefully for suicidal intentions.

Prevention of relapse and recurrence

Drug treatment

Continuation therapy

After recovery, the patient should be followed up for several months by the psychiatric team or general practitioner. If the recovery appears to have been brought about by an antidepressant drug, the drug should usually be continued for about 6 months and then gradually withdrawn over several weeks. If residual symptoms are still present, it is safer not to withdraw medication. At follow-up interviews, a careful watch should be kept for **signs of discontinuation reactions** or **relapse**. It is helpful to discuss with the patient possible early signs of relapse and to develop plan of action should any of these signs appear. If the patient is in agreement it is helpful to involve relatives in this plan.

Maintenance treatment

Major depression is often recurrent, and long-term maintenance treatment may need to be considered. The risk factors for recurrence have been noted above (p. 246). In addition, the clinician will need to take into account other individual factors:

- the likely impact of a recurrence on the patient's life;
- the previous response to drug treatment;
- the patient's view of long-term drug treatment.

It is estimated that, among patients who have had three episodes of major depression, the chance of another episode is 90 per cent. The usual recommendation is that maintenance drug treatment should be considered if a patient has had two previous episodes of depression in a 5-year period, particularly if there is a family history of recurrent major depression or personal and social factors predictive of recurrence (Anderson *et al.*, 2000b). Persistent residual symptoms are also an indication for maintenance treatment.

Choice of medication

In most patients, the choice of antidepressant will be derived from their response in the acute or continuation phase of treatment. In this case, the same medication can be continued, if possible at the same dose. As noted earlier, newer antidepressant drugs are better tolerated in the longer term and may be preferred for maintenance treatment. If a change needs to be made because of adverse effects (for example, sexual dysfunction with SSRIs), an alternative choice should be determined by side-effect profile.

Lithium can also be effective for long-term maintenance of recurrent depression in some patients. Its adverse effect profile and the need for plasma monitoring means that it will not be a first choice for most patients but its use should be considered if there is any history of manic episodes, even where these have been mild and transient. In addition, lithium will sometimes be effective in patients with recurrent depression who do not respond to maintenance treatment with antidepressants.

Other measures

If a depressive disorder was related to self-imposed stressors, such as overwork or complicated social relationships, the patient should be encouraged to change to a lifestyle that is less likely to lead to further illness. These readjustments may be helped by psychotherapy, which may be individual, marital, or group therapy. As noted above, cognitive behaviour therapy appears to be helpful in lowering the risk of relapse in patients with residual depressive symptomatology. Community nurses and nurse therapists can play a valuable role in delivering treatment of this kind.

General practitioners can play a key role in long-term monitoring of patients and should always be involved in treatment planning. This involvement can be particularly helpful if an intercurrent illness occurs.

The assessment of mania

In the assessment of mania, the steps are the same as those for depressive disorders, as outlined above:

- decide the diagnosis;
- assess the severity of the disorder;
- form an opinion about the causes;
- assess the patient's social resources;
- judge the effects on other people.

Diagnosis depends on a careful history and examination. Whenever possible, the history should be taken from relatives as well as from the patient because the latter may not recognize the extent of their abnormal behaviour. Differential diagnosis has been discussed earlier in this chapter. It is always important to remember that mildly disinhibited behaviour can result from frontal lobe lesions (such as tumours) as well as from mania. There should be a urine screen for illicit substances.

Severity is judged next. For this purpose, it is essential to interview an informant as well as the patient. Manic patients may exert some self-control during an interview with a doctor, and may then behave in a disinhibited and grandiose way immediately afterwards. At an early stage of mania, the doctor can easily be misled and may lose the opportunity to persuade the patient to enter hospital before causing himself long-term difficulties, for example, ill-judged decisions or unjustified extravagance. Where possible, it is important to identify any life events that may have provoked the onset of manic illness. Some manic episodes follow physical illness, treatment by drugs (especially steroids or antidepressants), or operations. **Sleep deprivation** may trigger mania in some susceptible individuals.

The patient's resources and the effect of the illness on other people are assessed in the ways described above for depressive disorders. Even for the most supportive family, it is extremely difficult to care for a manic patient at home for more than a few days unless the disorder is exceptionally mild. The patient's responsibilities in the care of dependent children or at work should always be considered carefully.

The management of mania

Acute episodes

The first decision is whether to **admit the patient to hospital**. In all but the mildest cases, admission is nearly always advisable to protect the patient from the consequences of their own behaviour. If the disorder is not too severe, the patient will usually agree to enter hospital after some persuasion. When the disorder is more severe, compulsory admission is likely to be needed.

Clinical management

Development of a **therapeutic alliance** with the manic patient is an important goal of treatment although lack of insight and anger at involuntary detention can make this a testing and timeconsuming process. It is best to use an understanding, yet firm, approach which minimizes confrontation. For example, it is often possible to avoid an argument by taking advantage of the manic patient's easy distractibility; instead of refusing demands, it is better to delay until the patient's attention turns to another topic that they can be encouraged to pursue. In hospital, nursing staff play a pivotal role in this kind of management where they attempt to provide manic patients with a low-stimulus and safe environment which limits confrontations and ill-judged sexual liaisons.

Supportive, reality-orientated psychotherapy is an important part of treatment and may need to be extended to partners and family who often will have suffered great strain through the manic episode.

Educational sessions are important when patients are more settled. Patients may need much practical help to limit financial, legal, and occupational repercussions of the illness.

Medication

Medication plays an important role in the acute management of mania. However, all current drug treatments have limitations in terms of efficacy and tolerability. In the UK, antipsychotic drugs are generally used as primary agents in acute mania, with mood stabilizers being reserved for longer-term prophylaxis or where the initial response to antipsychotic drugs is unsatisfactory. For patients not already taking mood-stabilizers, the drug management can summarized as follows:

- begin treatment with an atypical antispychotic drug (a modest dose of haloperidol is an alternative;
- where needed, use adjunctive high-potency benzodiazepines (for example, lorazepam or clonazepam) to prevent the need for high-dose antipsychotic therapy and to ensure satisfactory sleep;
- add a mood stabilizer if the response to this treatment is unsatisfactory (use lithium for 'classical' mania and valproate for mania with prominent dysphoric or mixed states or where lithium is contraindicated).

If it is decided to use a mood stabilizer as the initial treatment, the choice lies between lithium and valproate. Valproate is somewhat easier to use and has a faster onset of action. As before, benzodiazepines can be used as an adjunct to reduce overactivity and permit sleep, whilst antipsychotic agents can be reserved for patients unresponsive to these measures. If a patient presents with a manic episode and is already taking a mood stabilizer, the first step is to optimize the mood stabilizer treatment in terms of dosing and adherence. Concomitant treatment with antipsychotic drugs will then probably be needed; addition of a second mood-stabilizing drug is an alternative (Goodwin, 2003).

Progress of a manic episode can be judged not only by the **mental state** and **general behaviour**, but also by the **pattern of sleep** and the regaining of any weight lost during the illness. As progress continues, antipsychotic drug treatment is reduced gradually. It is important not to discontinue the drug too soon; otherwise, there may be a relapse and a return of all the original problems of management.

ECT was used to treat mania before antipsychotic drugs were introduced, but evidence about its effectiveness is still limited (see above). It is appropriate to consider the treatment for the unusual patients who do not respond to drug treatment even when given at maximum doses. In such cases, clinical experience suggests that ECT may often be followed by a significant reduction in symptoms sufficient to allow treatment to be continued with drugs. ECT may also be helpful for **mixed affective states** in which depressive symptoms are prominent.

Whatever treatment is adopted, a careful watch should be kept for symptoms of **depressive disorder**. It should be remembered that transient but profound depressive mood change, accompanied by depressive ideas, is common among manic patients (see Mixed states p. 224). The clinical picture may also change rapidly to a sustained depressive disorder. If either change happens, the patient may develop suicidal ideas. A sustained change to a depressive syndrome is likely to require additional treatment unless the disorder is mild.

Treatment of bipolar depression

Depressive episodes are common in bipolar illness. Treatment of depression in the context of a bipolar disorder can be problematic because standard antidepressant treatments carry a number of disadvantages:

- apparent lower efficacy than in unipolar depression;
- risk of inducing mania;
- risk of inducing rapid cycling.

Lithium can be a useful antidepressant in bipolar patients and does not cause mania. On the other hand, it is ineffective in a significant proportion of cases and many bipolar patients become depressed despite taking lithium. In these circumstances, the use of antidepressants is common and despite the problems outlined above, a recent systematic review (Gijsman *et al.*, 2004) showed that antidepressant treatment is effective in the treatment of bipolar depression. However, the rate of switching into mania with tricyclic antidepressants (10 per cent) was greater than that seen with either SSRIs (3.2 per cent) or placebo (4 per cent) suggesting that SSRIs are safer from this point of view. The treatment of bipolar depression with antidepressant medication should generally include a mood stabilizer because this probably lessens the risk of manic upswing (Goodwin, 2003).

Lamotrigine may also have a role in the acute management of bipolar depression (Calabrese *et al.*, 1999) and is probably free of the risk of inducing mania or rapid cycling. Atypical antipsychotic drugs have also been studied. Tohen *et al.* (2003) reported a randomized study of olanzapine and combined olanzapine and fluoxetine treatment in 833 patients with bipolar depression. Remission rates were best in the olanzapine–fluoxetine treatment group (48.8 per cent) followed by olanzapine alone (32.8 per cent) and then placebo (24.5 per cent). Rates of mania onset did not differ between any of the treatment groups. For a review of the treatment of bipolar depression see Frangou (2005).

Prevention of relapse and recurrence

Continuation treatment

Since the untreated duration of a manic episode can be several months (see above), some form of **continuation treatment**, as in the management of depression, is advisable for at least 6 months. As a guide, treatment should not be withdrawn finally until patients have been asymptomatic for at least 8 weeks. Withdrawal of lithium should be particularly cautious (for example, by not more than about 100 mg a week) because sudden discontination can lead to **'rebound' mania** (Goodwin, 2003).

Maintenance treatment

Medication

We have already seen that the majority of patients with bipolar disorder will experience recurrence, suffering both depressive and manic episodes, though the pattern in individual patients is variable. For patients who have had two or more episodes of illness in less than 5 years, particularly where the illnesses have proved personally disruptive or hazardous, longer-term maintenance treatment should be considered. This will usually involve long-term treatment with a mood stabilizer.

People with bipolar disorder are often reluctant to consider long-term treatment with medication. There are usually a number of reasons for this and it necessary to spend time in discussion with patients so that their point of view can be fully appreciated and understood. An excellent personal account is given by Jamison (1997). Among the reasons may be:

- Difficulties in accepting a diagnosis of a life-long condition and the need for maintenance treatment with medicines. Issues of stigma are usually important.
- A belief that it should be possible to control mood without medication and that the use of medication for this purpose signals personal weakness.
- A fear that medication will blunt emotional life, sometimes specifically that mood-stabilizing drugs will decrease feelings of joy and creativity. If the latter feelings are associated with hypomania it is indeed possible that they will be lessened by medication. For some individuals this can represent a significant loss which needs to balanced against the prevention of disabling episodes of depression.

In the UK, lithium is still regarded as the first choice of mood stabilizer, although in the USA valproate is the most popular because of its better tolerability. However, the evidence for its long-term prophylactic efficacy is less complete. In addition, there is evidence that the supervised use of lithium is associated with a decreased risk of suicidal behaviour in bipolar illness.

The practical aspects of using lithium to prevent further episodes are discussed on p. 560. There are two aspects of maintenance that require emphasis. First, patients should be seen and plasma lithium and renal and thyroid function assessed at regular intervals. Second, some patients stop lithium of their own accord because they fear that the drug may have harmful long-term effects or because it makes them feel 'flat'. The risk of stopping lithium suddenly is that it may well lead to relapse. Therefore, patients should be advised to discontinue lithium slowly under supervision.

With carefully supervised follow-up, the chances of relapse can be reduced substantially by maintenance treatment, though lesser degrees of mood change often continue. These mood changes often require adjunctive antidepressant or antipsychotic drug treatment. For patients who do not show a good response to lithium, alternative mood-stabilizing drugs can be used. It is possible to use combinations of mood stabilizers, although the risk of adverse reactions is increased.

Rapid-cycling disorder Some patients with bipolar disorder develop rapid-cycling mood disorder (see p. 224). Sometimes this disorder is apparently provoked by antidepressant treatment, in which case the best plan is to try to withdraw the antidepressant drug. Rapid cycling often requires treatment with combinations of mood stabilizers and occasionally atypical antipsychotic drugs can be helpful. In particularly resistant cases the use of high dose thyroid hormone has been advocated (For a review see Mackin and Young, 2004).

Psychosocial approaches

Bipolar disorder is often a life-long, disruptive illness which carries a substantial morbidity. There are several areas of psychosocial function where problems may arise:

- adjustment to diagnosis and need for lifestyle limitations;
- interpersonal and marital difficulties;
- occupational problems;

BOX 11.10 PSYCHOLOGICAL APPROACHES TO BIPOLAR DISORDER

- advice about lifestyle (regular social and sleep routines, avoidance of illicit drugs);
- identification and avoidance of triggers for relapse (for example, sleep deprivation, substance misuse);
- identification of early subjective signs of relapse (for example, feeling driven, sleeping badly) with contingency plans for action;
- education about the importance of medication. Sensitivity to side-effects and active measures to reduce them.

- misuse of both illegal and legal substances;
- problems relating to concordance with medication.

Psychological treatment approaches designed to help with these important problems employ a number of theoretical approaches. However, they have a number of features in common which centre around education about the illness and enhancing self-management (Goodwin, 2003) (Box 11.11).

Although there are some useful drug therapies for bipolar illness, the effectiveness of treatment in clinical practice is often disappointing. The use of the psychosocial measures outlined above should enhance the overall effectiveness of treatment plans and preliminary randomized trials are promising in this respect (Goodwin, 2003).

Further reading

Griez EJ, Faravelli C, Nutt DJ, Zohar J (2005) *Mood disorders: clinical management and research issues.* John Wiley, Chichester. (Multi-author textbook with comprehensive coverage of clinical research and management of mood disorders.)

Kraepelin, E (1921) *Manic-depressive insanity and paranoia* (transl. R. M. Barclay), Churchill Livingstone, Edinburgh, pp. 1–164. Reprinted in 1976 by Arno Press, New York. (The classical account. See especially the description of untreated mania - seldom seen today.)

Jamison, KR (1997) *An unquiet mind.* Picador, London. (A superb autobiographical account of the experience of bipolar illness and its treatment.)

Lewis, AJ (1934) Melancholia: a clinical survey of depressive states. *Journal of Mental Science* **80**, 277–378. Reprinted in Lewis, AJ (1967) *Inquiries in Psychiatry*, Routledge and Kegan Paul, London, pp. 30–117. (This landmark study contains a detailed account of the clinical picture of depressive disorder.)

CHAPTER 12

Schizophrenia

Chapter contents

Of all the major psychiatric syndromes, schizophrenia is the most difficult to define and describe. This largely reflects the fact that, over the past 100 years, widely divergent concepts have been held in different countries and by different psychiatrists. Although there is now a greater consensus, substantial uncertainties remain. Indeed, schizophrenia remains the best example of the fundamental issues with which psychiatry continues to grapple: concepts of disease, classification, and aetiology.

Having noted the complexities, we start with an introduction to two basic concepts – **acute schizophrenia** and **chronic schizophrenia**. The reader should bear in mind that these will be idealized descriptions and comparisons, but it is useful to oversimplify at first before introducing the controversial issues.

The predominant clinical features in acute schizophrenia are delusions, hallucinations, and interference with thinking (Table 12.1). Features of this kind are often called **positive symptoms**. Some patients recover from the acute illness, whilst others progress to the chronic syndrome; its main features are very different: apathy, lack of drive, slowness, and social withdrawal (Table 12.2). These features are often called **negative symptoms**. Once the chronic syndrome is established, few patients recover completely. In both phases of the disorder, there may also be cognitive and affective symptoms and other features (p. 271).

TABLE 12.2 The most frequent features in chronic schizophrenia

Characteristic	Frequency (%)
Social withdrawal	74
Underactivity	56
Lack of conversation	54
Few leisure interests	50
Slowness	48
Overactivity	41
Odd ideas	34
Depression	34
Odd behaviour	34
Neglect of appearance	30
Odd postures and movements	25
Threats or violence	25
Poor mealtime behaviour	13
Socially embarrassing behaviour	8
Sexually unusual behaviour	8
Suicidal attempts	4
Incontinence	4

Source: Creer and Wing (1975).

Clinical features

In this section, it is assumed that the reader has read the descriptions of symptoms and signs in Chapters 1 and 3, which include definitions of many of the cardinal features of schizophrenia.

TABLE 12.1 The most frequent symptoms of acute schizophrenia

Symptom	Frequency (%)
Lack of insight	97
Auditory hallucinations	74
Ideas of reference	70
Suspiciousness	66
Flatness of affect	66
Voices speaking to the patient	65
Delusional mood	64
Delusions of persecution	64
Thought alienation	52
Thoughts spoken aloud	50

Source: World Health Organization (1973).

The acute syndrome

The vignette in Box 12.1 illustrates several common features of acute schizophrenia: prominent persecut-

BOX 12.1 A VIGNETTE OF ACUTE SCHIZOPHRENIA

A previously healthy 20-year-old male student had been behaving in an increasingly odd way. At times he appeared angry and told his friends that he was being persecuted; at other times he was seen to be laughing to himself for no apparent reason. For several months he had seemed increasingly preoccupied with his own thoughts. His academic work had deteriorated. When interviewed, he was restless and awkward. He described hearing voices commenting on his actions and abusing him. He said that he believed that the police had conspired with his university teachers to harm his brain with poisonous gases and take away his thoughts. He also believed that other people could read his thoughts.

ory delusions, with accompanying hallucinations, gradual social withdrawal and impaired performance at work, and the odd idea that other people can read one's thoughts.

In appearance and behaviour some patients with acute schizophrenia are entirely normal. Others seem changed, although not always in a way that would immediately point to psychosis. They may be preoccupied with their health, their appearance, religion, or other intense interests. Social withdrawal may occur, for example spending a long time in their room, perhaps lying immobile on the bed. Some patients smile or laugh without obvious reason. Some appear to be constantly perplexed, whilst others are restless and noisy, or show sudden and unexpected variability of behaviour.

The speech often reflects an underlying thought disorder. In the early stages, there is vagueness in the patient's talk that makes it difficult to grasp his meaning. Some patients have difficulty in dealing with abstract ideas. Other patients become preoccupied with vague pseudoscientific or mystical ideas. When the thought disorder is more severe, two characteristic kinds of abnormality may occur. Disorders of the stream of thought include pressure of thought, poverty of thought, and thought blocking, described on p. 15. Thought withdrawal (p. 12) is also not uncommon. Disorders of the form of thought are reflected in the loosening of association between expressed ideas. This may be detected in illogical thinking (for example, 'knight's move') or talking past the point (*Vorbeireden*, p. 15). In the severest form of loosening, the structure and coherence of thinking is lost, so that utterances are jumbled (word salad or verbigeration). Some patients use ordinary words or phrases in unusual ways (metonyms or paraphrases), and a few coin new words (neologisms).

Abnormalities of mood are common and are of three main kinds. First, there may be sustained abnormalities such as anxiety, depression, irritability, or euphoria. Second, there may be blunting (or flattening) of affect (p. 5), the sustained emotional indifference or diminution of emotional response. Third, there is incongruity of affect (p. 5), in which the expressed mood is not in keeping with the situation or with the patient's own feelings.

Auditory hallucinations are among the most frequent symptoms. They may take the form of noises, music, single words, brief phrases, or whole conversations. They may be unobtrusive or so severe as to cause great distress. Some voices seem to give commands to the patient. Some patients hear their own thoughts apparently spoken out loud either as they think them (*Gedankenlautwerden*) or immediately afterwards (*echo de la pensée*). Some voices discuss the patient in the third person or comment on his actions. As described later, these last three symptoms have particular diagnostic value. Visual hallucinations are less frequent and usually occur together with other kinds of hallucination. Tactile, olfactory, gustatory, and somatic hallucinations are reported by some patients. They are often interpreted in a delusional way; for example, hallucinatory sensations in the lower abdomen are attributed to unwanted sexual interference by a persecutor.

Delusions are characteristic. Primary delusions (p. 10) are infrequent and are difficult to identify with certainty. Delusions may originate against a background of so-called primary delusional mood (*Wahnstimmung*, p. 10). Persecutory delusions are common, but are not specific to schizophrenia. Less common but of greater diagnostic value are delusions of reference and of control, and delusions about the possession of thought. The latter are delusions that thoughts are being inserted into or withdrawn from one's mind, or 'broadcast' to other people (p. 12).

Insight is almost always impaired. Most patients do not accept that their experiences result from illness, but usually ascribe them to the malevolent actions of other people.

Orientation is usually normal, although this may be difficult to determine if there is florid thought disorder or if the person is too preoccupied with their psychotic experience to attend to the interviewer's questions.

Finally, we emphasize the variability of the clinical picture. Few patients experience all the symptoms introduced above, whilst others already have features of the 'chronic' syndrome at first presentation. Moreover, the overall pattern, and duration, of features are also taken into account before making a diagnosis. These issues are discussed later in the chapter.

The chronic syndrome

In contrast with the 'positive' symptoms of the acute syndrome, the chronic syndrome is characterized by the 'negative' symptoms of underactivity, lack of drive, social withdrawal, and emotional apathy, and by thought disorder (Box 12.2).

This description illustrates several of the negative features of what is sometimes called a schizophrenic defect state. The most striking feature is diminished **volition**, that is, a lack of drive and initiative. Left to herself, the patient may be inactive for long periods, or may engage in aimless and repeated activity. She withdraws from social encounters and her social behaviour may deteriorate in ways that embarrass other people. Self-care may be poor and, particularly in women, the

BOX 12.2 VIGNETTE OF CHRONIC SCHIZOPHRENIA

A middle-aged man lives in a group home and attends a sheltered workshop. He spends most of his time alone. He is usually dishevelled and unshaven, and cares for himself only when encouraged to do so by others. His social behaviour seems odd and stilted. His speech is slow, and its content is vague and incoherent. He shows few signs of emotion. For several years this clinical picture has changed little except for brief periods of acute symptoms which are usually related to upsets in the ordered life of the hostel.

style of dress and presentation may be careful but somewhat inappropriate. Some patients collect and hoard objects, so that their surroundings become cluttered and dirty. Others break social conventions by talking intimately to strangers or shouting obscenities in public. These behavioural difficulties may be compounded by a worsening of cognitive impairment in elderly patients.

Speech is often abnormal, showing evidence of thought disorder of the kinds found in the acute syndrome described above. Affect is generally blunted; when emotion is shown, it is often incongruous. Hallucinations and delusions are common but by no means universal. They tend to be held with little emotional response. For example, patients may be convinced that they are being persecuted but show neither fear nor anger.

Various disorders of movement occur, including stereotypies, mannerisms and other catatonic symptoms, and dyskinesias (p. 16, Hamilton, 1984). The latter are common, primarily but not entirely due to antipsychotic medication (p. 534).

As with acute schizophrenia, the symptoms and signs of the chronic illness are variable. At any stage, positive symptoms may recur or become exacerbated; this may be in response to life events, or discontinuation of medication.

Subtypes of schizophrenia

Schizophrenia is conventionally divided into several subtypes, based upon the predominant clinical features.

- **Paranoid schizophrenia** is the commonest form. It is characterized by persecutory delusions, often systematized, and by persecutory auditory hallucinations. Thought disorder and affective, catatonic and negative symptoms are not prominent. Personality is relatively well preserved. It has a later age of onset, and better prognosis, than other subtypes.
- In **hebephrenic schizophrenia**, also called **disorganized schizophrenia**, thought disorder and affective symptoms are prominent. The mood is variable, with behaviour often appearing silly and unpredictable. Delusions and hallucinations are fleeting and not systematized. Mannerisms are common. Speech is rambling and incoherent, reflecting the thought disorder. Negative symptoms occur early, and contribute to a poor prognosis.
- In **catatonic schizophrenia**, the most striking features are motor symptoms, as noted on p. 16, and by changes in activity varying between excitement and stupor. At times the person may appear to be in a dream-like (**oneiroid**) state. Formerly common, it is now very rare, at least in industrialized countries. Possible reasons include a change in the nature of the illness, improvements in treatment, or past misdiagnosis of organic syndromes with catatonic symptoms.
- **Simple schizophrenia** is characterized by the insidious development of odd behaviour, social withdrawal, and declining performance at work. Delusions and hallucinations are not evident. Since clear schizophrenic symptoms are absent, simple schizophrenia is difficult to identify reliably, and the category is now infrequently used.
- **Undifferentiated schizophrenia** is the term for cases which do not fit readily into any of these subtypes, or where there are equally prominent features of more than one of them.

Two other categories have been introduced more recently. **Residual schizophrenia** refers to a stage of chronic schizophrenia when, for at least a year, there have been persistent negative symptoms but no recurrence of positive symptoms. **Deficit syndrome** describes a subtype of schizophrenia with early, severe and persistent negative symptoms (Carpenter *et al.*, 1988).

These various subtypes are primarily descriptive rather than delineating valid subsyndromes, although paranoid schizophrenia may have a somewhat different (and lesser) genetic loading. Hence other subclassifications of schizophrenia have been proposed, intended to reflect biologically more valid entities. Two prominent examples are given here.

Type I and type II schizophrenia

Crow (1985) described two syndromes of schizophrenia, based upon a combination of clinical and neurobiological factors. **Type I** has an acute onset, mainly positive symptoms, and preserved social functioning during remissions. It has a good response to antipsychotic drugs, associated with biochemical evidence of dopamine overactivity. By contrast, **type II** has an insidious onset, mainly negative symptoms, poor outcome and response to antipsychotic drugs, and without evidence of dopamine overactivity but with structural brain changes (especially ventricular enlargement). In practice, although some patients can be recognized to have type I syndrome, those with pure type II are much less common and most patients show a mixture of both. Moreover, subsequent research does not strongly support the biological subtypes and correlations which are predicted by the model. However, it was important as an example of the renewed focus on the neurobiological aspects of schizophrenia which occurred around that time.

Three clinical syndromes

Recent studies have proposed more complex delineations and correlates of psychopathology. The most important is that of Liddle (1987). He studied patients with chronic schizophrenia and described three overlapping clinical syndromes, which he called **reality disturbance**, **disorganisation**, and **psychomotor poverty** (Table 12.3). Later studies have essentially confirmed these findings. Notably, Liddle linked these symptom clusters to patterns of neuropsychological deficit and to regional cerebral blood flow (Liddle *et al.*, 1992). The most reproducible finding is the link between psychomotor poverty, impaired performance on frontal lobe tasks, and decreased frontal blood flow.

Other aspects of the clinical syndrome

Depressive symptoms

It has been recognized since the time of Kraepelin that depressive symptoms commonly occur in schizophrenia, at any phase of the illness, including before the florid positive symptoms become apparent. In addition, about a quarter of patients subsequently exhibit persistent and significant depression, called **post-schizophrenic depression**.

There are several reasons why depressive symptoms may be associated with schizophrenia:

- Depression may be an integral part of schizophrenia. This view is supported by the observation that about 50 per cent of patients with acute schizophrenia experience significant depressive symptomatology which improves as the psychosis remits.
- In the post-psychotic phase, depressive symptoms may be a response to recovery of insight into the nature of the illness and the problems to be faced. Again, this may happen at times, but it does not provide a convincing general explanation.
- Depression may be a side-effect of antipsychotic medication. This is not the only explanation since depressive symptoms can occur in the absence of antipsychotic drug therapy.

Depressive symptoms in schizophrenia should not be confused with motor side-effects of medication or negative symptoms. These distinctions are important but can be difficult to make. For a review of the relationship between depression and schizophrenia see Mulholland and Cooper (2000).

Cognitive features

Cognitive features are an important but neglected component of schizophrenia (Sharma and Harvey, 2000;

TABLE 12.3 Cerebral and psychological correlates of three symptom clusters

Syndrome	Symptoms	Regional cerebral bloodflow correlates	Impaired psychological performance
Reality disturbance	Delusions, hallucinations	Left medial temporal lobe, cingulate cortex	Disorders of self-monitoring
Disorganization	Formal thought disorder, inappropriate affect, bizarre behaviour	Anterior cingulate, right ventral frontal cortex, bilateral parietal regions	Tests of selective attention
Psychomotor poverty	Flat affect, poverty of speech, decreased spontaneous movement	Underactivity of frontal cortex	Word generation tasks, planning tests

Goldberg *et al.*, 2003). Impairments are seen in all domains of learning and memory, with disproportionate involvement of semantic memory, working memory, and attention. Such deficits average 1–2 standard deviations below expected performance. Selective deficits in working memory (suggestive of prefrontal cortex dysfunction) are seen even in patients with otherwise intact neuropsychological performance.

The time course of neuropsychological involvement in schizophrenia is complex and not entirely clear. People who develop schizophrenia already have reduced scores on IQ tests during childhood. The onset of illness is associated with further cognitive impairments, which may partially improve after resolution of the acute episode. However, most of the cognitive deficits appear to be trait rather than state features, largely independent of other symptom domains. In the seventh decade a proportion of patients undergo a substantial decline in cognitive performance and develop severe dementia, similar in nature to Alzheimer's disease, but without any detectable neuropathology. Like many other features of schizophrenia, cognitive deficits are seen in attenuated form in unaffected relatives, suggesting that they are related to the genetic predisposition.

Cognitive aspects of schizophrenia are currently being emphasized for several reasons. First, because they are a major determinant of poor functional outcome (Green *et al.*, 2000). Second, they are now viewed as potential therapeutic targets (see p. 300). Third, cognitive features are increasingly conceptualized as core symptoms or endophenotypes (p. 284) of schizophrenia. Reflecting the increasing relevance of cognitive dysfunction in schizophrenia, methods are being developed to allow its rapid assessment in routine practice, for example, the Repeatable Battery for the Assessment of Neuropsychological Status (RBANS; Gold *et al.*, 1999).

Neurological signs

Neurological signs are another neglected clinical feature of schizophrenia (Heinrichs and Buchanan, 1988). They are called 'soft signs' as they do not localize pathology to a particular tract or nucleus. They include abnormalities in sensory integration, coordination, and sequencing of complex motor acts; catatonic features and dyskinesias may also be considered under this category. Neurological signs are seen in unmedicated, first-episode patients (and are therefore separate from the effects of antipsychotic drugs in this regard) but are commoner in chronic schizophrenia. The presence of neurological signs correlates with cognitive dysfunction, evidence for developmental anomaly, and diffuse brain pathology, and they are thought to be a manifestation of the neurodevelopmental origins of schizophrenia. Neurological signs in schizophrenia can be assessed using the Neurological Evaluation Scale (Buchanan and Heinrichs, 1989). For a review, see Bombin *et al.*, 2005.

Olfactory dysfunction

Patients with schizophrenia have deficits in olfactory function, affecting the identification of, sensitivity to, and memory for, odours (Moberg *et al.*, 1999). The deficits are not attributable to medication or smoking. They are prominent in patients with the deficit syndrome, and are worse in the left than the right nostril, perhaps related to other evidence of lateralized pathology in schizophrenia (p. 284). Their clinical relevance is that they may contribute to the lack of social drive apparent in many patients (Malaspina and Coleman, 2003).

Water intoxication

A few patients with chronic schizophrenia drink excessive amounts of water, thus developing a state of water intoxication characterized by polyuria and hyponatraemia. When this condition is severe, it may give rise to cerebral oedema, seizures, coma, and sometimes death. The 'drive' to drink water may include unsuitable sources, such as toilet bowls. The reasons for this behaviour are unknown. Possible mechanisms include a response to a delusional belief, shared genetic factors, or abnormalities affecting hypothalamic regulation of thirst and antidiuretic hormone release (see Merceir-Guidez and Loas, 1998).

Factors modifying the clinical features

The social and cultural background of the patient may affect the content of symptoms. For example, religious delusions are less common now than a century ago, replaced by delusions concerned with cloning, satellites, or HIV. Age also seems to modify the clinical features of schizophrenia. In adolescents and young adults, the clinical features often include thought disorder, mood disturbance, passivity phenomena, thought insertion, and withdrawal. With increasing age paranoid symptomatology is more common, with more organized delusions.

Intelligence also affects the clinical features and the psychiatrist's ability to elicit them. Patients with learning disability usually present with a simple clinical picture, sometimes referred to as *pfropfschizophrenie*. In contrast, highly intelligent people develop complex delusional systems, and are also better able to articulate, or conceal, their experiences.

The amount of social stimulation has a considerable effect on the clinical picture. Understimulation is thought to increase negative symptoms, whereas overstimulation precipitates positive symptoms. Modern psychosocial approaches to treatment are designed to avoid both extremes: the understimulation associated with institutionalization, and the excess stimulation of high expressed emotion (p. 299).

Diagnosis and classification

This section is concerned mainly with the diagnostic criteria and classification of schizophrenia as specified in DSM-IV and ICD-10. However, the current approach - and its problems - can be understood better with some knowledge of the historical perspective.

Historical development of ideas about schizophrenia

The development of ideas about schizophrenia is discussed in Box 12.3. To a large extent, they mirror the development of ideas about psychiatric illness in general, reflecting the central position in psychiatry held by schizophrenia during the last century. For review, see Berrios (2000).

In the 1960s it was noticed that there were wide divergences in the use of the term schizophrenia, and marked differences in diagnostic practice. This was unsurprising, given the multiple views and traditions summarized in Box 12.3. For example, in the UK and continental Europe, psychiatrists generally employed Schneider's first rank symptoms to identify a narrowly delineated group of cases. In the USA, however, interest in psychodynamic processes led to diagnosis on the basis of mental mechanisms and to the inclusion of a much wider group of cases. First admission rates for schizophrenia were also much higher in the USA than in the UK.

These discrepancies prompted two major cross-national studies of diagnostic practice, introduced in Chapter 2, which proved highly influential not just for schizophrenia but for the development of diagnostic criteria and classificatory systems. The US-UK Diagnostic Project (Cooper *et al.*, 1972) confirmed that the concept of schizophrenia was much wider in New York than in the UK. In New York the concept included cases that were diagnosed in the UK as mood disorder or personality disorder. The International Pilot Study of Schizophrenia (IPSS) was concerned with the diagnosis of schizophrenia in nine countries (World Health Organization, 1973). The main finding was that similar criteria were adopted in seven of the nine countries: Colombia, Czechoslovakia, Denmark, India, Nigeria, Taiwan, and the UK. Broader criteria were used in the USA and the former USSR.

These findings led to a consensus that agreed diagnostic criteria were required, and development of standardized methods by which these criteria could be defined and identified. Three examples, all of which contributed to the current DSM-IV and ICD-10 criteria, are mentioned here. CATEGO is a computer program designed to process data from a standard interview known as the Present State Examination (p. 63). The narrowest syndrome (S+) is diagnosed mainly on the symptoms of thought intrusion, broadcast, or withdrawal, delusions of control, and voices discussing the patient in the third person or commenting on his actions. The Feighner criteria (Feighner *et al.*, 1972) were developed in St Louis to identify patients with a poor prognosis. They include symptomatic criteria that are less precise than those in CATEGO, 6 months' continuous illness, and exclude cases meeting diagnostic criteria for mood disorder or substance misuse. The criteria are reliable but restrictive, leaving many cases without a diagnosis. Patients with a poor prognosis are identified well (probably because of the criterion of 6 months' continuous illness). The Research Diagnostic Criteria (RDC) were developed from those of Feighner by Spitzer *et al.*, (1978). The main difference is that only a 2 week history is required to make the diagnosis. A structured interview, the Schedule of Affective Disorders and Schizophrenia (SADS), was developed for use with the RDC.

In summary, a wide range of views about schizophrenia have been held over the past century since Kraepelin and Bleuler established the concept. With the advent of current classificatory systems, the term now refers to a syndrome which can be diagnosed reliably, essential for rational clinical practice. However, as noted in Chapter 3, reliability is not in itself sufficient. For example, use of Schneider's first rank symptoms leads to high reliability in diagnosis but has no prognostic value, and nor do they delineate a syndrome with any apparent heritability even though the latter is the most established aetiological characteristic of schizophrenia (McGuffin *et al.*, 1984). Therefore, because the cause of schizophrenia is still largely unknown, the

BOX 12.3 DEVELOPMENT OF SCHIZOPHRENIA CONCEPTS AND TERMINOLOGIES

In the nineteenth century, one view was that all serious mental disorders were expressions of a single entity which Griesinger called *Einheitpsychose* (unitary psychosis). The alternative view, put forward by Morel in France, was that mental disorders could be separated and classified. Morel searched for specific entities, and argued for a classification based on cause, symptoms, and outcome. In 1852 he gave the name *démence précoce* to a disorder which he described as starting in adolescence and leading first to withdrawal, odd mannerisms, and self-neglect, and eventually to intellectual deterioration. Not long after, Kahlbaum (1863) described the syndrome of **catatonia**, and Hecker (1871) wrote an account of a condition he called **hebephrenia**.

Emil Kraepelin (1855–1926) derived his ideas from study of the course of the disorder as well as the symptoms. His observations led him to argue against the idea of a single psychosis, and to propose a division into **dementia praecox** and **manic-depressive psychosis**. This grouping brought together as subclasses of dementia praecox the previously separate entities of hebephrenia and catatonia. (His adoption of the word 'dementia' emphasizes the prominence he attributed to the cognitive impairments of the disease, noted on p. 272). Kraepelin's description of dementia praecox appeared for the first time in 1893, in the fourth edition of his textbook, and the account was expanded in subsequent editions. He described the illness as occurring in clear consciousness, and consisting of: 'a series of states, the common characteristic of which is a peculiar destruction of the internal connections of the psychic personality' (Kraepelin, 1919). Kraepelin originally divided dementia praecox into three subtypes (catatonic, hebephrenic, and paranoid) and later added a fourth (simple). Kraepelin separated the condition he named **paraphrenia** (see p. 513) from dementia praecox on the grounds that it started in middle life and seemed to be free from the changes in emotion and volition found in dementia praecox. It is commonly held that Kraepelin regarded dementia praecox as invariably progressing to chronic deterioration. However, he reported that, in his series of cases, 13 per cent recovered completely (though some relapsed later) and 17 per cent were ultimately able to live and work without difficulty.

Eugen Bleuler (1857–1959) based his work on that of Kraepelin, and in his own book wrote 'the whole idea of dementia praecox originates with Kraepelin' (Bleuler, 1911). He also acknowledged the help of his younger colleague, Carl Jung, in trying to apply some of Freud's ideas to dementia praecox. Compared with Kraepelin, Bleuler was concerned less with prognosis and more with the mechanisms of symptom formation. Bleuler proposed the name **schizophrenia** to denote a 'splitting' of psychic functions, which he thought to be of central importance. Bleuler believed in a distinction between **fundamental** and **accessory symptoms**. Fundamental symptoms included disturbances of associations, changes in emotional reactions, and autism (withdrawal from reality into an inner world of fantasy). It is interesting that, in Bleuler's view, some of the most frequent and striking symptoms were accessory (secondary), for example, hallucinations, delusions, catatonia, and abnormal behaviours. Bleuler was interested in the psychological study of his cases, but did not deny the possibility of a neuropathological cause for schizophrenia. Since Bleuler was preoccupied more with psychopathological mechanisms than with symptoms themselves, his approach to diagnosis was less precise than that of Kraepelin. Bleuler also took a more optimistic view of the outcome, but still held that one should not 'speak of cure but of far reaching improvement'. He also wrote: 'as yet I have never released a schizophrenic in whom I could not still see distinct signs of the disease, indeed there are very few in whom one would have to search for such signs' (Bleuler, 1911).

Kurt Schneider (1887–1967) – not to be confused with Carl Schneider, who categorized types of thought disorder – tried to make the diagnosis more reliable by identifying a group of symptoms characteristic of schizophrenia and rarely found in other disorders. Schneiderian **'first rank' symptoms** (Table 12.4) have a major role in the contemporary diagnosis of schizophrenia. However, unlike Bleuler's fundamental symptoms, Schneider's symptoms were not supposed to have any central psychopathological role; moreover, he noted that they were neither necessary nor sufficient for the diagnosis:

'Among the many abnormal modes of experience that occur in schizophrenia, there are some which we put in the first rank of importance, not because we think of them as basic disturbances, but because they have this special value in helping us to determine the diagnosis of schizophrenia. When any one of these

BOX 12.3 *(continued)*

modes of experience is undeniably present and no basic somatic illness can be found, we may make the diagnosis of schizophrenia ... Symptoms of first rank importance do not always have to be present for a diagnosis to be made.'

(Schneider 1959)

Several German psychiatrists tried to define subgroupings within schizophrenia. Karl Kleist, a pupil of the neurologist Wernicke, looked for associations between brain pathology and different subtypes of psychotic illness. He accepted Kraepelin's main diagnostic framework but used careful clinical observation in an attempt to distinguish various subdivisions within schizophrenia and other atypical disorders. His attempt to match these subtypes to specific kinds of brain pathology was ingenious but not successful.

Leonhard continued this approach of careful clinical observation, and published a complicated classification that distinguishes schizophrenia from the **'cycloid' psychoses**, a group of non-affective psychoses of good outcome (Leonhard, 1957). He also divided schizophrenia into two groups. The first is characterized by a progressive course, and is divided into catatonias, hebephrenias, and paraphrenias. Leonhard gave this group a name which is often translated as **systematic**. The second group, called **non-systematic**, is divided into **affect-laden paraphrenia**, **schizophasia**, and **periodic catatonia**. Affect-laden paraphrenia is characterized by paranoid delusions and the expression of strong emotion about their content. In schizophasia, speech is grossly disordered and difficult to understand. Periodic catatonia is a condition with regular remissions; during an episode, akinetic symptoms are sometimes interrupted by hyperkinetic symptoms.

Scandinavian psychiatrists were influenced by Jaspers' distinction between process schizophrenia and reactive psychoses. In the late 1930s, Langfeldt, using follow-up data on patients in Oslo, proposed a distinction between true schizophrenia, which had a poor prognosis, and **schizophreniform states**, which had a good prognosis (Langfeldt, 1961). True schizophrenia was defined narrowly and was similar to Kraepelin's dementia praecox. Schizophreniform states were described as often precipitated by stress and accompanied by confusional and affective symptoms. Langfeldt's distinction between cases with good and bad prognosis has been influential but research has not found that his criteria predict prognosis accurately. According to modern diagnostic criteria, most of Langfeldt's schizophreniform states would be classified as mood disorders (Bergen *et al.*, 1990). Note that in DSM-IV the term schizophreniform disorder is used in a different way (p. 278).

In Denmark and Norway, cases of psychosis arising after stressful events have received much attention. The terms **reactive psychosis** or **psychogenic psychosis** are commonly applied to conditions which appear to be precipitated by stress, are to some extent understandable in their symptoms, and have a good prognosis. In current diagnostic schemes such disorders would be classified as **brief psychotic disorder** or **schizophreniform disorder**. For historical review of concepts of brief psychosis, see Garrabé and Cousin (2000).

TABLE 12.4 Schneider's symptoms of the first rank

Hearing thoughts spoken aloud
Third-person hallucinations
Hallucinations in the form of a commentary
Somatic hallucinations
Thought withdrawal or insertion
Thought broadcasting
Delusional perception
Feelings or actions experienced as made or influenced by external agents

syndrome remains of uncertain validity. Until this fundamental question is answered, there will continue to be dispute as to its most important features, diagnostic boundaries, and internal subdivisions.

Classification of schizophrenia in DSM-IV and ICD-10

The classification of schizophrenia and schizophrenia-like disorders in ICD-10 and DSM-IV is outlined and compared in Table 12.5. The classifications are seen to be broadly similar.

DSM-IV

In this classification schizophrenia is defined in terms of the symptoms in the acute phase and also of the

TABLE 12.5 Classification of schizophrenia and schizophrenia-like disorders in ICD-10 and DSM-IV*

ICD–10	DSM-IV
Schizophrenia	**Schizophrenia**
◆ Paranoid	◆ Paranoid
◆ Hebephrenic	◆ Disorganized
◆ Catatonic	◆ Catatonic
◆ Undifferentiated	◆ Undifferentiated
◆ Residual	◆ Residual
◆ Simple schizophrenia	
◆ Post-schizophrenic depression	
◆ Other schizophrenia	
◆ Unspecified schizophrenia	
Schizotypal disorder	
Schizoaffective disorder	**Schizoaffective disorder**
Persistent delusional disorders	**Delusional disorder**
◆ Delusional disorder	
◆ Other persistent delusional disorders	
Acute and transient psychotic disorder	**Brief psychotic disorders**
◆ Acute schizophrenia-like psychotic disorder	**Schizophreniform disorder**
◆ Acute polymorphic psychotic disorder	
◆ Other acute psychotic disorders	
Induced delusional disorder	**Shared psychotic disorder**
Other non-organic psychotic disorders	
Unspecified non-organic psychosis	**Psychotic disorder not otherwise specified**

* The order of categories in the two systems has been changed slightly to show their comparable features more clearly.

course, for which the requirement is continuous signs of disturbance for at least 6 months (Table 12.6). The acute symptoms (criterion A) include delusions, hallucinations, disorganized speech or behaviour, and negative symptoms. At least two of these symptoms must have been present for a period of one month (unless successful treatment has occurred). Where subjects have major disturbances of mood occurring concurrently with the acute-phase symptoms, a diagnosis of a schizoaffective disorder or mood disorder with psychotic features should be made.

A further criterion for the diagnosis of schizophrenia in DSM-IV is that the patient must have exhibited deficiencies in their expected level of occupational or social functioning since the onset of the disorder. As noted above, for the diagnosis to be made there must have been at least 6 months of continuous disturbance; this can include prodromal and residual periods when acute-phase symptoms, as described above, are not evident. Patients whose symptom duration does not meet this criterion 6-month period will be classified as suffering from a schizophreniform disorder or a brief psychotic disorder.

In DSM-IV, schizophrenic disorders are divided into a number of subtypes, defined by the predominant symptomatology at the time of evaluation. After at least 1 year has elapsed since the onset of active phase symptoms, DSM-IV also allows the disorder to be classified by longitudinal course, and specification of the pattern of relapse and remission.

In DSM-IV, schizophrenia is distinguished from two other major categories: delusional disorder (Chapter 13) and the mixed group of psychotic disorders not elsewhere classified (discussed below).

ICD-10

The ICD-10 definition of schizophrenia (Table 12.7) places more reliance than DSM-IV on first-rank symptoms (Table 12.4), and requires a duration of only 1 month, excluding prodromal symptoms. There are several clinical subtypes; these differ most obviously from DSM-IV in the inclusion of categories of simple schizophrenia and post-schizophrenic depression. Like DSM-IV, cases in which symptoms of schizophrenia are accompanied by prominent mood disturbances are classified as schizoaffective disorders.

Certain aspects of personality are genetically associated with schizophrenia. ICD-10 includes **schizotypal disorder** among schizophrenic disorders, whereas in DSM-IV, this condition is classified as a personality disorder. Schizotypal disorder is associated with social isolation and restriction of affect; in addition there are perceptual distortions with disorders of thinking and speech and striking eccentricity or oddness of behaviour.

Similar to DSM-IV, ICD-10 classifies delusional disorders separately from schizophrenia (see Chapter 13). In addition, a group of acute and transient psychotic disorders are recognized that have an acute onset and complete recovery within 2–3 months (see below).

Summary of differences between DSM-IV and ICD-10

The main differences between the two systems in their diagnostic approach to schizophrenia are:

TABLE 12.6 Criteria for schizophrenia in DSM-IV

A Characteristic symptoms of the active phase

Two (or more) of the following, each present for a significant portion of time during a 1-month period (or less if successfully treated)

1. Delusions
2. Hallucinations
3. Disorganized speech (e.g. frequent derailment or incoherence)
4. Grossly disorganized or catatonic behaviour
5. Negative symptoms, i.e. affective flattening, alogia, or avolition

B Social/occupational dysfunction

For a significant portion of the time since the onset of the disturbance, one or more major areas of functioning such as work, interpersonal relations, or self-care are markedly below the level achieved prior to the onset (or when the onset is in childhood or adolescence, failure to achieve expected level of interpersonal, academic, or occupational achievement)

C Duration

Continuous signs of the disturbance persist for at least 6 months. This 6-month period must include at least 1 month of symptoms (or less if successfully treated) that meet criterion A (i.e. active-phase symptoms) and may include:

Periods of prodromal or residual symptoms, the signs of the disturbance may be manifested by only negative symptoms or two or more

Symptoms listed in criterion A present in an attenuated form (e.g. odd beliefs, unusual perceptual Experiences)

D Schizoaffective and mood disorder exclusion

Schizoaffective disorder and mood disorder with psychotic features have been ruled out because either (1) no major depressive, manic, or mixed episodes have occurred concurrently with the active-phase symptoms, or (2) if mood episodes have occurred during active phase symptoms, their total duration has been brief relative to the duration of the active and residual periods

E Substance/general medical condition exclusion

The disturbance is not due to the direct physiological effects of a substance (e.g. drug of abuse, a medication) or a general medical condition)

F Relationship to a pervasive developmental disorder

If there is a history of autistic disorder or another pervasive development disorder, the additional diagnosis of schizophrenia is made only if prominent delusions or hallucinations are also present for at least 1 month (or less if successfully treated)

TABLE 12.7 Criteria for schizophrenia in ICD–10

The normal requirement for a diagnosis of schizophrenia is that a minimum of one very clear symptom (and usually two or more if less clear-cut) belonging to any one of the groups listed as (a)–(d) below, or symptoms from at least two of the groups referred to as (e)–(h), should have been clearly present for most of the time *during a period of 1 month or more*

(a) Thought echo, thought insertion or withdrawal, and thought broadcasting

(b) Delusions of control, influence, or passivity, clearly referred to body or limb movements or specific thoughts, actions, or sensations; delusional perception

(c) Hallucinatory voices giving a running commentary on the patient's behaviour, or discussing the patient among themselves, or other types of hallucinatory voices coming from some part of the body

(d) Persistent delusions of other kinds that are culturally inappropriate and completely impossible

(e) Persistent hallucinations in any modality, when accompanied either by fleeting or half formed delusions without clear affective content, or by persistent overvalued ideas, or when occurring every day for weeks or months on end

(f) Breaks or interpolations in the train of thought, resulting in incoherence or irrelevant speech, or neologisms

(g) Catatonic behaviour, such as excitement, posturing, or waxy flexibility, negativism, mutism, and stupor

(h) 'Negative' symptoms such as marked apathy, paucity of speech, and blunting or incongruity of emotional responses, usually resulting in social withdrawal and lowering of social performance; it must be clear that these are not due to depression or to neuroleptic medication

(i) A significant and consistent change in the overall quality of some aspects of personal behaviour, manifest as loss of interest, aimlessness, idleness, a self-absorbed attitude, and social withdrawal

- ICD-10 places greater weight on Schneider's first rank symptoms. DSM-IV emphasizes course and functional impairment.
- ICD-10 requires a duration of illness of 1 month; DSM-IV requires 6 months.
- Schizotypal disorder is included in ICD-10, but categorized as a personality disorder in DSM-IV.
- ICD-10 includes some additional subtypes: simple schizophrenia, post-schizophrenic depression.
- Disorganized schizophrenia in DSM-IV is called hebephrenic schizophrenia in ICD-10.

Schizophrenia-like disorders

Whatever definition of schizophrenia is adopted, there will be cases that resemble schizophrenia in some respects and yet do not meet the criteria for diagnosis. In DSM-IV and ICD-10, these disorders are divided into four groups:

1. Delusional disorders (paranoid psychoses)
2. Brief disorders
3. Disorders accompanied by prominent affective symptoms
4. Disorders without all the required symptoms for schizophrenia.

Delusional disorders are discussed in Chapter 13. The latter three groups are discussed here.

Brief disorders

DSM-IV uses the term **brief psychotic disorder** for a syndrome characterized by at least one of the acute-phase positive symptoms shown in Table 12.6. The disorder lasts for at least 1 day but not more than 1 month, by which time full recovery has occurred. The disorder may or may not follow a stressor, but psychoses induced by the direct physiological effects of drugs or medical illness are excluded. **Schizophreniform psychosis** is a syndrome similar to schizophrenia (meeting criterion A) which has lasted more than 1 month (and so cannot be classified as brief psychotic disorder) but less than the 6 months required for a diagnosis of schizophrenia to be made. Social and occupational dysfunction are not needed to make the diagnosis.

In ICD-10, the grouping is **acute and transient psychotic disorder**. These disorders are of acute onset, and complete recovery within 2–3 months is the rule. The disorder may or may not be precipitated by a stressful life event. The category is then subdivided into several overlapping and somewhat confusing subtypes. In the first two, **acute polymorphic psychotic disorders, with or without symptoms of schizophrenia**, hallucinations, delusions, and perceptual disturbance are obvious but change rapidly in nature and extent. There are often accompanying changes in mood and motor behaviour. *Bouffée délirante* and **cycloid psychosis** (Box 12.3) are given as synonyms for these categories, although the Scandinavian school continues to argue that the latter comprise a distinct group. A third subtype, **acute schizophrenia-like psychotic episode**, is a non-committal term for cases meeting the symptom criteria for schizophrenia but lasting for less than a month. Residual cases that do not fit these subtypes of acute psychosis are called **other acute psychotic episodes**. Overall, the ICD-10 category identifies a heterogeneous group of disorders in terms of outcome (Singh *et al.*, 2004).

Disorders with prominent affective symptoms

Some patients have a more or less equal mixture of schizophrenic and affective symptoms. As mentioned earlier, such patients are classified under **schizoaffective disorder** in both DSM-IV and ICD-10.

The term schizoaffective disorder has been used in several distinct ways. It was first applied by Kasanin (1933) to a small group of young patients with severe mental disorders characterized by a very sudden onset in a setting of marked emotional turmoil. The psychosis lasted a few weeks and was followed by recovery.

The current definitions differ substantially from this description. DSM-IV requires that there should have been an uninterrupted period of illness during which, at some time there is either a major depressive episode, a manic episode or a mixed episode concurrent with symptoms that meet criterion A for schizophrenia. During this continuous episode of illness, the acute-phase psychotic symptoms must have been present for at least 2 weeks in the absence of prominent mood symptoms (or the diagnosis would be a mood disorder with psychotic features). However, the episode of mood disturbance must have been present for a substantial part of the illness. The definition of schizoaffective disorder in ICD-10 is similar. It specifies that the diagnosis should only be made when both definite schizophrenic and definite affective symptoms are equally prominent and present simultaneously, or within a few days of each other. (This is an important point: the label 'schizoaffective' should not be applied just because a patient has an isolated symptom or two consistent with both diagnoses, or because the assessment has not been sufficiently detailed to identify the primary diagnosis.)

ICD-10 classifies schizoaffective disorder by whether the mood disturbance is depressive, manic, or mixed. In DSM-IV schizoaffective disorder is specified either as depressive type or bipolar.

Family studies have shown that the more recent diagnostic concepts of schizoaffective disorder delineate a syndrome in which first-degree relatives have an increased risk of both mood disorders and schizophrenia. In addition, the outcome of schizoaffective disorder is generally thought to be better than that for schizophrenia, with negative symptoms rarely developing (Tsuang *et al.*, 2000).

As noted above, it is not uncommon for patients with schizophrenia to develop depression as the symptoms of acute psychosis subside. This is recognized in ICD-10 as post-schizophrenic depression, where prominent depressive symptoms have been present for at least 2 weeks while some symptoms of schizophrenia (either positive or negative) still remain.

Persistent disorders without all the required symptoms for schizophrenia

A difficult problem is presented by cases with long-standing schizophrenia-like symptoms but which do not fully meet diagnostic criteria. There are four groups:

1. Patients who have exhibited the full clinical picture of schizophrenia in the past but no longer have all the symptoms required to make the diagnosis. These cases are classified as **residual schizophrenia** in both DSM-IV and ICD-10.
2. People who from an early age have behaved oddly and shown features seen in schizophrenia, for example, ideas of reference, persecutory beliefs, and unusual types of thinking. When long-standing, these disorders can be classified as personality disorders in DSM-IV (**schizotypal personality disorder**), or with schizophrenia in ICD-10 (**schizotypal disorder**). Because of a suggested close relationship to schizophrenia, these disorders have also been called **latent schizophrenia**, or part of the **schizophrenia spectrum**.
3. People with social withdrawal, lack of initiative, odd behaviour, and blunting of emotion, in whom positive psychotic symptoms are never known to have occurred. A variety of terms may be applicable, including **simple schizophrenia** (p. 270), **schizoid personality disorder** (p. 135), and **Asperger's syndrome** (p. 671).
4. Finally, we note again the group of patients who have persistent, stable delusions but without other features of schizophrenia (Chapter 13).

Gjessing's syndrome

Gjessing (1947) described a schizophrenia-like disorder in which catatonic symptoms recurred in phases, together with changes in nitrogen balance, which were not always in phase with the symptoms. Gjessing believed that there were underlying changes in thyroid function and that the disorder could be treated successfully with thyroxine. The condition, if it exists, is exceedingly rare, and may have been a variant of rapid cycling bipolar disorder.

Differential diagnosis

We have already described how current classifications include schizophrenia-like disorders as well as schizophrenia, but that the boundary between them is blurred and to some extent arbitrary. Similarly, there is no clear distinction between disorders that are considered to be variants of schizophrenia, and some which are viewed as being part of its differential diagnosis (Adler and Strakowski, 2003). For example, delusional disorders are often included in both categories, whilst schizotypal disorder is classified as a personality disorder in DSM-IV but with schizophrenia in ICD-10. Such difficulties reflect the unknown validity of the syndrome(s), and are unlikely to be resolved until the classification is based upon aetiology or other empirically validated markers.

With these caveats in mind, current diagnostic practice requires schizophrenia to be distinguished from a number of other disorders:

- **Organic syndromes**. Acute schizophrenia can be mistaken for **delirium**, especially if there is pronounced thought disorder and mood disturbance. Careful observation is needed for clouding of consciousness, disorientation, and other features of delirium (Chapter 14). Schizophrenia-like disorders can also occur, in clear consciousness, in a range of neurological and medical disorders. These conditions are referred to as a **psychotic disorder secondary to a general medical condition** (DSM-IV) or an **organic delusional disorder** (ICD-10). Classic examples include temporal lobe epilepsy (complex partial seizures), general paralysis of the insane, and metachromatic leukodystrophy (see Chapter 14). Visual, olfactory and gustatory hallucinations are said to be suggestive of an organic disorder. The occurrence of organic schizophrenia-like disorders emphasizes the importance of a careful medical history and physical examination (and investigations, if indicated) in all such patients. One study in London found that 10 out of 268 cases (3.7 per cent) of 'first-episode schizophrenia' had an organic cause other than drug or alcohol misuse (Johnstone *et al.*, 1987).

- **Drug-induced states (including substance misuse).** Certain prescribed drugs, particularly steroids and dopamine agonists, can cause florid psychotic states. Psychoactive substance misuse, particularly with psychostimulants or phencyclidine, and also alcohol, should always be considered in the presentation of schizophrenia-like psychoses. Urine or hair testing can be helpful in diagnosis, as is the temporal association between drug use and symptoms. However, the high prevalence of recreational drug use in young adults means that a clear distinction between a drug-induced psychosis and schizophrenia is not always possible.
- **Mood disorder with psychotic features.** The distinction of schizophrenia (and schizoaffective disorder) from affective psychosis depends on the degree and persistence of the mood disorder, the relation of any hallucinations or delusions to the prevailing mood, and the nature of the symptoms in any previous episodes. The distinction from mania in young people can be particularly difficult, and sometimes the diagnosis can be clarified only by longer-term follow-up. A family history of mood disorder may be a useful pointer.
- **Delusional disorders.** These disorders (Chapter 13) are characterized by chronic, systematized paranoid delusions, and occasionally with hallucinations. They lack other symptoms of schizophrenia and many areas of the mental state are unremarkable.
- **Personality disorder.** Differential diagnosis from personality disorder, especially of the paranoid, schizoid or schizotypal forms, can be difficult when insidious changes are reported in a young person, or paranoid ideas are present. Prolonged observation may be required to detect genuine symptoms of psychosis, and for the additional features indicative of schizophrenia. Some patients with borderline personality disorder also exhibit psychotic symptoms, although the presence of affective instability and other features mean there should rarely be diagnostic confusion with schizophrenia.

Epidemiology

Schizophrenia is a disorder with a low incidence but a relatively high prevalence, and costs (Knapp *et al.*, 2004), reflecting its chronicity in many patients. Estimates of the incidence and prevalence of schizophrenia depend on the criteria for diagnosis and the population surveyed. The annual incidence using current diagnostic criteria is between 0.16 and 0.54 per 1000 population using a broad definition; for more restrictive diagnoses, the incidence is about two to three times lower (Jablensky, 2003). The prevalence of schizophrenia is about 1.4–4.6 per thousand population at risk (Jablensky, 2003) and is similar in different countries. For example, the British National Psychiatric Morbidity Survey found an annual prevalence of 'functional psychosis' of 4 per 1000 (Jenkins *et al.*, 1998). There are, however, exceptions to this general uniformity of rates, with high rates being reported in certain isolated communities in Sweden and Finland and in the Afro-Caribbean population in the UK (p. 290). By contrast, a consistently low prevalence of about 1.2 per 1000 has been reported among the Hutterites and the Anabaptist sect in the USA (Nimgaonkar *et al.*, 2000). These reported differences in prevalence may reflect differences in diagnostic criteria, genetic susceptibility, or migration (see below).

Some studies have suggested that the incidence of schizophrenia may be falling in industrialized countries. For example, Eagles and Whalley (1985) reported a 40 per cent fall in first admission rates for schizophrenia in Scotland between 1969 and 1978. This observation has been supported by some, but not all, subsequent investigations. Whether the observed decline represents a true fall in the inception rate for schizophrenia remains an open question; for example, Kendell *et al.*, (1993) found that in Scotland, at least, the apparent decline may be attributable to changing diagnostic criteria and inaccurate recording of true first admissions. Moreover, increased rates have also been reported (Jablensky, 2003).

The onset of schizophrenia characteristically occurs between the ages of 15 and 45. There are minor sex differences in age of onset, incidence, and mortality (see p. 305). Late onset schizophrenia is discussed in Chapter 20.

Aetiology

Overview

Views about the aetiology of schizophrenia have been inextricably linked with the controversies regarding its nature and classification (Chapter 2 and this chapter, p. 273). Schizophrenia therefore exemplifies the whole range of biological, psychological and social factors considered important in psychiatric causation (Chapter 5 and Table 12.8), and the methods which have been applied to try and identify them. This section summarizes the current knowledge and theories in each domain and also mentions some outdated but influential views. It takes a broad definition of aetiology, and includes pathogenesis and pathophysiological findings.

Key aspects of the present consensus regarding the aetiology of schizophrenia are summarized as follows. The most important influence is genetic, with about 80 per cent of the risk of schizophrenia being inherited. The mode of inheritance is complex and the genes, some of which have recently been identified, act as risk factors, not determinants of illness. A number of environmental factors contribute too, many of which appear to act prenatally, and which interact with the genetic predisposition. Together these and subsequent risk factors lead to a neurodevelopmental disturbance which either causes, or renders the individual vulnerable to, the later emergence of symptoms, and which manifests itself premorbidly in a range of behavioural, intellectual and neuroanatomical features. In schizophrenia, the brain is slightly smaller than normal, and there are localized differences in its structure and function, leading to the view that the syndrome is a disorder of connectivity within and between brain regions. Acute psychosis is associated with excess dopamine neurotransmission, whereas the persistent cognitive impairments may result from deficient dopamine function in the prefrontal cortex. Both may be secondary to abnormalities of the glutamate system. Psychosocial factors have been neglected recently, but significantly influence the onset and course of illness. Finally, it is emphasized that there are few certainties about the aetiology of schizophrenia, and even where facts are robust, their interpretation often remains unclear.

TABLE 12.8 Aetiological factors and theories in schizophrenia

Category	Examples
Genes	Neuregulin
	Dysbindin
Environmental	Obstetric complications
	Maternal influenza
	Winter birth
	Early cannabis use
	Paternal age
Social	Migration
	Urban birth and upbringing
	Recent life events
Structural	Smaller brain size
	Reduced synaptic markers
Functional imaging	Hypofrontality
Neurophysiological	Abnormal eye tracking
	Abnormal sensory evoked potentials
Neurochemical	Dopamine
	Glutamate
Psychological	Cognitive impairments
	Personality factors
	Psychodynamic theories
	Family dynamics and communication
Hypotheses	Neurodevelopmental
	Aberrant connectivity
	Stress-vulnerability

Genetics

As noted in Chapter 5, a genetic basis for a condition can be shown using family, twin and adoption studies. All three have been applied extensively in schizophrenia. For a review see Gottesman (1991).

Family studies

The first systematic family study was carried out in Kraepelin's department by Ernst Rudin, who showed that the rate of dementia praecox was higher among the siblings of probands than in the general population. More recent research has used better criteria for diagnosis in probands and relatives, and better ways of selecting the probands. These improved methods yield estimates of an average lifetime risk of about 5–10 per cent among first-degree relatives of schizophrenics, compared with 0.2–0.6 per cent among first-degree relatives of controls (Table 12.9). To some extent, the risk depends on the definition of the phenotype. For example, in a prospective study of over 200 children of mothers with schizophrenia, Parnas *et al.*, (1993) found not only a significant excess of schizophrenia (16.2 per cent versus 1.9 per cent in controls) but also an excess of schizotypal, paranoid, and schizoid personality disorders (21.3 per cent versus 5 per cent). Similar findings were reported by Kendler *et al.*, (1993b, c, d) in a study of first-degree relatives of patients with schizophrenia (Table 12.9). Taken together, the family studies provide clear evidence of a familial aetiology but do not distinguish between genetic effects and those of the family environment.

An additional value of family studies is to determine whether the liability to schizophrenia and mood disorders is transmitted independently, which should be the observed pattern if the two disorders are separate syn-

TABLE 12.9 Approximate lifetime risk of developing schizophrenia for relatives of a proband with schizophrenia

Relationship	Risk (%)	
	Definite cases only	Definite and probable cases
Parents	4.4	5.5
All siblings	8.5	10.2
Siblings (one parent schizophrenic)	13.8	17.2
Children	12.3	13.9
Children (both parents schizophrenic)	36.6	46.3
Half siblings	3.2	3.5
Nephews and nieces	2.2	2.6

Adapted from Shields (1980).

dromes with differing aetiology. However, the findings from the various studies have been contradictory, with some researchers arguing for separate familial transmission of mood disorders and schizophrenia, while others suggest that what is transmitted is a general vulnerability to psychosis (Crow, 1994). The following conclusions can be drawn from the more recent studies (Kendler *et al.*, 1993a, b, c, d; Maier *et al.*, 1993; Parnas *et al.*, 1993) (Table 12.10).

- The risk of schizophrenia, schizoaffective disorder, and schizotypal personality is increased in first-degree relatives of patients with schizophrenia.
- The risk of both schizophrenia and mood disorder is increased in first-degree relatives of patients with schizoaffective disorder.
- The risk of bipolar disorder is not increased in first-degree relatives of patients with schizophrenia.

Twin studies

The rationale, methods and problems of twin studies were introduced on p. 98. They have been of considerable importance in schizophrenia, providing unequivocal evidence of its heritability.

The first substantial twin study was carried out in Munich by Luxenberger (1928), who found concordance in 11 of his 19 MZ pairs and in none of his 13 DZ pairs. Subsequent investigations, though differing in concordance rates, all agree that concordance is several-fold higher in MZ than DZ twins, indicating a large heritable component. Representative figures for concordance are about 50 per cent for MZ pairs and about 10 per cent for DZ pairs (Cardno and Gottesman, 2000). For example, a recent analysis of 108 twin pairs from the Maudsley Twin Series gave concordance rates for ICD-10 schizophrenia of 42 per cent in MZ twins and 1.7 per cent in DZ twins.

Modern twin studies also produce estimates of heritability (the proportion of liability to schizophrenia in the population which can be attributed to genes, p. 98), and can decompose environmental factors into those that are unique to the individual and those which are shared with others (i.e. the co-twin). A recent meta-analysis (Sullivan *et al.*, 2003) thereby confirmed the substantial heritability of schizophrenia (81 per cent; 95 per cent confidence interval, 73–90 per cent). Although there are some caveats about the interpretation of precise heritability figures, these data unambiguously show that genes are the largest risk factor for schizophrenia. The meta-analysis also showed, less predictably, that most of the environmental contribution comes from shared rather than individual-specific influences (11 per cent; 95 per cent confidence interval,

TABLE 12.10 Lifetime risk of psychiatric disorder in first-degree relatives of probands with schizophrenia, schizoaffective disorder, and controls

Disorder	Diagnosis of proband		
	Schizophrenia (%)	Schizoaffective disorder (%)	Control (%)
Schizophrenia	6.5	6.7	0.5
Schizotypal disorder	6.9	2.8	1.4
Schizoaffective disorder	2.3	1.8	0.7
All affective illness	24.9	49.7	22.8
Psychotic affective illness	8.3	12.4	2.6
Bipolar disorder	1.2	4.8	1.4

From Kendler *et al.*, (1993b, c, d).

3–19 per cent). The shared influences might include the kinds of family factors proposed by earlier psychodynamic theories (p. 292), but equally includes biological factors, such as viral infections or nutrition, suggested by more recent epidemiological studies (p. 285).

It is worth noting that, amongst discordant MZ twins, the risk of schizophrenia is increased equally in children of the unaffected and the affected co-twin. This confirms that the unaffected co-twin had the same genetic susceptibility to developing schizophrenia as the affected twin but for some reason did not express the phenotype. This is most likely due to environmental protective factors or chance ('stochastic processes').

Adoption studies

Heston (1966) studied 47 adults who had been born to mothers with schizophrenia and separated from them within 3 days of birth. As children they had been brought up in a variety of circumstances, though not by the mother's family. At the time of the study their mean age was 36. Heston compared them with controls matched for circumstances of upbringing, but whose mothers had not suffered from schizophrenia. Amongst the offspring of the affected mothers, five were diagnosed as having schizophrenia compared with none of the controls. The rate for schizophrenia among the adopted-away children was comparable with that among children with a schizophrenic parent who remained with their biological family.

Further evidence has come from a series of studies started in 1965 by a group of Danish and American investigators, using Danish national registers of psychiatric cases and adoptions. In one major project (Kety *et al.*, 1975) two groups of adoptees were identified: 33 who had schizophrenia, and a matched group who were free from schizophrenia. Rates of disorder were compared in the biological and adoptive families of the two groups of adoptees. The rate for schizophrenia was greater among the biological relatives of the adoptees with schizophrenia than among the relatives of controls, a finding which supports the genetic hypothesis. Furthermore, the rate for schizophrenia was not increased amongst couples who adopted the affected children, suggesting that environmental factors were not of substantial importance. Follow-up studies using a national sample of adoptees in Denmark confirmed that biological first-degree relatives of patients with schizophrenia have an approximately tenfold increased risk of suffering from schizophrenia or a related ('spectrum') disorder (Kety *et al.*, 1994).

The data from adoption studies thus strongly support the view that genetic factors explain the familial clustering of schizophrenia. However, note that they cannot control for the prenatal environment, which other studies suggest is important (p. 285). Nor can they rule out an interaction between environmental causes in the adoptive family and genetic predisposition; indeed, Finnish data show that adoptees at high genetic risk of schizophrenia are more sensitive to adverse upbringing (Tienari *et al.*, 2004).

The mode of inheritance

The ratios of the frequencies of schizophrenia among people with different degrees of relationship with the proband do not fit any simple Mendelian pattern to be expected if the disorder were caused by a single major dominant or recessive gene. One possibility is that there is such a gene, but it exhibits variable penetrance. However, genetic linkage studies have made it highly unlikely that, whatever modifications of this kind are invoked, schizophrenia is associated with a single gene of main effect (Owen *et al.*, 2004). There are two main alternatives, which may both be correct:

1. Schizophrenia arises from the cumulative effect of several genes, as a so-called complex or non-Mendelian genetic disorder. The liability to schizophrenia lies on a continuum in the population, and is expressed when a certain threshold of genetic susceptibility is exceeded. None of the genes are either necessary nor sufficient, and they act as risk factors and not determinants of disease. That is, the variants are polymorphisms not mutations (p. 101).
2. Schizophrenia is a label for a group of disorders of different genetic make-up or perhaps with genetic and non-genetic forms. In other words, schizophrenia is genetically heterogeneous.

The identification of several susceptibility genes for schizophrenia, described below, provides positive support for the first theory. It is not yet clear whether the different genes are involved in different subgroups of patients, and thereby whether the findings also support the heterogeneity model.

Crow's lateralization hypothesis

A very different view of the genetic aetiology of schizophrenia has been proposed by Crow (see Crow, 2002). He argues that schizophrenia is due to a single gene, which is also responsible for two unique properties of the human brain: cerebral asymmetry and language. No other genes, nor environmental factors, are required. For various reasons, the gene is hypothesized to reside at a particular location on the sex chromosomes. Other aspects of schizophrenia, including the lack of a Mendelian pattern of inheritance, expected of a single gene disorder, are explained by epigenetic (p. 103) factors. The theory is ingenious, and draws attention to the reduced cerebral asymmetry seen in schizophrenia (Sommer *et al.*, 2001), but it awaits direct support in terms of identification of the putative gene, and a mechanism by which it could fulfil such a diverse range of normal and pathological roles.

What is heritable?

Identification of genes for a condition is much easier if the boundaries of the inherited phenotype are known. However, this is a circular argument since it is ultimately identification of causative genes that, whenever possible, defines diseases. The uncertain boundaries of schizophrenia with regard to schizophrenia spectrum disorders and mood disorders have already been mentioned.

Another possibility is that it is particular components of schizophrenia, or other features associated with it, which are actually being inherited. Much evidence suggests that there are such features, called endophenotypes or intermediate phenotypes (p. 100), which are more closely related to the genes, and therefore more aetiologically valid. A range of heritable endophenotypes of schizophrenia are known, including evoked potentials, working memory, brain structure, and eye-tracking dysfunction (pp. 289–90). It is also possible that different genes act upon different endophenotypes of the syndrome. Whether any of these endophenotypes become part of a redefined syndrome or syndromes of schizophrenia will depend upon confirmation of their genetic basis, and demonstration that they have reliability and utility, for example in predicting outcome or therapeutic responsiveness.

Velocardiofacial syndrome

Velocardiofacial syndrome (VCFS; di George syndrome) is caused by deletion of one copy of chromosome 22q11 (hence its alternative name of 22q11 deletion syndrome). The syndrome is a relatively common cytogenetic anomaly (1 in 4000 live births) and causes a range of physical abnormalities and cognitive impairment (Murphy, 2002). Of relevance here, it is also associated with psychosis (either schizophrenia-like or affective) in about 30 per cent of cases. Thus, even though VCFS is a rare cause of schizophrenia (~1 per cent of cases), 22q11 is implicated as a locus for schizophrenia genes in general, as outlined below.

Schizophrenia susceptibility genes

Despite its high heritability, and a large number of studies over the past twenty years, it has proven difficult to identify the chromosomal loci harbouring genes for schizophrenia, let alone the genes themselves. This difficulty likely reflects the various problems mentioned above, notably the uncertainty as to the phenotype being inherited, and the existence of multiple genes of small effect which are hard to detect. However, significant progress has been made in the past few years. For review, see Owen *et al.* (2004).

First, two meta-analyses have revealed chromosomal loci which are linked to schizophrenia, with either a high or very high probability, notably 2p, 8p, 13q and 22q (p and q refer to the short and long arm of the chromosome respectively). Second, several specific genes have been identified which are associated with schizophrenia. The findings are summarized in Table 12.11. It is emphasized that none of the genes cause schizophrenia (in the way that a gene causes a Mendelian disorder), but that variants (polymorphisms) of each gene are associated with a modestly (less than threefold) increased risk of the illness.

The best evidence is for neuregulin and dysbindin, and the evidence for both is now strong in terms of replications in different populations. Both genes are particularly complex, and their biology and functions are not well understood. Neuregulin is involved in many aspects of neuronal and glial growth and synaptic plasticity; dysbindin is also involved in synaptic functioning and signalling. The evidence for the other genes in Table 12.11 is less compelling, and some will likely prove to be false positives. Equally, more genes will undoubtedly be identified, for example underlying the locus on chromosome 2. At present it is not possible to state how many susceptibility genes for schizophre-

TABLE 12.11 Susceptibility genes for schizophrenia and their chromosomal location

Gene name	Alternative nomenclature	Locus
Neuregulin	NRG1	8p
Dysbindin	DTNBP1	6p
G72	D-amino acid oxidase activator	13q
RGS-4	Regulator of G protein signalling-4	1q
DISC-1	Disrupted in schizophrenia-1	1q
GRM3	Metabotropic glutamate receptor 3	7q
COMT	Catechol-O-methyl transferase	22q
DAAO	D-aminoacid oxidase	12q
HTR2A	5-HT2A receptor	13p
DRD3	Dopamine D3 receptor	3q

nia exist, nor their relative importance, nor how they operate or interact. For example, for neuregulin and dysbindin, the polymorphisms associated with schizophrenia differ from one study to another, and no amino-acid changes have been found in the encoded proteins. One possibility is that the variants associated with schizophrenia affect the expression of the genes, and that the genes function by converging upon the functioning of glutamate and dopamine circuits in the brain, as envisaged by existing theories of schizophrenia, discussed below (Harrison and Weinberger, 2005).

Environmental risk factors

The twin studies discussed earlier show that there is a small but clear environmental contribution to schizophrenia. A range of factors, especially pre- and perinatal, have been identified which may account for this. This section describes the main biological factors; social influences are covered in a subsequent section. Risk factors for schizophrenia have been reviewed by McGrath and Murray (2003).

Obstetric complications

Retrospective studies of schizophrenic patients have reported more obstetric complications than their unaffected siblings or normal controls. Meta-analyses suggest an odds ratio of about 2 (Geddes *et al.*, 1999), although several individual studies, including prospective ones, have been negative. It is possible that obstetric complications may be more relevant in individuals with a genetic predisposition to schizophrenia (McNeil *et al.*, 2000). It is also unclear which specific complications are relevant; Geddes *et al.* (1999) found significant effects for premature rupture of membranes, birth before 37 weeks, use of a resuscitator or incubator, and low birth weight. The association of obstetric complications with schizophrenia has many possible explanations: they might be directly causal (e.g. via fetal hypoxia), or a reflection of pre-existing fetal abnormality, or the fetus' genetic background, or even a reflection of maternal antenatal health behaviour.

Maternal influenza

Several studies have suggested that fetuses exposed during the second trimester to influenza, especially the 1957 influenza A2 pandemic, have an increased risk of schizophrenia. Some biological support for this association was provided by animal studies showing that prenatal influenza affects brain development. However, many other studies have been negative, and a relationship between influenza and schizophrenia has been hard to establish. Additional support has recently emerged with the demonstration that serological evidence of influenza infection during early pregnancy was associated with a seven-fold increase in risk of schizophrenia in the offspring (Brown *et al.*, 2004).

Several other maternal (and childhood) infections have also been associated with schizophrenia (e.g. Buka *et al.*, 2001), including toxoplasmosis, poliomyelitis, measles and varicella, but these remain unconfirmed.

Other prenatal factors

Other pregnancy factors reported to be associated with schizophrenia include rhesus incompatibility, malnutrition, and stress (McGrath and Murray, 2003; Neugebauer, 2005).

Winter birth

Schizophrenia is slightly more frequent among people born in the winter than among those born in the summer (Davies *et al.*, 2003). It has been shown in both Northern and Southern hemispheres and becomes more prominent at higher latitudes. Winter birth may be more common in patients without a family history of schizophrenia. The explanation for the winter birth effect is unknown. It has been linked to the prevalence of influenza earlier in the winter, and to sunshine and vitamin D levels around birth, but could also relate to the time of conception, via seasonal fluctuations in the genetic make-up of gametes.

Child development

Parnas *et al.*, (1982) reported a study of 207 children of mothers with schizophrenia who were first assessed when they were 8–12 years old and then again, as adults, 18 years later, by which time 13 had developed schizophrenia and 29 had 'borderline schizophrenia'. Of the measures made on the first occasion, those predicting schizophrenia were:

- Poor rapport at interview.
- Socially isolated from peers.
- Disciplinary problems mentioned in school reports.
- Reports by the parents that the person had been passive as a baby.

More recently, Done *et al.*, (1994) found that in a cohort of more than 16,000 children prospectively studied over a 16-year period, those who developed schizophrenia could be distinguished at age 11, if not earlier, by greater hostility towards adults and speech and reading difficulties. The difference was seen compared to those who grew up to develop neurotic illness as well as those who remained well. In a similar study, Jones *et al.* (1994), found that children who eventually developed schizophrenia showed delayed milestones and speech problems, together with lower education test scores and less social play. A relationship between delayed milestones (e.g. walking) and schizophrenia has been confirmed in a Dutch population-based study. Davidson *et al.* (1999) found that male adolescents who later developed schizophrenia exhibited defects in social functioning, organizational ability, and intellectual functioning. Finally, Walker and colleagues have shown that the behaviour of children (including motor acts in infants), as recorded in home movies and videotapes, also predicts schizophrenia (Schiffman *et al.*, 2004).

Overall, there is therefore good evidence that people who will develop schizophrenia show increased rates of intellectual and motor dysfunction and poor social competence in childhood. However, it is not clear how specific these changes are, nor how they may be related to the subsequent development of the illness. Most children destined to develop schizophrenia were not considered clinically abnormal at the time, and many children performing poorly on these indices do not develop schizophrenia. Nevertheless, the findings are supportive of an early neurodevelopmental contribution to schizophrenia.

Substance use

The relationship between use of drugs and alcohol and schizophrenia is controversial. If substance use is considered to have directly caused the psychosis, then it is diagnosed as such and not as schizophrenia (Chapter 18). However, there is evidence that use of some drugs is associated with a increased risk of subsequently developing schizophrenia. The evidence is strongest for cannabis. Andreasson *et al.* (1987) followed up over 45,000 Swedish conscripts for 15 years, and found that the relative risk of developing schizophrenia was 2.5 times greater in subjects who used cannabis, with a six-fold increase in risk for heavy users. These data had two interpretations: first, that cannabis misuse is indeed a risk factor for schizophrenia; second, that those predisposed to develop the illness (or in the prodrome of it) tend to misuse cannabis. Recent studies suggest a genuine causal contribution, with early onset of cannabis use conferring the greatest excess risk (Arsenault *et al.*, 2004). Moreover, the risk is much greater in those predisposed to psychosis for other reasons (Henquet *et al.*, 2005), including genetic factors (Caspi *et al.*, 2005).

Other risk factors

Rates of schizophrenia are elevated in people with **epilepsy** (Chapter 14) and those with a low IQ (Chapter 25). Schizophrenia is also associated with **paternal** age, in those without a family history of psychosis (Sipos *et al.*, 2004), perhaps because the frequency of *de novo* genetic mutations in sperm increases with age. Older studies suggested **head injury** is a risk factor for schizophrenia and other psychoses. However, the evidence is weak and inconclusive (David and Prince, 2005).

Structural brain changes

Whether there is a neuropathology associated with schizophrenia has been a matter of debate for over a century. The search began with Alzheimer, who spent a decade studying the brains of patients with dementia praecox before he reported the case of presenile dementia with which his name is associated. The failure of Alzheimer and others to identify reliable, characteristic brain changes was central to the view of schizophrenia as a functional rather than an organic disorder. However, evidence accrued over the past thirty years from both brain imaging and post-mortem studies methods, means that schizophrenia can now be considered unequivocally a 'brain disease' (Weinberger, 1995), albeit one where the details and interpretation of the neuropathology remain poorly understood. The main findings are summarized in Table 12.12.

TABLE 12.12 Summary of structural brain changes in schizophrenia

Brain imaging
◆ Decreased brain volume
◆ Enlarged lateral ventricles
◆ Enlarged third ventricle
◆ Smaller medial temporal lobes
◆ Decreased cortical grey matter
◆ Reduced cerebral asymmetry
Neuropathology
◆ Decreased brain weight
◆ Absence of neurodegenerative changes
◆ Absence of gliosis
◆ Decreased pre-synaptic markers
◆ Decreased markers of dendrites
◆ Decreased oligodendroglia
◆ Smaller pyramidal neurons in some areas
◆ Fewer thalamic neurons

Structural imaging

In a landmark study, Johnstone *et al.* (1976) used the then novel technique of computerized tomographic (CT) scanning, and found significantly larger ventricles in seventeen elderly hospitalized patients with schizophrenia than in eight normal controls. Lateral ventricular enlargement in schizophrenia had been reported decades previously using pneumencephalography, but it was the study of Johnstone and colleagues which stimulated renewed interest. A large number of subsequent imaging studies, mostly using MRI, have confirmed and extended the findings. For review, see Shenton *et al.* (2001).

A recent meta-analysis of MRI studies concluded that there are reliable and significant differences in the volumes of the whole brain, lateral and third ventricles, and hippocampus in schizophrenia (Wright *et al.*, 2000). The ventricular enlargement, and probably the other changes, shows a unimodal distribution in patients, indicating that the abnormality is not confined to an 'organic' subtype of schizophrenia. There is no clear association with gender. The differences are present in first episode and unmedicated patients, indicating that they are not due to treatment. However, the changes are modest (e.g. the difference in brain volume is about 3 per cent), and with significant overlap between patients and controls. Furthermore, they are not diagnostically specific; for example, enlarged ventricles and cerebral atrophy occur in Alzheimer's disease, whilst smaller hippocampi may also occur in mood disorder. There are few clear clinicopathological associations, although particular structural alterations have been associated with specific symptoms and cognitive deficits; for example, thought disorder with smaller superior temporal gyri.

Recent studies have attempted to identify the course of structural brain changes in schizophrenia. The results are complex and controversial (Weinberger and McClure, 2002). Some changes are present before the onset of symptoms, whilst others emerge during the first episode (Pantelis *et al.*, 2003). Thereafter, the majority of alterations appear non-progressive, but some studies indicate that further changes occur in a subgroup of patients, or at specific phases of illness.

First-degree relatives of patients with schizophrenia tend to show changes in regional brain volumes that intermediate between patients and unrelated healthy controls (Lawrie *et al.*, 1999), implying that some of the brain abnormalities are associated with genetic predisposition to the disorder.

Neuropathology

Post-mortem neuropathological studies have sought to explain the cellular and molecular basis for the neuroimaging findings (Harrison, 1999; Table 12.12). A few findings are noteworthy:

- Brain weight is decreased.
- There is no evidence of any neurodegenerative processes. This supports a neurodevelopmental origin of the pathology, and also argues that any progression of pathology during the illness, noted in some MRI studies, is not neurotoxic or degenerative in nature.
- The main positive findings are alterations in markers of synapses and dendrites, and in the density of specific populations of neurons and glia. These changes, which are present in the cerebral cortex, hippocampus, and thalamus, suggest differences in synaptic connections, and have contributed to the 'aberrant connectivity' hypothesis of schizophrenia (p. 293).
- An abnormal position or clustering of some neurons, notably in the entorhinal cortex or white matter, has been reported in several studies. Such findings are strongly suggestive of a prenatal abnormality in neuronal migration. However, these findings have not been well replicated.
- Studies of gene expression have shown differences in families of genes consistent with involvement of both neuronal and oligodendroglial cells in schizophrenia. The relationship between the molecular findings, structural neuropathology, and genetic factors is not clear (see Harrison and Weinberger, 2005).

Cerebral blood flow

As described in Chapter 5, a number of techniques, particularly positron emission tomography (PET), single-photon emission tomography (SPET), and functional magnetic resonance imaging (fMRI), have been used to assess cerebral blood flow and metabolic activity in schizophrenia. Three types of approach have been used:

1. Measurement of regional cerebral blood flow at rest.
2. Patterns of cerebral activation and deactivation associated with specific neuropsychological tasks.
3. Correlation of patterns of regional cerebral blood flow with the presence of specific symptomatology.

The first study was by Ingvar and Franzen (1974), who used injections of radioactive xenon, and found a decreased perfusion of frontal cortex compared to posterior regions in chronic, medicated patients with schizophrenia. This 'hypofrontality' has been considered a feature of schizophrenia since this time and, though many studies have been negative, was confirmed in a recent meta-analysis (Hill *et al.*, 2004). However, stronger relationships with hypofrontality are seen if the phase of illness and symptom profile are taken into account, for example, the association with psychomotor poverty mentioned above (Table 12.3). Alterations of frontal perfusion and activity are particularly apparent in schizophrenia during performance of cognitive tasks such as the Wisconsin Card Sorting Task (Liddle and Pantelis, 2003). However, the interpretation of the changes is difficult, since patients usually perform worse on these tasks, and therefore decreased activation may simply reflect failure to perform (or attend to) the task. Some data show that patients require more frontal cortex activation to achieve the same level of performance as controls, suggestive of a reduced 'efficiency' of cortical processing (Callicott *et al.*, 2003). Such abnormalities have been related to theories of aberrant connectivity and dopamine in schizophrenia, discussed below.

Other studies have looked at the cerebral correlates of specific symptoms. For example, using fMRI, it was found that when patients listened to externally generated speech, the presence of auditory hallucinations was linked to reduced activity of the temporal regions that normally process external speech. This could represent competition for a common neural substrate (see David and Busatto, 1999).

Neurochemical findings

Many neurotransmitter receptors, enzymes, and metabolites, have been measured in schizophrenia, and a wide range of abnormalities described. Research now uses increasingly sensitive and sophisticated methods to link neurochemistry with neuroanatomy, and build up a profile of the 'neurochemical anatomy' of schizophrenia (Fallon *et al.*, 2003). Efforts are also being made to link post-mortem findings with functional imaging studies *in vivo*, and most recently to relate the neurochemistry to genes. However, for many of the findings to be described here, their role in the aetiology of schizophrenia is still unclear, and hard to distinguish from alterations which are part of the brain's adaptive or maladaptive response to the illness, including the effects of medication.

Dopamine

Two early lines of research converged on dopamine, which has remained the neurotransmitter most implicated in schizophrenia for over thirty years (Seeman, 1987). The first concerns the effects of amphetamine which, among other actions, releases dopamine at central synapses. Repeated use of amphetamine at high doses can induce a disorder similar to acute schizophrenia in some normal people, and acute amphetamine administration worsens psychotic symptoms in people with schizophrenia. The second approach starts from the finding that all antipsychotic drugs are dopamine receptor antagonists, and that their affinity at dopamine D_2 receptors is the property which correlates best with their clinical potency (p. 530).

Although the evidence that dopamine is central to the action of antipsychotic drugs is strong, evidence that dopamine neurotransmission is abnormal in schizophrenia has, until recently, been much weaker, in part because of the difficulty distinguishing drug from disease effects in medicated patients. More recently, however, PET and SPET studies provide ways to investigate dopamine receptors and dopamine synthesis in the brain of unmedicated patients using appropriately radiolabelled ligands. Most of these studies have not found a simple difference in the number of dopamine receptors in schizophrenia. However, studies using more complex paradigms have shown convincing evidence of dopaminergic abnormality in schizophrenia (Harrison, 2000). As explained earlier (Chapter 5) it is possible to measure the release of dopamine *in vivo* following pharmacological challenge by measuring the displacement of a D_2 receptor radioligand such as $[^{11}C]$raclopride. In patients with acute schizophrenia, injection of amphetamine causes a two-fold greater decrease in $[^{11}C]$raclopride binding than is seen in control subjects; studies in monkeys indicate that this decrease corresponds to a three-fold greater increase of synaptic dopamine release (Laruelle and Abi-Dargham, 1999). Further studies have shown an excessive dopamine release in acute schizophrenia without using amphetamines, supporting the conclusion that **'hyperdopaminergia'** is a feature of the illness. In patients in remission, dopamine release returns to normal, suggesting that excess dopamine release is directly related to acute psychotic symptoms: the 'wind of the psychotic fire' (Laruelle and Abi-Dargham, 1999).

Other phases and aspects of schizophrenia may be associated with different abnormalities in dopamine function. In particular, various lines of evidence suggest that there is deficient dopaminergic regulation of the prefrontal cortex (Winterer and Weinberger, 2004), relevant to the enduring cognitive deficits of the illness (p. 272 and Box 5.3).

The mechanisms of dopaminergic involvment in schizophrenia are unclear. There may be a genetic component (Egan *et al.*, 2001), but current theories emphasize dysregulation secondary to glutamatergic abnormalities, as outlined below. A phenomenological approach to dopamine in schizophrenia has recently been proposed by Kapur (2003). He argues that the known roles of dopamine in cognition and behaviour suggest that it mediates the 'salience' of external events and internal representations, and that in schizophrenia the dopamine abnormalities lead the patient to misattribute stimuli and their meaning. Delusions and hallucinations are viewed as the consequence of these experiences and the patient's attempt to make sense of them.

Glutamate

There is increasing interest in the role of the amino-acid neurotransmitter glutamate in schizophrenia. The key finding was that antagonists of the N-methyl-D-aspartate (NMDA) type of glutamate receptor (such as phencyclidine and ketamine) can induce a schizophrenia-like psychosis; it was complemented by data showing that NMDA receptor modulators (such as glycine) have some antipsychotic effects (Goff and Coyle, 2001). Other lines of evidence support glutamate involvement in schizophrenia (Konradi and Heckers, 2003), including alterations in pre and post-synaptic indices of glutamate signalling, especially in the medial temporal lobe, wherein non-NMDA glutamate receptors are reduced.

There are several theories to explain glutamatergic involvement in schizophrenia. First, the '**NMDA receptor hypofunction**' model, which postulates that an abnormality in function of this receptor is an important developmental pathogenic factor in schizophrenia (Olney and Farber, 1995). Second, much research indicates that the dopaminergic dysfunction in schizophrenia is secondary to aberrant regulation by glutamatergic neurons (Laruelle *et al.*, 2003). Third, a primary role for glutamate in schizophrenia is now suggested by the fact that most of the identified susceptibility genes are involved in glutamate transmission (Harrison and Weinberger, 2005).

GABA (γ-aminobutyric acid)

GABA is the major inhibitory transmitter in the brain, and is implicated in schizophrenia for several reasons (Blum and Mann, 2002). First, there is a decrease in its synthetic enzyme, glutamic acid decarboxylase (GAD) in the cerebral cortex in the disease. Second, the density of a particular GABAergic neuron type (those which contain parvalbumin) and their synaptic terminals, are reduced. Third, there are alterations in expression of $GABA_A$ receptors. Together, these findings indicate impairment of GABA signalling in schizophrenia (Lewis *et al.*, 2005). However, its origin and relationship to the disturbances in other neurotransmitters mentioned is unclear; GABA may have a causal role, as there is preliminary evidence that one of the GAD genes is associated with the disorder.

Serotonin

A possible role of serotonin (5-HT) in schizophrenia has long been considered, because the hallucinogen, lysergic acid diethylamide (LSD), is an agonist at 5-HT_2 receptors. More recently it has become apparent that 5-HT_2 receptor antagonism may contribute to the atypical profile of some antipsychotics (p. 532), and allelic variation in the 5-HT_{2A} gene may be a minor risk factor for schizophrenia. Additional support for a pathophysiological role for 5-HT is provided by the decreased expression of frontal cortex 5-HT_{2A} receptors in schizophrenia seen in both post-mortem and functional imaging studies (Dean, 2003). Increased cortical 5-HT_{1A} receptor binding has also been reported. The findings are of interest because of the roles of 5-HT in neurodevelopment, and the many interactions between 5-HT, dopamine, and glutamate (Carlsson *et al.*, 2001).

Neurophysiological findings

Electroencephalography

The EEG in schizophrenia generally shows increased amounts of theta activity, fast activity, and paroxysmal activity. The significance of these findings is unknown. Recently, more sophisticated combinations of EEG and event-related potential analyses have been used. This work shows that there is a decreased synchronization or coherence of electrical activity in the prefrontal cortex, suggestive of 'noisy' or inefficient cortical processing in schizophrenia (Winterer and Weinberger, 2004).

Sensory evoked potentials: P300 and P50

The P300 response is an auditory evoked potential which occurs 300 milliseconds after a subject identifies a target stimulus embedded in a series of irrelevant stimuli. The response provides a measure of auditory information processing. In patients with schizophrenia, and a proportion of their first-degree relatives, the amplitude of the P300 wave is reduced.

Abnormalities in another evoked potential, the P50 wave, have also been reported in patients with schizophrenia and their relatives. Moreover, molecular genetic studies in families with schizophrenia have shown that P50 deficits are linked to the gene coding for a subunit of the nicotinic cholinergic receptor, implying that alterations in cholinergic neurotransmission could underlie abnormalities in information processing in schizophrenia. A recent meta-analysis confirms the presence of P300 and P50 deficits in schizophrenia (Bramon *et al.*, 2004).

Eye tracking

Over 50 per cent of patients with schizophrenia have defective performance in tests of eye tracking. A similar abnormality affects about 25 per cent of first-degree relatives. Holzman (2000) has proposed that eye-tracking dysfunction is a genetically transmitted and phenotypically mild variant of schizophrenia.

Social and psychosocial factors

Occupation and social class

Several studies have shown that schizophrenia is over-represented among people of lower social class. In Chicago, for example, Hollingshead and Redlich (1958) found both the incidence and the prevalence of schizophrenia to be highest in the lowest socioeconomic groups. At first, these findings were thought to be of aetiological significance, but they could be a consequence of schizophrenia. For instance, Goldberg and Morrison (1963) found that people with schizophrenia were of lower social status than their fathers and that this was usually because they had changed status after the illness began. However, Castle *et al.* (1993) found that, compared with controls, patients with schizophrenia were more likely to have been born into socially deprived households. The authors proposed that some environmental factor of aetiological importance was more likely to affect those of lower economic status living in inner cities.

Place of residence

Faris and Dunham (1939) studied the place of residence of mentally ill people in Chicago, and found that schizophrenics were over-represented in the disadvantaged inner-city areas. This distribution has been confirmed in other cities and it has been suggested that unsatisfactory living conditions can cause schizophrenia. These findings have often been ascribed to the occupational and social decline described above, or by a search for social isolation by people about to develop schizophrenia.

However, recent data suggest that schizophrenia is associated with place of birth and upbringing, findings which cannot be explained away as a consequence of illness. Specifically, population-based studies in several countries show that urban birth is associated with an increased risk of schizophrenia. Larger cities carry a higher odds ratio than small towns or suburban areas (Pedersen and Mortensen, 2001). The cause of the association remains unclear, and may relate to social deprivation, migration, infections, stress, or interactions between genetic vulnerability and urban environments (Peen and Dekker, 2004).

Migration

High rates of schizophrenia have been reported among migrants. In a study of Norwegians who had migrated to Minnesota, Ødegaard (1932) found that the inception rate for schizophrenia was twice that of Norwegians in Norway. The reasons for these high rates are not clear and have been attributed mainly to a disproportionate migration of people who are unsettled because they are becoming mentally ill. The effects of a new environment may also play a part in provoking illness in predisposed people. Thus 'social selection' and 'social causation' may both contribute to an excess of schizophrenia among migrants.

A recent meta-analysis of 18 studies confirms that migration is a risk factor for schizophrenia, and that this cannot be explained solely by selection (Cantor-Grae and Selten, 2005). The relative risk for migrants is 2.7 (95 per cent confidence interval, 2.3–3.2), with a higher risk for the children of migrants (4.5, 95 per cent confidence interval, 1.5–13.1). Risks were also higher for migrants from developing countries.

A particularly controversial aspect of migration and schizophrenia concerns the Afro-Caribbean population in the United Kingdom, reported to have a strikingly increased incidence of schizophrenia (about 6 per 1000; Harrison *et al.*, 1988), particularly in the 'second generation' born in the UK. By contrast, rates in the Caribbean are not appreciably increased. One possibility is that there is misdiagnosis, reflecting unfamiliarity with Caribbean beliefs or racial bias by primarily Caucasian psychiatrists. However, there is no evidence that this explains away the increased incidence, given the results of the meta-analysis by Cantor-Grae and Selten (2005). If the incidence of schizophrenia is indeed increased in the British Afro-Caribbean population, the same range of biological and psychosocial possibilities applies as for other migrant populations, including viral infections, cannabis use, psychosocial adversity, or the stress of racial discrimination (Sharpley *et al.*, 2001).

Social isolation

People with schizophrenia often live alone, unmarried, and with few friends. The findings reviewed above suggest the pattern of isolation may begin before the illness, sometimes in early childhood. Of course, some patients may choose to isolate themselves as a way of decreasing social stimulation. In this sense social isolation, though undesirable in a general sense, is not a straightforward stressor.

Life events and difficulties

Life events and difficulties have often been put forward as precipitants of schizophrenia, but few satisfactory studies have been carried out. In one of the most convincing, Brown and Birley (1968) used a standardized procedure to collect information from 50 patients newly admitted with a precisely datable first onset or relapse of schizophrenia. By comparison with a control group, the rate of 'independent' events in the schizophrenics was increased in the 3 weeks before the onset of the acute symptoms. When the events (which included moving house, starting or losing a job, and domestic crises) were compared with events preceding depression, neurosis, and suicide attempts, they were found to be non-specific. Paykel (1978) calculated that experiencing a life event doubles the risk of developing schizophrenia over the subsequent 6 months. Others have confirmed these findings for both first episodes and relapse of schizophrenia (e.g. Bebbington *et al.*, 1993). In a review, Norman and Malla (1993) concluded that in patients with chronic schizophrenia, the level of symptoms over time correlated with life events; however, there was little evidence that patients with schizophrenia suffered more life events than the general population.

Culture

If cultural factors were important in the aetiology of schizophrenia, differences in the incidence of the disorder might be expected in countries with contrasting cultures. As already explained, the incidence of schizophrenia is remarkably similar in widely different places and cultures (Jablensky, 2003).

Psychological factors

Personality factors

Several early writers, including Bleuler (1911), commented on the frequency of abnormalities of personality preceding the onset of schizophrenia. Kretschmer (1936) proposed that both personality and schizophrenia were related to the asthenic type of body build. He suggested a continuous variation between normal personality, schizoid personality and schizophrenia. He regarded schizoid personality as a partial expression of the psychological abnormalities that manifest in their full form in schizophrenia. Such ideas must be treated with caution, since it is difficult to distinguish between premorbid personality and the prodromal phase of slowly developing illness. However, his ideas are similar to the current concept of the schizophrenia spectrum, in which schizophrenia is the most severe end of a continuum. Taken together, the findings suggest that abnormal personality features are not uncommon among people who later develop schizophrenia and among their first-degree relatives. However, many people with schizophrenia have no obvious disorder of personality before the onset of the illness and only a minority of people with schizotypal or schizoid personalities develop schizophrenia.

Neuropsychological factors

As noted above, it is now well established that patients with schizophrenia have widespread cognitive deficits particularly in tasks involving learning and memory. Neuropsychological studies from a research perspective aim to answer two rather different questions:

1. What is the pattern of neuropsychological defects in schizophrenia and how might this reflect abnormalities in the various brain regions that subsume these psychological functions?
2. How might specific cognitive abnormalities account for the characteristic symptoms of schizophrenia?

A well-known neuropsychological model of schizophrenia is that by Gray *et al.* (1991), who proposed that positive symptoms arise from a failure to integrate stored memories with current stimuli. The theory was unusual at the time, in attempting to explain psychological features in terms of limbic circuits and dopamine projections.

Using a different model, Frith (1996) argued that in schizophrenia there is a breakdown in the internal representation of mental events. For example, a failure to monitor and identify one's own willed intentions might give rise to the idea that thoughts and actions arise from external sources, resulting in delusions of control.

The concept of **social cognition** – the role of cognitive factors in the impaired social functioning of schizophrenia – has become prominent recently. Abnormalities of emotional processing, face recognition, and theory of mind are postulated to be important, and to result from the involvement of neural circuits involving the frontal cortex and amgydala (Pinkham *et al.*, 2003).

Dynamic and interpersonal factors

From the point of view of evidence-based aetiology, these theories of schizophrenia are largely of historical interest (Box 12.4). However, they remain important both because they focus attention on interpersonal aspects, which are important in view of the evidence described above suggesting that patients with schizophrenia have abnormal social development during childhood, and also because some carers and health professionals continue to consider them relevant. For review, see Jackson and Cawley (1992).

BOX 12.4 PSYCHODYNAMIC AND FAMILY THEORIES OF AETIOLOGY

Psychodynamic theories

Freud's theory of schizophrenia was stated most clearly in his 1911 analysis of the Schreber case and in his 1914 paper 'On narcissism: an introduction'. According to Freud, in the first stage, libido was withdrawn from external objects and attached to the ego. The result was exaggerated self-importance. Since the withdrawal of libido made the external world meaningless, the patient attempted to restore meaning by developing abnormal beliefs. Because of libidinal withdrawal, the patient could not form a transference and therefore could not be treated by psychoanalysis. Although Freud developed his general ideas considerably after 1914, he elaborated his original theory of schizophrenia but did not replace it.

Melanie Klein (1952) believed that the origins of schizophrenia were in infancy. In the 'paranoid schizoid position' the infant dealt with innate aggressive impulses by splitting both his own ego and his representation of his mother into two incompatible parts, one wholly bad and the other wholly good. Only later did the child realize that the same person could be good at one time and bad at another. Failure to pass through this stage adequately was the basis for the later development of schizophrenia.

The family as a cause of schizophrenia

Two kinds of theory have been proposed about the family as a cause of schizophrenia: **deviant role relationships** (asssociated with Fromm-Reichmann and Lidz) and **disordered communication** (associated with Bateson and Wynne). The different role of the family in influencing the course of schizophrenia is discussed later.

The concept of the **'schizophrenogenic' mother** was suggested by the analyst Fromm-Reichmann in 1948. Lidz and his colleagues (1965) used intensive psychoanalytical methods to study the families of 17 patients with schizophrenia, of whom 14 were in social classes I or II. Two types of abnormal family pattern were reported:

- **Marital skew**, in which one parent yielded to the other's (usually the mother's) eccentricities, which dominated the family.
- **Marital schism**, in which the parents maintained contrary views so that the child had divided loyalties. It was suggested that these abnormalities were the cause rather than the result of the schizophrenia.

Investigations by other clinicians have not confirmed these findings. Even if they were confirmed, the abnormalities in the parents could be an expression of genetic causes, or secondary to the disorder in the patient. These and other speculations about the causative role of family relationships have had the unfortunate consequence of inducing unjustified guilt in parents.

Research on disordered communication in families originated from the idea of the **double bind** (Bateson *et al.*, 1956). A double bind is said to occur when an instruction is given overtly, but is contradicted by a second more covert instruction. For example, a mother may overtly tell her child to come to her, whilst conveying by manner and tone of voice that she rejects him. According to Bateson, double binds leave the child able to make only ambiguous or meaningless responses, and schizophrenia develops when this process persists. The theory is ingenious but not supported by evidence.

Studies of communication in families of patients with schizophrenia have given rather conflicting results (Singer and Wynne, 1965; Hirsch and Leff, 1975). However, it is worth noting that an association between abnormal social communication in parents and schizophrenic illness in children may, in fact, be a consequence of a shared genetic inheritance; for example, because the incidence of schizotypal disorder (characterized by abnormalities of thought and speech) is raised in first-degree relatives of patients with schizophrenia.

Current aetiological hypotheses about schizophrenia

The dopamine (p. 288), NMDA receptor (p. 289) and cerebral asymmetry (p. 283) hypotheses of schizophrenia have already been mentioned. Here we note three other current hypotheses, reflecting the various aetiological considerations discussed above.

Neurodevelopmental hypothesis

The leading hypothesis is that schizophrenia is a disorder of neurodevelopment. Original suggestions of this kind were made by Clouston in 1892 and by others, including Kraepelin, at the turn of the last century, but the current view can be traced to Murray and Lewis (1987) and Weinberger (1987). The hypothesis is simple: schizophrenia results from an abnormality in some aspect of brain development. This is implicitly contrasted with the alternative, that schizophrenia is a neurodegenerative disorder (McClure and Lieberman, 2003). Specific forms of the neurodevelopmental hypothesis implicate the prenatal period, adolescence, or an interaction between the two. Evidence in favour of the model has accrued from several sources (Lewis and Levitt, 2002) and is summarized in Table 12.13. Many of the factors have already been discussed. The others are briefly mentioned here. The frequency of minor physical anomalies, aberrant fingerprint patterns (dermatoglyphics; Bramon *et al.*, 2005) and cavum septum pellucidum (an uncommon feature seen on MRI scans) are all increased in schizophrenia; each is believed to be a sign of early neurodevelopmental abnormality (McGrath and Murray, 2003). The absence of gliosis (the proliferation and hypertrophy of astrocytes) is important, as it argues for a prenatal (second trimester) timing of the neuropathology.

TABLE 12.13 Findings supporting the neurodevelopmental hypothesis of schizophrenia

Structural brain lesions present at or before illness onset
Lack of progression of structural brain changes after onset
Cognitive and social impairments in childhood
Neuropathological changes without gliosis
'Soft' neurological signs at presentation
Minor physical anomalies and aberrant dermatoglyphics
Pre- and peri-natal risk factors
Increased frequency of cavum septum pellucidum
Animal models show delayed effects of early brain lesions

There are no serious challenges to the neurodevelopmental hypothesis as a pathogenic model of schizophrenia. This partly reflects its vagueness, which allows most findings to be interpreted as being consistent with it. Its other weaknesses include a failure to explain readily the onset or course of the disorder (Broome *et al.*, 2005), nor the proportion of cases which it can account for.

Aberrant connectivity

Bleuler conceptualized the fundamental symptoms of schizophrenia as reflecting 'psychic splitting' or a failure of integration of mental functions. This view is currently framed in terms of abnormal connectivity, whereby the activity of different brain regions or circuits is aberrant in schizophrenia (McGuire and Frith, 1996; Andreasen, 1999). Some variants of this model involve a structural component (i.e. changes in the 'wiring' of the brain; p. 286), such as the hypothesis that schizophrenia is a disorder of the synapse (Frankle *et al.*, 2003) or of white matter. However, connectivity could also be functionally abnormal (e.g. in terms of signalling characteristics) without a structural neuropathology being present. Most connectivity models assume that the abnormality arises developmentally, but this need not be the case.

Stress-vulnerability model

This model (also called the **stress-diathesis model**) incorporates development, but emphasizes the interaction of the early events (whether genetic, biological or social) with later stressors (e.g. substance use, life events). The early factors confer vulnerability to schizophrenia, whereas the latter explain its onset and course (Neuchterlein and Dawson, 1984). This model is therefore similar to the Brown and Harris theory of depression described in Chapter 11. It is useful in drawing attention to the later events, as these may be relevant for treatment. The emphasis on interactions between aetiological factors is also appropriate, as an increasing number of studies, including many mentioned above, indicate that environmental factors act primarily upon those who are already at risk, for genetic or other reasons. Future studies will need to be very large if such interactions are to be reliably identified.

Course and prognosis

Kraepelin initially believed that dementia praecox had an invariably poor outcome, although he later reported that in the long term, 17 per cent of his patients were socially well-adjusted. Although it remains generally agreed that the outcome of schizophrenia is worse than that of most psychiatric disorders, it is difficult to draw clear conclusions (Häfner and an der Heiden, 2003).

An important long-term study was carried out by Manfred Bleuler (1974), son of Eugen Bleuler, who personally followed up 208 patients who had been admitted to hospital in Switzerland between 1942 and 1943. Twenty years after admission, 20 per cent had a complete remission of symptoms, 35 per cent had a good outcome in terms of social adjustment, and 24 per cent were severely disturbed. When full recovery had occurred, it was usually in the first 2 years. When the illness was recurrent, each subsequent episode usually resembled the first in its clinical features. Bleuler's diagnostic criteria were narrow, and his findings suggest that the traditional view of schizophrenia as a generally progressive and disabling condition must be reconsidered. Nevertheless, 10 per cent of his patients suffered an illness of such severity that they required long-term sheltered care.

Bleuler's conclusions are broadly supported by Ciompi's larger but less detailed study of long-term outcome in Lausanne (Ciompi, 1980). The study was based on the well-kept records of 1642 patients diagnosed as having schizophrenia from the beginning of the century to 1962. The average follow-up was 37 years. A third of the patients were found to have a good or fair social outcome. Symptoms often became less severe in the later years of life.

More recent studies are in general agreement with these findings. For example, in a 3–13-year follow-up study of patients with schizophrenia discharged between 1975 and 1985, Johnstone (1991) found that almost half had a good social outcome. In a 15-year follow-up of 330 Chinese patients with first admission schizophrenia, almost one-third recovered, but 17 per cent remained unable to function outside hospital (Tsoi and Wong, 1991). Finally, a recent 15 and 25-year follow-up study of patient cohorts in 15 countries found that one-sixth of patients had achieved full recovery; importantly, late recovery was seen in a significant minority, challenging the therapeutic pessimism that such improvements are very rare (Harrison *et al.*, 2001).

Whether the outcome of schizophrenia has improved since Kraepelin's era remains unclear. A meta-analysis found a 'recovery rate' of 35 per cent prior to 1955, and 49 per cent for the period 1956–1985, a difference that may reflect the use of antipsychotics. However, the rate fell back to 36 per cent between 1986 and 1992 (Hegarty *et al.*, 1994). Any apparent time-trends must be interpreted very cautiously because of changes in diagnostic practice and outcome measures during the century.

Mortality in schizophrenia

All studies with prolonged follow-up report an increased mortality in patients with schizophrenia. In a meta-analysis of 36 000 patients Harris and Barraclough (1998) found that risk of death from all causes was increased 1.6-fold. Almost 40 per cent of the excess mortality was accounted for by unnatural causes, mainly suicide, the risk of which was increased ten-fold. The lifetime risk of suicide in schizophrenia is usually quoted at about 10 per cent, although longer-term follow-up suggests that the rate may be somewhat lower, perhaps about 4 per cent (Palmer *et al.*, 2005). This is probably because the highest risk of suicide in schizophrenia is soon after diagnosis and declines somewhat thereafter. Recent studies also suggest that suicide rates in schizophrenia may be declining (Nordentoft *et al.*, 2004). Deaths due to cardiovascular and respiratory causes are also substantially increased, presumably reflecting the high rates of smoking, as well as poor diets, sedentary lifestyle, and higher rates of obesity and type II diabetes.

Predictors of outcome

The outcome of a case of schizophrenia is remarkably heterogeneous and unpredictable (Häfner and an der Heiden, 2003). For example, in the International Pilot Study of Schizophrenia (World Health Organization, 1973), tests were made of the predictive value of several sets of criteria based on symptoms. All proved largely unsuccessful at predicting outcome at 2 years or 5 years. The best predictors of poor outcome appear to be the criteria used for diagnosis in DSM-IV, probably because they stipulate that the syndrome should have been present for 6 months before the diagnosis can be made.

Poor outcome in schizophrenia is associated with younger age of onset, male sex, poor premorbid functioning, and persistence of negative symptoms. There is also evidence that the duration of psychotic symptoms prior to treatment correlates with time to remission and level of remission (Marshall *et al.*, 2005). Whilst reluctance to seek treatment could be associated with other predictors of poor outcome, it is also possible that early treatment, either with drugs or psychological therapies, may improve the prognosis (see p. 304).

Some of the predictors that have emerged from the various studies are listed in Table 12.14 and may be taken as a moderately useful guide. However, it is wise to be cautious when asked to predict the outcome of individual cases.

So far this discussion has been concerned with factors operating before or at the onset of schizophrenia.

TABLE 12.14 Factors predicting the outcome of schizophrenia

Good prognosis	Poor prognosis
Sudden onset	Insidious onset
Short episode	Long episode
No previous psychiatric history	Previous psychiatric history
Prominent affective symptoms	Negative symptoms
Paranoid type of illness	Enlarged lateral ventricles
	Male gender
Older age at onset	Younger age at onset
Married	Single, separated, widowed, divorced
Good psychosexual adjustment	Poor psychosexual adjustment
Good previous personality	Abnormal previous personality
Good work record	Poor work record
Good social relationships	Social isolation
Compliance with treatment	Poor compliance

An account will now be given of factors acting after the illness has been established.

Geographical variation in course

As noted above, international studies suggest that the incidence of schizophrenia is broadly similar in different countries; however, the course and outcome are not. In the International Pilot Study of Schizophrenia (World Health Organization, 1973), two year outcome was better in India, Colombia, and Nigeria than in the other centres. This finding could not be explained by any recorded differences in the initial characteristics of the patients. The possibility of selection bias remains; for example, in these three countries patients with acute illness may be more likely to be taken to hospital than patients with illness of insidious onset. However, later studies designed to overcome these objections also found a more favourable course of illness in less developed countries (Jablensky, 2003). The major difference in outcome was that patients in developing countries were more likely to achieve a complete remission than those in developed countries, who tended to be impaired by continual residual symptoms.

The better outcome of schizophrenia in developing countries is unexplained. It does not appear to be due to differences in levels of expressed emotion; a 15 and 25 year follow-up study confirmed the stability of geographical differences in course, and suggested that a difference in the severity and type of illness at first presentation is an important contributory factor (Harrison *et al.*, 2001).

Life events

As explained above, some patients experience an excess of life events in the weeks before the onset of acute symptoms of schizophrenia. This applies not only to first illnesses but also to relapses (Bebbington *et al.*, 1993). In addition, patients with increased numbers of life events experience a more symptomatic course.

Social stimulation

In the 1940s and 1950s, clinicians recognized that among schizophrenics living in institutions many clinical features were associated with an unstimulating environment. Soon after this Wing and Brown (1970) investigated patients at three mental hospitals. One was a traditional institution, another had an active rehabilitation programme, and the third had a reputation for progressive policies and short admissions. The research team devised a measure of 'poverty of the social milieu' which took into account little contact with the outside world, few personal possessions, lack of constructive occupation, and pessimistic expectations on the part of ward staff. Poverty of social milieu was found to be closely related to three aspects of the patients' clinical condition: social withdrawal, blunting of affect, and poverty of speech. The causal significance of these social conditions was strongly supported by a further survey 4 years later; improvements had taken place in the environment of the hospitals, and these changes were accompanied by corresponding improvements in the three aspects of the patients' clinical state.

While an understimulating hospital environment is harmful, an overstimulating environment can precipitate positive symptoms and lead to relapse. Since factors in a hospital environment play an important part in determining prognosis, it seems likely that similar factors are important to patients living in the community.

Family life and expressed emotion

Brown *et al.* (1958) found that, on discharge from hospital, patients with schizophrenia returning to their families generally had a worse prognosis than those entering hostels. Brown *et al.* (1962) found that relapse rates were greater in families where relatives showed **high expressed emotion** ('high EE') by making critical comments, expressing hostility, and showing signs of emotional over-involvement. In such families the risk of relapse was greater if the patients were in contact with their close relatives for more than 35 hours a week. The work was confirmed and extended when Leff and Vaughn (1981) investigated the interaction between expressed emotion in relatives and life events in the 3 months before relapse. The onset of illness was associated either with a high level of expressed emotion or with an independent life event.

Vaughn and Leff (1976) also suggested an association between expressed emotion in relatives and the patient's response to antipsychotic medication. Among patients who were spending more than 35 hours a week in contact with relatives showing high emotional expression, the relapse rate was 92 per cent for those not taking antipsychotics and only 53 per cent for those who were. Patients taking antipsychotic drugs and spending less than 35 hours in contact with relatives showing high emotional expression had a 15 per cent relapse rate.

Further studies (Leff *et al.*, 1985) strongly suggested that high expressed emotion has a causal role. Twenty-four families were selected in which a schizophrenic patient had extended contact with relatives showing high emotional expression. All patients were on medication. Half the families were randomly assigned to routine outpatient care. The other half took part in a programme including education about schizophrenia, relatives' groups, and family sessions for relatives and patients. The relapse rate was significantly lower in this group than in the controls. Apart from providing further evidence of the importance of relatives' expressed emotion in relapse, this study showed the effectiveness of combined social intervention and drug treatment.

Expressed emotion has now been widely investigated as a predictor of psychotic relapse, and overall it appears that patients living in families with high levels of expressed emotion have a two- to three-fold increased risk. An associated finding is that relatives with low levels of expressed emotion are more likely to regard schizophrenia and its associated behaviour as an illness beyond the control of the patient, and the nature of these causal attributions are also predictors of outcome (Barrowclough *et al.*, 1994).

Effects of schizophrenia on the family

With the increasing care of patients in the community rather than in hospital, difficulties have arisen for some families. Relatives of patients with schizophrenia describe two main groups of problems. The first group relates to social withdrawal. Patients tend not to interact with other family members; they seem slow, lack conversation, have few interests, and neglect themselves. The second group relates to more obviously disturbed or socially inappropriate behaviour, and threats of violence. These problems are likely to play a part in the development of high expressed emotion in relatives, which in turn may worsen the situation.

Relatives of patients with schizophrenia may feel anxious, depressed, guilty, or bewildered. They may be understandably uncertain of how to deal with difficult and odd behaviour. Further difficulties can arise from differences in opinion between family members, and from a lack of understanding and sympathy among neighbours and friends. The effects on the lives of relatives and families are often serious. Unfortunately, community services and support for patients with schizophrenia and their relatives are often less than adequate. Improving help, advice, and services to carers of patients is a priority of the UK National Service Framework for Mental Health (Department of Health, 1999). Leff (1998) has commented:

> 'Relatives should be respected for the caring they undertake day and night for years on end. They do not want to be considered pathogenic and suitable cases for treatment. Instead they wish to be regarded as partners in the struggle against schizophrenia'.

Working with patients with schizophrenia and their carers is discussed further in the section on management, and on p. 306.

Conclusion

Social factors play a role in the onset of schizophrenia and the level of symptomatology in established cases. The emotional involvement of relatives can affect the risk of relapse, and it is possible that a lower degree of expressed emotion in families in developing countries could play a part in the improved prognosis of schizophrenia in these cultures. In terms of the general environment in which patients live, too much stimulation appears to precipitate relapse into positive symptoms, whilst understimulation can worsen negative symptoms.

Treatment

The treatment of schizophrenia is concerned with both the acute illness and chronic disability. In general, the best results are obtained by combining antipsychotic drugs and certain psychosocial treatments. This section is concerned with evidence about the efficacy of the individual treatments. The section on management deals with the use of these treatments in clinical practice. Pharmacological aspects of antipsychotic drugs are discussed in Chapter 21. The organization of community care and care planning is discussed in Chapter 23.

For recent treatment guidelines, see National Institute for Clinical Excellence (2002) and Lehman *et al.* (2004).

Antipsychotic drugs

Acute schizophrenia

The effectiveness of antipsychotic medication in the treatment of acute schizophrenia is well established. For example, the National Institute of Mental Health Collaborative Project (Cole *et al.*, 1964) compared chlorpromazine, fluphenazine and thioridazine with placebo. Three-quarters of the patients receiving antipsychotic treatment for 6 weeks improved, whilst half of those receiving placebo worsened. In a meta-analysis, Thornley *et al.* (1997) reviewed 42 randomized acute trials of chlorpromazine. Relative to placebo, chlorpromazine was more likely to lead to global clinical improvement at 8 weeks (55 per cent versus 37 per cent, NNT = 6).

Drug treatment has most effect on the positive symptoms of schizophrenia, such as hallucinations and delusions, and least effect on the negative and cognitive symptoms. The sedative action may be immediate, but the antipsychotic effect, though not delayed in onset as sometimes believed (Agid *et al.*, 2003), develops more slowly, sometimes taking several weeks to be clearly apparent.

Treatment after the acute phase

Since the original demonstration by Pasmanick *et al.* (1964), many controlled trials have shown the effectiveness of continued antipsychotic therapy in preventing relapse (Gilbert *et al.*, 1995). In a systematic review, Thornley *et al.*, (2003) showed that chlorpromazine reduces the risk of relapse over 6–24 months (relative risk = 0.65, NNT = 3) and improves global functioning (relative risk = 0.76; NNT = 7). Intermittent treatment, where antipsychotics are given at the first sign of relapse, is less effective than continuous prophylaxis (Jolley *et al.*, 1990).

Some patients with chronic schizophrenia do not respond even to long-term medication, whilst other patients remain well without drugs. Unfortunately, there has been no success in predicting which patients benefit from longer-term drug treatment, nor good evidence as to how long such prophylaxis should continue. The general consensus is that even long periods of remission do not protect patients from relapse once medication is withdrawn (see Cunningham Owens and Johnstone, 2000). Whenever antipsychotic treatment is discontinued, withdrawal should be carried out slowly, and with careful monitoring of mental state for several months afterwards.

There is a widespread clinical impression, supported by some data, that depot injections are more successful than continued oral medication in preventing relapse (Davis *et al.*, 1994), presumably due to improved compliance. A greater range of depot atypical antipsychotics is therefore to be desired; currently, only risperidone is available in this form.

Differences between antipsychotic drugs

There are no clear differences in efficacy between one typical antipsychotic and another, nor, with the exception of clozapine, between one atypical antipsychotic and another. Whether there are differences between typical and atypical antipsychotics has been more controversial. Meta-analyses of acute treatment trials differ in their conclusions as to whether atypical antipsychotics have greater efficacy or greater tolerability and, if so, the size and clinical relevance of the benefit. For example, Geddes *et al.* (2000) concluded that any benefits were trivial, whereas Davis *et al.* (2003) reported significantly greater efficacy for several atypical antipsychotics. A recent large long-term trial comparing several atypical antipsychotics and the typical agent perphenazine also found relatively minor differences (Lieberman *et al.*, 2005). Current British guidelines implicitly recommend atypical antipsychotics as the first-line drug treatment, but also recognize a continuing role for typical antipsychotics (National Institute for Clinical Excellence, 2002).

The superiority of atypical antipsychotics compared to conventional antipsychotics in prevention of relapse in schizophrenia also continues to be a matter of controversy. However, the balance of evidence is swinging in favour of the newer agents. The first substantive randomized controlled trial was by Csernansky *et al.* (2002) who compared the effect of risperidone with haloperidol in 365 stable patients with chronic schizophrenia over a 12 month period. Relapse occurred in 25 per cent of those treated with risperidone compared with 40 per cent treated with haloperidol, a highly significant difference both statistically and clinically. A recent systematic review (Leucht *et al.*, 2003) confirmed that atypical antipsychotics are effective in relapse prevention compared to placebo (NNT = 3–5), and produce modestly lower rates of relapse than do typical antipsychotics (NNT = 9–13), although the data were heavily weighted by the Csernansky *et al.* study, with other studies being much less impressive.

In clinical practice, atypical antipsychotics are usually chosen for treatment of new cases of schizophrenia, or if there is inadequate response to, or intolerance of, typical antipsychotics. The choice of individual drug, with the exception of clozapine, is then determined by a range of other factors, described in the section on management (p. 301).

Treatment resistant schizophrenia

About 30 per cent of patients do not respond to antipsychotics, or are intolerant to them, usually because of extrapyramidal side-effects. The only proven drug intervention for this group is clozapine, which is effective in between a third and a half of such patients, as shown by the key trial of Kane *et al.* (1988), and confirmed in subsequent analyses (Figure 12.1; Wahlbeck *et al.*, 1999). There is no evidence that any other atypical antipsychotic shares this greater efficacy (Chakos *et al.*, 2001). Clozapine may also have unique benefits against suicide in schizophrenia (see p. 305). It should therefore be recommended to all patients who do not respond to or cannot tolerate at least two other antipsychotics. However, its use is limited by the need for regular blood monitoring and the risks of agranulocytosis and other side effects, notably weight gain, sedation and hypersalivation (p. 536). Suggestions that clozapine should be used earlier in the illness in order to improve prognosis were not supported by a one-year trial which did not find clear superiority over chlorpromazine in first-episode or treatment-naïve patients (Lieberman *et al.*, 2003).

There is little guidance as to the appropriate drug treatment of patients unresponsive to, or unable to take, clozapine. A common augmentation strategy, for which there is some evidence, is to use an antipsychotic which has a high affinity for the D_2 dopamine receptor, such as sulpiride, amisulpride or risperidone. This is the only situation in which antipsychotic polypharmacy is currently justified (Freudenreich and Goff, 2002). There is also weak evidence in favour of augmentation with lamotrigine or valproate.

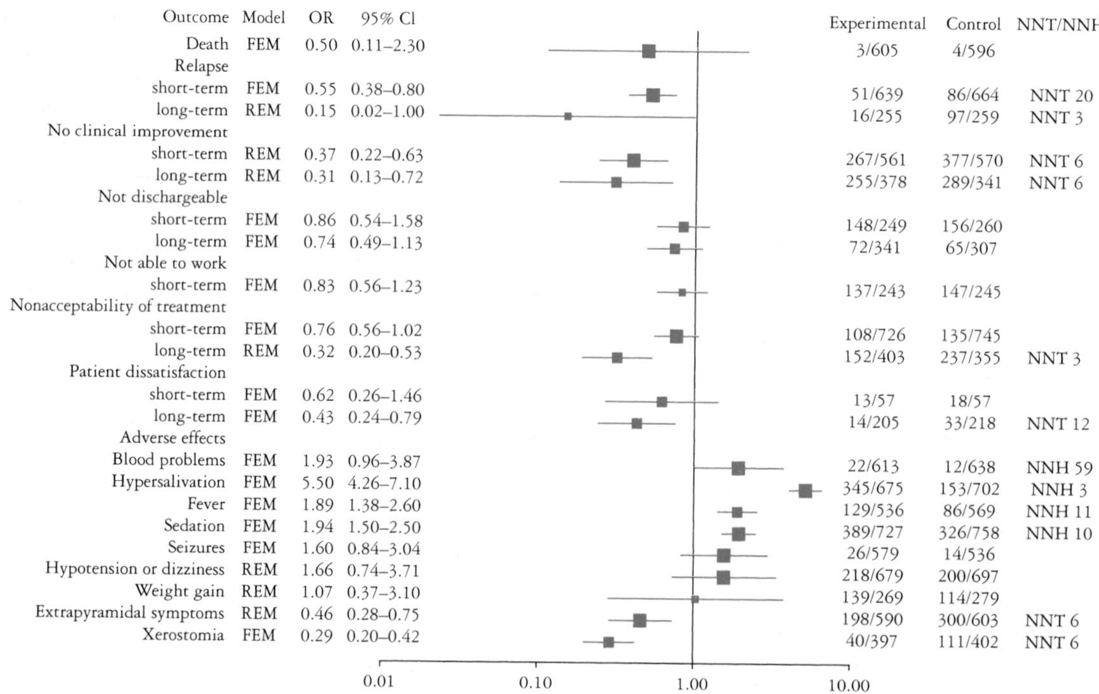

Fig. 12.1 Outcomes of schizophrenic patients randomly assigned to short- or long-term treatment with clozapine (experimental) or conventional neuroleptics (control) in 30 trials. OR, odds ratio; CI, confidence interal; NNT, number needed to treat; NNH, number needed to harm; FEM, fixed effects model; REM, random effects model. Columns with headings Experimental and Control refer to numbers of subjects. See Chapter 5 for explanation of terms.

For a review of treatment-resistant schizophrenia, see Barnes *et al.* (2003).

Antidepressants and mood stabilizers

As already explained, symptoms of depression occur commonly in schizophrenia. Since it is not easy to distinguish between depressive and negative symptoms, it is difficult to assess the effects of antidepressants in schizophrenia, and there have been few satisfactory clinical trials (Whitehead *et al.*, 2003).

Siris *et al.* (1987) carried out a placebo-controlled trial of imipramine in schizophrenic patients receiving fluphenazine in whom a depressive episode became apparent following resolution of the psychotic symptoms. Imipramine was significantly better than placebo, improving depressed mood but not altering psychotic symptoms. A second study by the same group confirmed the beneficial effect of imipramine. In patients where depressive symptoms coexist with an active psychosis, antidepressants do not seem to be helpful and in fact there is some evidence that they may worsen psychotic symptoms (Plasky, 1991). Newer antidepressants, notably SSRIs, are now widely used to treat depressive symptoms in schizophrenia but have not been rigorously evaluated.

The value of lithium and other mood stabilizers in treating schizophrenia is uncertain. There is no evidence that they have an antipsychotic effect, and the beneficial effects seen in some trials could be due to treatment of affective symptoms. For example, in the Northwick Park Functional Psychosis study, lithium decreased elevated mood, whatever the diagnosis, but had no significant effect on positive or negative symptoms (Johnstone *et al.*, 1988). A recent systematic review confirmed that lithium's benefits in schizophrenia occur primarily in patients with affective symptoms (or with schizoaffective disorder), and that there is no clear evidence for its efficacy in schizophrenia without these symptoms (Leucht *et al.*, 2004). The use of mood stabilizers for clozapine augmentation was mentioned above.

Electroconvulsive therapy

In the treatment of schizophrenia, the traditional indications for ECT are catatonic stupor and severe depressive symptoms. The effects of ECT are often rapid and striking in both these conditions. There is also some evidence that it is rapidly effective in acute episodes, and may enhance response to antipsychotics in treatment-resistant cases. Overall, however, the evidence base is weak (Tharyan and Adams, 2002) and ECT is seldom used for schizophrenia in the UK, although it remains more widely used in some other countries.

Psychosocial approaches

The development of community-based services has led to increasing emphasis on psychosocial interventions in the treatment of schizophrenia. These interventions are of several different kinds but share similar purposes:

- Enhancement of interpersonal and social functioning.
- Promotion of independent living in the community.
- Attenuation of symptom severity and associated comorbidity (for example, substance misuse).
- Improvement in personal illness management.

There is evidence in favour of a range of psychosocial interventions (Table 12.15).

Family therapy

As noted above, schizophrenia places a considerable burden on patients' families, and family therapy of various kinds is often employed at various stages of treatment. The most systematically evaluated family intervention is that designed to decrease expressed emotion in family members. The procedure is usually combined with education about the illness and its consequences, together with practical advice on management (Table 12.16). A recent meta-analysis confirmed that such interventions lower rates of hospitalization (NNT = 7) and improve medication compliance; however, the studies showed a wide range of outcomes, with more recent investigations showing less effect (Pharoah *et al.*, 2003). Psychoeducation and family therapy are currently advocated in the management of schizophrenia for patients who live with, or are in close

TABLE 12.15 Effective psychosocial interventions for schizophrenia

Family therapy (psychoeducation)
Cognitive behaviour therapy
Cognitive remediation
Social skills training
Supported employment
Illness management skills
Integrated treatment for comorbid substance misuse
Assertive community treatment

Adapted from Mueser and McGurk (2004).

TABLE 12.16 Elements in family intervention in schizophrenia

Education about schizophrenia
Improving communication
Lowering expressed emotion
Expanding social networks
Adjusting expectations
Reducing hours of daily contact

Source: Leff (1998)

contact with, their family (Pilling *et al.*, 2002b; National Institute for Clinical Excellence, 2002).

Cognitive–behaviour therapy

The use of cognitive–behaviour therapy (CBT) in schizophrenia is based on the rationale that positive psychotic symptoms are amenable to structured reasoning and behavioural modification. With delusional beliefs, for example, individual ideas are traced back to their origin and alternative explanations are explored. However, direct confrontation is avoided. Similarly, it may be possible to modify a patient's beliefs about the omnipotence, identity, and purpose of auditory hallucinations, with a resulting decrease in the distress that accompanies the experience and, perhaps, in its frequency.

Several controlled trials have reported that CBT is effective in schizophrenia. Tarrier *et al.*, (1998) found that CBT was more effective than supportive counselling in decreasing positive symptoms. Another study found that both CBT and a less specific 'befriending' intervention led to significant reductions in both positive and negative symptoms over 9 months of treatment but that gains were more enduring in the CBT group (Sensky *et al.*, 2000). Turkington *et al.* (2004) concluded that CBT has a robust effect on positive, negative, and overall symptoms in schizophrenia, and could be delivered as a brief intervention by community psychiatric nurses. However, other reviews have come to more cautious conclusions about its efficacy and value, especially in routine clinical settings (Pilling *et al.*, 2002a; Turkington and McKenna, 2003). Nevertheless, CBT should now be considered part of an integrated treatment package for patients with schizophrenia.

Social skills training and illness self-management

Social skills training uses a variety of approaches to teach complex interpersonal skills, including behavioural rehearsal, feedback, and training. Skills training may be combined with illness self-management in which patients learn to adjust their own medication and organize their lives to minimize troublesome symptoms. The results of these interventions are generally positive but concerns remain about whether the gains are maintained when treatment ends and whether benefit is restricted to patients who have a good prognosis. Indeed, a meta-analysis concluded that social skills training does not produce reliable benefits and it was not recommended for routine use (Pilling *et al.*, 2002b).

Treating cognitive impairments

As noted above, cognitive impairments are important determinants of poor outcome in schizophrenia. Both pharmacological and psychological approaches are now being used to try and ameliorate them.

Conventional antipsychotics have minimal beneficial effects on cognitive symptoms (Mishara and Goldberg, 2004), and high doses, especially of drugs with anticholinergic properties, impair performance. Atypical antipsychotics may produce slightly greater improvements in some domains (Harvey and Keefe, 2001), although this remains unclear, there is no convincing evidence that individual drugs differ in their overall cognitive benefits. Various drugs are being tested or developed with the aim of specifically improving cognition in schizophrenia, independent of any antipsychotic actions.

A range of psychological treatments for cognitive deficits have also been trialled. Most rely on exercises and training to improve performance through practice. One of the most extensively tested is **cognitive remediation therapy**. However, results are unclear; one meta-analysis and a subsequent long-term trial were positive (Krabbendam and Aleman 2003; Hogarty *et al.*, 2004), but another meta-analysis concluded that it did not produce reliable benefits (Pilling *et al.*, 2002b).

Dynamic psychotherapy

In the past, dynamic psychotherapy was used quite commonly for schizophrenia, more so in the USA than in the UK. Evidence from clinical trials is sparse, but it does not support the use of this kind of psychological treatment. May (1968) found that psychotherapy had little benefit, although the treatment was short and provided by relatively inexperienced psychiatrists. Apart from the lack of convincing evidence that individual psychotherapy is effective in schizophrenia, there may be some danger that the treatment will cause overstimulation and relapse (see Malmberg and Fenton, 2000).

Interaction of drug and psychosocial treatments

Psychosocial treatments are usually given in conjunction with antipsychotic medication, and both are now integral parts of the care package. It is unclear to what extent successful psychosocial treatment works because it improves compliance with medication. It is worth noting that a psychological intervention designed specifically to improve adherence with medication is itself a useful treatment adjunct (Kemp *et al.*, 1996).

Management

Success in management of schizophrenia depends on first establishing a good relationship with the patient. This can be difficult because of the nature of the illness, but with skill and patience progress can usually be made. It is important to make plans that are realistic, especially for the more disabled patient, and acceptable to the patient and their carers. Explaining the benefits of medication, but also discussion and limitation of its side-effects, are important. Finally, novel treatments and modes of service delivery are likely to impact on management of schizophrenia substantially over the next few years, and it is important to keep up to date with developments in this respect.

Table 12.17 summarizes some key elements of the management of schizophrenia (National Institute for Clinical Excellence, 2002). For general review, see Cunningham Owens and Johnstone (2000).

The acute illness

Admission to hospital for assessment and treatment is usually needed for first episodes of schizophrenia and acute relapses, although with adequate resources home treatment is possible and carries some advantages, including patient preference (Dedman, 1993). This is reflected in recent development of crisis teams which aim to treat and support acutely ill patients at home. However, hospital admission has advantages: it allows a thorough assessment, provides a safe environment, and gives a period of relief to the family, who have often experienced considerable distress during the prodromal phase of the illness.

TABLE 12.17 Components and principles in the management of schizophrenia

Therapeutic partnership with patient and carers
Integrated, multidisciplinary working, involving primary and secondary care
Antipsychotic drugs for treatment and prophylaxis – at lowest effective dose
Cognitive behavioural therapy
Family interventions
Early interventions
Assertive outreach for vulnerable patients
Regular assessment of needs
Crisis resolution and home treatment teams as alternatives to admission
Maintain realistic therapeutic optimism

A drug-free observation period is desirable, although acutely disturbed patients may require immediate treatment. It allows thorough evaluation of the patient's mental state and behaviour, helpful in making the diagnosis, and distinguishing schizophrenia from other conditions, notably organic disorders, and drug-induced psychosis (p. 279). Investigations may also be needed for this purpose. In practice, the main difficulty is often to elicit all the symptoms from a withdrawn or suspicious patient. This procedure may require several interviews as well as information from relatives or close friends, and careful observations by nursing staff.

While the diagnosis is being established, a social assessment should be carried out. This includes a history of the patient's personality, level of functioning, work record, accommodation, and leisure pursuits, and the attitudes to the patient of relatives and any close friends. The current social functioning and capabilities can be assessed by other members of the multidisciplinary team, notably occupational therapists, social workers and nurses.

Antipsychotic medication is the mainstay of the treatment of schizophrenia, and other psychoses. It will usually be initiated soon after the diagnosis is made, and will often continue for many years. Thus, decisions about the use of medication, and appropriate involvement of the patient and the carer, are a key aspect of management. In the acute phase, the priority is to suppress the positive symptoms and control agitation, without producing unnecessary side-effects, notably acute dystonias. To achieve this, a combination of a moderate dose of an antipsychotic with a benzodiazepine is useful (e.g. haloperidol 2–10 mg/d or risperidone 2–6 mg/d, plus lorazepam 2 mg four hourly as required). Haloperidol and lorazepam can both be given intramuscularly if necessary. Alternatively, a more sedative antipsychotic, such as olanzapine, 10–20 mg per day, or chlorpromazine (200–400 mg per day) can be used. Oral medication is always preferable, although occasional intramuscular doses may be needed for patients who exhibit acutely disturbed behaviour and are unwilling to comply with oral treatment. If there are doubts about whether the patient is swallowing tablets, the drug can be given as syrup or orally dispersible tablet. An alternative is to give a short-acting depot preparation of zuclopenthixol acetate or olanzapine, but this approach must be used with caution, and it has been recommended that zuclopenthixol acetate should not be given to patients whose tolerance of antipsychotics is undetermined (Royal College of Psychiatrists, 1993). Anticholinergic drugs should be prescribed if parkinsonian side-effects are troublesome, but should not be given routinely or for sustained periods. Issues affecting the choice of individual antipsychotic drug are considered further in the next section.

The acute symptoms of excitement, restlessness, irritability, and insomnia can be expected to improve within days of instituting treatment. Delusions, hallucinations and other psychotic symptoms respond more slowly, often persisting for several weeks. Lack of improvement at this stage suggests inadequate dosage or failure to take the drugs prescribed, but a few cases resist all efforts at treatment. Once there is undoubted evidence of sustained improvement, dosage can be reduced cautiously while careful watch is kept for any return of symptoms. This reduced dose is continued then for a further period (see below).

As soon as the patient's mental state permits, it is essential to explain the need for drug treatment and to obtain their full consent, especially because of the risk of serious and long-term side-effects such as tardive dyskinesia (see pp. 530–8). Where a patient is not judged able to make decisions of this nature, the appropriate legal safeguards under the Mental Health Act and its code of practice should be employed. The patient's family should be involved as far as possible in decisions about treatment, both as a matter of principle but also because they will have a role in encouraging compliance. The use of patient advocates is also helpful.

By the time that symptomatic improvement has taken place, the team should have formulated a provisional plan for continuing care, based upon the social assessment which has been carried out. Although it is difficult to predict the long-term prognosis at this stage, a judgement has to be made about the likely immediate outcome. The judgement is based on the degree and speed of response to treatment, the history of previous episodes, and on the factors listed in Table 12.14. The aim is to decide how much aftercare patients will require, and to make realistic plans accordingly.

Choice of antipsychotic drug

The evidence regarding efficacy of antipsychotics was discussed above, and the broad similarity between drugs and classes noted. Thus, in practice, other factors determine choice of drug. The key factors are: the patient's past drug response and preference; the availability of different preparations (i.e. dispersible tablets, intramuscular, depot), and the anticipated side-effects, which do vary markedly between drugs determined largely by their pharmacological profile (p. 530). Important side-effects to consider when choosing an antipsychotic include:

- **Extra-pyramidal side effects**. The reduced liability of atypical antipsychotics to cause these side-effects is the one advantage agreed by all the meta-analyses. There is also increasing evidence that the risk of tardive dyskinesia is lower than with typical antipsychotics (Correll *et al.*, 2004).
- **Hyperprolactinaemia**, induced by antipsychotics with a high D_2 dopamine receptor affinity. This includes some atypical (e.g. amisulpride, risperidone) as well as typical antipsychotics. Other atypical antipsychotics are 'prolactin-sparing' and, in the case of aripiprazole, may lower prolactin levels. Raised prolactin is important not only because of the immediate effects on menstrual function and galactorrhoea, but because of concerns about increased risks of malignancy and osteoporosis (Wieck and Haddad, 2004). Note that both the extrapyramidal and hyperprolactinaemic effects of antipsychotics are dose-related, emerging at doses (and D_2 receptor occupancies) higher than that required for the antipsychotic effect (Kapur *et al.*, 1999). Their occurrence in a patient thus implies that the dose is already too high; if therapeutic response is not adequate, the antipsychotic should be changed to one with less propensity to cause these side-effects.
- **Sedation**. Some antipsychotics are very sedative, especially those with high affinity for histamine and muscarinic receptors. For example, chlorpromazine, olanzapine and clozapine. This property is often desirable in the acute situation to control agitation, but may be problematic in the longer-term, impairing normal levels of functioning.
- **Weight gain** is an important side-effect of many typical and atypical antipsychotics, notably those with histamine and 5-HT_{2C} receptor blocking effects and associated in part with genetic variation at the 5-HT_{2C} receptor. For example, three months' treatment with

olanzapine increases weight on average by about 5kg. Of the atypical antipsychotics, amisulpride, aripiprazole and risperidone have less of a propensity to increase weight.

- **Type II diabetes mellitus** is of increasing concern. It is unclear to what extent it is actually caused by antipsychotics, rather than being related to illness factors (e.g. shared genetic predisposition; lifestyle). Neither is it clear whether some antipsychotics are worse in this regard than others; some data suggest that the risks are greatest with clozapine and olanzapine (e.g. Lieberman *et al.*, 2005). In light of the current uncertainties, regular monitoring for diabetes should become a routine part of prescribing with all antipsychotics, along with measuring weight and blood lipids (American Diabetes Association and others, 2004).
- **Cardiovascular risk factors**. Antipsychotics have been associated with increased risks of cardiovascular and cerebrovascular events, in part via their influence on weight and insulin resistance, and dyslipidaemia. Some drugs also prolong the QTc interval on the electrocardiogram, a risk factor for cardiac arrythmia. An antipsychotic with low tendency to produce these changes should therefore be chosen in patients with any cardiac or vascular risk factors. This includes the elderly, in whom antipsychotics should be prescribed with great caution (Chapter 20).

Taking these factors into account, the clinician should become thoroughly familiar with a few antipsychotics, including both typical and atypical agents, and drugs with differing side-effect profiles. Familiarity with parenteral as well as oral use of antipsychotics is also important, and their combination and interaction with other drug classes.

Aftercare of 'good prognosis' patients

After a first episode of schizophrenia, patients who have responded well and who are judged to have a good immediate prognosis have two principal needs. The first is to take medication, at the smallest effective dose, for several months after recovery. The second is to be given advice about avoiding obviously stressful events. The patient should be seen regularly as an outpatient or at home by a member of the community mental health team, often a psychiatric nurse, until a few months after medication has been stopped and symptoms have ceased. Thereafter, a cautiously optimistic prognosis can be given, but patient and family should be warned to seek medical help quickly if there is any suggestion of the condition returning. The patient's GP has an important role to play in this phase of treatment.

Aftercare of 'poor prognosis' patients without major impairments

In the majority of cases, further relapse will be considered likely and continuing care will be required.

Sustained use of antipsychotic medication is an important component of treatment. It may be better to give such medication by depot injection since some patients fail to take oral medication regularly over long periods. However, this currently precludes all atypical antipsychotics except risperidone. The dosage, which should be the minimum required to suppress symptoms, can be determined by cautiously varying its size and frequency while observing the patient's clinical state. If response is partial at maximum tolerated dose of the first antipsychotic, swap to another drug, perhaps with a different receptor profile. However, there is little evidence to guide this common situation. Clozapine remains the only antipsychotic with evidence for effectiveness in this group and should be considered in all such patients, taking into account its potential risks (p. 538). Presence of high suicide risk also argues for an early trial of clozapine (p. 305). If available, CBT directed at the residual positive symptoms is a useful adjunct (p. 300).

The follow-up plan should include regular review of mental state and medication, social adjustment, and occupation. It may be helpful for advice to be given about stressful situations and family problems. Specific interventions may be needed to help the family understand the patient's illness, to have realistic expectations of what the patient can accomplish, and to decrease their emotional involvement where appropriate. Work of this nature can be undertaken by community psychiatric nurses, social workers, psychiatrists, and GPs working together. Some patients understandably tend to withdraw from treatment and follow-up after recovery. In those judged at continuing risk of relapse, assertive community treatment has a useful role to play (see Chapter 23) (Marshall and Lockwood, 2000).

Some patients fail to return to their premorbid level of functioning and activities despite resolution of positive symptoms. This may be due to negative symptoms, depressive symptoms, cognitive impairments, or the sedative or anticholinergic side-effects of medication. These possibilities should all be considered, and appropriate action taken as described previously in this chapter. Each is at least partially treatable, by optimizing the use of medication and psychosocial interventions.

Patients with poor prognosis and significant impairments

When patients have prominent negative symptoms, poor social adjustment and behavioural defects, characteristic of chronic schizophrenia, they require more elaborate and indefinite aftercare. The components of a community service for chronic schizophrenia are described in Chapter 23.

Maintenance drug therapy continues to play an important part, but the main emphasis is on a programme of rehabilitation, psychosocial interventions, and social support, tailored to the needs of the individual patient. Contributions from an occupational therapist and clinical psychologist can be particularly helpful. Particular issues that require attention are:

- Living accommodation and circumstances. Will the patient be able to live alone or will she return to live with parents or other relatives? Will a group home or hostel be needed?
- Occupational activities. Will the patient be able to undertake some form of paid employment or voluntary work?
- Activities of everyday living. Patients often need help to re-learn basic living skills such as cooking, budgeting, shopping, housework, and personal hygiene.
- Social skills training and leisure activities.
- If available, the newer therapies mentioned above, aimed at improving cognition and social functioning.
- Optimizing antipsychotic medication, in terms of choice of drug and dose.

When a patient has persisting abnormalities of behaviour, particular attention needs to be given to the problems of their carers. Relatives may be helped by joining a voluntary group and meeting others who have learned to deal with similar problems. They also need to know that professional help will be provided whenever problems become too great. Advice is needed about the best ways of responding to abnormal behaviour, and about the expectations that they should have of the patient. Such advice is often given best by community psychiatric nurses (see Gournay, 2000). Social workers also have a part to play in advising and helping relatives.

Other aspects of management

Care plans

Care plans are important in the management of psychiatric disorders, largely because of the need for coordinated multidisciplinary working, risk management, and clear documentation of responsibilities for their delivery (Chapter 23). While this approach is applicable to all patients, it is particularly appropriate for those with schizophrenia who often require complex and long-term support. The essential elements of a care plan are to identify and record:

- A systematic assessment of health and social needs.
- A treatment plan agreed by the relevant staff, the patient, and the relatives.
- The allocation of a key worker whose task is to maintain contact with patient, monitor progress, and ensure that the treatment programme is being delivered.
- Regular review of the patient's progress and needs.

Early intervention

There is growing interest in the idea that early treatment of schizophrenia may improve the long-term prognosis, particularly from the work of McGorry in Australia (McGorry and Killackey, 2002). This is based on a number of pieces of evidence:

- Patients with a longer duration of untreated psychosis have a worse longer-term prognosis (Marshall *et al.*, 2005).
- There is an increasing time of response to treatment during subsequent psychotic episodes.
- Much of the deterioration in social function takes place in the first 2 years after diagnosis.

These observations imply that it may be worthwhile recognizing patients with psychosis as early as possible so that effective treatment can be instituted. Early interventions being tested include both low-dose, atypical antipsychotic medication, and psychological interventions; there is preliminary evidence in favour of both (Marshall and Lockwood, 2004). Whilst few would disagree with the principle of early, effective treatment, it is being extended to those thought to be in the prodrome of illness but who do not have overt psychotic symptoms, and even to those who are well but at high risk of schizophrenia (for example, children of parents with schizophrenia). The feasibility and desirability of starting treatment in these groups remains under active debate; for example, how to identify 'patients', and the risks and costs of labelling and treating people who may never become ill (Warner 2002; Pelosi and Birchwood, 2003).

Substance misuse

Many patients with schizophrenia misuse psychoactive substances, both legal and illegal. For example, the Epidemiological Catchment Area Study in the USA found that patients with schizophrenia had a four- to five-fold increased risk of substance misuse. The reasons for this are likely to be complex but might include:

- Exposure to socioeconomic factors associated with substance misuse in the general population.
- Relief of personal distress, induced by psychiatric symptoms or by medication.
- Shared genetic susceptibility.

Patients who misuse substances tend to have a worse course symptomatically and be more difficult to engage in treatment. Also, substance misuse is associated with increased risks of homelessness, violent behaviour, and poor general health. Recent studies suggest that benefit can be obtained with comprehensive out-patient and assertive community programmes that address both substance misuse and psychotic illness in an integrated way (Drake *et al.*, 1998). CBT may also be valuable in this group (Haddock *et al.*, 2003).

The violent patient

Overactivity and disturbances of behaviour are common in schizophrenia, and although major violence towards others is not common, it certainly does occur. For example, Humphreys and Johnstone (1992) found that, in a group of 253 patients with a first schizophrenic episode, 52 behaved in a way threatening to the lives of others. In about half the patients, the behaviour was directly attributable to psychotic symptoms, usually delusions. As noted above, substance misuse increases the risk of violence (see Citrome and Volavka, 1999).

General management for the potentially violent patient is the same as that for any other patient with schizophrenia, although a compulsory order is more likely to be required. Whilst medication is often needed to bring disturbed behaviour under immediate control, much can be done by providing a calm, reassuring, and consistent environment in which provocation is avoided. Threats of violence should be taken seriously, especially if there is a history of such behaviour, whether or not the patient was ill at the time. The danger usually resolves as acute symptoms are brought under control, but a few patients pose a continuing threat. The management of violence is considered further in Chapter 26.

Suicide risk

We have already seen that the rate of suicide is markedly increased in schizophrenia. As in other psychiatric disorders, demographic risk factors apply, such as male gender, social isolation, unemployment, and a previous episode of suicidal behaviour. Other risk factors include:

- depression and hopelessness
- frequent exacerbations of psychosis
- good premorbid functioning
- early in the course of the disorder
- during hospitalization or shortly after discharge.

Patients with pronounced negative symptoms are less likely to make suicide attempts. Whilst suicide may be associated with active positive symptoms such as delusions of control or auditory hallucinations, more often suicide occurs in those with previously high educational attainment in a relatively non-psychotic stage of their illness. Such patients often have depressive symptoms in the context of high premorbid expectations of themselves and a negative appraisal of the way their illness has damaged their future prospects.

Lowering the risk of suicide in schizophrenia means being aware of the relevant risk factors (De Hert and Peuskens, 2000), and treating depressive symptoms vigorously. A randomized trial suggested that clozapine treatment may significantly reduce suicide risk in schizophrenia (Meltzer *et al.*, 2003), but the size and mechanism of this effect requires further study (Hennen and Baldessarini, 2005).

Other issues

Women and schizophrenia

There are important gender differences in several aspects of schizophrenia and its treatment. For review see Castle *et al.* (2000).

Several epidemiological features show gender differences. First, the age of onset distribution. Many studies since Kraepelin have shown a later mean age of onset in women, with fewer cases presenting in the second and third decades, and a second peak around the fifth decade. Second, the incidence of schizophrenia is higher in men than women (incidence risk ratio 1.42; 95 per cent confidence interval 1.30–1.56; Aleman *et al.*, 2003). The male preponderance is more pronounced in severe forms of the disorder. The gender difference in incidence is not due to differences in referral, identification, or age of onset. It has been attributed to the neuroprotective effects of oestrogen, but the evidence is poor. Gender differences in genetic and epigenetic risk factors may also be relevant. Third, the mortality rate in men with schizophrenia is twice that of women.

Gender differences also affect treatment (Seeman, 2004). First, the pharmacokinetics of antipsychotics, including clozapine, is different in women and men.

Second, the raised prolactin and lowered oestrogen levels induced by many antipsychotics is of potentially greater harm to women, not only because of the interference with menstrual function, but because of concern about increased risks of osteoporosis and some cancers (Wieck and Haddad, 2003).

Race and schizophrenia

Increased rates of the diagnosis and compulsory treatment of schizophrenia amongst ethnic minority groups has led to controversy, particularly with regard to Afro-Caribbeans in the United Kingdom (p. 290; see Morgan *et al.*, 2005), and has fostered claims of 'institutional racism' in British psychiatry (Sashidharan, 2001). It goes without saying that this is to be abhorred. The diagnosis of schizophrenia should always be based strictly upon the criteria used in ICD-10 or DSM-IV, paying due attention to cultural factors when determining if a belief is a delusion (p. 8). Conversely, behavioural manifestations (e.g. aggression), which might be erroneously considered to show racial differences, should not in isolation influence diagnostic judgement. Similarly, the use of medication or compulsory treatment should adhere to the same principles outlined in this book, regardless of the patient's race. See Bhui *et al.* (2003) for a review of ethnic variation in service pathways and utilization.

Discussing schizophrenia with patients and their carers

There is probably more stigma and misunderstanding associated with schizophrenia than any other psychiatric diagnosis. It is therefore particularly important that the term is used carefully and sensitively, and all patients and their carers should have regular opportunities to ask questions, express views, and raise concerns.

There should be discussion about the nature of the illness, identification of any misapprehensions, and an explanation of the current meaning of the term schizophrenia (see Barrowclough *et al.*, 2001). The prospects for recovery should be portrayed realistically but optimistically, given that some people wrongly believe schizophrenia is untreatable and inevitably follows an unremitting or deteriorating course. The key role of medication, together with psychosocial factors (e.g. family environment, substance misuse), in influencing outcome should be emphasized. Equally, full discussion as to the risks and benefits of antipsychotics is necessary. It is worth discussing what is known about the aetiology of schizophrenia, in part to ensure that misconceptions do not lead to unnecessary guilt. For example, some parents worry that their behaviour may have caused the illness, and are relieved to be informed that there is no evidence for this. Mention of its heritability may lead to questions about risks of schizophrenia in other relatives or future generations; these can be answered clearly using the figures in Table 12.9, acknowledging the increased risk whilst emphasizing the probability that unaffected relatives will remain well. If, after discussion, the family continue to have very different concepts of schizophrenia from those of the clinical team, such views should be respected.

A further area in which there may be a difference in emphasis between psychiatrist and carer or patient is the focus upon the content rather than the nature of the patient's beliefs (McCabe *et al.*, 2002). That is, the psychiatrist is usually more concerned as to whether a thought is or is not delusional, or a perception is or is not a hallucination, whereas the patient wishes to discuss the thought or percept itself and its meaning for them. The psychiatrist should give the patient or carer adequate time to voice these concerns, whilst also explaining why it is necessary to ask detailed questions about the nature of the experiences.

Other than noting these broad themes, there can be no one procedure for discussing schizophrenia and its implications with patients and their carers. The timing, content, and participation in meetings are influenced by their needs and wishes, and by the patient's mental state, past history, and the family's background. The psychiatrist must be prepared to adapt to the circumstances of each case. Involvement of patients and their carers fully should be an integral part of the management of schizophrenia. It is reasonable to assume that establishing and maintaining a genuine therapeutic alliance in this way will increase the likelihood that a patient maintains contact with psychiatric services, is adherent with treatment, and thereby has an improved prognosis.

Further reading

Bleuler, E (1911) *Dementia praecox or the group of schizophrenias* (English edition 1950). International University Press, New York.

Kraepelin, E (1919) *Dementia praecox and paraphrenia*. Churchill Livingstone, Edinburgh.

Hirsch SR, Weinberger D (2003) *Schizophrenia*, 2nd edn. Blackwell Scientific, Oxford. (Definitive and up-to-date reference on all aspects of schizophrenia.)

CHAPTER 13

Paranoid symptoms and delusional disorders

Chapter contents

The term **paranoid** can be applied to symptoms, syndromes, or personality types. **Paranoid symptoms** are overvalued ideas or delusions which are most commonly persecutory but not always so (Box 1.2, p. 11). **Paranoid syndromes** are those in which paranoid delusions form a prominent part of a characteristic constellation of symptoms, such as pathological jealousy or erotomania. In **paranoid personality disorder**, there is excessive self-reference and undue sensitiveness to real or imaginary humiliations and rebuffs, often combined with self-importance and combativeness. Thus the term paranoid is descriptive; if we recognize a symptom or syndrome as paranoid, this is not making a diagnosis, but it is a preliminary to doing so. In this respect it is like recognizing stupor or depersonalization.

Paranoid syndromes present considerable problems of classification and diagnosis. The difficulties can be reduced by dividing them into two distinct groups:

1. Paranoid symptoms occurring as part of another psychiatric disorder, such as schizophrenia, mood disorder, or an organic mental disorder.
2. Paranoid symptoms occurring without evidence for any underlying disorder. This group of disorders has gone by a variety of names, commonly **paranoid states** or **paranoid psychosis**, but the ICD-10 and DSM-IV category is **delusional disorder**. It is this second group that has caused persistent difficulties in several respects; for example, regarding its terminology, relationship to schizophrenia, and forensic implications.

This chapter begins with definitions of the common paranoid symptoms, expanding upon their descriptions in Chapter 1, and then reviews the causes of such symptoms. Next comes a short account of paranoid personality. This is followed by discussion of primary psychiatric disorders with which paranoid symptoms are frequently associated, and the differentiation of these disorders from delusional disorders. The general features of delusional disorder, and its major subtypes are then reviewed. A historical perspective is also given, with particular reference to paranoia and paraphrenia. The chapter finishes with a summary of the assessment and treatment of patients with paranoid symptoms.

Paranoid symptoms

It was pointed out above that the commonest paranoid delusions are persecutory. The term paranoid is also applied to the less common delusions of grandeur and jealousy, and sometimes to delusions concerning love, litigation, or religion. It may seem puzzling that such varied delusions should be grouped together. The reason is that the central abnormality implied by the term paranoid is a morbid distortion of beliefs or attitudes concerning relationships between oneself and other people. If someone believes falsely or on inadequate grounds that he is being victimized, or exalted, or deceived, or loved by a famous person, then in each case he is construing the relationship between himself and other people in a morbidly distorted way.

The varieties of paranoid symptom were discussed in Chapter 1, but important ones are also outlined in Box 13.1 for convenience. The definitions are derived from the glossary to the Present State Examination (p. 63; Wing *et al.*, 1974).

BOX 13.1 SOME PARANOID SYMPTOMS

Ideas of reference Ideas of reference are held by people who are unduly self-conscious. The subject cannot help feeling that people take notice of him in buses, restaurants, or other public places, and that they observe things about him that he would prefer not to be seen. He realizes that this feeling originates within himself and that he is no more noticed than other people, but all the same he cannot help the feeling, quite out of proportion to any possible cause.

Delusions of reference Delusions of reference consist of an elaboration of ideas of reference, to the point that the beliefs become delusional. The whole neighbourhood may seem to be gossiping about the subject, far beyond the bounds of possibility, or she may see references to herself in the media. She may hear someone on the radio say something connected with a topic she has just been thinking about, or she may seem to be followed, her movements observed, and what she says tape-recorded. The importance of distinguishing a delusion of reference from an idea of reference is that the former is a symptom of psychosis.

Delusions of persecution When a person has delusions of persecution he believes that a person, organization, or power, is trying to kill him, harm him in some way, or damage his reputation. The symptom may take many forms, ranging from the direct belief that he is being hunted down by specific people to vague, bizarre, or impossible plots.

Delusions of grandeur These may be divided into delusions of grandiose ability and delusions of grandiose identity. The subject with delusions of grandiose ability thinks that she is chosen by some power, or by destiny, for a special purpose because of her unusual talents. She may think that she is able to read people's thoughts, is much cleverer than anyone else, or has invented machines or solved mathematical problems beyond most people's comprehension.

The subject with delusions of grandiose identity believes that she is famous, rich, titled, or related to prominent people. She may believe that she is a changeling and that her real parents are royalty.

Causes of paranoid symptoms

When paranoid symptoms occur as part of another psychiatric disorder, the main aetiological factors are those determining the primary illness. However, the question still arises as to why some people develop paranoid symptoms, whilst others do not. It has usually been answered in terms of premorbid personality, and social isolation.

Premorbid personality

Many writers, including Kraepelin, have held that paranoid symptoms are most likely to occur in patients with premorbid personalities of a paranoid type (see next section). Kretschmer (1927) also believed this, and thought that such people developed sensitive delusions of reference (*sensitive Beziehungswahn*) as an understandable psychological reaction to a precipitating event. Modern studies of so-called late-onset paraphrenia have supported these views (see Box 3.2). Thus Kay and Roth

(1961) found paranoid or hypersensitive personalities in over half of their group of 99 subjects with late-onset paraphrenia.

Freud (1911) proposed that, in predisposed people, paranoid symptoms could arise through the defence mechanisms of denial and projection. He held that a person does not consciously admit his own inadequacy and self-distrust, but projects them onto the outside world. Freud also held that paranoid symptoms could arise when denial and projection were being used as defences against unconscious homosexual tendencies. These ideas were derived from his study of Daniel Schreber, the presiding judge of the Dresden appeal court (Freud, 1911). Freud never met Schreber, but read the latter's autobiographical account of his paranoid illness (now generally accepted to be paranoid schizophrenia), together with a report by Weber, the physician in charge. Freud thought that Schreber could not consciously admit his homosexuality, and so the idea 'I love him' was dealt with by denial and changed by a reaction formation to 'I hate him'; this was further changed by projection into 'it is not I who hate him, but he who hates me', and this in turn became transformed to 'I am persecuted by him'. Freud believed that all paranoid delusions could be represented as contradictions of the idea 'I (a man) love him (a man)'. He went so far as to argue that delusions of jealousy could be explained in terms of unconscious homosexuality; the jealous husband was unconsciously attracted to the man whom he accused his wife of loving. In this case the formulation was 'it is not I who love him; it is she who loves him'. At one time these ideas were widely taken up, but nowadays they gain little acceptance. They are not supported by clinical experience.

Social isolation and deafness

Social isolation may also predispose to the emergence of paranoid symptoms. Prisoners (especially those in solitary confinement), refugees, and migrants have all been considered to be prone to paranoid symptoms and syndromes, with social isolation being the common factor. The findings and their interpretation with regard to migration were discussed in Chapter 12 (p. 290).

There is evidence that deafness increases the risk of paranoid symptoms, as originally noted by Kraepelin, and usually attributed to the social isolation produced by deafness. Houston and Royse (1954) found an association between deafness and paranoid schizophrenia, whilst Kay and Roth (1961) found hearing impairment in 40 per cent of patients with late-onset paraphrenia. Subsequent studies confirm that hearing impairment is a risk factor for disorders in which paranoid symptoms occur, and that this relationship is stronger in but not limited to the elderly (David *et al.*, 1995; Prager and Jeste, 1993). However, it should be remembered that the great majority of deaf people do not become paranoid, and many deaf people may not be socially isolated.

Paranoid personality disorder

The concept of personality disorder was discussed in Chapter 7, and paranoid personality disorder was briefly described there. It is characterized by:

- extreme sensitivity to setbacks and rebuffs
- suspiciousness
- a tendency to misconstrue the actions of others as hostile or contemptuous
- a combative and inappropriate sense of personal rights.

This definition embraces a wide range of types. At one extreme is the excessively sensitive youth who shrinks from social encounters and thinks that everyone disapproves of him. At the other is the assertive and challenging woman who flares up at the least provocation. A recent American study found a 4.4 per cent prevalence of DSM-IV paranoid personality disorder, which is higher than previous estimates; the study also showed that the disorder had a significant impact on social and role functioning (Grant *et al.*, 2004).

Because of the implications for treatment, it is important to distinguish paranoid personality disorder from the paranoid syndromes (delusional disorders) to be described later. The distinction can be very difficult to make, and is based on the fact that in paranoid personality disorder there are no delusions (only overvalued ideas), and no hallucinations. Separating paranoid ideas from delusions calls for considerable skill. The criteria for doing so were given in Chapter 1, and exemplified by the comparison made in Box 13.1 between ideas of reference and delusions of reference. In reality, the conditions are likely on a continuum. Thus, family studies indicate a genetic relationship between paranoid personality disorder and delusional disorder (p. 313), whilst individuals with paranoid personality traits are at increased risk of developing a delusional disorder. It has been suggested that this may have happened to the philosopher, Jean Jacques Rousseau and the dictator, Joseph Stalin (Hachinski, 1999).

Paranoid symptoms in psychiatric disorders

Paranoid symptoms are often secondary to an underlying or primary psychiatric disorder. Thus, when paranoid symptoms, especially persecutory delusions, are elicited it is important to assess for the other features of these disorders. The diagnosis of delusional disorder, to be considered below, is in many respects a 'residual' category, used for patients whose delusions cannot be attributed to one of these other conditions. As the primary disorders are described at length in other chapters, they are mentioned only briefly here.

Paranoid symptoms in delirium and dementia

Paranoid symptoms are common in delirium. Impaired grasp of what is going on around the patient may give rise to apprehension and misinterpretation, and so to suspicion. Delusions may then emerge which are usually transient and disorganized; they may lead to disturbed behaviour, such as querulousness or aggression. Similarly, persecutory delusions occur commonly at some stage in dementia, and are occasionally the presenting feature. Organic causes of paranoid symptoms and states were reviewed by Gorman and Cummings (1990).

Paranoid symptoms in substance misuse disorders

Paranoid symptoms occur in many substance misuse disorders, especially those associated with amphetamines, cocaine and alcohol. An important example is the association between alcohol misuse and morbid jealousy, described below. Some therapeutic drugs can also precipitate paranoid symptoms, such as L-DOPA (Gorman and Cummings, 1990).

Paranoid symptoms in mood disorders

Paranoid symptoms are not uncommon in patients with severe depressive disorders, and paranoid delusions are a feature of psychotic depression.

It is sometimes difficult to determine whether the paranoid symptoms are secondary to depressive disorder, or vice versa. Both scenarios are common. The distinction is of some importance as the two disorders differ in treatment and prognosis. A depressive disorder is likely if the mood changes occurred earlier and are of greater intensity than the paranoid features. Previous psychiatric history and family history may also be useful pointers. Finally, in depressive disorder, the patient typically accepts the persecution as justified by his own guilt or wickedness. This is a useful point clinically, since it contrasts with non-affective psychoses, wherein such persecutions are resented bitterly.

Paranoid symptoms also occur in mania, and are typically mood-congruent and thus grandiose rather than persecutory.

Paranoid symptoms and paranoid schizophrenia

Paranoid schizophrenia was described in Chapter 12. Its distinction from delusional disorders has been particularly problematic, both conceptually and practically (see Box 13.2), but the difficulties can be decreased by noting the differences in their core features (compare Table 12.6 with Table 13.1). Three features help in making the distinction in cases of doubt:

- The diagnosis of paranoid schizophrenia rather than delusional disorder is suggested if the paranoid delusions are particularly odd in content (often referred to by psychiatrists as **bizarre delusions**). Except in extreme cases, judgment as to how bizarre they are must be arbitrary (Flaum *et al.*, 1991). DSM-IV defines non-bizarre delusions as involving situations that could conceivably occur in real life, for example, being followed, poisoned, or loved at a distance. ICD-10, perhaps recognizing the difficulty of defining bizarre, omits this criterion.
- In schizophrenia, delusions tend to be fragmented and multiple, whereas in delusional disorder they are **systematized** and based around a single, internally consistent, theme. In delusional disorder, the delusional system is also characteristically **encapsulated**, such that the rest of the mental state can appear remarkably normal, in contrast to schizophrenia.
- Patients with paranoid schizophrenia often have auditory hallucinations, and the content of these seems unrelated to their delusions. In delusional disorder, hallucinations are rare, and when they do occur are fleeting and clearly related to the delusions.

Paranoid symptoms in schizophrenia-like syndromes

Paranoid symptoms are features of several schizophrenia-like syndromes discussed in Chapter 12 (and listed in Table 12.5). These include the DSM-IV categories of 'brief psychotic disorders' and 'schizophreniform disorder', and the ICD-10 categories grouped under the heading 'acute and transient psychotic disorders'.

Delusional disorders (paranoid psychoses)

As mentioned in the introduction, the terminology and classification of psychoses which are neither affective, organic, nor schizophrenia, has been disputed for many years. Box 13.2 summarizes the main historical

BOX 13.2 HISTORICAL BACKGROUND: PARANOIA AND PARAPHRENIA

The terms **paranoia** and **paraphrenia** have played a prominent part in psychiatric thought. Much can be learned from reviewing the conceptual difficulties associated with them

The term **paranoia**, from which the modern adjective paranoid is derived, has a long and chequered history. It has probably given rise to more controversy and confusion of thought than any other term used in psychiatry. A comprehensive review of the large body of literature, which is mostly German, and from the period before the 1970s has been provided by Lewis (1970); see also Box 1.2. The word is derived from the Greek *para* (beside) and *nous* (mind). It was used in ancient Greek literature to mean 'out of mind', i.e. of unsound mind or insane. This broad usage was revived in the eighteenth century, but when it came into prominence in the second half of the nineteenth century, in German psychiatry, it became particularly associated with conditions characterized by delusions of persecution and grandeur. The German term *Verrucktheit* was often applied to these conditions, but eventually was superseded by **paranoia**. There were many different conceptions of these disorders. The main issues, most of which remain today, can be summarized as follows:

- Did these conditions constitute a primary disorder, or were they secondary to another disorder?
- Did they persist unchanged for many years, or were they a stage in an illness which later manifested deterioration of intellect and personality?
- Could they occur in the absence of hallucinations?
- Were there forms with good prognosis?

Kahlbaum raised these issues as early as 1863, when he classified paranoia as an independent primary condition which would remain unchanged over the years. Kraepelin had a strong influence on the conceptual history of paranoia, although he was never comfortable with the term, and his views changed strikingly over the years. In 1896 he used the term only for incurable, chronic, and systematized delusions without severe personality disorder. In the sixth edition of his textbook he wrote:

'The delusions in dementia praecox [schizophrenia] are extremely fantastic, changing beyond all reason, with an absence of system and a failure to harmonize them with events of their past life; while in paranoia the delusions are largely confined to morbid interpretations of real events, are woven together into a coherent whole, gradually becoming extended to include even events of recent date, and contradictions and objects are apprehended and explained'.

(Kraepelin 1904, p. 199)

In later descriptions, Kraepelin (1919) used the distinction made by Jaspers (1913) between personality development and disease process. He proposed paranoia as an example of the former, in contrast to the disease process of dementia praecox. In his final account, Kraepelin (1919) developed these ideas by distinguishing between dementia praecox, paranoia, and a third paranoid psychosis, **paraphrenia**. He suggested that:

- Dementia praecox had an early onset and a poor outcome ending in mental deterioration, and was fundamentally a disturbance of affect and volition.
- Paranoia was restricted to patients with the late onset of completely systematized delusions and a prolonged course, usually without recovery but not inevitably deteriorating. An important point was that the patients did not have hallucinations.
- Paraphrenia was somewhat intermediary, in that the patient had unremitting systematized delusions but did not progress to dementia. The main difference from paranoia was that the patient with paraphrenia had hallucinations.

Bleuler's concept of the paranoid form of dementia praecox (which he later called paranoid schizophrenia) was broader than that of Kraepelin (Bleuler 1906, 1911). Thus Bleuler did not regard paraphrenia as a separate condition, but as part of dementia praecox. However, he accepted Kraepelin's view of paranoia as a separate entity, although he differed from Kraepelin in maintaining that hallucinations could occur in many cases. Bleuler was particularly interested in the psychological development of paranoia; at the same time he left open the question of whether paranoia had a somatic pathology.

From this time, two views of paranoia predominated. The first theme was that paranoia was distinct from schizophrenia and psychogenic in origin. The second theme was that paranoia was part of schizophrenia. Some celebrated studies of individual cases appeared to support the first theme. For example, Gaupp (1974) made an intensive study of the diaries

BOX 13.2 *(continued)*

and mental state of the mass murderer Wagner who murdered his wife, four children, and eight other people as part of a careful plan to revenge himself on his supposed enemies. Gaupp concluded that Wagner suffered from paranoia in the sense described by Kraepelin. At the same time, he believed that Wagner's first recognizable delusions developed as a psychogenic reaction. The most detailed argument for psychogenesis was put forward by Kretschmer (1927) in his monograph *'Der Sensitive Beziehungswahn'*. Kretschmer believed that paranoia should not be regarded as a disease, but as a psychogenic reaction occurring in people with particularly sensitive personalities. However, many of Kretschmer's cases would nowadays be classified as schizophrenia. In 1931, Kolle put forward evidence for the second view, that paranoia is part of schizophrenia. He analysed a series of 66 patients with so-called paranoia, including those diagnosed by Kraepelin. For several reasons, including symptomatic and genetic factors, Kolle came to the conclusion that paranoia was really a mild form of schizophrenia.

Considerably less has been written about paraphrenia. However, it is interesting that Mayer (1921), following up Kraepelin's series of 78 paraphrenic patients, found that 50 of them had developed schizophrenia. He found no difference in original clinical presentation between those who developed schizophrenia and those who did not. Since then paraphrenia has increasingly been regarded as late-onset schizophrenia or schizophrenia-like disorder of good prognosis. Kay and Roth (1961) used the term late paraphrenia to denote paranoid conditions in the elderly that were not due to primary organic or affective illnesses. These authors found that a large majority of their 99 patients had the characteristic features of schizophrenia.

In current classifications, the term paranoia has, in effect, been replaced by delusional disorder. Paraphrenia does not feature either, but it continues to be used clinically to describe chronic, atypical, paranoid psychoses of middle and late life (see p. 513).

terms and themes, and provides the backdrop to the way in which the disorders are currently categorized. In this section, the core features of delusional disorders – the current terminology for these conditions – are described. The specific types of delusional disorder are covered in the following section.

Classification of delusional disorder

DSM-IV uses **delusional disorder** to describe a disorder with persistent, non-bizarre delusions that is not due to any other disorder. It is synonymous with the widely used term **paranoid psychosis**, and includes the non-specific term of **paranoid states**. ICD-10 has a similar category of **persistent delusional disorders**. The essence of the modern concept of delusional disorder is that of a stable delusional system developing insidiously in a person in middle or late life. The delusional system is encapsulated, and there is no impairment of other mental functions. The patient can often go on working, and his social life may be maintained fairly well.

The criteria for delusional disorder in DSM-IV are summarized in Table 13.1, with the subsequent description of five specific subtypes of delusional disorder and two other categories:

- persecutory
- jealous
- erotomanic
- somatic
- grandiose
- mixed
- unspecified.

ICD-10 gives a similar definition for the principal category (F22.0) of persistent delusional disorders. Unlike

TABLE 13.1 DSM-IV criteria for delusional disorder

A	Non-bizarre delusions (i.e. involving situations that occur in real life, such as being followed, poisoned, infected, loved at a distance, or deceived by spouse or lover, or having a disease) of at least 1 month's duration
B	Criterion A for schizophrenia has never been met. **Note:** Tactile and olfactory hallucinations may be present in delusional disorder if they are related to the delusional theme
C	Apart from the impact of the delusion(s) or its ramifications, functioning is not markedly impaired and behaviour is not obviously odd or bizarre
D	If mood episodes have occurred concurrently with delusions, their total duration has been brief relative to the duration of the delusional periods
E	The disturbance is not due to the direct physiological effects of a substance (e.g. a drug of abuse, a medication) or a general medical condition

DSM-IV, the symptoms must have been present for at least 3 months, and the delusions are not required to be 'non-bizarre.' ICD-10 also includes litigious and self-referential subtypes, and has a separate sub-category (F22.8) of 'other persistent delusional disorders' (see below).

For reviews of delusional disorder, see Sedler (1995) and Munro (2000).

Epidemiology of delusional disorder

Delusional disorder is regarded as being an uncommon illness, although there are relatively few data. In a community survey of over 5000 people aged 65 and over, Copeland *et al.* (1998) found a prevalence of 0.04 per cent for delusional disorder. In a retrospective study of over 10,000 outpatients, Hsiao *et al.* (1999) diagnosed 86 (0.83 per cent) as meeting DSM-IV criteria for delusional disorder of various kinds (Table 13.2). The disorder was a little more common in women than men and the mean age of onset of symptoms was 42 years. About 5 per cent of psychiatric inpatients with a diagnosis of functional psychosis met criteria for delusional disorder (Kendler and Walsh, 1995).

Significant depressive symptoms are common in delusional disorder (note category D in Table 13.1), being present in about a third of subjects (Hsaio *et al.*, 1999; Serretti *et al.*, 2004).

Aetiology of delusional disorder

What little is known of the aetiology of delusional disorder is based upon its relationship to, and comparison with, schizophrenia and paranoid personality disorder. This question has been addressed by family and neurobiological studies. However, the relatively small sample sizes and varying diagnostic definitions mean that few conclusions can be drawn. Psychological explanations for delusional disorder centre upon the delusions themselves, and are mentioned elsewhere (pp. 308–9).

TABLE 13.2 Subtypes of delusional disorder in 86 Chinese outpatients

Subtype	Number
Persecutory	61
Mixed	12
Jealous	7
Somatic	2
Erotomanic	1
Grandiose	1
Unspecified	2

Family studies of delusional disorder

First-degree relatives of patients with delusional disorder have an increased incidence of paranoid personality disorder (Kendler *et al.*, 1985). The familial relationship of delusional disorder to schizophrenia is less clear. At present it appears that the risk of delusional disorder is increased in first-degree relatives of patients with schizophrenia, but relatives of patients with delusional disorder do not have an increased risk of schizophrenia or schizotypal personality (Kendler *et al.*, 1995; Kendler and Walsh, 1995; Tienari *et al.*, 2003). This familial association pattern has been called asymmetric co-aggregation and may be due to a number of factors:

- Differences in the incidence rates of the two disorders in the general population.
- Differences in diagnostic error rate between probands and relatives (probands are usually subject to more intensive assessment).
- A higher genetic loading for severe illness in those who come to medical attention (and are therefore assessed as probands).

Overall, there appears to be a weak genetic link between delusional disorder and, on the one hand, schizophrenia and, on the other, paranoid personality disorder. However, the extent of genetic overlap between these conditions is unclear. Most authorities would include delusional disorder as part of the schizophrenia spectrum (Kendler, 2003).

There is a familial association between alcoholism and delusional disorder (Kendler and Walsh, 1995), which could explain the association between morbid jealousy and alcohol misuse (see below).

Neurobiological studies

Structural MRI studies suggest that elderly patients with delusional disorder have enlarged cerebral ventricles similar to patients with schizophrenia (Howard *et al.*, 1995). The two groups may also show similar abnormalities in tasks of eye tracking (Campana *et al.*, 1998). There are inconsistent and inconclusive reports that delusional disorder may be associated with polymorphisms in dopaminergic genes (e.g Morimoto *et al.*, 2002).

Specific delusional disorders

As noted above, specific subtypes of delusional disorder are recognized, based on the content of the predominant delusion(s) (Table 13.3). Historically, these symptoms have been of particular interest to French psychiatrists.

Classification in this area is confusing for several reasons:

- Some of the disorders are often referred to by older, eponymous terms.
- Some of the syndromes can be viewed as symptoms (e.g. delusional misidentification), or can occur secondary to other psychiatric disorders.
- Not all of the categories are included in DSM-IV or ICD-10, but are mentioned here because of continuing usage.

In this section we also consider stalking and persistent litigants, since both behaviours may be secondary to delusional disorder.

Pathological jealousy

Pathological or **morbid jealousy** (other synonyms are given in Table 13.3) is described first and in most detail as it is the archetypal delusional disorder; it is also the commonest (other than 'persecutory delusional disorder, not otherwise specified') and, importantly, appears to carry the greatest risk of dangerousness.

The essential feature is an abnormal belief that the patient's partner is being unfaithful. The condition is called pathological because the belief, which may be a delusion or an overvalued idea, is held on inadequate grounds and is unaffected by rational argument. The belief is often accompanied by strong emotions and characteristic behaviour, but these do not in themselves constitute pathological jealousy. A man who finds his wife in bed with a lover may experience extreme jealousy and may behave in an uncontrolled way, but this should not be called pathological jealousy. The term should be used only when the jealousy is based on unsound evidence and reasoning.

TABLE 13.3 Types of delusional disorder

Type	Synonymous with, or includes
Jealous	Morbid jealousy; pathological jealousy; erotic jealousy; sexual jealousy; Othello syndrome
Erotic	Erotomania; De Clérambault's syndrome
Somatic	Monosymptomatic hypochondriacal psychosis; delusional body dysmorphic disorder
Querulous	
Persecutory	
Shared	Induced delusional disorder; *folie à deux*; communicated insanity
Other	Delusional misidentification syndrome; Capgras syndrome; Fregoli delusion; intermetamorphosis; syndrome of subjective doubles

The main sources of information about pathological jealousy come from the classic paper by Shepherd (1961) and surveys by Langfeldt (1961), Vaukhonen (1968), and Mullen and Maack (1985). Shepherd examined the hospital case notes of 81 patients in London and Langfeldt did the same for 66 patients in Norway. Vaukhonen made an interview study of 55 patients in Finland; Mullen and Mack examined the hospital case notes of 138 patients.

The frequency of pathological jealousy in the general population is unknown, although jealous feelings are ubiquitous (Mullen and Martin, 1994). Pathological jealousy is not uncommon in psychiatric practice, and most full-time clinicians probably see one or two cases a year. They merit careful attention, not only because of the great distress that they cause within marriages and families, but also because they may be highly dangerous.

It is likely that pathological jealousy is more common in men than in women. For example, the surveys noted above found that about two men are affected for every woman. However, the precise sex ratio may depend on the particular group studied and in particular whether the jealousy is secondary to another disorder. For example, in a retrospective survey of in-patients, Soyka *et al.* (1991) found that amongst patients with paranoid schizophrenia more females than males had delusions of jealousy, whilst amongst patients with alcoholic psychosis more men developed delusional jealousy (even allowing for the fact that more men than women were affected with alcoholic psychosis).

Clinical features of pathological jealousy

As indicated above, the main feature is an abnormal belief in the partner's infidelity. This may be accompanied by other abnormal beliefs, for example, that the partner is plotting against the patient, trying to poison him, taking away his sexual capacities, or infecting him with venereal disease. The mood of the pathologically jealous patient may vary with the underlying disorder, but often it is a mixture of misery, apprehension, irritability, and anger.

Typically, the behaviour involves an intensive search for evidence of the partner's infidelity, for example, by looking through diaries and by examining bed linen and underwear for signs of sexual secretions. The patient may follow the partner about, or engage a private detective. The jealous person often cross-questions the partner incessantly. This may lead to violent quarrelling and paroxysms of rage in the patient. Sometimes the partner becomes exasperated and worn out, and is finally goaded into making a false confession. If this happens, the jealousy is inflamed rather than assuaged.

An interesting feature is that the jealous person often has no idea as to who the supposed lover may be, or what kind of person he or she may be. Moreover, he may avoid taking steps that could produce unequivocal proof one way or the other.

Behaviour may be strikingly abnormal. A successful city businessman carried a briefcase that contained not only his financial documents but also a machete for use against any lover who might be detected. A carpenter installed an elaborate system of mirrors in his house so that he could watch his wife from another room. A third patient avoided waiting alongside another car at traffic lights, in case his wife in the passenger seat might surreptitiously make an assignation with the other driver.

Aetiology of pathological jealousy

Pathological jealousy – as with other paranoid symptoms and syndromes – is associated with a range of primary disorders (Table 13.4). In the surveys mentioned, the frequencies of disorders varied, probably reflecting the population studied and the diagnostic scheme used. For example, paranoid schizophrenia was reported in 17–44 per cent of patients, depressive disorder in 3–16 per cent, neurosis and personality disorder in 38–57 per cent, alcoholism in 5–7 per cent, and organic disorders in 6–20 per cent.

The role of personality in the genesis of pathological jealousy should be stressed. It is often found that the patient has a pervasive sense of inadequacy, together with low self-esteem. There is a discrepancy between his ambitions and his attainments. Such a personality is particularly vulnerable to anything that may heighten this sense of inadequacy, such as loss of status or advancing age. In the face of such threats the person may project the blame onto others, and this may take the form of jealous accusations of infidelity. As mentioned earlier, Freud believed that unconscious homosexual urges played a part in all jealousy, but clinical studies do not support an association between homosexuality and pathological jealousy. Similarly, though pathological jealousy has sometimes been attributed to the onset of sexual difficulties, Langfeldt (1961) and Shepherd (1961) found little or no evidence of an association.

TABLE 13.4 Disorders associated with pathological jealousy

Schizophrenia
Mood disorder
Organic disorder
Substance misuse (especially alcohol)
Paranoid personality disorder

Prognosis of pathological jealousy

Little is known about the prognosis of pathological jealousy. It likely depends on a number of factors, including the nature of any underlying psychiatric disorder and the patient's premorbid personality. When Langfeldt (1961) followed up 27 of his patients after 17 years, he found that over half of them still had persistent or recurrent jealousy. This confirms a general clinical impression that the prognosis is often poor.

Risk of violence

Although there are no good estimates of the risks of violence, there is no doubt that people with pathological jealousy can be dangerous (Silva *et al.*, 1998). Three out of 81 patients in Shepherd's (1961) series had shown homicidal tendencies. In addition to homicide, the risk of physical injury inflicted by jealous patients is considerable. In Mullen and Maack's (1985) series, a quarter had threatened to kill or injure their partner, and 56 per cent of men and 43 per cent of women had been violent to or threatened the supposed rival. Recently, Schanda *et al.* (2004), studying convicted murderers in Austria, confirmed that delusional disorder (subtype not specified) is associated with homicide, with an odds ratio of 6. There is also a risk of suicide, particularly when an accused partner finally decides to end the relationship.

Assessment of pathological jealousy

The assessment of a patient with pathological jealousy should be particularly thorough, and should always include the partner, who should be interviewed separately whenever possible.

The partner may give a much more detailed account of the patient's morbid beliefs and actions than can be elicited from the patient. The doctor should try to find out tactfully how firmly the patient believes in the partner's infidelity, how much resentment he feels, and whether he has contemplated any vengeful action. What factors provoke outbursts of accusations and questioning? How does the partner respond to such outbursts? How does the patient respond in turn to the partner's behaviour? Has there been any violence so far? Has there been any serious injury?

In addition to these enquiries, the doctor should take a detailed marital and sexual history from both partners, and assess for underlying psychiatric disorder, as this will have implications for treatment.

Treatment of pathological jealousy

The treatment of pathological jealousy, as with other delusional disorders, is in principle fairly straightforward - the mainstay being antipsychotic drugs - but in practice can be very difficult because of lack of insight and reluctance to collaborate in the treatment plan.

Adequate treatment of any associated disorder such as schizophrenia or a mood disorder is a first requisite. If alcohol or other substance misuse is present, specific treatment will be needed. In other cases the pathological jealousy may be the symptom of a delusional disorder, or an overvalued idea in a patient with low self-esteem and personality difficulties.

When the jealousy seems to be delusional in nature, a careful trial of an antipsychotic drug is worthwhile, though results are often disappointing. When the jealousy is an overvalued idea, treatment with selective serotonin re-uptake inhibitors (SSRIs) may be useful (Stein *et al.*, 1994); however, no randomized trials have yet been reported. As noted above, even when depressive disorder is not the primary diagnosis, it frequently complicates pathological jealousy and may worsen it. Treatment with an antidepressant may help in these circumstances.

Psychotherapy may be given to patients where the jealousy appears to arise from personality problems. One aim is to reduce tensions by allowing the patient (and partner) to ventilate feelings. Behavioural methods include encouraging the partner to produce behaviour that reduces jealousy, for example, by refusal to argue, depending on the individual case. A study of cognitive therapy, in which patients were encouraged to identify faulty assumptions and taught strategies of emotional control, gave superior results relative to a waiting list control group (Dolan and Bishay, 1996).

If there is no response to outpatient treatment or if the risk of violence is high, inpatient care may be necessary. Not uncommonly, however, the patient appears to improve as an inpatient, only to relapse on discharge.

If there appears to be a risk of violence, the doctor should warn the partner even if this involves a breach of confidentiality (see Chapter 4). In some cases the safest procedure is to advise separation. It is not uncommon for feelings of pathological jealousy to wane once a relationship has ended. Sometimes, however, the problem re-emerges if the patient enters a new relationship.

Erotomania and erotic delusions

Erotic delusions can occur in any psychotic disorder, especially paranoid schizophrenia, but they are the predominant and persistent symptom in a form of delusional disorder called **erotomania**. It was a French psychiatrist, De Clérambault who, in 1921, proposed that a distinction should be made between paranoid delusions and delusions of passion. The latter differed in their pathogenesis and in being accompanied by excitement. This distinction is of historical interest only, but the syndrome is still known as **De Clérambault's syndrome**. It is rare and occurs almost entirely in women, although Taylor *et al.* (1983) reported four cases in a series of 112 men charged with violent offences.

In erotomania, the subject, usually a single woman, believes that an exalted person is in love with her. The supposed lover is usually inaccessible, as he is already married, or famous as an entertainer or public figure. According to De Clérambault, the infatuated woman believes that it is the supposed lover who first fell in love with her, and that he is more in love than she. She derives satisfaction and pride from this belief. She is convinced that the supposed lover cannot be a happy or complete person without her.

The patient often believes that the supposed lover is unable to reveal his love for various unexplained reasons, and that he has difficulties in approaching her, has indirect conversations with her, and has to behave in a paradoxical and contradictory way. The woman may be a considerable nuisance to the supposed lover, who may complain to the police and the courts. Sometimes the patient's delusion remains unshakeable, and she invents explanations for the other person's paradoxical behaviour. She may be extremely tenacious and impervious to reality. Other patients turn from a delusion of love to a delusion of persecution, become abusive, and make public complaints about the supposed lover. This was described by De Clérambault as two phases - hope followed by resentment.

The concept of erotomania has been reviewed by Berrios and Kennedy (2002).

Stalking

A proportion of 'stalkers' appear to suffer from delusional disorders, including erotomania, which is why the topic is mentioned here.

There is no clear consensus about the definition of stalking. Most formulations contain the following elements:

- A pattern of intrusive behaviour.
- The intrusive behaviour is associated with implicit or explicit threats.

- The person being stalked experiences fear and distress.

Stalkers typically follow their victim around and loiter outside their house or place of work. Unwanted communications by telephone, letter, graffiti, and, more recently, e-mail, are very common. Behaviour can then become more threatening with hoax advertisements or orders for services, scandalous rumour-mongering, damage to the victim's property, threats of violence, and actual assault.

Stalkers are a heterogenous group with differing underlying psychopathologies. Some, usually women, have erotomania or erotic delusions secondary to other psychotic disorders. Patients with pathological jealousy can also stalk their victims (Silva *et al.*, 2000). More commonly, stalkers suffer from personality disorder, predominantly with borderline, narcissistic, and sociopathic traits. They have often had a relationship with their victim that may have been quite superficial; in other cases, however, a serious relationship has cooled. A previous history of domestic violence in the relationship puts the victim at particularly high risk of assault and injury. Whether or not victims suffer actual assault, they invariably experience severe psychological stress, which can lead to anxiety and mood disorders and post-traumatic stress disorder. (For a review of stalking see Kamphuis and Emmelkamp, 2000 or Mullen *et al.*, 2000; see also Chapter 26.)

Somatic delusional disorder

People with somatic delusional disorder believe that they suffer from a physical illness or deformity. The term encompasses monosymptomatic hypochondriacal psychosis, where there is a single delusional belief of this kind. Somatic delusional disorder needs to be distinguished from the hypochondriacal delusions that occur in severe depression and schizophrenia. It must also be distinguished from patients with severe body dysmorphic disorder (also called dysmorphophobia; see p. 209), in whom the overvalued ideas can approach delusional intensity. In fact, there appears to be much overlap clinically, and perhaps therapeutically, between delusional and non-delusional forms of body dysmorphic disorder (Phillips, 2004). Specific drug treatments for somatic delusional disorder have been advocated, as discussed below.

Querulant delusions and reformist delusions

Querulant delusions were the subject of a special study by Krafft-Ebing (1888). Patients with this kind of delusion indulge in a series of complaints and claims lodged against the authorities. Closely related to querulant patients are paranoid litigants, who undertake a succession of lawsuits; they become involved in numerous court hearings, in which they may become passionately angry and may make threats against the magistrates. The characteristics of persistent litigants have been reviewed by Rowlands (1988) and Lester *et al.* (2004).

Baruk (1959) described 'reformist delusions', which are centred on religious, philosophical, or political themes. People with these delusions constantly criticize society and sometimes embark on elaborate courses of action. Their behaviour may be violent, particularly when the delusions are political. Some political assassins fall within this group. It is extremely important that this diagnosis is made on clear psychiatric grounds rather than political grounds, as occurred in the Soviet Union (see Chapter 2; Bloch and Chodoff, 1981).

Delusional misidentification syndrome

Another group of delusions involve different aspects of misidentification, either of the self or others. They often occur in other psychotic disorders, especially schizophrenia and organic disorders, but they can also occur in isolation, and have been given the collective label of delusional misidentification syndrome (Ellis and Young, 1990; Christodoulou, 1991). This category is not named in ICD-10 or DSM-IV, but constitutes an example of 'other persistent delusional disorders' coded in the former. One argument for bringing them together is that they all appear to be 'face processing disorders', and associated with abnormalities in the posterior part of the right hemisphere wherein systems subserving face recognition are located (Cutting, 1991; Breen *et al.*, 2000). Note also the seemingly close relationship of these disorders to the neurological category of **prosopagnosia**, the inability to recognize familiar faces. Interestingly, the delusions are specific to a few, usually familiar, people, and recognition of other faces (and objects) is not impaired. Although the beliefs are delusional, the patient is aware that something is wrong with the 'replacement' person. The patient may be extremely distressed, and occasionally act against persons they believe to be impostors.

As outlined here, four main variants of delusional misidentification are recognized. In each case, there has been debate as to whether they constitute a symptom or a syndrome.

Capgras syndrome

Although there had been previous case reports, the condition now known as **Capgras syndrome** was well described by Capgras and Reboul-Lachauz in 1923. They called it *l'illusion des sosies* **(illusion of doubles)**, but it is a delusion not an illusion, hence the alternative term of **Capgras delusion**.

The patient believes that a person closely related to her has been replaced by a double. She accepts that the misidentified person has a great resemblance to the familiar person, but still believes that they are different people. It is a rare condition, seen more often in women than men. A history of depersonalization, derealization, or déjà vu is not unusual. Schizophrenia is the commonest diagnosis (Berson, 1983). The misidentified person is usually the patient's partner or another relative. Some patients with Capgras syndrome may behave dangerously by attacking the presumed doubles. The syndrome is an example of a reduplicative paramnesia (Lishman, 1998). For review, see Edelstyn and Oyebode (1999).

Fregoli syndrome

Also called the **Fregoli delusion**, it derives its name from an actor called Fregoli who had remarkable skill in changing his facial appearance. It was originally described by Courbon and Fail in 1927. The condition is even rarer than the Capgras delusion. The patient believes that one or more people have changed their appearance to resemble familiar people, usually in order to persecute her. She maintains that, although there is no physical resemblance between the familiar person and the others, nevertheless they are psychologically identical. This symptom is usually associated with schizophrenia or with organic brain disease (Portwich and Barocka, 1998).

Intermetamorphosis

In this syndrome, the patient believes that a person (or persons) has been transformed, both physically and psychologically, into another person, or that people have exchanged identities with each other. As with the other forms of delusional misidentification, note that intermetamorphosis is not a hallucination; the abnormality is one of interpretation not misperception.

The syndrome of subjective doubles

In the syndrome of subjective doubles, the patient has the delusion that another person has been physically transformed into his own self, like a *Doppelganger.*

Shared (induced) delusional disorder

Sometimes a person in a close relationship with someone who already has an established delusional system develops similar ideas. The commonest term is a ***folie à deux***, although the ICD-10 category is **shared delusional disorder**, and the DSM-IV term is **induced delusional disorder**. It has also been called **communicated insanity**. The frequency of induced psychosis is not known, but it is low. Sometimes more than two people are involved (*folie à plusieurs*), but this is exceedingly rare. It has been speculated that some apocalyptic cults involve phenomena of this kind.

Over 90 per cent or more of reported cases are members of the same family. Usually there is a dominant partner with fixed delusions who appears to induce similar beliefs in a dependent or suggestible partner, sometimes after initial resistance. The beliefs in the recipient may or may not be truly delusional. Generally the two people have lived together for a long time in close intimacy, often in isolation from the outside world. Once established, the condition runs a chronic course.

It is usually necessary to advise separation of the affected people. This may lead to resolution of the quasi-delusional state in the recipient; the original patient should be treated in the usual fashion for delusional disorder. See Silveira and Seeman (1995) for review.

Assessment of paranoid symptoms

In the assessment of paranoid symptoms there are two stages: the recognition of the symptoms themselves, and the diagnosis of the underlying condition.

Sometimes it is obvious that the patient has persecutory ideas or delusions. At other times recognition of paranoid symptoms may be exceedingly difficult. The patient may be suspicious or angry. They may be very defensive, say little, or speak fluently about other topics whilst steering away from persecutory beliefs or denying them completely. Considerable skill may be needed to elicit the false beliefs. The psychiatrist should be tolerant and impartial, acting as a detached but interested listener who wants to understand the patient's point of view. The interviewer should show compassion and ask how they can help, but without colluding in the delusions or giving promises that cannot be fulfilled. Tact is required to avoid any argument that may cause the patient to take offence. Despite skill and tact, experienced psychiatrists may interview a patient for a long time without detecting the morbid thoughts. When an apparently false belief is disclosed, considerable time and effort may be needed to determine whether or not it meets the criteria for a delusion rather than an overvalued idea or other form of belief. This is of crucial diagnostic significance, since the presence of a delusion is likely to be the symptom upon which a diagnosis of psychotic disorder is based, whereas non-delusional thoughts which may be similar in content are consistent with a personality disorder or a neurotic disorder (e.g. hypochondriasis) depending on the other features of the history and mental state examination.

If delusions are detected, the next step is to diagnose the underlying psychiatric disorder. This means looking for the diagnostic features of the disorders noted earlier in this chapter (p. 310), and described in detail in other chapters. It is important to determine whether the patient is likely to try to harm any alleged persecutor. This calls for close study of the patient's personality and the characteristics of his delusions and any associated hallucinations. Hints or threats of homicide should be taken seriously, in the same way as for suicide. A full risk assessment is needed. The doctor should be prepared to ask tactfully about possible homicidal plans and preparations to enact them. In many ways the method of enquiry resembles the assessment of suicide risk: 'Have you ever thought of doing anything about it?' 'Have you made any plans?' 'What might prompt you to do it?'

The assessment of dangerousness is discussed further in Chapter 26.

Treatment of paranoid symptoms

General principles

Management of paranoid symptoms and delusional disorder is frequently difficult. The patient may be suspicious and distrustful, believing that psychiatric treatment is intended to harm them. Or, regarding their delusional beliefs as justified, see no need for treatment. The same tact and skill needed to encourage them to describe their symptoms fully is also necessary to persuade them then to accept treatment. Sometimes treatment can be made acceptable by offering to help non-specific symptoms such as anxiety or insomnia, or by pointing out the harmful consequences of the beliefs. Thus a patient who believes that he is surrounded by persecutors may agree that his nerves are being strained as a result, and that this needs treatment.

A decision must be made whether to admit the patient for inpatient care. This may be indicated if there is a significant or immediate risk of violence to others, or of suicide. When assessing such factors, consult other informants and to obtain a history of the patient's behaviour. If voluntary admission is refused, compulsory admission may be justified to protect the patient or other people, although this is likely to add to the patient's resentment.

Psychological treatment

Patients with paranoid symptoms require support, encouragement, and reassurance. This form of non-specific psychological treatment is an integral part of management, and essential if the patient is to be persuaded of the benefits of more targeted interventions. Of the latter, drugs are the mainstay of treatment (see below), but specific psychological therapies may have a role too. In particular, cognitive therapy, as used for the treatment of delusions in schizophrenia, may be worth trying if a sufficiently good therapeutic rapport exists. Interpretative psychotherapy and group psychotherapy are unsuitable.

Drug treatment

Paranoid symptoms in delusional disorder are treated with antipsychotic drugs just as in other psychoses. The importance of establishing a good therapeutic relationship to improve collaboration with treatment has already been emphasized.

Antipsychotics for delusional disorder

Munro has advocated pimozide as the drug of choice, particularly for monosymptomatic hypochondriacal psychosis (delusional disorder, somatic type in DSM-IV) and pathological jealousy (Munro, 2000); however, there is no good randomized evidence that it is more effective than other antipsychotics (Sultana and McMonagle, 2000). Also, pimozide's potential cardiotoxicity should be taken into account. Newer antipsychotics may be better tolerated. A non-sedating drug is usually preferable. Whichever is chosen, it is important to start with a low dose, and to take into account the patient's age, coexistent medical conditions, and prior treatment response.

Antidepressants for delusional disorder

Some randomized controlled trial data suggest that SSRIs rather than antipsychotics should be used as first line for treatment of the delusional form of body dysmorphic disorder, with antipsychotic augmentation for those who do not respond (Phillips, 2004). The role of antidepressants in other delusional disorders remains unclear, although they are often used at some stage in treatment, reflecting the frequency of comorbid depressive symptoms, and their emergence during treatment. The risk of suicide should be monitored regularly.

Signs of improvement, notably a decrease in preoccupation with the delusion(s) and reduction in agitation, may be seen within a few days of starting medication. There are few long-term outcome data. Clinical impression suggests that the prognosis in delusional disorder is poor, although Munro (2000) claims that, in compliant patients, full recovery occurs in 50 per cent with substantial improvement in another 30 per cent. In some patients, medication can be reduced or stopped without ill effects, whilst in others - probably the majority - delusions recur rapidly on discontinuation, and treatment must be maintained for prolonged periods. This issue can be judged only by a careful clinical trial with regular monitoring of mental state, and it requires discussion with the patient as to the risks and benefits of long-term medication.

Further reading

Enoch MD, Ball HN (2001) *Uncommon psychiatric syndromes*, 4th edn. London, Edward Arnold. (Fascinating descriptions of many delusional disorders, and other uncommon and eponymous psychiatric syndromes.)

Hirsch, SR and Shepherd, M (eds) (1974) *Themes and variations in European psychiatry*. John Wright, Bristol. (See the following sections: E Strömgren, Psychogenic psychoses; R Gaupp, The scientific significance of the case of Ernst Wagner and The illness and death of the paranoid mass murderer schoolmaster Wagner: a case history; E Kretschmer, The sensitive delusion of reference; H Baruk, Delusions of passion; H Ey,)

Lewis, A (1970) Paranoia and paranoid: a historical perspective. *Psychological Medicine* **1**, 2–12. (A searching and scholarly review of the origin and development of the term paranoid and related concepts.)

Munro A (1999) *Delusional disorder*. Cambridge, Cambridge University Press.

CHAPTER 14

Dementia, delirium, and other neuropsychiatric disorders

Chapter contents

Neuropsychiatry comprises psychiatric disorders that arise from demonstrable abnormalities of brain structure and function. Cognitive impairments are the most prominent feature, especially in dementia and delirium, but behavioural and emotional disturbances are also common, and may be the sole manifestations.

The term 'neuropsychiatry' is sometimes used interchangeably with **organic psychiatry** (see Lishman, 1998). However, the latter category is broader, including psychiatric disorders that arise from general medical disorders with their basis outside the brain (e.g. endocrine and metabolic disorders). These disorders are covered in Chapter 16. Moreover, the term 'organic' has the fundamental problem that it wrongly implies that other psychiatric disorders do not have any such basis (see Chapter 2); neuroscience increasingly shows the falsity of this dichotomy. Both terminologies run the risk that psychological and social factors are neglected because the disorder is considered to be 'physical'.

We have retained the term 'neuropsychiatry' here, and cover the range of types of disorder conventionally considered under this heading:

- **Delirium**: acute, generalized cognitive impairment in the setting of altered consciousness.
- **Dementia**: chronic, generalized cognitive impairment in clear consciousness. As with delirium, the syndrome of dementia can be caused by many separate disease processes. This chapter covers the clinical features and aetiology of the major dementias. *The treatment and management of dementia is covered in Chapter 20, since it is almost entirely carried out by old age psychiatrists, even when it occurs in younger patients.*
- **Amnestic** (or **amnesic**) **syndromes**: circumscribed deficits in memory.
- **Epilepsy**.
- **Head injury**.
- **Other neuropsychiatric disorders**, including focal cerebral syndromes, infections, tumours, and multiple sclerosis.
- **Secondary or symptomatic neuropsychiatric disorders**. That is, disorders such as depression and anxiety which in particular cases can be attributed directly to a neuropsychiatric cause; for example, psychosis due to cerebral vasculitis. (Psychiatric disorders secondary to diseases elsewhere in the body are covered in Chapter 16.)

Classification

In ICD-10, organic psychiatric disorders are termed **'organic, including symptomatic, mental disorders'**, and in DSM-IV, **'delirium, dementia, amnestic and other cognitive disorders'**. The two classifications are

TABLE 14.1 Classification of organic mental disorders

DSM-IV	ICD-10
Delirium, dementia, amnestic and other cognitive disorders	***Organic, including symptomatic mental disorders***
Delirium ◆ Delirium due to a general medical condition ◆ Substance-induced delirium ◆ Substance-withdrawal delirium ◆ Delirium due to multiple aetiologies ◆ Delirium, not otherwise specified	**Delirium, not induced by alcohol and other drugs**
Dementia ◆ Dementia in Alzheimer's type with early onset ◆ Dementia of Alzheimer's type with late onset	**Dementia of Alzheimer's disease** (early or late onset)
◆ Vascular dementia	**Vascular dementia**
◆ Dementia due to Pick's disease	**Dementia in other diseases classified elsewhere** ◆ Dementia in Pick's disease
◆ Dementia due to Parkinson's disease	◆ Dementia in Parkinson's disease
◆ Dementia due to Huntington's disease	◆ Dementia in Huntington's disease
◆ Dementia due to Creutzfeldt–Jakob disease	◆ Dementia in Creutzfeldt–Jakob disease
◆ Dementia due to HIV disease	◆ Dementia in HIV disease
◆ Dementia due to substance abuse	
◆ Dementia due to head trauma	
◆ Dementia due to multiple causes	
◆ Dementia, not otherwise specified	**Unspecified dementia**
Amnestic disorders	**Organic amnestic syndrome, not induced by alcohol or other psychoactive substance**
◆ Amnestic disorder due to general medical condition ◆ Substance-induced persisting amnestic disorder	

TABLE 14.1 Classification of organic mental disorders *(continued)*

DSM-IV	ICD-10
	Other mental disorders due to brain damage and dysfunction and to physical disease ◆ Organic hallucinosis ◆ Organic delusional (schizophrenia-like) disorder ◆ Organic mood disorders ◆ Organic anxiety disorder
Cognitive disorder not otherwise specified ◆ Postconcussional disorder	**Personality and behavioural disorders due to brain disease, damage, and dysfunction** ◆ Organic personality disorder ◆ Postencephalitic syndrome ◆ Post-concussional syndrome **Unspecified organic or symptomatic mental disorder**

compared in Table 14.1. The main differences are as follows:

- The decision by the authors of DSM-IV to omit the word organic from the section title has led to rearrangement of the classification of some conditions formerly grouped under the heading organic. Thus major depression with organic aetiology is classified under mood disorders as secondary to a general medical condition, or as substance induced. As a result of these changes, DSM-IV avoids the problems within ICD-10 of the definition of the terms organic, symptomatic, and secondary (Spitzer *et al.* 1992).
- In both classifications the specific medical conditions causing the mental disorder can be coded in addition to the latter disorder. In DSM-IV, this additional code is recorded on Axis III.
- In ICD-10, the section on organic disorder includes subcategories for mental disorders due to brain damage and dysfunction and to physical disease, and for personality and behavioural factors due to brain disease, damage, and dysfunction. For example, 'organic anxiety disorder, thyrotoxicosis'. In DSM-IV these conditions are classified under the relevant psychiatric disorder with the addition of a code to indicate that the disorder is secondary to a medical condition.
- DSM-IV includes categories of substance-induced delirium, dementia, and amnestic disorders. In ICD-10 these conditions are recorded in the section on mental and behavioural disorders due to psychoactive substance abuse. Thus, for example, amnestic syndrome is coded in ICD-10 in this section, but amnestic syndrome due to alcohol (Korsakov's syndrome) is classified as a psychoactive substance abuse disorder.

Symptoms associated with regional brain pathology

Before considering the various syndromes, it is helpful to consider the characteristic features associated with lesions in different regions of the brain, and the neuroanatomical basis of memory. Knowledge of the regional affiliation of neurological and psychopathological findings is relevant when attempting to localize neuropsychiatric conditions. However, the clinical features are not diagnostically specific and the clinicopathological correlations are often modest rather than strong. We do not consider in detail the dysphasias, agnosias, and dyspraxias, as these lie traditionally in the domain of neurologists.

For a comprehensive review, see Lishman (1998). See also pp. 50–1 for an introduction to neuropsychiatric assessment.

Frontal lobe

The frontal lobes, together with their reciprocal connections to other cortical and subcortical regions, have a crucial role in personality and judgement (Dolan, 1999). Patients with a frontal lobe syndrome may present with a variety of clinical syndromes. They may:

- be disinhibited, overfamiliar, tactless, and garrulous, make fatuous jokes and puns (*Witzelsucht*), commit errors of judgement and sexual indiscretions, and disregard the feelings of others.
- Appear inert (abulic) and apathetic, with a paucity of spontaneous speech, movement, and emotional expressions.
- Engage in obsessive, ritualistic behaviours with perseveration of thought and gesture.

Measures of formal intelligence are generally unimpaired in frontal lobe disease; however, there may be difficulties in abstract reasoning ('How are glass and ice different?') and cognitive estimates are typically inaccurate but precise ('364 miles from London to New York'). Concentration and attention are reduced. Insight is often markedly impaired. Verbal fluency, assessed using word generation by letter (for example, number of words beginning with 's' in one minute) and category (for example, number of animals), is reduced and unusual (low-frequency) examples may be volunteered. The patient has difficulty switching between tasks (perseveration), carrying out sequenced movements, and understanding rules. Utilization behaviour (for example, donning several pairs of spectacles) may be evident.

Posterior extension of a dominant frontal lobe lesion may involve Broca's area and produce an expressive (non-fluent) dysphasia. Encroachment on the motor cortex or deep projections may result in a contralateral hemiparesis. Other signs may include ipsilateral optic atrophy or anosmia, a grasp or other primitive reflexes and, if the process is bilateral or in the midline, incontinence of urine.

See Ron (1989) and Garrard and Hodges (2000) for a review of psychiatric aspects of frontal lobe pathology.

Parietal lobe

Lesions of the parietal lobe may cause various neuropsychological disturbances which are easily mistaken for conversion disorder (p. 206). Involvement of the non-dominant parietal lobe characteristically gives rise to visuospatial difficulties, with neglect of contralateral space, constructional and dressing **apraxias**. Lesions of the dominant lobe may be associated with receptive dysphasia, limb apraxia, body image disorders, right-left disorientation, dyscalculia, finger agnosia and agraphia. Other signs may include contralateral sensory loss, **astereognosis** and **agraphaesthesia**, and (with more extensive lesions) a contralateral hemiparesis or homonymous inferior quadrantanopia.

Persistent unawareness of neurological deficit (**anosognosia**) is not uncommon, especially with non-dominant parietal lesions. In extreme cases, the patient may deny that paretic limbs belong to him. This should be distinguished from denial due to a psychological unwillingness to recognize disability and its consequences.

Temporal lobe

The temporolimbic syndromes are characterized by complex and wide-ranging neuropsychiatric clinical pictures (Trimble, 1997). There may be personality change resembling that of frontal lobe lesions, but more often accompanied by specific cognitive deficits and neurological signs. The relatively florid behavioural disturbances which characterize the frontotemporal dementias reflect the combined temporal and frontal involvement, and their interconnections.

Unilateral medial temporal lobe lesions, especially those involving the hippocampus, produce lateralizing memory deficits: left hippocampal damage impairs verbal memory (and can cause semantic impairment and fluent dysphasia), whilst right hippocampal damage affects non-verbal (spatial) aspects of memory. Some evidence also suggests that left medial temporal lobe lesions are more likely to produce psychotic symptoms, and right-sided lesions produce affective ones.

Occipital lobe

Occipital lobe lesions may cause disturbances of visual processing which are easily misinterpreted as being of psychological origin. Such phenomena occasionally accompany migraine or occipital lobe seizures. Complex visual hallucinations may occur with lesions involving visual association areas, sometimes referred to a hemianopic field. These include multiple visual images (**polyopia**), persistent aftertraces of the features of an image (visual perseveration or **palinopsia**), and distortions of the visual scene (**metamorphopsia**). Lesions which impinge anteriorly on the parietal or temporal lobes may produce visual disorientation (inability to localize objects in space under visual guidance) with **asimultagnosia** (difficulty perceiving the visual scene as a unity), or **prosopagnosia** (inability to recognize familiar faces). In patients with suspected occipital lobe pathology, the visual fields should be mapped using perimetry, and neuropsychological tests performed to delineate visual agnosias and other higher-order derangements of visual processing. Some patients who are blind due to occipital lobe damage deny they are blind (**Anton's syndrome**).

Corpus callosum

Corpus callosum lesions (classically, the 'butterfly glioma') typically extend laterally into both hemispheres. They then produce a picture of severe and rapid intellectual deterioration, with localized neurological signs varying with the degree and direction of extension into adjacent structures. Pure callosal lesions (usually iatrogenic, following surgery for intractable epilepsy), can be surprisingly difficult to identify, and require specialized neuropsychological testing to expose a 'disconnection syndrome', reflecting disruption of interhemispheric communication. These unique 'split brain' patients raise intriguing questions concerning the mechanisms which normally bind the two hemispheres together to generate a consistent, unitary sense of the self (see Gazzaniga, 2000). Callosal degeneration is a hallmark of the rare Marchiafava–Bignami syndrome, seen in severe alcohol dependence.

Subcortical structures and cortico–subcortical circuits

The regional cortical associations with cognitive, affective and behavioural features reflect the classic 'locationist' approach to neurology and neuropsychiatry. Increasingly, this is being complemented, if not replaced, by a 'connectionist' approach, in which emphasis is placed on distributed neural systems in which cortical regions are linked with subcortical structures. The latter are also important in their own right for memory and other aspects of higher functions (Brown and Marsden, 1998).

Thalamus and basal ganglia

A variety of cognitive and psychiatric consequences have been described following lesions of subcortical grey matter structures. These include memory, language, and mood disturbance. Reduced initiation of actions is also characteristic.

Rostral brainstem

Behavioural disturbances frequently accompany lesions of the rostral brainstem. The most characteristic features are an amnestic syndrome (see below), hypersomnia, and the syndrome of 'akinetic mutism' ('vigilant coma') or stupor.

Cortico–subcortical networks

There are now several networks and systems which have been hypothesized to underlie higher functions of the human brain. Mesulam (1998) describes five networks:

1. A right hemisphere spatial awareness network including posterior parietal cortex and frontal eye fields.
2. A left hemisphere language network including Broca's and Wernicke's areas.
3. A memory–emotion network including hippocampus, amygdala and cingulate cortex.
4. A working memory–executive function network including prefrontal cortex and posterior parietal cortex.
5. A face and object recognition network in temporoparietal and temporo–occipital cortex.

Another influential model is that by Alexander and Crutcher (1990), who proposed four parallel circuits linking different parts of the cerebral cortex with specific basal ganglia and thalamic nuclei. Each circuit mediates different functions. For example, the 'limbic' circuit, involved in emotional and motivational processes, links anterior cingulate cortex and medial prefrontal cortex with ventral striatum, ventral pallidum, and mediodorsal thalamus.

White matter

There is increasing interest in the neuropsychiatric and behavioural consequences of subcortical and periventricular white matter damage (Filley, 1998). For example, degeneration of the white matter (leukodystrophy) can produce a schizophrenia-like syndrome (Hyde *et al.*, 1992), whilst multiple focal areas of white matter damage are associated with increased risks of mood disorder and dementia. These clinicopathological relationships are believed to result from partial disconnections between brain regions.

Memory systems and their neuroanatomy

Clinical, neuropsychological, and brain imaging studies (both structural and functional) support the existence of multiple memory systems in the human brain. These functions may all be affected more or less selectively by brain lesions. The most basic division lies between implicit (e.g. procedural) and explicit (declarative) memory. The former includes a range of phenomena not usually subject to conscious analysis, such as motor skills, conditioned behaviours, and repetition priming. Explicit memory is subclassified into episodic (autobiographical events) and semantic (knowledge of the world) functions.

The short-term store underpins working memory (for example, when dialling an unfamiliar telephone number). Distinct anatomical substrates for short-term storage of verbal and visuospatial information, both controlled by a central executive, have been proposed. In neuropsychological terms, short-term refers to immediate recall. By contrast, the concept of 'short-term' memory as sometimes applied by clinicians to recall over minutes and days, does not correspond to an anatomical substrate.

Specific types of memories, such as faces and topographical information, may engage dedicated subsystems. Episodic memory has both anterograde (new learning) and retrograde (recall of past events) components. It appears to be mediated by a network of cortical and subcortical structures, which include the hippocampus, parahippocampal and entorhinal cortices, amygdala, mammillary bodies, fornix, cingulate, thalamus, and frontobasal cortex, whereas semantic memory may be subserved by a partly independent network overlapping the language areas. Broadly speaking, verbal memories are mediated by the left (dominant) hemisphere and non-verbal by the right.

For review of the classification and neuroanatomical basis of memory and its dysfunction, see Hodges (1994) and Budson and Price (2005).

Assessment of the patient with cognitive impairment

The assessment of cognitive function was introduced in Chapters 1 and 3 as part of the general psychiatric assessment, and in this chapter the evaluation of amnesia, delirium and dementia will be discussed in turn. In this section, we introduce key aspects of the initial approach to the patient with suspected cognitive impairment. For a review, see Kipps and Hodges (2005). See also Chapter 20 for discussion of assessment in the elderly.

History and mental state examination

First, although physical examination and laboratory investigations play a much larger role than elsewhere in psychiatry, the history remains essential. The informant is especially important, since the presence of cognitive impairment will necessarily impair the patient's ability to provide a full and accurate history. Key points in the history include the onset, duration and progression of the impairment; for example, an acute onset suggests delirium or, if it began after a fall, may indicate a subdural haematoma. The neurological, medical, and family history are all important too, since many causes of cognitive impairment are secondary to pre-existing disorders, or have a genetic basis. The physical examination needs to be comprehensive and careful, since signs may not be conspicuous. Particular attention should be paid to the nervous system, as well as searching for peripheral stigmata of systemic disease and alcohol dependence.

A question to be addressed early is whether there is clouding of consciousness, since this defines delirium, and the assessment can proceed to determine its cause. If there is no impaired consciousness, then the main diagnostic possibilities are amnesia, dementia, or a 'functional' cause for cognitive impairment. The key feature of an amnestic syndrome is a specific deficit in episodic memory, as outlined above. Although rare, amnestic syndrome always needs consideration in a person presenting with memory impairment, especially in those with alcohol dependence. A functional cause should always be considered, since apparent memory impairment may occur secondary to many psychiatric disorders. In particular, depression in the elderly may present as **'pseudodementia'** (p. 511). Distinction between organic and functional causes requires positive evidence to be sought for both forms of disorder, and is an important distinction to make since it impacts significantly upon treatment and prognosis. Once these other causes of cognitive impairment (delirium, amnestic syndrome, functional disorder) have been ruled out, attention can turn to determining the type and severity of dementia from which the patient is suffering.

Investigations

The choice and extent of investigations will depend on the findings from the history, mental state examination, and physical examination, but usually includes a core set of tests, such as the cognitive tests and blood tests used in evaluation of dementia noted below. In difficult or atypical cases, and in younger people, investigations may be extensive, and the opinion and assistance of a neurologist, physician or neurosurgeon required.

Some examples of specialized investigations used in neuropsychiatric evaluation are:

- **Structural brain imaging** with CT or MRI. Neuroimaging can detect focal and diffuse pathologies, and longitudinal scans can map progressive changes which mirror clinical decline. MRI is superior to CT for most purposes, including evaluation of white matter disease, and the ability to perform volumetric measurements.
- **Neuropsychological testing** to determine the nature and severity of cognitive deficits is less widely used than previously, in part because of the increasing availability of brain imaging; however, it can still play a valuable part in characterization of the impairment (e.g. the cognitive domains most affected), inferred localization of the lesion, and in measuring progression.
- **EEG** studies are less commonly used, but retain a valuable role in several situations where EEG findings are characteristic: in delirium, prion disease, and detection of non-convulsive status epilepticus. It is also useful in the differential diagnosis of stupor, since a normal EEG would suggest a dissociative state.
- **Cerebrospinal fluid (CSF)** examination after lumbar puncture is essential if an inflammatory or infective process is suspected. It may also become more widely used in evaluation of dementia, as different proteins are being found which have diagnostic or prognostic value.
- **Brain biopsy**, usually of the right frontal lobe, is occasionally indicated as a last resort in diagnosis of

unexplained cognitive impairment, for example in suspected prion disease. However, the risks of this procedure must always be weighed against the diagnostic and prognostic information which will result.

Amnestic syndromes

Amnesia is loss of memory, and **amnestic syndromes** or **amnestic disorders** are those in which memory is specifically and persistently affected (Table 14.2). An amnestic disorder is defined by DSM-IV as a specific impairment of episodic memory, manifesting as inability to learn new information (anterograde amnesia) and to recall past events (retrograde amnesia) accompanied by 'significant impairment in social or occupational functioning' and with evidence of a general medical condition 'aetiologically related to the memory impairment'. Unlike dementia, the memory deficit occurs in the absence of evidence for generalized intellectual dysfunction. **Korsakov syndrome** is sometimes erroneously used as synonymous with amnestic syndrome, but is really a specific form of it, as described below.

For review, see Kopelman (2000) and Berrios and Hodges (2000).

Clinical features

The cardinal feature is a profound deficit of episodic memory. The full clinical picture is striking. There is disorientation for time, loss of autobiographical information (often extending back for many years), severe anterograde amnesia for verbal and visual material, and lack of insight into the amnesia. Events are recalled immediately after they occur, but forgotten a few minutes later. Thus digit span, testing the short-term memory store, is typically normal. New learning is grossly defective, but retrograde memory is variably preserved and shows a temporal gradient, with older memories better preserved. Other cognitive functions are relatively intact, although some emotional blunting and inertia are often observed.

The other classic feature, seen particularly in Korsakov syndrome, is **confabulation**, in which gaps in memory are filled by a vivid and detailed but wholly fictitious account of recent activities which the patient believes to be true. The confabulating patient is often highly suggestible.

TABLE 14.2 Causes of amnesia

Transient
◆ Transient global amnesia
◆ Transient epileptic amnesia
◆ Head injury
◆ Alcoholic blackouts
◆ Post-electroconvulsive therapy
◆ Post-traumatic stress disorder
◆ Psychogenic fugue
◆ Amnesia for criminal offence
Persistent (Amnestic syndrome)
◆ Korsakov syndrome
◆ Encephalitis
◆ Posterior cerebral artery and thalamic strokes
◆ Head injury

Aetiology and pathology

Amnesia results from lesions in the medial thalamus, other midline diencephalic structures, or medial temporal lobes (hippocampus and adjacent temporal cortex). Cases due to damage in medial temporal lobe typically produce the 'purest' amnesia, with little in the way of disorientation or confabulation; these latter features are characteristic of thalamic and diencephalic lesions.

Neuropsychologically, the information processing defect in the amnestic syndrome is likely to involve the encoding of new material, consolidation of this material into long-term storage, and subsequent retrieval, to a variable degree dependent on the precise anatomy of the causative lesion (Hodges, 1994).

Korsakov syndrome

The commonest cause of amnestic syndrome is **Korsakov syndrome**, named after the Russian neuropsychiatrist (sometimes spelt as Korsakoff) who described it in 1889. The alternative term **Wernicke–Korsakov syndrome** was proposed by Victor *et al.* (1971), because the syndrome often follows an acute neurological syndrome called **Wernicke's encephalopathy**, (described by Wernicke in 1881) comprising delirium, truncal ataxia, pupillary abnormalities, ophthalmoplegia, nystagmus, and a peripheral neuropathy. Korsakov syndrome is usually caused by thiamine deficiency, secondary to alcohol abuse, though it occasionally results from hyperemesis gravidarum and severe malnutrition. Post-mortem findings typically include petechial haemorrhages with astrocytic degeneration in the mammillary bodies, the region of the third ventricle, the periaqueductal grey matter, pons, and mediodorsal thalamic nuclei. Other causes of amnestic syndrome include tumours and infarcts in the medial thalamus (diencephalic amnesia), and encephalitis (see p. 355).

Investigation and management

Alertness to the possibility of the amnestic syndrome is essential; the patient may not fit the stereotype of chronic alcohol misuse associated with Korskov syndrome, and this is a potentially reversible condition. Useful findings from investigations include a reduced red cell transketolase level, which is a marker of thiamine deficiency, and an increased MRI signal in midline structures.

In practice, Korsakov syndrome should be assumed to be the cause of amnestic syndrome until another aetiology (Table 14.2) can be demonstrated, and treated urgently with thiamine without awaiting the results of investigations. Thiamine is given parenterally in an acute presentation, together with rehydration, general nutritional support, and treatment of supervening alcohol withdrawal. Thiamine replacement should always precede administration of intravenous glucose-containing solutions. Close liaison with physicians and neurologists is important.

In the longer-term, persistent amnestic syndrome may require substantial rehabilitation and support, since the condition markedly impairs normal activities and ability to self-care.

Course and prognosis of amnestic syndrome

In the series of Victor *et al.* (1971) comprising 245 patients with Wernicke–Korsakov syndrome, 96 per cent presented with Wernicke's encephalopathy. Mortality was 17 per cent in the acute stage, and 84 per cent of survivors developed amnestic syndrome. There was no improvement in half, complete recovery in a quarter, and partial recovery in the remainder. Favourable prognostic factors were a short history before diagnosis, and prompt commencement of thiamine replacement.

The prognosis is poor in cases of amnestic syndrome due to encephalitis and other causes of irreversible bilateral hippocampal or diencephalic damage; however, amnestic syndrome due to head injury has a better outlook. Progressive amnesia suggests a slowly expanding structural lesion, such as a midbrain tumour.

Transient global amnesia

The syndrome of **transient global amnesia** is important in the differential diagnosis of paroxysmal neurological and psychiatric disturbance (see Table 14.3). It occurs in middle or late life. The clinical picture is of sudden onset of isolated anterograde amnesia in a clear sensorium generally lasting less than 24 hours. Functional imaging studies during transient global amnesia have demonstrated localized transient hypo- or hyperperfusion consistent with dysfunction of circuits mediating episodic memory.

The patient appears bewildered, and requires repeated reorientation, only to ask the same questions moments later; however, there is no disturbance of alertness and (in contrast to psychogenic fugue) personal identity is retained. Procedural memory is spared (for example, the patient may carry on driving competently during the episode). Apart from the memory disturbance, the neurological examination is entirely normal.

Complete recovery, with amnesia for the period of the episode, is usual and recurrence is rare. However, investigation is always indicated since the condition may be exactly mimicked by a temporal lobe tumour. Other causes of amnestic syndrome (see above and Table 14.2) must also be excluded. Patients with transient global amnesia often present as emergencies to general practitioners and casualty departments, and the syndrome may be misdiagnosed as a dissociative fugue.

TABLE 14.3 Differential diagnosis of paroxysmal neuropsychiatric symptoms

Organic
◆ Syncope (cardjogenic, vasovagal, reflex)
◆ Transient ischaemic attacks
◆ Migraine
◆ Epileptic seizure
◆ Hypoglycaemia, other metabolic encephalopathies, phaeochromocytoma
◆ Transient global amnesia
◆ Narcolepsy, cataplexy, somnambulism, parasomnias
◆ Tonic spasms of multiple sclerosis
◆ Treatment-related complications in Parkinson's disease
◆ Drug abuse (covert)
Functional
◆ Panic attacks and hyperventilation
◆ Dissociative disorder
◆ Schizophrenia
◆ Bipolar affective disorder
◆ Aggressive outburst in personality disorder
◆ Temper tantrums (children)
◆ Breath-holding spells (children)

Delirium

Delirium is characterized by global impairment of consciousness (**clouding of consciousness**), resulting in reduced levels of alertness, attention, and perception of the environment. A number of other terms such as '**confusional state**' and '**acute organic syndrome**' have also been used, but delirium is the preferred term in both ICD-10 and DSM-IV. Delirium occurs in 15–30 per cent of patients in general medical or surgical wards, and a higher proportion of patients in intensive care units (Lipowski, 1990). It is more common in the elderly and other individuals with diminished 'cerebral reserve', notably those with pre-existing dementia. The prognosis is related to the underlying cause. Many cases recover rapidly, but there is a 25 per cent mortality at 3 months. There is no evidence that delirium progresses to dementia. For review of delirium and its management, see Burns *et al.* (2004).

Clinical features

The cardinal feature is disturbed consciousness. It is manifested as drowsiness, decreased awareness of surroundings, disorientation in time and place, and distractibility. At its most severe the patient may be unresponsive (stuporose), but more commonly the impaired consciousness is quite subtle. Indeed the first clue to the presence of delirium is often one of its other features, which include mental slowness, distractibility, perceptual anomalies, and disorganization of the sleep–wake cycle.

Symptoms and signs vary widely between patients, and in the same patient at different times of day, typically being worse at night. For example, some patients are hyperactive, restless, irritable and have psychotic symptoms; others are hypoactive, with psychomotor retardation and perseveration. Repetitive, purposeless movements are common in both forms. Thinking is slow and muddled, but often rich in content ('dream-like'). Ideas of reference and delusions (often persecutory) are common, but usually transient and poorly elaborated. Visual perception is often distorted, with illusions, misinterpretations, and visual hallucinations, sometimes with fantastic content. Tactile and auditory hallucinations also occur. Anxiety, depression, and emotional lability are common. Patients may be frightened, or perplexed. Experiences of depersonalization and derealization are sometimes described. Attention and registration are particularly impaired, and on recovery there is usually amnesia for the period of the delirium.

Aetiology

The main causes of delirium are shown in Table 14.4. Old age, frailty, and prior medical and neurological disorders lower the threshold for developing delirium.

The pathophysiological basis of delirium is unclear. The severity of clinical disturbance correlates with the degree of slowing of cerebral rhythms on EEG, and the neurotransmitters dopamine and acetylcholine are implicated in a final common pathway (Trzepacz, 2000).

TABLE 14.4 Causes of delirium

Drugs
◆ Alcohol intoxication
◆ Alcohol withdrawal and delirium tremens
◆ Opiates
◆ Prescribed drugs
◆ Any drug with anticholinergic properties
◆ Any sedative
◆ Digoxin
◆ Diuretics
◆ Lithium
◆ Steroids
Medical conditions
◆ Febrile illness (e.g. urinary tract infection)
◆ Septicaemia
◆ Organ failure (cardiac, renal, hepatic)
◆ Hypo- or hyper-glycaemia
◆ Post-operative hypoxia
◆ Thiamine deficiency
Neurological conditions
◆ Epileptic seizure (post-ictal)
◆ Head injury
◆ Space occupying lesion
◆ Encephalitis
◆ Cerebral haemorrhage
Other
◆ Constipation
◆ Dehydration
◆ Pain
◆ Sensory deprivation

Management of delirium

General principles

Delirium is a medical emergency. It is essential to identify and treat the underlying cause. As delirium is often due to drugs (either as side-effects or withdrawal effects), these should always be suspected until there is evidence of another cause. As well as urgent investigation, general measures are necessary to relieve distress, control agitation, and prevent exhaustion. These include frequent explanation, reorientation, and reassurance. Unnecessary changes in staff caring for the patient should be avoided. The patient should ideally be nursed in a quiet single room. Relatives should be encouraged to visit regularly. At night, lighting should be sufficient to promote orientation, while not preventing sleep. See American Psychiatric Association (1999) and Burns *et al.* (2004) for review.

Drug treatment

Drug treatment of the underlying physical problem should be reviewed to ensure that it is the minimum required. Despite the above interventions, which should always be tried first, many patients with delirium require medication to control agitation and distress, and permit adequate sleep. The drug of choice is usually an antipsychotic. Haloperidol is conventionally used, in a dose carefully titrated to achieve the desired calming without excess sedation or side-effects, generally between 2 and 10 mg/day. If necessary, the first dose can be given intramuscularly. Some causes of delirium require avoidance of, or particular caution with, antipsychotics. This includes all patients with dementia, especially dementia with Lewy bodies, who are particularly sensitive to antipsychotics. Antipsychotics should be avoided in delirium associated with alcohol withdrawal (delirium tremens), or with epilepsy, because of the risk of seizures. In delirium tremens, a reducing regimen of the benzodiazepine chlordiazepoxide is the standard treatment. All sedative drugs should be used sparingly in liver failure because of the danger of precipitating hepatic coma.

Dementia

Dementia is an acquired global impairment of intellect, memory and personality, but without impairment of consciousness (Lishman, 1998). It is usually but not always progressive. The syndrome of dementia is caused by a range of diseases (Table 14.5), of which Alzheimer's disease (accounting for 50–60 per cent of cases), vascular dementia (20–25 per cent), and dementia with Lewy bodies (15–20 per cent) are the commonest. For review, see Ritchie and Lovestone (2002).

Although dementia is a global or generalized disorder, it often begins with focal cognitive or behavioural disturbances, but both DSM-IV and ICD-10 definitions require impairment in two or more cognitive domains

TABLE 14.5 Causes of dementia

Primary neurodegenerative disorders
Alzheimer's disease*, dementia with Lewy bodies, Pick's disease and other frontotemporal dementias,* Parkinson's disease*, prion diseases*, Huntington's disease*
Vascular
Vascular dementia, multiple strokes, focal thalamic and basal ganglia strokes, subdural haematoma
Inflammatory and autoimmune
SLE and other vasculitides with CNS involvement, Behçet's disease, neurosarcoidosis, Hashimoto's encephalopathy, multiple sclerosis
Traumatic
Severe head injury, or repeated head trauma in boxers ('dementia pugilistica') and others
Infections and related conditions
HIV, iatrogenic and variant CJD (prion disease), neurosyphilis, post-encephalitic, Lyme disease
Metabolic and endocrine
Sustained uraemia, renal dialysis, liver failure, hypothyroidism, hyperthyroidism ('apathetic' or masked), hypoglycaemia, Cushing's syndrome, hypopituitarism, adrenal insufficiency
Neoplastic
See Table 14.21
Post-radiation
See Table 14.21
Post-anoxic
Severe anaemia, post-surgical (especially cardiac bypass), carbon monoxide poisoning, cardiac arrest, chronic respiratory failure
Vitamin and other nutritional deficiency
Sustained lack of vitamin B12, folate
Toxic
Alcohol, poisoning with heavy metals, organic solvents, organophosphates
Other
Normal pressure hydrocephalus

*Causes asterisked exist in genetically determined forms.

(memory, language, abstract thinking and judgement, praxis, visuoperceptual skills, personality, and social conduct), sufficient to interfere with social or occupational functioning. Deficits may initially be too mild or circumscribed to fulfil this definition, and are called **mild cognitive impairment** (see p. 334). The fluctuations in alertness which characterize delirium are usually absent, except that fluctuating impairment of consciousness is a feature of dementia with Lewy bodies (see below).

In this section, the main features of dementia as a clinical syndrome are described, followed by the principles of assessment. We then discuss the individual clinical, epidemiological, aetiological and neuropathological features of the major diseases that produce dementia. Note in Table 14.5 that many other neuropsychiatric disorders can also produce cognitive impairment (e.g. multiple sclerosis; normal pressure hydrocephalus) as a less common or subsidiary clinical feature; these conditions are considered later in the chapter. Table 14.5 also shows that dementia occurs in a range of medical disorders (e.g. systemic lupus erythematosus), covered in Chapter 16, and as a result of substance misuse, especially alcohol, as discussed on p. 345 and in Chapter 18.

Finally, note that the treatment and management of dementia, and the relationships between dementia and ageing, are deferred until Chapter 20.

Clinical features of dementia

The presenting complaint is usually of poor memory. Other features include disturbances of behaviour, language, personality, mood, or perception. Dementia is often exposed by a change in social circumstances or an intercurrent illness; indeed, patients with dementia are especially susceptible to superimposed delirium.

The clinical picture is much determined by the patient's premorbid personality. People with good social skills may continue to function adequately despite severe intellectual deterioration. The elderly, socially isolated, or deaf are less likely to compensate for failing intellectual abilities; however, their difficulties may be unrecognized or dismissed.

Forgetfulness is usually early and prominent, but may sometimes be difficult to detect in the early stages. Poor memory is not anatomically localizing: it may reflect disrupted registration (frontotemporal interactions), encoding (mesial temporal lobes), or retrieval (frontal lobes). Impaired attention and concentration are common and nonspecific features. Difficulty in new learning is usually the most conspicuous feature. Memory loss is more evident for recent than for more remote material. Disturbed episodic memory manifests as forgetfulness for recent day-to-day events, with relative preservation of procedural memory (for instance, riding a bicycle), and, at least initially, general knowledge about the world at large. By contrast, words and, ultimately, the very objects to which they refer, lose their meaning for patients with semantic memory impairment (as in certain frontotemporal dementias).

Loss of flexibility and adaptability in new situations, with the appearance of rigid and stereotyped routines ('organic orderliness'), and, when taxed beyond restricted abilities, sudden explosions of rage or grief ('catastrophic reaction') are frequent. As dementia worsens, patients are less able to care for themselves and they neglect social conventions. Disorientation for time, and later for place and person, is common. Behaviour becomes aimless, and stereotypies and mannerisms may appear. Thinking slows and becomes impoverished in content and perseverative. False ideas, often of a persecutory kind, gain ground easily. In the later stages, thinking becomes grossly fragmented and incoherent. This is reflected in the patient's speech, with syntactical and dysnomic errors. Eventually, the patient may become mute. Mortality is increased, with death often following bronchopneumonia and a terminal coma.

Behavioural, affective and psychotic features often accompany the cognitive deficits during dementia. They appear to be part of the underlying biology of the disease process, although in the early stages, whilst insight is retained, they may also be a psychological response to the realisation of cognitive decline. Mood disturbances are particularly common, together with distress, anxiety, irritability and sometimes aggression. Later, emotional responses become blunted, and sudden, apparently random mood changes occur. Psychotic symptoms are also a common and fluctuating feature during dementia.

The balance of these core symptoms and signs, together with some additional features, forms the basis for the clinical differentiation between the various causes of dementia, as summarized in Table 14.6 and described in the following sections.

Subcortical and cortical dementia

A clinical distinction is sometimes drawn between cortical and subcortical dementia, based upon their putative neuroanatomical basis (Cummings, 1990).

TABLE 14.6 Clinical features helpful in distinguishing between major causes of dementia

	Prominent symptoms and signs	Other clinical features
Alzheimer's disease	Memory loss, especially short-term	Relentlessly progressive
	Dysphasia and dyspraxia	Survival 5–8 years
	Sense of smell impaired early	
	Behavioural changes – e.g. wandering	
Vascular dementia	Personality change	Stepwise progression
	Labile mood	Signs of cerebrovascular disease
	Preserved insight	History of hypertension
		Commoner in men, smokers
Dementia with Lewy bodies	Fluctuating alertness	Sensitive to antipsychotics
	Parkinsonism	
	Visual hallucinations	
	Falls and faints	
Frontotemporal dementia	Prominent behavioural change	Onset usually before age 70
	Expressive dysphasia	Range of clinical subtypes
	Early loss of insight	
	Early primitive reflexes	
Huntington's disease	Schizophrenia-like psychosis	Presents in third to fifth decade
	Abnormal movements (choreiform)	Strong family history
	Depression and irritability	
	Dementia occurs later	
Prion disease	Myoclonic jerks	Often early onset
	Seizures	Rapid onset and progression
	Cerebellar ataxia	Transmissible
	Psychiatric symptoms (vCJD)	
Normal pressure hydrocephalus	Mental slowing, apathy, inattention	Commonest in 50–70 year olds
	Urinary incontinence	Commonest reversible dementia
	Problems walking (gait apraxia)	

Although the distinction is blurred, clinically and pathologically, the terms have descriptive utility (Turner *et al.*, 2002). The key features are summarized in Table 14.7, and examples of the diseases given in Table 14.8. The term 'subcortical dementia' is seen to refer to a syndrome of slowness of thought, difficulty with complex, sequential intellectual tasks, impoverishment of affect and personality, with relative preservation of language, calculation, and learning. It contrasts with the spectrum of dysfunction (including early, prominent impairments of memory, word finding, or visuospatial abilities) seen in 'cortical dementias', notably Alzheimer's disease.

Presenile and senile dementia

A clear distinction used to be drawn between dementia occurring in those under 65 (presenile or early-onset dementia) from those beginning later in life (senile or late-onset dementia), in part because of the belief that the major causes were different - Alzheimer's disease in the former, vascular dementia in the latter. The distinction is now much less important with the realization that Alzheimer's disease is the commonest form of dementia in both groups. However, there are several related aspects of presenile dementia that are different from the senile form (Greicius *et al.*, 2002). Frontotemporal dementia and prion disease are relatively more com-

TABLE 14.7 Features of cortical and subcortical dementias

	Subcortical dementia	Cortical dementia
Memory impairment	Moderate	Severe, early
Language	Normal	Dysphasias, early
Mathematical skills	Preserved	Impaired early
Personality	Apathetic, inert	Indifferent
Mood	Flat, depressed	Normal
Co-ordination	Impaired	Normal
Cognitive and motor speed	Slowed	Normal
Abnormal movements	Common, choreiform or tremor	Rare

TABLE 14.8 Examples of cortical, subcortical and mixed causes of dementia

Cortical
◆ Alzheimer's disease
◆ Frontotemporal dementias
◆ Creutzfeldt-Jacob disease
Subcortical
◆ Normal pressure hydrocephalus
◆ Huntington's disease
◆ Parkinson's disease
◆ Focal thalamic and basal ganglia lesions
◆ Multiple sclerosis
Mixed
◆ Vascular dementia
◆ Dementia with Lewy bodies
◆ Corticobasal degeneration
◆ Neurosyphilis

mon, vascular dementia rarer, and a higher proportion of cases are due to genetic diseases. These factors influence management. Patients with presenile dementia are more likely to be referred to and investigated by neurologists, before involvement of psychiatrists in their care. Investigations are more intensive and extensive because of the importance in making a definite diagnosis and providing a clear prognosis; the results will also have implications for relatives if a genetic aetiology is discovered (Sampson *et al.*, 2004).

Assessment of dementia

Assessment of a patient presenting with cognitive impairment has several stages. A key question to be addressed initially is whether the impairment is due to dementia. This involves ruling out other causes, notably delirium, amnesia, and pseudodementia, as outlined on p. 326, and using the principles of assessment described in Chapter 3.

Having established the probable diagnosis of dementia, its characteristics (including severity, symptom and behaviour profile, and associated risks) are considered, together with assessment of its cause. For review, see Fleminger (2000a) and Ross and Bowen (2002).

Assessing the severity and profile of dementia

Screening tests are useful in the assessment of dementia and its severity, and for monitoring progression. Different scales are available to assess cognition, behav-

TABLE 14.9 Screening tests for dementia

Cognitive function
◆ Mini-mental state examination (MMSE)
◆ Seven-minute screen
◆ Clock drawing test
◆ Hopkins verbal learning test (HVLT)
◆ Mental test score (MTS)
◆ Alzheimer's Disease Assessment Scale – cognitive section (ADAS-Cog)
◆ Cambridge Mental Disorders of the Elderly Examination, cognitive section (CAMCOG)
Behavioural and psychological features
◆ Neuropsychiatric inventory
◆ MOUSEPAD
◆ BEHAVE-AD
◆ Cohen-Mansfield aggression inventory
Activities of daily living
◆ Bristol scale
◆ Alzheimer's Disease Functional Assessment and Change Scale
◆ Disability Assessment for Dementia
Depression
◆ Cornell scale
◆ Geriatric Depression Rating Scale
Global assessment
◆ Clinical dementia rating (CDR)

Adapted from Burns *et al.* (2002)

ioural symptoms, global functioning, and activities of daily living, and depression; the latter is useful as depression can coexist with dementia and worsen functioning. Some commonly used ones are shown in Table 14.9. For cognitive impairment, the benchmark is the MMSE (Appendix to Chapter 3), which has a sensitivity and specificity for dementia of around 80 per cent when a cut-off score of 23 is chosen. The 'seven-minute screen' and clock test are valuable and brief alternatives. The ADAS-Cog is particularly designed for suspected Alzheimer's disease, and widely used in clinical trials to monitor treatment response. The CAMCOG is largely a research tool.

Careful evaluation of the behavioural symptoms of dementia are an integral part of the assessment, and need to be repeated during the illness, since they are common and pose as many difficulties for carers as the cognitive symptoms. This issue is discussed in detail in Chapter 20 (p. 507).

Assessment of risk in dementia

Patients with dementia are at risk from self-neglect, poor judgement, wandering, and abuse. Their physical health is often a problem. Risks to others may occur because of aggressive or disinhibited behaviour. Fitness to drive is a specific issue to consider, and may be difficult to determine in the early stages of dementia (Brown and Ott, 2004); current British regulations allow those with 'sufficient skills' and whose 'progression [of dementia] is slow' to continue to drive subject to annual review. Thus, risk assessment is part of a full assessment of dementia. A good history from carers and other informants is essential, and an occupational therapist has an important role to play in assessment of functional ability.

Early detection of dementia

Mild cognitive impairment

Increasing attention is being given to the earlier diagnosis of dementia in those with equivocal evidence, or subjective complaints, of worsening memory (Petersen *et al.*, 2001). This intermediate category, introduced in ICD-10, is called **mild cognitive impairment**. About 10–20 per cent of cases are thought to develop dementia within a year, although neuropsychological tests may be able to detect such subjects with a higher accuracy (Blackwell *et al.*, 2004). Neuropathologically, mild cognitive impairment is associated with Alzheimer-type changes, and with vascular pathology (Bennett *et al.*, 2005). For review of mild cognitive impairment, see Davis and Rockwood (2004).

Presymptomatic diagnosis

There is increasing evidence that dementia, especially Alzheimer's disease, can be detected premorbidly, long before overt symptoms are present. Longitudinal studies show that there are selective and characteristic neuropsychological impairments, detectable up to 20 years before the onset of symptoms, as well as functional brain changes (e.g. in regional glucose metabolism) and structural and neuropathological abnormalities that precede symptoms by several years (Scheltens *et al.*, 2002; Nestor *et al.*, 2004). For example, hippocampal atrophy at the rate of about 2 per cent per annum begins several years before symptoms of Alzheimer's disease; this contrasts with normal age related decreases of 0.5 per cent. There are also characteristic profiles of proteins in the cerebrospinal fluid with good sensitivity and specificity (e.g. reduced β-amyloid and increased tau; see below) (Blennow and Hampel, 2003). Finally, it is now possible to image β-amyloid deposits in the brain by PET using a ligand called PIB; this will enhance the ability to diagnose Alzheimer's disease early, and differentiate it from other dementias.

Presymptomatic diagnosis of dementia will become clinically important in the near future if potential preventative or disease-retarding treatments emerge (Chapter 20).

Assessing the cause of dementia

Definitive diagnosis of the cause of dementia can only be made neuropathologically or, in rare cases, by iden-

TABLE 14.10 Baseline investigations for dementia

In all patients
◆ Full blood count
◆ Erythrocyte sedimentation rate
◆ Urea and electrolytes
◆ Liver function tests
◆ Calcium and phosphate
◆ Thyroid function tests
◆ Syphilis serology
◆ Urinalysis
◆ B12 and folate
Worth considering
◆ HIV status
◆ Chest radiograph
◆ ECG
◆ CT or MRI brain scan
◆ EEG
◆ Neuropsychological assessment

Adapted from Fleminger (2000a)

tification of genetic mutations. However, the differing profiles of the various dementias allow 'probable' diagnoses to be made by experienced clinicians with reasonable accuracy. For example, Burns *et al.* (1990) found 88 per cent of cases of clinically diagnosed Alzheimer's disease were confirmed at autopsy. Use of biochemical, radiological and genetic investigations adds only modestly to the diagnostic accuracy of common dementias, but is important in ruling out rarer and potentially reversible causes (Lovestone, 2000; Scheltens *et al.*, 2002). Table 14.10 summarizes baseline investigations for dementia. More specialized tests are needed on occasion, depending on the patient's age, history, results of the initial tests, and the subsequent differential diagnosis. As noted above, young patients require particularly extensive investigation.

Alzheimer's disease

In 1907, Alzheimer reported the case of Auguste D, a woman with presenile dementia whose brain exhibited unusual neuropathological features. It was Alzheimer's colleague, Kraepelin, who named the disease (Maurer *et al.*, 1997). For many years, the disease was thought to be rare and limited to presenile forms of dementia, but classic studies by Roth and colleagues (Blessed *et al.*, 1968) showed that it is in fact the commonest cause of senile dementia. This is confirmed by a recent population-based autopsy study, which showed that 64 per cent of subjects with dementia had Alzheimer's disease (Neuropathology Group of the MRC Cognitive Function and Aging Study, 2001). Prevalence rates for populations over 65 years old range from 2–7 per cent for moderately or severely affected people. Age-specific prevalence rates approximately double with every additional 5 years of age from about 1 per cent at 65, rising to about 8–10 per cent at age 80 and 30–40 per cent at age 90 (Nussbaum and Ellis, 2003; see Fig. 20.3, p. 499). See Jorm (2000) for review of the epidemiology of Alzheimer's disease.

Clinical features of Alzheimer's disease

The main features of dementia have been described above, and Table 14.11 summarizes the clinical features of Alzheimer's disease (strictly, 'dementia of the Alzheimer type', since formal diagnosis awaits neuropathology). See also Table 14.6.

The first evidence of the condition is often minor forgetfulness which may be difficult to distinguish from normal ageing. The condition progresses gradually for the first 2–4 years, with increasing memory disturbance and lack of spontaneity. Memory is lost for recent events first. Language is usually affected early, with difficulty in finding words or naming objects, and

TABLE 14.11 Key clinical features of Alzheimer's disease (from DSM-IV)

Memory impairment
Gradual onset and continuing decline
One or more of: ◆ Aphasia ◆ Apraxia ◆ Agnosia ◆ Disturbance in executive functioning (e.g. planning, reasoning)
Exclusion of other disorders causing dementia

impairments in the ability to construct fluent and informative sentences. Visuospatial skills may be affected with difficulties in tasks such as copying pictures or learning the way round unfamiliar environments, for example, on holiday or in an unfamiliar house. Disorientation in time gives rise to poorly kept appointments and changes in the diurnal pattern of activity.

Depression

The relationship between Alzheimer's disease and depression is complex: depression is a risk factor for the disease, may be confused with it, or occur as part of the syndrome. Regarding the latter point, major depression occurs in about 10 per cent of cases, with less marked episodes and symptoms occurring in over 50 per cent. Patients who experienced depression have greater decreases in serotonin and noradrenergic markers at autopsy than other patients with Alzheimer's disease.

Psychotic symptoms

Delusions and hallucinations occur in a significant minority of patients at some stage in the illness. Their prevalence is unclear since many studies did not distinguish Alzheimer's disease from dementia with Lewy bodies (see below). Recent estimates suggest rates of 10–50 per cent for delusions and 10–25 per cent for hallucinations. The commonest delusions are persecutory, concerning theft (however, as this idea often arises from the patient's forgetfulness it is questionable whether it is helpful to regard this as a true delusion). Treatment of psychosis in Alzheimer's disease must take into account its transience, and the sensitivity of patients to medication (pp. 507–9).

Behaviour

Changes in behaviour are common and are of particular concern to carers. Patients may be restless and wake at night, disorientated and perplexed. Motor activity may increase in the evening ('**sundowning**'), and eventually the sleep–wake cycle may become totally disorganized. **Aggression** is common, both verbal and physical, and often takes the form of resistance to help with personal care. Serious physical violence to others is rare. Both increases and reductions in level of activity are common, involving varying degrees of purposefulness. **Wandering** can refer to a variety of different behaviours, but patients may place themselves at risk by going into unsafe environments. Patients with dementia may under- or overeat, with associated change in weight and nutritional state. Changes in sexual behaviour occur, usually with reduction in drive, although sexual disinhibition occasionally occurs. All these issues should be addressed in risk assessments, as outlined on p. 333 and in Chapter 20.

Self-care and social behaviour decline, although some patients maintain a good social façade despite severe cognitive impairment, particularly if carers are able to assist with these functions.

Course

In the early stages of Alzheimer's disease, the clinical features are modified by the person's premorbid personality, and their traits tend to be exaggerated. In the middle and later stages of the illness, the cognitive impairments increasingly predominate, together with the neurological and behavioural features noted above. Incidental physical illness may cause a superimposed delirium resulting in a sudden deterioration in cognitive function. Median survival from diagnosis is 5–8 years, slightly less in men than women. Shorter survival is also associated with an older age of onset, and with a rapid rate of cognitive decline.

Differential diagnosis of Alzheimer's disease

Clinical features

Careful clinical evaluation allows Alzheimer's disease to be distinguished reasonably reliably from other causes of dementia (Table 14.6), bearing in mind that mixed dementias are common (p. 345). As Alzheimer's disease is the commonest dementia, and the clinical profile to which others are compared, much of the differential diagnosis is based on recognition of the positive features of another dementia. Thus, distinction from vascular dementia is based largely on the stepwise progression, fluctuating course, focal motor signs, and other evidence of vascular disease and its risk factors. At a comparable stage of dementia, episodic memory is more affected in Alzheimer's disease, with semantic memory and attentional deficits commoner in vascular dementia (Graham *et al.*, 2004).

Distinction from dementia with Lewy bodies is similarly based upon the positive features of the latter syndrome which, compared to Alzheimer's disease, has more prominent, earlier, and more persistent visual hallucinations and delusions, as well as parkinsonism, a greater degree of fluctuation in alertness and cognitive impairment, and unexplained falls.

Investigations

Brain imaging and genetic tests can help in differentiation of Alzheimer's disease from other dementias, although neither are yet carried out routinely in most countries. Hippocampal atrophy and ventricular enlargement are characteristic CT or MRI findings, as is the rapid progression of these changes during the early stages of the dementia. Genetic testing can help in two ways, based upon the research findings outlined below. First, in the rare cases of familial Alzheimer's disease, discovery of a causative mutation can be diagnostic. Second, apoE4 status (the major genetic risk factor for the disease; see Box 5.3 and p. 338) modestly increases the diagnostic accuracy in patients with early dementia. However, the clinical value, and ethical implications, of genetic testing for Alzheimer's disease (and other dementias) are still controversial, and it is not currently recommended (van der Cammen *et al.*, 2004). See Liddell *et al.* (2001) for review of genetic testing for Alzheimer's disease, and the implications for relatives. There is agreement that there is currently no place for genetic screening of healthy subjects to predict future dementia.

Neuropathology of Alzheimer's disease

On gross examination the brain is shrunken with widened sulci and enlarged ventricles. Brain weight is reduced. On microscopic examination, the cardinal diagnostic features are **neurofibrillary tangles** and **senile plaques** (also called **amyloid plaques**) in the cerebral cortex and many subcortical regions. Although these features occur in normal aging, and some other disorders, they are more widespread and abundant in Alzheimer's disease, and the diagnostic criteria are based upon their abundance and distribution: the Consortium to Establish a Registry for Alzheimer's Disease (CERAD) criteria (Mirra *et al.*, 1991).

In addition to the tangles and plaques, there is selective loss of neurons in the hippocampus and entorhinal cortex, proliferation of astrocytes (gliosis), and loss of synapses. The latter is the strongest neuropathological correlate of cognitive impairment. Other histological findings include amyloid deposits in blood vessel walls ('**vascular amyloid**' or '**congophilic angiopathy**'), **Hirano bodies** (intracellular, crystalline deposits) and **granulovacuolar accumulation** (vacuoles or 'holes' within neurons).

For review of the neuropathology of Alzheimer's disease, see Morris and Nagy (2004).

Progression of Alzheimer's disease

The disease starts in the entorhinal cortex, before spreading to the hippocampus, association areas of the parietal lobe, and to some subcortical nuclei; six neuropathological stages based upon β-amyloid deposition, are recognized, called Braak stages, which correlate with clinical severity (Braak and Braak, 1991). The spread of pathology along corticocortical projections leads to an effective 'disconnection' between affected regions.

Senile (amyloid) plaques.

Senile plaques are deposits of insoluble proteins, together with degenerating neurites (neuronal processes) and glia. They occur in the space between neurons (the neuropil). Both neuritic and diffuse plaques are recognized, depending on their appearance using silver stains; neuritic plaques have a dense staining core, whereas diffuse plaques have been likened to cotton wool. The neuritic plaques are pathologically more significant. The protein at the heart of all senile plaques is **β-amyloid** (also called Aβ or A4), a 39–42 amino-acid peptide. This molecule and its encoding gene are central to the aetiology of the disease (see below).

Neurofibrillary tangles

Neurofibrillary tangles occur within the cell body of neurons, especially pyramidal neurons of the cerebral cortex and hippocampus. They are formed of paired helical filaments, which in turn are comprised of the microtubule-associated protein **tau**. The normal function of tau is in axonal transport and maintenance of the neuronal cytoskeleton. Tangles are thought to occur because tau becomes hyperphosphorylated, rendering it insoluble. The presence of a tangle causes dysfunction and death of the neuron.

Aetiology of Alzheimer's disease

Familial Alzheimer's disease

In rare families, usually those with an early onset of illness (before age 60), an autosomal dominant mode of inheritance can be discerned. Mutations in three genes have been identified: **amyloid precursor protein** (APP, on chromosome 21), **presenilin 1** (PS1, on chromosome 14) and **presenilin 2** (PS2, on chromosome 1). Discovery of APP as the first 'Alzheimer gene' was a seminal event in psychiatry (Box 14.1). These three genes together account for the majority of familial cases of the disease; equally, at least one other gene is likely to exist. Different mutations are known in each gene, and the age of onset, features, and progression of disease vary depending on the causative mutation.

Genetic factors in sporadic Alzheimer's disease

The vast majority of Alzheimer's disease, and virtually all cases in the elderly, are not inherited in a Mendelian fashion, and it is often called 'sporadic'. However, first-degree relatives of patients with late-onset Alzheimer's disease have a risk of developing the disorder which is three times that of the general population, and the implication of a genetic predisposition is supported by studies showing an association between polymorphisms in several genes, notably **apoE**, with all forms of Alzheimer's disease. As discussed in Box 5.3 (p. 103), the apoE4 variant of this gene accounts for about half of the vulnerability to late onset Alzheimer's disease.

BOX 14.1 DISCOVERY OF APP GENE MUTATIONS IN FAMILIAL ALZHEIMER'S DISEASE

In 1984, the protein which accumulates in vasculature, senile plaques and meninges in Alzheimer's disease was discovered to be the β-amyloid peptide. Knowledge of its amino-acid sequence allowed the encoding gene, called amyloid precursor protein (APP) to be identified, and localized to chromosome 21. It was already known that there was a relationship between Alzheimer's disease and Down's syndrome (trisomy 21; Holland and Oliver, 1995), suggesting that APP was a 'candidate gene' for Alzheimer's disease. Researchers collected DNA from families with autosomal dominant Alzheimer's disease to test this hypothesis. The work culminated in the landmark discovery in 1991 of an APP mutation (a point mutation changing valine to isoleucine at position 717) which caused Alzheimer's disease, reported by a group in London (Goate *et al.*, 1991). Since then, different APP mutations have been found in other families. Any doubt that the APP mutations are causative for the disease was removed by the demonstration that transgenic mice containing a mutated APP gene become cognitively impaired and deposit β-amyloid (Games *et al.*, 1995). APP mutations are pathogenic primarily because they affect metabolism of APP, promoting the formation of β-amyloid. APP mutations explain only a tiny fraction of cases of Alzheimer's disease. However, mismetabolism of APP, caused by a range of other factors, appears to be central to much if not all Alzheimer's disease, as described in the text.

Its main effect is to promote an earlier onset of disease, by about a decade. Other data suggest that apoE4-positive cases may have some differences in pathology, course, and response to medication. In Caucasians, the apoE2 variant reduces the risk of Alzheimer's disease, but this does not hold in African-Americans. The role of genetic testing for apoE4 was mentioned above. It is stressed that apoE4 is not a determinant of disease; at least a third of patients with Alzheimer's disease are apoE4 negative, and some apoE4 homozgyotes never develop the disease.

It is not known how apoE4 elevates risk of Alzheimer's disease, but it is likely to reflect its interaction with β-amyloid metabolism, cholesterol, and many other cellular functions in the brain. It may also modify susceptibility to the environmental risk factors (Lahiri *et al.*, 2004).

Many other genetic risk factors for Alzheimer's disease have been implicated, but all remain to be confirmed. One candidate is ubiquilin 1, on chromosome 9 (Bertram *et al.*, 2005). Ubiquilin 1 is involved in protein degradation.

Environmental factors

Various environmental factors are associated with an altered risk for developing Alzheimer's disease (Table 14.12). However, for many of them, it is not clear to what extent they are causal, act independently, or whether they interact with genetic predisposition.

The negative associations with exposure to NSAIDs (Szekely *et al.*, 2004) and HRT (LeBlanc *et al.*, 2001) are quite strong, and for both classes of drug there is a plausible biological explanation. For example, NSAIDs reduce risk by 50 per cent, and have specific effects on APP metabolism. However, it is premature to argue that any of these drugs should be given preventatively, in part because the causality of the associations are not clear. For example, the inverse association with HRT may be confounded by the fact that HRT users are more likely to be well-educated and healthy. Raised homocysteine is increasingly recognized as an important, independent risk factor, and may explain some of the shared features of Alzheimer's disease and vascular dementia (Seshadri *et al.*, 2002). The finding that levels of educational attainment, as well as cognitive and physical activity, predict lower rates of Alzheimer's disease supports a 'use it or lose it' hypothesis, by which such attributes increase cerebral reserve (Wilson *et al.*, 2002). A past history of depression is now a well-established risk factor, but the mechanism is not known (Green *et al.*, 2003). The same applies to diabetes mellitus, which also predisposes to vascular dementia (Schnaider Beeri *et al.*, 2004). Aluminium exposure has been implicated, but the evidence is weak and it is not generally considered to be an established risk factor.

TABLE 14.12 Environmental factors and Alzheimer's disease

Risk factors
◆ Low educational attainment
◆ Past head injury
◆ Cerebrovascular disease
◆ History of depression
◆ High homocysteine levels
◆ Diabetes mellitus
Protective factors
◆ Use of non-steroidal anti-inflammatory drugs (NSAIDs)
◆ Hormone replacement therapy (HRT)
◆ Use of statins (possible)
◆ Cognitive and physical activity in mid-life

The amyloid cascade hypothesis

The APP research summarized in Box 14.1 led to the **'amyloid cascade hypothesis'** (Hardy and Higgins, 1992), which has become the dominant molecular model for the disorder, and the basis for most ongoing therapeutic research (see Chapter 20). It proposes that the central pathogenic event is an increased formation and deposition of β-amyloid, particularly the 42 amino acid variant (Hardy and Selkoe, 2002). APP is a transmembrane protein, which can be cleaved by one of three enzymes, called secretases. Normally, α-secretase activity predominates, and this does not give rise to β-amyloid. However, in Alzheimer's disease, more APP is processed via β- and γ-secretase pathways, leading to increased β-amyloid formation. The presenilins are part of the γ-secretase complex, emphasizing the common pathogenic effects of the genes which cause familial Alzheimer's disease. The increased production of β-amyloid leads to disease because it tends to aggregate, becomes insoluble, and is neurotoxic. It is still controversial how the amyloid pathology relates to the tau protein and neurofibrillary tangles, but the consensus is in favour of the latter being downstream.

Additional hypotheses for the pathogenesis of Alzheimer's disease include the role of oxidative stress, inflammation, apoptosis (programmed cell death), and disturbances of the cell cycle (Mattson, 2004). Most of these theories still involve β-amyloid mis-metabolism in some way.

Neurotransmitter changes: the cholinergic hypothesis

Prior to the amyloid hypothesis, the prevailing view was the '**cholinergic hypothesis**' of Alzheimer's disease, based on findings in the 1970s that there is a severe and widespread loss of acetylcholine in the cerebral cortex, which exceeds that of other neurotransmitters. The loss occurs because of pathology and atrophy in the cells of origin, in the nucleus basalis of Meynert. The findings led to the development of cholinergic replacement therapies for the disease (p. 509). However, although cholinergic deficits may well explain some of the cognitive impairment, they are no longer considered to have a causal role. For review, see Francis *et al.* (1999). Cholinergic pathology may in fact be of more relevance in dementia with Lewy bodies, and it is possible that the earlier studies of Alzheimer's disease included patients in this category.

Vascular dementia

The dementia caused by cerebrovascular disease was in the past referred to as 'atherosclerotic psychosis'. Following the separation of distinct syndromes of psychiatric disorder in late life (Roth, 1955), it became apparent that dementia was often associated with multiple infarcts, and Hachinski *et al.* (1974) suggested the term multi-infarct dementia. Although this is still used, subsequent research has shown that patients with **multi-infarct dementia** are a subgroup of a larger group of patients with dementia due to vascular disease. Hence the term vascular dementia is now preferred. The pathogenic mechanisms are varied, and include large or small vessel arteriosclerosis, embolus, vasculitis, amyloid angiopathy, and intracranial haemorrhage. Complicating the issue further, additional terms have been used to describe subgroups of cerebrovascular disease, including *état lacunaire*, leucoariosis and Binswanger's disease.

Vascular dementia is the second commonest cause of dementia. It is slightly more common in men than in women. The prevalence increases with age, approximately doubling every 5 years. There appear to be geographical differences, with high rates reported in China, Japan, and the Russian Federation.

For reviews of vascular dementia, see Roman (2002) and O'Brien *et al.* (2003).

Clinical features of vascular dementia

Onset is usually in the seventh or eighth decade. It is often relatively acute and follows a stroke. Emotional and personality changes may appear first, followed by impairments of memory and intellect that characteristically progress in steps. Depression is frequent, and episodes of emotional lability and confusion are common, especially at night. Transient ischaemic attacks or mild strokes may recur from time to time. Insight is often maintained to a late stage. Behavioural retardation and anxiety are more common than in Alzheimer's disease. Several sets of diagnostic criteria are available, with differing pathological correlates (Gold *et al.*, 2002).

The course of vascular dementia is usually a stepwise progression, with periods of deterioration that are sometimes followed by partial recovery for a few months. About 50% of the patients die from ischaemic heart disease, and others from cerebral infarction or renal complications. From the time of diagnosis the life span varies widely; most studies show somewhat shorter survival in than in Alzheimer's disease.

The diagnosis is difficult to make with confidence unless there is a clear history of strokes or localizing neurological signs. Suggestive features are patchy psychological deficits, erratic progression, and relative preservation of the personality. On physical examination there are usually signs of hypertension and of arteriosclerosis in peripheral and retinal vessels, and there may be neurological signs such as pseudobulbar palsy, rigidity, akinesia, and brisk reflexes. The Hachinski scale is sometimes used. See Erkinjuntti (2000) for a review.

Aetiology of vascular dementia

It is assumed that vascular dementia results from the neuronal dysfunction and death which follow from the cumulative effects of focal ischaemia. The risk factors for vascular dementia are essentially those of cerebrovascular disease. However, recent research is also emphasizing similarities and overlaps with Alzheimer's disease; for example, in terms of shared risk factors and pathophysiological findings (Jagust, 2001; see p. 345).

Dementia with Lewy bodies

Since the late 1980s, a new type of dementia with a relatively distinct pathology and clinical course has been described under various terms: dementia with Lewy bodies, Lewy body dementia, cortical Lewy body disease, diffuse Lewy body disease and Lewy body variant of Alzheimer's disease. Dementia with Lewy bodies is now the consensus term. Neuropathological studies have found dementia with Lewy bodies in ~15–20 per cent of all cases, suggesting that it is the third, if not the second, most frequent cause of dementia. As the name suggests, the cardinal feature neuropathologically is Lewy bodies in the cerebral cortex; it also has a characteristic clinical profile. The recent 'discovery' of dementia with Lewy bodies may reflect sampling bias of earlier studies (e.g. under-representation in patients having an autopsy) and the fact that cortical Lewy bodies are hard to see using routine stains.

See McKeith *et al.* (2004) for review.

Clinical features of dementia with Lewy bodies

The core clinical features, agreed by a consensus panel (McKeith *et al.*, 1996) are summarized in Table 14.13. The fluctuating level of dementia with recurrent delirium-like phases, together with parkinsonism and visual hallucinations is characteristic. Use of the criteria allows dementia with Lewy bodies to be diagnosed with good specificity and sensitivity. Average survival is about 5 years.

Neuropathology of dementia with Lewy bodies

The characteristic histopathological feature is the presence of Lewy bodies in the cerebral cortex. As in Parkinson's disease, they are also seen in the substantia nigra, and their composition is the same in both diseases; the key protein is **α-synuclein**, although routine detection of Lewy bodies is currently based on the presence of another protein, **ubiquitin**. It is not clear whether dementia with Lewy bodies is separable from the dementia of Parkinson's disease (p. 341), nor whether dementia with Lewy bodies and Parkinson's disease are aetiologically or neuropathologically distinct (McKeith *et al.*, 2004; Singleton and Gwinn-Hardy, 2004). Senile plaques are present and can be abundant, but neurofibrillary tangles are sparse. Dementia with Lewy bodies is associated with widespread reductions in choline acetyltransferase in the neocortex (perhaps more so than Alzheimer's disease) and there is also loss of dopaminergic markers in the caudate nucleus. These neurochemical changes may contribute to the high incidence of psychiatric symptoms. Brain atrophy is less marked than in Alzheimer's disease, especially in the hippocampus.

TABLE 14.13 Abbreviated clinical criteria for dementia with Lewy bodies

Key features
◆ Progressive cognitive decline, especially in attention and visuospatial ability
◆ Pronounced fluctuations in cognition and attention
◆ Recurrent visual hallucinations, usually well formed and detailed
◆ Motor features of parkinsonism
Supportive features
◆ Repeated falls
◆ Syncope
◆ Transient loss of consciousness
◆ Sensitivity to antipsychotics
◆ Systematized delusions
◆ Non-visual hallucinations
Diagnosis made less likely in the presence of
◆ Evidence of cerebrovascular disease or stroke
◆ Evidence of other disorder sufficient to account for the clinical picture

Aetiology of dementia with Lewy bodies

Dementia with Lewy bodies is closely related to Parkinson's disease, and both are characterized as 'synucleinopathies' reflecting the abnormal aggregation of α-synuclein protein present in Lewy bodies. There does not appear to be a strong genetic component, although there is an association with apoE4. No environmental risk factors have been well established, although factors relevant to Parkinson's disease, discussed below, may prove applicable.

Parkinson's disease

Parkinson's disease is considered here since, though not a recognized major cause of dementia, it is a neurodegenerative disorder closely related to dementia with Lewy bodies.

Dementia and psychiatric disturbances are features of several diseases traditionally classified as extrapyramidal disorders: idiopathic Parkinson's disease, progressive supranuclear palsy, and other related syndromes. All produce rigidity, slowness, and impoverishment of voluntary movement, hence their designation as akinetic-rigid syndromes. Olfactory deficits help distinguish idiopathic Parkinson's disease from the related syndromes. Note also the importance of distinguishing parkinsonian syndromes from the parkinsonian side-effects of antipsychotic medication (p. 534).

Clinical features

The cardinal neurological features of idiopathic Parkinson's disease are tremor at rest, rigidity, and bradykinesia. The main psychiatric consequences are cognitive impairment, subcortical in type, and depression (Table 14.14). For review, see Lauterbach (2004).

Dementia

Estimates of the prevalence of dementia in Parkinson's disease vary widely, probably because different populations have been studied and diagnostic criteria have

TABLE 14.14 Neuropsychiatric manifestations in Parkinson's disease

Delirium, stupor (often due to drugs or intercurrent infection)
Cognitive decline (subcortical dementia)
Depression, mania
Hallucinations (chiefly visual)
Delusions
Sleep attacks, REM sleep behaviour disorder
Sexual disorders

varied, and because of the increasing recognition of dementia with Lewy bodies. The convention is that the former category ('dementia in Parkinson's disease') is used if the dementia begins more than 12 months after onset of parkinsonism (Emre, 2003). By this definition, dementia occurs in up to 40 per cent of cases of Parkinson's disease, especially later onset cases and those with severe bradykinesia. L-DOPA does not improve the dementia; cholinesterase inhibitors may (Press, 2004).

Depression

The association of Parkinson's disease with depression is well established, with a prevalence of approximately 40 per cent. It is most common in the early and in the very advanced stages of the disease. The mechanism is uncertain; depression correlates poorly with degree of disability and disease duration, and may be related to frontal lobe abnormalities and disturbed dopaminergic mechanisms. Antidepressants must be used with care, to avoid exacerbation of cognitive impairment or induction of delirium. SSRIs and newer generation agents, with less anticholinergic activity, are preferable to tricyclics.

Psychotic symptoms

Psychotic symptoms occur at some stage in 20 per cent of patients. Visual hallucinations are associated with dopaminergic medication, increasing age, disease duration and severity, depression, cognitive impairment, and reduced visual acuity. Delusions are less frequent and are usually paranoid in content. Antiparkinsonian drugs have been implicated as causes; whenever possible these should be reduced. If antipsychotic medication is necessary, newer drugs, notably clozapine or quetiapine, should be used.

Other neuropsychiatric manifestations

Excessive somnolence, a disordered sleep–wake cycle, sleep attacks, and REM sleep behaviour disorder are more common in Parkinson's disease. As a result, patients with Parkinson's disease must be counselled about the risks of driving, even in the absence of dementia (Schrag, 2005).

Aetiology of Parkinson's disease

Idiopathic Parkinson's disease is an important disorder of later life, occurring in ~1 per cent of the population over the age of 55 (Nussbaum and Ellis, 2003). It results primarily from degeneration of dopaminergic neurons in the zona compacta of the substantia nigra, although the first site of pathology is in the IX/X cranial nerve nuclei, and it later extends to other dopamine pathways. The pathological hallmark is Lewy bodies, inclusions within dopaminergic and some other neurons. The composition of Lewy bodies was mentioned above.

Parkinson's disease occurs in a rare autosomal dominant form, caused by mutations in α-synuclein, UCHL1, NR4A2 and LRRK2 (dardarin) genes; there is also an autosomal recessive form, due to mutations in several other genes (parkin, DJ-1, and Pink1). Polymorphisms in these and other genes also contribute to sporadic Parkinson's disease. For review, see Hardy *et al.* (2003). Environmental risk factors include exposure to some toxins, solvents, carbon monoxide, and possibly well water, whereas smoking and perhaps caffeine have a protective effect (Di Monte, 2003). Pathophysiologically, the disease process is thought to be due to impairment of mitochondrial and synaptic functioning, and oxidative stress (Moore *et al.*, 2005).

Frontotemporal dementias

Frontotemporal dementias are the second most common form of presenile dementia, and also underlie about 7 per cent of late life dementias. Presentation is usually between 45 and 70 years. The term was proposed in 1994 when criteria were developed (the Lund–Manchester criteria, later updated; Neary *et al.*, 1998). The grouping is based upon the shared clinical features (Table 14.15) and regional neuropathology of a range of hitherto diverse syndromes (Table 14.16); the concept has gained validity as evidence has accumulated that many or all types of frontotemporal dementia result from a disease process in which tau (p. 343) is central. For review, see Neary *et al.* (2005).

Clinical features and subtypes

Frontotemporal dementias comprise a broader and more heterogeneous range of clinical presentations (Table 14.16), than the other common dementias. The prominence of behavioural rather than cognitive features is emphasized (Perry and Miller, 2001).

TABLE 14.15 Some clinical criteria for frontotemporal dementias

Behavioural features
◆ Insidious onset, slow progression
◆ Early loss of insight
◆ Early signs of disinhibition and lack of judgement
◆ Mental inflexibility
◆ Stereotyped and imitative behaviour
◆ Hyperorality (e.g. craving for sweet foods)
◆ Distractibility and impulsivity
Language and speech features
◆ Progressive decrease in speech output
◆ Perseveration
◆ Echolalia
Affective features
◆ Depression
◆ Apathy
◆ Emotional blunting
◆ Hypochondriasis
Physical signs
◆ Early primitive reflexes
◆ Early incontinence
◆ Late parkinsonism
◆ Low and labile blood pressure

Frontal and temporal variants are recognized, reflecting the predominant features of pathology in the two lobes (pp. 323–4). Thus, the frontal form presents with behavioural and personality change, whereas language disorder occurs in the temporal form. There is often asymmetry of cortical involvement, with left temporal atrophy associated with language deficits, and right-sided disease producing a behavioural disorder. Other subdivisions can be made based on familial versus sporadic cases, and on the presence of parkinsonism, or features of motor neuron disease.

Pick's disease

Arnold Pick described the disease bearing his name in 1892. The key clinical features he noted were aphasia with dementia; the striking pathological findings were focal **'knife-blade' atrophy** of the frontal and temporal poles, with ballooned neurons (**Pick cells**) containing inclusions called **Pick bodies**. Pick bodies also occur in other areas, notably the hippocampus. They are comprised of tau, ubiquitin and other proteins. Features of Alzheimer's disease are absent. Pick's disease remains the archetypal frontotemporal dementia, and is sometimes used as synonymous with it, but if defined properly (including the neuropathological features), it explains only a small proportion of cases.

TABLE 14.16 Diagnostic categories subsumed within frontotemporal dementia

Pick's disease
Lobar atrophy
Frontal lobe degeneration of non-Alzheimer type
Dementia lacking distinctive histology
Motor neuron disease with dementia
Semantic dementia
Progressive aphasic syndrome
Frontotemporal dementia with parkinsonism
Corticobasal degeneration*
Progressive supranuclear palsy*
Parkinsonism-dementia complex of Guam*

*Not always included

Familial forms of frontotemporal dementia

About a third of cases have a first-degree relative with the disorder, but the heritability and genetic architecture of frontotemporal dementia as a whole (and of Pick's disease in particular) remains unknown (Bird *et al.*, 2003). However, subgroups show autosomal dominant inheritance. One such form is frontotemporal dementia with parkinsonism linked to chromosome 17 (FTDP-17), which can be caused by tau gene mutations. However, tau mutations are not always found, and they have also been found occasionally in other forms of frontotemporal dementia. Other familial frontotemporal dementias are linked to chromosome 3, and frontotemporal dementia–motor neuron disease complex is linked to chromosome 10.

Semantic dementia

Semantic dementia refers to a syndrome distinguished by selective, progressive loss of meaning for verbal and non-verbal material, accompanied by striking difficulty in naming, categorization and comprehension (Garrard and Hodges, 2000). It is usually considered to be a frontotemporal dementia because it is associated with a reasonably selective, often left-predominant, anterior temporal lobe atrophy. Autobiographical memory is relatively preserved (though it may be difficult to access). When asked to demonstrate an object or action, patients typically stare at the examiner uncomprehendingly, repeating the instruction as if it had been asked in a foreign language. Associated cognitive, psychiatric or neurological signs are minimal in the early stages, and the increasingly severe semantic impairment may remain circumscribed for many years.

Differential diagnosis and investigations

A study in 1993 found that 18 out of 21 patients with Pick's disease had been misdiagnosed clinically as having Alzheimer's disease. Although the situation has probably improved with the development of diagnostic criteria and greater awareness, frontotemporal dementia remains difficult to diagnose, reflecting its heterogeneity and its relative neglect by researchers. The behavioural features are more useful than the neuropsychological profile in making the distinction from Alzheimer's disease and other dementias (Perry and Miller, 2001). There are few investigations to aid diagnosis (Pasquier *et al.*, 2003), although both neuroimaging and EEG may help: there is focal, often asymmetric atrophy of temporal and frontal poles, without the medial temporal lobe atrophy of Alzheimer's disease, and the EEG is usually normal in frontotemporal dementia but diffusely slowed in Alzheimer's disease.

Neuropathology of frontotemporal dementia

The classic features of Pick's disease were summarized above. Other forms of frontotemporal dementia lack such specific neuropathological correlates. All show the gross atrophy of the temporal and frontal lobes, with neuronal loss, gliosis, spongiform change in superficial layers of the cortex, and often ballooned cells and neuronal inclusions which stain for ubiquitin, tau, and phosphorylated neurofilaments. However, the pattern is variable, and the relationship between pathological findings and clinical phenotype remains somewhat unclear (Munoz *et al.*, 2003).

Neurochemically, frontotemporal dementia differs from Alzheimer's disease in not showing cholinergic deficits. Dopamine also appears unaffected, but serotonin markers are reduced in affected brain areas (Perry and Miller, 2001).

Aetiology of frontotemporal dementia

The aetiology of frontotemporal dementias remains largely unknown, with the exception of the familial subgroups mentioned above which can be attributed to mutations in tau. Genetic factors may well be relevant in other cases too, but this remains uncertain.

Although mutations in the tau gene are rare, and tau involvement in the neuropathology is not invariable, tau is viewed as central to the pathogenesis of frontotemporal dementias, perhaps via alterations in processing of the protein. There multiple variants ('isoforms') of the protein, containing differing numbers of 'repeats', some of which are associated with frontotemporal dementias. For example, Pick's disease is characterized by 'three-repeat' tau, whereas 'four-repeat' tau is characteristic of progressive supranuclear palsy and corticobasal degeneration (Table 14.16). The differing forms of tau pathology in frontotemporal dementia from that in Alzheimer's disease remains unexplained, but are likely due to the variable number of tau repeats and degrees of hyperphosphorylation which occur in the two disorders. For review, see Lee *et al.* (2001).

Prion diseases

Prion diseases are a unique group of diseases. They can be inherited, or acquired infectiously or iatrogenically, whilst other cases are sporadic (Collins *et al.*, 2004). They are grouped together because of the central role of a protein, called **prion protein** (PrP; described below), as well as by common neuropathological features: diffuse spongiosis (hence the older term **transmissible spongiform encephalopathies**), neuronal loss, gliosis and, in many cases, amyloid plaques (Johnson, 2005). The latter are composed of PrP, not the β-amyloid protein of Alzheimer's disease.

Creutzfeldt–Jakob disease

Creutzfeldt–Jakob disease (CJD) is the main prion disease, with an approximate annual incidence of one case per million. A small number of cases are inherited as an autosomal dominant disorder due to point or length mutations in the PrP gene (see below). Other cases have been transmitted iatrogenically, via pituitary-derived growth hormone, contaminated neurosurgical instruments or graft material, and possibly by blood transfusion. The incubation time in these cases can exceed 20 years. Because of the potential infectivity, no patients with dementia should be organ or blood donors.

Sporadic CJD affects both sexes equally. Onset is typically between 50 and 65 years. It is usually heralded by memory impairment, which may be accompanied by prominent behavioural abnormalities or personality change, prompting initial referral to a psychiatrist. Visual symptoms, cerebellar signs, involuntary movements, myoclonic jerks, and other motor features are frequent. Seizures occur later in the course. There is usually a relentless and rapid progression to death, often within 6 months, but some patients have a more protracted illness. The EEG classically shows a triphasic 1–2Hz discharge which, together with the history and rapid course is diagnostically characteristic. The biochemical profile of the CSF, notably the presence of '14-3-3 proteins' is also strongly suggestive. However, definitive diagnosis in life requires a brain biopsy.

In the UK, all cases of suspected prion disease should be referred to the National Surveillance Centre in Edinburgh.

Variant Creutzfeldt–Jakob disease

Intense interest in prion disease has followed the description of variant Creutzfeldt-Jakob disease (vCJD), first identified in the UK in 1996, and with about 150 cases since reported. This is linked with bovine spongiform encephalopathy (BSE), epidemic in British dairy herds at that time. BSE and vCJD are caused by the same prion strain, and it is beyond reasonable doubt that vCJD occurred from eating contaminated bovine products (Harrison, 1997). Whether the existing cases herald a larger human epidemic is unknown; current projections suggest this will not occur. There is a polymorphism at codon 129 of the PrP gene that encodes either methionine or valine; all vCJD patients except one have been homozygous for methionine (compared with 40 per cent in the population) suggesting that this genetic subgroup are more susceptible to vCJD.

Compared to other forms of CJD, vCJD has an earlier onset, slower course, and usually presents with psychiatric symptoms, including depression and personality change (Spencer *et al.*, 2002); EEG abnormalities are less common. The **'pulvinar' sign** on MRI (hyperintensity over the posterior thalamus) is a useful and non-invasive diagnostic sign. Diagnosis of vCJD is possible via tonsil biopsy, but the role of this in clinical practice remains unclear.

Other prion diseases

Kuru, described in the Fore tribe of New Guinea highlanders, was transmitted by ritual cannibalism; the disease has virtually disappeared since this practice was abolished in the 1950s. Transmission of kuru to monkeys in 1970 was the first experimental proof of the infectivity of prion disease.

Other inherited prion diseases are **Gerstmann-Sträussler-Scheinker syndrome** and **fatal familial insomnia**. Like familial CJD, both are caused by autosomal dominant mutations of the prion protein gene, although there is not perfect correspondence between the precise mutation, the nature of the clinical syndrome, and the neuropathological findings. Both are extremely rare.

Aetiology of prion diseases

The name 'prion' denotes proteinaceous infectious particles. It was coined in 1982 by Prusiner, who received the 1999 Nobel Prize for Medicine (Prusiner, 2001). As noted above, prion protein (PrP) is encoded by a gene on chromosome 20. The functions of 'normal' PrP (denoted PrP^{C}) are unknown, but it is expressed by neurons and may serve as a receptor and influence synaptic properties. Prion diseases are caused when PrP^{C} takes on an abnormal conformation, called PrP^{Sc} (named after scrapie, the prion disease which affects sheep). PrP^{Sc} is both the core molecular marker of, and presumed causative agent for, prion diseases. Compared to PrP^{C}, PrP^{Sc} is resistant to breakdown by proteases, is insoluble, and tends to self-aggregate and deposit in the brain. PrP^{Sc} is also thought to promote synaptic and neuronal loss and gliosis, and produce the resulting spongiform appearance of the brain.

In familial cases, the mutated PrP is presumed to be intrinsically more likely to self- aggregate. In acquired forms (iatrogenic or through diet), it is hypothesized that the normal PrP^{C} becomes 'corrupted' by the acquired PrP^{Sc} which changes the conformation of PrP^{C} into PrP^{Sc}, thus propagating ever more PrP^{Sc}. The molecular details of this remarkable process remain obscure. In the case of peripheral acquisition, PrP^{Sc} may spread via nerves, lymphatics and blood to reach the brain. Different PrP conformations and modifications (glycosylation patterns) give rise to various disease 'strains'. The aetiology of 'sporadic' prion disease is unknown; it may result from spontaneous mutation or conversion of PrP^{C} to PrP^{Sc}, or it may arise from occult environmental sources. It is not known why PrP^{Sc} is infectious, when other misfolded, amyloidogenic proteins (such as β-amyloid) are not. Prion diseases are not caused by slow viruses, as was formerly believed.

Huntington's disease

This disease, also called **Huntington's chorea**, was described by the New England physician George Huntington in 1872 (reproduced in Huntington, 2003). It has a worldwide distribution, with estimated prevalence 4–7 per 100 000. Onset is typically in middle life, though adolescent cases are well recognized. There is relentless progression of cognitive and behavioural decline in most cases. The tell-tale choreiform movements may be subtle, taking the form of excessive, purposeless 'fidgeting' which the patient may attempt to disguise.

The disease may present to the psychiatrist, since these patients commonly become depressed early in the course while insight is retained, and later often become withdrawn, 'eccentric', and socially isolated. The clinical features of depression are similar to those of major depression, and both biological and reactive components probably contribute. Paranoid symptoms are common, with a schizophrenia-like or affective psychosis. Cognitive impairment with subcortical features is usual in the later stages, but its severity and progression vary widely (Ho *et al.*, 2003). Distractibility is characteristic, with reduced ability to regulate attention and psychomotor speed, and apathy later in the course. A gaze apraxia and inability to sustain tongue protrusion ('serpentine tongue') are typically found. See Tost *et al.* (2004) for review of the psychiatric aspects of Huntingdon's disease.

Neuropathology of Huntington's disease

The pathological changes mainly affect the caudate nucleus and frontal lobes. The caudate nucleus is markedly atrophic and gliotic. Pyramidal neuronal loss occurs in the frontal cortex, with thinning of the grey matter. Polyglutamine nuclear inclusions are present within some cells, reflecting the causative mutation described below. Neurochemically, there is a decreased concentration of the inhibitory transmitter gamma-aminobutyric acid (GABA) in the caudate nucleus.

Aetiology of Huntington's disease

Huntington's disease is one of the few single gene, autosomal dominant disorders in psychiatry. Penetrance is complete (that is, all carriers of the mutation develop the disease), and new mutations are very rare; most apparently sporadic cases reflect an incomplete family history or lack of knowledge of true paternity. The gene, on chromosome 4p, encodes a protein called **huntingtin**. The mutation, identified in 1993, is a 'triplet repeat' or '**trinucleotide repeat**' of the codon CAG, which codes for glutamine. Normal subjects have less than 30 repeats of this 'polyglutamine' sequence; disease occurs in individuals with more than 36 copies. The expansion tends to increase in succeeding generations, leading to an earlier age of onset, a feature called **anticipation**, characteristic of trinucleotide repeat diseases (Everett and Wood, 2004). The normal function of huntingtin and the pathogenic mechanism by which the mutation causes disease remains a topic of intense research (Li and Li, 2004). Diagnostic and predictive genetic testing is now widely available. Because of the severe implications for sufferer and descendants, genetic counselling is required (Harper *et al.*, 2004).

There is no specific therapy. Dopaminergic blockade may occasionally be required to suppress severe chorea if it is producing exhaustion or limiting mobility. Antidepressants are useful for major depressive symptoms.

Dementia due to HIV disease

See Chapter 16.

Dementia due to alcohol misuse

See Chapter 18.

Emerging concepts of dementia

Classification and clinical practice is based on the dementia syndromes described above. However, epidemiological and biological research is increasingly calling current diagnostic concepts into question.

Mixed dementia

First, the frequency and importance of 'mixed dementia' is becoming apparent, particularly the coexistence of Alzheimer's disease and vascular dementia. This occurs in about 20 per cent of cases of dementia. Their coexistence worsens the severity of dementia (Nagy *et al.*, 1997), and has treatment implications (Langa *et al.*, 2004). The clinical overlap is now complemented by the increasing evidence that risk factors for Alzheimer's disease and vascular dementia overlap (e.g. apoE, homocysteine; Mattson and Shea, 2003), and suggestions that Alzheimer's disease has a vascular basis (de la Torre, 2004).

Molecular classification of neurodegenerative diseases

The blurring of diagnostic boundaries is furthered at the molecular level, in that the same core biochemical process – misfolding and accumulation of proteins – appears to be central to all major neurodegenerative disorders, e.g., β-amyloid in Alzheimer's disease, PrP in prion disease, and huntingtin in Huntington's disease. (Lovestone and McLoughlin, 2001; Soto, 2003). Equally, it is apparent that there is not a one-to-one correspondence between protein and syndrome, as exemplified by the involvement of tau in both Alzheimer's disease and frontotemporal dementia. These factors are leading to the molecular reclassification of dementias as '**amyloidopathies**, '**tauopathies**' and '**synucleinopathies**' (Hardy and Gwinn-Hardy, 1998; Forman *et al.*, 2004); prion disease is already defined in this way. At the same time, identification of subtypes of individual dementia syndromes (e.g. Alzheimer's disease caused by APP, PS1 or PS2 mutations) has led to the suggestion that, from a genetic perspective, these are separate diseases. All these issues remain in the research domain, but are likely to influence clinical thinking and practice in the near future, as their prognostic and treatment implications become clear (Chapter 20).

Epilepsy

Epilepsy is the tendency to recurrent seizures, a seizure consisting of a paroxysmal electrical discharge in the brain and its clinical sequelae. The tendency to recurrent seizures, which defines epilepsy, must be distinguished from isolated seizures; these may be provoked by many factors, including drugs, hypoglycaemia, and intercurrent illnesses. Epilepsy is managed primarily by neurologists, and for a full description the reader is referred to a neurology textbook. However, epilepsy also has several important psychiatric aspects, reflecting its description as the 'bridge' between psychiatry and neurology:

- The differential diagnosis of episodic disturbances of behaviour (particularly 'atypical' attacks, aggressive behaviour, and sleep problems).
- The treatment of the psychiatric and social complications of epilepsy.
- Seizures caused by psychotropic medication.
- The side-effects of anticonvulsant drugs.

Types of seizures

The current classification of seizures was proposed by the International League Against Epilepsy in 1969, later revised (Dreifuss *et al.*, 1981). A simplified outline is shown in Table 14.17. The principal distinction is between focal onset seizures, called partial seizures, and seizures which are generalized from the start. Since focal onset seizures may become generalized, an accurate description of the onset is essential. It is also necessary to distinguish between types of epilepsy and types of seizure. Traditional terms such as '*petit mal*' and '*grand mal*' are ambiguous, and are best avoided. It should be remembered that an 'aura' is in fact a partial seizure; most so-called 'absences' and '*petit mal*' are actually complex partial seizures, implying a focal rather than generalized disturbance, as in true absences.

A brief clinical description of the more common seizure types follows.

Simple partial seizures

The content depends upon the site of the focus. They include Jacksonian motor seizures and a variety of sensory seizures in which the phenomena are relatively unformed. Awareness is not impaired. Focal neurological or cognitive dysfunction may persist for a variable period following the seizure.

Complex partial seizures

Complex partial seizures are characterized by altered awareness of self and environment, and include a wide range of 'psychiatric' features (Table 14.18), hence the earlier term '**psychomotor epilepsy**', and making them the form of epilepsy of most importance to psychiatrists, and frequently forming part of the differential diagnosis of psychiatric disorder.

Consciousness is not lost, unless secondary generalization occurs. However, the subject appears out of touch with the surroundings, and often has great difficulty in describing their experiences later. The seizures arise most commonly in the temporal lobe, reflecting the additional former term of **temporal lobe epilepsy**, but the latter is not an appropriate term as

TABLE 14.17 Classification of seizures

Seizures beginning focally
◆ Simple motor or sensory (without impaired consciousness)
◆ Complex partial (with impaired consciousness)
◆ Partial seizures with secondary generalization
Generalized seizures without focal onset
◆ Tonic-clonic
◆ Myoclonic
◆ Atonic
◆ Absence
◆ Unclassified

TABLE 14.18 Clinical features of complex partial seizures

Domain	Features
Consciousness	Altered
Autonomic and visceral	'Epigastric aura', dizziness, flushing, tachycardia, and other bodily sensations
Perceptual	Distorted perceptions, *déjà vu*, *jamais vu*, visual, auditory, olfactory, gustatory, somatic hallucinations
Cognitive	Disturbances of speech, thought, and memory, derealization, depersonalization
Affective	Fear and anxiety; occasionally, euphoric or ecstatic states
Psychomotor	Automatisms, grimacing and other bodily movements; repetitive or more complex stereotyped behaviours

complex partial seizures can also begin in the frontal lobes and other sites. Seizures originating in the latter region are particularly likely to be misdiagnosed as functional, since they are frequently accompanied by bizarre posturing and other semi-purposeful, complex motor behaviours. Complex partial seizures of temporal lobe origin are often heralded by an **aura**, which may take the form of olfactory, gustatory, auditory, visual, or somatic hallucinations. Particularly common is the 'epigastric aura', a sensation of churning in the stomach which rises toward the neck. The patient may also experience odd disturbances of thought or emotion, including an intense sense of familarity (*déjà vu*) or unfamiliarity (*jamais vu*), depersonalization or derealization, or, rarely, vivid hallucinations of past experiences ('experiential phenomena'). The sequence of events in the seizure tends to be stereotyped in the individual patient, an important diagnostic aid. The whole ictal phase usually lasts up to 1–2 minutes. After recovery, only the aura may be recalled. Non-convulsive status epilepticus may take the form of a prolonged single seizure, or a rapid succession of brief seizures. In such cases, a protracted period of automatic behaviour may be mistaken for a dissociative fugue or other psychiatric disorder.

Absences

The key feature of an absence attack is loss of awareness which starts suddenly, without an aura, lasts for seconds, and ends abruptly. Simple automatisms (such as eyelid fluttering) often accompany the attack. There are no post-ictal abnormalities. For purposes of diagnosis and treatment, it is essential to distinguish between absence seizures and complex partial seizures. The latter last longer, automatisms during the episode are more complex, recovery occurs more slowly, and the patient may subsequently recall an aura. Absence attacks in children were previously called '*petit mal*', and are classically associated with 3 per second 'spike and wave' EEG discharges.

Generalized tonic–clonic seizures

This is the familiar epileptic convulsion with a sudden onset, tonic and clonic phases, and a succeeding period of variable duration (up to many hours) in which the patient may be unrousable, sleepy, or disorientated. Incontinence, tongue-biting, or other injuries may occur during the seizure. In the post-ictal phase, the patient may present with delirium, which may cause diagnostic uncertainty if the convulsion was not witnessed. Generalized tonic–clonic seizures may be initiated by a partial seizure, implying localized brain disease, often overlooked. This is an issue of importance, since primary and secondary generalized seizures differ in significance and management.

Myoclonic, atonic, and other seizure types

There are several types of seizures with predominantly motor symptoms, including myoclonic jerks and drop attacks with loss of postural tone. They are unlikely to present to the psychiatrist.

Epidemiology of epilepsy

In the UK, general practice data indicate the prevalence of epilepsy in adults is about 6 per 1000. The inception rate is highest in early childhood, and there are further peaks in adolescence and over the age of 65. Epilepsy is usually of short duration and only becomes a chronic condition in about a fifth of subjects. This means that regular attenders at specialist clinics are a minority of all those with epilepsy, and include those especially likely to suffer from its medical and social complications. Childhood epilepsies are more often associated with significant cognitive impairment.

Aetiology of epilepsy

Age at onset is an important clue to aetiology. For example, in the newborn, birth injury, congenital brain malformations, and metabolic disorders are common causes. Infantile febrile convulsions, especially status epilepticus, are classically associated with later complex partial epilepsy, via damage to the hippocampus (hippocampal sclerosis). An increasing number of genetic mutations causing epilepsy are being identified, but to date account for only a small proportion of cases (Gutirriez-Delicado and Serratosa, 2004). In adults, identifiable causes include cerebrovascular disease, brain tumours, head injury, and neurodegenerative disorders. Patterns of alcohol and other drug use should always be established, particularly in young adults. Seizure threshold may be lowered by drug therapy, including antipsychotics and tricyclic antidepressants. Sudden withdrawal of substantial doses of any drug with anticonvulsant properties, most commonly diazepam and alcohol, can precipitate seizures and, not infrequently, status epilepticus.

Making the diagnosis

Epilepsy is essentially a clinical diagnosis that depends upon detailed accounts of the attacks given by witnesses as well as by the patient. The background history, physical examination, and special investigations are directed to establishing aetiology. The extent of investigation is guided by the initial findings, the type of attack, and the patient's age. Only an outline can be given here; for a full account the reader is referred to a neurology or epilepsy textbook. An EEG can confirm but cannot exclude the diagnosis. It is more useful in determining the type of epilepsy and site of origin. The standard EEG recording may be supplemented by sleep recording, ambulatory monitoring, and split-screen video (telemetry) techniques. Although neuroimaging has an increasing clinical role (Koepp and Duncan, 2004), no specific brain abnormality (or other cause) is found in the majority of patients with epilepsy.

Epilepsy can be erroneously diagnosed as the cause of paroxysmal neurological and psychiatric symptoms, and it is important to keep in mind the extensive differential diagnosis (see Table 14.3). A clear description of the circumstances surrounding the episode and the mode of onset is fundamental. The most important differential diagnosis of generalized seizures are vasovagal syncope (commonly associated with involuntary movements, a fact not always appreciated) and cardiac arrhythmias. Hyperventilation (of which the patient is often unaware) and panic attacks frequently produce symptoms similar to complex partial seizures, and may lead to actual loss of consciousness if prolonged. Sudden changes in motor activity, affect, and cognition can occur in schizophrenia.

Factors that together suggest a seizure include an abrupt onset, a stereotyped course lasting many seconds to a few minutes, tongue-biting, urinary incontinence, cyanosis, sustaining injury during the attack, and prolonged post-ictal drowsiness or confusion; however, none alone is necessary or sufficient to make the diagnosis. Some forms of frontal lobe epilepsy are particularly likely to be misdiagnosed as psychogenic. If the diagnosis remains uncertain, and attacks are frequent, close observation in hospital, including video recording and EEG telemetry and ambulatory monitoring, may be worthwhile.

Non-epileptic attacks (**'pseudoseizures'**) and dissociative states can be very difficult to distinguish from epilepsy; indeed, up to 50 per cent of patients referred to epilepsy services have non-epileptic attacks exclusively or in combination (Brown and Trimble, 2000). A detailed description and careful history of the background of the attacks are crucial. Features that suggest non-epileptic episodes include identifiable psychosocial precipitants, a past history of physical or sexual abuse, a personal or family history of psychopathology, an unusual or variable pattern of attacks, occurrence only in public or while alone, and absence of autonomic signs or change in colour during 'generalized' attacks. The patient may be suggestible, or betray other evidence of retained awareness during the episode. Complex, purposeful behaviour is more often seen in dissociative states. Ambulatory EEG may be helpful; however, some types of seizure may not be reflected in the surface EEG and conversely, EEG abnormalities occur in perhaps 3 per cent of healthy individuals. Post-ictal serum prolactin is useful in a minority of cases (it is elevated after a generalized seizure) but should not be relied upon to make the distinction. See Brown and Trimble (2000) for review of the differentiation between epilepsy and psychiatric causes of episodic behavioural abnormalities.

Psychiatric aspects of epilepsy

Psychiatric comorbidity is common in people with epilepsy, with overall rates increased at least two-fold, and higher amongst those in specialist care. Many different types of psychiatric disorder are associated with epilepsy, including cognitive, affective, emotional, and behavioural disturbances. These can occur before, during, after, or between seizures (Table 14.19). The rela-

TABLE 14.19 Associations between epilepsy and psychological disturbance

Psychiatric disorders associated with the underlying cause
Behavioural disturbances associated with seizures
◆ **Pre-ictal:** prodromal states and mood disturbance
◆ **Ictal:** complex partial seizures (affective disturbances, hallucinations, experiential phenomena, automatisms); absence seizures (altered awareness, automatisms)
◆ **Post-ictal:** impaired consciousness; delirium; psychosis; Todd's paresis (hemiparesis, dysphasia, other focal signs)
Epileptic pseudodementia (non-convulsive status)
Inter-ictal disorders
Cognitive
Psychoses
Sexual behaviour
◆ Depression and emotional disorder
◆ Suicide and deliberate self-harm
◆ Crime and other antisocial behaviour (disputed, see p. 350)
◆ Personality change (disputed, see p. 349)

tionship between epilepsy and psychiatric disorder may reflect several factors:

- A shared aetiology or pathophysiology. For example, temporal lobe pathology appears to predispose to epilepsy and to psychosis.
- The stigma and psychosocial impairments associated with epilepsy.
- The side-effects of antiepileptic drugs.

For review of the psychiatric aspects of epilepsy, see Marsh and Rao (2002) and Gaitatzis *et al.* (2004).

Pre-ictal psychiatric disturbances

Increasing tension, irritability, anxiety, and depression are sometimes apparent as prodromata for several hours or even days before a seizure, generally increasing in intensity as the seizure approaches.

Ictal psychiatric disturbances

Ictal psychiatric disturbances (i.e. those directly related to seizure activity) are common and diverse, as noted above. During seizures, transient confusional states, affective disturbances, anxiety, automatisms, and other abnormal behaviours often occur (especially in partial seizures). On occasion, an abnormal mental state may be the only sign of non-convulsive (complex partial or absence) status epilepticus, and the diagnosis is easily overlooked.

Psychoses may occur as an ictal phenomenon. Clues to this possibility include sudden onset and termination of the disturbance, olfactory or gustatory hallucinations (especially with partial seizures), a relative lack of first-rank symptoms, and amnesia for the period of the disturbance.

Ictal violence is extremely rare (less than 0.3 per cent in one large series; Delgado-Escueta *et al.* 1981) and crimes committed during epileptic automatisms are probably even rarer, an important medico-legal finding (Treiman, 1999).

Post-ictal disturbances

Psychiatric disturbances may occur in the hours following a seizure. Psychotic symptoms are seen in about 10 per cent of cases, and are associated with bilateral seizure foci, long duration of epilepsy, and structural brain lesions. These transient psychoses are distinct from the inter-ictal psychoses described below. Diverse motor, sensory, cognitive and autonomic dysfunction can also occur and, as with the psychoses, may occur as part of a delirium, or in clear consciousness. Post-ictal violence is rare, but commoner than during the seizure, and may be secondary to psychotic experiences. Extreme post-ictal violence may be recurrent, stereotyped, and more likely to occur in men, after a cluster of seizures (Gerard *et al.*, 1998). There is usually amnesia for the event.

Inter-ictal psychiatric disturbances

Cognitive impairments

In the nineteenth century, it was widely held, based on experience with institutionalized populations, that epilepsy was associated with an inevitable decline in intellectual functioning. However, it is now established that relatively few people with epilepsy show cognitive changes. When these do occur, they are likely to reflect concurrent brain damage, unrecognized non-convulsive seizures, or the effects of antiepileptic drugs. A few epileptic patients show a progressive decline in cognitive function. In such cases, careful investigation is required to exclude an underlying progressive neurological disorder; this is a particular concern in paediatric practice.

Personality

The historical concept of an 'epileptic personality', characterized by egocentricity, irritability, religiosity, quarrelsomeness, and 'sticky' thought processes, has been discarded. Community surveys indicate that only a minority of patients have serious personality difficulties and these probably reflect the adverse consequences of brain damage on education, employment, and social life rather than a specific association with epilepsy (Trimble, 1997). It has been suggested that behavioural abnormalities (including hypergraphia) are particularly associated with medial temporal lobe lesions.

Depression and emotional disorders

Depression is particularly common in people with epilepsy, for both biological and psychosocial reasons, and the rate of depression may be higher than in other chronic neurological disorders (Kanner, 2003). The rate of mood disorder, especially unipolar depression, is increased several-fold, with prevalence rates of 22–77 per cent reported. Many subjects meet criteria for dysthymia rather than major depression, and the term 'interictal dysphoric disorder' is sometimes used. Risk factors for depression in epilepsy are summarized in Table 14.20.

Inter-ictal psychosis

The nature and prevalence of inter-ictal psychosis has long been controversial, including the fundamental question about whether the two coexist more or less

TABLE 14.20 Risk factors for depression in epilepsy

Biological
◆ Family history of mood disorder
◆ Focus in temporal or frontal lobe
◆ Left-sided focus
Psychosocial
◆ Perceived stigma
◆ Fear of seizures
◆ Learned helplessness
◆ Pessimistic attributional style
◆ Decreased social supports
◆ Unemployment
Iatrogenic
◆ Epilepsy surgery
◆ Antiepileptic drugs, especially polypharmacy and high serum levels

Adapted from Marsh and Rao (2002).

often than expected. For review, see Mace (1993). Following the important study by Slater *et al.* (1963), the evidence supports the view that epilepsy is associated with an increased risk of psychosis, especially but not exclusively schizophrenia-like in presentation (Sachdev, 1998). Religious and paranoid delusions appear to be particularly common and affect tends to be preserved. Risk factors include complex partial seizures, especially with the focus in the mesial temporal lobe or frontal lobe, a lesion which is prenatal in origin, and in the left hemisphere (Flor-Henry, 1969), and seizure onset in adolescence. These biological associations contributed to neurodevelopmental, lateralized, and temporal lobe-based theories of schizophrenia (Roberts *et al.*, 1990a).

Suicide

Suicide is four times, and deliberate self-harm six times, more frequent among people with epilepsy than among the general population. The rate is higher still in those with temporal lobe epilepsy (twenty-five times increased), and after surgical treatment for epilepsy (Harris and Barraclough, 1997). Suicide risk factors in epilepsy include the same range of risk factors as in the general population.

Social aspects of epilepsy

The consequences for quality of life correlate with the severity of the seizure disorder and the presence of structural brain pathology. The social implications and stigma attached to a diagnosis of epilepsy can be far-reaching, as is the unpredictability of seizure occurrence. In counselling patients and their families, it is important to be sensitive to these issues and to allay groundless fears and misconceptions. Restrictions on driving are a major burden for many patients, whose livelihood may be at stake. To obtain a British driving licence, the patient must have had at least 1 year with no seizures while awake, whether or not she is still taking antiepileptic drugs. Those who suffer seizures only while asleep may hold a licence if this pattern has been stable for at least 3 years.

It is often stated that there is an association of epilepsy with crime (e.g. Toone, 2000), either for biological or, more likely, psychosocial reasons. However, the association may be another myth about epilepsy, since a meta-analysis found that rates of epilepsy amongst prisoners were not increased (Fazel *et al.*, 2002).

Treatment of epilepsy

The drug treatment of epilepsy is undertaken by neurologists (McCorry *et al.*, 2004). Here, discussion will be restricted to some key points of psychiatric relevance.

It is important to distinguish between peri-ictal and inter-ictal psychiatric disorders when planning treatment. For peri-ictal psychiatric disorders, treatment is aimed at control of the seizures. Treatment of inter-ictal psychiatric disorders is similar to that in non-epileptic patients, though it should be remembered that psychotropic drugs may increase seizure frequency. Suitable antidepressants for use in epilepsy are the SSRIs or MAOIs, whilst amisulpride, risperidone or haloperidol are useful antipsychotics.

Anticonvulsant drugs can cause a variety of cognitive and psychiatric symptoms (Ovsiew, 2004). For example, vigabatrin and topiramate can give rise to psychotic and mood disorders. Topiramate also frequently produces marked but reversible cognitive impairment, particularly affecting language. Finally, there are pharmacokinetic interactions between antiepileptic drugs and psychotropic medications that necessitate careful attention to dosing to avoid toxicity or subtherapeutic levels (Monaco and Cicolin, 1999).

Head injury

The psychiatrist is likely to see two main groups of patients who have suffered a head injury:

- The relatively small group with persistent, serious, cognitive and behavioural sequelae.

- A larger group with emotional symptoms and personality change.

The severity of non-penetrating (closed) head injury is best assessed by the duration of **post-traumatic amnesia** (PTA); the interval between the injury and the return of normal day to day memory. The measure has the advantage of being reasonably accurate even when assessed retrospectively, i.e. by asking the patient several months later what they remember of the immediate post-injury period. A PTA of less than a week is associated with reasonable outcome (e.g. return to work) in the majority, but a PTA of more than a month often results in failure to return to work. **Retrograde amnesia** (i.e. prior to the injury) is much less predictive of outcome. An MRI scan is useful in defining the extent of brain injury, but a normal MRI scan does not preclude some degree of brain damage. A CT scan is less sensitive.

The vast majority of closed head injuries are due to acceleration and deceleration forces. When loss of consciousness occurs for a few seconds it is thought to be due to disruption of cholinergic transmission in the brainstem. With more severe injuries, haemorrhagic areas of damage, and diffuse axonal injury and shearing in white matter, are the two main pathological events. Both contribute to coma duration. Other complications include extra- and subdural haemorrhage and anoxia. Deposition of β-amyloid occurs in some, which may explain the link between head injury and later Alzheimer's disease (Fleminger *et al.*, 2003), and with dementia pugilistica (see below). There is some evidence that apolipoprotein E4 (apoE4) genotype increases the risk of death or cognitive deficits after head injury.

For review of the psychiatry of head injury, see Fleminger (2000b).

Acute psychological effects

After severe injury, a phase of delirium may follow awakening from coma. Prolonged delirium may be accompanied by a transient confabulatory state. Occasionally, delusional misidentification or reduplicative paramnesia (p. 317) is observed; for example, ward staff may be identified as old friends, or the ward as being a duplicate in a distant town. Agitation and disinhibition, often sexual, are often present, and may take days or weeks to resolve.

Chronic psychological effects

Both primary and secondary (the effects of brain swelling and raised intracranial pressure) damage determine the neurological and cognitive deficits. Long-term outcome is also influenced by premorbid personality traits, occupational attainment, availability of social supports, and compensation issues. Post-traumatic epilepsy may be a further significant complicating factor in more serious injuries. The risk of suicide is increased three-fold after head injury.

Post-concussional syndrome

After head injury, many patients describe a group of symptoms known as the post-concussional syndrome. The main features are anxiety, depression, and irritability, accompanied by headache, dizziness, fatigue, poor concentration, and insomnia. The duration and severity of these symptoms are highly variable. Since this syndrome often occurs after mild head injury, it has been suggested that it is partly or largely psychologically based (Lishman, 1988; see also Jacobson, 1995). Most cases resolve without specific medical intervention.

Lasting cognitive impairment

The particular vulnerability of frontal and temporal lobes to closed head injury hints at the usual pattern of neuropsychological deficits, with memory and executive function being most affected. The patient may show significant impairments in these domains (e.g. organizing and planning activities) without an overall decline in performance in terms of IQ. Newer and more sensitive measures to detect these deficits are being developed, such as the Behavioural Assessment of Dysexecutive Syndrome (BADS).

Personality change

Personality change is common after severe injuries, particularly if there is frontal lobe damage, when there may be irritability, apathy, loss of spontaneity and drive, disinhibition and occasionally reduced control of aggressive impulses. ICD-10 has a category of 'organic personality disorder' to describe this group. Management is difficult, demanding considerable social support and, in some cases, prolonged rehabilitation. Such resources are scarce and often unavailable.

Emotional disorder

Depression, anxiety, and emotional lability are very common after head injury. Persistent depression and anxiety occur in about a quarter of cases, a frequency similar to that in other serious physical disorders. Left frontal lesions appear to carry a greater risk of depression, but an association with the right frontal damage has been reported for penetrating injuries. Post-head injury mania, also linked to right frontal damage, is much less common, and can be mistaken for personality change.

Psychosis

Transient psychotic symptoms are common during the delirium after head injury. Whether there is also an increased risk of schizophrenia-like psychosis developing long after this phase has passed is controversial. Davison and Bagley (1969) found a 2-3-fold greater risk in survivors of war head injuries. However, more recent data do not support head injury as a risk factor for psychosis (David and Prince, 2005).

Boxing and head injury

Ten to twenty per cent of professional boxers develop a chronic traumatic encephalopathy, sometimes called punch drunk syndrome or **dementia pugilistica** (Roberts, 1969), related to the cumulative extent of head injuries suffered during the career.

The syndrome typically develops and progresses after retirement from the ring, and appears to interact with the effects of age. The principal early features are executive dysfunction, bradyphrenia, mild dysarthria and incoordination, followed by parkinsonism, spasticity, and ataxia. The fully developed syndrome may comprise cerebellar, pyramidal, and extrapyramidal features, mixed cortical and subcortical cognitive deficits, and a variety of behavioural manifestations.

At post-mortem examination, there is loss of neurons in cortex, substantia nigra and cerebellum, together with neurofibrillary tangles and diffuse amyloid plaques (Roberts *et al.*, 1990b).

Treatment of head injury

Prospective studies demonstrate that early assessment of the extent of neurological signs provides a useful guide to the likely pattern of long-term physical disability. Neuropsychiatric problems should be assessed and their impact anticipated, and a comprehensive social assessment is crucial. The clinical psychologist can sometimes contribute behavioural and cognitive techniques (see Wilson, 1999). If psychotropic drugs are necessary, always start with a low dose and choose agents with less potential for seizure generation, anticholinergic or extra-pyramidal side-effects. Practical support is needed for family and carers. Issues of compensation and litigation should be settled as quickly as possible. See National Institutes of Health Consensus Development Panel (1999) for a review of the management of head injury.

Other neuropsychiatric syndromes

Dystonias

Dystonias are uncontrolled focal muscle spasms leading to involuntary movements of the eyelids, face, neck, jaw, shoulders, larynx, hands, and, rarely, other parts of the body. They are uncommon but disabling. The aetiology is uncertain. In the past, dystonias were regarded as conversion phenomena (p. 206); now there is strong evidence that they are genetic, idiopathic or drug-induced neurological disorders, and that psychogenic cases are rare (Trost, 2003). However, psychiatric factors may exacerbate symptoms and disability. Clinical types include blepharospasm, torticollis, writer's cramp, and laryngeal dystonia. The most effective treatment is the injection of botulinum toxin directly into the affected muscles. Deep brain stimulation is also being used. Psychiatric symptoms secondary to the physical disorder can be treated with antidepressants or behavioural therapy.

Occupational dystonia

Muscular problems are common amongst musicians and may threaten to end their careers. There are many causes, including overuse injury, pressure on peripheral nerves, and focal dystonias. These problems should be assessed by a physician with experience in the field. Performance anxiety is also frequent, and may impair or prevent performance. Beta-blockers alleviate this symptom and are used by many musicians, sometimes without medical supervision. Anxiety management is effective in some cases. Other occupations and activities also have their characteristic afflictions, for example 'auctioneer's jaw' and 'golfer's hip'. See Frucht *et al.* (1999) for a review.

Tics

Tics are purposeless, stereotyped, and repetitive jerking movements occurring most commonly in the face and neck. They are much more common in childhood than in adult life, though a few cases begin at ages of up to 40 years. The peak of onset is about 7 years, and the onset is often at a time of emotional disturbance. They are especially common in boys. Most sufferers have just one kind of abnormal movement, but a few people have more than one (multiple tics). Like almost all involuntary movements, tics are worsened by anxiety. They can be controlled briefly by voluntary effort, but this results in an increasing unpleasant feeling of tension. Many tics occurring in childhood last only a few weeks; others last longer but 80–90 per cent of cases improve within 5 years. Tics in children are associated with a range of psychiatric disorders, notably obsessive–compulsive disorder, attention deficit hyperactivity disorder, and anxiety disorders (Kurlan *et al.*, 2002). Tics can be treated with antipsychotics or alpha-2 adrenergic agonists.

Gilles de la Tourette syndrome

This condition was described first by Itard in 1825 and subsequently by Gilles de la Tourette in 1885. It is said to be the most common tic disorder. The main clinical features are multiple tics beginning before the age of 16, together with vocal tics (grunting, snarling, and similar ejaculations). About a third of the people affected show **coprolalia** (involuntary uttering of obscenities), but few of these are children. Between 10 and 40 per cent show **echolalia** or **echopraxia**. There may be stereotyped movements such as jumping and dancing. The tics are often preceded by premonitory sensations. Associated features include overactivity, difficulties in learning, emotional disturbances, and social problems. Obsessive–compulsive symptoms occur frequently, and more often among the families of patients than in the general population. Attention-deficit hyperactivity disorder has also been reported to be more frequent in these patients.

The reported prevalence of the condition varies according to the criteria for diagnosis and method of enquiry. A generally accepted figure is about 0.5 per 1000 population. The disorder is three to four times more common in males than in females, and ten times more prevalent in children and adolescents than in adults.

The aetiology of the syndrome is uncertain. There is a substantial genetic contribution, and an overlap with the genetic predisposition to obsessive-compulsive disorder. Altered dopamine function and aberrant cortico-striatal connectivity have also been implicated (Pringsheim *et al.*, 2003). Autoimmune abnormalities are also suspected in a subgroup (Hoekstra *et al.*, 2002).

Mild cases may not require specific treatment. Many treatments have been tried. Antipsychotics, especially haloperidol, have been widely used and are effective, but the side-effects can be troublesome. There are also randomized trials showing efficacy of risperidone, desipramine, and clonidine. Treatment of comorbid psychiatric disorder, such as obsessive-compulsive disorder and attention-deficit hyperactivity disorder, may be more valuable than treatment of the core features of the syndrome.

There are few good outcome data. Clinical experience suggests that two-thirds of patients can expect improvement or lasting remission in early adult life, but the outcome is frequently poor. Coprolalia disappears in one-third of patients, but the tics and obsessive–compulsive symptoms may be lifelong. For review, see Robertson (2000).

Multiple sclerosis

Multiple sclerosis is the most common cause of chronic neurological disability in young adults in developed countries, and imposes a heavy burden on families and carers in its later stages. Its consequences for work and relationships may be profound. The disease is difficult to diagnose early in the course, and physical symptoms are sometimes misinterpreted as psychiatric. Psychological symptoms are rarely the presenting feature but two-thirds of patients will experience them at some stage, especially depression (see below), euphoria, emotional lability and fatigue. Such symptoms probably result both directly from the disease process, and from the disbilities associated with it. There is a several-fold increase in the risk of suicide.

Depression is more common in multiple sclerosis than in most other neurological disorders, with a lifetime risk of 50 per cent. It does not appear to be closely related to the severity of the clinical syndrome or the site of lesions; nevertheless, biological factors may play a role (Siegert and Abernethy, 2005). Depression may also be a side-effect of beta-interferon, sometimes used to treat multiple sclerosis.

Cognitive impairment is present in 40 per cent of patients from community samples. It may be an early manifestation of the illness, and occasionally a rapidly progressive dementia occurs (Zarei *et al.*, 2003). In most cases, however, intellectual deterioration begins later, is less severe and progresses slowly. Well-practised verbal skills are often preserved despite deficits in problem solving, abstraction, memory, and learning. Cogniive impairment correlates with total lesion load and degree of callosal atrophy on MRI and probably reflects axonal loss rather than demyelination per se.

See Feinstein (2004) for a review of psychiatric aspects of multiple sclerosis.

Normal pressure hydrocephalus

The characteristic clinical triad in this condition, described by Adams and Hakim (Adams *et al.*, 1965), comprises an early, striking 'gait apraxia' (a broad-based, small-stepped gait with difficulty in initiation) on which supervenes a progressive frontal subcortical syndrome with bradyphrenia and, later, urinary incontinence. Frank dementia is rare. The prevalence is uncertain, ranging from 0–6 per cent of cases of late-life dementia in published series. The condition is more common in the elderly, but sometimes occurs in middle life, and in children with congenital abnormalities.

The pathogenesis has been thought to be a block to cerebrospinal fluid flow within the ventricular system due to aqueduct stenosis, or in the subarachnoid space; however, often no cause can be discovered. Ventricular pressure is generally normal or low, though episodes of raised pressure may occur, leading to the suggestion that the disorder should be renamed (Bret *et al.*, 2002). Ventricular enlargement out of proportion to the degree of cortical atrophy, often with periventricular signal change, is the hallmark finding on brain imaging.

It is important to differentiate this condition from a degenerative dementia, and from depression with pseudodementia. Cases with a short history and prominent gait disturbance with relative sparing of intellect may be amenable to a neurosurgical shunt procedure to improve the circulation of cerebrospinal fluid; however, the outcome is variable and difficult to predict. The presence of hippocampal atrophy on imaging suggests associated Alzheimer's disease and predicts a poor response to shunting.

Anoxia, hypoglycaemia, and carbon monoxide poisoning

Anoxia (e.g. due to cardiac arrest), hypoglycaemia, and carbon monoxide poisoning produce similar patterns of brain injury. Cerebral and cerebellar atrophy may occur, with hippocampus and globus pallidus especially vulnerable. Clinical experience suggests that the recovery trajectory is relatively brief compared with traumatic brain injury, and that neurological sequelae are less disabling. Parkinsonism is not infrequent after a latent interval. The commonest cognitive impairment is memory loss. For review see Caine and Watson (2000) and Auer (2004).

Carbon monoxide poisoning usually arises from deliberate self-harm by car exhaust fumes, and, more recently, from burning charcoal in the Far East. However, it can also occur accidentally from badly ventilated gas boilers and fires. The prevalence of complications after carbon monoxide poisoning is unclear, with a wide range of figures reported. It is also unclear if brain damage ever occurs if the poisoning was insufficient to cause loss of consciousness, although many sufferers complain of problems with memory, concentration fatigue and headache. See Ernst and Zibrak (1998) for review.

Stroke

Cognitive deficits

Strokes, which may or may not have presented acutely, may lead to vascular dementia, as described above (p. 339; Leys *et al.* 2005). However, strokes have other neuropsychiatric implications too. Overt strokes usually present as a neurological emergency, with hemiparesis, dysphasias and other focal signs. Subsequently, survivors may be left with these impairments, in addition to a range of psychiatric symptoms which depend largely on the site and size of the vascular event.

Personality change

Irritability, apathy, lability of mood, and occasionally aggressiveness may occur. Inflexibility in coping with problems is common and may be seen in extreme form as a catastrophic reaction (p. 331). These behavioural changes are often as disabling, and as distressing to carers, as residual hemiplegia or dysphasia. They are probably due more to associated widespread arteriosclerotic vascular disease than to a single stroke; and they may continue to worsen even when the focal signs of a stroke are improving.

After a stroke, some people become abnormally emotional, with mixtures of spontaneous laughter and crying, and the emotional display frequently at odds with the patient's apparent mood. Antidepressants are said to be helpful.

Mood disorder

Depressed mood is common after stroke and may contribute to the apparent intellectual impairment or impede rehabilitation (Robinson, 2003). Estimates of prevalence range from 12–64 per cent. Its development is influenced by the premorbid psychological and social factors demonstrated for all mood disorders (Sharpe *et al.*, 1994). It has been claimed that the risk of depression is related to the location of the stroke, being associated with a left anterior or right posterior hemisphere stroke (Starkstein and Robinson, 1993), but the findings remain controversial. Post-stroke depression is associated with an increased mortality rate.

Treatment of post-stroke depression depends in part on active rehabilitation. A trial of an antidepressant is often used, but should be done cautiously as side-effects are frequent. Moreover, a systematic review found no clear evidence that either medication or psychotherapy improves outcome (Hackett *et al.,* 2004). Patients who have suffered strokes are at increased risk of suicide (Stenager *et al.,* 1998).

Subdural haematoma

Subdural haematoma may follow a fall in elderly patients, and especially those associated with alcoholism. However, a history of head trauma is commonly lacking. Acute haematomas may cause coma or fluctuating impairment of consciousness, associated with hemiparesis and oculomotor signs. The psychiatrist is more likely to see the chronic syndromes, in which patients present with headache, poor concentration, vague physical complaints, and fluctuating consciousness, but often few localizing neurological signs. It is particularly important to consider this possibility as a cause for accelerated deterioration in patients with a neurodegenerative dementia. Treatment is by surgical evacuation, which may reverse the symptoms.

Subarachnoid haemorrhage

Subarachnoid haemorrahge usually results from rupture of a berry aneurysm located on the Circle of Willis. If not fatal, cognitive impairment and personality change are common, either from damage at the time of the bleed or as a result of clipping or embolization of the aneurysm. Aneurysms of the anterior communicating artery are particularly likely to cause an amnestic syndrome with confabulation, perhaps due to disruption to the basal forebrain.

Intracranial infections

Many intracranial infections cause cognitive impairment, and effective treatment is available for the majority. HIV infection is considered in Chapter 16. Unusual infections should always be considered as a cause of otherwise unexplained cognitive and psychiatric symptoms.

Neurosyphilis

Neurosyphilis, a manifestation of the tertiary stage of infection with the spirochaete *Treponema palidum*, is now rare in Western countries; however, increasing numbers of cases have been reported in Eastern Europe and in association with HIV. Because of its protean manifestations, the possibility of neurosyphilis should be considered in all 'neuropsychiatric' patients, especially those with delirium or dementia, and appropriate blood or CSF serological tests ordered. Prior treatment with antibiotics may produce partial and atypical syndromes.

An asymptomatic stage precedes clinical disease with variable latency. Symptomatic neurosyphilis takes three forms:

1. **Meningovascular syphilis**, which appears within 5 years of primary infection. It presents with strokes, or with personality changes, emotional lability and headache. Dementia may occur subsequently, accompanied by psychotic symptoms.
2. **General paresis** (also called **general paralysis of the insane**, or **dementia paralytica**) begins about 20 years after infection. Presentation is with dementia, personality change, dysarthria and motor symptoms and signs. Affective and psychotic symptoms may be florid, classically with euphoria and grandiose delusions. Discovery of the cause of general paresis was an important landmark in the history of psychiatry, stimulating a search for organic causes of other psychiatric syndromes (Hare, 1959).
3. **Tabes dorsalis** is a degeneration of spinal cord pathways and is unlikely to present to psychiatrists.

In the early stages, treatment with penicillin reverses the condition, and halts progression later in the illness. Untreated, death usually occurs within five years.

Encephalitis

Encephalitis may occur with primary (generally viral) infection of the brain parenchyma, or as a complication of bacterial meningitis, septicaemia, or a cerebral abscess. A great many viral causes of encephalitis have been identified, notably herpes simplex. Effective treatment (intravenous acyclovir) is available. The sequelae of the untreated disease may be devastating. In the acute stage, headache, vomiting, and impaired consciousness are usual, and seizures are common. Presentation may be with delirium. The psychiatrist may be involved in initial diagnosis but is more likely to see chronic complications which include prolonged anxiety and depression, a profound amnestic syndrome, personality change, or complex partial epilepsy.

Other significant encephalitides in adults include those produced by arthropod-borne viruses (including Japanese B and Murray Valley) and (especially in the immunocompromised) varicella zoster.

Encephalitis lethargica

A small outbreak of encephalitis lethargica (also called **post-encephalitic parkinsonism**) was first reported in

1917 by Von Economo at the Vienna Psychiatric Clinic (Von Economo, 1929). The condition attained epidemic proportions in the 1920s. By the 1930s, it had largely disappeared, although rare sporadic cases still occur (Howard and Lees, 1987). It is thought to be caused by the influenza virus or the immune reaction to it. Parkinsonism is the most disabling complication; another is personality change with antisocial behaviour. Some patients develop a clinical state resembling schizophrenia. Sacks (1973) gave a vivid description of such cases, and the striking but temporary 'awakening' brought about in some by L-dopa. Neuropathologically, the condition is similar to progressive supranuclear palsy.

Brain tumours

Many brain tumours cause psychological and cognitive symptoms at some stage in their course, and a significant proportion present with such symptoms (Ron, 1989; Jarquin-Valdivia, 2004). Psychiatrists are likely to see patients with slow-growing tumours in 'silent' (especially frontal) areas which produce psychological effects, but few neurological signs, for example, subfrontal meningioma or glioma of the corpus callosum. The nature of psychological symptoms is influenced by the global effects of raised intracranial pressure, in addition to tumour location. The rate of tumour growth is also important; rapidly expanding tumours can present as delirium, whereas slower growing tumours are more likely to cause chronic cognitive deficits. The latter are more common with dominant hemisphere tumours. Craniopharyngiomas and other tumours around the hypothalamus are often associated with personality changes and apathy.

Cognitive impairments in cancer

In addition to the direct effects of brain tumours, neoplasms both within and outside the cranium can impair cognition via a range of mechanisms (Table 14.21; Taphoorn and Klein, 2004). Cognitive impairments can be the presenting feature, particularly for primary CNS lymphomas, they emerge later in the illness, often as a complication of radiotherapy.

TABLE 14.21 Some causes of cognitive decline in patients with cancer

Direct tumour effects
◆ Mass effects (primary and metastatic brain tumours)
◆ Obstructive hydrocephalus
◆ Diffuse tumour infiltration of brain parenchyma
◆ Gliomatosis cerebri
◆ Carcinomatous meningitis
◆ En plaque meningioma
Indirect tumour effects
◆ Paraneoplastic syndromes (e.g. limbic encephalitis)
◆ Hypercalcaemia
◆ Hyponatraemia
◆ Hypoglycaemia
◆ Seizures
Secondary to opportunistic infections
◆ Herpes zoster
◆ Cryptococcus and other fungal infections
◆ Progressive multifocal leucoencephalopathy
Treatment effects
◆ Radiotherapy (radionecrosis, thromboangiopathy, leudodystrophy)
◆ Chemotherapy
◆ Neurosurgery

Secondary or symptomatic neuropsychiatric syndromes

All the disorders discussed in this chapter so far are either defined by their underlying pathology (e.g. the dementias), or have an undisputed biological basis (e.g. epilepsy). However, by convention, neuropsychiatry also includes disorders that are usually not in this category (i.e. are 'functional' or idiopathic) but which can on occasion be explained in the same fashion. They are called secondary, symptomatic, or organic. ICD-10 and DSM-IV code these disorders in different ways and use differing terminologies (p. 322); as noted earlier (p. 322), in this book we cover psychiatric disorders secondary to brain diseases in this chapter, whereas those resulting from systemic diseases are covered in Chapter 16. Examples of secondary neuropsychiatric disorders are given in Table 14.22.

The clinical features of these secondary disorders are generally indistinguishable from those in the equivalent primary psychiatric disorder. Thus, recognition of a secondary syndrome depends on associated features. The following guidelines, adapted from ICD-10, suggest that the disorder is secondary to a physical condition:

- Evidence of cerebral disease, damage or dysfunction, or of physical disease, known to be associated with one of the listed syndromes.

TABLE 14.22 Some causes of symptomatic or secondary psychiatric syndromes

Syndrome	Causes
Psychosis	Temporal lobe disorders, Huntington's disease, focal basal ganglia lesions, dementias, endocrinopathies, metabolic disorders, cerebral vascultidies, neurosyphilis
Mood disorder	Alzheimer's disease, stroke, head trauma, Parkinson's disease, multiple sclerosis, Huntington's disease, CJD, paraneoplastic limbic encephalitis, endocrinopathies, metabolic disorders (especially hypercalcaemia), neurosyphilis
Personality change	Frontotemporal dementias, frontal lesions, Huntington's disease, focal basal ganglia lesions, neurosyphilis, CJD, paraneoplastic limbic encephalitis
Obsessive–compulsive behaviours	Frontotemporal dementias, complex partial seizures, basal ganglia disorders, Rett syndrome
Self-mutilation	Lesch–Nyhan syndrome

- A temporal relationship (of weeks or a few months) between the development of the underlying disease and the onset of the psychiatric syndrome.
- Recovery from the psychiatric disorder following removal or improvement of the presumed cause.
- Absence of evidence suggesting an alternative 'psychological' cause of the psychiatric disorder. For example, in the case of depression, no evidence of family history of mood disorder, relevant personality traits, previous episodes of mood disorder, recent life events, etc.

Further reading

Lishman, WA. (1998) *Organic psychiatry,* 3rd edn. Blackwells, Oxford. (The standard textbook on neuropsychiatry - an essential reference work. A new edition is due shortly.)

Asbury AK, McKhann GM, McDonald WI, *et al.* (2002) *Diseases of the nervous system. Clinical neuroscience and therapeutic principles,* 3rd edn. Cambridge University Press, Cambridge. (A two volume reference text which includes neurological as well as neuropsychiatric disorders, and up to date reviews of their neurobiological basis).

CHAPTER 15

Eating disorders and sleep disorders

Chapter contents

In psychiatry, eating disorders are characterized by abnormalities in the pattern of eating which are determined primarily by the attitude a person takes to their weight and shape. The disorders covered in this chapter include anorexia nervosa and bulimia nervosa and a number of related conditions. Obesity is dealt with briefly but it is not regarded as psychiatric disorder, though it can, of course, have adverse psychological consequences as well as medical complications. For convenience sleep disorders are also described in this chapter.

Eating disorders

Until the late 1970s, eating disorders were believed to be uncommon. Following the description of bulimia nervosa, they have increasingly been seen as conspicuous and disabling. It remains uncertain whether the rapid rise in presentation and diagnosis reflects a true increase in incidence or rather increased detection and diagnosis (Curren *et al.*, 2005). Many eating disorders go clinically unrecognized and it is estimated that only about half of the cases of anorexia nervosa in the population are detected in primary care; for bulimia nervosa the figure is substantially less and most individuals with bulimia are untreated.

Anorexia nervosa and bulimia nervosa appear to be subgroups of a larger range of eating disorders which include those that are clinically very similar to the two main diagnoses, but fail to meet their precise diagnostic criteria. These disorders are classified within DSM-IV as Eating Disorders Not Otherwise Specified (EDNOS).

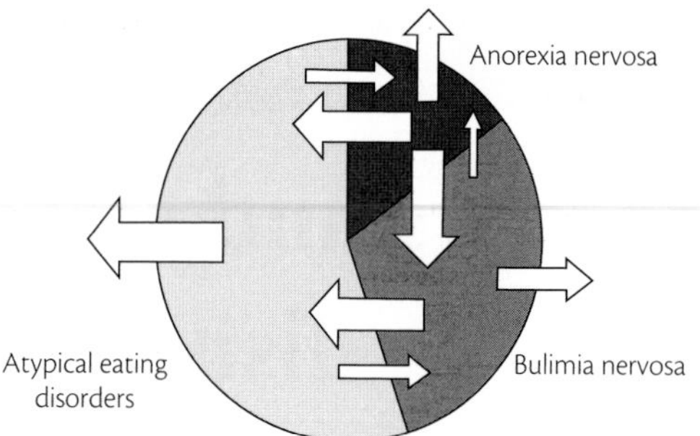

Fig. 15.1 Schematic representation of temporal movement between the eating disorders. The size of the arrow indicates likelihood of movement in shown direction. Arrows that point outside of the circle indicate recovery. (Reproduced with permission from Fairburn and Harrison, 2003.)

They are also known as Atypical Eating Disorders and in community samples are actually more frequent than either anorexia nervosa or bulimia nervosa. In fact, many patients with EDNOS have previous histories of anorexia or bulimia nervosa and some patients with EDNOS will eventually meet criteria for one of the two latter diagnoses. The fact that patients with eating disorders tend to 'migrate' between these various diagnoses (Figure 15.1) suggests that anorexia and bulimia nervosa and EDNOS have a common pathophysiology. The three conditions certainly share a distinctive core psychopathology which is best described as 'overevaluation' of weight and shape. That is to say, patients with these eating disorders 'judge their self-worth largely, or even exclusively, in terms of their shape and weight and their ability to control them' (Fairburn and Harrison, 2003).

Anorexia nervosa

Although there were many previous case histories, anorexia nervosa was named in 1868 by the English physician William Gull, who emphasized the psychological causes of the condition, the need to restore weight, and the role of the family. The other key description at this time was by Charles Lasegue in Paris (see Palmer, 2000). The main features are very low body weight (defined as being 15 per cent below the standard weight or body mass index [BMI] below 17. 5), an extreme concern about weight and shape characterized by an intense fear of gaining weight and becoming fat, a strong desire to be thin and, in women, amenorrhoea (see Box 15.1 for DSM-IV criteria).

Most patients are young women (see epidemiology, below). The condition usually begins in adolescence, although childhood-onset and older onset cases are encountered. It generally begins with ordinary efforts at dieting, which then get out of control. The central psychological features are the characteristic overvalued ideas about body shape and weight. The patient may have a distorted image of her body, believing herself to be too fat even when severely underweight. This belief explains why most patients do not want to be helped to gain weight.

The **pursuit of thinness** may take several forms. Patients generally eat little and set themselves very low daily calorie limits (often between 600 and 1000 kcal). Some try to achieve weight loss by inducing vomiting, excessive exercising, and misusing laxatives. Patients

BOX 15.1 DSM-IV CRITERIA FOR ANOREXIA NERVOSA

- Refusal to maintain body weight at or above a minimally normal weight for age and height (e.g. weight loss leading to maintenance of body weight less than 85 per cent of that expected; or failure to make expected weight gain during a period of growth, leading to body weight less than 85 per cent of that expected).
- Intense fear of gaining weight or becoming fat, even though underweight.
- Disturbance in the way in which one's body weight or shape is experienced, undue influence of body weight or shape on self-evaluation, or denial of the seriousness of the current low body weight.
- In postmenarchal females, amenorrhoea, i.e. the absence of at least three consecutive menstrual cycles. (A woman is considered to have amenorrhoea if her periods occur only following hormone, e.g. oestrogen, administration.)

Types

Restricting type During the current episode of anorexia nervosa, the person has not regularly engaged in binge-eating or purging behaviour (i.e. self-induced vomiting or the misuse of laxatives, diuretics or enemas).

Binge-eating/purging type During the current episode of anorexia nervosa, the person has regularly engaged in binge-eating or purging behaviour (i.e. self-induced vomiting or the misuse of laxatives, diuretics, or enemas).

are often preoccupied with thoughts of food, and sometimes enjoy cooking elaborate meals for other people. Some patients with anorexia nervosa admit to stealing food, either by shoplifting or in other ways.

Binge eating A subgroup of patients have repeated episodes of binge eating (uncontrollable overeating). This behaviour becomes more frequent with chronicity and increasing age. During binges, the patients typically eat foods that are usually avoided. After overeating they feel bloated and may induce vomiting. Binges are followed by remorse and intensified efforts to lose weight. If other people encourage them to eat, patients are often resentful; they may hide food or vomit secretly as soon as the meal is over. In DSM-IV, anorexia nervosa with binge eating and purging (self-induced vomiting or the misuse of laxatives or diuretics) is recognized as a distinct type, differing from the restricting type.

Amenorrhoea is one of several physical abnormalities that have traditionally been incorporated in diagnostic criteria. It occurs early in the development of the condition, and in about a fifth of cases it precedes obvious weight loss, although careful history taking generally reveals that these patients had already started dieting. Some cases first come to medical attention with amenorrhoea rather than disordered eating.

Other symptoms Depressive, anxiety and obsessional symptoms, lability of mood, and social withdrawal are all common. Lack of sexual interest is usual.

Physical consequences

A number of important symptoms and signs of anorexia nervosa are secondary to starvation. Several body systems can be affected (Table 15.1).

Epidemiology

Incidence Estimates of incidence of anorexia nervosa based on case registers in the UK and the USA range from 0.37–4.06 per 100, 000 population per year. These are likely to be underestimates. Reported incidence rates increased from the beginning of the twentieth century up to the 1970s but have probably been fairly stable since then (Hoek and van Hoeken, 2003; Currin *et al.*, 2005) (Figure 15.2).

Prevalence It is difficult to determine the true prevalence of anorexia nervosa because many people with the condition deny their symptoms. Surveys have suggested prevalence rates of around 0.7 per cent among schoolgirls and female university students.

Gender, social class and ethnicity As noted above, many more young women have restricted eating and overevaluation of weight and shape without meeting strict criteria for the diagnosis of anorexia nervosa.

TABLE 15.1 Main physical features of anorexia nervosa

Physical symptoms
◆ Heightened sensitivity to cold
◆ Gastrointestinal symptoms – constipation, fullness after eating, bloatedness
◆ Dizziness and syncope
◆ Amenorrhoea (in females not taking an oral contraceptive) low sexual appetite, infertility
◆ Poor sleep with early morning wakening
Physical signs
◆ Emaciation; stunted growth and failure of breast development (if preprubertal onset)
◆ Dry skin; fine downy hair (lanugo) on the back, forearms and side of face; orange discolouration of the skin and palms and soles
◆ Swelling of parotid and submandibular glands (especially in bulimic patients)
◆ Erosion of inner surface of front teeth (perimylolysis) in those who vomit frequently
◆ Cold hands and feet; hypothermia
◆ Bradycardia; hypotension; cardiac arrhymias (especially in underweight patients and those with electrolyte abnormalities)
◆ Dependent oedema (complicating assessment of body weight)
◆ Weak proximal muscles (elicited as difficulty rising from a squatting position)
Abnormalities on physical investigation
◆ Endocrine abnormalities
◆ Low concentrations of leutenizing hormone, follicle stimulating hormone, and oestradiol
◆ Low T_3 with T_4 in low normal range, normal concentrations of thyroid stimulating hormone (low T_3 syndrome)
◆ Increase in plasma cortisol and dexamethsaone non-suppression
◆ Raised growth hormone concentration
◆ Hypoglycaemia (rare)
Cardiovascular
◆ ECG abnormalities (especially in those with electrolyte disturbance)
◆ Conduction defects, especially prolongation of the Q-T interval
Gastrointestinal
◆ Delayed gastric emptying
◆ Decreased colonic motility (secondary to chronic laxative misuse)
◆ Acute gastric dilatation (rare, secondary to binge eating or excessive re-feeding)

TABLE 15.1 Main physical features of anorexia nervosa (*continued*)

Haematological
◆ Moderate normocytic normochromic anaemia
◆ Mild leucopenia with relative lymphocytosis
◆ Thrombocytopenia
Other metabolic abnormalities
◆ Hypercholesterolaemia
◆ Raised serum carotene
◆ Hypophosphataemia (exaggerated during re-feeding)
◆ Dehydration
◆ Electrolyte disturbance (varied in form; present in those who vomit frequently or misuse large quantities of laxatives or diuretics)
◆ Hypokalaemia
Other abnormalities
◆ Osteopenia and osteoporosis (with heightened fracture risk)

Reproduced with permission from Fairburn and Harrison (2003).

Amongst patients with anorexia nervosa seen in clinical practice only 5–10 per cent are male. The condition is more common in the upper than the lower social classes, and is reported to be rare in non-Western countries or in the non-white population of Western countries (Hoek and van Hoeken, 2003).

Genetics

Among the female siblings of patients with established anorexia nervosa, 5–10 per cent suffer from the condition compared with the 0.5–1.0 per cent found in the general population of the same age. Siblings also have an increased risk of other eating disorders such as bulimia nervosa and EDNOS suggesting a common familial liability. This increase in risk might be due to family environment or to genetic influences, however, twin studies have shown much higher concordance rates for anorexia nervosa in monozygotic twins (about 55 per cent) than dizygotic twins (about 5 per cent) suggesting a substantial genetic component to the condition (Treasure and Holland, 1989).

The nature of the genetic contribution to anorexia nervosa remains unclear. Some association studies have implicated a polymorphism in the promoter region of the 5-HT_{2A} receptor but a significant number of studies have failed to replicate this observation. Similarly a genome-wide linkage analysis of nearly 200 families in which at least one pair of relatives suffered from anorexia nervosa found only weak evidence for linkage to a site on chromosome 1p (Grice *et al.*, 2002). It is possible that the inherited liability to anorexia nervosa might involve relevant personality traits such as perfectionism and obsessionality (see below). In addition, family studies show an association between eating disorders and mood disorders but this seems unlikely to be due to a single, shared, aetiological factor for the two conditions (see Lilenfeld and Kaye, 1998).

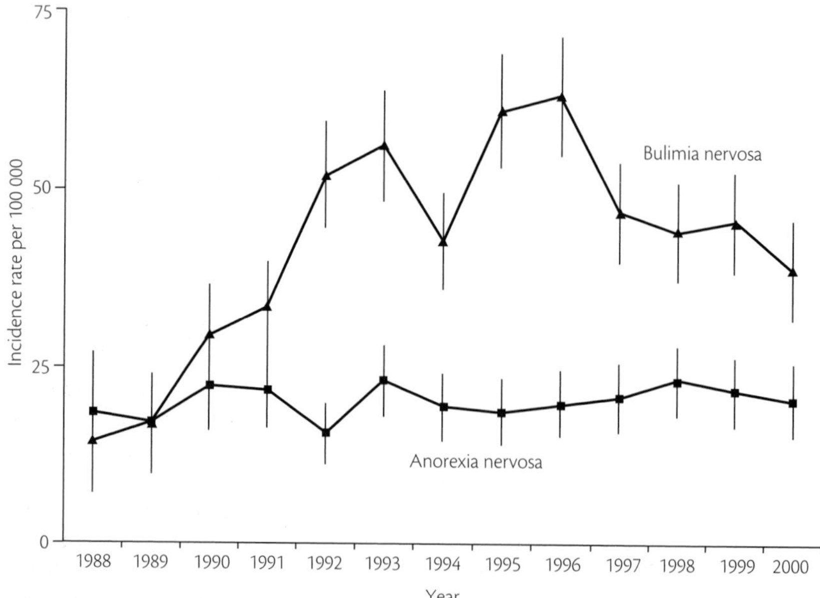

Fig 15.2 Annual incidence of anorexia and bulimia nervosa in women aged 10–39 years from 1988–2000 (error bars represent 95% confidence intervals). (Reproduced with permission from Currin *et al.*, 2005).

Social factors

The fact that anorexia nervosa is more common in certain societies suggests that cultural factors play a part in its development. Important among such factors is likely to be the notion that thinness is desirable and attractive. Surveys in more affluent societies show that most schoolgirls and female college students diet at one time or another. However, once other risk factors are taken account, people who develop anorexia nervosa have no greater exposure to factors that increase the risk of dieting. This suggests that the problem is more in how an individual reacts to dieting than in dieting per se (Fairburn *et al.*, 1999).

Individual psychological causes

Bruch (1974) was one of the first writers to discuss the psychological antecedents to anorexia nervosa. She suggested that these patients are engaged in 'a struggle for control, for a sense of identity and effectiveness with the relentless pursuit of thinness as a final step in this effort'. These clinical observations are supported by epidemiological studies, which implicate low self-esteem and perfectionism in the development of the disorder (Fairburn *et al.*, 1999). It has been suggested that these premorbid personality traits can make it particularly difficult for individuals to negotiate the demands of adolescence. Certainly the timing of onset of the disorder suggests that developmental issues are important, an idea now demonstrated epidemiologically in case-control designs (Fairburn *et al.*., 1999) (see below).

Causes within the family

Disturbed relationships are often found in the families of patients with anorexia nervosa, and some authors have suggested that they have an important causal role. Minuchin *et al.* (1978) held that a specific pattern of relationships could be identified, consisting of 'enmeshment, over protectiveness, rigidity and lack of conflict resolution'. They also suggested that the development of anorexia nervosa in the patient served to prevent dissent within the family.

Epidemiological studies suggest that people who develop anorexia nervosa are more likely than healthy controls to be exposed to a range of childhood adversities, including poor relationships with parents and parental psychiatric disorder, particularly depression. However, these risk factors are not specific to anorexia nervosa because they are found with equal frequency among people who subsequently develop other psychiatric disorders, such as mood disorders (Fairburn *et al.*, 1999). It seems likely that these general risk factors interact with specific factors within the individual, such as perfectionism and low self-esteem, to increase the risk of developing anorexia nervosa.

Course and prognosis

In its early stages, anorexia nervosa often runs a fluctuating course with exacerbations and periods of partial remission. Full recovery is not uncommon in cases with a short history. The long-term prognosis is difficult to judge because most published series are based on selected cases or are incomplete in their follow-up. Outcome is very variable but the following general findings are reported:

1. Although weight and menstrual functioning usually improve, eating habits and attitudes to weight and shape often remain abnormal and some patients develop bulimia nervosa or EDNOS.
2. Anorexia nervosa does not evolve into other forms of psychiatric disorder.
3. Although the disorder may run a chronic course, recovery can occur even after many years
4. Reported mortality rates from long-term follow-up studies of severe cases are high at around 15 per cent; this represents a sixfold increase in the standardized mortality rate. The usual causes of death are suicide or a direct result of medical complications. It is believed that the mortality rate is lower in more representative community samples and may be falling with improved methods of treatment (see Nielsen *et al.*, 1998).
5. About a fifth of patients make a full recovery, and another fifth remain severely ill; the remainder show some degree of chronic or fluctuating disturbance.
6. The main **predictors** of better outcome are a short history and starting at a younger age. Childhood obesity, low self-esteem and personality disturbances are associated with a worse outcome (Sullivan *et al.*, 1998).

Assessment

Most patients with anorexia nervosa are reluctant to see a psychiatrist, and so it is important to try to establish a good relationship. This means listening to the patient's views, explaining treatment alternatives, and being willing to contemplate compromises. A thorough history should be taken of the development of the disorder, the present pattern of eating and weight control, and the patient's ideas about body weight (see Boxes 15.2 and 15.3). In the mental state examination, particular attention should be given to depressive

BOX 15.2 ASSESSMENT OF EATING: SOME TOPICS TO BE INCLUDED

What is a typical day's eating? To what degree is the patient attempting restraint?

Is there a pattern? Does it vary? Is eating ritualized?

Does she avoid particular foods? And if so why?

Does she restrict fluids?

What is the patient's experience of hunger or of any urge to eat?

Does she binge? Are these objectively large binges? Does she feel out of control?

Are the binges planned? How do they begin? How do they end? How often?

Does she make herself vomit? If so how? Does she vomit blood? Does she wash out with copious fluids afterwards?

Does she take laxatives, diuretics, emetics, appetite suppressants? With what effects?

Does she chew and spit? Does she fast for a day to more?

Can she eat in front of others?

Does she exercise? Is this to 'burn off calories'?

Reproduced with permission from B. Palmer, B. (ed.) (2000) *Helping people with eating disorders. A clinical guide to assessment and treatment.* John Wiley, Chichester

BOX 15.3 ASSESSMENT OF PSYCHOLOGICAL ISSUES: SOME TOPICS TO BE INCLUDED

What does the patient feel about her body and her weight?

If she is restraining her eating, what is her motivation?

Does she feel fat? Does she dislike her body? If so, in what way?

Does she have a distorted body image? If so, in what way?

What does she feel would happen if she did not control her weight or eating?

Does she fear loss of control? Is she able to say what she means by this?

Does she feel guilt or self-disgust? If so, what leads her to feel this?

Does anything about her disorder lead her to feel good?

If she binges, what are her feelings before, during, and after bingeing?

What has she told others about her eating disorder – if anything?

How does she think about her disorder? What does she make of it?

Reproduced with permission from Palmer, B. (ed.) (2000) *Helping people with eating disorders. A clinical guide to assessment and treatment.* John Wiley, Chichester

symptoms. More than one interview may be needed to obtain this information and gain the patient's confidence. The parents or other informants should be interviewed whenever possible. It is essential to perform a physical examination, with particular attention to the degree of emaciation, cardiovascular status, and signs of vitamin deficiency. Other wasting disorders, such as malabsorption, endocrine disorder, or cancer, should be excluded. Electrolytes should be measured if there is any possibility that the patient has been inducing vomiting or abusing purgatives.

Evidence about treatment

Psychotherapy

There is a lack of good evidence about treatment and management. In part, this reflects the wide range in severity and the difficulty of evaluating complex interventions. This means that many current views about treatment depend upon clinical experience and opinion. Several forms of psychotherapy have been tried. It is generally agreed that intensive psychoanalytical methods are not helpful. Clinical experience suggests that there is some value in measures directed to improving personal relationships and increasing the patient's sense of personal effectiveness.

In recent years, **family therapy** has been advocated. The results of a controlled evaluation suggest that there may be benefits with younger patients but do not support the general use of family therapy (Russell *et al.*, 1987). If this treatment is used, it should be for selected cases in which family problems seem particularly relevant and the family members are willing to participate. There are various forms of family therapy and which is best in the treatment of anorexia nervosa is unclear. **Cognitive-behaviour therapy** has also been used with the aim of modifying abnormal cognitions about shape, weight, and eating, but it has yet to be formally evaluated (Hay *et al.*, 2003). The difficulty of this area is shown by a recent randomized trial in which neither cognitive behaviour therapy nor interpersonal therapy was superior to non-specific clinical management (McIntosh *et al.*, 2005).

Medication

Medication does not have primary role in the treatment of anorexia nervosa; however, many patients have significant symptoms of depression and SSRIs are sometimes used for this indication. Usually, however, depressive symptoms will improve as weight is restored. There is a preliminary report that fluoxetine may help maintain recently restored weight but this requires confirmation (Kaye *et al.*, 2001). There are also anecdotal accounts that the atypical antipsychotic agent olanzapine may provide benefit but no randomized trials have yet been reported (Powers and Santana, 2004).

Management

Starting treatment

Success largely depends on establishing a good relationship with the patient. It should be made clear that achieving an adequate weight is essential in order to reverse the physical and psychological effects of starvation. It is important to agree a definite dietary plan but not to become involved in wrangles about it. At the same time, it should be emphasized that weight control is only one aspect of the problem, and help should be offered with the accompanying psychological problems.

Educating the patient and family about the disorder and its treatment is important. Most cases may be treated on a day patient or outpatient basis. Admission to hospital is indicated if:

1. The patient's weight is dangerously low;
2. There is severe depression and suicidal risk;
3. Outpatient care has failed.

Admission to a medical ward is appropriate if the main reason for admission is life-threatening consequences of weight loss such as electrolyte disturbance, hypoglycaemia or severe infection.

Restoring weight

Outpatient treatment Weight restoration is normally accomplished on an outpatient basis. A reasonable aim is an increase of 0.5Kg a week, which will usually require an extra 500–1,000 calories a day. The target weight usually has to be a compromise between a healthy weight (a BMI above 20) and the patient's idea of what her weight should be. A balanced diet of about 3000 kcal should be taken as three or four meals a day. It is good practice to monitor the patient's physical state regularly and to prescribe vitamin supplements if indicated. It is also important to assess and modify other weight-reducing strategies that the patient may employ, for example over-exercising and laxative misuse.

Inpatient treatment For those requiring inpatient treatment, there should be an understanding that the patient will stay in hospital until her agreed target weight has been reached and maintained and there is a comprehensive, mutually agreed, treatment plan for subsequent outpatient care. Successful inpatient treatment depends on good nursing care, with clear aims and a carefully structured treatment plan. In the past, strict behavioural regimens were used. However, these had no advantage and often appeared punitive.

Eating must be supervised by a nurse, who has three important roles: to reassure the patient that she can eat without the risk of losing control over her weight; to be clear about agreed targets; and to ensure that the patient does not induce vomiting or take purgatives. It is reasonable to aim for a weight gain of between 0.5 and 1.0 kg each week and weight restoration usually takes between 8 and 12 weeks. Some patients demand to leave hospital before their treatment is finished, but with patience the staff can usually persuade them to stay.

Rarely, the patient's weight loss is so severe as to pose an immediate threat to life. If such a patient cannot be persuaded to enter hospital, compulsory admission is necessary (see Box 15.4). For guidelines on the treatment of anorexia nervosa see The National Institute of Clinical Excellence (2004b) (Box 15.5).

BOX 15.4 **COMPULSORY TREATMENT**

Laws about compulsory treatment require evidence of mental illness to enable involuntary treatment. Their application to anorexia nervosa is controversial. Is anorexia a mental illness in the legal sense? Is successful treatment possible without consent?

In practice, compulsory treatment is used rarely and as a last resort when the patient is in physical danger. In these circumstances it may save the patient's life and gain the time to establish long-term voluntary treatment.

Compulsory treatment has many disadvantages, including losing the possibility of the patient ever cooperating with any reasonable treatment plan.

BOX 15.5 GUIDELINES FOR MANAGEMENT OF ANOREXIA NERVOSA

- Most people with anorexia nervosa should be managed on an outpatient basis, with psychological treatment and monitoring of physical condition.
- Psychological therapies for anorexia nervosa include cognitive analytic therapy (CAT), cognitive -behaviour therapy (CBT), interpersonal psychotherapy (IPT), focal psychodynamic therapy and family interventions focused explicitly on eating disorders.
- Outpatient psychological treatment for anorexia nervosa should normally be of at least 6 months' duration. Failure to improve or deterioration should lead to more intensive forms of treatment (for example, a move from individual therapy to combined individual and family work; or day-care or inpatient care). Dietary counselling should not be provided as the sole treatment for anorexia nervosa.
- For inpatients with anorexia nervosa it is important to monitor the patient's physical status during refeeding. Psychological treatment should be provided which has a focus both on eating behaviour and attitudes to weight and shape, and on wider psychosocial issues with the expectation of weight gain. Rigid inpatient behaviour modification programmes should not be used in the management of anorexia nervosa.
- Following inpatient weight restoration, people with anorexia nervosa should be offered outpatient psychological treatment that focuses both on eating behaviour and attitudes to weight and shape, and on wider psychosocial issues, with regular monitoring of both physical and psychological risk.

Adapted from the National Institute for Clinical Excellence (2004b)

Bulimia nervosa

The term bulimia refers to episodes of uncontrolled excessive eating, sometimes called 'binges'. As mentioned above, the symptom of bulimia occurs in some cases of anorexia nervosa. The syndrome of bulimia nervosa was first described by Russell (1979) in a highly influential paper in which he named the condition and described the key clinical features in 30 patients seen between 1972 and 1978. However, Russell's cases also suffered from concomitant anorexia nervosa and were therefore unlike the cases we now think of as bulimia nervosa. Thereafter the syndrome 'bulimia' was included in DSM-III and it soon became evident that bulimia nervosa was common in the general population among people who did not have anorexia nervosa (see Palmer, 2004, for a review).

Although the syndrome was described by Russell

BOX 15.6 DSM-IV CRITERIA OF BULIMIA NERVOSA

Recurrent episodes of binge eating An episode of binge eating is characterized by both of the following:

- eating, in a discrete period of time (e.g. within any 2-hour period) an amount of food that is definitely larger than most people would eat during a similar period of time and similar circumstances;
- a sense of lack of control over eating during the episode (e.g. a feeling that one cannot stop eating or control what or how much one is eating).

Recurrent inappropriate compensatory behaviour in order to prevent weight gain such as self-induced vomiting; misuse of laxatives, diuretics, enemas, or other medication; fasting; or excessive exercise. The binge eating and inappropriate compensatory behaviour both occur, on average, at least twice a week for 3 months. The disturbance does not occur exclusively during episodes of anorexia nervosa.

Types

Purging type During the current episode of bulimia nervosa the person has regularly engaged in self-induced vomiting or the misuse of laxatives, diuretics, or enemas.

Non-purging type During the current episode of bulimia nervosa, the person has used other inappropriate compensatory behaviours, such as fasting or excessive exercise, but has not regularly engaged in self-induced vomiting or the misuse of laxatives, diuretics, or enemas.

as an 'ominous variant' of anorexia nervosa, only a quarter have a history of preceding anorexia nervosa. The central features are:

1. an irresistible urge to overeat
2. extreme measures to control body weight
3. overvalued ideas concerning shape and weight of the type seen in anorexia nervosa.

Two subtypes of bulimia nervosa are recognized in DSM-IV (see Box 15.5), the purging type characterized by the use of self-induced vomiting, laxatives, and diuretics to prevent weight gain, and the non-purging type in which 'purging' symptoms do not occur regularly but the person uses other behaviours to avoid weight gain, such as fasting and excessive exercise. Patients with bulimia nervosa are usually of normal weight; patients who are substantially underweight usually qualify for a diagnosis of anorexia nervosa, which takes precedence. Most patients are female and they often have normal menses.

Patients have a profound loss of control over eating. Episodes of bulimia may be precipitated by stress or by the breaking of self-imposed dietary rules, or may occasionally be planned. In the episodes large amounts of food are consumed, on average over 2000 kcal per episode; for example, a loaf of bread, a whole pot of jam, a cake, and biscuits. This voracious eating usually takes place alone. At first it brings relief from tension, but relief is soon followed by guilt and disgust. The patient may then induce vomiting or take laxatives. There may be many episodes of bulimia and purging each day.

Depressive symptoms are more prominent than in anorexia nervosa, and are probably secondary to the eating disorder. A high proportion of patients meet criteria for major depression. The depressive symptoms usually remit as the eating disorder improves. A few patients appear to suffer from a depressive disorder of sufficient severity and persistence to require treatment with antidepressant medication.

Physical consequences

Repeated vomiting leads to several complications. Potassium depletion is particularly serious, resulting in weakness, cardiac arrhythmia, and renal damage. Rarely, urinary infections, tetany, and epileptic fits may occur. The teeth become pitted by the acid gastric contents in a way that dentists can recognize as characteristic.

Epidemiology

The **prevalence** of bulimia nervosa is around 1 per cent among women aged between 16 and 40 years in Western societies. It is at least ten times less common in men. Bulimia nervosa has only been identified in developed countries. The dramatic increase in presentation and diagnosis seen in the UK in the early 1990s has been followed by a modest decline (see Figure 15.2). It is possible that the earlier increase represented increased detection of relatively long-standing cases (Currin *et al.*, 2005).

Development of the disorder

Bulimia nervosa usually has an onset in late adolescence (i.e. several years later than anorexia nervosa). It often follows a period of concern about shape and weight and a quarter of patients have a history of a previous episode of anorexia nervosa. There is usually an initial period of dietary restriction which, after a variable length of time, but usually within 3 years, breaks down with increasingly frequent episodes of overeating. As the overeating becomes more frequent, the body weight returns to a more normal level. At some stage self-induced vomiting and laxative misuse are adopted to compensate for the overeating. However, this may result in even less control of eating.

Aetiology

General risk factors Like anorexia nervosa bulimia nervosa appears to be the result of exposure to general risk factors of psychiatric disorder including a family history of psychiatric disorder, especially depression and substance misuse, and a range of adverse childhood experiences. It used to be thought that sexual abuse was especially common but the evidence now suggests the rate is no higher than amongst those who develop other types of psychiatric disorder (Fairburn *et al.*, 1999).

Specific risk factors Epidemiological studies also suggest that unlike anorexia nervosa, patients with bulimia nervosa have increased exposure to factors that specifically promote dieting such as childhood obesity, parental obesity and early menarche. Perfectionism also appears to be a risk factor but to a lesser extent than in anorexia nervosa (Fairburn *et al.*, 1999).

Genetic risk factors The magnitude and identity of genetic factors in bulimia nervosa remains unclear, with contradictory evidence. Overall it seems likely that there is a significant genetic component, particularly in view of the cross-familial transmission of anorexia and bulimia nervosa noted above (Fairburn and Harrison, 2003), but no individual genes have yet been identified.

5-HT neurotransmission A number of experimental paradigms, including neuroendocrine challenge tests and brain imaging studies, suggest that brain 5-HT function is abnormal in bulimia nervosa (Kaye *et al.*, 2001). The procedure of tryptophan depletion causes an acute relapse in both mood and cognitions about weight and shape in recovered, asymptomatic bulimic subjects. This suggests that people with a history of bulimia nervosa have neuropsychological vulnerability to lowered brain serotonin levels. Interestingly, weight loss through dieting lowers tryptophan availability suggesting a mechanism whereby excessive dieting could trigger symptoms of bulimia nervosa in those at risk of the disorder (see Smith *et al.*, 1999).

Course and prognosis

This is uncertain since there have been few long-term studies. The course and outcome in those who do not present for treatment is unknown. The average length of history at clinical presentation is about five years, indicating that among this subgroup the disorder is already chronic. The overall outcome is very variable. The evidence to date suggests that cases of clinical severity tend to run a chronic course. Thus even five to ten years later between one third and a half of individuals still have a clinical eating disorder although in many it will take an atypical form (Fairburn *et al.*, 2000). There is no evidence that bulimia nervosa is associated with the onset of any other psychiatric disorder.

The mortality rate in bulimia nervosa is less than that of anorexia nervosa but whether it is increased relative to the general population is uncertain (Keel *et al.*, 2003). However, bulimia nervosa is certainly strongly associated with depression and substance misuse, both of which do carry a burden of raised mortality (Harris and Barraclough, 1995). The disorder tends to improve during pregnancy but subsequent relapse is common. No convincing predictors of course or outcome have been identified though childhood obesity and low self-esteem may be associated with a worse prognosis (Fairburn *et al.*, 2000).

Evidence about treatment effectiveness

The most extensively studied psychological treatment is a manual-based, cognitive-behaviour therapy which helps patients regain control over their eating. There have also been numerous trials of antidepressant medication, particularly SSRIs. The overall efficacy of available treatments has recently been summarized (Bacaltchuk *et al.* 2000; Wilson and Fairburn, 2002):

- The most effective current treatment for bulimia nervosa is a specific cognitive behaviour therapy that focuses on modifying the behaviours and ways of thinking that maintain the eating disorder.
- With this form of cognitive behaviour therapy between one third and a half of patients make a complete and lasting recovery.
- Antidepressant drugs such as SSRIs decrease the frequency of binge eating and purging, and improve mood. The effect is not as great as cognitive behaviour therapy and benefit may not be as sustained.
- The combination of cognitive behaviour therapy and antidepressant medication offers no clear advantage over psychotherapy alone.
- Interpersonal psychotherapy may be as effective as cognitive behaviour therapy but takes longer to work.
- Simple self-help treatments may be tried initially but are not usually sufficient for the majority of patients.

Management

The management of bulimia nervosa is easier than that of anorexia nervosa because the patient is more likely to wish to recover and a good working relationship can often be established. Also, there is no need for weight restoration. It is necessary to assess the patient's physical state and to measure electrolyte status in those who are vomiting frequently or misusing laxatives.

As with many common disorders, a 'stepped-care' approach appears to be the best way of providing appropriate care to large numbers of people with varying degrees of severity of disorder. The management of bulimia nervosa has recently been the subject of a review by the National Institute for Clinical Excellence (2004b):

Step one Identify the small minority (less than 5 per cent) who require specialist treatment because of severe depression, physical complications requiring inpatient or day patient care, or severe substance abuse requiring treatment in its own right.

Step two Guided cognitive-behavioural self-help as appropriate using a self-help book and with the guidance of a non-specialist facilitator. Treatment usually takes about 4 months and requires eight to ten meetings with the facilitator. Such treatment is appropriate for primary care and appears to lead to good progress in about a third of patients.

Step three Patients who do not show benefit within around 6 weeks of step two require full cognitive-behavioural therapy. In a minority of cases, where concomitant depressive symptoms are severe, it is worthwhile adding an antidepressant drug such as fluoxetine in doses of up to 60 mg daily. Most depressive symptoms, however, will resolve with successful cognitive-behaviour therapy.

BOX 15.7 QUESTIONS PATIENTS AND THEIR FAMILIES ASK ABOUT EATING DISORDERS AND THEIR TREATMENT

Patient

1. What kind of eating problem do I have?
2. What does it mean for my health, daily life, work or schooling?
3. Why have you decided to offer me this kind of treatment?
4. Are there other treatments that might suit me better?

Family

1. How can we help with the problem?
2. Should we be more directly involved in supervising how the person eats?
3. Can you let us know how treatment is progressing?
4. Might we benefit from support as a family?

See National Institute for Clinical Excellence (2004b)

Step four Patients who do not improve with cognitive-behavioural therapy require comprehensive specialist reassessment. In some cases, measures to provide better cognitive therapy or an antidepressant drug may be useful. It is important to review the initial treatment with the patient with the aim of agreeing a treatment approach that the patient finds acceptable (Box 15.7).

Eating disorder not otherwise specified (atypical eating disorders)

These DSM-IV and ICD categories are for disorders of eating that do not meet the criteria for anorexia nervosa or bulimia nervosa, but are of clinical severity. As noted above, they are frequent, and are diagnosed in at least a third of referrals. Little is known about the course of atypical eating disorders although what evidence is available suggests that the eating disorder persists in most cases with about half evolving into anorexia nervosa or bulimia nervosa. The treatment of atypical eating disorders has received very little research attention. It has been advised that clinicians follow guidelines for the treatment of anorexia nervosa in instances where weight is low and those for bulimia nervosa where the problem is more concerned with binge-eating (see Fairburn and Harrison, 2003).

Binge eating disorder

A subgroup within EDNOS is recognized in DSM-IV as 'requiring further study'. It has been named **binge-eating disorder**; its definition and validity remain unclear because relatively little is known about it. It is characterized by recurrent bulimic episodes in the absence of the other diagnostic features of bulimia nervosa, particularly counter-regulatory measures such as vomiting and purging. Patients may have depressive symptoms and some dissatisfaction with their weight and shape; however the latter are usually less severe than are seen in bulimia nervosa.

Binge eating disorder appears to be associated with exposure to risk factors for psychiatric disorder in general and for obesity. About 25 per cent of patients who present for treatment for obesity have features of binge eating disorder. The condition generally affects an older age group than bulimia nervosa and up to a quarter of those presenting for treatment are men. Unlike the other eating disorders described here binge eating disorder has a high spontaneous remission rate and seems reasonably responsive to cognitive-behaviour therapy and treatment with SSRIs (for a review see Dingemans *et al.*, 2002).

Obesity

Obesity is a medical condition characterized by excess body fat. It is diagnosed when the BMI (weight in kg/height in m^2) exceeds 30. At least 20 per cent of the adults in the UK meet this criteria and the figure is rising. Obesity is associated with an increased mortality, and severe obesity (BMI greater than 40) is associated with a 12-fold increase of risk in those aged 25–35 years. It has been estimated that in the USA, 300,000 deaths each year can be attributed to obesity, making it a public health problem second only to smoking as a potentially preventative cause of death (see Zohrabian, 2005).

Aetiology

Most obesity is attributable to genetic factors exacerbated by social circumstances that encourage overeating of high calorie foods and lack of exercise. Psychological causes do not seem to be of great importance in most cases, but psychiatrists are sometimes asked to see obese people whose excessive eating seems to be deter-

BOX 15.8 SOME PSYCHOTROPIC DRUGS ASSOCIATED WITH EXCESSIVE WEIGHT GAIN

Antidepressants Amitriptyline, imipramine, mianserin, mirtazapine, phenelzine

Antipsychotic agents Chlorpromazine, clozapine, olanzapine, quetiapine

Mood-stabilizing drugs Lithium, valproate

mined by emotional factors. It is important for psychiatrists to be aware that certain psychoptropic drugs can promote excessive weight gain together with associated metabolic consequences (Box 15.8).

Psychological consequences

Although there have been many reports of emotional disturbance amongst the obese, numerous careful studies have shown little difference in psychopathology as compared with non-obese people in the general population. Concern appears to be most common in teenage and young women of upper and middle socioeconomic status who are likely to live in social circumstances in which prejudice and discrimination are frequent.

One form of psychopathology that is specific to obesity is a distortion of body image, feeling grotesque, and a belief that others feel contempt. This disorder, which is associated with self-consciousness and social limitations, occurs only in the minority of obese people who have been obese since childhood and also have low self-esteem. See Stunkard and Waddon (2000).

Course

Obesity is a chronic, indeed lifelong, problem. Obese children and adolescents are unlikely to grow out of their obesity unless treated. Most untreated adults continue to gain weight at the rate of approximately 1 kg per year.

Treatment

It is now widely accepted that the goal of treatment should be one of reduction of body weight by as little as 5–10 per cent rather than unrealistically attempting to attain an ideal weight which is unlikely to be achieved or maintained. Such more modest goals may have medical benefits and also improve mood and body image. They are also appropriate to attaining long-term weight management. The main treatment options are:

- **Behaviour modification.** This consists of a package which aims to change both eating patterns and the nature of the food consumed while at the same time producing an overall modest reduction in calorie intake. Physical activity is gradually increased. There is consistent evidence that although this approach is effective in the short term, weight is then gradually regained.
- **Pharmacological treatments.** Two treatments are in use currently in the UK. Orlistat is a lipase inhibitor which decreases fat absorption. Sibutramine in a mixed monoamine re-uptake inhibitor, which decreases appetite centrally. Both drugs produce a modest benefit in terms of weight loss which is sustained for up to a year (Padwal *et al.*, 2003). It is recommended that sibutramine should not be given with antidepressant or antipsychotic drugs.

The long-term results of all kinds of treatment are disappointing, whether supervised by a doctor or not. Group therapy and self-help groups based on principles of behaviour modification produce short-term benefit but do not improve long-term results. The same is true for appetite-suppressing drugs and behavioural methods (see Eckel, 2002).

Surgical treatment

Surgical treatment is for very severe obesity (BMI >40) or for those with a slightly lower BMI >35 and significant medical complications that will benefit if weight reduction if achieved.

Two kinds of surgery are employed. The first is gastric restriction which limits stomach size by stapling, thereby increasing feelings of fullness. The second method creates an intestinal bypass so that the length of gut available for food absorption is decreased. Both these operations carry significant risks and should be offered only when other treatments have failed (see National Institute for Clinical Excellence, 2002).

Management

Most treatment is provided in primary care and medical clinics. Psychiatrists need to be aware of the standard treatments for obesity, including the role of self-help and commercial programmes such as Weight Watchers. Whilst the effectiveness of the latter remains unclear, the dependence of Weight Watchers and some other programmes on sound principles of nutrition and activity mean that they are probably helpful to those with moderate degrees of obesity and health risk.

Mildly overweight people can be helped by simple advice about diet and exercise while those with a greater degree of obesity will probably need a more structured behavioural programme with pharmacological treatment if the former treatment is not successful. Patients should be encouraged to reduce consumption of refined sugar and flour and eat more fibre-rich carbohydrates. Typically calorie intake will need to be reduced by about 500 kcal a day to produce weight loss at the recommended rate of about 1lb per week. Physical activity should also be increased because it will promote weight loss and improve cardiovascular fitness. Although there has been concern that dieting may be associated with adverse physiological and psychological consequences, this does not seem to be a problem in obese individuals undergoing modest dieting. (Hitchcock and Pugh, 2002).

Severely overweight people require assessment and treatment in specialized clinics. For a review of obesity see Stunkard and Wadden (2000) and Eckel (2002).

Psychogenic vomiting

Psychogenic vomiting is chronic and episodic vomiting without an organic cause which commonly occurs after meals and in the absence of nausea. It should be distinguished from the more common syndrome of bulimia nervosa, in which self-induced vomiting follows episodes of binge eating (uncontrolled overeating). Psychogenic vomiting appears to be more common in women than in men and usually presents in early or middle adult life. It is reported that both psychotherapeutic and behavioural treatments can be helpful.

Sleep disorders

Psychiatrists may be asked to see patients whose main problem is either difficulty in sleeping or, less often, excessive sleep. Such problems are important:

- As primary sleep disorders, the focus of this section.
- As causes of psychological symptoms.
- As symptoms of psychiatric disorder, especially depression and anxiety disorders, covered in other chapters.

Many patients who sleep badly complain of tiredness and mood disturbance during the day. Although prolonged sleep deprivation leads to some impairment of intellectual performance and disturbance of mood, loss of sleep on occasional nights is of little significance except in those whose responsibilities or activities require maximum alertness. The daytime symptoms of people who sleep badly are probably related more to the cause of their insomnia (often a depressive disorder or anxiety disorder) than to insomnia itself.

Classification

Table 15.2 shows the DSM-IV classification of sleep disorders, which is compatible with the considerably more elaborate International Classification of Sleep Disorders.

TABLE 15.2 Classification of primary sleep disorders in DSM-IV

Dyssomnias
◆ Primary insomnia
◆ Primary hypersomnia
◆ Narcolepsy
◆ Breathing-related sleep disorder
◆ Circadian rhythm sleep disorder
◆ Dyssomnia not otherwise specified
Parasomnias
◆ Nightmare disorder (dream anxiety disorder)
◆ Sleep terror disorder
◆ Sleepwalking disorder
◆ Parasomnia not otherwise specified
Sleep disorder related to another mental disorder
◆ Insomnia
◆ Hypersomnia
Other sleep disorders
◆ Secondary sleep disorder due to a general medical condition
◆ Substance-induced sleep disorder

Classification in ICD-10 is rather different, with sleep disorders occurring in three different parts of the classification.

Epidemiology

Sleep disorders are common. There is a wide range of variation in estimates of the prevalence of insomnia depending on the definition and on the population studied. Up to 30 per cent of adults complain of insomnia, a third of these as a chronic problem. Excessive sleepiness occurs in 5 per cent of adults, and possibly 15 per cent of adolescents and 14 per cent of the adult population suffer some form of chronic sleep–wake disorder.

In the Epidemiologic Catchment Area Study (Ford and Kamerow, 1989), 10.2 per cent of the community sample reported insomnia and 3.2 per cent reported hypersomnia. Forty per cent of those who suffered insomnia and 46.5 per cent of those with hypersomnia had a psychiatric disorder compared with 16.4 per cent of those with no sleep complaints. Groups at special risk of persistent sleep problems include young children, adolescents, the physically ill, those with learning disability, and those with dementia.

BOX 15.9 ASSESSMENT OF SLEEP DISTURBANCE

Screening questions

Do you sleep well enough and long enough?
Are you very sleepy during the day?
Is your sleep disturbed at night?

Sleep history

Detailed history of the sleep complaint
Pattern of occurrence, factors making sleep better or worse
Consequences for mood, everyday life, family
Past and present treatment
Typical 24-hour sleep–wake schedule

Sleep diary

Systematic 2 week or longer record

History from bed partner

Investigation

Video recording
Wrist scintigraphy (monitoring body movement)
Polysomnography (EEG, EMG)

(See Stores, 2000)

Assessment

Assessment requires a full psychiatric and medical history, together with detailed enquiries about the sleep complaint (Box 15.9). In several cases specialist investigation is necessary (see Stores 2000).

Insomnia

Transient insomnia occurs at times of stress or as 'jet lag'; short-term insomnia is often associated with personal problems, for example, illness, bereavement, relationship difficulties, or stress at work. Insomnia in clinical practice is usually secondary to other disorders, notably painful physical conditions, depressive disorders, and anxiety disorders; it also occurs with excessive use of alcohol or caffeine, and in dementia. Sleep may be disturbed for several weeks after stopping heavy drinking. Sleep problems are also common in association with any medical illness that results in significant pain or discomfort or is associated with metabolic disturbances. They may also be provoked by prescribed drugs. In about 15 per cent of cases of insomnia, no cause can be found (**primary insomnia**). People vary in the amount of sleep they require, and some of those who complain of insomnia may be having enough sleep without realizing it. For review of insomnia, see Sateia and Nowell (2004).

Assessment of insomnia

Usually the diagnosis of insomnia is made on the account given by the patient, focusing both on the nature of the sleep problem and its daytime consequences, as well as screening for psychiatric and medical disorders and use of drugs and alcohol. Sleep studies are rarely used.

Treatment of insomnia

Both pharmacological and non-pharmacological treatments can help insomnia (Sateia and Nowell 2004). Drugs have been more widely used, but are not now recommended as first-line treatment.

Sleep hygiene refers to a series of steps which are useful for all patients with insomnia and can be applied in primary care (Box 15.10). For more serious or persistent insomnia, a range of specific non-pharmacological treatments have been shown to be effective (Table 15.3). Cognitive therapy (also called **cognitive restructuring**) identifies and changes distorted cognitions about insomnia. **Stimulus control therapy** focuses on the principle that one only goes to bed when sleepy, and if not asleep within twenty minutes, to get up and engage in relaxing activity before returning to bed.

Although it may sometimes be justifiable to give a hypnotic for a few nights, demands for prolonged medication should be resisted. This is because withdrawal of hypnotics may lead to insomnia that is as distressing as

BOX 15.10 PRINCIPLES OF SLEEP EDUCATION (HYGIENE)

Sleep environment

Familiar and comfortable
Dark
Quiet

Encourage

Bedtime routines
Consistent bedtime and waking up time
Going to bed only when tired
Thinking about problems *before* going to bed
Regular exercise

Avoid

Overexcitement before going to bed
Late evening exercise
Caffeine-containing drinks late in the day
Excessive alcohol and smoking
Excessive daytime sleep
Large late meals
Too much time in bed lying awake

TABLE 15.3 Treatments for insomnia

Non-pharmacological treatments
◆ Sleep hygiene
◆ Cognitive therapy
◆ Stimulus control therapy
◆ Sleep restriction
◆ Progressive muscle relaxation
Pharmacological treatments
◆ Benzodiazepines, e.g. temazepam
◆ 'Z drugs' – zolpidem, zalepon, zopiclone
◆ Low dose sedative antidepressants, e.g. trazodone

the original sleep disturbance. Continuation of hypnotics may be associated with impaired performance during the day, tolerance to the sedative effects, and dependency. The use of hypnotic drugs is described further on p. 529. Sedative antidepressants, such as trazodone, are an alternative for short term treatment of insomnia, for example in the early stages of SSRI treatment.

Hypersomnia and excessive daytime sleepiness

Excessive daytime sleepiness is common (with a reported prevalence between 3–5 per cent) and underdiagnosed. Many cases are secondary to loss of night-time sleep. Table 15.4 shows the principal causes. For review, see Zeman *et al.* (2004). Treatment of excessive daytime sleepiness is covered in Anonymous (2004).

TABLE 15.4 Causes of excessive daytime sleepiness

Insufficient night-time sleep
Unsatisfactory sleep routines or circumstances
Circadian rhythm sleep disorders
Frequent parasomnias
Chronic physical illness
Psychiatric disorders
Pathological sleep
Narcolepsy
Obstructive sleep apnoea
Other central nervous system disease
Drug effects
Kleine–Levin syndrome
Depressive illness

Narcolepsy

Narcolepsy usually begins between the ages of 10 and 20 years, though it may start earlier. Onset is rare after middle age. The prevalence is about 5 per 10,000. The key features are **cataplexy** (sudden, brief episodes of paralysis with loss of muscle tone), which occurs in most cases, and sleep paralysis and hypnagogic hallucinations, which occur in only a quarter of patients. It usually presents with excessive sleepiness or the consequences of cataplexy (e.g. collapse), and has major effects on lifestyle. For review, see Zeman *et al.* (2004).

Aetiology of narcolepsy

Many aetiological theories have been advanced. Evidence favours a complex genetic predisposition, although occasional families with apparent autosomal dominant transmission are known. The strongest genetic association is with HLA DR2 tissue type; specifically, the HLA DQB1*0602, present in over 85 per cent of cases compared with 18–35 per cent in the general population. The association suggests an autoimmune mechanism.

The **hypocretins** (also called **orexins**) are hypothalamic neuropeptide transmitters which regulate the sleep–wake cycle. Recent evidence strongly implicates them in narcolepsy, especially cases with cataplexy. In these individuals, concentrations of hypocretin-1 and hypocretin-2 are decreased in the brain and cerebrospinal fluid, and there are fewer hypocretin-positive cells in the hypothalamus.

Assessment of narcolepsy

Narcolepsy usually presents to neurologists. The differential diagnosis is from other causes of excessive daytime sleepiness, and occasionally epilepsy, schizophrenia, or chronic fatigue syndrome. Psychiatric referral may occur if the latter are suspected. A full history, especially a sleep history, is the main assessment tool. The Epworth sleepiness scale is often used. Sleep laboratory studies, if available, are valuable. Measurement of HLA status or hypocretin levels in CSF are not routine.

Psychiatric aspects of narcolepsy

Strong emotions sometimes precipitate cataplexy. Patients with narcolepsy often have secondary emotional and social difficulties, and their difficulties are increased by other people's lack of understanding.

Treatment of narcolepsy

Patients need considerable help in adjusting to a disabling chronic illness. They should be encouraged to follow a regular routine with planned naps during the day. If stressful events or other factors (e.g. fatigue) seem to provoke cataplexy, efforts should be made to avoid them or to arrange lifestyle to minimize their impact.

Most patients require treatment with stimulant drugs, such as dexamfetamine, which decreases sleepiness and moderately reduce the frequency of sleep attacks. More recently, modafinil, a non-amfetamine stimulant, has been introduced; it also reduces daytime sleepiness and has fewer side-effects; it has not been compared directly with amfetamines. Clomipramine and other antidepressants can also be used to decrease cataplexy.

Breathing-related sleep disorder

This syndrome consists of daytime drowsiness together with periodic respiration, recurrent apnoeas, and excessive snoring at night. It is usually associated with upper airways obstruction, hence **obstructive sleep apnoea syndrome**. The prevalence is about 4 per cent in the male population. The typical patient is a middle-aged overweight man who snores loudly. Treatment consists of relieving the cause of the respiratory obstruction and encouraging weight loss. Continuous positive pressure ventilation using a face mask is often effective. Compliance with advice is often poor. Obstructive sleep apnoea is a risk factor for stroke.

Kleine–Levin syndrome

This very rare secondary sleep disorder consists of episodes of somnolence and increased appetite, often lasting for days or weeks and with long intervals of normality between them. The combination of appetite disorder and sleep disturbance suggests a hypothalamic disorder, and an autoimmune basis has been postulated; however, there is no convincing evidence. Case series suggest that lithium may decrease the severity of the episodes.

Idiopathic hypersomnia

In this uncommon condition patients complain that they are unable to wake completely until several hours after getting up. During this time they feel confused and possibly disorientated ('sleep drunkenness'). They usually report prolonged and deep night-time sleep. Almost half have periods of daytime automatic behaviour, the aetiology of which is obscure. Most patients respond well to small doses of stimulant drugs.

Circadian rhythm sleep disorder (sleep–wake schedule disorders)

There are several forms of circadian sleep disorder of which jet lag is the most familiar. Shift-work type is a common and increasing problem whose consequences are widely underestimated. Fatigue and transient difficulties in sleeping accompany regular changes of shift, or the irregular alternation of night work and days off may lead to chronic problems of poor sleep, fatigue, impaired concentration, and an increased liability to accidents as well as adverse effects on family life. Modafinil has efficacy in these disorders, but the 'medicalization' of these conditions is controversial (Anonymous, 2004).

Parasomnias

Parasomnias are characterized by abnormal behaviour or physiological events occurring in association with sleep, specific sleep stages, or sleep-wake transitions. For review, see Mahowald *et al.* (2004).

Nightmares (dream anxiety disorder)

A nightmare is an awakening from REM sleep to full consciousness with detailed dream recall. Children experience nightmares with a peak frequency around the ages of 5 or 6 years. Nightmares may be stimulated by frightening experiences during the day, and frequent nightmares usually occur during a period of anxiety. Other causes include post-traumatic stress disorder, fever, psychotropic drugs, and alcohol detoxification.

Night terror disorder

Night terrors are much less common than nightmares. They are sometimes familial. The condition begins in childhood and usually ends there, but occasionally persists into adult life. A few hours after going to sleep, the child, whilst in stage 3–4 non-REM sleep, sits up and appears terrified. They may scream and usually appear confused. There are marked increases in heart and respiratory rates.

After a few minutes the child slowly settles and returns to normal calm sleep. There is little or no dream recall. A regular bedtime routine and improved sleep hygiene have been shown to be helpful. Benzodiazepines and imipramine have been shown to be effective in preventing night terrors, but their prolonged use should be avoided.

Sleepwalking disorder

Sleepwalking is an automatism occurring during deep non-REM sleep, usually in the early part of the night. It is most common between the ages of 5 and 12 years, and 15 per cent of children in this age group walk in their sleep at least once. Occasionally, the disorder persists into adult life. Sleepwalking may be familial. Most children do not actually walk, but sit up and make repetitive movements. Some walk around, usually with their eyes open, in a mechanical manner but avoiding familiar objects. They do not respond to questions and are very difficult to wake. They can usually be led back to bed. Most episodes last for a few seconds or minutes, but rarely as long as an hour.

As sleepwalkers can occasionally harm themselves, they need to be protected from injury. Doors and windows should be locked and dangerous objects removed. Adults with severe problems should be given advice about safety, avoidance of sleep deprivation, and any other circumstances that might make them excessively sleepy (for example, drinking alcohol before going to bed).

Other parasomnias

Rapid eye movement (REM) sleep behaviour disorder is a parasomnia which should be considered when behavioural problems, particularly agitation or aggression, occur during the night. It is thought to occur when the normal atonia of REM sleep is lost so that dreams are acted out. It is more common in the elderly, particularly men, and is associated with neurological disorders, particularly those associated with parkinsonism. Clonazepam and donepezil may be effective.

Sleep paralysis is an inability to perform voluntary movements in the transitions between sleep and wakefulness, either at sleep onset (hypnagogic) or awakening (hypnopompic). The episodes are often accompanied by extreme fear.

Further reading

Cooper M (2003) *A psychology of bulimia nervosa: a cognitive perspective*. Oxford University Press, Oxford. (Highly readable account of key cognitive psychological issues in bulimia.)

Fairburn C and Brownell K (2001) *Eating disorders and obesity. a comprehensive handbook*. Guilford Press, London. (Comprehensive and authoritative coverage of all eating disorders.)

Kryger MH, Roth T, Dement WC (2000) *Principles and practice of sleep medicine*. Saunders, Philadelphia. (Covers methodology and major areas of sleep medicine including psychiatric aspects.)

Palmer, B (2000) *Helping people with eating disorders*. (A clinical guide to assessment and treatment.) John Wiley, Chichester.

CHAPTER 16

Psychiatry and medicine

Chapter contents

Introduction

This chapter considers the relevance of psychiatry to the rest of medical practice. It is organized as follows:

1. Psychiatry, medicine and the concept of mind–body dualism
2. Epidemiology of psychiatric disorder in medical settings
3. Comorbidity: the co-occurrence of psychiatric and medical conditions
4. Medically unexplained symptoms: somatic symptoms unexplained by medical conditions
5. Services and consultation–liaison psychiatry
6. Psychiatric aspects of specific medical conditions.

This chapter should be read in conjunction with other chapters, especially the chapters on stress related and adjustment disorders, and neuropsychiatry.

Psychiatry, medicine, and mind–body dualism

Patients usually attend their doctors because they are concerned about symptoms which are causing distress and/or dysfunction, that is, when they have an illness. Medical assessment is directed to making a diagnosis for the illness, and this diagnosis is used to guide the plan of management. The diagnosis is conventionally defined as either medical or psychiatric.

Medical diagnosis

Most medical diagnoses are based symptoms and physical signs and the results of biological investigations that together indicate the presence of bodily pathology (abnormal structure and/or function) which is referred to as disease. Not all medical diagnoses are arrived at in this way (e.g. migraine) and ultimately a medical diagnosis is a label for a condition that is conventionally treated by medical doctors and listed in classifications of disease such as ICD-10.

Psychiatric diagnosis

Psychiatric diagnosis was discussed earlier and the following brief account is intended to remind the reader of that discussion. A psychiatric diagnosis, like a medical one, is essentially a label for a condition that is conventionally treated by doctors, sometimes psychiatrists but also other practitioners. Psychiatric diagnoses are listed in the classifications of disease, along with medical diagnoses, but although some have associated physical pathology, many do not. Because they generally lack known pathology, they are generally referred to as disorders rather than diseases.

In the past, psychiatric diagnoses have been regarded as 'mental' in nature, in contrast to the 'physical' nature of medical diagnoses. This distinction reflects the absence of gross pathology in most psychiatric disorders, and the fact that these conditions usually present with disturbed mental states or behaviour rather than physical symptoms. (Presentations with physical symptoms are considered later in this chapter).

Medicine, psychiatry, and dualism

Underlying this division of illnesses into physical and mental, is the assumption that a parallel distinction can be made in healthy people – that there is 'mind–body dualism', an idea commonly attributed to the philosopher Descartes. So-called Cartesian dualism has and continues to exert a profound influence on Western medical thinking (see Brown, 1989). Whilst this division has some utility it can also be problematic.

Limitations of dualism

Dualism is at best an oversimplification as it can be convincingly argued that there are no such things as purely physical or psychological conditions, whether in health or illness. The associated assumption that psychological symptoms indicate psychopathology and physical symptoms physical pathology leads to the categories shown in Table 16.1. Two of these, disease and disorder have been considered, the other two – comorbidity and somatization – will be considered next.

Comorbidity means the co-occurrence of two disorders. The term has been extended in the table to describe the co-occurrence of prominent mental symptoms and bodily pathology since these patients are usually given a psychiatric and a physical diagnosis (Kisely and Goldberg, 1996). In practice neither of these diagnoses may lead to effective treatment because a focus on either may lead to neglect of the other. An example

TABLE 16.1 Traditional 'dualistic' categories of mental and physical illness

	Psychological symptoms	**Physical symptoms**
Bodily pathology	*Comorbidity*	Medical disease
Psychopathology	Psychiatric disorder	*Somatization*

is the widespread neglect of depression in patients with medical disease (Sharpe *et al.*, 2004).

Somatization Some patients have somatic symptoms but no evidence of bodily pathology (DeGucht and Fischler, 2002) It is then unclear whether their illness should be categorized as medical (with presumed but unidentified somatic pathology) or as psychiatric (with assumed psychopathology). In the past these conditions were generally given the medical diagnosis of **functional illness** (function is abnormal but there is no pathology). Now these conditions are usually given the psychiatric diagnosis of **somatoform disorder**. This diagnosis implies that (i) the somatic symptoms are caused by psychopathology; and (ii) there is a hypothetical process – somatization – by which the psychopathology has caused the bodily symptoms. Such patients can therefore receive both a medical diagnosis (functional disorder) and a psychiatric diagnosis (somatoform disorder) and the resulting confusion and controversy is well illustrated by literature about the condition called Chronic Fatigue Syndrome (CFS) or Myalgic Encephalomyelitis (ME) (Sharpe, 2002).

Practical consequences of dualism

One of the consequence of this way of thinking is the professional and organizational separation of medicine and psychiatry, which makes it is difficult to provide integrated care for patients with comorbidity and those with somatoform disorders. One organizational response to this problem has been the establishment of liaison psychiatry services to general hospitals (see below).

An integrated approach

New scientific knowledge, such as the demonstration of a neural basis to many psychiatric disorders, has shown that crude dualistic thinking is untenable. Recent evidence for the effect of psychiatric disorder on the outcome of medical conditions such as myocardial infarction (Frasure-Smith, *et al.*, 1993) has pointed to the same conclusion. Mind and brain are now increasingly regarded as two sides of the same coin – the mind/brain (Granville-Grossman, 1993). This paradigm shift implies that psychiatric disorders are no more distinct from medical conditions than the higher nervous system is from the rest of the body (Sharpe and Carson, 2001). As Eisenberg (1986a) put it, psychiatry has to become less 'brain-less' and medicine less 'mindless'. Correspondingly medical and psychiatric care need to be more integrated (Mayou *et al.*, 2004).

TABLE 16.2 The biopsychosocial formulation

Biological factors
Disease
Physiology
Psychological factors
Cognition
Mood
Behaviour
Social factors
Interpersonal
Social and occupational
Relating to the health care system

For the present, however, dualism continues to shape everyday thinking and practice. Illnesses are given separate medical and psychiatric diagnoses linked to separate knowledge bases and distinct systems of care. The psychiatrist working in medical settings needs to be aware of these problems and help to address them by ensuring that not only the biological, but also the psychological and social aspects of illness are considered in every case. This is the 'biopsychosocial' approach proposed many years ago by Engel (1977). The factors to consider in a biopsychosocial formulation are shown in Table 16.2. They can be divided further into predisposing, precipitating and perpetuating causes. The last group of causes is the usual target for treatment while the first two are relevant to prevention.

Epidemiology of psychiatric disorder in medical settings

Though common in all settings, the type and presentation of psychiatric disorders differs from one medical setting to another. The most common diagnoses in each setting are shown in Table 16.3

General practice

The most common psychiatric disorders in general practice are the somatoform disorders, depression, anxiety and stress-related disorders, and substance misuse. Patients with psychosis are uncommon (Ansseau *et al.*, 2004).

Casualty departments

Deliberate self-harm is the major psychiatric problem in casualty departments. Although only a minority of

TABLE 16.3 The relative prevalence of common psychiatric disorders in medical settings other than psychiatry

	General practice	Casualty	Medical/surgical outpatients	Medical /surgical inpatients
Depression/anxiety	++	++	+++	+++
Delirium	–	+	–	+++
Alcohol misuse	++	+++	++	+++
Psychosis	+	+	–	–
Somatoform disorders	+++	+	+++	++

- rare; + uncommon; ++ common; +++ very common.

these patients have persistent psychiatric disorders, many have stress-related disorders and some have depressive disorders. Intoxication and delirium related to alcohol and drugs are also common, particularly in inner city hospitals and among people involved in accidents. Some patients with somatoform disorders and a few with factitious disorders (see p. 388) are frequent attenders at casualty departments (E. R. Williams *et al.*, 2001).

Medical and surgical outpatient clinics

About a third of people attending medical and surgical outpatient clinics have a psychiatric disorder (Carson *et al.*, 2000; Maiden *et al.*, 2003). Half of these have depressive and anxiety disorders, and most of the remainder have somatoform disorders. In both these groups, adequate recognition and treatment of the psychiatric disorder should be an integral part of management, since it has been shown to improve outcome: depression is a common cause of apparent worsening of a medical condition.

Medical and surgical wards

About 20 per cent of medical and surgical inpatients have a depressive or anxiety disorder coexisting with their medical disease; ten per cent have a significant alcohol misuse problem; and a quarter of elderly inpatients have an episode of delirium (Mayou *et al.*, 1991). Some patients with severe somatoform disorders undergo multiple investigations and even surgery before the diagnosis is made.

The presentation of psychiatric disorder in medical settings

Although psychiatric disorders commonly present in medical settings with psychological symptoms or behavioural disturbance other less obvious presentations are common. These are as: (a) somatic symptoms; (b) a medical management problem; (c) an apparent exacerbation of a medical condition.

Psychiatric disorder presenting with somatic symptoms

A significant minority of patients seen in general practice and in hospital outpatient clinics have somatic symptoms which cannot be explained by medical disease, and many of these have a psychiatric disorder (Gureje *et al.*, 1997a).

Somatic symptoms due to depressive and anxiety disorders Depression is associated with somatic symptoms, such as fatigue, weigh loss and pain, which may lead to referral to a medical specialty. Anxiety is associated with symptoms of autonomic arousal, such as palpitations, and with breathlessness and sensory symptoms. A WHO collaborative study of patients presenting to primary care in 14 countries, found a strong association between somatic symptoms and depressive and anxiety disorders in all centres, despite different cultures and health services. Also, there was a linear relationship between number of somatic symptoms and the presence of depression and anxiety disorder (Simon *et al.*, 1999). Among the anxiety disorders, panic disorder is an especially important cause of medically unexplained symptoms such as chest pain, dizziness and tingling (Katon, 1996).

Somatoform disorders Medically unexplained somatic symptoms in the absence of a depressive or anxiety disorder, are mostly diagnosed somatoform disorder (see above).

Psychiatric disorder presenting as apparent worsening of a medical condition

An exacerbation of complaints about symptoms or disablity associated with a chronic medical condition is sometimes caused by a comorbid depressive disorder.

Refusal of treatment is sometimes the first pointer to a psychiatric disorder.

Comorbidity: the co-occurence of psychiatric and medical conditions

Comorbidity of psychiatric disorders with medical conditions is important. For example, an eating disorder may greatly complicate the treatment of diabetes, and depression is a risk factor for increased mortality and morbidity following myocardial infarction.

Epidemiology

Psychiatric disorder is present in as many as a third of patients with serious acute, recurrent, or progressive medical conditions. It is difficult to ascertain the exact proportion because standard criteria for the diagnosis of psychiatric disorder incude some symptoms that can also be caused by medical illness, for example fatigue and poor sleep. Although modifications have been suggested to make the criteria more appropriate for use with people with physical as well as psychiatric disorder, none is wholly satisfactory. It is best to start with standard criteria and then use knowledge of the medical condition to decide which of the symptoms that point to psychiatric disorder could have originated in this other way. However, this approach requires skilled interviewers and is difficult to achieve on a large scale.

Suicide is easier to identify and there is an increased risk in the medically ill as compared with the general population. Asociations have been reported with cancer, multiple sclerosis, and a number of other conditions (see Harris and Barraclough, 1995).

TABLE 16.4 Psychiatric disorders that are common in the medically ill

Adjustment disorder
Major depression
Anxiety disorder:
Generalized anxiety disorder
Panic disorder
Phobic disorder
Acute stress disorder
Post-traumatic stress disorder
Somatoform disorder
Substance misuse
Eating disorder
Sleep disorder
Factitious disorder
Sexual disorders

Common associations between psychiatric and physical illness are shown in Table 16.4. See Mayou and Sharpe (1995) for a review of the epidemiology of psychiatric disorder in association with medical illness.

The importance of psychiatric comorbidity in the medically ill

A comorbid psychiatric disorder can greatly affect the impact and outcome of medical conditions, for example, in patients with ischaemic heart disease (Lesperance et al 1996) and diabetes (Ludman *et al.*, 2004). Anxiety and depression are also risk factors for non-compliance with medical treatment (see above and DiMatteo *et al.*, 2000).

The causes of psychiatric comorbidity in the medically ill

Psychiatric disorder may be present in medical patients for three main reasons:

1. by chance, as both are common.
2. the psychiatric disorder may have caused the medical condition, for example alcohol dependence causing cirrhosis of the liver.
3. the medical condition may have caused the psychiatric disorder, either through an action of the disease or its treatment on the brain; or as a reaction to the psychological impact of the medical condition or its treatment; or as a result of the social effects of the medical condition or its treatment, for example loss of employment. These factors interact with the person's premorbid vulnerability.

The medical condition and its treatment

Biological mechanisms

In addition to delirium and dementia, a number of other psychiatric disorders may be caused by effect of the medical condition on the brain. Conditions that may act in this way include acute infection, endocrine disorders, and some forms of malignancy. This resulting psychiatric condition is referred to in DSM as organic mental disorder. The principal medical conditions that may act in this way are listed in Table 16.5.

Medical treatment may also cause psychiatric disorder by its effect on the brain. Table 16.6 list some commonly used drugs that may produce psychiatric disorder as a side-effect. Other treatments associated with psychiatric disorder include radiotherapy, cancer chemotherapy, and mutilating operations such as mastectomy.

Psychological and social mechanisms

The most common means by which a medical condition can cause psychiatric disorder is by its psychologi-

TABLE 16.5 Medical conditions that may cause psychiatric disorder directly

Depression
Carcinoma
Infections
Neurological disorders (see Chapter 14)
Diabetes, thyroid disorder, Addison's disease
Systemic lupus erythematosus
Anxiety
Hyperthyroidism
Hyperventilation
Phaeochromocytoma
Hypoglycaemia
Drug withdrawal
Some neurological disorders (see Chapter 14)

TABLE 16.6 Some drugs with psychological side-effects

Drug	Side-effect
Antiparkinsonian agents	
Anticholinergic drugs (benzhexol, benztropine, procyclidine)	Disorientation, agitation, confusion, visual hallucinations
L-Dopa	Acute organic syndrome, depression psychotic symptoms
Antihypertensive drugs	
Methyldopa	Tiredness, weakness, depression
Calcium-channel blockers	
Clonidine	
Sympathetic blockers	Impotence, mild depression
Digitalis	Disorientation, confusion, and mood disturbance
Diuretics	Weakness, apathy, and depression (due to electrolyte depletion)
Analgesics	
Salicylamide	Confusion, agitation, amnesia
Phenacetin	Dementia with chronic abuse
Antituberculous therapy	
Isoniazid	Acute organic syndrome and mania
Cycloserine	Confusion, schizophrenia-like syndrome
Steroids	

cal impact. Certain types of medical condition are particularly likely to provoke serious psychiatric consequences. These include life-threatening acute illnesses and recurrent progressive conditions. Psychiatric disorder is more common in chronic medical illness when there are distressing symptoms such as severe pain, persistent vomiting, and severe breathlessness; and where there is severe disability (Mayou and Sharpe, 1995).

Patients at risk for both acute and persistent psychiatric disorder in the course of medical illness include those who:

- have developed psychological problems in relation to stress in the past
- have suffered other recent adverse life events
- are in difficult social circumstances.

The reactions of family, friends, employers, and doctors may affect the psychological impact of a medical condition. They may reduce the consequences by their support, reassurance, and other help, or they may increase it by their excessive caution, contradictory advice, or lack of sympathy.

Prevention of psychiatric disorder in the medically ill

There are three main strategies. First to **identify those at risk**, second to **minimize the negative effect** of illness by providing good medical and nursing care, and third to **detect early and treat effectively the early stages** of any psychiatric disorder. Prevention should focus on those suffering illnesses or undergoing treatments which are known to be associated with the development of psychiatric disorder, and on patients who are psychologically vulnerable as evidenced, for example, by a previous history of psychiatric disorder.

Effectiveness of psychiatric treatments in the medically ill

Clinical experience indicates that psychiatric treatments are generally effective in patients who are also medically ill. There is, however, little evidence from randomized controlled trials because comorbid patients are usually excluded - although there are a few trials of antidepressants in medically ill patients (Gill and Hatcher, 1999). Clinical experience also suggests that psychological treatments such as cognitive-behaviour therapy are effective in medically ill patients but again there is little evidence from clinical trials. There is better evidence for the benefits of 'collaborative care' in which medical and psychiatric treatment are coordinated, especially in the management of chronic medical conditions such as diabetes mellitus (Katon *et al.*, 2004).

Management of psychiatric disorder in the medically ill

Assessment

Assessment is like that for psychiatric disorder in other circumstances but with the additional need to

- be well informed about the medical condition and its treatment.
- distinguish anxiety and depressive disorders from normal emotional responses to physical illness and its treatment. Symptoms that seldom occur in normal distress (such as hopelessness, guilt, loss of interest, and severe insomnia) help to make the distinction.
- be aware that medical conditions and their treatment may cause symptoms such as fatigue and loss of appetite that are used to diagnose psychiatric disorder.
- discover each person's understanding and fears of the medical condition and its treatment.

General considerations

The nature of the medical condition and its treatment should be explained clearly and the opportunity provided for patients to express their worries and fears. The treatment for the associated psychiatric disorder is conducted using the methods appropriate for the same disorder in a physically healthy person. Careful consideration should be given to possible interactions between the proposed psychiatric treatment and the medical condition and its treatment. Treatment can often usually be given by the general practitioner or medical specialist, but more complex cases require the skills of a psychiatrist.

Medication

Hypnotic and anxiolytic drugs can give valuable short term refief when distress is severe. The indications for antidepressants are the same as those for patients who are not physically ill. The side-effects and possible interactions of the psychotropic drugs with other medication should be considered carefully before prescribing.

Psychological treatments

Explanation and advice are be part of the treatment of every patient. Cognitive behaviour therapy may be chosen to reduce distress, increase adherence to treatment, reduce disproportionate disability, and to modify lifestyle risk factors.

Somatic symptoms unexplained by somatic pathology

Somatic symptoms which are not clearly associated with physical pathology are common in the general population and in patients in all medical settings (Mayou and Farmer, 2002). Although most of these symptoms are transient, a minority are persistent and disabling, and a cause of frequent medical consultations. Some conditions that may give rise to somatic symptoms are shown in Table 16.7.

As noted already, the most common association with psychiatric disorder is with anxiety and depressive disorders, and some conditions meet the criteria for a somatoform disorder (see p. 204). A few of these patients have a factitious disorder, and a very small number are malingering. However, many of those who present to doctors with unexplained somatic symptoms do not meet the diagnostic criteria for any of these conditions. Even in these undiagnosed cases, however, psychological and social factors are often important as causes of the symptoms and as reasons for seeking help, and psychological measures are often helpful.

Terminology

Many terms have been used to describe medically unexplained somatic symptoms, and none is wholly satisfactory. These terms include hysteria, hypochondriasis, somatization, somatoform symptoms, functional somatic symptoms, and functional overlay. Some of these terms will now be considered further.

- **Somatization** The term was introduced at the beginning of the twentieth century by Stekl, a German psychoanalyst, to describe the expression of emotional distress as bodily symptoms. More recently, the term has been used to describe the disorder as well as the process producing it. Some current usage is even broader, covering the **perception** of bodily sensations as symptoms and the behaviour of consulting about them. Most usage accepts, explicitly or implicitly, Stekl's original idea that physical symptoms are an expression of psychopathology, for example 'a tendency to experience and communicate psychological distress in the form of somatic symptoms and to seek medical help for them' (Lipowski, 1988). Some definitions of somatization reject Stekl's view and use criteria that require physical symptoms to be accompanied by anxiety or mood disorder diagnosed according to standard criteria. Also, current research suggests that emotional distress and somatic symptoms are positively related rather than inversely related as they would be if they were alternative expressions of an underlying psychopathology. Because there is no agreed definition, and because of the unsubstantiated aetiological assumptions, the term somatization is unsatisfactory.

- **Somatoform disorder** is a term used originally in DSM-III to describe a group of disorders including traditional psychiatric diagnoses such as hysteria and hypochondriasis, and newly proposed categories, including somatization disorder. The somatoform disorders are discussed on pp. 204–11.
- **Functional somatic symptoms** is the term used often by physicians. It refers to a condition caused by a disturbance of bodily function without any structural pathology. The term is relatively acceptable to patients but the use of word functional (as opposed to organic) has been criticized.
- **Medically unexplained symptoms** This term has the advantage of describing a clinical problem without impying any assumptions about its causes. However it has been criticized as implying that understanding of the condition is not possible. Despite this limitation we use it in this chapter.

Epidemiology

Medically unexplained symptoms are common in the general population and in people attending primary care; and they are more frequent in women than in men (Gureje *et al.*, 1997b). Although most of these symptoms are recognized as not serious and although most are short-lived, a sizeable minority lead to distress, taking time off work, consulting doctors, and taking medication (Kroenke *et al.*, 1994).

Aetiology

Although unexplained by any physical pathology, something is known about the causes of medically unexplained symptoms. Most arise from misinterpretation of the significance of normal bodily sensations: they are interpreted as a sign of disease. Concern leads to the focusing of attention on the sensations and this leads to even greater concern, apprehension and anxiety which exacerbate and maintain the symptom. For example, awareness of increased heart rate when excited or anxious may lead to worry about heart disease, restriction of daily activities, and repeated requests for investigation and reassurance. Good communication by clinical staff can help to counter the effects of such misinterpretations.

TABLE 16.7 Some physiological sources of bodily sensations

Sinus tachycardia and benign minor arrhythmias
Effects of fatigue
Hangover
Effects of overeating
Effects of prolonged inactivity
Autonomic effects of anxiety
Effects of lack of sleep

Table 16.7 lists sources of bodily sensations that may be misinterpreted as symptoms of disease.

Predisposing factors include:

- *Beliefs about illnesss* shape a person's response to sensations and symptoms. These beliefs may be related to personal experience of illness in earlier life, to involvement in the illness of family or friends, or to portrayals of illness in the media (see Table 16.8).
- *Adverse experiences in childhood* Adults with medically unexplained symptoms commonly report adversities in childhood, for example, poor parenting and various forms of abuse.
- *Social circumstances* Medically unexplained symptoms are associated with poor socioeconomic circumstances and acute or chronic adversity.
- *Personality* Some people with medically unexplained symptoms have had concerns about bodily health going back to adolescence or earlier and these can be viewed as part of their personality.

Perpetuating factors include:

- *Behavioural factors* such as repeatedly seeking information about illness, and inactivity
- *Emotional factors* especially chronic anxiety and depression
- *The reactions of others* including doctors as well as family and friends. Doctors may inadvertently prolong the problem by failing to give clear, relevant information which takes account of the patient's individual fears and other concerns.

See Mayou and Farmer (2002) for a review of the causes of unexplained symptoms.

The classification of medically unexplained symptoms

The classification of medically unexplained symptoms has been considered from two perspectives.

TABLE 16.8 Experiences which may affect the interpretation of bodily sensations

Childhood illness, with encounters with medical services, and absence from school
During childhood, illness of close family members
Physical illness in adult life
In adult life, illness among family and friends
Accounts of illness in the media
Other sources of information about illness

1. **The medical approach** has been to identify patterns of physical symptoms such as irritable bowel syndrome and fibromyalgia. The syndromes differ somewhat in different countries, for example, low blood pressure syndrome is accepted in Germany, and *mal de foie* in France, but neither is accepted in England. These are descriptive syndromes, not aetiological entities and they overlap with other disorders (Wessely *et al.*, 1999). **Diagnostic criteria** have been produced for some of these syndromes and these criteria are useful in research and service planning.
2. **The psychiatric approach** The alternative approach is to attempt to identify psychiatric syndromes that are the basis of the symptoms. These include **anxiety and depressive disorders, somatoform disorder, and factitious disorder**. A psychiatric and a medical diagnosis can be made in the same patients: for example a patient with chest pain and no heart disease may receive a medical diagnosis of 'non-cardiac chest pain' and a psychiatric diagnosis of panic disorder, both describing the same symptoms.

Prevention of medically unexplained symptoms

Until we know more of the causes of medically unexplained symptoms, there is no solid basis for preventation. While a reduction in predisposing factors in the population such as childhood abuse and poor parenting might have some effect, if they were achievable, it is more plausible to address factors such as poor communication by doctors (Ring *et al.*, 2004) and inadequate treatment of depression and anxiety in patients who present with somatic complaints. See Hotopf (2004) for a fuller discussion of prevention.

Treatment of medically unexplained symptoms

There is rather little evidence about the effectiveness of treatments for medically unexplained symptoms. There have been some trials of medication and of cognitive-behaviour therapy, some of which are cited in the course of this chapter.

Antidepressant medication have been shown to benefit several kinds of medically unexplained symptoms including fibromyalgia and irritable bowel syndrome. Facial pain may be helped by tricyclics. This benefit is especially but not exclusively for patients with medically unexplained symptoms accompanied by marked depressive symptoms (O'Malley *et al.*, 1999).

Cognitive-behaviour therapy is moderately effective in the treatment of non-cardiac chest pain, irritable bowel, and chronic fatigue syndrome (Kroenke and Swindle, 2000).

Management of medically unexplained symptoms

Assessment

An adequate medical assessment is essential. At the end of this the physician should explain:

- the purpose and results of all investigations carried out, and why it has been concluded that there is no medical cause for the symptoms.
- That the symptoms are nevertheless accepted as real and that it makes sense to seek for other causes.

If the patient is then referred to a psychiatrist, the latter should be informed about the results of the investigations and of the way these have been explained to the patient.

The psychiatrist explores the nature and significance to the patient of the unexplained symptoms, and completes the usual psychiatric history and a mental state examination, with particular attention to:

- Previous concerns about illness
- Current beliefs about illness
- Personality
- Social and psychological problems
- Detection of a depressive or anxiety disorder.

Information should be sought from other informants as well as from the patient.

Management

The basic plan of management is the same for all medically unexplained symptoms but individual treatment plans should take account of the patient's special concerns, the type of unexplained symptoms, and any associated psychiatric disorder.

The management of chronic fatigue syndrome and some other special functional medical syndromes is dis-

BOX 16.1 BASIC PROCEDURES FOR MEDICALLY UNEXPLAINED SYMPTOMS

Emphasize that the symptoms are real and familiar to the clinician

Explain the role of psychosocial factors in all medical conditions

Offer and discuss a psychosocial explanation of the symptoms

Allow adequate time for the patient and partner/family to ask questions

Agree a treatment plan to include:

- Treatment of any minor medical problem contibuting to the symptoms
- Treatment of any associated psychiatric disorder (commonly anxiety or depression)
- If appropriate, improve fitness by graded activity
- If appropriate, diary keeping to explore the relationship between symptoms and possible psychosocial causes

cussed below. The management of somatoform disorders is described in Chapter 10.

After completing the basic procedures outlined in Box 16.1, many patients will be reassured. Those who are not reassured may seek repeated investigation and reassurance. Therfore, when all medically necessary investigations have been completed, the clinician should explain thoroughly why no further investigation is required. After this initial discussions, it is seldom helpful to engage in repeated arguments about the causes. Most patients are willing to accept at least that psychological as well as biological factors may influence their symptoms, and this acceptance can provide a basis for psychological management.

When the problem is of recent onset, explanation and reassurance are often enough. When the symptoms have been present for longer, reassurance is seldom enough, and repeated reassurance may lead to increasing requests for still more reassurance. Keeping a diary to explore the relationship of symptoms to psychosocial causes can be more convincing than further explanation.

Further treatment should be based on the formulation of the person's individual problems. The treatment plan might include, for example, antidepressant medication, anxiety management, and cognitive therapy to change the inaccurate beliefs about the origin and significance of symptoms.

Much can usually be achieved by the primary care team, and by the physicians using the basic procedures. However, chronic and recurrent problems may need to be referred to a psychiatrist or clinical psychologist for further treatment of any associated psychiatric disorder, or for cognitive therapy or dynamic psychotherapy. The psychiatrist can also help to coordinate any continuing medical care, especially when this involves several specialties and professions.

Prognosis

The prognosis for the less complex cases of fairly recent onset is good but the prognosis for chronic, multiple, or recurrent conditions is much less good. For such cases the realistic goal may be to limit disabilty and requests for unnecessary medical investigation.

For a fuller information about the management of medically unexplained symptoms, see Richardson and Engel (2004) and Mayou *et al.* (1995).

Chronic fatigue syndrome

Many terms have been used to describe this syndrome whose most prominent feature is chronic disabling fatigue: the terms include post-viral fatigue syndrome, neurasthenia, and myalgic encephalomyelitis (ME). The descriptive term chronic fatigue syndrome (CFS) is now preferred. The diagnosis requires that the illness must have lasted for least six months and that other causes of fatigue have been excluded (Fukuda *et al.*, 1994).

Chronic fatigue syndrome has a long history. In the nineteenth century the symptoms were diagnosed as neurasthenia (Wessely, 1990) and in ICD-10 the syndrome can still be recorded in this way, an option that is chosen widely in China and some other countries. The diagnostic criteria for chronic fatigue syndrome overlap with those for number of other psychiatric disorders, including depression, anxiety, and somatoform disorders.

Clinical features

The central features are fatigue at rest and prolonged exhaustion after minor physical or mental exertion. These features are accompanied by muscular pains, poor concentration, and other symptoms from the list in Table 16.9. People with this condition are commonly most concerned to avoid activity. Frustration, depression, and loss of physical fitness are common.

Epidemiology

Surveys of the general population indicate that persistent fatigue is reported by up to a quarter of the population at any one time. The complaint is common amongst people attending primary care and medical outpatient clinics. However, only a small proportion of people who complain of excessive fatigue meet the diagnostic criteria for chronic fatigue syndrome. Estimates of prevalence are between 0.3–1 per cent of the general population (Jason *et al.*, 1999).

Aetiology

The aetiology of chronic fatigue syndrome is controversial. Suggested factors include:

- *Biological causes.* Several biological causes have been proposed, including chronic infection, immune dysfunction, a muscle disorder, neuroendocrine dysfunction, and ill-defined neurological disorders. There is no convincing evidence for any of these causes, except infection which may act as a precipitating factor.
- *Psychological and behavioural factors.* These appear to be important, especially concerns about the significance of symptoms, the resulting focusing of attention on symptoms, and avoidance of physical mental and social activities that worsen them. Many patients are depressed and/or anxious.
- *Social factors.* Stress at work is sometimes important. Belief that there must be a physical cause may be influenced by the stigma attached to a psychiatric diagnosis; and by some of the information provided by patient groups and practitioners.

TABLE 16.9 Case definition of chronic fatigue syndrome (Fukuda *et al.*, 1994)

Inclusion criteria
Clinically evaluated, medically unexplained fatigue of at least 6 months that is: ◆ of new onset (not lifelong) ◆ not result of ongoing exertion ◆ not substantially alleviated by rest ◆ a substantial reduction in previous level of activities
The occurrence of 4 or more of the following symptoms: ◆ subjective memory impairment ◆ sore throat ◆ tender lymph nodes ◆ muscle pain ◆ joint pain ◆ headache ◆ unrefreshing sleep ◆ post-exertional malaise lasting more than 24 hours
Exclusion criteria
Active, unresolved or suspected disease
Psychotic, melancholic or bipolar depression (but not uncomplicated major depression)
Psychotic disorders
Dementia
Anorexia or bulimia nervosa
Alcohol or other substance misuse
Severe obesity

An alternative approach to aetiology is to consider predisposing, precipitating, and perpetuating factors:

- **Predisposing** factors include a past history of major depressive disorder and perhaps personality characteristics such as perfectionism.
- **Precipitating factors** include viral infection and life stresses.
- **Perpetuating factors** may include neuroendocrine dysfunction, emotional disorder, attribution of the whole disorder to physical disease, coping by avoidance, chronic personal and social difficulties, and misinformation from the media and other sources.

See Wessely *et al.* (1998) for more information. Chronic fatigue syndrome in children is considered on p. 686.

Course and prognosis

For established cases, the long-term outcome is poor. However, it must be remembered that the most studies of prognosis relate to patients referred to specialist centres who may have experienced fatigue for a long time before the referral. Also, most studies refer to prognosis before modern treatments (see below) were widely used.

Treatment

Many treatments have been suggested but very few are of proven efficacy. There have been several randomized controlled trials of cognitive-behavioural therapy and of graded exercise regimes which have shown the benefits of these procedures over standard medical care alone, and over relaxation therapy (Whiting *et al.*, 2001).

Management

Assessment

As with all medically unexplained conditions, assessment should exclude treatable medical or psychiatric cause of chronic fatigue. It is important to enquire carefully about depressive symptoms, especially as patients may not at first reveal them. Although extensive medical investigations are unlikely to be rewarding, the psychiatrist can usefully collaborate with a physician when assessing these patients. The formulation should refer to any relevant aetiological factors (see above).

Starting treatment

The six basic steps are to:

1. acknowledge the reality of the patient's symptoms and the disability associated with them;
2. provide appropriate information about the nature of the syndrome to the patient and to the family;
3. present the aetiological formulation as a working hypothesis to be tested, not argued over;
4. treat identifiable depression and anxiety;
5. encourage gradual return to normal functioning by overcoming avoidance and regaining the capacity for physical activity;
6. help with any occupational and other practical problems.

Medication

When there is a definite evidence of a depressive disorder, antidepressant drugs should be prescribed in usual doses. Clinical experience suggests that selective serotonin re-uptake inhibitor (SSRI) drugs are best tolerated. Antidepressant drugs are also useful in reducing anxiety, improving sleep, and reducing pain.

Psychological treatment

On the simplest level, these include education about the condition, and the correction of misconceptions about cause and treatment. Cognitive behavioural methods include addressing misconceptions about the nature of the condition and excessive concerns about activity; and encouraging a gradual increase in activity. Associated personal or social difficulties can be addressed using a problem-solving approach.

See Afari and Buchwald (2003) and Wessely *et al.* (1998) for reviews of chronic fatigue syndrome.

Irritable bowel syndrome

Irritable bowel syndrome is characterized by abdominal pain or discomfort, with or without an alteration of bowel habits, persisting for longer than three months in the absence of any demonstrable disease. There are operational diagnostic criteria - the Rome criteria (Thompson *et al.*, 1999).

Epidemiology The condition occurs in as many as ten percent of the general population (Wilson *et al.*, 2004), the majority of whom do not consult a doctor.

Aetiology The cause of the syndrome is uncertain although there appears to be a disturbance of bowel function and sensation. Depressive and anxiety disorders are common among people who attand gastroenterology clinic with irritable bowel syndrome, especially among those who fail to respond to treatment.

Treatment People with mild symptoms usually respond to education, reassurance about the absence of serious pathology, change in diet and, when required, antimotility drugs. More severe and chronic symptoms may need additional treatment. Both dynamic psychotherapy and cognitive–behavioural therapy have been shown to be of benefit, and so have antidepressant drugs (Raine *et al.*, 2002).

See Ringel *et al.*(2001) for a review of irritable bowel syndrome.

Fibromyalgia

The term fibromyalgia refers to a syndrome of generalized muscle aching, tenderness, stiffness, and fatigue, often accompanied by poor sleep. An operational definition has been published by the American College of Rheumatology (Wolfe *et al.*, 1990). A physical sign of multiple specific tender points has been described but it is probably non-specific. Women are affected more than men, and the condition is more common in middle age. The aetiology is uncertain but there is a marked association with depression and anxiety. Controlled trials have shown the value of antidepressants (O'Malley *et al.*, 2000) and of behavioural interventions, especially those including increased exercise (Sim and Adams, 2002).

See Thompson *et al.* (2003) for review of fibromyalgia.

Factitious disorder

DSM-IV defines factitious disorder as the 'intentional production or feigning of physical or psychological symptoms which can be attributed to a need to assume the sick role'. The category is divided further into cases with psychological symptoms only, those with physical symptoms only, and those with both. In factitious disorder, symptoms are feined to enable the person

TABLE 16.9 Some other symptoms and syndromes that may be medically unexplained

Facial pain
Back pain
Non-cardiac chest pain
Palpitation
Vertigo
Non-ulcer dyspepsia
Environmental allergy
Forearm pain (repetitive strain injury)
Gulf War syndrome

to adopt a sick role and obtain medical care (in malingering symptoms are feigned to obtain other kinds of advantage - see below). The term **Munchausen's syndrome** denotes an extreme form of this disorder (described below).

Epidemiology The prevalence of factitious disorder is not known with certainty, but it accounts for about one percent of referrals to consultation liaison services. The disorder usually begin before the age of 30.

Aetiology The cause is uncertain, in part because many of these people give histories that are inaccurate. There is often a history of of parental abuse or neglect; of chronic illness in early life with many encounters with the medical services, sometimes long periods in hospital, and sometimes alleged medical mismanagement. Previous substance misuse, mood disorder, and personality disorder are other common features. Many patients have worked in medically related occupations.

Prognosis is variable but the condition is usually long lasting. Few patients accept psychological treatment, but some improve during supportive medical care. In some cases there is evidence of other disturbed behaviours, including abuse of children and (on the part of those working in health professions), harm to patients.

Management

Assessment When factitious disorder is suspected, the available information should be reviewed carefully, including the history given by informants as well as that provided by the patient. A psychiatrist may be able to assist in this assessment, and in cases of doubt further specialist medical investigation may be needed. Additional evidence may be obtained by careful observation of the patient, but the ethical and legal aspects of any proposal to make covert observations should be considered most carefully.

Starting treatment When the diagnosis has been made, the doctor should explain to the patient the findings and discuss their implications. This should be done in a way that conveys an understanding of the patient's distress and makes possible a discussion of potential psychosocial causes. Although some patients admit at this point that the symptoms are self-inflicted, others persistently deny this. In the latter cases, management should still be directed to helping the patient identify and overcome associated psychological and social difficulties, in the hope that improvement in such problems may be followed eventually by a lessening of the factitious disorder. Staff who have been caring for the patient while the investigations were being carried out, may become angry when they discover that the patient has deceived them. Such feelings make management more difficult and the psychiatrist should play a part in resolving them through discussion, and by explaining the nature and severity of the patient's psychosocial problems. All closely involved staff should be involved in agreeing a treatment plan which defines what future medical care, and what help with the associated problems is needed, both for the patient and or the family. Special risks and difficult ethical problems may arise when the patient is a healthcare worker - see Box 16.2.

See Bass and Gill (2000) for a review of factitious disorder

BOX 16.2 HEALTHCARE WORKERS WITH FACTITIOUS DISORDER

Highly publicized cases of serious physical harm to patients caused by a small number of healthcare workers with factitious disorder, or by those producing fictitious disorder by proxy, have aroused great public concern. It is essential, therefore, in the management of these patients to consider the risk to others if the patient continues to work in healthcare.

These infrequent cases can present difficult medicolegal problems. If the diagnosis is in doubt, it may be judged necessary to seek additional evidence by searching the patient's belongings for items (such as needles or medication) that could have been used to simulate symptoms. In general it is it unethical to search patients' belongings without first explaining the reason and obtaining permission. If the patient refuses to be searched, and there is a serious risk to others should the diagnosis be missed, it usually appropriate to obtain advice from one or more experienced professionals, including a medico-legal opinion. Advice may be needed also when judging risk and, when the risk is serious and, when the patient refuses to allow discussion with the employers, in deciding whether to breach confidentiality.

Munchausen's syndrome

Richard Asher (Asher, 1951) suggested the term Munchausen's syndrome for an extreme form of factitious disorder in which patients attend hospital with a false but plausible and often dramatic history suggesting serious acute illness. Often the person is found to have attended and deceived the staff of many other hospitals, and to have given a different false name at each. Many of these people have scars from previous (negative) exploratory operations.

People with this disorder may obstruct efforts to obtain information about them and some interfere with diagnostic investigations. When further information is obtained,especially that about previous hospital attendence, the patient often leaves. The aetiology and long-term outcome of this puzzling disorder are unknown.

Factitious disorder by proxy

In 1977, Meadow described a form of child abuse in which parents (or other carers) give false accounts of symptoms in their children, may fake signs of illness and seek repeated medical investigations and needless treatment for the children (Meadow 1985). (Despite the name, it is not a factitious disorder as defined in DSM-IV.)

The signs reported most commonly are neurological signs, bleeding, and rashes. Some children collude in the production of the symptoms and signs. The perpetrators usually have severe personality disorder and some have a factitious disorder. Hazards for the children include disruption of education and social development. The prognosis is probably poor for both children and perpetrators, and there is a significant mortality. Occasional cases of murder of children by professional carers have been described as an extreme form of this disorder; some of these people had factitious disorder (see Box 16.2).

The condition is rare and diagnosis should be made with great caution and only after the most careful investigation. In the UK, a number of high profile legal cases have highlighted the danger of diagnosis on insufficient positive evidence and without adequate exclusion of other causes of the child's symptoms.

Malingering

Malingering is not a medical diagnosis but a description of behaviour. The term denotes the deliberate simulation or exaggeration of symptoms for the purpose of obtaining some gain such as financial compensation. The distinction from factitious disorder and from somatoform disorder can be difficult because it requires an accurate understanding the person's motives.

Malingering is infrequent and most often encountered among prisoners, the military, and people seeking compensation for accidents. Several kinds of clinical picture have been described:

- malingered medical conditions and disability;
- malingered psychosis, seen in those wishing to obtain admission to hospital for shelter or to prolong their stay in hospital; and in criminal defendants trying to avoid standing trial or to influence sentencing;
- malingered or exaggerated post-traumatic stress disorder;
- malingered cognitive deficit;

Ganser's syndrome (p. 215) is thought by some to be a form of malingering.

Assessment

Assessment depends on careful history taking and clinical examination, and a watch for discrepancies in the person's behaviour. Lawyers or insurers sometimes use surveillance by video or other means to detect the behaviour but, for ethical reasons, clinicians seldom do. Psychological tests have been used to aid detection, but none is of proven validity.

Management

When malingering is certain, the patient should be informed tactfully and his situation discussed non-judgementally. He should be encouraged to deal more appropriately with any problems that led to the behaviour, and in appropriate cases offered some brief face-saving intervention as a way to give up the symptoms.

See (Sharpe 2003) for a review of malingering.

Services

Psychiatric services for general hospitals are named and organized in several ways:

Consultation-liaison psychiatry (sometimes known as C-L psychiatry or as **liason psychiatry**) is the traditional term. In **consultation** work, the psychiatrist is available to give opinions on patients referred by physicians and surgeons. In **liaison** work the psychiatrist is a member of a medical or surgical team, and offers advice about any patient to whose care he feels able to contribute. The liaison psychiatrist also assists other staff to deal with day-to-day psychological problems encountered in their work, including the problems of patients whom staff have discussed but the psychiatrist has not interviewed.

Psychological medicine is a general term for the use of consultation and liaison methods with help to enable medical and nursing staff to provide basic psychological and psychiatric care (see Mayou *et al.*, 2004).

Behavioural medicine is the term for similar arrangements provided by clinical psychologists rather than psychiatrists.

Psychosomatic medicine is a term used widely in the past in the US and elsewhere, and still current in Germany. It has been revived in the USA as the name for consultation–liaison psychiatry as a recognized subspeciality of psychiatry (Gitlin *et al.*, 2004).

The make-up of services

Consultation and liaison units vary in their size and organization. Some are staffed entirely by psychiatrists, and others by a multidisciplinary team of psychiatrists, nurses, social workers, and clinical psychologists. A few liaison services have inpatient beds for patients who are both medically and psychiatrically ill. In a few North American hospitals with large consultation–liaison services, up to 5 per cent of all admissions are referred to psychiatrists. In the UK and many other countries, a smaller proportion of inpatients are referred, most being emergencies especially deliberate self-harm (see Chapter 17). Most of the literature on consultation–liaison psychiatry has focused on inpatients, but most of the patients referred are from outpatient clinics and emergency departments.

Consultation–liaison psychiatry is increasingly concerned with the provision of psychiatric and psychological assessment, and the collaborative management of patients with either medically unexplained symptoms or psychiatric disorders comorbid with chronic medical illness. A major challenge is to find ways of extending these overstretched services to similar patients treated in primary care.

For further information about consultation and liaison psychiatry and psychosomatic medicine see Kornfeld (2002).

Psychiatric consultation in a medical setting

The consultation has two parts: the **assessment** of the patient and **communication** with the patient and with the doctor making the referral. Assessment is similar to that of any other patients referred for a psychiatric opinion with the addition that it is necessary to take into account their medical condition and treatment, and their willingness to see a psychiatrist.

First steps

Having received the request for a consultation, the psychiatrist should make sure that the referring doctor has adequately discussed the psychiatric referral with the patient and that the latter has agreed to see the psychiatrist. Before interviewing the patient, the psychiatrist should read the relevant medical notes and ask the nursing staff about the patient's mental state and behaviour. The psychiatrist should find out what treatment the patient is receiving, and if necessary consult a work of reference about the side-effects of any drugs.

The assessment interview

At the start of the interview the psychiatrist should make clear to the patient the purpose of the consultation. It may be necessary to discuss the patient's concerns about seeing a psychiatrist (for example, it does not imply that they are mad) and to explain how the interview may contribute to the treatment plan (by adding another kind of expertise to their medical care).

Next, an appropriately detailed history is obtained and the mental state examined. Usually the medical status is already recorded in the case notes. Occasionally it will be necessary to perform some physical examination, for example of the nervous system.

After the interview, it may be necessary to ask further questions of the ward staff or a social worker, to interview relatives, or to telephone the family doctor and enquire about the patient's social background and any previous psychiatric disorder.

Clinical notes

The psychiatrist should keep separate full notes of the examination of the patient and of interviews with informants. The entry in the medical notes should be different from these psychiatric notes. It should be brief and free from psychiatric jargon, and should contain only information essential for those caring for the patient. As far as possible it should omit confidential information, focus on practical issues, and answer the questions raised by the referring doctor.

Writing the response to the referral

It is often appropriate to discuss the proposed plan of management with the consultant, ward doctor, or nurse in charge before writing a final opinion. In this way the psychiatrist can make sure that recommendations are feasible and acceptable, and that answers have been given to the questions asked about the patient.

The entry the medical notes should be along the lines of a letter to a general practitioner (see p. 62). It is important to make clear the nature of any immediate treatment that is recommended, and who is to carry it out. If the assessment is provisional until other informants have been interviewed, the psychiatrist should state when the final opinion will be given. The note should be signed legibly, and should tell the ward staff where the psychiatrist or a deputy can be found should further help be required.

Management

Treatment is similar to that of a similar psychiatric disorder in a medically well patient. However, when psychiatric drugs are prescribed, special attention should be paid to the possible effects of the patient's medical condition on their metabolism and excretion, and to any possible interactions with other drugs that the patient is taking. The plan should be based on a realistic assessment of the amount of supervision available on a medical or surgical ward, for example, for a depressed patient with suicidal ideas. With support from a psychiatrist the nursing staff can manage most brief psychiatric disorders that arise in a general hospital although some support may be needed from a psychiatric nurse (who may be a member of the consutation–liason team).

Continuing care

The psychiatrist may need to review the patient' progress whilst in hospital. After discharge it is important to attempt to ensure continuity of care by speaking or writing to the general practitioner. According to the needs of the case, care may be continued by the general practitioner, or the liason psychaitrist may continue to see the patient, or care may be transferred to the community psychiatric team.

Some common emergency problems

General approach

The successful management of any psychiatric emergency depends importantly on the initial clinical interview. The aims are those of any assessment interview: to establish a good relationship with the patient, elicit information from the patient and other informants, and observe the patient's behaviour and mental state. A relaxed, sympathetic and firm approach helps to calm the situation enough for the doctor to reach an understanding of the patient's concerns and suggest a plan that the patient will agree. In an emergency, it may not be possible to conduct a full assessment interview, but the assessment should be as systematic and as complete as the circumstances permit (see also p. 53).

The anxious patient

Panic attacks The somatic symptoms of a panic attack are frequent reasons for an emergency presentation. Common features include non-cardiac chest pain, tingling in the extremities, and the effects of hyperventilation (see p. 192). Most patients can be talked through an episode of panic, and **hyperventilation** responds to rebreathing into a paper bag. Occasionally a small dose of a benzodiazepine is needed to control the anxiety. Follow up with treatment for panic disorder (see p. 194) may be required.

Severe generalized anxiety may complicate any medical presentation. Attendance at an emergency department can be a frightening experience and the consequent anxiety may be made worse by the response of unaware staff. It is usually possible to reduce the anxiety by explaining what is happening in a sympathetic manner. Occasionally a small dosage of a benzodiazepine may be required to control the anxiety.

The angry patient

It can be very upsetting to clinicians and other carers when the person they are trying to help responds with anger. When this happens, it is essential to keep calm and avoid doing or saying anything that may increase the person's anger, and to be careful about physical safety (see below). The clinician should try to find out and understand why the person is angry. Sometimes it is helpful to comment on the anger and to ask directly why the person is so upset. It is always unwise either to show anger in return or to be unduly submissive. It may be necessary to apologize for the problem that has caused the anger, for example, if the patient has been kept waiting for a long time.

The aggressive or violent patient

If the patient is actually or potentially violent, it is essential to arrange for adequate but unobtrusive help to be available. Physical contact (including physical examination) should not be attempted unless the purpose has been clearly understood by and agreed with the patient. If restraint cannot be avoided, it should be accomplished quickly by an adequate number of people using the minimum of force. Staff should not attempt single-handed restraint. Extreme caution is, of course, required if the patient could be in possession of an offensive weapon. Aggressive and violent patients are discussed also on p. 52.

Emergency drug treatment of disturbed or violent patients

Diazepam (5–10 mg) may be useful for a patient who is frightened. For a more disturbed patient, rapid calming is best achieved with 2–5 mg haloperidol injected intramuscularly and repeated, if necessary, up to a usual maximum of 30 mg in 24 hours depending upon the patient's body size and physical condition. When distress and agitation are particularly severe, it may be helpful to combine haloperidol with a benzodiazepine. When the patient has become calm, haloperidol may be continued in smaller doses, usually three to four times a day and preferably by mouth, using syrup if the patient will not swallow tablets. The dosage depends on the patient's weight and on the initial response to the drug. Careful observations by nurses of the physical state and behaviour are necessary during this treatment. Extrapyramidal side-effects may require treatment with an antiparkinsonian drug (see p. 534).

Problems in consent to treatment

General principles relating to consent to treatment are discussed in Chapter 4. Psychiatrists are sometimes asked to advise about patients who are refusing to accept medical or surgical treatment. There are several reasons why patients may be unwilling to accept treatment that is recommended to them. They may not have understood the information they have been given, they may be frightened or angry or, occasionally, they may have a mental illness that interferes with their ability to make an informed decision.

It has to be accepted that a conscious mentally competent adult has the right to refuse treatment even after a full and rational discussion of the reasons for carrying it out. When the patient's condition is such that he cannot give consent, then in the UK and many other countries, the doctor in charge of the patient has the right to give immediate treatment in life-threatening emergencies The medico-legal issues are summarized in Box 16.3.

See Boland *et al.* (2000) for a review of the management of psychiatric syndromes in intensive care units. See Strain *et al.* (2000) for a review of ethical issues in the care of the medically ill.

BOX 16.3 MEDICO-LEGAL AND ETHICAL ISSUES: PATIENTS WHO REFUSE TO ACCEPT ADVICE ABOUT EMERGENCY TREATMENT

- *In life-threatening emergencies* where it is not possible to obtain the patient's consent (consciousness is impaaired, or there is evidence of psychiatric disorder which cannot be immediately assessed), opinions should be obtained from medical and nursing colleagues, and, if possible, from the patient's relatives. Detailed records should be kept of the reasons for the decision. It is essential for all doctors to know the law about these matters in the country in which they are practising.
- If a patient has a *mental disorder that impairs the ability to give informed consent*, it may be appropriate to use legal powers of compulsory assessment and treatment of the mental disorder. In the UK, the powers for compulsory treatment of a mental disorder do *not* give the doctor a right to treat concurrent physical illness against the patient's wishes. However, after successful treatment of the psychiatric disorder, the patient may decide to give informed consent for the treatment of the physical illness.

Psychiatric aspects of medical procedures and conditions

Genetic counselling

Genetic counselling about the reproductive risks of hereditary disease is mainly given to couples contemplating marriage, or planning or expecting a child. Such counselling is made easier if the prior testing was carried out in ways that minimize distress (see Box 16.14). Counselling includes:

- providing information about risks,
- helping people to cope with concerns about the diagnosis,
- enabling patients to take informed decisions about family planning.

Counselling should be non-directive, allowing those counselled to make decisions for themselves after receiving complete and up-to-date information. Counselling may be required also for anxiety felt while awaiting the results of prenatal tests, for distress before and after termination of pregnancy for medical reasons, for concerns about being a carrier, and for worry about any children at risk of an inherited disorder.

Usually, counselling is an opportunity to allay anxiety and to reassure, but sometimes it is necessary to help a couple to confront distressing facts and make difficult decisions. The latter kind of counselling requires an awareness of the couple's circumstances and beliefs, and knowledge of the likely effects of the information provided.

After giving information about risk, the counsellor should discuss alternative actions with the couple. These actions include effective contraception and, where possible, prenatal diagnosis with the posibility of termination. Decisions about termination can be very distressing, especially for couples who have experienced a previous abnormal pregnancy. Many of these couples choose to keep the pregnancy, accepting that their future children will be at high risk.

While those who find that they or their possible children have a genetic predisposition to disease may be very distressed, it is uncommon for this distress to be of the severity of a psychiatric disorder. Nevertheless, some need counselling and this may be needed also by family members who have been told the results of the testing.

Decisions about this and other aspects of genetic counselling should be guided by an understanding of the ethical issues. Some common ethical problems are listed in Box 16.5.

BOX 16.4 GOOD PRACTICE IN GENETIC TESTING

Good practice of genetic testing includes the following:

- *A written protocol* for the testing programme that sets out how the laboratory tests are to be conducted, and how communication with patients is to be arranged.
- *Clear information* Before people are asked to decide whether to be tested, they should receive clear information about the advantages and disadvantages of testing, and the meaning of any possible test result.
- *Enough time* to decide. The initial offer of a test should be separated by a day or more from the taking of a biological sample.
- *Explain the results* and offer support to those tested and to their relatives.
- *Assess the programme* The testing programme should be assessed for its effectiveness in achieving good understanding and facilitating behaviours that reduce risk, without producing high levels of distress or false reassurance.

BOX 16.5 GENETIC COUNSELLING: SOME ETHICAL AND LEGAL ISSUES

- *Consent* to testing.
- *Confidentiality* of test results.
- *Children*: It is generally thought wise to delay testing until an age at which the young person is mature enough to make the decisions.
- Safeguards about the storage and use of genetic information.
- *Wider implications* of the results, for example for life insurance.

See Svenson and Folstein (2000) for a review of the psychological aspects of testing for genetic disorders.

Screening for disease

Presymptomatic screening include prenatal screening for foetal abnormalities, and screening for breast and cervical cancers and for hypertension. The success of any programme depends in part upon the psychological factors which determine whether people attend for screening, and whether those who attend are distressed by the experience. Most people cope well with a positive result. A negative result does not always allay anxiety, and screening may increase fears about health, especially in people recalled for further assessment. Psychiatrists can contribute to screening programmes by assisting in staff training, by helping in the production of information for patients, and by assessing and treating the most distressed patients.

See Rimes and Salkovskis (2000) for a review.

Psychiatric aspects of surgical treatment

Pre-operative problems

Patients about to undergo surgery are often anxious, and those who are most anxious before operation are likely to be anxious afterwards. Most studies of psychological preparation for surgery have shown that it can reduce post-operative distress, especially when the preparation includes measures to improve coping.

Psychiatrists may be asked to assess patients before surgery. Common reasons for such a request include:

- clarification of the role of emotional factors in the patient's physical complaints;
- uncertainty about the patient's cognitive state and capacity to provide informed consent;
- help in the management of current psychiatric problems;
- help in predicting the patients' response to surgery and their capacity to cooperate with post-operative treatment and rehabilitation.

Psychiatric problems in the post-operative period

Delirium

Delirium is common after major surgery, especially in the elderly (Brown and Boyle, 2002). Whether delirium develops depends on the type of surgery, the type of anaesthetic, the presence of post-operative physical complications, and the type of medication. Delirium is associated with increased mortality and longer stay in hospital.

Pain

Psychiatrists are sometimes asked to advise on the management of patients with unusually severe post-operative pain. Patients who are given greater control over the timing of analgesia usually experience less pain and make less use of analgesia Some are helped by anxiety management, and others by help in resolving anger arising, for example, from disagreements with the staff who are caring for them.

Long-term psychological problems after surgery

Adjustment problems are particularly common after mastectomy and laryngectomy, and after surgery that has not led to the expected benefit. Psychiatrists can sometimes contribute to the management of such problems, especially when the surgery is part of the treatment of a relapsing, chronic, or progressive disorder. The psychiatrist may help to discover psychosocial factors that are impeding adjustment, and to help the patient resolve or come to terms with the problems. Some patients require antidepressant medication.

See Rodin and Abbey (2000) and Stoddard *et al.* (2000) for reviews.

Plastic surgery

People with physical deformities often suffer embarrassment and distress and this may markedly restrict their lives as children and as adults. When such patients are psychiatrically healthy, plastic surgery usually gives good results. Even when there is no major objective defect to match the concerns about appearance, cosmetic surgery to the nose, face, and breasts is usually successful. Nevertheless, psychological assessment can contribute to assessment before plastic surgery: the outcome is likely to be poor in patients who have delusions about their appearance, dysmorphobia or greatly unrealistic expectations, or have been dissatisfied with previous surgery. See Sarwer *et al.* (1998) for a review.

Limb amputation

Limb amputation has different psychological consequences for young and for elderly people. Young adult amputees, such as those losing a leg in a road accident or in military action, characteristically show denial at first, and may later experience depression and phantom limb pains which resolve slowly. Children and adolescents seem to have a similar outcome. Older people usually undergo amputation after prolonged problems associated with vascular disease. Such patients do not commonly report severe distress immediately after the operation, but they often develop phantom limb pain. Some have difficulty with the prosthesis and show a degree of functional incapacity disproportionate to their physical state.

Organ transplantation

These operations have considerable associated psychiatric consequences related to the nature of the surgery, the need for continuing intensive medical care.

Selection for transplantation The selection process can be stressful, and so can the wait for a suitable organ, though the latter tends to be less so for kidney transplants because there is the alternative of continuing dialysis during the waiting period. There are few psychological contraindications for these operations, mostly relate to inability to cope with the demands of the necessary long-term post-operative care. After operation, transplantation is associated with the same psychiatric and emotional problems that occur after other major surgery, especially anxiety, delirium and depression. There are also some problems specific to a particular type of transplant; for example, liver transplantation has the highest rate of pre- and post-operation neuropsychiatric complications.

These problems are sufficiently frequent and serious to justify psychiatric liaison with transplant units in order to support staff and train them to recognize and respond appropriately to patients who have such problems.

See Trzepacz and DiMartini (2000) and House (2000) for reviews of psychiatric aspects of transplantation.

Diabetes

Diabetes mellitus

Diabetes is a chronic condition requiring prolonged medical supervision and informed self-care, and many physicians emphasize the psychological aspect of treatment.

Psychological factors and diabetic control

Psychological factors are important in established diabetes because they influence its control, and it is now generally accepted that good control of blood glucose is the most important single factor preventing long-term complications. Psychological factors can impair control in two ways. First, stressful experiences can lead to endocrine changes. Second, many diabetics do not adhere well to their treatment regime, especially at times of stress, and this is an important cause of 'brittle' diabetes.

Problems of being diabetic

Psychological and social problems may be caused by restrictions of diet and activity, the need for self-care, and the possibility of serious physical complications such as vascular disease and impaired vision. Although most diabetic people overcome or adapt to such problems, an important minority have difficulties. Adherence to regimes for testing, diet, and insulin is often unsatisfactory so that glycaemia control is less than optimal. Problems of this kind are particularly likely in adolescence.

Other problems

Associated eating disorder Control of diabetes is more difficult when the diabetic person has an eating disorder. Also, some women with diabetes and eating disorders misuse insulin to lose weight.

Associated medical complications Psychosocial problems are more than usually common in diabetics who have severe medical complications such as loss of sight, renal failure, and vascular disease.

Sexual problems are common among diabetics. Two kinds of impotence occur in diabetic men. The first is psychogenic impotence of the kind found in other chronic debilitating diseases. The second kind is more common in diabetes, and may predate other features of the disease. It is thought to be associated with pelvic autonomic neuropathy and vascularity, while endocrine factors may play a part.

Pregnancy is a difficult time for diabetic women with problems in the control of diabetes and increased risks of miscarriage and foetal malformations.

Organic psychiatric syndromes in diabetic patients

Delirium The first evidence of developing diabetic coma is sometimes an episode of disturbed behaviour, starting either abruptly or insidiously. The cause of the behaviour becomes clearer as other prodromal symptoms develop, including thirst, headaches, abdominal pain, nausea, and vomiting. The pulse is rapid and blood pressure is low. Dehydration is marked and acetone may be smelt on the breath.

Chronic cognitive impairement Mild dementia is not uncommon among those with chronic diabetes. It may be caused by recurrent attacks of hypoglycaemia or by cerebral arteriosclerosis. More severe dementia may develop in patients with associated cerebrovascular disease.

Psychiatric aspects of management

Possible measures include treatment for depressive disorder; blood glucose awareness training to improve the ability to recognize and act on fluctuations in blood glucose concentrations; weight management programmes; cognitive–behavioural approaches to improve self-care; help with psychosocial problems; and treatment of sexual dysfunction. Tricyclic antidepressants may be helpful in relieving the pain of neuropathy. See Jacobson (1996) for a review of psychological care of patients with insulin-dependent diabetes.

Other endocrine disorders

Many endocrine disorders, and most conspicuously thyroid dysfunction, have been associated with psychiatric complications. Box 16.6 summarizes some of the more common associations, together with aspects of steroid therapy.

See Kornstein *et al.* (2000) for a review of the psychiatric aspects of endocrine disorder.

BOX 16.6 PSYCHIATRIC ASPECTS OF OTHER ENDOCRINE DISORDERS AND STEROID THERAPY

Hyperthyroidism (thyrotoxicosis) May present with psychiatric symptoms such as anxiety, irritability, emotional lability, and difficulty in concentrating. These, together with hyperactivity, fatigue and tremor, may make differential diagnosis from anxiety disorder difficult. Treatment of thyroid dysfunction usually results in improvement of the psychiatric symptoms.

Hypothyroidism (myxoedema) Cognitive impairment and other psychiatric disorders are common. Mood disorder may take a rapid-cycling form (see p. 225). Replacement therapy may reverse the mood symptoms but neuropsychiatric problems may persist. See Dugbartey (1998) for a review.

Hyper-adrenalism (Cushing's syndrome) Depressive symptoms are common. Their severity is not closely related to plasma cortisol concentrations, and personality and stressful circumstances may play a part. Psychological symptoms usually improve quickly when the medical condition is controlled. Paranoid symptoms also occur, especially in those with the most severe illness. See W. F. Kelly (1996) and Sonino and Fava (1998).

Steroid therapy Affective symptoms, especially euphoria or mild mania, are frequent. Paranoid symptoms are less common. The **severity of the mental disorder is not** closely associated with dosage. Symptoms usually improve when the dosage is reduced but, when severe, lithium prophylaxis should be considered for patients who need to continue steroid treatment after a mood disorder has been controlled. Withdrawal of corticosteroids may cause lethargy, weakness, and joint pain.

Anabolic steroids Anabolic-androgenic steroids are widely used by athletes. Mood disturbances and increased aggression have been reported. (See Wroblewska, 1997; W. F. Kelly, 1996; Sonino and Fava, 1998).

Other metabolic and auto-immune disorders

Psychiatric aspects of the porphyrias, sarcoidosis, systemic lupus erythematosis, and myaesthenia gravis are considered in section 5.3.4 of the *New Oxford Textbook of Psychiatry* (Gelder *et al.*, 2000).

Cardiac disorders

For many years, it has been suggested that emotional disorder predisposes to ischaemic heart disease and Dunbar (1954) described a 'coronary personality'. Recent research has concentrated on several possible risk factors including chronic emotional disturbance, social and economic disadvantage, overwork and other chronic stress, and the so-called type A behaviour pattern. The latter consists of hostility, excessive competitive drive, ambitiousness, a chronic sense of urgency, and a preoccupation with deadlines (Friedman and Rosenman, 1959). Although type A behaviour has been widely accepted as an independent risk factor for ischaemic heart disease, recent evidence has cast doubt on this conclusion.

Angina

Angina is often precipitated by emotions such as anxiety, anger, and excitement. It is a frightening symptom, and some patients become overcautious despite reassurance and encouragement to resume normal activities. Angina is sometimes accompanied by atypical chest pain and breathlessness caused by anxiety or hyperventilation, and it is important to identify this rather than increasing medical anti-angina therapy.

Myocardial infarction

Patients often respond to the early symptoms of myocardial infarction with denial, and consequently delay in seeking treatment. In the first few days in hospital, acute organic mental disorders and anxiety symptoms are common.

Recent research has concentrated on the replicated finding that depression, anxiety, and social isolation are important risk factors for both a lower quality of life (Ruo *et al.*, 2003) and for death after MI (Frasure-Smith *et al.*, 1993, 2000).

Some survivors of cardiac arrest suffer cognitive impairment. When such impairment is mild, it may show up later as apparent personality change or as behavioural symptoms which may be attributed wrongly to an emotional reaction to the illness.

When patients return home from hospital, they commonly report non-specific symptoms such as fatigue, insomnia, and poor concentration, as well as excessive concern about somatic symptoms and an unnecessarily cautious attitude to exertion. Most patients overcome these problems and return to a fully active life. A few continue with emotional distress and social disability out of proportion to their physical state, often accompanied by atypical somatic symptoms. Such problems are more common in patients with long-standing psychiatric or social problems, overprotective families, and myocardial infarction with a complicated course.

The finding that depression and social isolation are associated with increased mortality after MI has led to research to evaluate interventions to treat depression and to reduce social isolation. In the large trials so far completed, nursing support to combat social isolation was ineffective. Cognitive–behaviour therapy (Berkman *et al.*, 2003) and antidepressant drugs (Glassman *et al.*, 2002) are effective in treating depression after MI but do not increase survival (Frasure-Smith *et al.*, 1997).

Non-cardiac chest pain

During the American Civil War, Da Costa (1871) described a condition which he called 'irritable heart'. This syndrome consisted of a conviction that the heart was diseased, together with palpitations, breathlessness, fatigue, and inframammary pain. This combination has also been named 'disorderly action of the heart', 'effort syndrome', and 'neurocirculatory asthenia'. The symptoms were originally thought to indicate a functional disorder of the heart.

Non-cardiac chest pain, in the absence of heart disease and often associated with complaints of breathlessness and palpitations, is very common among patients in primary care and in cardiac outpatient clinics. Most patients with the symptoms are reassured by a thorough assessment, but a significant minority continue to complain of physical and psychological symptoms and to limit their everyday activities. Follow-up studies of patients with chest pain and normal coronary angiograms have consistently found subsequent mortality and cardiac morbidity to be little greater than expectation, but persistent disability to be common.

Many causes have been suggested for atypical cardiac symptoms including pain originating in the chest wall, oesophageal reflux and spasm, microvascular angina, mitral valve prolapse, and psychiatric disorder. In most patients chest pain appears to be due to minor non-cardiac physical causes or to hyperventilation, which are misconstrued as heart disease and associated with anxiety. The aetiology is as for other medically unexplained symptoms (see p. 384). The most common psychiatric concomitant is panic disorder; less common are depressive disorder and hypochondriasis.

Management should follow the general principles described on p. 385 with a particular emphasis on the treatment of hyperventilation, graded increase in activity, and discussion of beliefs about the cause of the pain. Cognitive-behaviour therapy may be effective in the management of anxiety with hyperventilation. Depressive disorder should be treated with antidepressant medication. See Chambers *et al.* (1999) for a review.

Sensory disorders

Deafness

Deafness may develop before speech is learned (prelingual deafness) or afterwards. Profound early deafness interferes with speech and language development, and with emotional development. Prelingually deaf adults often keep together in their own social groups and communicate by sign language. When they have problems, it appears that these are more often behaviour problems and social maladjustment than emotional disorder. These problems are managed best by those with special knowledge of the effects of deafness.

Deafness of later onset has less severe effects than those just described. However, the acute onset of profound deafness can be extremely distressing, whilst milder restriction of hearing may cause depression and considerable social disability.

Kraepelin was the first to suggest that deafness is an important factor in the development of persecutory delusions.Subsequent evidence supports an association between deafness and paranoid disorders in the elderly (see p. 309). See Hindley and Kitson (1999) for a review.

Tinnitus

Tinnitus is very common, but few patients seek treatment and most are able to live a normal life. Persistent tinnitus may be associated with low mood. Some patients are helped by devices that mask tinnitus with a more acceptable sound. Antidepressant medication may improve mood and reduce the intensity of the tinnitus (Sullivan *et al.*, 1993). Cognitive and behavioural methods may enable people to accept their tinnitus and to minimize their social handicaps.

Blindness

Although it imposes many difficulties, blindness in early life need not lead to abnormal psychological development in childhood or to unsuccessful later development. In previously sighted people, the later onset of blindness often causes considerable distress. Initial denial and subsequent depression are common, as are prolonged difficulties in adjustment. See Fitzgerald and Parkes (1998).

Infections

Acute infections Psychological factors may affect the course of recovery from an acute infection (Hotopf *et al.*, 1996). In a classic early study, psychological tests were completed by 600 people who subsequently developed Asian influenza. Delayed recovery from the influenza was no more common among people whose initial illness had been severe, but it was more frequent among those who had obtained more abnormal scores on the psychological tests before the illness (Imboden *et al.*, 1961). More recent findings of research on viral illness in general practice and infectious mononucleosis have reported similar conclusions (see White *et al.*, 1998). The role of infection as a cause of chronic fatigue syndrome is discussed on p. 387.

Viral encephalitis is often accompanied by psychiatric symptoms. In addition, some infectious diseases, for example hepatitis A, influenza, and brucellosis, are frequently followed by periods of depression and fatigue.

HIV infection

HIV infection affects the brain at an early stage and the disease has a chronic progressive course associated with a wide range of psychiatric consequences. Even so, many patients with AIDS manage to lead relatively normal lives for substantial periods. The nature of the physical symptoms, their progressive course, and the reactions of other people all explain why emotional distress is common in people with HIV infection. A further reason is that some of those at high risk for HIV (for example, drug abusers) may have other psychological problems. Effeccts on the family may be considerable, especially where the partner and or one or more of the children are infected. Women may be concerned about the effects of the infection on childbearing. Psychiatrists can contribute to the care of AIDS patients by providing counselling and specialist treatment for neuropsychiatric and other psychiatric complications

Reactions to testing Although HIV antibody testing is worrying for most of those who undergo it, the distress is usually short-lived whatever the outcome of the test. People who have persistent and unjustified worries about having AIDS require psychiatric help of the kind appropriate for other illness fears (see p. 184).

Psychiatric problems including adjustment disorder, depressive disorder, and anxiety disorder are frequent at the time of diagnosis though they may occur at any stage of the disease. People with previous psychological problems, long-standing social difficulties, or lack of social support are especially vulnerable.

Suicide and deliberate self-harm may occur in people who are concerned about the possibility of HIV infection as well as in people with proven disease. Among the latter, the risk is greater in those with advanced symptoms. However, it is not certain how much greater is the risk of suicide and deliberate self-harm in AIDS patients than in the general population.

Neuropsychiatric disorders are common, both secondary to the complications of immune suppression and as direct effects of HIV on the brain. Minor cognitive disorders are frequent. HIV associated dementia (AIDS-dementia complex), HIV encephalopathy, and subacute encephalitis occur late in the illness in around a third of patients. There is usually an insidious onset with progression to profound dementia. HIV infection can also result in neurological symptoms and dementia in those who do not have AIDS. Delirium may occur when there is an opportunistic infection or cerebral malignancy. See Maj (2000) for a review of dementia associated with HIV infection.

Social consequences are considerable because of the public fears of the condition and stigma. Cultural differences in acceptance or rejection, and in the availability of family and other support are major determinants of quality of life.

Problems in relation to illicit drug use are considered on p. 453. The disorganized way of life of some drug users and their personal and social problems make the treatment of HIV difficult.

Ethical problems are related to confidentiality: the importance of maintaining confidentiality; disclosure to third parties who are at risk of infection; disclosure to insurers and to employers; and protection of the public from risk of transmission from HIV-infected healthcare workers.

See Bialer *et al.* (2000) and Grant and Atkinson (2000) for reviews of the psychiatric aspects of HIV infection.

Cancer

The psychological consequences of cancer are similar to those of any other serious physical illness:

- Delay in seeking medical help because fear or denial.
- *Response to the diagnosis* which may be anxiety, shock, anger, disbelief or depression. Sometimes the response is severe enough to meet the criteria for a psychiatric disorder, usually an adjustment disorder or sometimes a depressive disorder. The risk of suicide is increased (Harris and Barraclough, 1995).
- *Later consequences* Major depression occurs throughout the course of cancer affecting 10–20 per cent of patients and appears to be more frequent in those suffering pain. The rate is similar to that among other physically ill patients (Holland, 1998).
- *The progression and recurrence* of cancer are often associated with increased psychiatric disturbance, which may result from a worsening of physical symptoms such as pain and nausea, from fear of dying, or from the development of an organic psychiatric syndrome.
- *Delirium and dementia* may arise from brain metastases, which originate most often from carcinoma of the lung, but also from tumours of the breast and alimentary tract, and from melanomas. Occasionally, brain metastases produce psychiatric symptoms before the primary lesion is discovered. (See also Chapter 14.)
- *Neuropsychiatric problems (para-neoplastic syndromes)* are sometimes induced by certain kinds of cancer in the absence of metastases, notably by carcinoma of the lung, ovary, breast, stomach and Hodgkin's lymphoma. The aetiology is thought to be an autoimmune response to the tumour. (See also Chapter 14.)

Treatment for cancer may cause psychological disorder. Emotional distress is particularly common after mastectomy and other mutilating surgery. *Radiotherapy* causes nausea, fatigue, and emotional distress. *Chemotherapy* often causes malaise and nausea, and anxiety about chemotherapy may cause anticipatory nausea before the treatment. The latter may be helped by behavioural treatments in addition to anti-emetic medication.

Family and other close relatives of cancer patients may experience psychological problems, which may persist even if the cancer is cured. Nevertheless, many patients and relatives make a good adjustment to cancer. The extent of their adjustment depends partly on the information they receive.

Treatment for psychological consequences

In the past doctors were reluctant to tell patients that the diagnosis was cancer, but most patients prefer to know the diagnosis and how it will affect their lives. However, the information must be communicated well, otherwise there may be problems in achieving a psychological adjustment. Depression and anxiety disorders are often missed in these patients and systematic screening has been recommended (Sharpe *et al.*, 2004).

Cognitive behavioural approaches can help these patients adjust (Sheard and Maguire, 1999). Patients most likely to need such help include those with a history of previous psychiatric disorder or poor adjustment to other problems, and those who lack a supportive family.

Childhood cancer

Childhood cancer presents special problems. Communication of the diagnosis is particularly difficult but it is generally better to explain the diagnosis in terms appropriate to the child's stage of development. The child often reacts to the illness and its treatment with behaviour problems. Many parents react at first with shock and denial, and may take months to accept the full implications of the diagnosis. Some mothers develops an anxiety or depressive disorder and other family members may be affected. In the early stages of the illness parents are usually helped by advice about practical matters, and later by discussions of their feelings, which often include guilt. Adult survivors of cancer in childhood or adolescence appear to be at risk of social difficulties.

See Rouhani and Holland (2000), Roth *et al.* (2000), and Holland (1998) for reviews of psychiatric aspects of cancer.

Accidents

Psychiatric associations

Psychiatric disorder predisposing to accidents This is often through cognitive impairment occuring , for example, in alcohol or drug intoxication, delirium or dementia.

Psychiatric disorder caused by accidents includes adjustment disorder, anxiety and depressive disorders, and post-traumatic stress disorder. Avoidance of situations associated with the accident is common and may be severe enough to meet diagnostic criteria for phobic anxiety disorder. **Head injury** may cause specific cognitive disorders (see p. 351).

Associations with particular kinds of accident

Criminal assault can have especially severe and persistent consequences for victims (Acierno *et al.*, 1997). Victims' problems are discussed further on p. 162.

Road traffic accidents are the leading cause of death in people aged under 40 and a major cause of physical morbidity. ***Psychiatric factors contributing*** to road accidents include the misuse of alcohol and drugs, psychiatric illness, suicidal and risk-taking behaviour, and the side-effects of some prescribed psychotropic drugs. **Psychiatric consequences** include acute stress disorder, anxiety and depressive disorders, post-traumatic stress disorder, phobias of travel, and disorders caused by brain injury. Some of these conditions are transient, but others persist and may cause considerable disability. Most of those affected do not seem to have been psychologically vulnerable before the accident (see Hickling and Blanchard, 1999).

Occupational injury The psychiatric consequences of occupational injury resemble those of other accidents. It is sometimes alleged that hopes of compensation or other benefits help to maintain the symptoms and disability – see Compenation neurosis below.

Spinal cord injury Around a quarter of patients admitted to a spinal injury unit suffer from psychiatric problems requiring treatment. Depression is common in the period immediately after a spinal cord injury but usually improves with time. Nevertheless, suicide appears to be more common among these patients than in the general population.

Burns In children, burns are associated with overactivity, learning disability, child abuse and child neglect. In adults, burns are associated with alcohol and drug misuse, deliberate self-harm, and dementia. Severe burns and their protracted treatment may cause severe psychological problems. Hamburg *et al.* (1953) described three stages:

- *Stage 1* lasts days or weeks; denial is common. The most frequent psychiatric disorders are organic syndromes. At this stage the relatives often need considerable help.
- *Stage 2* is prolonged and painful; here denial recedes and emotional disorders are more common. Patients need to be helped to withstand pain, to express their feelings, and gradually accept disfigurement.
- *Stage 3* the patient leaves hospital and has to make further adjustments to deformity or physical disability and the reaction of other people to his appearance.

Post-traumatic stress disorder is common among those with severe burns and persistent anxiety and depression occur in more than a third. The outcome is worse for patients with burns affecting the face. Such patients are likely to withdraw from social activities. These patients need considerable support from the staff of the burns unit, but only a minority also require referral to a psychiatrist.

See Bernstein (2000) for a review.

'Compensation neurosis'

The term compensation neurosis (or accident neurosis) refers to psychologically determined physical or mental symptoms occurring when there is an unsettled claim for compensation. From his experience as a neurologist, Miller (1961) claimed that such psychological factors were important in claims for persistent physical disability after occupational injuries and road accidents. He emphasized the role of the compensation claim in prolonging symptoms and suggested that settlement was followed by recovery. More recent evidence has failed to substantiate this extreme view.

In fact many accident victims do not claim compensation, and few become involved in prolonged litigation. However, it does appear that time off work and disability are affected by the type of accident, social factors, and the prospect of compensation, social security, or other benefits. It has usually been assumed that settlement of a compensation claim is followed by improvement. However, this assumption is not supported by follow-up studies (Mendelson, 1995).

See Malt (2000) for a review of the psychiatric aspects of accidents, burns, and other trauma.

Psychiatric aspects of obstetrics and gynaecology

Pregnancy

Psychiatric disorder is more common in the first and third trimesters of pregnancy than in the second. In the *first trimester* unwanted pregnancies are associated with anxiety and depression. In the *third trimester* there may be fears about the impending delivery or doubts about the normality of the foetus. Psychiatric symptoms in pregnancy are more common in women with a history of previous psychiatric disorder and probably also in those with serious medical problems affecting the course of pregnancy, such as diabetes. Although minor affective symptoms are common in pregnancy, serious psychiatric disorders are probably less common than in non-pregnant women of the same age.

Some **women who had chronic psychological problems before being pregnant** report improvement in these problems during pregnancy whilst others require extra psychiatric care. The latter are often late or poor attenders at antenatal care, thus increasing the risk of obstetric and psychiatric problems. Misuse of alcohol, opiates, and other substances should be strongly discouraged in pregnancy, especially in the first trimester when the risk to the foetus is greatest (see p. 524). Eating disorders do not appear to be precipitated by pregnancy, and bulimic symptoms may improve.

Great care must be taken in the use of psychotropic drugs during pregnancy and while breastfeeding – see Chapter 21 (p. 524).

Hyperemesis gravidarum

About half of all pregnant women experience nausea and vomiting in the first trimester. Some authors have suggested that these symptoms, as well as the severe condition of hyperemesis gravidarum, are primarily of psychological aetiology but this has not been established. It is, however, probable that psychological factors influence the severity and course of the symptoms.

Pseudocyesis

Pseudocyesis is a rare condition in which a woman believes that she is pregnant when she is not, and develops amenorrhoea, abdominal distension, and other changes similar to those of early pregnancy. The condition is more common in younger women. Pseudocyesis usually resolves quickly once diagnosed, but some patients persist in believing that they are pregnant. Recurrence is common. Only rarely is the condition associated with a psychiatric disorder.

Couvade syndrome

In this syndrome, the husband of the pregnant woman reports that he is himself experiencing some of the symptoms of pregnancy. This condition may occur in the early months of the woman's pregnancy, when the man complains usually of nausea and morning sickness and often of toothache. These complaints generally resolve after a few weeks.

Termination of unwanted pregnancy

In the past, psychiatrists in the UK were often asked to see pregnant women who were seeking a therapeutic abortion on the grounds of mental illness. The provisions of current legislation in the UK and many other countries now make it generally more appropriate for decisions to be made by the family doctor and the gynaecologist, without involving a psychiatrist. Nevertheless, psychiatric opinions are still sought at times, not only about the grounds for termination of pregnancy but also for an assessment of the likely psychological effects of termination in a particular patient. Most of the evidence suggests that the psychological consequences of termination are usually mild and transient, although they are greater for mothers who have cultural or religious beliefs against termination (see Major *et al.*, 2000). See p. 393 for termination after genetic testing.

Spontaneous abortion

Approximately a fifth of diagnosed pregnancies do not progress beyond 20 weeks, mainly because of foetal defects. Friedman and Gath (1989) interviewed women 4 weeks after spontaneous abortion and found that half were psychiatric cases of depression (a rate four times higher than in the general population of women). Many women showed features typical of grief. Depressive symptoms were most frequent in women with a history of previous spontaneous abortion. Although most improve with time (Janssen *et al.*, 1996), the extent of morbidity indicates the importance of recognizing the needs of those who suffer miscarriage.

Antenatal death

Antenatal death (stillbirth) causes an acute bereavement reaction and, for some women, long-term psychiatric problems, as well as concern about future pregnancy. The parents should be helped to mourn by encouraging them to see and hold the baby, to name it, and to have a proper funeral. They may need further support after the funeral and the next pregnancy may be a particularly worrying time.

Caesarian section

Caesarian section has been said to have adverse psychological consequences for parents and infants. Most of the research has failed to test this association because it has not separated the effects of surgery from other adverse factors. However, it would seem sensible to pay particular attention to parental support and to initial bonding.

See Brockington (1998, 2000) for reviews of the psychiatric aspects of pregnancy.

Post-partum mental disorders

These disorders can be divided into minor mood disturbance (maternity blues), puerperal psychosis, and chronic depressive disorders of moderate severity.

Minor mood disturbance – 'maternity blues'

Amongst women delivered of a normal child, between half and two-thirds experience brief episodes of irritability, lability of mood, and episodes of crying. Lability of mood is particularly characteristic, taking the form of rapid alternations between euphoria and misery. The symptoms reach their peak on the third or fourth day post partum. Patients often speak of being 'confused', but tests of cognitive function are normal. Although frequently tearful, patients may not be feeling depressed at the time but tense and irritable.

'Maternity blues' is more frequent among primigravida. The condition is not related to complications at delivery or to the use of anaesthesia. 'Blues' patients have often experienced anxiety and depressive symptoms in the last trimester of pregnancy; they are also more likely to give a history of premenstrual tension, fears of labour, and poor social adjustment.

Both the frequency of the emotional changes and their timing suggest that maternity blues may be related to readjustment in hormones after delivery although this has not been established. No treatment is required because the condition resolves spontaneously in a few days.

Post-partum psychosis

In the nineteenth century, puerperal and lactational psychoses were thought to be specific entities distinct from other mental illnesses (Esquirol, 1845). Later psychiatrists such as Bleuler and Kraepelin regarded the puerperal psychoses as no different from other psychoses. This latter view is widely held today.

Epidemiology The incidence of post-partum (puerperal) psychoses has been estimated in terms of admission rates to psychiatric hospital (Kendell *et al.*, 1987). The reported rates vary, but a representative figure is one admission per 500 births. This incidence is substantially above the expected rate for psychoses in non-puerperal women of the same age. Puerperal psychoses are more frequent in primiparous women, those who have suffered previous major psychiatric illness, those with a family history of mental illness, and probably in unmarried mothers. There is no clear relationship between psychosis and obstetric factors. Puerperal illnesses are reported to be more common in developing than in developed countries, and the excess may be of cases with an organic aetiology.

Aetiology The early onset of puerperal psychoses has led to speculation that they might be caused by hormonal changes such as those discussed above in relation to the blues syndrome. There is, however, no evidence that hormonal changes in women with puerperal psychoses differ from those in other women in the early puerperium. Hence if endocrine factors do play a part, they would seem to act only as precipitating factors in predisposed women. Genetic factors, related to those involved in bipolar disorder, have been reported (Chaudron and Pies, 2003).

Clinical features

The onset of puerperal psychosis is usually within the first 1–2 weeks after delivery, but rarely in the first 2 days. Three types of clinical picture are observed: delirium, mood disorder, and schizophreniform disorder. **Delirium** was common in the past, but is now much less frequent since the incidence of puerperal sepsis was reduced by antibiotics. Nowadays **mood disorders** predominate; either bipolar disorder or schizoaffective disorder. **Schizophreniform** disorders presenting for the first time are rare. The clinical features of these syndromes are generally regarded as being much the same as those of corresponding non-puerperal syndromes.

Insomnia and overactivity are often early features. Perplexity and confusion are common.

Management

Assessment As well as the usual psychiatric assessment it is essential to ascertain the mother's **ideas concerning the baby**. Severely depressed patients may have delusional ideas that the child is malformed or otherwise imperfect. These false ideas may lead to attempts to kill the child to spare it from future suffering. Schizophrenic patients may also have delusional beliefs about the child; for example, they may be convinced that the child is abnormal or evil. Again, such beliefs may point to the risk of an attempt to kill the child. Patients with depression or schizophrenia may also make **suicide attempts**.

Treatment is given according to the clinical syndrome, as described in other chapters. Admission to hospital is normally required. It has been argued that this should be in a special mother and baby unit where the child can remain with the mother to minimize adverse effects on maternal bonding. However, it is very difficult to ensure the safety and care of the infant, and the benefits of such units for outcome have not been established. Once the admission is arranged, all contacts between mother and baby should be supervised, at first, by nursing staff and thereafter reviewed in the light of clinical progress.

Electroconvulsive therapy (ECT) is often the best treatment for patients with depressive or manic disorders of marked or moderate severity, because it is rapidly effective and enables the mother to resume the care of her baby quickly. For less urgent depressive disorders, antidepressant medication may be tried first. If the patient has predominantly schizophrenia-like symptoms, an antipsychotic drug may be prescribed; if definite improvement does not occur within a short period, ECT should be considered, especially if the onset was acute.

Prognosis

Most patients recover fully from a puerperal psychosis, but some of those with a schizophrenic disorder remain chronically ill. After subsequent childbirth the recurrence rate for depressive illness in the puerperium is approximately 20–30 per cent. According to Protheroe (1969), at least half of women who have suffered a puerperal depressive illness will later suffer a depressive illness that is not puerperal. All mothers who have suffered post-partum psychosis should be considered for special psychiatric review during any further pregnancies so that post-partum problems can be identified early and treated promptly and effectively.

Postnatal depression of mild or moderate severity

Less severe depressive disorders are much more common than the puerperal psychoses, occurring in 10 per cent of women in the early weeks post partum. Tiredness, irritability, and anxiety are often more prominent than depressive mood change, and there may be phobic symptoms. Most patients recover after 2–6 months.

Aetiology Clinical observation suggests that these disorders are often precipitated in vulnerable mothers by the psychological adjustment required after childbirth, as well as by the loss of sleep and hard work involved in the care of the baby. There is little evidence of a biological basis. The main risk factors are a previous history of depression (especially when accompanied by obstetric complications) and indications of social adversity.

Management Despite the medical and other care given to women after childbirth, many post-partum depressions are undetected or, if detected, untreated. Therefore those providing care to mother and baby need to be alert to the possibility of depression. In treatment, psychological and social measures are usually as important as antidepressant drugs. Most women can be treated effectively in primary care with support, help with solving practical problems. A small proportion need antidepressant medication, and a few with severe or complex problems require referral to the psychiatric services.

Effects on the child Postnatal depression adversely affects the infant's relationship with its mother and its early cognitive and emotional development (Stein *et al.*, 1991). Evidence of negative consequences later in childhood is less clear (See Murray and Cooper, 1997).

See Cooper and Murray (1998) for a review of postnatal depression. See Brockington (1998, 2000) for reviews of all aspects of post-partum psychological complications. See Viguera and Cohen (2000) for a review of psychopharmacology during pregnancy and the post-partum period.

Psychiatric aspects of gynaecology

Premenstrual syndrome

This term denotes a group psychological and physical symptoms starting a few days before and ending shortly after the onset of a menstrual period. The psychological symptoms include anxiety, irritability, food cravings, and depression; the physical symptoms include breast tenderness, abdominal discomfort, and a feeling of distension. Premenstrual syndrome is not included in current classifications of psychiatric disorder, although premenstrual dysphoric disorder is listed as a condition for future study in DSM-IV. The syndrome should be distinguished from the much more frequent occurrence of similar symptoms that are not strictly premenstrual in timing.

Epidemiology Estimates of the frequency of the premenstrual syndrome in the general population vary widely from 30–80 per cent of women of reproductive age. There are three main reasons for this wide variation. First, there is a problem of **definition**. Mild and brief symptoms are frequent premenstrually, and it is difficult to decide when they should be classified as premenstrual syndrome. Second, **information** about symptoms is often collected retrospectively by asking women to recall earlier menstrual periods, and this is an unreliable way of establishing the time relations. Third, the description of premenstrual symptoms is **subjective** and may be influenced by knowledge that the enquiry is concerned specifically with the premenstrual syndrome.

Aetiology The aetiology is uncertain. Biological explanations have been based on ovarian hormones (excess oestrogen, lack of progesterone), pituitary hormones, and disturbed fluid and electrolyte balance. None of these theories has been proved. Various unproven psychological explanations have been based on possible associations of the syndrome with neuroticism or with attitudes towards menstruation.

Treatment The syndrome has been widely treated with progesterone, and also with oral contraceptives, bromocriptine, diuretics, and psychotropic drugs. There is no convincing evidence that any of these is effective, and treatment trials suggest a high placebo response (up to 65 per cent). Psychological support and encouragement may be as helpful as medication. There have been encouraging reports of the effectiveness of SSRI antidepressants during the vulnerable period and of cognitive behavioural treatment.

See Blake *et al.* (1995) for a review of the syndrome and its psychological treatment.

The menopause

In addition to the physical symptoms of flushing, sweating, and vaginal dryness, menopausal women often complain of headache, dizziness, and depression. It is not certain whether depressive symptoms are more common in menopausal women than in non-menopausal women. Nevertheless, amongst patients who consult general practitioners because of emotional symptoms, a disproportionately large number of women are in the middle-age group that spans the menopausal years.

Depressive and anxiety-related symptoms at the time of the menopause could have several causes. Hormonal changes have often been suggested, notably deficiency of oestrogen. In some countries, notably the USA, oestrogen has been used to treat emotional symptoms in women of menopausal age, but the results of trials of treatment with oestrogens have been disappointing (see Pearce *et al.*, 1995). Psychiatric symptoms at this time of life could equally well reflect changes in the woman's role as her children leave home, her relationship with her husband alters, and her own parents become ill or die. It seems best to treat depressed menopausal women with methods that have been shown to be effective for depressive disorder at any other time of life

Hysterectomy

Several retrospective studies have indicated an increased frequency of depressive disorder after hysterectomy. An important prospective investigation using standardized methods (Gath *et al.*, 1982a, 1982b). showed that patients who are free from psychiatric symptoms before hysterectomy seldom develop them afterwards. Some patients with psychiatric symptoms before hysterectomy lose them afterwards, but in others they persist. It is likely that these latter, who have symptoms before and after surgery, are identified in the retrospective studies, leading to the erroneous conclusion that hysterectomy causes depressive disorder. This finding provides a general warning about inferring the effects of treatment from the results of retrospective investigations.

Sterilization

Considerations similar to those for hysterectomy apply to these procedures. Although retrospective studies suggested that sterilization leads to psychiatric disorder and sexual dysfunction, prospective enquiry has contradicted this. Indeed sexual relationships are more likely to improve than worsen, and definite regrets are reported by fewer than one person in 20.

See Robinson (2000) and Brockington (2000) for reviews of the psychological aspects of gynaecology.

Further reading

Gelder, MG, López-Ibor, JJ Jr and Andreasen, NC (eds) (2000) *The new Oxford textbook of psychiatry*. Oxford University Press, Oxford. (See Section 5 on Psychiatry and medicine by various authors.)

Rundell, JR and Wise, MG (eds) (1999) *Essentials of consultation liaison psychiatry*. American Psychiatric Press, Washington, DC. (A short reference work with brief accounts of the basic clinical issues.)

Stoudemire, A, Fogel, BS and Greenbury, D (eds) (2000) *Psychiatric care of the medical patient*, 2nd edn. Oxford University Press, New York. (A comprehensive reference book.)

Levenson, JL (ed.) (2004) *Textbook of psychosomatic medicine*. American Psychiatric Publishing, Washington DC. (A comprehensive textbook.)

Mayou, R, Sharpe, M and Carson, A (2003) *ABC of psychological medicine*. BMJ Books, London. (A collection of brief practical reviews.)

CHAPTER 17

Suicide and deliberate self-harm

Chapter contents

Suicide is among the ten leading causes of death in most countries for which information is available. In the UK it is the third most important contributor to life years lost after coronary heart disease and cancer. Over the last two decades several countries have reported a considerable increase in the number of young men who kill themselves, though in recent years there have been some signs that this trend may be reversing. The subject is important to all doctors who may at times encounter people who are at risk for suicide, and who may at times be involved in helping family or others after a suicide. The importance of the subject is reflected in national and international initiatives for suicide prevention (World Health Organization, 1998; Department of Health, 2002).

For every suicide it is estimated that that more than 30 non-fatal episodes of self-harm occur. Depression, substance misuse, and other mental health problems are more common in people who deliberately harm themselves and the rate of suicide in the year following an episodes of deliberate self-harm is some 60–100 times that of the general population (Hawton *et al.*, 2003a). The rate of suicide is also raised in the period following discharge from inpatient psychiatric care. For these reasons psychiatrists need to be particularly well informed about the nature of deliberate self-harm and suicidal behaviour, and about strategies aimed at its prevention. For reviews of all aspects of suicide and deliberate self-harm see Hawton and van Heeringen (2000).

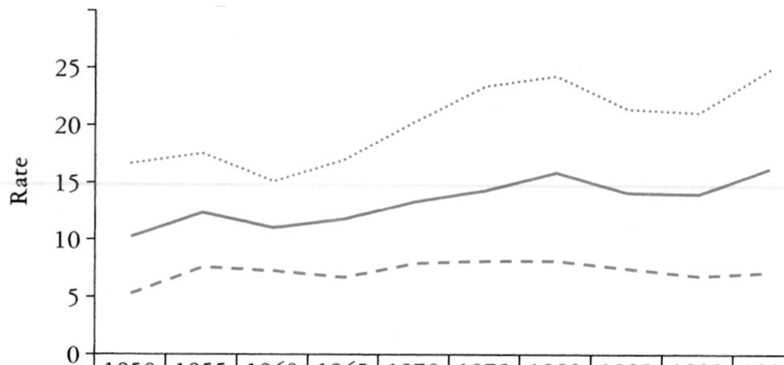

	1950	1955	1960	1965	1970	1975	1980	1985	1990	1995
········ Total	10.1	12.3	10.9	11.6	13.2	14.1	15.8	14	13.9	16
—— Males	16.6	17.5	14.9	16.7	20	23.2	24.1	21.4	21	24.7
- - · Females	5.2	7.4	7	6.7	7.7	8	8	7.4	6.8	6.9

Fig. 17.1 Global suicide rates (per 100 000), by gender, 1950–95 (selected countries indicated in Table 17.1). Reproduced with permission *World Health Organization Figures and Facts about Suicide*, World Health Organization, Geneva, 1999.

Suicide

The act of suicide

Suicide has been defined as an act with a fatal outcome, that is deliberately initiated and performed by the person in the knowledge or expectation of its fatal outcome. People who take their lives do so in several different ways. In England and Wales, in 2001, hanging was the most commonly used method for suicide by men, accounting for almost 40 per cent of all deaths, followed by drug overdose (20 per cent) and self-poisoning by car exhaust fumes (almost 10 per cent) drowning and jumping. The commonest methods for women were drug overdose (46 per cent), hanging (almost 27 per cent), and drowning (7 per cent) (Brock and Griffiths, 2003). In the USA, gunshot and other violent methods are more frequent than in the UK.

Most completed suicides have been planned. Precautions against discovery are often taken, for example, choosing a lonely place or a time when no one is expected. However, in most cases a warning is given. In a US study, suicidal ideas have been expressed by more than two-thirds of those who die by suicide, and clear suicidal intent by more than a third. Often the warning had been given to more than one person. In an important British study of people who had committed suicide (Barraclough *et al.*, 1974), two-thirds had consulted their general practitioner for some reason in the previous month, and 40 per cent had done so in the previous week. A quarter were seeing a psychiatrist, of whom half had seen the psychiatrist in the week before their suicide. More recent evidence has confirmed generally high rates of contact with mental health services in the period before suicide, though the rates among young men are lower.

The epidemiology of suicide

The accuracy of the statistics Accurate statistics about suicide are difficult to obtain because information about the exact cause of a sudden death is not always available. For example, in England and Wales, official figures depend on the verdicts reached in coroners' courts. A verdict of suicide is recorded by a coroner only if there is clear evidence that the injury was self-inflicted and that the deceased intended to kill himself. If there is any doubt about either point, a verdict of accidental death or an open verdict is recorded. Open verdicts are more often recorded when the method of self-harm is less active (e.g. drowning compared with hanging) and when the deceased is young rather than old (Neeleman and Wessely, 1997). For these reasons it is accepted that official statistics underestimate the true rates of suicide. Barraclough (1973) demonstrated that amongst people whose deaths are recorded as accidental, many have recently been depressed or dependent on drugs or alcohol, thus resembling people who commit suicide. For example, in Dublin at that time, psychiatrists ascertained four times as many suicides as did coroners, and similar discrepancies have been reported elsewhere. An attempt has been made to overcome these problems by reporting 'probable suicides', which combine deaths attributed to suicide and 'open verdicts' (Schapira *et al.*, 2001).

Differences in suicide rates For the reasons considered above, caution should be exercised when comparing rates of suicide in different time periods and between different countries. Despite this, long-standing and fairly stable differences in rates of suicide between different countries are apparent. Sainsbury and Barraclough (1968) presented indirect evidence that differences in rates of suicide among different nations are real by demonstrating that, within the USA, the rank order of suicide rates among immigrants from 11 different nations was similar to the rank order of national rates within the 11 countries of origin. The official suicide rate in the UK is in the lower range of those reported in Western countries. Generally, higher rates are reported in eastern and northern European countries, and lower rates in Mediterranean countries. Reported suicide rates are very low in Islamic countries. The sex differences are less in Asian than in Western countries. Some methods of suicide reflect local culture, for example self-immolation or ritual disembowelment (Cantor, 2000; Cheng and Lee, 2000). In Hong Kong, poisoning from carbon monoxide produced by burning charcoal has become one of the frequent methods of suicide in recent years (Leung *et al.*, 2002).

Changes in suicide rates

Suicde rates have changed in several ways since the beginning of the last century. Recorded rates for both men and women fell during each of the two world wars. There were also two periods during which rates increased. The first, 1932–33, was a time of economic depression and high unemployment; the second, between the late 1950s and the early 1960s, was not. Following this, from 1963–74, rates declined in England and Wales but not in other European countries (with the exception of Greece) nor in North America. The decline in England and Wales seems to have resulted mainly from a change in the domestic gas supply from a toxic form derived from coal to a non-toxic form from wells in the North Sea. Before this change, suicide using domestic gas had been the most frequent method of suicide.

Figure 17.2 shows changes in the rates of suicide in England and Wales from 1979 to 2001, analysed by gender and by method of suicide. It shows the higher rates in men, the increase in the category 'hanging, strangulation and suffocation' (mainly hanging), and the decrease in the category 'other poisoning' (mainly car exhaust fumes).

Variations with the seasons

In England and Wales, suicide rates have been highest in spring and summer for every decade since 1921–30. A similar pattern has been found in other countries in the northern hemisphere. In the southern hemisphere, a similar rise occurs during the spring and early summer, even though these seasons are in different months of the year. The reason for these fluctuations is not known though it has been suggested that they relate to changes in the incidence of mood disorders. In any case, there is some evidence that in England and Wales, and in some other countries, the seasonal variations have diminished in the last decade (Yip *et al.*, 2000).

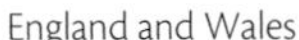

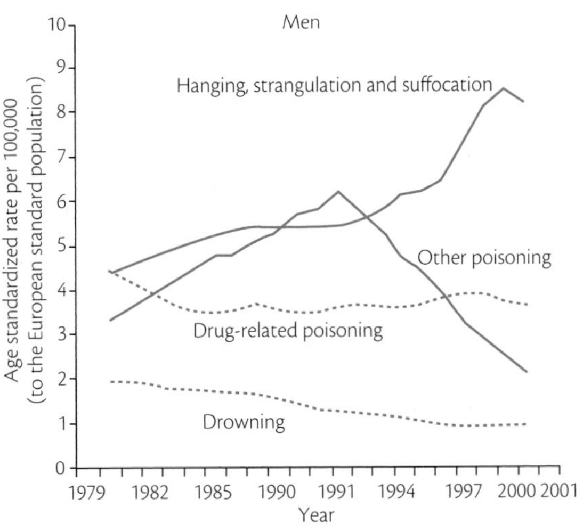

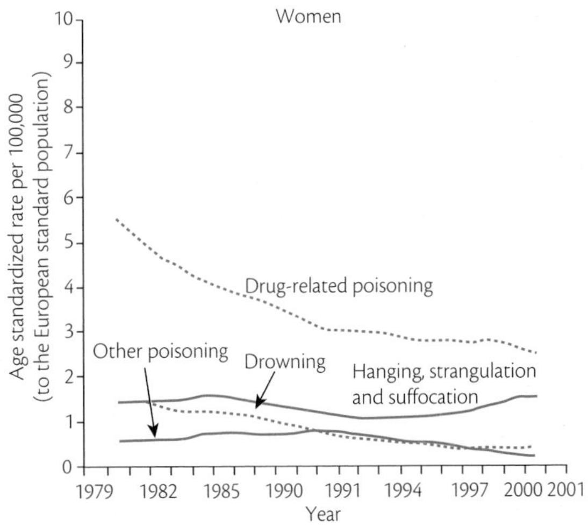

Fig. 17.2 Age-standardized rates for suicide by method of injury and sex, ages 15 and over, 1979–2001 (3-year moving average). From Brock, A and Griffiths, C (2003) Trends in suicide by method in England and Wales 1979–2001. Health Statistics Quarterly 20, 7–18.

Demographic characteristics

Suicide is about three times as common in men as in women. The highest rates of suicide in both men and women are in the elderly. Suicide rates are lower among the married than the never married, and increase progressively through widowers, widows and the divorced. Rates are higher in the unemployed than in the employed. In terms of **social class**, the highest rates are seen in social class V (unskilled workers) followed by social class I (professional), in which rates are higher than in social classes II, III, and IV. Rates of suicide are high among prisoners, especially amongst those on remand.

Rates are particularly high in certain **professions**. Veterinary surgeons have three times the expected rate, and pharmacists and farmers have double the expected rate (Charlton *et al.*, 1993). Suicide rates are also higher in doctors with higher rates among female doctors than males (Hawton *et al.*, 2001a; Schernhammer and Colditz, 2004). Suicide among doctors is discussed further on p. 413.

The causes of suicide

Methods of investigation

Investigations into the causes of suicide face several difficulties. Information concerning the health and well-being of the deceased at the time of suicide cannot be obtained directly. Prospective studies of suicide are difficult to arrange because of its relative rarity and the consequent need to study very large groups. Two strategies have been used to overcome these difficulties.

1. Retrospective studies have pieced together the circumstances that surrounded the suicide by examining records and interviewing doctors, relatives, and friends who knew the deceased well.
2. Epidemiological studies have examined associations between social and demographic factors and rates of suicide in different populations at different times.

Each approach has methodological problems. However, the first type of study, which has become known as 'psychological autopsy' study, has helped identify factors that precede suicide. The second approach has informed our understanding of social circumstances that may give rise to increased rates of suicide.

Individual psychiatric and medical factors

The most consistent finding of studies of individual factors (Table 17.1) is that the large majority of those who die from suicide have some form of mental disorder at the time of death (Barraclough *et al.*, 1974). Similar results have been reported in other countries (Cheng and Lee, 2000). The most freqent conditions are:

- **Personality disorder** which is diagnosed in up to a third to half of people who commit suicide (Foster *et al.*, 1997).
- **Mood disorder** About 6 per cent of those who suffer from a mood disorder will die by suicide. Depressed patients who die by suicide are more likely than other depressed patients to have a past history of self-harm and to have experienced a sense of hopelessness (Fawcett *et al.*, 1990). They are also more often single, separated or widowed, are older, and are more often male.
- **Alcohol misuse** Follow-up studies of patients dependent on alcohol show a continuing risk of suicide, with a lifetime risk of 7 per cent (Inskip *et al.*, 1998). Among those who are alcohol dependent, suicide is more likely when the patient is male, of older age, has a long history of drinking, and a history of depression, and of previous suicidal attempts. Suicide risk is also increased among those whose drinking has caused physical complications, marital problems, difficulties at work, or arrests for drunkenness offences.
- **Drug misuse** is relatively common among those who die by suicide, particularly in the young (Oyefeso *et al.*, 1999).
- **Schizophrenia** Suicide rate is increased among young men early in the course of the disorder, particularly when (i) there have been relapses, (ii) when there are depressive symptoms, and (iii) when the illness has turned previous academic success into failure. The lifetime risk of suicide in this group has been estimated at 7 per cent (Inskip *et al.*, 1998).

TABLE 17.1 Rates (%) of mental disorders in five psychological autopsy studies on completed suicides using DSM-III or DSM-III-R criteria

Depressive disorders	36–90
Alcohol dependence or abuse	43–54
Drug dependence or abuse	4–45
Schizophrenic disorders	3–10
Organic mental disorders	2–7
Personality disorders	5–44

From Lonnqvist, JK (2000) Epidemiology and causes of suicide. In MG Gelder, JJ López-Ibor Jr, and NC Andreasen (eds) *The new Oxford textbook of psychiatry*, Chapter 4.15.1. Oxford University Press, Oxford.

Other factors associated with suicide are a **past history of deliberate self-harm** (see p. 421) and **poor physical ill-health**, especially **epilepsy**. (See Harris and Barraclough, 1995 and Stenager and Stenager, 2000 for reviews.)

Social factors associated with suicide.

Comparisons of rates of suicide between and within different countries have been conducted over many years. None has been more influential than that conducted by Emile Durkheim at the end of the nineteenth century (Durkheim, 1951). Durkheim examined variations in the rate of suicide within France and between France and other European countries. He demonstrated that a range of social factors impact on rates of suicide. Rates were lower at times of war and revolution, and increased during periods of both economic prosperity and economic depression. This led him to the conclusion that social integration and social regulation were central to the rate of suicide. Durkheim described four types of suicide, of which one, '**anomic**' **suicide**, is most important for this discussion. It describes suicide by a person who lacks ties with other people and no longer feels part of society. (Durkheim's other types of suicide were egoistic, altruistic and fatalistic.)

More recent studies have repeatedly demonstrated that areas with **high unemployment, poverty** (Gunnel *et al.*, 1995), **divorce**, and **social fragmentation** (Whitley *et al.*, 1999) have higher rates of suicide. Whilst the results of such studies cannot be used as a means of examining the characteristics of individuals who kill themselves, they provide important information about factors within society that may affect the rate of suicide. **Cross-cultural evidence** indicates wide variation in the meaning of suicide and social attitudes to it which appear to be associated with differences in suicide rates.

Another social factor that seems to affect rates of suicide is **media coverage of suicide**. Suicide and attempted suicide rates were shown to increase after the showing of fictional television programmes and films depicting suicide (Hawton *et al.*, 1999b). Sometimes the means and timing of a suicide seem to have been influenced by the circumstances of a previous suicide that attracted attention in a community or in the newspapers or on television (Eisenberg, 1986b; Gould *et al.*, 1990).

Biological factors

A family history of suicide is associated with suicide, and adoption studies (Wender at al., 1986) indicate that this mechanism is genetic. The genetic mechanism may be independent of those giving rise to any psychiatric disorder (Roy *et al.*, 2000) and perhaps related to personality traits of impulsivity and aggression.

Suicidal behaviour has also been linked with decreased activity of brain 5-HT pathways. For example, pre-synaptic markers of 5-HT function such as CSF 5-HIAA and the density of 5-HT transporter sites are lowered in suicide victims. In contrast the density of post-synaptic 5-HT_{1A} and 5-HT_{2A} receptors is increased in prefrontal cortex; this may represent a compensatory upregulation in response to lowered 5-HT release (see Mann, 2003). The association between underactivity of 5-HT pathways and suicidal behaviour seems to extend across diagnostic boundaries and may be related to increased impulsivity and aggression in those with low brain 5-HT function (Mann, 2003). The link between 5-HT function and suicidality has prompted genetic association studies of polymorphisms in genes coding for 5-HT receptors in people with suicidal behaviour. However, reliable associations are yet to emerge (Arango *et al.*, 2003).

Psychological factors

Psychological factors in suicide have been derived mainly by extrapolation from studies of non-fatal deliberate self-harm, but the factors may not be the same. An exception is the work by Beck and colleagues who followed more than 200 patients who had been hospitalized because of suicidal ideation (Beck *et al.*, 1985). They demonstrated that people who scored highly on a measure of **hopelessness** had very high rates of suicide over the following 5–10 years. More recent work indicates other psychological variables that may be associated with suicidal behaviour – impulsivity, dichotomous thinking, cognitive constriction, problem-solving deficits, and overgeneralized autobiographical memory. All these could act by predisposing to act impulsively (Williams and Pollock, 2000).

Conclusion

The associations considered above do not, of course, establish causation. Nevertheless, they suggest three sets of interacting influences: (i) medical factors, including depressive disorder alcohol misuse, and abnormal personality, (ii) psychological factors, of which hopelessless is the strongest, (iii) social factors, especially social isolation and poverty. Personality traits of impulsivity and aggression could be important, and these may have a biological basis, possibly related to dysregulation of the 5HT system.

Special groups

Suicide among those in contact with psychiatric services

Given the strong association between mental disorder and suicide, it is no surprise that many people who kill themselves are in contact with psychiatric services. A National Confidential Inquiry set up in England and Wales collected information on all patients who, in the previous 12 months, had committed suicide while in contact with the mental health services (Appleby *et al.*, 2001). Suicide rates were higher during treatment in hospital with about a quarter of inpatient suicides occuring during the first week in hospital. About a third occured while the patient was on planned leave, and about a quarter occur within three months of discharge, most in the first two weeks and most before the first follow-up appointment. Suicides were particularly likely to occur following short admissions and when patients had taken discharge against medical advice.

Almost half of the suicide patients in the enquiry had been cared for using the Care Programme Approach (see p. 637) with multidisciplinary reviews of their progress. However, about a quarter were not collaborating with the approach at the time and a fifth were not taking prescribed medication. In nearly two-thirds, the mental health team had made special efforts to re-establish cooperation. Many of these non-cooperative patients had schizophrenia.

These findings indicate the need to:

- *Support patients intensively* during the first few weeks after discharge from hospital, with the first follow-up generally within a few days of discharge or of going on leave.
- *Plan in advance* the steps that should be taken if a patient ceases to cooperate with the treatment regime.
- *Monitor side-effects* of drugs and change to one with fewer side-effects if these seem likely to lead to refusal to take more.
- *Ward design:* Since hanging is a common method of suicide by inpatients, ensure that wards do not contain structures from which this could be effected.

To these general points can be added some specific ones concerning depressive disorder and schizophrenia.

Depressive disorder Among patients treated for depressive disorder, the risk of suicide may be increased following initial treatment as psychomotor retardation decreases. However, most patients who kill themselves have probably not been taking their antidepressant medication at the time of their death (Isacsson *et al.*, 1994). The possibility that some antidepressants may increase the risk of suicidal behaviour is considered on p. 546.

Schizophrenia The factors associated with suicide among people treated for schizophrenia include mood disorder, suicidal thoughts, concerns about the impact of the illness on mental functioning, loss events, poor compliance with medication, and drug misuse. The features of the schizophrenic illness itself appear to be less important as risk factors, except indirectly through their effect on the factors mentioned above (see Hawton *et al.*, 2005.)

Rational' suicide

Despite the findings reviewed above, suicide is occasionally the rational act of a mentally healthy person. Also, mass suicides have been described, for example by the members of a closely knit religious community, and it is unlikely that all those who died had a mental disorder. Despite these exceptions, it is a good general rule to assume, until further enquiry has proved otherwise, that a person who talks of suicide has an abnormal state of mind. If the assumption is correct - and it is sometimes difficult to identify a depressive disorder when the person is first seen - the patient's urge to die is likely to diminish when the abnormal mental state recovers. Moreover, even when the decision to die was arrived at rationally, it is still reasonable to attempt to prevent the person from self-harm. This is because the decision about suicide may have been made rationally but on false premises, and will change when the person is better informed - for example, that death from cancer need not be as painful as formerly believed.

Older people

In most countries the highest rate of suicide is among people aged over 75 years. The most frequent methods are hanging among men, and drug overdose among women (Harwood *et al.*, 2000a). In addition to active self-harm, some older adults die from deliberate self-neglect, for example by refusing food or necessary treatment. As in younger age groups, depression is a strong predictor of suicide in the elderly. Others are social isolation and impaired physical health, though the latter may act in part through causing depression (Conwell *et al.*, 2002). Personality is also important, especially anxious and obsessional traits (Harwood *et al.*, 2000b). For further information about suicide in the elderly see Harwood and Jacoby (2000).

Children and adolescents

Children Suicide is rare in children. In 1989, the suicide rate for children aged 5–14 years was estimated as

0.7 per 100 000 in the USA and 0.8 per 100 000 in the UK. Little is known about factors leading to suicide in childhood, except that it is associated with severe personal and social problems. Children who died by suicide have usually shown antisocial behaviour, and suicidal behaviour and depressive disorders are common among their parents and siblings (Shaffer, 1974). Shaffer distinguished two groups of children. The first comprised children of superior intelligence who seemed to be isolated from less educated parents. Many of their mothers were mentally ill. Before death, the children had appeared depressed and withdrawn, and some had stayed away from school. The second group consisted of children who were impetuous, prone to violence, and resentful of criticism (Pfeffer, 2000; Shaffer *et al.*, 2000).

Adolescents Suicide rates among adolescents have increased in recent years. In England and Wales the increase has been mainly in males aged 15–19 years (McClure, 2000) and the principal methods among males have been hanging and poisoning with car exhaust fumes (Hawton *et al.*, 1999a). A psychological autopsy study (Houston *et al.*, 2001) showed that about 70 per cent of adolescents who killed themselves had psychiatric disorders, mainly depressive and personality disorders which were sometimes comorbid. Many misused alcohol or drugs. The suicide was often the culmination of long-term difficulties with relationships and other psychosocial problems. Approximately two-thirds had made a previous suicide attempt. For further information see de Wilde (2000).

Ethnic groups

Rates amongst immigrants closely reflect those of their countries of origin. In the UK, there is particular concern about possible high rates amongst Asian women.

High-risk occupational groups

Doctors The suicide rate among doctors is greater than that in the general population and the excess is greater among female doctors that among males (Hawton *et al.*, 2000; Schernhammer and Colditz, 2004). Many reasons have been suggested for the excess, including the ready availability of drugs, increased rates of addiction to alcohol and drugs, extra stresses of work, reluctance to seek treatment for depressive disorders, and the selection into the medical profession of predisposed personalities. A psychological autopsy study of 38 working doctors who had died by suicide (Hawton *et al.*, 2004a) found psychiatric disorder – mainly depressive disorder and/or drug or alcohol misuse – in about two-thirds, and problems at work in a similar proportion. About a third had relationship problems, and about a quarter had financial problems. Among the methods used, self-poisoning with drugs was more common than in the general population, and half of the anaesthetists used anaesthetic agents. Both sets of factors are relevant to programmes of prevention.

Compared with doctors in general medicine, rates have been reported to be higher in anaethetists, community health doctors, general practitioners and psychiatrists (Hawton *et al.*, 2000). It is not known whether these higher rates are related more to factors in the invidual (contributing to specialty choice and to suicide rate) or to the nature of work.

Farmers also have high rates of suicide. Possible causes include the ready availability of means of self-harm (such as poisons and guns), together with stress related to work and financial difficulties (Malmberg *et al.*, 1999).

In contrast to many suggestions that **students** are a high-risk group, suicide rates are generally close to expectations for the age group in the wider population.

Suicide pacts

In suicide pacts two, or occasionally more, people agree that at the same time each will take his or her own life. Completed suicide pacts are uncommon. In Far Eastern countries, those involved are usually lovers aged less than 30 years, and in Western countries usually interdependent couples aged more than 50 years. Suicide pacts have to be distinguished from cases where murder is followed by suicide (especially when the first person dies but the second is revived), or where one person aids another person's suicide without intending to die himself.

The psychological causes for these pacts are not known with certainty. Usually the two people have a particularly close relationship but are socially isolated from others. Often a dominant partner initiates the suicide.

Mass suicide is occasionally reported, for example, 913 followers of the Peoples Temple cult died at Jamestown, Guyana in 1978 and 39 members of the Heavens Gate cult in California in 1997. These tragic events are generally initiated by a charismatic leader who has strong convictions and is sometimes deluded. Sometimes there is evidence to suggest murder followed by suicide within the group.

Recently there has been concern about the use of the internet to arrange suicide pacts (Rajagopal, 2004). See Nock and Marzuk (2000) for a review of suicide pacts.

The assessment of suicidal risk

General issues

Every doctor should be able to assess the risk of suicide. There are two requirements. The first is a willingness to make direct but tactful enquiries about a patient's intentions. There is convincing evidence that asking a patient about suicidal inclinations makes suicidal behaviour more likely. On the contrary, someone who has already thought of suicide is likely to feel better understood when the doctor raises the issue and this feeling may reduce the risk.

The second requirement is to be alert to factors that predict suicide. However, prediction based on these factors has a rather low sensitivity and specificity, and even when the risk is correctly assessed as high, it is difficult to predict when the suicide will take place. The limitations of prediction are illustrated by the study of Goldstein *et al.* (1991) who tried to develop a statistical model to predict the occurrence of 46 suicides from amongst a group of high-risk hospital patients, but failed to identify a single patient who later committed suicide.

Assessing risk

The most obvious warning sign is a direct statement of intent. It cannot be repeated too often, that there is no truth in the idea that people who talk of suicide do not enact it. On the contrary, two-thirds of those who die by suicide have told someone of their intentions. The difficulty arises with people who talk repeatedly of suicide. In time their statements may no longer be taken seriously, but instead discounted as threats intended to influence other people. However, some people who repeatedly make such threats do eventually kill themselves. Just before the act, there may be a subtle change in their way of talking about dying, sometimes in the form of oblique hints instead of former more open statements.

Risk is assessed further by considering factors that have shown to be associated with suicide (see p. 410). Factors pointing to greater risk include:

- marked hopelessness
- **previous suicide attempts**: 40–60 per cent of those who die by suicide have made a previous attempt
- social isolation
- older age
- **depressive disorder**, especially with severe mood change with insomnia, anorexia, and weight loss
- **alcohol dependence**, especially with physical complications or severe social damage
- drug dependence
- **schizophrenia**, especially among young men with recurrent severe illness, depression, intellectual deterioration, and a history of a previous suicide attempt (see pp. 305, 412).
- chronic painful illness
- epilepsy
- abnormal personality.

Completing the history

When these general risk factors have been assessed, the rest of the history should be evaluated. The interview should be conducted in an unhurried and sympathetic way that allows the patient to admit any despair or self-destructive intentions. It is usually appropriate to start by asking about current problems and the patient's reaction to them. Enquiries should cover losses, both personal (such as bereavement or divorce) and financial, as well as loss of status. Information about conflict with other people and social isolation should also be elicited. Physical illness should always be asked about, particularly any painful condition in the elderly. (Some depressed suicides have unwarranted fears of physical illness as a feature of the psychiatric disorder.)

In assessing previous personality, it should be borne in mind that the patient's self-description might be coloured by depression. Whenever possible, another informant should be interviewed. The important points include mood swings, impulsive or aggressive tendencies, and attitudes towards religion and death.

Mental state examination

The assessment of mood should be particularly thorough, and cognitive function must not be overlooked. The interviewer should then assess suicidal intent. It is usually appropriate to begin by asking whether patients think that life is too much for them, or whether they no longer want to go on. This first question can lead to more direct enquiries about thoughts of suicide, specific plans, and preparations such as saving tablets. It is important to remember that severely depressed patients occasionally have homicidal ideas; they may believe that it would be an act of mercy to kill other people, often the spouse or a child, to spare them intolerable suffering. Such homicidal ideas should always be taken extremely seriously.

Assessment of risk among inpatients

The suicide of a hospital inpatient is always of particular concern and it is highly desirable therefore to be able to identify those at risk. Unfortunately it is difficult to do this because the general risk factors noted above are present in so many of those who have been admitted to hospital so they do not differentiate well between degrees of risk. The problem is illustrated by the results of a retrospective case control study of inpatients who had committed suicide (Powell *et al.*, 2000). The authors identified five predictors: (i) suicidal ideation, (ii) recent bereavement, (iii) delusions, (iv) chronic mental illness, and (v) family history of suicide. An inpatient with all five risk factors would have a risk of about 30 per cent but only about 1 in 100 had all five. For the rest, the sensitivity and specificity of the predictors was low, identifying correctly only 2 per cent of those with a risk of 1 in 20, while most of those who died had predicted risks of 1 per cent or less. Therefore the patients at risk can be identified only in company with many false positives, with the consequent close supervision of large numbers of patients who will not commit suicide and effect on them of this unnecessary supervision, as well as the extra staffing requirements.

The management of suicidal patients

General issues

Having assessed the suicidal risk, the clinician should make a treatment plan and try to persuade the patient to accept it. The first step is to decide whether the patient should be admitted to hospital or treated as an outpatient or day patient. This decision depends on the intensity of the suicidal intention, the severity of any associated psychiatric illness, and the availability of social support outside hospital. If outpatient treatment is chosen,patients should be given a telephone number with which they can, at all times, obtain help if they feel worse. Frustrated attempts to find a doctor can be the last straw for a patient with suicidal inclinations.

If the immediate risk of suicide is judged to be high, inpatient care is likely to be required unless there is (i) an effective crisis management team in the community, or (ii) the patient lives with reliable relatives who wish to care for the patient themselves, understand their responsibilities, and are able to fulfil them. Such a decision requires an exceptionally thorough knowledge of the patient and his problems and of the relatives. If hospital treatment is essential and the patient refuses it, admission under a compulsory order will be necessary. Readers should be aware of and follow the legal requirements of the place in which they work.

TABLE 17.2 Care of the potentially suicidal patient in the community

Full assessment of patient and proposed carers
Organization of adequate social support
Regular review of the suicide risk and the arrangements
Safe psychiatric treatments given in adequate dosage using less toxic drugs
Small prescriptions
Involve relatives in the safe keeping of tablets
Arrangements for immediate access to extra help for patient and carers

Management in the community

The management of patients identified as being at risk of suicide but not requiring admission requires continuing assessment of the suicidal risk, and agreed plans for appropriate treatment and support (see Table 17.2). Where available and the patient consents,relatives or other carers should be involved. The key worker should liaise closely with other members of the community team to ensure that there will be a prompt and appropriate response if the patient or the carers asks for additional help. If medication is required, for example to treat a depressive disorder, a drug should be chosen that is least dangerous in overdose, the choice should be discussed with the general practitioner, and small quantities should be prescribed on each occasion. When appropriate, medication should be kept safely by the carer. Both patients and carers need to know how to obtain immediate help should there be an emergency.

Management in hospital

The obvious first requirement is to prevent patients from harming themselves. These arrangements require adequate staffing and a safe ward environment. A policy (Table 17.3) should be agreed with all staff members when the patient is admitted.

Ward arrangements. Wards design should minimize the availability of means of self-harm. These include (i) preventing access to open windows and other places where jumping could lead to serious injury or death; (ii) removing ligature points from which hanging could take place (e.g. by boxing in pipes); (iii) preventing access to ward areas in which self-injury would be easier to enact; and (iv) removing potentially dangerous personal possessions such as razors and belts. When the

TABLE 17.3 Care of the suicidal patient in hospital

(i) Safe ward environment
(ii) An adequate number of well-trained staff
(iii) Good working relationships between staff and between staff and patients
(iv) Agreed policies for the observation, assessment, and review of patients
On admission
Assess risk
Agree the level of observation
Remove objects which might be used for suicide
Discuss and agree plans with the patient
Agree a policy for visitors (number, duration of visit, what they need to know)
During admission
Regular review of risk and plans
Agreed plans for the level of supervision
Clear communication of assessments and plans between staff, especially when shifts change
Agree action to be taken if the patient leaves the ward without notice or permission
At discharge
Agree date and plan for aftercare in advance of discharge
Discuss and agree the plan with the patient and thiose involved in care
Prescribe in adequate but non-dangerous amounts
Arrange follow-up, and agree action to be taken if the patient does not attend

risk is high, special nursing arrangements may be needed to ensure that the patient is never alone.

The **management policy** (Table 17.3) should be:

- **reviewed** carefully at frequent intervals until the danger passes
- **explained to and agreed with each new shift of staff** especially when the review has led to changes in the plan
- **explained to and if possible agreed with the patient.** If the patient does not agree to necessary parts of the plan, the reasons for them should be carefully explained. If the patient still refuses to collaborate, and the risk is high, compulsory treatment may be required, using the legal powers available in the country at which treatment is being carried out.

When intensive supervision is needed for more than a few days, patients may become irritated by, and resentful of, the constant supervision and may try to evade it. Staff should anticipate such problems, ensure that treatment of any associated mental illness is not delayed, and support the patient intensively while waiting for treatment to have an effect. However determined the patient is to die, there is usually some small remaining wish to go on living. If staff adopt a caring and hopeful attitude, the patient's remaining positive feelings can be encouraged, and they can be helped towards a more positive view of their future. At the same time, they can be helped to see how an apparently overwhelming accumulation of problems can be dealt with one by one.

The risk of suicide is greater during any period of home leave arranged to test the patient's readiness for discharge. It is greater also in the period immediately before discharge, and in the first few weeks after discharge (see p. 412). Therefore the discharge plan should include early reassessment, effective psychological and social support, and rapid response to any need for extra help. Plans for leave and for discharge should be discussed with patients and their concerns elicited; and, if appropriate, the plans should be modified.

However carefully patients are cared for, occasionally a patient will die by suicide despite all the efforts of the staff. The doctor then has an important role in supporting other staff, particularly any nurses who have come to know the patient particularly well. While it is essential to review every suicide carefully to determine whether useful lessons can be learned, this process should never become a search for a scapegoat.

The relatives

When a patient has died by suicide, the relatives require not only the support that is appropriate for any bereaved person, but also help with particular problems such as anger, guilt, and a feeling that they could have done more to prevent the suicide. In a noteworthy study by Barraclough and Shepherd (1976), the relatives usually reported that the police conducted their enquiries in a considerate way, but nearly all found the public inquest distressing. The subsequent newspaper publicity caused further grief, reactivating the events surrounding the death and increasing any feelings of stigma. Sympathetic listening, explanation, and counselling are likely to help relatives with these difficulties. It is essential to understand that anger is often a part of grief and that it should be met by a patient willingness to listen and to provide full information. See

Wertheimer (2001) for a review of consequences of suicide for relatives.

Suicide prevention

In population terms, suicide is a rare event; in western Europe this approximates to between one and two deaths per every 10 000 people per year. Therefore, a controlled trial to show the effect of an intervention in reducing the number of people who commit suicide, would need to include many thousands of participants, and such trials have not been completed. There is, however, some evidence from observational studies to suggest measures (listed in Table 17.4) that could affect the rate of suicide in the population. Such possible measures are discussed next; for more information see Hawton (2000b).

Service changes

Educating primary care physicians The effectiveness of interventions based in primary care is equivocal. In a frequently quoted study, Rutz and colleagues conducted an intervention study involving all general practitioners on the Swedish island of Gotland in 1983 and 1984. The study aimed to evaluate the impact of teaching the island's GPs about the diagnosis and treatment of affective disorder. After the programme was introduced, the suicide rate dropped to an extent that was significantly different from both the long-term suicide trend on Gotland and that for Sweden as a whole. A further study found that by 1988, 3 years after the project had ended, the suicide rate had returned almost to baseline values (Rutz *et al.*, 1992). The researchers concluded that the programme had been effective but that it would need to be repeated every 2 years to have long-term benefits. Also, it appeared to benefit only females. These findings have, so far, not been replicated.

Improving psychiatric services Earlier recognition and better treatment of the psychiatric disorders might be expected to reduce suicide rates. Published studies have not shown this effect conclusively but there are, of course, other reasons for improving services.

TABLE 17.4 Suicide prevention
Better and more available psychiatric services
Restricting the means of suicide
Encouraging responsible reporting
Educational programmes
Improved care for high risk groups
Crisis centres and 'hot lines'

Targetting high risk groups The usual clinical approach is to provide additional help for high-risk groups such as patients who have recently received inpatient psychiatric treatment, and those who have recently deliberately harmed themselves. (Crisis centres are discussed below.)

Long-term medication Although the continued prescribing of **antidepressants** in the period following an episode of depression reduces the risk of a subsequent episode of depression, reduction in suicidal behaviour has not been demonstrated. However, there is accumulating evidence that lithium prophylaxis reduces suicide rates (Cipriani *et al.*, 2005c), and some evidence that clozapine may reduce suicide attempts by people with schizophrenia or schizoaffective disorder (see the fuller discussion on p. 305).

Prescribing less toxic antidepressants Selective serotonin re-uptake inhibitors **(SSRIs)** are less toxic in overdose than tricyclic antidepressants. On the other hand, SSRIs have been reported to cause the emergence or worsening of suicidal ideas, possibly because the drugs can cause agitation and insomnia when first taken. Although it is not possible to reach a decisive conclusion with the available evidence, it seems that the overall risk of suicide associated with SSRIs is similar to that with tricyclics (Cipriani *et al.*, 2005b). Nevertheless there is some evidence from epidemiological studies that increased prescribing of less toxic antidepressants is associated with a decrease in suicide rate (see Grunebaum *et al.*, 2004). The nature of this association, if it is reliably confirmed, remains to be determined. Until the evidence is conclusive, the most appropriate drug should be decided for each patient with progress monitored and support provided in the first few weeks of treatment. For further discussion of the risks of SSRIs see p. 546.

Counselling services In the UK, the best known service for people who are suicidal is the Samaritan organization founded in London in 1953 by the Reverend Chad Varah. People in despair are encouraged to contact a widely publicized telephone number. The help offered ('befriending') is provided by non-professional volunteers, trained to listen sympathetically without attempting to take on tasks that are in the province of a professional. An often quoted survey found that, amongst people who telephone the Samaritans, the suicide rate in the ensuing year is higher than in the general population (Barraclough and Shea, 1970). This finding suggests that the organization attracts people at risk for suicide, but it also sheds doubt on the efficacy of the help offered. Comparisons of matched towns with and without services suggest little difference in suicide rates (Jennings *et al.*, 1978). Even if this is so, the Samaritans provide valuable support for many lonely and despairing people.

Population strategies

Reducing the availability of methods of suicide

The ease with which people can access lethal methods of self-harm may affect the rate of suicide using these methods, and may have some effect on rates in general. If the available methods are less are less harmful, more people will be resuscitated. No matter what changes are made, however, people who are determined to kill themselves can eventually find the means to do so. Several changes have been made:

Detoxifying gas In Britain, in the period 1948–50, poisoning by domestic coal gas accounted for 40 per cent of reported suicides among men and 60 per cent among women. Following the introduction of less toxic North Sea gas, the number using this method reduced dramatically, and the national rate of suicide also fell. It has been argued that the removal of coal gas was responsible for this change.

Detoxifying car exhaust fumes The fitting of catalytic converters to motor vehicles to reduce the toxicity of car exhaust fumes may have reduced the deaths from this method.

Restricting amounts of analgesics In the UK, government legislation has limited the amount of paracetamol, salicylates and their compounds that people can buy at one time. There is evidence that this legislation has reduced suicides using overdoses of these drugs (Hawton *et al.*, 2004b).

Removing and preventing access to hazards In hospital wards and police and prison cells, ligature points from which hanging could take place, should be removed or enclosed (see p. 415). Physical barriers on bridges, train platforms, and other potentially dangerous places, may reduce suicide at these places.

Other measures

More responsible media reporting Sometimes people copy methods of suicde that have received wide media attention. For this and other reasons, reporters and editors should be encouraged to report suicide responsibly.

Social policy Given the repeatedly demonstrated association between unemployment and suicide, Lewis and colleagues have argued that policies aimed at reducing rates of unemployment may be help to reduce the rate of suicide (Lewis *et al.*, 1997). Others have argued that other factors such as increasing social isolation also need to be tackled in this way. While the means to achieve such strategies are far from clear and it would be difficult to evaluate their effectiveness, such calls are a reminder of the relationship between social policy and health.

Public education Campaigns to educate the public about mental illness and its treatment have included approaches in schools, with teaching about solving problems and seeking help when distressed. The value of such approaches is uncertain.

Deliberate self-harm

Until the 1950s little distinction was made between people who killed themselves and those who survived after an apparent suicidal act. In the UK, Stengel (1952) was the first to identify epidemiological differences between the two groups. He proposed the term 'attempted suicide' to describe self-injury that the person could not be sure to survive. Subsequent studies investigated the motivation for such episodes and found that the intention of many of the survivors had not been to die. As a result the terms 'deliberate self-poisoning', 'parasuicide' and 'deliberate self-harm' were introduced to describe episodes of intentional self-harm that did not lead to death and may or may not have been motivated by a desire to die. Kreitman (1977) defined this behaviour as 'a non-fatal act in which an individual deliberately causes self-injury or ingests a substance in excess of any prescribed or generally recognized dosage'. This definition is useful because it does not specify the extent of suicidal intent. In this chapter, the term deliberate self-harm will be used to describe such incidents.

Acts ending in suicide and acts of deliberate self-harm overlap on another. Some people who had no intention of dying succumb to the unintended effects of an overdose. Others who intended to die are revived. Importantly, many people were ambivalent at the time, uncertain whether they wished to die or survive. It should be remembered that, among people who have been involved in deliberate self-harm, the suicide rate in the subsequent 12 months is about a hundred times greater than in the general population and remains high for many years. Therefore, deliberate self-harm should not be regarded lightly.

The act of deliberate self-harm

Methods of deliberate self-poisoning.

In the UK, about 90 per cent of the cases of deliberate self-harm referred to general hospitals involve a drug overdose, and most of them present no serious threat to life. The type of drug used varies somewhat with age, local prescription practices, and the availability of drugs. The most commonly used drugs are the non-opiate analgesics, such as paracetamol and aspirin. Paracetamol is particularly dangerous because it damages the liver and may lead to the delayed death of patients who had not intended to die. It is particularly worrying that younger patients who are usually unaware of the serious risks often take this drug. Antidepressants, both tricyclic and SSRI, are taken in about a quarter of episodes. About a third of males and about a quarter of females consume alcohol in the 6 hours before the act (Hawton *et al.*, 2003b).

Methods of deliberate self-injury

Deliberate self-injury accounts for about 10 per cent of all deliberate self-harm presenting to general hospitals in Britain. The commonest method of self-injury is laceration, usually of the forearm or wrists; it accounts for about four-fifths of the self-injuries referred to a general hospital. (Self-laceration is discussed further below.) Other forms of self-injury are jumping from heights or in front of a train or motor vehicle, shooting, and drowning. These violent acts occur mainly among older people who intended to die (Harwood and Jacoby, 2000).

Deliberate self-laceration

There are three forms of deliberate self-laceration: (i) deep and dangerous wounds inflicted with serious suicidal intent, more often by men; (ii) self-mutilation by schizophrenic patients (often in response to hallucinatory voices) or people with severe learning difficulties; and (iii) superficial wounds that do not endanger life, more often by women. Only the last group will be described here.

Usually, the act of laceration is preceded by increasing tension and irritability, and these diminish afterwards. After the act, the patient often feels shame and disgust. Some of these people say that they lacerated themselves while in a state of detachment from their surroundings, and that they experienced little or no pain. The lacerations are usually multiple, made with glass or a razor blade, on inflicted on the forearms or wrists. Some of these people also injure themselves in other ways, for example by burning with cigarettes or inflicting bruises.

Self-cutters who attend hospital are more often men (Hawton *et al.*, 2004c). People who cut themselves superficially do not always seek help from the medical services and many of these people are young females, often with personality problems characterized by low self-esteem, impulsive or aggressive behaviour, unstable moods, difficulty in interpersonal relationships, and problems of alcohol and drug misuse.

The epidemiology of deliberate self-harm

In the early 1960s a substantial increase in deliberate self-harm began in most Western countries. In the UK, the rates of admission to general hospitals increased about fourfold in the 10 years up to 1973. The rates continued to increase more slowly in the mid-1970s, but then fell in

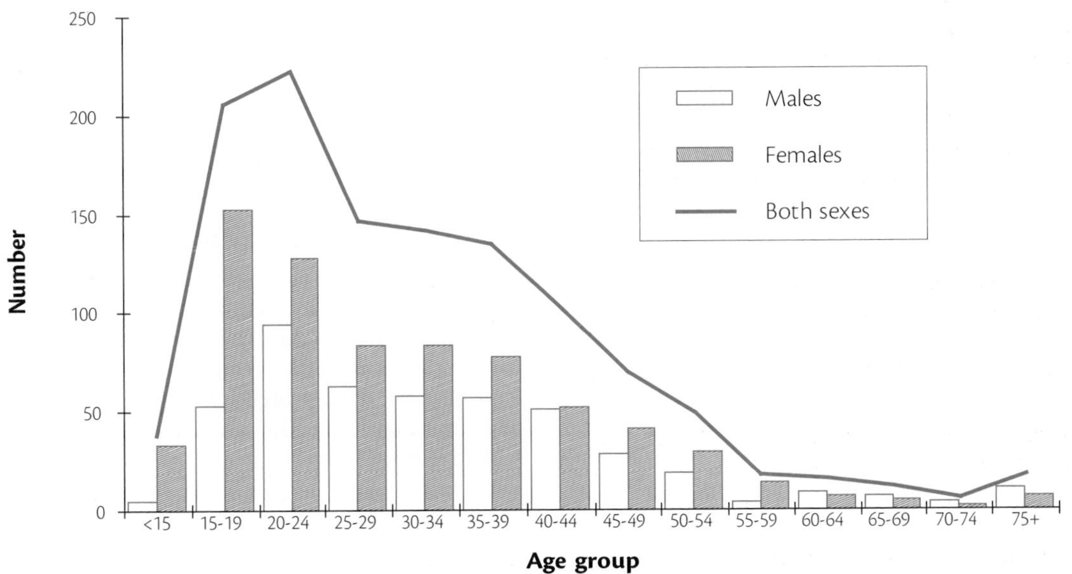

Fig. 17.3 Age groups of deliberate self-harm patients by gender in 2002. Reproduced by permission of Professor KE Hawton, Oxford University.

the late 1970s. Rates then increased again. Current estimates of the rate of deliberate self-harm in Britain suggest a figure of about 3 per 1000 per year. Rates in most European countries are lower (see Kerkhof, 2000).

Variations according to personal characteristics

Deliberate self-harm is more common among younger people, with the rates declining sharply in middle age (Figure 17.3). Over recent years, the proportion of men presenting following deliberate self-harm has risen. In the 1960s and 1970s the female-to-male ratio was about 2:1; recent studies show much smaller differences. The peak age for men is older than that for women. For both sexes, rates are very low under the age of 12 years. Deliberate self-harm is more prevalent in the lower social classes. There are also differences related to marital status. The highest rates for both men and women are among the divorced; high rates are found also among teenage wives, and younger single men and women (see Hawton *et al.*, 2003b).

Rates of deliberate self-harm in the elderly have changed little in recent years. The characteristics of such people seem to be rather more similar to those of people who kill themselves than do those of younger people who harm themselves deliberately (Harwood and Jacoby, 2000).

Variations according to place of residence

High rates are found in areas characterized by high unemployment, overcrowding, many children in care, and substantial social mobility (Gunnel *et al.*, 1995).

Causes of deliberate self-harm

Precipitating factors

Compared with the general population, people who harm themselves deliberately have experienced four times as many **stressful life problems** in the 6 months before the act (Paykel *et al.*, 1975). The events are various, but a recent quarrel with a spouse, girlfriend, or boyfriend is common. Other events include separation from or rejection by a sexual partner, the illness of a family member, recent personal physical illness, and appearance in a court of law.

Predisposing factors

Familial and developmental factors may predispose to deliberate self-harm (Statham *et al.*, 1998). There is some evidence that early parental loss through bereavement, or a history of parental neglect or abuse, is more frequent among cases of deliberate self-harm.

Personality disorder In the UK (Haw *et al.*, 2001) and other countries (eg. Suominen *et al.*, 1996) personality disorder is present in almost a half of patients with deliberate self-harm. Borderline personality disorder has been reported to be common but studies using standard methods for assessment have found anxious, anankastic (obsessional) and paranoid personality disorders more frequently (see Haw *et al.*, 2001). Poor skills in solving interpersonal problems, and impulsiveness may also predispose to deliberate self-harm.

Long-term problems with partners In an important early study, (Bancroft *et al.*, 1977) about two-thirds of the deliberate self-harm patients had a problem in their relationship with a partner

Economic and social environment Rates of deliberate self-harm are higher among the unemployed. However, unemployment is related to other social factors associated with deliberate self-harm, such as financial difficulties, and it is difficult to determine whether unemployment is a direct cause. Rates of deliberate self-harm are also higher in areas of socio-economic deprivation (Gunnell *et al.*, 1995; Hawton *et al.*, 2001b).

Ill health A background of poor physical health is common.

Psychiatric disorder

It used to be held that, with the exception of adjustment disorder, psychiatric disorder was uncommon among people who harmed themselves deliberately. However, when standardized assessments have been used, psychiatric disorder has been detected in about 90 per cent of deliberate self-harm patients seen in hospital (Haw *et al.*, 2001; Suominen *et al.*,1996). Depressive disorder is the most frequent diagnosis, followed in men by dependency on and harmful use of alcohol and drugs. Among women, anxiety disorders are in second place. Comorbidity is frequent, especially between psychiatric disorder and personality disorder.

Motivation and deliberate self-harm

The motives for deliberate self-harm are usually mixed and often difficult to identify with certainty. Even when patients know their own motives, they may try to hide them from other people. For example, people who have taken an overdose in response frustration and anger may feel ashamed and say instead that they wished to die. Conversely, people who truly intended to kill themselves may deny it. For this reason, when individuals are assessed, more emphasis should be placed on a common-sense evaluation of their actions leading up to self-harm than on their subsequent accounts of their motives.

TABLE 17.5 Reasons given for deliberate self-harm

To die
To escape from unbearable anguish
To get relief
To change the behaviour of others
To escape from a situation
To show desperation to others
To get back at other people/make them feel guilty
To get help

From Hawton, K. (2000). Treatment of suicide attempters and prevention of suicide and attempted suicide. In MG Gelder, JJ López-Ibor Jr, and NC Andreasen (eds) *The new Oxford textbook of psychiatry*, Chapter 4.15.4. Oxford University Press, Oxford.

Despite this limitation, useful information has been obtained by questioning groups of patients about their motives. Indeed a study in 13 European countries found similar reported motives in all the study sites (Hjelmeland *et al.*, 2002). The motives are listed in Table 17.6. Only a few say that the act was premeditated. About a quarter say that they wished to die. Some say that they are uncertain whether they wanted to die or not, others that they were leaving it to 'fate' to decide, and others that they were seeking unconsciousness as a temporary escape from their problems. Another group admit that they were trying to influence someone, for example, that they were seeking to make a relative feel guilty for having failed them in some way. This motive of influencing other people was first emphasized by Stengel and Cook (1958), who wrote that these people hoped to call forth 'action from the human environment'. This behaviour has since been referred to as 'a cry for help'. Although some acts of deliberate self-harm result in increased help for the patient, others may arouse resentment, particularly when they are repeated.

The outcome of deliberate self-harm

Repetition of self-harm

In the weeks after deliberate self-harm, many patients report changes for the better. People with psychiatric symptoms often report that they have become less intense. This improvement may result from help provided by professionals or from improvements in the person's relationships, attitudes, and behaviour. Some people do not improve and harm themselves again, in some cases fatally. A systematic review of 90 studies by Owens *et al.* (2003) concluded that among people who have engaged in deliberate self-harm:

TABLE 17.6 Factors associated with risk of repetition of attempted suicide

Previous attempt(s)
Personality disorder
Alcohol or drug abuse
Previous psychiatric treatment
Unemployment
Lower social class
Criminal record
History of violence
Age 25–54 years
Single, divorced, or separated

From Hawton, K. (2000a). Treatment of suicide attempters and prevention of suicide and attempted suicide. In MG Gelder, JJ López-Ibor Jr, and NC Andreasen (eds) *The new Oxford textbook of psychiatry*, Chapter 4.15.4. Oxford University Press, Oxford.

- About 1 in 6 repeats the deliberate self-harm within 1 year
- About 1 in 4 repeats the deliberate self-harm within 4 years.

Factors associated with repetition of deliberate self-harm (Kreitman, 1977; Appleby, 1993) are listed in Table 17.6.

Suicide following deliberate self-harm

People who have intentionally harmed themselves have a much increased risk of later suicide.The same systematic review (Owens *et al.*, 2003) concluded that among these people:

- Between 1 in 200 and 1 in 40 commit suicide within 1 year
- About 1 in 15 commits suicide within 9 years or more.

These risks are compiled from several countries so that they cannot be compared directly with the general population rate of about 1 in 10 000 people per annum in the UK. Nevertheless the risk is clearly much increased.

Among people who deliberately harm themselves, the risk of eventual suicide is even greater among people who are older, male, depressed, or alcoholic. A dangerous or violent method also indicates a high risk. However, a non-dangerous method of self-harm does not necessarily indicate a low risk of subsequent suicide, partly because patients may have incomplete knowledge of the dangerousness of the available methods.

It is difficult to predict which patients will die by suicide following previous self-harm because of the rate of suicide, although greater than that in the population, is still quite low, and the predictive factors have low specificity. Although designed to assess immediate suicide risk, the Beck Suicide Intent Scale (Beck *et al.*, 1974) is of some value in assessing suicide risk over the first year following the original self-harm (Harris *et al.*, 2005).

Results of treatment after deliberate self-harm

Although randomized controlled studies have shown decreases in psychopathology and improvements in social problems after various treatments, there is less evidence that treatment prevents the repetition of deliberate self-harm. One reason for this lack of evidence is that different kinds of treatment have been investigated, and the numbers in most studies have been rather low. A meta-analysis has been carried out of 20 randomized controlled trials in which repetition of deliberate self-harm was an outcome measure. These 20 trial were concerned with 10 types of intervention so that the conclusions are provisional (Hawton *et al.*, 1998). The conclusions were:

- For people who have repeated deliberate self-harm many times, depot flupenthixol was superior to placebo in reducing further repetition (this conclusion was based on a single trial).
- For those with borderline personality disorder, rates of repetition were lower with dialectical behaviour therapy than with standard aftercare (based on a single trial).
- Trends towards greater reduction of repetition were found for: (i) problem-solving therapy, (ii) the provision of emergency contact cards allowing immediate access to help, and (iii) community outreach when compared with standard aftercare. However, the effectiveness of contact cards was not confirmed by M. O. Evans *et al.* (1999).

Brief psychodynamic interpersonal therapy (see p. 601) has been shown, in one randomized controlled trial, to reduce self reported attempts at self-harm more than did treatment as usual (Guthrie *et al.*, 2001).

Special groups

Mothers of young children

Mothers of young children require special consideration because of the known association between deliberate self-harm and child abuse. It is important to ask about the mother's feeling towards her children, and to enquire about their welfare. In the UK, information about the children can usually be obtained from the general practitioner, who may ask his health visitor to investigate the case.

Children and adolescents

Deliberate self-harm amongst children and adolescents increased in the 1990s in many parts of the developed world. It is difficult to obtain the exact rates because many of the acts are minor drug overdoses or self-injuries that do not reach the medical services (Hawton *et al.*, 2002). It is generally agreed that deliberate self-harm is rare among pre-school children, and becomes increasingly common after the age of 12. Except at the youngest ages, it is more common amongst girls. It is less common among Asian than white females (Hawton *et al.*, 2003c).

Methods Drug overdose is the most common method among those attending hospital; self-cutting is common especially among females though it less often leads to attendence at hospital. More dangerous forms of self-injury are more frequent amongst boys (Hawton *et al.*, 2003c).

Motivation It is difficult to determine the motivation of self-harm in young children, especially as a clear concept of death is not usually developed until around the age of 12. It is probable that only a few of the younger children have any serious suicidal intent. Their motivation may be more often to communicate distress, to escape from stress, or to influence other people. Epidemics of deliberate self-harm occasionally occur as a result of imitative behaviour amongst adolescents in psychiatric hospitals and other institutions: see de Wilde (2000).

Causes Deliberate self-harm in adolescents is associated with broken homes, family psychiatric disorder, and child abuse. It is often precipitated by social problems; for younger adolescents most often family problems, for older ones difficulties with boy- or girlfriends, and for both age groups problems with schoolwork. Deliberate self-harm among adolescents is associated also with alcohol and drug misuse especially among males, violence and being the victim of violence, with mood disorder and personality disorder (Hawton *et al.*, 2003c).

Outcome For most children and adolescents, the outcome of deliberate self-harm is relatively good, but an important minority continue to have social and psychiatric problems, and to repeat acts of deliberate self-harm. A poor outcome is associated with poor psychosocial adjustment, a history of previous deliberate self-harm, and severe family problems. There is a significant risk of suicide amongst these adolescents, especially boys.

Management When children harm themselves, it is better for them to be assessed by child psychiatrists rather than members of the adult services for deliberate self-harm. Treatment usually involves the family and is directed to the causal problems and to the adolescent's coping skills (see Shaffer *et al.*, 2000).

The management of deliberate self-harm

The organization of services

The care of deliberate self-harm patients involves a variety of services including primary care teams, ambulance services, emergency department staff, and social services. All these staff require training to enable them to respond appropriately and to make necessary decisions including how to assess immediate risk, obtain informed consent; and to assess capacity to consent and in what circumstances necessary care can be given without consent. The organization of the medical and surgical response to these patients is beyond the scope of this book: readers requiring information should consult National Institute for Clinical Excellence (2004c).

Arrangements for psychosocial assessment vary. In some centres this is done by psychiatrists, in others suitably trained staff, who may be medical staff, nurses, or social workers carry out the assessments. Whatever arrangement is made, it is important to ensure that all patients receive a psychosocial assessment as well as an assessment of the medical effects of the self-harm (see below). Each hospital site should have a code of practice detailing the arrangements for psychosocial assessment agreed by general medical and psychiatric services and known to those who work there.

Facilities should be available for the special needs of patients from ethnic minorities. Children and adolescents should whenever possible be assessed by staff trained in the assessment and care of young people and familiar with the problems of confidentiality and consent that can arise in such cases. If possible patients over the age of 65 years should be assessed by staff familiar with the special probems of the elderly, and aware of the greater risk of completed suicide in this age group.

The assessment of patients after deliberate self-harm

General aims

Assessment is concerned with three main issues:

1. the immediate risks of suicide,
2. the subsequent risks of further deliberate self-harm,
3. current medical or social problems.

The assessment should be carried out in a way that encourages patients to undertake a constructive review of their problems and of the ways in which they could deal with them themselves. It is important to encourage self-help, because many of these people are unwilling to be seen again by a psychiatrist.

Usually the assessment has to be carried out in an accident and emergency department or a ward of a general hospital, in which there may be little privacy. Whenever possible, the interview should be in a side room so that it will not be overheard or interrupted. If the patient has taken an overdose, the interviewer should first make sure that the patient has recovered sufficiently to be able to give a satisfactory history. If consciousness is still impaired, the interview should be delayed. Information should also be obtained from relatives or friends, the family doctor, and any other person (such as a social worker) already attempting to help the patient. Wide enquiry is important because sometimes information from other sources may differ substantially from the account given by the patient. See Hawton (2000b) for reviews of general hospital assessment.

Specific enquiries

The interview is directed to five questions:

1. What were the patients' intentions when they harmed themselves?
2. Do they now intend to die?
3. What are their current problems?
4. Is there a psychiatric disorder?
5. What helpful resources are available?

Each question will be considered in turn.

What were the patient's intentions when he harmed himself?

As mentioned already, patients sometimes misrepresent their intentions. For this reason the interviewer should reconstruct, as fully as possible, the events that led up to the act of self-harm in order to find the answers to five subsidiary questions:

1. **Was the act planned or carried out on impulse?** The longer and more carefully the plans have been made, the greater is the risk of a fatal repetition.
2. **Were precautions taken against being found?** The more thorough the precaution, the greater is the risk of a further fatal overdose. Of course, events do not always take place as the patient expected; for example, a spouse may arrive home earlier than usual so that the patient is discovered alive. In such circumstances it is the patient's reasonable expectations that count in predicting the future risk.
3. **Did the patient seek help?** Serious intent can be inferred if there were no attempts to obtain help after the act.
4. **Was the method thought to be dangerous?** If drugs were used, what were they and what amount was taken? Did the patient take all the drugs available? If self-injury was used, what form did it take? (As noted above, the greater the suicidal intent the greater is the risk of a further suicide attempt.) Not only should the actual dangerousness be assessed, but also that anticipated by the patient, which may be inaccurate. For example, some people wrongly believe that paracetamol overdoses are harmless or that benzodiazepines are dangerous.
5. **Was there a 'final act'** such as writing a suicide note or making a will? If so, the risk of a further fatal attempt is greater.

By reviewing the answers to these questions, the interviewer makes a judgement of the patient's intentions at the time of the act (Table 17.7).

A similar approach has been formalized in Beck's Suicide Intent Scale (Box 17.2).

Does the patient now intend to die?

The interviewer should ask directly whether the patient is pleased to have recovered or wishes that he had died. If the act suggested serious suicidal intent and if the patient now denies such intent, the interviewer should try to find out by tactful questioning whether there has been a genuine change of resolve.

What are the current problems?

Many patients will have experienced a mounting series of difficulties in the weeks or months leading up to the act. Some of these difficulties may have been resolved by the time that he is interviewed, sometimes as a result of the act of self-harm, for example a partner who had threatened to leave the patient may have decided to stay. The more serious the problems that remain, the greater is the risk of a fatal repetition. This risk is particularly strong if the problems include loneliness or ill-health. The review of problems should be systematic and should cover the following:

- intimate relationships with the spouse or another person;
- relations with children and other relatives;
- employment, finance, and housing;
- legal problems;
- social isolation, bereavement, and other losses;
- physical health.

Drug and alcohol problems can be considered at this stage of the assessment or later when the psychiatric state is reviewed.

Is there psychiatric disorder?

It should be possible to answer this question from the history and from a brief but systematic examination of the mental state. Particular attention should be directed to depressive disorder, alcoholism, anxiety disorder and personality disorder. Schizophrenia and dementia should also be considered, though they will found less often.

What are the patient's resources?

These include capacity to solve problems, material resources, and the help that others are likely to pro-

TABLE 17.7 Factors that suggest high suicidal intent

Factors that suggest high suicidal intent
Act carried out in isolation
Act timed so that intervention unlikely
Precautions taken to avoid discovery
Preparations made in anticipation of death (e.g. making Will, organizing insurance)
Preparations made for the act (e.g. purchasing means, saving up tablets)
Communicating intent to others beforehand
Extensive premeditation
Leaving a note
Not alerting potential helpers after the act
Admission of suicidal intent

From Hawton, K (2000) Treatment of suicide attempters and prevention of suicide and attempted suicide. In MG Gelder, JJ López-Ibor Jr, and NC Andreasen (eds) *The new Oxford textbook of psychiatry*, Chapter 4.15.4. Oxford University Press, Oxford.

BOX 17.2 BECK SUICIDE INTENT SCALE

Circumstances related to suicidal attempt

Isolation

0 Somebody present
1 Somebody nearby or in contact (as by phone)
2 No-one nearby or in contact

Timing

0 Timed so that intervention is probable
1 Timed so that intervention is not likely
2 Timed so that intervention is highly unlikely

Precautions against discovery and/or intervention

0 No precautions
1 Passive precautions as: avoiding others but doing nothing to prevent their intervention (alone in a room with unlocked door)
2 Active precaution as: locked door

Acting to gain help during/after attempt

0 Notified potential helper regarding the attempt
1 Contacted but did not specifically notify potential helper regarding the attempt
2 Did not contact or notify potential helper

Final acts in anticipation of death

0 None
1 Partial preparation or ideation
2 Definite plans made (changes in Will, giving of gifts, taking out insurance)

Degree of planning for suicide attempt

0 No preparation
1 Minimal preparation
2 Extensive preparation

Suicide note

0 Absence of note
1 Note written but torn up
2 Presence of note

Overt communication of intent before act

0 None
1 Equivocal communication
2 Unequivocal communication

Purpose of attempt

0 Mainly to change environment
1 Components of '0' and '2'
2 Mainly to remove self from environment

Self-report

Expectations regarding fatality of act

0 Patient thought that death was unlikely
1 Patient thought that death was possible but not probable
2 Patient thought that death was probable or certain

Conception of method's lethality

0 Patient did less to himself than he thought would be lethal
1 Patient wasn't sure, or did what he thought might be lethal
2 Act equalled or exceeded patient's concept of its medical lethality

'Seriousness of attempt'

0 Patient did not consider act to be a serious attempt to end his life
1 Patient was uncertain whether act was a serious attempt to end his life
2 Patient considered act to be a serious attempt to end his life

Ambivalence towards living

0 Patient did not want to die
1 Patient did not care whether he lived or died
2 Patient wanted to die

Conception of reversibility

0 Patient thought that death would be unlikely if he received medical attention
1 Patient was uncertain whether death could be averted by medical attention
2 Patient was certain of death even if he received medical attention

Degree of premeditation

0 None, impulsive
1 Suicide contemplated for 3 hours or less prior to attempt
2 Suicide contemplated for more than 3 hours prior to attempt

Reprinted with permission from Beck, A. T. *et al* (1974). *The prediction of suicide*. Charles Press, Philadelphia

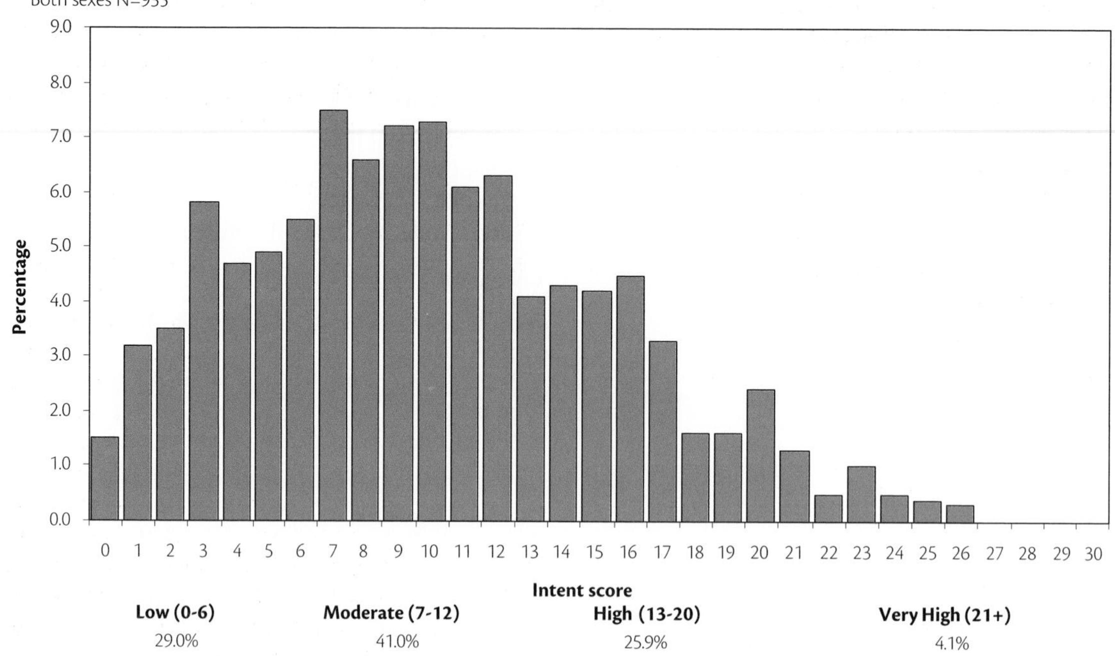

Fig. 17.4 Scores on the Beck Suicide Intent Scale in 2002. From *Deliberate self harm patients presenting to hospital*. Reproduced by permission of Professor KE Hawton, Oxford.

vide. The best guide to patients' ability to solve future problems is their record of dealing with difficulties in the past, for example, the loss of a job or a broken relationship. The availability of help should be assessed by asking about friends and confidants, and about any support the patient is receiving or can be expected to receive from the general practitioner, social workers, or voluntary agencies.

Is there a continuing risk of suicide?

The interviewer now has the information required to answer this important question. The answers to the first four questions outlined above are reviewed:

- Did the patient originally intend to die?
- Does he intend it now?
- Are the problems which provoked the act still present?
- Is there a psychiatric disorder?
- Is additional support available, and is the patient likely to accept it?

Having reviewed the answers to these questions, the interviewer compares the patient's characteristics with those that found in people who have died by suicide.

These characteristics are summarized in Table 17.7.

Is there a risk of further non-fatal self-harm?

The predictive factors are summarized in Table 17.6. The interviewer should consider all the points before deciding the risk.

What treatment is required and will the patient agree to it?

If the risk of suicide is judged to be high, the procedures are those outlined in the first part of this chapter (see p. 415). About 5–10 per cent of deliberate self-harm patients require admission to a psychiatric unit; most need treatment for depression or alcoholism, and a few for schizophrenia. Some need a period of respite from overwhelming stress.

When admission to hospital is not indicated, a plan of management has to be agreed with the patient and any potential carers. If the patient refuses the offer of help, their care should be discussed with the general practitioner before they are allowed to return home (see below and Box 17.3). For some patients it is useful to provide an emergency telephone number providing immediate access to advice or an urgent appointment should there be a further crisis.

Management after the assessment

Patients who have harmed themselves are often reluctant to accept further help and it is important to carry out the assessment interview in a way that fosters a therapeutic relationship. Plans should be discussed with the patient, and they are not agreed an alternative mutually acceptable plan should be negotiated. Patients' needs fall into three groups:

1. A small minority (perhaps 5–10 per cent) need admission to a psychiatric unit for treatment.
2. About a third have a psychiatric disorder requiring treatment from a primary care, or psychiatric team in the community .
3. The remainder need help with various psychosocial problems and help to improve their ways of coping with stressors. This help is needed even when the risk of immediate suicide or non-fatal repetition is low since continuing problems increase the risk of later repetition. Apart from practical help, problem-solving is usually the best approach, starting with the problems identified during the assessment interview. Unfortunately, such help is often refused.

Where the episode of self-harm is associated with problems in a specific interpersonal relationship, it is often helpful to interview the other person involved, first alone and then with the patient if the latter agrees. This joint interview can lead to an improved dialogue between the couple and this may help decrease the risk of acure repetition. For a review of treatment see Hawton (2000a).

Some special problems of management

Patients who refuse assessment

After deliberate self-harm, some patients refuse to be interviewed, and others seek to discharge themselves before the assessment is complete. Such patients have very high rates of repetition of self harm (Crawford and Wessely, 1998). In these cases it is essential to gather as much information as possible from other sources in order to exclude serious suicidal risk of psychiatric disorder before letting the patient leave hospital. It is important to inform and discuss the problem with the general practitioner and with the community mental health team if they are already involved with the case. If the risk of suicide is judged to be high, it may be necessary to keep the patient until an assessment is made for detention under a compulsory order.

BOX 17.3 PATIENTS WHO HARM THEMSELVES AND REFUSE TREATMENT

Note that there are international differences in laws and practices.

- The most senior experienced doctor available should see the patient and discuss the proposed treatment, the alternatives, and the patient's concerns. It is often helpful to involve relatives or close friends. Sympathetic, patient discussion of the patient's concerns is often followed by consent.
- A patient who has harmed himself but is alert and conscious should be presumed the mental capacity to refuse medical advice unless shown to be otherwise. This capacity should be assessed (see p. 75), as soon as possible. All staff should be able to perform this assessment but where possible incapacity should be confirmed by a psychiatrist. If appropriate, assessment for compulsory treatment should be arranged.
- When a patient is assessed as mentally incapable (for example, because of persistent intoxicating effects of overdose) staff have a responsibility under common law to act in that person's best interests. This may include taking the person to hospital, keeping them there for assessment, and giving immediate life-saving treatment (see p. 74).
- Staff should remember that mental capacity may change over time, and attempts should be made to explain each new procedure or treatment and to obtain consent before it is carried out.
- When, after full discussion, a competent patient continues to refuse to consent and there are no grounds for compulsory treatment, a further attempt should be made to find an acceptable alternative plan. If the attempt does not succeed, the consequences of the decision should be explained clearly, and the discussions recorded fully in the notes. If the patient insists on leaving he has to be allowed to go, but should be encouraged to return, and given an emergency contact number and options for the further treatment. The situation should be discussed as soon as possible with the general practitioner.
- It is generally appropriate to attempt to contact the patient on the following day and repeat the offer of help. The case should be discussed with the general practitioner to decide who should make the contact.

For further guidance see National Institute for Clinical Excellence (2004c).

Frequent repeaters

Some patients take overdoses repeatedly at times of stress. Often the behaviour seems intended to reduce tension or gain attention. However, when overdoses are taken repeatedly, relatives often become unsympathetic or even overtly hostile, and staff of hospital emergency departments may feel frustrated. These patients usually have a personality disorder and many insoluble social problems, but neither counselling nor intensive psychotherapy is usually effective. All those involved in management should agree a care plan which should seek to reward constructive behaviour. An opportunity for continuing support by one person should be arranged. However, whatever help is arranged, the risk of eventual death by suicide is high.

Repeated self-cutting

The management of self-laceration presents many problems. Patients often have difficulty in expressing their feelings in words, and so formal psychotherapy may not be helpful. Simple efforts to gain the patients' confidence and increase their self-esteem are more likely to succeed. Assessment should include a behavioural analysis of the sequences of events that lead to self-cutting. This may help to formulate ways in which treatment could either interrupt the chain of events which leads to self-cutting, or replace the cutting by an alternative method of relieving methods.

Medication appears to have a limited role, although atypical antipsychotic agents such as rsiperidone or olanazapine in low dose may be valuable as a short-term measure to reduce tension. Many people who cut themselves have severe personality difficulties. Treatment should be directed towards these problems, although it may be difficult and prolonged. Admission to a psychiatric unit is occasionally necessary, and it is essential that a clear and detailed policy is agreed by those involved since self-cutting is very often difficult to manage in an inpatient unit and, indeed, may be imitated by other patients.

Further reading

Gelder, MG, López-Ibor, JJ Jr and Andreasen NC (eds) (2000) *The new Oxford textbook of psychiatry*, Section 4.1.5, Suicide. Oxford University Press, Oxford. (The four chapters in this section review comprehensively deliberate self harm and suicide.)

Hawton, KE and van Heeringen, K (2000) *The international handbook of suicide and attempted suicide*. John Wiley, Chichester. (Highly authoritative reviews on all aspects of suicide and attempted suicide by leading writers.)

CHAPTER 18

The misuse of alcohol and drugs

Chapter contents

The presentation of alcohol and drug misuse is not limited to any particular psychiatric or indeed medical specialty. Alcohol and drug use may play an important part in all aspects of psychiatric practice, and are relevant for example, to the assessment of a patient with acute confusion on a medical ward, a suicidal patient in the accident and emergency department, the elderly patient whose self-care has deteriorated, the troubled adolescent, or a disturbed child who may be inhaling volatile substances.

The phrases **substance use disorder** (DSM-IV) or **disorders due to psychoactive drug use** (ICD-10) are used to refer to conditions arising from the misuse of alcohol, psychoactive drugs, and other chemicals such as volatile substances. In this chapter, problems related to alcohol will be discussed first under the general heading of alcohol use disorders; problems related to drugs and other chemicals will be discussed second under the general heading of other substance use disorders.

Classification of substance use disorders

The two classification systems, DSM-IV and ICD10, use similar categories for substance use disorders but group them in different ways. Both schemes recognize the following disorders: Intoxication, abuse (or harmful use), dependence, withdrawal states, psychotic disorders, amnestic syndromes. These and some additional categories are shown in Table 18.1.

In both diagnostic systems the first step in classification is to specify the **substance or class of substance** that is

TABLE 18.1 Substance-related disorders

DSM-IV	ICD-10
Intoxication	Intoxication
Abuse	Harmful use
Dependence	Dependence syndrome
Withdrawal	Withdrawal state
Withdrawal delirium	Withdrawal state with delirium
Psychotic disorders	Psychotic disorder
Dementia	
Amnestic disorder	Amnestic syndrome
Mood disorders	Residual and late onset psychotic disorder
Anxiety disorders	Other mental and behavioural disorders
Sexual dysfunctions	
Sleep disorders	

involved (Table 18.2); this provides the primary diagnostic category. Although many drug users take more than one kind of drug, the diagnosis of the disorder is made on the basis of the most important substance used. Where this judgement is difficult or where use is chaotic and indiscriminate, the categories **polysubstance-related disorder** (DSM-IV) or **disorder due to multiple drug use** (ICD-10) may be employed. Then the relevant disorder listed in Table 18.1 is added to the substance misused. In this system any kind of disorder can, in principle, be attached to any drug, though in practice certain disorders do not develop with individual drugs. ICD-10 also has a specific category **residual and late-onset psychotic disorder**, which describes physiological or psychological changes that occur when a drug is taken but then persist beyond the period during which a direct effect of the substance would reasonably be expected to be operating. Such categories might include hallucinogen-induced flashbacks or alcohol-related dementia.

TABLE 18.2 Classes of substances

DSM-IV	ICD-10*
Alcohol	Alcohol
Amphetamines	Other stimulants, including caffeine
Caffeine	
Cannabis	Cannabinoids
Cocaine	Cocaine
Hallucinogens	Hallucinogens
Inhalants	Volatile solvents
Nicotine	Tobacco
Opioids	Opioids
Phencyclidine	
Sedatives, hypnotics or anxiolytics	Sedatives or hypnotics
Polysubstance	Multiple drug use
Other	

* The order of entries in the classification has been amended to show parallels with DSM-IV.

Definitions in DSM-IV and ICD-10

Intoxication Both DSM-IV and ICD-10 provide definitions of intoxication. In both systems, intoxication is seen as a transient syndrome due to recent substance ingestion

TABLE 18.3 Criteria for substance abuse (DSM-IV) and harmful use (ICD-10)

DSM-IV	ICD-10
A A maladaptive pattern of substance use leading to clinically significant impairment or distress, or mental health as manifested by one (or more) of the following occurring within a 12-month period	A A pattern of psychoactive substance use that is causing damage to health; the damage may be to physical or mental health
(1) Recurrent substance use resulting in a failure to fulfil major role obligations at work, school, or home	
(2) Recurrent substance abuse in situations that are physically hazardous	
(3) Recurrent substance abuse-related legal problems	
(4) Continued substance abuse despite having persistent or recurrent social or interpersonal problems caused by or exacerbated by the effects of the substance	
B Has never met the criteria for substance dependence for this class of substance	

that produces clinically significant psychological and physical impairment. These changes disappear when the substance is eliminated from the body. The nature of the psychological changes varies with the person as well as with the drug; for example, some people intoxicated with alcohol become aggressive, but others become maudlin.

Abuse The term **abuse** in DSM-IV and **harmful use** in ICD-10 refer to maladaptive patterns of substance use that impair health in a broad sense (Table 18.3). (The widely used term **misuse** carries a similar meaning.) The DSM and ICD criteria differ somewhat, with the emphasis on negative social consequences of substance use in DSM-1V and on adverse physical and psychological consequences in ICD-10. Some individuals show definite evidence of substance abuse but do not meet criteria for substance dependence (Table 18.4). However, if they do, the diagnosis of dependence should be made and not that of abuse or harmful use.

Dependence The term **dependence** refers to certain physiological and psychological phenomena induced by the repeated taking of a substance; the criteria for diagnosing dependence are similar in DSM-IV and ICD-10, and include:

- a strong desire to take the substance;
- progressive neglect of alternative sources of satisfaction;
- the development of tolerance;
- a physical withdrawal state (see Table 18.4).

Tolerance is a state in which, after repeated administration, a drug produces a decreased effect, or increasing doses are required to produce the same effect.

Withdrawal state: a group of symptoms and signs occurring when a drug is reduced in amount or withdrawn, which last for a limited time. The nature of the withdrawal state is related to the class of substance used.

TABLE 18.4 Criteria for dependence in DSM-IV and ICD-10

DSM-IV	ICD-10
A Diagnosis of dependence should be made if three (or more) of the following have been experienced or exhibited at any time in the same 12-month period	A Diagnosis of dependence should be made if three or more of the following have been experienced or exhibited at some time during the last year
(1) Tolerance defined by either need for markedly increased amounts of substance to achieve intoxication or desired effect, or markedly diminished effect with continued use of the same amount of the substance	(1) A strong desire or sense of compulsion to take the substance
(2) Withdrawal, as evidenced by either of the following: the characteristic withdrawal syndrome for the substance, or the same (or closely related) substance is taken to relieve or avoid withdrawal symptoms	(2) Difficulties in controlling substance-taking behaviour in terms of its onset, termination, or levels of use
(3) The substance is often taken in larger amounts over a longer period of time than was intended	(3) Physiological withdrawal state when substance use has ceased or been reduced, as evidenced by either of the following: the characteristic withdrawal syndrome for the substance, or use of the same (or closely related) substance with the intention of relieving or avoiding withdrawal symptoms
(4) Persistent desire or repeated unsuccessful efforts to cut down or control substance use	(4) Evidence of tolerance, such that increased doses of the psychoactive substance are required in order to achieve effects originally produced by lower doses
(5) A great deal of time is spent in activities necessary to obtain the substance, use the substance, or recover from its effects	(5) Progressive neglect of alternative pleasures or interests because of psychoactive substance use and increased amount of time necessary to obtain or take the substance or to recover from its effects
(6) Important social, occupational, or recreational activities given up or reduced because of substance use	(6) Persisting with substance use despite clear evidence of overtly harmful consequences (physical or mental)
(7) Continued substance use despite knowledge of having had a persistent or recurrent physical or psychological problem that was likely to have been caused or exacerbated by the substance	

Alcohol-related disorders

Terminology

Alcoholism In the past, the term **alcoholism** was generally used in medical writing. Although the word is still widely used in everyday language, it is unsatisfactory as a technical term because it has more than one meaning. It can be applied to habitual alcohol consumption that is deemed excessive in amount according to some arbitrary criterion. Alcoholism may also refer to damage, whether mental, physical, or social, resulting from such excessive consumption. In a more specialized sense, alcoholism may imply a specific disease entity that is supposed to require medical treatment. However, to speak of an alcoholic often has a pejorative meaning, suggesting behaviour that is morally bad. For most purposes it is better to use four terms that relate to the classifications outlined above:

1. **Excessive consumption of alcohol**. Excessive consumption of alcohol refers to a daily or weekly intake of alcohol exceeding a specified amount (see below). Excessive consumption of alcohol is also known as hazardous drinking.
2. **Alcohol misuse**. Alcohol misuse describes drinking that causes mental, physical, or social harm to an individual. It does not, however, include those with formal alcohol dependence.
3. **Alcohol dependence**. The term alcohol dependence can be used when the criteria for a dependence syndrome listed in Table 18.4 are met.
4. **Problem drinking**. Problem drinking is a term applied to those in whom drinking has caused an alcohol-related disorder or disability. Its meaning is essentially similar to alcohol misuse but it can also include drinkers who are dependent on alcohol.

The term alcoholism, if it is used at all, should be regarded as a shorthand way of referring to some combination of these four conditions. However, since these specific terms have been introduced fairly recently, the term alcoholism has to be used in this chapter when referring to the older literature.

At this point it is appropriate to examine the **moral** and **medical** models of alcohol misuse.

The moral and medical models

According to the moral model, if someone drinks too much, they do so of their own free will, and if their drinking causes harm to themselves or their family, their actions are morally bad. The corollary of this attitude is that public drunkenness should be punished. In many countries this is the official practice; public drunks are fined and if they cannot pay the fine, they go to prison. Many people now believe that this approach is too harsh and unsympathetic. Whatever the humanitarian arguments, there is little practical justification for punishment, since there is little evidence that it influences the behaviour of excessive drinkers.

According to the medical model, a person who misuses alcohol is *ill* rather than wicked. Although it had been proposed earlier, this idea was not strongly advocated until 1960 when Jellinek published an influential book, *The disease concept of alcoholism*. The disease concept embodies three basic ideas:

1. Some people have a specific vulnerability to alcohol misuse.
2. Excessive drinking progresses through well-defined stages, at one of which the person can no longer control his drinking.
3. Excessive drinking may lead to physical and mental disease of several kinds.

One of the main consequences of the disease model is that attitudes towards excessive drinking become more humane. Instead of blame and punishment, medical treatment is provided. The disease model also has certain disadvantages. By implying that only certain people are at risk, it diverts attention from two important facts. First, anyone who drinks a great deal for a long time may become dependent on alcohol. Second, the best way to curtail the misuse of alcohol may be to limit consumption **in the whole population**, and not just among a predisposed minority.

Perhaps a useful way to resolve these two approaches is to apply the moral model to excessive drinking in the population in the hope of decreasing the number of people who put themselves at risk of alcohol-related disability. Once dependence has occurred, however, with its attendant loss of control over drinking, a medical approach may be more appropriate.

Excessive alcohol consumption

In many societies the use of alcohol is sanctioned and even encouraged by sophisticated marketing techniques. Therefore the level of drinking at which an individual is considered to demonstrate excessive alcohol consumption is a somewhat arbitrary concept, usually defined in terms of the level of use associated with significant risk of alcohol-related health and social problems. It is usually expressed in units of alcohol consumed per week (Austoker 1994) (Table 18.5).

TABLE 18.5 Alcohol consumption in men and women and risk of social and health problems

Alcohol intake (units/week)	Risk of problems
Men 0–21	Low
Women 0–14	
Men 22–50	Increasing, particularly in smokers
Women 15–35	
Men >50	High, particularly in smokers
Women >35	

Source Austoker (1994).

Whilst there is reason to suppose that anyone may become dependent on alcohol if he or she drinks a sufficiently large amount for long enough, because of substantial individual variation no exact threshold can be specified. However, **women are more sensitive than men** to the harm-inducing effects of alcohol.

If the concept of excessive alcohol consumption is to be understood and accepted, it is necessary to explain the units in which it is assessed. In everyday life, this is done by referring to conventional measures such as pints of beer or glasses of wine. These measures have the advantage of being widely understood, but they are imprecise because both beers and wines vary in strength (Table 18.6). Alternatively, consumption can be measured as the amount of alcohol (expressed in grams). This measure is precise and useful for scientific work, but is difficult for many people to relate to everyday measures.

For this reason, the concept of a **unit of alcohol** has been introduced for use in health education. A unit can be related to everyday measures for it corresponds to half a pint of beer, one glass of table wine, one conventional glass of sherry or port, and one single bar measure of spirits. It can also be related to average amounts of alcohol (see Table 18.6); thus on this measure a can of beer (450 ml) contains nearly 1.5 units, a bottle of table wine contains about 7 units, a bottle of spirits about 30 units, and 1 unit is about 8 g of alcohol.

TABLE 18.6 Alcohol content of some beverages

Beverage	Approximate alcohol content (%)	Grams alcohol per conventional measure	Units of alcohol per conventional measure (approximate)
Beer and cider			
Ordinary beer	3	16 per pint	2 per pint
		12 per can	1.5 per can
Strong beer	5.5	32 per pint	4 per pint
		24 per can	3 per can
Extra-strong beer	7	40 per pint	5 per pint
		32 per can	4 per can
Cider	4	24 per pint	3 per pint
Strong cider	6	32 per pint	4 per pint
Wine			
Table wine	8–10	8 per glass	1 per glass
		56 per bottle	7 per bottle
Fortified wines	13–16	8 per measure	1 per measure
(sherry, port, vermouth)		120 per bottle	15 per bottle
Spirits	32	8–12 per single	1–1.5 per measure*
(whisky, gin,		Measure	
Brandy, vodka)		240 per bottle	30 per bottle

* Somewhat larger measures are used in Scotland and Northern Ireland (12 grams).

Epidemiological aspects of excessive drinking and alcohol misuse

Epidemiological methods can be applied to the following questions concerning excessive drinking and alcohol misuse.

- What is the annual per capita consumption of alcohol for a nation as a whole, and how does this vary over the years and between nations?
- What is the pattern of alcohol use of different groups of people within a defined population?
- How many people in a defined population misuse alcohol?
- How does alcohol misuse vary with such characteristics as gender, age, occupation, social class, and marital status?

Unfortunately, we lack reliable answers to these questions, partly because different investigators have used different methods of defining and identifying alcohol misuse and 'alcoholism', and partly because excessive drinkers tend to be evasive about the amounts that they drink and the symptoms that they experience.

Consumption of alcohol in different countries

In the UK, the annual consumption of alcohol per adult (calculated as absolute ethanol consumption) has doubled between 1950 and 2000, rising from about four litres to over eight litres. Consumption in Western Europe has generally been higher than this, particularly in France. High levels of consumption are also seen in the former Soviet Union while in the Eastern Mediterrean and in Muslim countries consumption is much less (see Rehm *et al.*, 2003).

Recent changes in the UK can be usefully considered in a historical perspective. For example, in Great Britain between 1860 and 1900 the consumption of alcohol was about 10 litres of absolute alcohol per head of population over 15 years old. Consumption then fell until the early 1930s, reaching about 4 litres per person over 15 years per annum. Consumption then increased slowly until the 1950s when it began to rise more rapidly.

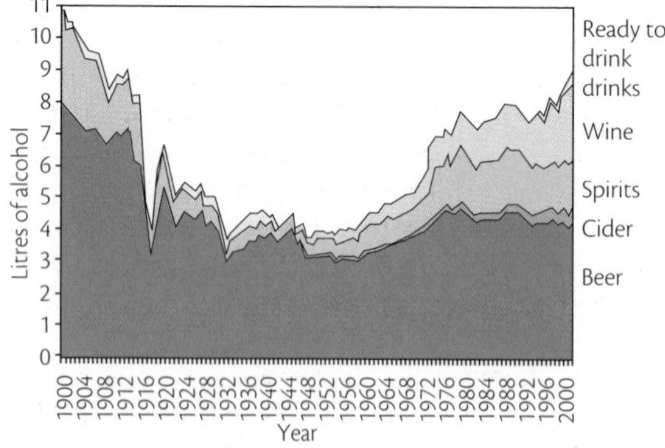

Fig 18.1 Average annual consumption of alcohol in the UK between 1900 and 2000. BBPA Statistical Handbook (2001).

These changes have been accompanied by alterations in the kinds of alcoholic beverages consumed. In Britain in 1900 beer and spirits accounted for most of the alcohol drunk; in 1980 the consumption of wine had risen about four times and accounted for almost as much of the consumption of alcohol as did spirits, though most alcohol was still consumed as beer (Figure 18.1).

Drinking habits in different groups Surveys of drinking behaviour generally depend on self-reports, a method that is open to obvious errors. Enquiries of this kind have been conducted in several countries including the UK and the USA.

Such studies show that the highest reported consumption of alcohol is generally amongst **young men** who are **unmarried, separated, or divorced**. However, over the last 15 years drinking by women has increased. From population estimates in 2001, men in England drank on average 16.9 units of alcohol a week, while women drank on average 7.5 units per week. The alcohol consumption of 27 per cent of men and 15 per cent of women exceeded recommended limits; therefore these subjects could be considered at risk of developing an alcohol-related disorder, including alcohol dependence. Thirteen per cent of men and 6 per cent of women drank more than 35 units a week (Office for National Statistics, 2003).

The prevalence of alcohol misuse

This can be estimated in three ways: from hospital admission rates, from deaths from alcoholic cirrhosis, and by surveys in the general population.

Hospital admission rates These give an inadequate measure of prevalence because a large proportion of excessive drinkers do not enter hospital.

- In England in 2000–2001 there about 30,000 **NHS psychiatric hospital admissions** with a primary diagnosis of mental and behavioural disorders due to alcohol (Office for National Statistics, 2003).
- Alcohol misuse also figures prominently in **admissions to general hospitals**, where screening questionnaires identify alcohol misuse in about 20–30 per cent of male admissions and 5–10 per cent of female admissions.
- Alcohol is estimated to be a causal factor in about one third of attendances at **Accident and Emergency Services** (Academy of Medical Sciences, 2004).

Deaths from alcoholic cirrhosis About 10–20 per cent of people who drink alcohol excessively develop cirrhosis of the liver, and there are correlations in a population between rates of liver cirrhosis and mean alcohol consumption. Therefore deaths from cirrhosis can be used as a means of estimating rates of alcohol misuse. Rates of mortality from liver cirrhosis are showing a decline in a number of developed countries. For example, in southern Europe there has been a sustained decrease in deaths from cirrhosis, probably as a result of sustained fiscal, law enforcement, and health promotion policies. On the other hand alcoholic liver cirrhosis appear to be increasing in England with a rise in recorded hospital admissions from 14,100 in 1995–1996 to 24,300 in 2000–2001 (Academy of Medical Sciences, 2004).

General population surveys One method of ascertaining the rate of alcohol misuse in a population is by seeking information from general practitioners, social workers, probation officers, health visitors, and other agencies who are likely to come in contact with heavy drinkers. Another approach is the community survey in which samples of people are asked about the amount they drink and whether they experience symptoms. Two epidemiological investigations in the USA (the Epidemiological Catchment Area Programme and the National Comorbidity Survey) suggested a combined 1-year prevalence rate for alcohol misuse and dependence of 7–10 per cent. The corresponding lifetime risks were about 14–20 per cent (Kessler *et al.*, 1994; Regier *et al.*, 1994).

The British Psychiatric Morbidity Survey, reporting in 2002, classified 26 per cent of adults living in households as hazardous drinkers, and 7 per cent as alcohol dependent (Coulthard *et al.*, 2002). However, an 18 month follow-up of these subjects showed considerable fluctuation over time with a substantial proportion of people moving from hazardous drinking towards safer drinking, and others moving into the hazardous drinking category (Farrell 2003).

Surveys based on households are likely to miss certain groups at high risk of alcohol misuse and dependence. The British Psychiatric Morbidity Survey has previously sampled separately from homeless populations and from those in institutions such as prisons. Among people living in night shelters or sleeping rough, 40 per cent were found to drink more than 50 units of alcohol a week and about 35 per cent of those sleeping rough were estimated to have severe alcohol dependence (Gill *et al.*, 1996). High rates of alcohol misuse were also found in prisoners, especially among white males (Singleton *et al.*, 1997).

In a cross-national study of ten different cultural regions, lifetime prevalence rates for alcohol misuse and dependence varied from about 0.5 per cent in Shanghai to 22 per cent in Korea (Helzer and Canino, 1992). Whilst there are undoubtedly wide variations between countries in the real prevalence of alcohol misuse and dependence, some of the apparent differences may stem from contrasting cultural perspectives on what constitutes alcohol misuse and the extent to which people chose to reveal their drinking habits to investigators.

Alcohol misuse and population characteristics

Gender Rates of alcohol misuse and dependence are consistently higher in men than in women but the ratio of affected men to women varies markedly across cultures. In Western countries, about three times as many men as women suffer from alcohol misuse and dependence, but in Asian and Hispanic cultures over ten times as many men are affected (Helzer and Canino, 1992). In the National Comorbidity Survey in the USA, the 1-year prevalence of alcohol misuse and dependence in men (14.1 per cent) was almost three times that in women (5.3 per cent) (Kessler *et al.*, 1994). Similarly, in the British Psychiatric Morbidity Survey, prevalence of alcohol dependence was three times higher among men than among women (Coulthard *et al.*, 2002). However, perhaps because of changing social attitudes, the gap between men and women in terms of excessive drinking seems to be narrowing in many Western countries (Marshall, 2000). This is of concern because studies indicate that women are more susceptible than men to many of the damaging effects of alcohol (see below).

Age We have seen that the heaviest drinkers are men in their late teens or early twenties. In most cultures the prevalence of alcohol misuse and dependence is lower in those aged over 45 years (Helzer and Canino, 1992; Coulthard *et al.*, 2002).

Ethnicity and culture The followers of certain **religions** which proscribe alcohol, for example, Islam, Hinduism, and the Baptist Church, are less likely than the general population to misuse alcohol. It is also worth noting that the non-white population in the UK and the USA are less likely to drink excessively than the white population and therefore have a lower rate of alcohol-related disorders (Kessler *et al.*, 1994, Coulthard *et al.*, 2002).

In some instances, the low consumption of alcohol in a particular ethnic group may be due to a **biologically determined** lack of tolerance to alcohol. For example, Asians and Orientals with a particular variant of the isoenzyme of aldehyde dehydrogenase experience flushing, nausea, and tachycardia due to accumulation of acetaldehyde when they drink alcohol. Such subjects are likely to be at reduced risk of excess drinking and the consequent development of alcohol-related disorders. Thus, although the aldehyde dehydrogenase variant that causes the flushing reaction was present in 35 of the general Japanese population, it was found in only 7 per cent of Japanese patients with alcoholic liver disease (Shibuya and Yoshida, 1988).

Occupation The risk of alcohol misuse is much increased among several **occupational groups** chefs, kitchen porters, barmen, and brewery workers, who have easy access to alcohol, executives and salesmen who entertain on expense accounts, actors and entertainers, seamen, and journalists and printers. Doctors are another important group with an increased risk of problem drinking, and they are often particularly difficult to help (Chick, 1992).

Syndromes of alcohol dependence and alcohol withdrawal

Patients are described as alcohol dependent when they meet the criteria for **substance dependence** described in Table 18.4. The presence of withdrawal phenomena are not necessary for the diagnosis of dependence and a substantial minority of subjects who meet dependence criteria do not experience any withdrawal phenomena when their intake of alcohol diminishes or stops. However, about 5 per cent of dependent subjects experience severe **withdrawal symptomatology** including **delirium tremens** and **grand mal seizures**.

Course of alcohol misuse and dependence

Schuckit *et al.* (1993) reviewed the course of over 600 men with alcohol dependence who received inpatient treatment at a single facility in the USA between 1985 and 1991. These subjects showed a general pattern of escalation of heavy drinking in their late twenties followed by evidence of serious difficulties in work and social life by their early thirties. In their middle to late thirties, following the perception that they could not control their drinking, subjects experienced increasing social and work problems together with a significant deterioration in physical health.

Vaillant (2003) described a 60 year follow-up of 194 men who had exhibited misuse of alcohol at some point in their adult lives. By the age of 70 over half the cohort had died and about 20 per cent were abstinent. Ten per cent were drinking in a controlled way while a further ten per cent continued to misuse alcohol. In a number of subjects alcohol misuse had apparently persisted for decades without remission, death, or progression to formal dependence. For alcohol-dependent men, however, periods of controlled drinking were invariably followed by return to a pattern of alcohol dependence. Attendance at Alcholics Anonymous was the best predictor of good outcome. This study suggests that the prognosis of alcohol misuse is very variable. However, once an individual has become alcohol-dependent the prognosis is poor unless abstinence can be maintained.

The alcohol withdrawal syndrome

Withdrawal symptoms occur across a spectrum of severity, from mild anxiety and sleep disturbance to the life-threatening state known as **delirium tremens**. The symptoms generally occur in people who have been drinking heavily for years and who maintain a high intake of alcohol for weeks at a time. The symptoms follow a drop in blood concentration. They characteristically appear on waking, after the fall in concentration during sleep. **Dependent drinkers** often take a **drink on waking** to stave off withdrawal symptoms. In most cultures, **early-morning drinking** is diagnostic of dependency. With increasing need to stave off withdrawal symptoms during the day, the drinker typically becomes secretive about the amount consumed, hides bottles, or carries them in a pocket. Rough cider and cheap strong beers may be drunk regularly to obtain the most alcohol for the least money.

The earliest and commonest feature of alcohol withdrawal is acute tremulousness affecting the hands, legs, and trunk ('the shakes'). The sufferer may be unable to sit still, hold a cup steady, or do up buttons. He is also agitated and easily startled, and often dreads facing people or crossing the road. Nausea, retching, and sweating are frequent. Insomnia is also common. If alcohol is taken, these symptoms may be relieved quickly; if not, they may last for several days (Table 18.7).

TABLE 18.7 Symptoms and signs of acute alcohol withdrawal

Anxiety, agitation, insomnia
Tachycardia and sweating
Tremor of limbs, tongue and eyelids
Nausea and vomiting
Seizures
Confusion and hallucinations

From Ritson (2005).

As withdrawal progresses, **misperceptions** and **hallucinations** may occur, usually only briefly.

Objects appear distorted in shape, or shadows seem to move; disorganized voices, shouting, or snatches of music may be heard. Later there may be **epileptic seizures**, and finally after about 48 hours delirium tremens may develop (Victor and Adams 1953) (see below).

Other alcohol-related disorders

The different types of damage – **physical, psychological**, and **social** – that can result from alcohol misuse are described in this section. A person who suffers from these disabilities may or may not be suffering from alcohol dependence.

Physical damage

Excessive consumption of alcohol may lead to physical damage in several ways. First, it can have a direct toxic effect on certain tissues, notably the brain and liver. Second, it is often accompanied by poor diet which may lead to deficiency of protein and B vitamins. Third, it increases the risk of accidents, particularly head injury. Fourth, it is accompanied by general neglect which can lead to increased susceptibility to infection.

Gastrointestinal

Gastrointestinal disorders are common, notably liver damage, gastritis, peptic ulcer, oesophageal varices, and acute and chronic pancreatitis. Damage to the liver, including fatty infiltration, hepatitis, cirrhosis, and hepatoma, is particularly important. For a person who is dependent on alcohol, the risk of dying from liver cirrhosis is almost ten times greater than the average. However, only about 10–20 per cent of alcohol-dependent people develop cirrhosis.

Nervous system

Alcohol also damages the nervous system. Neuropsychiatric complications are described later; other neurological conditions include **peripheral neuropathy, epilepsy**, and **cerebellar degeneration**. The last of these is characterized by unsteadiness of stance and gait, with less effect on arm movements or speech. Rare complications are optic atrophy, central pontine myelinolysis, and **Marchiafava–Bignami syndrome**. The last of these results from widespread demyelination of the corpus callosum, optic tracts, and cerebellar peduncles. Its main features are dysarthria, ataxia, epilepsy, and marked impairment of consciousness; in the more prolonged forms, dementia and limb paralysis occur. **Head injury** is also common in alcohol-dependent people.

Cardiovascular system

Alcohol misuse is associated with **hypertension** and increased risk of **stroke**. Paradoxically, men who drink moderate amounts of alcohol (up to about 10 units a week) appear less likely than non-drinkers to die from coronary artery disease (see Goldberg *et al.*, 1999). Alcohol misuse has also been linked to the development of certain cancers, notably of the mouth, pharynx, oesophagus, liver and breast.

Other physical complications of excessive consumption of alcohol are too numerous to detail here. Examples include anaemia, myopathy, episodic hypoglycaemia, haemochromatosis, cardiomyopathy, vitamin deficiencies, and tuberculosis. They are described in textbooks of medicine, for example the *Oxford Textbook of Medicine* (Warrell *et al.*, 2003).

Alcohol misuse in women

Studies suggest that women progress more rapidly than men to problem drinking, and tend to suffer the medical consequences of alcohol use after a shorter period of exposure to a smaller amount of alcohol. As well as the expected medical complications noted above, female drinkers also show elevated rates of breast cancer and reproductive pathology including amenorrhoea, anovulation, and possibly early menopause.

Damage to the fetus

There is evidence that a **fetal alcohol syndrome** occurs in children born to mothers who drink excessively. In France, Lemoine *et al.* (1968) described a syndrome of **facial abnormality, small stature, low birth-weight, low intelligence, and overactivity**. In a ten year follow-up of children with fetal alcohol syndrome, Spohr *et al.* (1993) found that, whilst the characteristic craniofacial malformations decreased with time, many had evidence of persisting learning disability.

Fetal alcohol syndrome is associated with clearly excessive alcohol use during pregnancy. However, subsequent research has suggested that even moderate or low levels of alcohol consumption at this time can produce adverse consequences for childhood development. For example, increased rates of behavioural disturbance in infants have been reported where mothers have consumed as little as one drink a week (see Mukherjee *et al.*, 2005). At the moment therefore, it is not known if there is, in fact, a 'safe level' of alcohol consumption during pregnancy and abstinence is the safest option.

Mortality

People with a low level of alcohol consumption (about one unit daily) have decreased mortality rates compared to non-drinkers (Doll *et al.*, 2005). This is mainly attributable to lowered cardiovascular mortality (see above). Not surprisingly, however, the mortality rate is increased in those who misuse alcohol. Follow-up investigations have studied mainly middle-aged men drinking excessively in whom overall mortality is at least twice the expected rate and mortality in women who drink excessively appears substantially higher than this (Harris and Barraclough, 1998).

Even allowing for the fact that heavy drinkers also tend to be heavy smokers, alcohol itself is almost certainly responsible for a substantial part of this increased mortality. In the UK it is estimated that excess alcohol consumption leads to about 33 000 premature deaths a year, mainly from cardiovascular disorders, cirrhosis, accidents, and cancer (Ashworth and Gerada, 1997).

Psychiatric disorders

Alcohol-related psychiatric disorders fall into four groups:

1. intoxication phenomena
2. withdrawal phenomena
3. toxic or nutritional disorders
4. associated psychiatric disorders.

Intoxication phenomena

The severity of the symptoms of alcohol intoxication correlate approximately with the blood concentration. As noted above, there is much individual variation in the psychological effects of alcohol, but certain reactions such as lability of mood and belligerence are more likely to cause social difficulties. At high doses, alcohol intoxication can result in serious adverse effects such as falls, respiratory depression, inhalation of vomit, and hypothermia.

The **molecular mechanisms** that underlie the acute effects of alcohol are not clear. An influential view has been that alcohol interacts with neuronal membranes to **increase their fluidity**, an action also ascribed to certain anaesthetic agents. This action gives rise to more specific changes in the release of a range of neurotransmitters leading to the characteristic pharmacological actions of alcohol. For example, the pleasurable effects of alcohol use could be mediated by release of **dopamine and opioids** in mesolimbic forebrain, whilst the anxiolytic effects could reflect facilitation of brain **gamma-aminobutyric acid** (GABA) activity (Lingford-Huges *et al.*, 2003).

The term **idiosyncratic alcohol intoxication** has been applied to marked maladaptive changes in behaviour, such as aggression, occurring within minutes of taking an amount of alcohol insufficient to induce intoxication in most people (with the behaviour being uncharacteristic of the person). In the past, these sudden changes in behaviour were called pathological drunkenness, or ***manie à potu***, and the descriptions emphasized the explosive nature of the outbursts of aggression. There is doubt, however, whether behaviour of this kind really is induced by small amounts of alcohol. The term idiosyncratic alcohol intoxication does not appear in DSM-IV or ICD-10.

Memory blackouts or **short-term amnesia** are frequently reported after heavy drinking. At first the events of the night before are forgotten, even though consciousness was maintained at the time. Such memory losses can occur after a single episode of heavy drinking in people who are not dependent on alcohol; if they recur regularly, they indicate habitual excessive consumption. With sustained excessive drinking, memory losses may become more severe, affecting parts of the daytime or even whole days.

Withdrawal phenomena

The general withdrawal syndrome has been described earlier under the heading of alcohol dependence. Here we are concerned with the more serious psychiatric syndrome of **delirium tremens**. Delirious states are described generally in Chapter 14 but delirium tremens is discussed here because of its prevalence and mortality, and its somewhat different treatment.

Delirium tremens This occurs in people whose history of alcohol misuse extends over several years. Following alcohol withdrawal there is a dramatic and rapidly changing picture of disordered mental activity, with clouding of consciousness, disorientation in time and place, and impairment of recent memory. Perceptual disturbances include misinterpretations of sensory stimuli and vivid hallucinations, which are usually visual but sometimes occur in other modalities. There is severe agitation, with restlessness, shouting, and evident fear. Insomnia is prolonged. The hands are grossly tremulous and sometimes pick up imaginary objects; truncal ataxia may occur. Autonomic disturbances include sweating, fever, tachycardia, raised blood pressure, and dilatation of pupils. Dehydration and electrolyte disturbance are characteristic. Blood testing shows leucocytosis and impaired liver function.

The condition lasts 3 or 4 days, with the symptoms characteristically being worse at night. It often ends with deep prolonged sleep from which the patient awakens with no symptoms and little or no memory of the period of delirium. Delirium tremens carries a

significant risk of mortality and should be regarded as a medical emergency.

Toxic or nutritional conditions

These include **Korsakov's psychosis** and **Wernicke's encephalopathy** (see also Chapter 14) and **alcoholic dementia**, which is described next.

Alcoholic dementia In the past there has been disagreement as to whether alcohol misuse can cause dementia. This doubt may have arisen because patients with general intellectual defects have been wrongly diagnosed as having Korsakov's psychosis. However, it is now generally agreed that chronic alcohol misuse can cause cognitive impairment, particularly in tests of memory and executive function (Zinn *et al.*, 2004).

Attention has also been directed to the related question of whether chronic alcohol misuse can cause structural brain atrophy. Both CT scanning and magnetic resonance imaging (MRI) have shown that excess alcohol consumption is associated with **enlarged lateral ventricles**. Furthermore, MRI scans have shown focal deficits with **loss of grey matter** in both cortical and subcortical areas. Subcortical changes are more likely to be found in patients with Korsakov's syndrome. Thinning of the **corpus callosum** has also been reported in patients with alcohol dependence.

Many of the changes noted above occur in patients without obvious neurological disturbance, though, as noted above, psychological testing usually reveals deficits in **cognitive function**. The changes in brain structure and cognitive impairment seen in excessive drinkers remit to some extent with cessation of alcohol use; however, many abnormalities can still be detected after long periods of abstinence. (For a review of brain imaging studies of the effects of alcohol see Lingford-Hughes *et al.*, 2003.)

Associated psychiatric disorder

Personality deterioration As the patient becomes more and more concerned with the need to obtain alcohol, interpersonal skills and attendance to usual interests and responsibilities may deteriorate. These changes in social and interpersonal functioning should not be confused with personality disorder, which should be diagnosed only when the appropriate features have been clearly present prior to the development of alcohol dependence.

Mood disorder The relationship between alcohol consumption and mood is complex. On the one hand, some depressed patients drink excessively in an attempt to improve their mood; on the other hand, excess drinking may induce persistent depression or anxiety. In hospital populations, recurrent mood disorder frequently coexists with alcohol misuse and dependence. In community samples, however, depression seems to be more often associated with interpersonal and social problems occurring as a result of alcohol misuse. The relationship between depression and alcohol misuse appears clearer in women and a follow-up study indicated that the risk of excessive drinking was increased at least twofold in women by a history of depressive disorder (Dixit and Crum, 2000).

Suicidal behaviour Suicide rates amongst people with alcohol use disorders are much higher than among people who do not misuse alcohol. For a review, and an argument for a focus on alcohol in global suicide prevention, see Foster (2001). There are many reasons for high suicide rates. For example, in a study of 50 alcohol misusers who had committed suicide, Murphy *et al.* (1992) identified a number of risk factors for suicidal behaviour, including continued drinking, comorbid major depression, serious medical illness, unemployment, and poor social support. It is worth noting that suicide in young men is associated with a high rate of substance misuse, including alcohol.

Impaired psychosexual function Erectile dysfunction and delayed ejaculation are common. These difficulties may be worsened when drinking leads to marital estrangement, or if the wife develops a revulsion for intercourse with an inebriated partner.

Pathological jealousy Excessive drinkers may develop an overvalued idea or delusion that the partner is being unfaithful. This syndrome of pathological jealousy is described on p. 314.

Alcoholic hallucinosis This is characterized by **auditory hallucinations**, usually voices uttering insults or threats, occurring in clear consciousness. The patient is usually distressed by these experiences, and appears anxious and restless. The hallucinations are not due to acute alcohol withdrawal and can indeed persist after several months of abstinence. There has been considerable controversy about the aetiology of the condition. Some follow Kraepelin and Bonhoffer in regarding it as a rare organic complication of alcoholism; others follow Bleuler in supposing that it is related to schizophrenia. Most recent reviewers have concluded that alcoholic hallucinosis is an alcohol-induced organic psychosis, which is distinct from schizophrenia and has a good prognosis if abstinence can be maintained (see Greenberg and Lee, 2001).

In both DSM-IV and ICD-10, **alcoholic hallucinosis** is subsumed under the heading of **substance-induced psychotic disorder**.

Social damage (see Box 18.1)

Family problems

Excessive drinking is liable to cause profound social disruption particularly in the family. Marital and family tension is virtually inevitable. The *divorce rate* amongst heavy drinkers is high, and the wives of such men are likely to become anxious, depressed, and socially isolated; the husbands of *'battered' wives* frequently drink excessively, and some women admitted to hospital because of self-poisoning blame their husband's drinking. The home atmosphere is often detrimental to the children because of quarrelling and violence, and a drunken parent provides a poor role model. Children of heavy drinkers are at risk of developing emotional or behaviour disorders, and of performing badly at school.

Work difficulties and road accidents

At work, the heavy drinker often progresses through declining efficiency, lower-grade jobs, and repeated dismissals to lasting unemployment. There is also a strong association between road accidents and alcohol misuse. In the USA in 1990, 44 529 people were killed in traffic accidents, with alcohol being involved in 41 per cent of these fatalities (Zobeck *et al.*, 1994). A remarkably similar figure of 44 per cent was reported in drivers killed in road accidents in Spain between 1991 and 2000 (Carmen del Rio *et al.*, 2002).

Crime

Excessive drinking is also associated with **crime**, mainly petty offences such as larceny, but also with fraud, sexual offences, and crimes of violence including murder. Studies of recidivist prisoners in England and Wales have shown that many of them had serious drinking problems before imprisonment. It is not easy to know how far alcohol causes the criminal behaviour and how far it is just part of the lifestyle of the criminal. In addition, there is a link between certain forms of alcohol misuse and **antisocial personality disorder** (see below and p. 136).

BOX 18.1 MEDICAL AND SOCIAL CONSEQUENCES OF EXCESSIVE ALCOHOL CONSUMPTION IN THE UK

1. Annual alcohol-related costs of crime and public disorder £7.3 billion, work-place costs £6.4 billion, health costs £1.7 billion.
2. Up to one third of all accident and emergency attendances.
3. 2.9 million (7 per cent) of the adult population dependent on alcohol.
4. Forty-seven per cent of victims of violence believe that their assailant was under the influence of alcohol.
5. Between 1993–2000 the number of casualties from road accidents involving alcohol rose by 20 per cent.
6. Between 30–60 per cent of child protection cases involve alcohol. Up to 1.3 million children adversely affected by family drinking.

Source: Prime Minister's Strategy Unit (2003)

The causes of excessive drinking and alcohol misuse

Despite much research, surprisingly little is known about the cause of excessive drinking and alcohol dependence. At one time it was believed that certain people were particularly predisposed, either through personality or an innate biochemical anomaly. Nowadays this simple notion of specific predisposition is no longer held. Instead, alcohol misuse is thought to result from a variety of interacting factors which can be divided into individual factors and those in society.

Individual factors

Genetic factors

Alcohol use Twin studies provide an opportunity to investigate the role of genetic and familial factors in patterns of alcohol use. A study employing this approach has suggested that liability to lifetime alcohol use is **environmentally determined**. However, the risk **of illicit, under-age drinking** has strong genetic determinants (Maes *et al.* 1999).

Alcohol misuse and dependence Most genetic studies of alcoholism have investigated subjects with evidence of alcohol dependence. If less severe diagnostic criteria are involved, for example, fairly broadly defined alcohol misuse, the relative genetic contribution is somewhat less.

It is well established that alcohol dependence **aggregates in families**. If this is partly the result of genetic factors (rather than social influences in the family), rates of dependence should be higher in monozygotic (MZ) than dizygotic (DZ) twins. Generally, results of MZ–DZ comparisons have shown a **higher MZ concordance** for alcohol dependence in male and female twins. These studies have suggested that the heritability for alcohol dependence is about 50 per cent for males and 25 per cent for females (Ball, 2004).

Support for a genetic explanation also comes from investigations of **adoptees**. A number of studies have indicated an increased risk of alcohol misuse and dependence in the adopted-away sons of alcohol-dependent biological parents than in the adopted-away sons of non-alcohol-dependent biological parents. Such studies suggest a genetic mechanism but do not indicate its nature.

Adoption studies in Sweden have led to the suggestion that there are two separate kinds of alcohol dependence, which have been called **type 1 and type 2** (Cloninger *et al.*, 1988). Type 2 alcoholism is strongly genetic, has an early age of onset and is associated with criminality and sociopathic disorder in both adoptee and biological father. By contrast, type 1 alcoholism has a later age of onset and is only mildly genetic (Gurling and Cook, 1999).

If a genetic component to aetiology were confirmed, it would still be necessary to discover the mechanism. The latter might be biochemical, involving the metabolism of alcohol or its central effects, or psychological, involving personality. In addition, it is important to note that a predisposition to misuse alcohol and develop dependence will be expressed only if a person consumes excessive amounts of alcohol. Here non-genetic familial factors are likely to play a major role (Ball, 2004).

Linkage and association studies are the two main molecular genetic approaches that have been used to study the genetic contribution to alcohol misuse and dependence. Allelic association studies have focused particularly on the alleles of the dopamine D_2 receptor. Results of studies have been contradictory, perhaps because of ethnic differences in the frequency of D_2 receptor polymorphisms, and the proneness of this kind of case-control study to produce false positives (see p. 102). Although the debate continues, the dopamine D_2 receptor gene now appears most likely to be falsely implicated (Ball, 2004).

Collaborative studies screening the entire human genome have indicated potential loci predisposing to alcohol dependence on several chromosomes, particularly chromosome 4. This is of interest because of the proximity of genes coding for GABA receptors. For a review of genetic approaches to alcohol dependence, see Ball (2004).

Other biological factors

Several possible biochemical factors have been suggested to predispose to alcohol misuse and dependence, including abnormalities in alcohol dehydrogenase or in neurotransmitter mechanisms. As mentioned above, a significant proportion of Oriental subjects, who possess a particular allele of the isoenzyme aldehyde dehydrogenase, develop unpleasant reactions to alcohol and therefore are less likely to misuse it.

The **sons of men with alcohol dependence** are at increased risk of developing alcohol dependence themselves, and a number of studies have attempted to find biological abnormalities that may antedate and predict the development of alcohol dependence in these subjects. A variety of impairments have been described, including abnormal performance on cognitive tasks and on the P300 visual evoked response, which is a measure of visual information processing (Carlson *et al.*, 2002). There is also reasonably consistent evidence that sons of alcohol-dependent men are less sensitive to the acute intoxicating effects of alcohol (Heath *et al.*, 1999). Presumably, if subjects experience less subjective response to alcohol, they may tend to drink more, thus putting themselves at risk of developing alcohol dependence. While plausible, this hypothesis is not supported by direct evidence.

Learning factors

Alcohol use Children tend to follow their parents' drinking patterns and from an early age boys tend to be encouraged to drink more than girls. Non-genetic familial factors appear to be important in determining levels of alcohol use. Nevertheless, it is not uncommon to meet people who are abstainers although their parents drank heavily.

Alcohol dependence It has also been suggested that learning processes may contribute in a more specific way to the development of alcohol dependence. For example, recent formulations that combine biochemical and cognitive approaches emphasize the role of dopamine release in mesolimbic pathways in mediating incentive learning. In this way drugs such as alcohol which increase dopamine levels in this brain region stimulate motivational behaviours focused on the need to secure further drug supplies. These behaviours may be outside conscious control and are difficult to extinguish (see Robbins and Everitt, 1999).

Personality factors

Little progress has been made in identifying personality factors that contribute to alcohol misuse and dependence. In clinical practice it is common to find that excessive alcohol consumption is associated with chronic anxiety, a pervading sense of inferiority, or self-indulgent tendencies. However, many people with personality problems of this kind do not resort to excessive drinking or become alcohol dependent. More recent surveys have emphasized the role of personality traits that lead to risk-taking and novelty seeking (Kampov-Polevoy *et al.*, 2004). It seems likely that these characteristics apply to those with antisocial personality disorder who are known to be at increased risk of misusing alcohol and developing alcohol dependence. However, the majority of alcohol-dependent subjects do not have an antisocial personality disorder.

Psychiatric disorder

Alcohol misuse is commonly found in conjunction with other psychiatric disorders and sometimes appears to be secondary to them. For example, some patients with **depressive disorders** take to alcohol in the mistaken hope that it will alleviate low mood. Those with anxiety disorders, particularly **panic disorder** and **social phobia**, are also at risk. Alcohol misuse is also seen in patients with bipolar disorder and schizophrenia. (The treatment of patients with severe mental illness and comorbid substance misuse is discussed on p. 457.)

Alcohol consumption in society

There is now general agreement that rates of alcohol dependence and alcohol-related disorders are correlated with the **general level of alcohol consumption** in a society. Previously it had been supposed that levels of intake amongst excessive drinkers were independent of the amounts taken by moderate drinkers. The French demographer Ledermann (1956) challenged this idea, proposing instead that the distribution of consumption within a homogeneous population follows a logarithmic normal curve. If this is the case, an increase in the average consumption must inevitably be accompanied by an increase in the number of people who drink an amount that is harmful.

Although the mathematical details of Ledermann's work have been criticized, there are striking correlations between average annual consumption in a society and several indices of alcohol-related damage among its members. For this reason, it is now widely accepted that the proportion of a population drinking excessively is largely determined by the average consumption of that population.

What then determines the average level of drinking within a nation? **Economic, formal**, and **informal** controls must be considered. The **economic control** is the price of alcohol. There is now ample evidence from the UK and other countries that the real price of alcohol (i.e. the price relative to average income) profoundly influences a nation's drinking. Also, heavy drinkers as well as moderate drinkers reduce their consumption when the tax on alcohol is increased.

The main **formal controls** are the licensing laws, but these do not seem to influence drinking behaviours in a consistent way when comparisons are made between different countries. **Informal controls** are the customs and moral beliefs in a society that determine who should drink, in what circumstances, at what time of day, and to what extent. Some communities seem to protect their members from alcohol misuse despite general availability of alcohol; for example, alcohol-related problems are uncommon among Jews even in countries with high rates in the rest of the community. For a discussion of economic and social aspects of alcohol consumption see The Academy of Medical Sciences (2004).

Recognition of alcohol misuse

Detection

Only a small proportion of alcohol misusers in the community are known to specialized agencies. When special efforts are made to screen patients in medical and surgical wards, between 10–30 per cent are found to misuse alcohol, with the rates being highest in accident and emergency wards.

Screening questionnaires Alcohol misuse often goes undetected because subjects conceal the extent of their drinking. However, doctors and other professionals often do not ask the right questions. It should be a standard practice to ask all patients – medical, surgical, and psychiatric – about their alcohol consumption. Brief screening questionnaires can be helpful, for example the CAGE questionnaire which consists of the following four questions.

- Have you ever felt you ought to cut down on your drinking?
- Have people annoyed you by criticizing your drinking?
- Have you ever felt guilty about your drinking?
- Have you ever had a drink first thing in the morning (an 'eye-opener') to steady your nerves or get rid of a hangover?

Two or more positive replies are said to identify alcohol misuse. Some patients will give false answers, but others find that these questions provide an opportunity to reveal their problems. Overall the CAGE has a good sensitivity but only modest specificity (Warner, 2004; see p. 123).

An alternative is the AUDIT, a ten-item structured interview designed at the request of the World Health

BOX 18.2 AUDIT QUESTIONNAIRE: SCREEN FOR ALCOHOL MISUSE

1. How often do you have a drink containing alcohol?
   - Never
   - Monthly or less
   - 2–4 times a month
   - 2–3 times a week
   - 4 or more times a week
2. How many standard drinks containing alcohol do you have on a typical day when drinking?
   - 1 or 2
   - 3 or 4
   - 5 or 6
   - 7 to 9
   - 10 or more
3. How often do you have six or more drinks on one occasion?
   - Never
   - Less than monthly
   - Monthly
   - Weekly
   - Daily or almost daily
4. During the past year, how often have you found that you were not able to stop drinking once you had started?
   - Never
   - Less than monthly
   - Monthly
   - Weekly
   - Daily or almost daily
5. During the past year, how often have you failed to do what was normally expected of you because of drinking?
   - Never
   - Less than monthly
   - Monthly
   - Weekly
   - Daily or almost daily
6. During the past year, how often have you needed a drink in the morning to get yourself going after a heavy drinking session?
   - Never
   - Less than monthly
   - Monthly
   - Weekly
   - Daily or almost daily
7. During the past year, how often have you had a feeling of guilt or remorse after drinking?
   - Never
   - Less than monthly
   - Monthly
   - Weekly
   - Daily or almost daily
8. During the past year, have you been unable to remember what happened the night before because you had been drinking?
   - Never
   - Less than monthly
   - Monthly
   - Weekly
   - Daily or almost daily
9. Have you or someone else been injured as a result of your drinking?
   - No
   - Yes, but not in the past year
   - Yes, during the past year
10. Has a relative or friend, doctor or other health worker been concerned about your drinking or suggested you cut down?
    - No
    - Yes, but not in the past year
    - Yes, during the past year

Scores for each question range from 0 to 4, with the first response for each question scoring 0, and the last response scoring 4. For questions 9 and 10, which only have three responses, the scoring is 0, 2 and 4.

People who score in the range (8–15) should receive a brief intervention based on their risk for developing alcohol-related harm. Those scoring (16–19) need a brief intervention and regular monitoring, including referral for a more formal diagnostic assessment if heavy drinking continues. Those scoring in the range (20–40) should receive a diagnostic assessment and, depending on the severity of physical dependence, detoxification and other treatments (Room *et al.*, 2005).

Organization for screening for both currently harmful and potentially hazardous drinking. It shows good sensitivity and specificity, can identify mild dependence, and is probably the most useful screening questionnaire for clinicians and researchers in primary care (Box 18.2).

General 'at risk'associations The next requirement is for the doctor to be suspicious about 'at-risk' associations. In general practice, alcohol misuse may come to light as a result of problems in the **marriage and family**, at **work**, with **finances**, or with **the law**. The alcohol misuser is likely to have many more days off work than the moderate drinker, and repeated absences on Monday are highly suggestive. The at-risk occupations should also be remembered.

Medical 'at risk' associations In hospital practice, the alcohol-dependent subject may be noticed if they develop withdrawal symptoms after admission. Florid delirium tremens is obvious, but milder forms may be mistaken for an acute organic syndrome, for example, in pneumonia or postoperatively. In both general and hospital practice, at-risk factors include physical disorders that may be alcohol related. Common examples are **gastritis, peptic ulcer**, and **liver disease**, but others such as **neuropathy** and **seizures** should be borne in mind. **Repeated accidents** should also arouse suspicion.

Psychiatric at-risk associations include anxiety, depression, erratic moods, impaired concentration, memory lapses, and sexual dysfunction. Alcohol misuse should be considered in all cases of **deliberate self-harm**.

Drinking history

If any of the above factors raise suspicion about alcohol misuse, the next stage is to take a comprehensive drinking history (Box 18.3). This should be carried out sensitively, with understanding that the patient may have difficulty giving a clear history. The clinician should aim to build up a picture of what and how much the patient drinks throughout a typical day for example, when and where do they have the first drink of the day? The patient should be asked how they feel if they go without a drink for a day or two, and how they feel **on waking**. This can lead on to enquiries about the typical features of dependence and the range of physical, psychological and social problems associated with it.

To get an idea of the duration of alcohol problems, key points in the history may include establishing when the patient first began **drinking every day**, when they began drinking **in the mornings** and when, if ever, they first experienced **withdrawal symptoms**. It is useful to ask about periods of abstinence from alcohol, what factors helped maintain this state of affairs and what led to a resumption of drinking. This can lead on to enquiries about past attempts at treatment.

BOX 18.3 **ALCOHOL USE HISTORY**

- Describe a typical day's drinking. What time is first drink of the day?
- When did daily drinking start?
- Presence of withdrawal symptoms in morning or after abstinence
- Previous attempts at treatment
- Medical complications
- Patient's attitude towards drinking

It is necessary to gain a clear understanding of the patient's own view of their drinking behaviour, because there are a number of possible treatment goals. In this situation the **patient's attitude** to their problems plays a key role in deciding which approaches are likely to be most beneficial (see section on motivational interviewing).

Laboratory tests

Several laboratory tests can be used to detect alcohol misuse, though none gives an unequivocal answer. This is because the more sensitive tests can give 'false positives' when there is disease of the liver, heart, kidneys, or blood, or if enzyme-inducing drugs, such as anticonvulsants, steroids, or barbiturates, have been taken. However, abnormal values point to the possibility of alcohol misuse. For the most useful tests see Box 18.4. For a review of biological markers of alcohol misuse, see Sharpe (2002).

The treatment of alcohol misuse (Box 18.5)

Early detection and treatment

Early detection of excessive consumption of alcohol and alcohol misuse is important because treatment of established cases is difficult, particularly when dependence is present. Many cases can be detected early by general practitioners, physicians, and surgeons when patients seek treatment for another problem.

Brief intervention

General practitioners are well placed to provide early treatment of alcohol problems, and they are likely to know the patient and his family well. It is often effective if the general practitioner gives simple advice in a frank matter-of-fact way, but with tact and understanding.

Brief intervention studies generally involve simple education and advice about safe levels of alcohol consumption. The aim is to promote safer drinking rather

BOX 18.4 LABORATORY TESTS FOR ALCOHOL DEPENDENCE

Gamma-glutamyl-transpeptidase (GGT) Estimations of GGT in blood provide a useful screening test. The level is raised in about 70 per cent of alcohol misusers, both men and women, whether or not there is demonstrable liver damage. The heavier the drinking, the greater is the rise in GGT.

Mean corpuscular volume (MCV) MCV is raised above the normal value in about 60 per cent of alcohol misusers, and more commonly in women than in men. If other causes are excluded, a raised MCV is a strong pointer to excessive drinking. Moreover, it takes several weeks to return to normal after abstinence.

Carbohydrate deficient transferrin This is a variant of a serum protein which transports iron, and levels are increased in response to heavy drinking. It is probably more specific than GGT (Salaspuro, 1999).

Blood alcohol concentration A high concentration does not distinguish between an isolated episode of heavy drinking and chronic misuse. However, if a person is not intoxicated when the blood alcohol concentration is well above the legal limit of driving, he is likely to be unusually tolerant of alcohol. This tolerance suggests persistent heavy drinking. Alcohol is eliminated rather slowly from the blood and can be detected in appreciable amounts for 24 hours after an episode of heavy drinking. In clinical practice, breath alcohol is often used as a proxy measurement for blood alcohol.

than abstinence. Generally brief interventions lead to significant reductions in alcohol consumption over the next year but it is uncertain how far these gains are maintained. It is generally agreed that brief interventions are not effective for people with severe problem drinking, particularly those who are alcohol dependent (Room *et al.*, 2005).

Motivational interviewing (Box 18.6)

Patients with problems of alcohol misuse, particularly those detected by screening methods, may be unsure whether or not to engage in treatment programmes. An appropriate interviewing style, particularly during the first assessment, can help to persuade the patient to engage in a useful review of their current pattern of drinking.

BOX 18.5 APPROACH TO TREATMENT OF ALCOHOL MISUSE

- Raise awareness of problem
- Increase motivation to change
- Support and advice
- Withdraw alcohol (or controlled drinking)
- Cognitive–behaviour therapy (social skills, relapse prevention)
- Couple therapy
- Alcoholics Anonymous
- Medication (disulfiram, acamprosate)

Confrontation is avoided in motivational interviewing, and a less directive approach is taken during which patients are helped to assess the balance of the positive and negative effects of alcohol on their lives. The clinician can help in this exercise by providing feedback to the patient on the personal risks that alcohol poses both to them and to their family, together with a number of options for change. The aim of motivational interviewing is to persuade the patients to argue their own case for changing their pattern of substance use (Box 18.6). (For a review of motivational interviewing and its role in the treatment of substance misuse in general see Treasure, 2004).

Treatment plans for more established alcohol misuse and dependence

Where patients have significant alcohol-related disorders, particularly in the presence of alcohol dependence, treatment may need to be more intensive (Figure 18.2). Any intervention should be preceded by a full assessment and should include a drinking history and an appraisal of current medical, psychological, and social problems. An intensive and searching enquiry often helps the patient gain a new recognition and

BOX 18.6 MOTIVATIONAL INTERVIEWING

- Express empathy
- Avoid arguing; don't be judgmental
- Detect and 'roll with' resistance
- Point out discrepancies in history
- Raise awareness about contrast between substance user's aims and behaviour

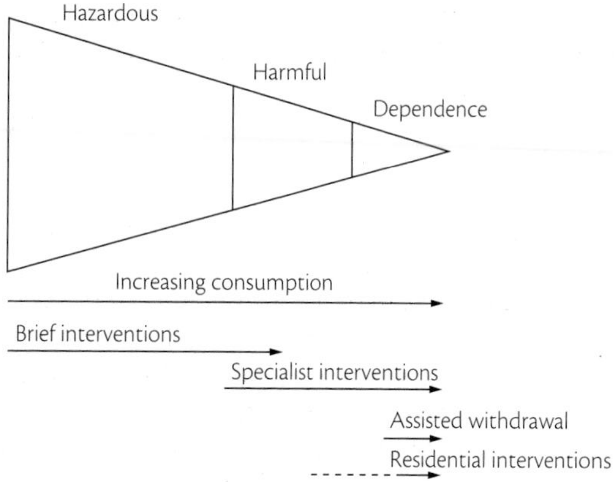

Fig. 18.2 Relationship between extent of alcohol misuse and level of intervention required. Lingford-Hughes *et al.* (2004).

understanding of their problem, and this is the basis of treatment. As noted above, however, it is important to avoid confrontation as this will only alienate someone who is likely to have very mixed feelings about the prospect of life without alcohol. It is usually desirable to involve the husband or wife in the assessment, both to obtain additional information and to give the spouse a chance to unburden feelings.

An explicit treatment plan should be worked out with the patient (and partner if appropriate). There should be specific goals and the patient should be required to take responsibility for realizing them. These goals should deal not only with the drinking problem, but also with any accompanying problems in health, marriage, job, and social adjustment. In the early stages they should be short term and achievable, for example, complete abstinence for 2 weeks. In this way the patient can be rewarded by early achievement.

Longer-term goals can be set as treatment progresses. These will be concerned with trying to change factors that precipitate or maintain excessive drinking, such as tensions in the family. In drawing up this treatment plan, an important decision is whether to aim at total abstinence or at limited consumption of alcohol (**controlled drinking**).

Total abstinence versus controlled drinking

The disease model of alcoholism proposes that an alcohol-dependent person must become totally abstinent and remain so, since a single drink would lead to relapse. Alcoholics Anonymous have made this a tenet of their approach to treatment.

The issue of abstinence versus controlled drinking remains unresolved. A prevalent view is that controlled drinking may be a feasible goal for people whose alcohol misuse has been detected early and who are not dependent or physically damaged. Abstinence is a better goal for others and those who have attempted controlled drinking unsuccessfully. While there are few controlled studies of this issue, recent investigations have supported the idea that controlled drinking can be a realistic goal in patients without alcohol dependence and lesser levels of alcohol-related disorders. If controlled drinking is to be attempted, then the doctor should advise the patient clearly about safe levels (see p. 432).

Withdrawal from alcohol

For patients with the dependence syndrome, withdrawal from alcohol is an important stage in treatment which should be carried out carefully. In the less severe cases, withdrawal may be at home provided there is adequate support and clinical monitoring (Table 18.8). This should involve daily assessment by the general practitioner, practice nurse, or specialist alcohol worker to check the patient's physical state and supervise medication (Box 18.7). In uncomplicated cases withdrawal symptoms usually resolve in 4–6 days. However, any patient likely to have severe withdrawal symptoms, especially if there is a history of delirium tremens or seizures, should be admitted to hospital (see Ritson, 2005).

The extensive research on pharmacological treatment for alcohol withdrawal has been systematically

TABLE 18.8 Considerations before alcohol detoxification

1. What are the medical risks?
2. What setting is appropriate?
3. What does the patient want from detoxification?
4. What kind of aftercare is needed to help maintain abstinence?

From Lingford-Hughes *et al.* (2004).

BOX 18.7 GENERAL MANAGEMENT OF ALCOHOL DETOXIFICATION

1. Explanation of process to patient and family
2. Patient should stay off work and rest. They should not drive
3. Take plenty of fluids but avoid caffeinated drinks
4. Daily visit by health professional
5. Maintain abstinence
6. Reducing course of benzodiazepines over 5–7 days (see text)

reviewed by Lingford-Hughes *et al.* (2004). The most important concern is the prevention of major complications of withdrawal such as seizures or delirium tremens; treatment with benzodiazepines is usually the most suitable choice.

Benzodiazepines differ in their duration of action. Whilst the longer-acting compounds may carry the risk of oversedation in the elderly or in those with significant liver disease, they also have the advantage of smoother withdrawal and generally better relief of withdrawal symptoms. **Chlordiazepoxide** is often used. A typical outpatient regimen would be 20–30 mg four times daily, reducing and stopping over 5–7 days. In more severe cases, particularly inpatients, higher doses are commonly used. If convulsions occur, the dose of benzodiazepine should be reviewed and increased if necessary. Administration of a benzodiazepine that is well-absorbed parenterally (such as lorazepam) may be useful to relieve severe acute withdrawal, though oral medication can usually be resumed promptly.

Carbamazepine has also been found to be effective in treatment of alcohol withdrawal, and although not often used in the UK, it is a good alternative to a benzodiazepine. There is no added benefit from using carbamazepine and a benzodiazepine together (see Lingford-Hughes *et al.*, 2004).

Clomethiazole was frequently used in the management of alcohol withdrawal in the past but is now not recommended because of its toxicity when combined with alcohol. It is occasionally used for the most severe withdrawal states where intensive inpatient medical monitoring is available, but there is no clear advantage compared with adequate doses of a benzodiazepine.

Antipsychotic drugs lower the seizure threshold and are less effective than benzodiazepines in preventing delirium. They are sometimes used to reduce agitation during alcohol withdrawal, but use of adequate doses of a benzodiazepine is a safer strategy.

Vitamin supplements, particularly thiamine, should also be given to prevent the Wernicke–Korsokov syndrome (p. 327). Parenteral thiamine should be given to patients at high risk (those with alcohol dependence and a poor diet). In the treatment of delirium tremens or Wernicke's encephalopathy, thiamine treatment should always precede glucose administration (Royal College of Physicians, 2001).

Psychological treatment

As noted above, **provision of information and advice** about the effects of excessive drinking is an important first stage in treatment. The information given should relate to the specific problems of the individual patient, both those that have occurred already and those likely to develop if drinking continues. The technique of **motivational interviewing** can be useful (Box 18.6).

Group therapy The aim of group therapy is to enable patients to observe their own problems mirrored in other problem drinkers and to work out better ways of coping with their problems. They gain confidence, whilst members of the group jointly strive to reorganize their lives without alcohol. Until recently, the most common plan of treatment in specialist alcohol units was an inpatient programme of group therapy lasting about 8 weeks; this treatment could be preceded by detoxification if required. However, because of the lack of evidence that this kind of intensive treatment approach is particularly beneficial, most clinics now offer a broader range of care including outpatient and day patient programmes that utilize a variety of psychotherapeutic approaches including marital and family therapy and cognitive-behavioural methods of treatment (see below). Group therapy is discussed further on p. 603.

Cognitive-behavioural therapy Cognitive-behavioural methods of treatment tackle the drinking behaviour itself rather than the presumed underlying psychological problems. Such approaches stress the role of **education** and the improvement of **social and interpersonal skills** as these relate to alcohol misuse.

For example, it may be helpful to identify situational or interpersonal triggers that cause an individual to drink excessively, and then to plan and rehearse new methods of coping with these situations. This is called **relapse prevention**. The use of **cue exposure** to alcoholic drinks, without subsequent consumption, may also lessen the risk of subsequent relapse when subjects have to contend with the ready availability of alcohol in social settings. It is important for the patient to appreciate that a **lapse** in drinking behaviour does not have to progress to a full-blown **relapse**. Many patients who misuse alcohol have general deficiencies in problem-solving skills, and appropriate training may help reduce relapse rates. Where patients are in a relatively stable relationship with a partner, **couple therapy** can produce improvements in drinking behaviour as well as marital adjustment (for a review of psychological treatments see Miller and Wilbourne, 2002).

Pharmacological treatments to help maintenance of abstinence

Disulfiram Disulfiram (**Antabuse**) acts by blocking the oxidation of alcohol so that acetaldehyde accumulates. Some patients find it useful because the anticipation of an unpleasant reaction acts as a deterrent to impulsive drinking. The reaction includes facial flushing, throbbing headache, hypotension, palpitations, tachycardia, and nausea and vomiting. In vulnerable patients, cardiac arrhythmias and collapse may occur.

The main **contraindications** to the use of disulfiram are a history of heart failure, coronary artery disease, hypertension, psychosis, and pregnancy. Patients should be given clear verbal and written instructions along with a list of substances to be avoided that contain alcohol. Common **side-effects** are drowsiness, bad breath, nausea, and constipation. Disulfiram is given in a single dose of 800 mg on the first day of treatment, reducing over 5 days to 100–200 mg daily.

The efficacy of disulfiram depends on **compliance**. The treatment is likely to be more successful if a partner or health worker is able to supervise treatment. In general, disulfiram appears to lower drinking frequency but without necessarily improving abstinence (Garbutt *et al.*, 1999).

Acamprosate (calcium acetyl homotaurinate) Acamprosate appears to suppress the urge to drink in response to learned cues, and produces modest but useful reductions in drinking behaviour in alcohol-dependent subjects. It is believed to act by stimulating GABA inhibitory neurotransmission and decreasing the excitatory effects of glutamate. There are a number of meta-analyses and systematic reviews of randomized controlled trials. Abstinence rates appear to be approximately doubled, with some evidence that the benefit continues after stopping the drug. It is unclear, however, which patients are most likely to benefit from acamprosate treatment.

The usual dose of acamprosate is two tablets (each 333 mg) three times daily with meals. In lighter subjects (>60 kg), four tablets daily are recommended. Acamprosate is not metabolized in the liver and is excreted by the kidney. Therefore it is unlikely to cause drug interactions. Adverse effects include diarrhoea, and, less frequently, nausea, vomiting, and abdominal pain. Skin rashes may occur as can fluctuations in libido.

Naltrexone The opioid antagonist, naltrexone, is believed to block some of the reinforcing effects of alcohol and in this way decrease the likelihood of relapse after detoxification. Not all trials have found significant benefit over placebo. However, a Cochrane review (Srisurapont and Jarusuraisin, 2003) concluded naltrexone is effective in the short-term treatment of alcohol dependence, but there is no clear benefit over acamprosate or disulfiram. It is possible that the main effect of naltrexone is to prevent a 'lapse' from becoming a full-blown 'relapse': hence it follows that naltrexone should not be stopped if the patient has a drink. Its effects may be enhanced by concomitant cognitive--behaviour therapy (Garbutt *et al.*, 1999). Side-effects of naltrexone treatment include headache, dizziness, and weight loss.

Antidepressant drugs Antidepressant medication is useful in patients who experience persistent symptoms of major depression after detoxification. However, tricyclic antidepressants are not recommended because of potentially serious interactions, including cardiotoxity and death following overdose (Lingford-Hughes *et al.*, 2004). Some studies have suggested that selective serotonin reuptake inhibitors (SSRIs) such as citalopram can reduce drinking in non-depressed alcohol-dependent patients but not all studies are in accord (see Chick, 2000). Re-analyses of some trials suggest that the effects of SSRIs may vary according to the 'Type 1' and 'Type 2' categories described by Cloningen *et al.* (1998). SSRIs may improve drinking outcome in Type 1 alcohol dependence (later age of onset, anxious traits) but may worsen outcome in Type 2 alcohol dependence (early age of onset, positive family history, impulsive/antisocial personality traits) (Lingford-Hughes *et al.*, 2004).

Other agencies concerned with drinking problems

Alcoholics Anonymous (AA) This is a self-help organization founded in the USA by two alcoholic men, a surgeon and a stockbroker. It has since spread to most countries of the world. Members attend group meetings, usually twice weekly on a long-term basis. In crisis they can obtain immediate help from other members by telephone. The organization works on the firm belief that abstinence must be complete. At present there are about 1200 groups in the UK.

Alcoholics Anonymous does not appeal to all problem drinkers because the meetings involve an emotional confession of problems. However, the organization is of great value to some problem drinkers, and anyone with a drink problem should be encouraged to try it.

A treatment approach similar to that provided by Alcoholics Anonymous coupled with encouragement to attend Alcoholic Anonymous meetings was one of the psychological therapies employed in project MATCH (see below). In general all the treatments employed appeared to be roughly equal in efficacy; however, patients with fewer psychiatric problems at entry tended have a better outcome with the Alcoholic Anonymous type of treatment.

Al-Anon This is a parallel organization providing support for the spouses of excessive drinkers. Al-Ateen does the same for their teenage children.

Non-statutory agencies These are voluntary bodies that provide a range of services including advice for problem drinkers and their families, counselling, and help with occupational and social activities for those who have recovered.

Hostels These are intended mainly for homeless problem drinkers. They provide rehabilitation and counselling. Usually abstinence is a condition of residence.

Results of treatment

In a controlled trial with 100 male alcoholics, Edwards *et al.* (1977) compared simple advice with intensive treatment that included introductions to Alcoholics Anonymous, medication, repeated interviews, counselling for their wives, and, where appropriate, inpatient treatment as well. The advice group received a 3-hour assessment together with a single session of counselling with the spouse present. The two groups were well matched. After 12 months there was no significant difference between them in drinking behaviour, subjective ratings, or social adjustment.

Similar findings with regard to drinking behaviour were reported by Chick *et al.* (1988) who found that at a 2-year follow-up there was no difference in stable abstinence rates between patients who received a minimal treatment intervention, consisting mainly of advice, and those offered a broad range of therapies, including inpatient care and group therapy. However, the group offered the broad range of therapies suffered **less alcohol-related harm**, particularly in relation to family life.

Some have argued that abstinence rates by themselves do not provide a useful measure of treatment outcome. For example, whilst subjects may still be drinking, the amount consumed may decrease. This can be associated with reductions in aspects of alcohol-related harm as shown by the study by Chick *et al.* (1988). From this viewpoint, harm reduction, even where people continue to drink, is a worthwhile achievement. The principles of the harm-reduction approach have been applied to the misuse of other substances (see below).

Interest in the effectiveness of structured psychological treatments has been reinforced by Project MATCH, a large randomized controlled trial of three psychological treatments for alcohol problems (Project MATCH Research Group 1997). The three treatments studied were a cognitive- behavioural intervention, a motivational therapy and a treatment that aimed to help people make use of the '12 step' philosophy of Alcoholics Anonymous. The main aim of the study was to attempt to find patient characteristics that predicted response to particular treatments. There were no important differences between the treatments and few strong correlations were found between effectiveness and patient characteristics. However, in general, the outcome was favourable and the authors concluded that structured psychological treatments of various kinds were helpful in the management of alcohol misuse.

There are likely to be factors within the patient that will predict a good response to a number of different kinds of treatment. There is some disagreement as to what these factors are, but the following generally predict a better prognosis whatever treatment is used: good insight into the nature of the problems; social stability in the form of a fixed abode, family support, and ability to keep a job; ability to control impulsiveness, to defer gratification, and to form satisfactory emotional relationships.

For a review of effectiveness of a broad range of treatment approaches for alcohol use disorders, see Miller and Wilbourne (2002).

Prevention of alcohol misuse and dependence

In seeking to prevent excessive drinking and alcohol-related disorders, two approaches are possible. The first is to improve the help and guidance available to the individual, as already described. The second is to introduce social changes likely to affect drinking patterns in the population as a whole might be reduced by four methods:

1. The pricing of alcoholic beverages. Putting up the price of alcohol would probably reduce the consumption (see above).
2. Controlling advertising. Controlling or abolishing the advertising of alcoholic drinks might be another preventive measure. It is unclear how far advertising encourages use of particular brands of alcohol rather than overall consumption. However, in the UK annual expenditure on alcohol advertising rose from £150 million to £250 million between 1989 and 2000 and during that time there was a very high correlation between advertising expenditure and mean weekly alcohol consumption by children age 11–15 years (Academy of Medical Sciences, 2004).

3. Controls on sale. Another preventive measure might be to control sales of alcohol by limiting hours or banning sales in supermarkets. While relaxation of restrictions has been shown to lead to increased sales of alcohol in some countries, it does not follow that increased restrictions would reduce established rates of drinking. However, there is evidence that a higher minimum age of legal drinking is associated with decreased alcohol consumption, car accidents, and suicide in recent school leavers (see Links, 2000). There is growing concern about the heavy-drinking, night-life culture of many UK cities.
4. Health education. It is not known whether education about alcohol misuse is effective. Little is known as to how attitudes are formed or changed. Although education about alcohol seems desirable, it cannot be assumed that classroom lectures or mass media propaganda would alter attitudes. In general, there is little convincing evidence that such approaches are effective (Room *et al.*, 2005).

Other substance use disorders

Under this heading we shall consider the use and misuse of substances other than alcohol. Although these substances include agents such as volatile substances (inhalants), the general term **drug** will be employed because it is in common use. In this discussion the term **misuse** will be applied to what is classified as **harmful use** in ICD-10 and **abuse** in DSM-IV (Table 18.3).

BOX 18.8 SOME RECOMMENDATIONS BY THE ACADEMY OF MEDICAL SCIENCES (2004) FOR DECREASING ALCOHOL-RELATED HARM IN THE UK

- Increase taxes on alcohol to restore its affordability relative to income to that obtaining in early 1970s
- Reduce duty-free allowance of alcohol to travellers
- Review advertising and promotion of alcoholic drinks, particularly to young people
- Improve medical research on damaging effects of alcohol
- Inform public and encourage debate about extent of alcohol-related harm (see Box 18.1)
- Reduce statutory blood alcohol concentration level for drivers from 80 mg per cent to 50 mg per cent. Impose zero statutory blood alcohol level for young drivers up to the age of 21

Epidemiology

Illicit drug use

The 2003 National Household Survey on Drug Use and Health (NSDUH) in the USA found that 14.7 per cent of the population aged 12 and over had used an illicit substance in the past year (Substance Abuse and Mental Health Services Administration [SAMHSA], 2004). Lifetime use of any illicit substance was 46.4 per cent. Use was highest in unemployed people in the age range 16–25. The most commonly used illicit drug was cannabis with about 55 per cent of illicit drug-takers using cannabis only. The British Crime Survey reported similar figures; in the UK, 12 per cent of adults had taken an illicit drug in the last year, most commonly cannabis. About 3 per cent of the UK population had used a class A drug (opiate, cocaine, lysergic acid diethylamide, injected stimulant) in the previous year (Aust *et al.*, 2002).

In a survey of 7722 school pupils aged 15 and 16 in the UK (part of a broader European survey), Miller and Plant (1996) found that 42 per cent said that they had at some time tried illicit drugs, mainly cannabis. This cross-sectional study does not provide information on regular use, though it indicates that **experimentation** with illicit drugs is common among young people in this age group. There was a strong association between **cigarette smoking** and the use of cannabis. Boys were more likely to have used an illicit drug than girls but the differences were not large (43 per cent of the boys and 38 per cent of the girls reported having used cannabis). Findings from a later phase of the European survey show little change in the UK data on drug use. Of the 35 countries included in the 2003 phase of the survey, the UK sample was substantially above average in terms of the proportion of young people reporting cannabis and other illicit drug use. A significant number of young people in the UK are part of the 'club scene' where polydrug misuse is common. About a quarter of 18-year-olds have used two or more illegal drugs (see Robson, 2000).

Drug misuse and dependence

Little is known for certain about the **prevalence** of different types of drug misuse and drug dependence. In the UK, information comes from several sources: **criminal statistics**, mainly based on offences involving the use and misuse of illicit drugs, **special surveys**, and **hospital admissions**. The UK Home Office for many years kept a national register of persons notified by doctors as dependent on certain drugs, but the register was discontinued in 1997. None of these sources is satisfactory since much drug misuse goes undetected.

Reported national prevalence rates of drug misuse and drug dependence vary widely, partly because different methods of ascertainment have been used. The National Comorbidity Survey in the USA (Kessler *et al.*, 1994) found that the 1-year prevalence for drug misuse and drug dependence (excluding alcohol misuse) was 3.6 per cent, whilst the lifetime prevalence was 11.9 per cent. The 1-year prevalence of drug misuse and dependence in men (5.1 per cent) was more than twice that in women (2.2 per cent).

In the British Psychiatric Morbidity Survey (Coulthard *et al.*, 2002), 4 per cent of adults living in private households met criteria for drug dependence, the majority meeting criteria in relation only to cannabis use. Men were twice as likely to be drug dependent as women and drug dependence was most common amongst young adults, especially men aged 16–24. Among the homeless population sampled in an earlier phase of the survey (Gill *et al.* 1996), 24 per cent of people sleeping rough met criteria for drug dependence. The sample for **prisoners** in the UK showed the highest rates of drug use with the majority of subjects reporting a history of illicit drug use (Singleton *et al.*, 1997). Among remand prisoners, 51 per cent of men and 54 per cent of women reported dependence on drugs before coming into prison, whereas among sentenced prisoners, 43 per cent of men and 41 per cent of women reported drug dependence.

Rates of drug misuse and dependence are high in disadvantaged areas of large cities. Adolescents are at risk, particularly around school-leaving age. A high proportion of attenders at drug-dependence clinics in large cities are unemployed with few stable relationships and leading disorganized lives. However, many young drug users remain in employment and apparently regard their drug taking as part of recreational activity for their particular peer group.

Causes of drug misuse

There is no single cause of drug misuse. It is generally argued that four factors are important:

1. Availability of drugs
2. A vulnerable personality
3. Adverse social environment.
4. Pharmacological factors

The widespread availability of illicit drugs means that occasional use in a young person can no longer be regarded as abnormal behaviour. However, about 10 per cent of those who experiment with drugs will go on to develop problems with them (Robson, 2000). Once drug-taking has started, personal, social and pharmacological factors play a role in determining misuse and dependence. Studies of the aetiology of misuse of substances other than alcohol are still at an early stage. For example, it is unclear whether similar risk factors predict misuse of a range of substances, including alcohol, or whether there is some specificity in the mechanisms, which leads certain individuals to misuse particular substances.

Availability of drugs

Drugs involved in misuse can be obtained from three main sources:

1. by taking drugs that can be bought legally without prescription. Nicotine and alcohol are obvious contemporary examples, and in the nineteenth century much dependence on opioids arose from taking freely available remedies containing morphia.
2. by taking drugs prescribed by doctors. In the first part of the twentieth century much of the known dependence on opioids and barbiturates in Western countries was of this kind; more recently, benzodiazepine dependence was often acquired in this way.
3. by taking drugs that can be obtained only from illicit sources ('street drugs').

Personal factors

Of those who experiment with drugs, the users who go on to develop problems appear to have some degree of personality vulnerability before taking drugs. They may live in disrupted families and have started taking drugs at a relatively young age. Associated behaviours include a **poor school record, truancy**, or **delinquency**. Traits such as **sensation seeking** and **impulsivity** are also common. Many of those who misuse drugs report depression and anxiety, but it is seldom clear whether these are the causes or the consequences of drug misuse and dependence. Some give a history of mental illness or personality disorder in the family.

Social environment

The risk of drug misuse is greater in societies that **condone drug use** of one sort or another. Within the immediate group, there may be **social pressures** for a young person to take drugs to achieve status. Thus drug use by individuals is influenced by the substance use of their peers. There are also links between drug misuse and indices of social deprivation such as **unemployment and homelessness** (Gill *et al.*, 1996).

Neurobiology of drug use, misuse, and dependence

Use, misuse and dependence Many subjects use drugs without misusing them, and not all drug misusers become drug dependent. Therefore it is useful to study the biological mechanisms underlying drug use, misuse, and dependence separately. Drugs are used and misused because they have the ability to serve as **positive reinforcers**, that is they increase the frequency of behaviours that lead to their use (Robbins and Everitt, 1999). Drugs act as positive reinforcers because they cause positive subjective experiences such as euphoria or reduction in anxiety.

Neurobiological mechanisms An important neurological substrate that mediates such effects is the **midbrain dopamine system**, whose cell bodies originate in the ventral tegmental area and innervate the forebrain, particularly the **nucleus accumbens.** It has been proposed that these dopamine pathways form part of a physiological reward system, which has the property of increasing the frequency of behaviours that activate it. Therefore it is of interest that administration of different kinds of drugs of misuse, including alcohol, nicotine, and opioids, to animals increases dopamine release in the nucleus accumbens. This suggests that activation of midbrain dopamine pathways may be a common property of drugs that have a propensity to be used and misused. While this hypothesis may explain in part the social use of particular drugs, it does not account for the misuse of drugs in some circumstances. Presumably this is a consequence of interactions between the pharmacological properties of the drug, the biological disposition and personality of the user, and the social environment. Current neurobiological formulations of drug dependence implicate changes in gene expression and synaptic connectivity in prefrontal cortical regions as well as the limbic areas involved in reward and motivation. The former might explain the ability of repeated drug administration to 'hijack' executive behaviour almost exclusively to serve the needs of the drug habit and the poor judgement and decision making shown by people with substance dependence (Volkow and Li, 2004).

Physiological and non-physiological dependence **Dependence** on drugs has traditionally been described as either psychological or physiological. In DSM-IV, dependence is separated into whether or not it is physiological in nature. **Physiological dependence** is diagnosed when a substance user demonstrates either **tolerance** to the pharmacological effects of the drug or a characteristic **withdrawal syndrome** when use of the drug is diminished. A cardinal feature of both physiological and non-physiological dependence is desire for the drug and drug-seeking behaviour. These features probably result from the continued need to obtain the reinforcing properties of the drug, as described above. Learning and conditioning factors are likely to be important here (Robbins and Everitt, 1999).

It is important to note that, even in non-physiological dependence, phenomena such as craving and dysphoria are associated with altered brain function. For example, in experimental studies the discontinuation of cocaine after a period of administration results in a sharp decline in dopamine release in the nucleus accumbens. It is possible that such an effect could correspond clinically to symptoms such as anhedonia and a desire to obtain more supplies of the drug.

Neurobiology of tolerance and dependence The phenomena of **tolerance** and **withdrawal** are believed to be a result of neuroadaptive changes in the brain. These are part of a homeostatic process that counteracts the acute pharmacological effects that occur when a drug is administered. For example, many drugs that are misused for their anxiolytic and hypnotic properties, such as barbiturates, benzodiazepines, and alcohol, have, among their acute pharmacological effects, the ability to **enhance brain GABA function**. During continued treatment with these agents, adaptive changes occur in GABA and benzodiazepine receptor sensitivity that tend to offset the effect of the drugs to facilitate GABA neurotransmission. Such an effect could account for the phenomenon of tolerance, with the result that an individual needs to take more of the drug to produce the same pharmacological effect.

If the drug is abruptly discontinued, persistence of the adaptive changes in receptor function could lead to a sudden decline in GABA activity. In fact, many of the clinical features of withdrawal from anxiolytic drugs, such as anxiety, insomnia, and seizures, can be explained on the basis of **diminished brain GABA** function. Such an effect can also explain the well-known phenomenon of cross-tolerance between anxiolytics and hypnotics and alcohol, which makes it possible, for example, to treat alcohol withdrawal with a benzodiazepine.

Similar kinds of adaptive changes have been proposed to account for the tolerance and withdrawal phenomena seen with other drugs of misuse. For example, whilst acute administration of opioids decreases the firing of noradrenaline cell bodies in the brainstem, tolerance to this effect occurs during repeated treatment, probably because of adaptive changes in the sensitivity of opioid receptors. If opioids are now suddenly withdrawn, there is a sudden increase in the firing of noradrenaline neurons and in the release of noradrenaline in terminal regions. Increased noradrenergic activity may account for several of the clinical features of acute opioid withdrawal, including sweating, tachycardia, hypertension, and anxiety. These studies have led to the use of the noradrenaline autoreceptor agonists, clonidine and lofexidine in the management of opioid withdrawal (see p. 459).

While the positive reinforcing actions of drugs are seen as the major factor in promoting continued drug use, withdrawal effects are also likely to play a part because they are invariably unpleasant and individuals are likely to try to prevent them by taking more drug. It is worth noting that for many months following the cessation of a clear-cut withdrawal syndrome, dependent subjects may experience a sudden intense desire to consume the drug. Often, particular **psychological and social stimuli** previously associated with drug use may trigger intense craving associated with symptoms resembling a withdrawal state. It has been proposed that a single exposure to the drug during this period may rapidly lead to a full relapse to drug dependence, the so called **reinstatement effect**. An analogous effect has been shown in previously drug-dependent animals where a single priming dose of the drug concerned can lead to a full recovery of drug-seeking behaviours that had previously been extinguished. For reviews of brain mechanisms involved in drug misuse and their implications for treatment see Robbins and Everitt (1999). For a review of brain imaging studies, see Daglish and Nutt (2003).

Adverse effects of drug misuse

Drug misuse has many undesirable effects both for the individual and society.

Physical health

Drug misuse can lead people to neglect their health in addition to the direct physical consequences of the substance itself. These are discussed in more detail under the heading of individual drugs.

Intravenous drug use poses particular health risks. This practice is very common with opioid use, but barbiturates, benzodiazepines, amphetamines, and other drugs may be taken in this way. Intravenous drug use has important consequences, some local and others general (Table 18.9).

The most serious complications of intravenous drug use include **HIV infection** and **hepatitis**. Rates of HIV infection among UK drug users are lower than those found in some other European countries and some attribute this to the vigorous harm reduction policies in the UK (methadone prescribing, needle exchanges, and education for drug users). However, hepatitis C is a major concern as preliminary studies suggest that this infection has a prevalence of between 50–80 per cent amongst UK users who inject drugs. Rates of hepatitis B are lower but still significant (30–50 per cent). Accidental drug overdose can occur by any route, but there is a far higher risk of death from heroin overdose when the intravenous route is used.

TABLE 18.9 Some consequences of intravenous drug misuse

Local
◆ Vein thrombosis
◆ Infection of injection site
◆ Damage to arteries
Systemic
◆ Bacterial endocarditis
◆ Hepatitis B and C
◆ HIV infection
◆ Accidental overdose

Substance dependence in women

Substance misuse treatment services, including those for alcohol-related disorders, are not usually designed to meet the special needs of women because existing treatment models have been developed for men (Marsh *et al.*, 2000). Swift *et al.* (1996) have emphasized that in the treatment of women patients, clinicians need to take into account factors such as:

- Social and parenting responsibilities
- Possible history of victimisation and sexual abuse
- Social barriers to obtaining medical care
- Availability of female therapists.

Drug misuse in pregnancy and the puerperium

Often drug misusers do not take up healthcare services until late into the pregnancy, which increases the health risk to both mother and baby. When a pregnant woman misuses drugs, the **fetus** may be affected. When drugs are taken in early pregnancy, there is a risk of increased rates of fetal abnormality. Opioids may directly decrease fetal growth. When drugs are taken in late pregnancy, the fetus may become dependent on them. The risk of fetal dependence is great with heroin and related drugs, and after delivery the neonate may develop serious withdrawal effects requiring skilled care. If the mother continues to take drugs after delivery, the infant may be neglected. Intravenous drug use may lead to infection of the mother with HIV or other conditions that can affect the fetus. Engagement in treatment and good antenatal care reduce the risks to mother and baby.

Psychiatric comorbidity

There is a strong association between between substance misuse and psychiatric comorbidity (often described as **dual diagnosis**). For example, people with substance misuse often have additional diagnoses of personality disorder, depression, and anxiety. Sometimes symptoms of mood disturbance may be a direct result of drug use. For example, people who use stimulants can experience depression subsequently.

In other cases the relationship is more complex with premorbid psychiatric disorder interacting with substance misuse. Thus patients with primary psychiatric disorders such as schizophrenia, bipolar disorder, and sociopathic personality disorder frequently misuse alcohol and illicit drugs. This practice increases the morbidity of the underlying disorder and heightens the risk of violence and self-harm. There is debate regarding the best ways of delivering treatment services to such patients, but as yet little firm evidence to provide guidance (see Cochrane review by Jeffrey *et al.*, 2000). The general consensus is that an integrated service, where the same clinical team deal with both psychiatric and substance misuse disorders, is likely to be the best approach. However, implementing such a service model poses difficulties (see Abou-Saleh, 2004). See below for a summary of management approaches to dual diagnosis patients.

Social consequences of drug misuse

There are three reasons why drug misuse can lead to undesirable social effects:

1. Chronic intoxication may affect behaviour adversely, leading to unemployment, motoring offences, accidents, and family problems including neglect of children.
2. Illicit drugs are generally expensive; the user may steal or sell sexual favours to obtain money.
3. Drug misusers often keep company with one another, and those with previously stable social behaviour may be under pressure to conform to a group ethos of antisocial or criminal activity.

The economic costs of problem drug use in the UK have been estimated by Godfrey *et al.* (2002) to be between £10.1 and £17.4 billion annually (Box 18.9).

BOX 18.9 SOCIAL COSTS OF DRUG MISUSE IN UK

- **Users:** Premature death, physical and mental illness, low educational achievement, unemployment
- **Families:** Adverse effect on children, poverty and deprivation
- **Others:** Victims of dangerous driving, victims of crime, victims of assault
- **Community:** Criminal activity related to drug-dealing, environmental impoverishment, health and crime risks to community
- **Industry:** Sickness absence, theft in the work place, productivity losses, costs of security
- **Public sector:** Healthcare expenditure, criminal justice expenditure, social services care and benefits.

Diagnosis of drug misuse

It is important to diagnose drug misuse early, at a stage when **dependence** may be less established and behaviour patterns less fixed, and the complications of intravenous use may not have developed. Before describing the clinical presentations of the different types of drugs, some general principles will be given. The clinician who is not used to treating people who misuse drugs should remember that they are in the unusual position of trying to help a patient who may be attempting to deceive them. Patients misusing heroin may overstate the daily dose to obtain extra supplies for their own use or for sale to others. Also, many patients **take more than one drug** but may not say so. It is important to try to corroborate the patient's account of the amount he takes by asking detailed questions about the duration of drug-taking, and the cost and source of drugs; by checking the story for internal consistency, and by external verification whenever possible.

Physical signs

Certain physical signs lead to the suspicion that drugs are being injected. These include **needle tracks and thrombosis of veins**, especially in the antecubital fossa, wearing garments with long sleeves in hot weather, and scars. Intravenous use should be considered in any patient who presents **with subcutaneous abscesses or hepatitis**.

Behavioural signs

Behavioural changes may also suggest drug misuse. These include absence from school or work and occupational decline. Dependent people may also neglect their appearance, isolate themselves from former friends, and adopt new friends in a drug culture. Minor criminal offences, such as petty theft and prostitution, may also be indicators.

Medical presentation

Dependent people may come to medical attention in several ways. Some declare that they are dependent on drugs. Others conceal their dependency, and ask for controlled drugs for the relief of pain such as renal colic or dysmenorrhoea. It is important to be particularly wary of such requests from temporary patients. Others present with drug-related complications, such as cellulitis, pneumonia, hepatitis, or accidents, or for the treatment of acute drug effects, overdose, withdrawal symptoms, or adverse reactions to hallucinogenic drugs. A few are detected during an admission to hospital for an unrelated illness.

Taking a drug history

When taking a **drug history** (Box 18.10) from a patient who is misusing drugs, the clinician should ask the patient to describe his drug use the previous day and also to describe a **typical drug-using day** (which drug, how often, and which route of use). A typical week can be described if drugs are not used every day. The clinician should ask about craving, withdrawal symptoms, and other features of the dependence syndrome such as increased tolerance to the drug and the priority of drug seeking over other duties and pleasures. The patient should be asked specifically about **risky behaviour** such as dangerous injecting (into groin or neck or infected injection sites), and sharing injection equipment.

A **chronological history** of the development of use of each drug can then be taken. Useful milestones can include the first use of the drug, when the patient began to use the drug daily, when withdrawal symptoms were first experienced, and when the patient first injected drugs. A history of sharing injection equipment will be important in estimating the risk of **HIV or hepatitis**.

If the patient has had periods of **abstinence**, it is useful to ask which influences helped them achieve this and what factors led to **relapse**. A history of complications should include adverse effects of the drug itself as well as complications of the route of administration. Any history of accidental overdose should also be elicited. The patient should be asked about family, occupational, and legal problems. Any past history of treatment should be elicted. There are several possible goals in the treatment of drug misusers. Abstinence is one but safer drug use (**harm reduction**) may be a more realistic aim for many. It is therefore important to obtain the patient's views on their drug use and the changes they would like to make.

BOX 18.10 DRUG-USE HISTORY

- Typical drug day or week
- Types and quantities of drugs taken (including alcohol and nicotine)
- Symptoms experienced when drugs unavailable
- Tolerance and primacy of drug habit
- Risky behaviour
- Developmental history of drug misuse
- Abstinence and relapse triggers
- Medical and social complications
- Psychiatric and forensic history

Laboratory diagnosis

Whenever possible, the diagnosis of drug misuse should be confirmed **by laboratory tests**. Urine testing is most commonly used, as it is easier and less invasive than repeated blood testing. However, saliva, blood and hair analysis can be useful in certain circumstances. The laboratory should be provided with as complete a list as possible of drugs that are likely to have been taken, including those prescribed (for a review of laboratory investigations see Wolff *et al.*, 1999).

Prevention, treatment, and rehabilitation – general principles

Prevention

Because treatment is difficult, considerable effort should be given to **prevention**. For many drugs, important preventive measures such as restricting availability and lessening social deprivation depend on government, not medical, policy. However, the reduction of over-prescribing by doctors is important, especially with benzodiazepines and other anxiolytic drugs.

Whilst education programmes by themselves do not seem effective in prevention, it is important that **information** about the dangers of drug misuse should be available to young people in the school curriculum and through the media. Another aspect of prevention is the identification and treatment of family problems that may contribute to drug-taking. In all these preventive measures, the general practitioner has an important role.

Treatment

Motivation and change

When drug misuse has begun, treatment is more effective before **dependence** is established. At this stage, as at later stages, the essential step is to **motivate** the person to control his drug-taking. This requires a combination of advice about the likely effects of continuing misuse and help with any concurrent psychological or social problems. The techniques of motivational interviewing (Miller and Rollnick, 1991) (Box 18.6) may be useful here. The **stages of change model** described by Prochaska and Diclemente (1986) can help the clinician to encourage motivation effectively (Box 18.11).

Aims of treatment

The ultimate aim of the treatment of the drug dependent person is the **withdrawal** of the drug of dependence. However, drug withdrawal (or detoxification) by itself has no effect on long-term outcome (Vaillant, 1988), and so this process should be part of a **wider treatment programme**. If withdrawal cannot be achieved, continued prescribing of certain drugs, for example, opioids, may be considered as part of a **harm reduction** programme (see below). In addition, psychological treatment and social support are required. At this point in the chapter, the general principles of treatment are outlined. In later sections, treatment specific to individual drugs will be considered.

BOX 18.11 STAGES OF CHANGE MODEL

Pre-contemplation
Misuser does not believe there is a problem, though others recognize it

Contemplation
Individual weighs up pros and cons and considers that change might be necessary

Decision
Point reached where decision is made to act (or not to act) on issue of substance misuse

Action
User chooses a strategy for change and pursues it

Maintenance
Gains are maintained and consolidated. Failure may lead to relapse

Relapse
Return to previous pattern of behaviour
However, relapse may be a positive learning experience, with lessons for the future

Treatment setting

In the UK, drug misusers are treated in a variety of settings. Most clinics are associated with psychiatric treatment facilities based in psychiatric hospitals or community bases. Inpatient care is provided in psychiatric hospitals, in psychiatric units in general hospitals, or in a small number of specialist inpatient units. Individual counselling, group therapy, and therapeutic communities are provided by a variety of charitable organizations. General practitioners may manage drug-dependent patients with the support of specialist services and models of shared care between primary and secondary services have been developed (Department of Health, 1999). All doctors in the UK treating drug misusers for their drug problems should provide information on the standard form to their local Regional Drug Misuse Database. Contact numbers are in the British National Formulary.

Physical complications

The complications of self-injection may need treatment in a general hospital. They include accidental overdose, skin infections, abscesses, septicaemia, hepatitis, and HIV infection. Drug misusers will also need help with general health issues such as nutrition and dental care. Immunization against hepatitis B may be advisable.

Principles of withdrawal

The withdrawal of misused drugs is sometimes called **detoxification**. For many drugs, particularly opioids, withdrawal may be most effectively carried out in hospital (see below). Withdrawal from stimulant drugs and benzodiazepines can often be an outpatient procedure provided that the doses are not very large and that barbiturates are not taken as well. Nevertheless, the risk of depression and suicide should be remembered.

Drug maintenance

Some clinicians undertake to prescribe certain drugs to dependent people who are not willing to give them up. The usual procedure is to prescribe a drug which has a slower action (and therefore is less addictive) than the 'street' drug. Thus methadone is prescribed in place of heroin. When this procedure is combined with help with social problems and a continuing effort to bring the person to accept withdrawal, it is called **maintenance therapy**.

The rationale of this approach is twofold:

1. Prolonged prescribing will remove the need for the patient to obtain 'street' drugs, and will thereby reduce the associated physical and social damage.

2. Social and psychological help will give the person the confidence and skills to be able to give up drugs eventually.

Maintenance drug treatment is used particularly for people with **opioid dependence**. If maintenance drug therapy is used, it should be remembered that some drug-dependent people convert tablets or capsules into material for injection, which is a particularly dangerous practice. Also, some attend a succession of general practitioners in search of supplementary supplies of drugs. They may withhold information about attendance at clinics or pose as temporary residents.

Some patients who receive maintenance drugs achieve a degree of social stability, but others continue heavy drug misuse and deteriorate both medically and socially. Subjects on maintenance methadone are more likely to be retained in treatment than those in drug-free programmes. This may be important because the length of time spent in treatment, regardless of type, is the best predictor of favourable outcome. (The use of methadone maintenance treatment in the management of opioid dependence is considered in more detail below.)

Harm reduction

The increase in HIV and hepatitis C infection has emphasized the importance of **harm-reduction programmes**, of which prescribing maintenance may be one component. Such programmes have the aim of increasing the number of substance misusers who enter and comply with treatment. The aim is to identify intermediate treatment goals, which though short of total abstinence, nevertheless reduce the risk of drug misuse to the individual and society. For example, even if subjects continue to misuse drugs, the risk of hepatitis and HIV infection can be lessened by appropriate education and practical help. Such interventions may lead to the drug misuser using safer routes of drug administration or sterile injection equipment. Counselling and screening for hepatitis and HIV may also be worthwhile and hepatitis B vaccination should be offered to non-immune patients.

Psychological treatments

Some drug-dependent patients are helped by simple measures such as counselling. In many units, group psychotherapy is provided to help patients develop insight into personal and interpersonal problems. Some patients benefit from treatment in a therapeutic community in which there can be a frank discussion of the effects of drug-taking on the person's character and relationships within the supportive relationship of the group (see p. 607 for an outline of community therapy).

Cognitive–behavioural methods of treatment as described for the management of alcohol misuse (see p. 447) are also helpful but probably not more so than other psychological approaches (Luty, 2003). The aim of such treatment is to increase recreational and personal skills so that the individual becomes less reliant on drugs and the drug culture as a source of satisfaction. Involvement of family and partners is often helpful. As with alcohol dependence, cognitive behavioural techniques can be used can be used to identify, in advance, situations that contain triggers for drug use; in this way alternative methods of coping can be planned. It has already been mentioned that when a drug misuser is confronted with a situation that contains personal cues for drug use, he can experience acute discomfort associated with a **strong desire** to use the drug. The technique of cue exposure aims, through repeated exposure, to desensitize drug misusers to these effects and thus improve their ability to remain abstinent.

Rehabilitation

Many drug takers have great difficulty in establishing themselves in normal society. The aim of rehabilitation is to enable the drug-dependent person to leave the drug subculture and to develop new social contacts. Unless this can be achieved, any treatment is likely to fail.

Rehabilitation may be undertaken after treatment in a therapeutic community (see p. 607). Patients first engage in work and social activities in sheltered surroundings, and then take greater responsibility for themselves in conditions increasingly like those of everyday life. Hostel accommodation is a useful stage in this gradual process. Continuing social support is usually required when the person makes the transition to normal work and living.

Dual-diagnosis patients

As noted above, the management of patients with both substance misuse and serious psychiatric illness such as schizophrenia and bipolar disorder poses several additional challenges. Such comorbidity is associated with an increased risk of violence and suicide and worse clinical and social outcomes (Department of Health, 2002). Patients with dual diagnoses are particularly hard to retain in treatment and frequently present in crisis with many unmet social needs. Drake and Mueser (2000) identified a number of common components of integrated treatment for patients with substance misuse and serious psychiatric illness.

- Multidisciplinary case management with assertive outreach to engage and retain patients in treatment

- Ready availability of crisis intervention
- Emphasis on motivational interviewing and harm reduction
- Use of coercion where applicable and appropriate (for example Drug Treatment and Testing Orders)
- Close monitoring with medication supervision and urine screening
- Long-term community support including day care and residential care
- Supported housing
- Pharmacotherapy with particular consideration of clozapine for those with schizophrenia and substance misuse.

Misuse of specific types of drug

Opioids

This group of drugs includes morphine, heroin, codeine, and synthetic analgesics such as pethidine, methadone, and dipipanone. The pharmacological effects of opioids are mediated primarily through interaction with specific opioid receptors, with morphine and heroin being quite selective for the μ-opioid receptor type. The medical use of opioids is mainly for their powerful analgesic actions; they are misused for their euphoriant and anxiolytic effects.

In the past morphine was misused widely in Western countries, but has been largely replaced as a drug of misuse by **heroin**, which has a particularly powerful euphoriant effect, especially when taken intravenously.

Epidemiology

The 2003 NHSDUS survey in the USA estimated that 0.1 per cent Americans had used heroin at least once in the previous month; the rate of lifetime use was about 1.6 per cent (SAMHSA, 2004). When the UK Home Office Addicts Index was still in operation, the numbers of subjects registered in 1997 was about 40,000. Of course many more users were not registered. The British household survey showed average levels of opiate use of about 1 per cent in the previous year in the adult population (Coulthard *et al.*, 2002). The United Kingdom has one of the higher prevalences of **problem opiate use** in Europe with a rate of about six per thousand (Kraus *et al.*, 2003). Higher rates would be expected in the homeless and in prisons.

Use and misuse

The epidemiological data indicate that many people use heroin without becoming dependent on it. However, there is no doubt that repeated heroin use can lead to the rapid development of **dependence** and marked **physiological tolerance**. As well as the intravenous route, opioid users may employ other methods of administration, for example, **subcutaneous administration** ('skin-popping') or **sniffing** ('snorting'). Heroin may also be heated on a metal foil and inhaled ('chasing the dragon'). Heroin users may change their customary method of drug administration from time to time. From the perspective of harm reduction, methods that avoid intravenous administration are preferable.

Clinical effects

As well as **euphoria and analgesia**, opioids produce respiratory depression, constipation, reduced appetite, and low libido. Tolerance develops rapidly, leading to increasing dosage. Tolerance does not develop equally to all the effects, and constipation often continues when the other effects have diminished. When the drug is stopped, tolerance diminishes rapidly so that a dose taken after an interval of abstinence has greater effects than it would have had before the interval. This loss of tolerance can result in dangerous – sometimes fatal – respiratory depression when a previously tolerated dose is resumed after a drug-free interval, for example, after a stay in hospital or prison.

Withdrawal from opioids

Withdrawal symptoms from opioids may include the following:

- intense craving for the drug
- restlessness and insomnia
- pain in muscles and joints
- running nose and eyes
- abdominal cramps, vomiting, diarrhoea
- piloerection, sweating dilated pupils, raised pulse rate
- disturbance of temperature control.

These features usually begin about 6 hours after the last dose, reach a peak after 36–48 hours, and then wane. Withdrawal symptoms rarely threaten the life of someone in reasonable health, though they cause great distress and so drive the person to seek further supplies.

Methadone

Methadone is approximately as potent, weight for weight, as morphine. It causes cough suppression, constipation, and depression of the central nervous system and of respiration. Pupillary constriction is less marked. The withdrawal syndrome is similar to that of heroin and morphine, and is at least as severe. Because methadone has a long half-life (1–2 days), symptoms of withdrawal may begin only after 36 hours and reach a peak after 3–5 days. For this reason, methadone is often used to replace heroin in patients dependent on the latter drug.

The natural course of opioid dependence

Longer-term follow-up studies of opioid misusers have revealed that in most the disorder appears to run a chronic relapsing and remitting course with a significant mortality (10–20 per cent) over 10 years. Nevertheless, up to 50 per cent of opioid users have been found to be abstinent at 10-year follow-up, which suggests a trend towards natural remission in survivors (Robson, 2000).

Deaths are not infrequently due to accidental overdosage, often related to loss of tolerance after a period of enforced abstinence. Suicide is also a common cause of death. Deaths from HIV infection and hepatitis have also become more frequent in recent years. Pointers to a good outcome include substantial periods of employment and marriage. Abstinence is often related to changed circumstances of life. This point is reflected in the report of 95 per cent abstinence among soldiers who returned to the USA after becoming dependent on opioids during service in the Vietnam War (Robins, 1993).

Prevention

Because dependence develops rapidly and treatment of dependent opioid misusers is unsatisfactory, preventive measures (see p. 455) are particularly important with this group of drugs.

Treatment of crisis

Opioid misusers present in crisis to a doctor in three circumstances. First, when their supplies have run out, they may seek drugs either by requesting them directly or by feigning a painful disorder. Although **withdrawal symptoms** are very unpleasant, so that the misuser will go to great lengths to obtain more drugs, they are not usually dangerous to an otherwise healthy person. Therefore it is best to offer drugs only as the first step of a planned maintenance or withdrawal programme. This programme is described in the following sections. The second form of crisis is **drug overdose**. This requires medical treatment, directed particularly to any respiratory depression produced by the drug. The third form of crisis is an **acute complication of intravenous drug usage** such as local infection, necrosis at the injection site, or infection of a distant organ, often the heart or liver.

Planned withdrawal (detoxification) (Box 18.12)

The severity of withdrawal symptoms depends on psychological as well as pharmacological factors. Therefore the **psychological management** of the patient during withdrawal is as important as the drug regimen. The speed of withdrawal should be discussed with the patient to establish a timetable which is neither so rapid that the patient will not collaborate, nor so protracted that the state of dependence is perpetuated. During withdrawal, much personal contact is needed to reassure the patient; the relationship formed in this way can be important in later treatment.

When the dose is low, opioids can be withdrawn rapidly while giving symptomatic treatment for the withdrawal effects. Drugs such as **loperamide** or **metoclopramide** can be useful for gastrointestinal symptoms. **Non-steroidal analgesics** may be useful for aches and pains. Another drug that may be useful is the α_2-adrenoceptor agonist, **lofexidine**. Lofexidine has a similar action to clonidine but causes less hypotension. Some studies suggest that it is as effective in ameliorating the withdrawal syndrome as methadone (see Gowing *et al.*, 2004).

When the daily dose of heroin is high, it may be necessary to prescribe an opioid, reducing the dose gradually. One approach is to use **methadone**, which has a more gradual action. The difficulty is to judge the correct dose of methadone because patients may either overstate their use of heroin because they fear the withdrawal symptoms, or understate it in an attempt to avoid censure. In addition, as noted below, the strength of street drugs varies.

Methadone should be given in a liquid form to be taken by mouth. The initial methadone dose is normally between 10 and 40 mg daily depending on the patient's usual consumption. Users with evidence of opioid tolerance may require dosing at the higher end of this range. If 4 hours after an initial dose there is evidence of withdrawal symptoms, a supplementary dose may be given but caution should be employed because methadone is long acting and accumulation and toxicity could result. Street heroin varies in potency in different places and at different times. Therefore, if possible, advice about the equivalent dose of methadone should be obtained from a clinician experienced in treating drug dependence. The rate of methadone reduction depends on the clinical circumstances and the patient's clinical responses. The most rapid regimen may take about 10 days to 3 weeks but slower reductions over several months may sometimes be appropriate.

Buprenorphine, a partial agonist at opioid receptors, can also be used to manage opioid withdrawal (Gowing *et al.*, 2004). Again, tapering doses are used at a rate agreed with the patient. Buprenorphine is often well-tolerated but care needs to be taken in starting treatment, especially for patients who are transferring from methadone. This is because the partial agonist action of the drug may precipitate acute withdrawal in patients transferring from higher doses of methadone (more than 30 mg) or heroin. It can usually be avoided by beginning treatment when the patient is already in mild withdrawal.

The opioid antagonist, naltrexone, has been procedure known as **rapid opioid detoxification** in conjunction with heavy sedation and sometimes general anaesthesia. The safety and efficacy of this procedure are not established (Spanagel, 1999).

When opioid drugs are prescribed to drug-dependent patients, there is the possibility of diversion of the medication to the illicit market. This can be avoiding by supervision of consumption of each daily dose, for example by nursing or pharmacy staff. This practice also reduces the risk of overdose, and the daily personal contact probably also has other therapeutic benefits. It is generally regarded as good practice at least while treatment is being established, though daily attendance can be difficult for patients who are in full-time employment.

Pregnancy and opioid dependence

The babies of women who misuse opioids are more likely than other babies to be **premature** and of **low birth-weight**. They may also show withdrawal symptoms after birth, including irritability, restlessness, tremor, and a high-pitched cry. These signs appear within a few days of birth if the mother was taking heroin, but are delayed if she was taking methadone, which has a longer half-life in the body. Low birth-weight and prematurity are not necessarily related directly to the drug, since poor nutrition and heavy smoking are common among heroin misusers. Women in **methadone maintenance programmes** have pregnancies with a better outcome than those who are not (Ward *et al.*, 1999).

Later effects have been reported, with the children of opioid-dependent mothers being more likely, as toddlers, to be overactive and to show poor persistence. However, these late effects may result from the unsuitable family environment rather than from a lasting effect of the intrauterine exposure to the drug.

Maintenance treatment for opioid dependence

As described above, withdrawal from opioids is the preferred treatment option, but if this is not possible, **maintenance treatment**, usually with methadone, may lessen the physical and social harm associated with the intravenous use of illicit drug supplies. The principle of this treatment is explained on p. 453. Instead of heroin, methadone is prescribed as a liquid preparation formulated to discourage attempts to inject it.

Methadone maintenance treatment has been extensively evaluated (see the Cochrane review by Mattick *et al.*, 2003a). There is good evidence from randomized studies that methadone maintenance decreases the use of illicit opioids and reduces criminal activity. In addition, subjects in methadone maintenance programmes show less risky injecting behaviours and lower rates of HIV infection. Overall subjects receiving methadone maintenance have an approximately three times greater likelihood of staying in treatment and are about two-thirds less likely to use illicit heroin (Mattick *et al.*, 2003a).

Methadone doses of 20–40 mg daily have been widely advocated as appropriate for maintenance treatment, but there is some evidence that higher doses (60–100 mg daily) are associated with lower rates of illicit opioid use and improved retention in the therapeutic programme (Faggiano *et al.*, 2003). The latter is associated with an improved therapeutic outcome. The best approach is probably to have a flexible dosing policy, bearing in mind the potential toxicity of methadone in subjects whose tolerance is unknown or hard to assess. Generally it is better to start treatment with lower doses initially (not more than 40 mg daily) and increase over a number of weeks, titrating against the presence of withdrawal symptoms. It should be remembered that methadone

BOX 18.12 PHARMACOLOGICAL MANAGEMENT OF OPIOID WITHDRAWAL

- If short-term, non-opiate treatment is desired, use an a_2-adrenoceptor agonist
- Buprenorphine can be used for short-term opioid withdrawal and has a better outcome than clonidine
- Methadone treatment for withdrawal can be successful but needs to be carried out slowly with a gradual tapering of dose
- Methadone may be preferable in pregnancy because of the greater experience with its use.

From Lingford-Hughes *et al.* (2004)

levels will go on increasing for about 5 days following the last dosage adjustment. (For practical advice on methadone treatment see Department of Health, 1999).

Evaluation of methadone clinics has shown that the more effective programmes have methadone maintenance treatment rather than abstinence as a primary goal of therapy. The more effective clinics were also characterized by high-quality counselling and a wide range of medical services (see Ward *et al.* 1999). There is also a growing evidence-base for the use of buprenorphine as an alternative to methadone for maintenance treatment for opioid users (Mattick *et al.*, 2003b). The same principles of treatment apply.

The concerns about diversion of prescribed opioid drugs, and about risk of overdose, have been described above in the section on management of opioid withdrawal (see above). These also apply in maintenance treatment, and daily supervised consumption is commonly continued for a proportion of patients in maintenance treatment.

Naltrexone is a long-acting opioid antagonist which is used to help prevent relapse in detoxified opioid-dependent subjects. While naltrexone treatment may have a role in certain dependent subjects with high motivation, such as doctors recovering from opioid dependence, or patients engaged in structured programmes associated with the criminal justice system, its benefit in the wider community of opioid users is less well-established (Kirchmayer *et al.*, 2003).

Therapeutic community methods

These forms of treatment aim to produce abstinence by effecting a substantial change in the patient's **attitudes and behaviour**. Drug-taking is represented as a way of avoiding pre-existing personal problems and as a source of new ones. Group therapy and communal living are combined in an attempt to produce greater personal awareness, more concern for others, and better social skills. In most therapeutic communities, some of the staff have previously been dependent on drugs and are often better able than other staff to gain the confidence of the patients in the early stages of treatment.

Anxiolytic and hypnotic drugs

The most frequently misused drugs of this group are now the **benzodiazepines**. **Barbiturates** are little prescribed and misuse has fallen. Other drugs of this group that are currently misused include clomethiazole and chloral. The clinical effects of these drugs are thought to result from their ability to facilitate brain **GABA function**. Benzodiazepines produce these effects by binding to a specific benzodiazepine receptor.

Benzodiazepines

These drugs were in therapeutic use for many years before it became apparent that their prolonged use could lead to tolerance and dependence with a characteristic **withdrawal syndrome**. The withdrawal syndrome includes:

- anxiety symptoms – anxiety, irritability, sweating, tremor, sleep disturbance,
- altered perception – depersonalization, derealization, hypersensitivity to stimuli, abnormal body sensations, abnormal sensation of movement,
- other features (rare) – depression, suidicidal behaviour, psychosis, seizures, delirium tremens.

Epidemiology Benzodiazepine use is extremely widespread; for example, it has been estimated that about 10 per cent of the population of Europe and the USA use benzodiazepines as anxiolytics or hypnotics. Over the last few years the prescription of benzodiazepines for anxiety has shown a decline. Most long-term users are older women; however, there is a significant misuse problem in younger people, often associated with intravenous adminstration and **polysubstance misuse**. A significant proportion of people who are **dependent on alcohol** are also dependent on benzodiazepines.

Dependence Dependence on benzodiazepines often results from prolonged medical use but may also result from the availability of benzodiazepines as street drugs because of their euphoriant and calming effects. The withdrawal syndrome closely resembles the anxiety symptoms for which the drugs are usually prescribed; hence if symptoms appear after the dose of benzodiazepine has been reduced, the doctor may revert to a higher dosage in the mistaken belief that these symptoms indicate a persistent anxiety disorder. It has been estimated that about one-third of subjects who take a benzodiazepine at therapeutic doses for more than 6 months may become dependent (see Lingford-Hughes *et al.*, 2004).

Treatment Treatment of dependence usually consists of gradual withdrawal over at least 8 weeks combined with supportive counselling. Withdrawal appears to be more severe from benzodiazepines that have **short half-lives and high potency** at the benzodiazepine receptor. For this reason it is often suggested that patients on such compounds should be switched to longer-acting drugs such as diazepam before withdrawal is attempted. For patients who have difficulty withdrawing with these measures, anxiety management may be useful (see p. 181).

Current advice is that the dose of benzodiazepine be lowered by about one-eighth every fortnight. However, if a patient experiences troublesome withdrawal symptoms, the dose can be maintained or even temporarily increased until symptoms settle. When patients have been misusing benzodiazepines and taking very high doses, it may be difficult to identify an appropriate starting dose. In general, patients should not be given more than 40–60 mg diazepam daily. This dose should gradually be reduced by about half over 6 weeks (Department of Health, 1999).

Many patients experience their most troublesome withdrawal symptoms once the benzodiazepine dose has been fully tapered off. Symptoms usually subside over the next few weeks, although the time course can be irregular and some symptoms such as muscle spasm may not appear until other features of withdrawal have largely disappeared. A few patients continue to experience withdrawal-like symptoms for months or even years after cessation of benzodiazepines ('prolonged withdrawal syndrome').

Prevention The prevention of benzodiazepine dependence lies in the restriction of prescribing. **Psychological treatments** are effective for most anxiety disorders (see p. 181) and non-pharmacological approaches to insomnia are also beneficial (p. 372). If benzodiazepines are prescribed, it should be for the short-term relief of symptoms that are severely disabling or distressing. In some patients who are already long-term users, the balance of benefit and risk will favour continued prescribing, but patients should be regularly reviewed and the daily dose of diazepam should not exceed 30 mg (Department of Health, 1999). Advice from a general practitioner can be sufficient to persuade between 20–40 per cent of long-term benzodiazepine users to reduce their daily dose or discontinue treatment. See Lingford-Hughes *et al.* (2004) for further information about benzodiazepine dependence and its treatment.

Barbiturates

Barbiturate prescribing has greatly diminished over the last decade as newer anxiolytic and antidepressant agents are preferred. Thus illicit use is becoming rare. Previously many people dependent on barbiturates began taking the drug because it had been prescribed as a hypnotic. Some barbiturates reached young drug misusers who administered them intravenously by dissolving capsules. Polysubstance misuse with barbiturates was common.

Withdrawal Abrupt withdrawal of barbiturates from a dependent person is dangerous. It may result in a delirium, like that after alcohol withdrawal, and may lead to seizures and sometimes to death through cardiovascular collapse. Hence if it is necessary to withdraw a person who has been taking doses substantially in excess of the therapeutic range, inpatient detoxification is advisable. If, however, a patient has been taking a therapeutic dose, slow outpatient withdrawal may be considered.

Cannabis

Cannabis is derived from the plant *Cannabis sativa*. It is consumed either as the dried vegetative parts in the form known as marijuana or grass, or as the resin secreted by the flowering tops of the female plant. Cannabis contains several pharmacologically active substances of which the most powerful psychoactive member is ***d-9-tetrahydrocannabinol***. It seems likely that the pharmacological effects of cannabinols are mediated through interaction with a specific cannabinoid receptor in the central nervous system. The endogenous ligand for these receptors is probably anandamide (for a review of the pharmacology of cannabis, see Howlett *et al.*, 2004).

Epidemiology In some parts of North Africa and Asia, cannabis products are consumed in a similar way to alcohol in Western society. In North America and Britain the intermittent use of cannabis is widespread. For example, as noted above it has been estimated that about 40 per cent of the population of the USA have used cannabis at least once in their lifetimes and about 8 per cent are current users. In the UK the corresponding figures are 27 per cent and 6 per cent (Ramsay *et al.*, 2001). It appears that most users do not take any other illegal drug, but some are given to high consumption of alcohol.

Clinical effects The effects of cannabis vary with the dose, the person's expectations and mood, and the social setting. Users sometimes describe themselves as 'high' but, like alcohol, cannabis seems to exaggerate the pre-existing mood, whether exhilaration or depression. Users report an increased enjoyment of aesthetic experiences and distortion of the perception of time and space. There may be reddening of the eyes, dry mouth, tachycardia, irritation of the respiratory tract, and coughing. Cannabis intoxication can lead to dangerous driving.

Adverse effects No serious adverse effects have been proved among those who use cannabis intermittently at small doses. Although there is no positive evidence of teratogenicity, cannabis has not been proved safe in the first 3 months of pregnancy. Inhaled cannabis smoke irritates the respiratory tract and is potentially carcinogenic. The most common adverse psychological effect of acute cannabis consumption is **anxiety**. Mild paranoid ideation is also not uncommon. At higher doses, toxic confusional states and occasionally psychosis in clear consciousness may rarely occur.

Cannabis and mental illness It is well-established that cannabis can modify the course of an established schizophrenic illness, with evidence from a number of studies that users are more likely to experience psychotic episodes and relapse (Hall and Solowij, 1998). The question as to whether cannabis use can predispose to the later development of schizophrenia has been more controversial. Andreasson *et al.* (1987) followed up 45 570 Swedish conscripts for 15 years. They found that the relative risk of developing schizophrenia was 2.5 times greater in subjects who used cannabis, and the relative risk for heavy users was six times greater. Whilst these data suggest that cannabis could be a risk factor for the development of schizophrenia, it is also possible that those predisposed to develop schizophrenia are also predisposed to misuse cannabis. However, a recent prospective cohort study found that evidence of predisposition for psychosis did not predict subsequent cannabis use in young people (Henquet *et al.*, 2005). In this study, cannabis use moderately increased the risk of psychotic symptoms in young people, but had a much stronger effect in those with additional risk factors for psychosis. In a review of the literature Arseneault *et al.* (2004) concluded that cannabis use in adolescence increased the risk of developing schizophrenia about twofold. They calculated that the removal of cannabis from society would prevent about 8 per cent of cases of schizophrenia.

There has also been concern that cannabis use in teenagers might increase the risk of subsequent depression, particularly in females (Patton *et al.*, 2005). However, a systematic review found that the evidence for cannabis causing psychosocial harm in young people was inconsistent and likely to be confounded by other factors such as childhood adversity (MaCleod *et al.*, 2004). It is also said that chronic use of cannabis can lead to a state of apathy and indolence (an amotivational state). However, this proposal has not been confirmed by epidemiological studies. It is possible that the symptoms and signs of the amotivational state could reflect chronic intoxication (see Hall and Solowij, 1998).

Tolerance and dependence There is evidence that tolerance to cannabis can occur in subjects exposed to high doses for a prolonged period of time, but it is much less evident in those who use small or intermittent dosing. Some subjects, however, do report inability to control cannabis use despite personal and social harm resulting from it. Withdrawal from high doses of cannabis gives rise to a syndrome of irritability, nausea, insomnia, and anorexia. These symptoms are generally mild in nature. The epidemiological data suggest the great majority of cannabis users do not misuse the drug or become dependent on it. For a review of the adverse effects of cannabis use see Hall (2000).

Stimulant drugs

These drugs include **amphetamines**, related substances such as phenmetrazine, and methylphenidate. **Cocaine** is also a stimulant drug, but is considered separately in the next section.

Amphetamine

Amphetamines have been largely abandoned in medical practice, apart from their use for the hyperkinetic syndrome of childhood (p. 675) and for narcolepsy (p. 374). The psychomotor stimulant effects of amphetamines are believed to result from their ability to release and block the re-uptake of dopamine and noradrenaline.

Epidemiology Amphetamines are probably the most frequently used stimulant in the UK, although cocaine is more commonly used in the USA. The NSDUH survey reported that in 2003 about 9 per cent of the US population had used a stimulant agent at least once in their lives whilst 0.5 per cent could be regarded as current users (SAMHSA, 2004).

In the UK, about 22 per cent of 16–29 year olds have used amphetamines at least once with a further 2 per cent having used them in the last year (Ramsay *et al.*, 2001). About 10 per cent of those presenting to specialist drug misuse services use amphetamine as their main drug whilst a further 10 per cent use it as a secondary drug usually in conjunction with opiates. Almost half of these users were injecting amphetamine and thereby exposed to the health risks of intravenous administration (see Seivewright and McMahon, 1996).

In the past, addiction to stimulant drugs arose chiefly from injudicious prescribing. However, most amphetamines are now illicitly synthesized and used as a 'street drug', known as 'speed' or 'whizz'. As well as being taken orally or intravenously, amphetamines can also be 'snorted' (taken like snuff). A pure form of amphetamine ('ice'), can be smoked or injected. It is said to produce particularly powerful effects.

Clinical effects Apart from their immediate effect on mood, the drugs produce over-talkativeness, overactivity, insomnia, dryness of lips, mouth, and nose, and anorexia. The pupils dilate, the pulse rate increases,

TABLE 18.10 Some complications of amphetamine and cocaine misuse

Medical
Cardiovascular – hypertension, stroke, arrhythmias, myocardial infarction
Infective – abscesses, septicaemia, hepatitis, HIV
Obstetric – reduced fetal growth, miscarriage, premature labour, placental abruption
Other – weight loss, dental problems, epilepsy, general neglect
Psychiatric
Anxiety, depression, antisocial behaviour, paranoid psychosis

and blood pressure rises. With large doses there may be **cardiac arrhythmia**, severe hypertension, cerebrovascular accident, and occasionally circulatory collapse. At increasingly high doses, neurological symptoms such as seizures and coma may occur. Acute adverse psychological effects of amphetamines include dysphoria, irritability, insomnia, and confusion. Anxiety and panic can also be present. **Obstetric complications** include miscarriage, premature labour, and placental abruption (Table 18.10).

Amphetamine-induced psychosis Prolonged use of high doses of amphetamines may result in repetitive stereotyped behaviour, for example, repeated tidying. A **paranoid psychosis** that has been likened to paranoid schizophrenia may also be induced by prolonged high doses. The features include persecutory delusions, auditory and visual hallucinations, and sometimes hostile and dangerously **aggressive behaviour** (Connell, 1958). Usually the condition subsides in about a week, but occasionally it persists for months. It is not certain whether these prolonged cases are true drug-induced psychoses, schizophrenia provoked by the amphetamine, or merely coincidental. Whatever the nature of the association, it is not uncommon for patients with amphetamine misuse to present to general psychiatric services. The ability of amphetamines to provoke psychosis has been one of the observations that has supported the dopamine hypothesis of schizophrenia (see Chapter 12).

Tolerance and dependence From the epidemiology of amphetamine use, it seems that many recreational users do not progress to misuse and dependence. In more persistent users tolerance to amphetamines leads to users taking higher doses of the drug. A withdrawal syndrome ('crash') of varying severity follows cessation of amphetamine use. In mild cases it consists mainly of low mood and decreased energy. In some cases, particularly in heavy users, depression can be severe, and accompanied by anxiety, tremulousness, lethargy, fatigue, and nightmares. Craving for the drug may be intense and suicidal ideation prominent. Dependence on amphetamines can develop quickly. Dependence on stimulant drugs may be recognized from the history of overactivity and high spirits alternating with inactivity and depression. Whenever amphetamine use is at all likely, a urine sample should be taken for analysis as soon as possible because these drugs are quickly eliminated.

Prevention and treatment Prevention of amphetamine misuse depends on restriction of the drugs and careful prescribing. Doctors should be wary of newly arrived patients who purport to suffer from narcolepsy.

Treatment of acute overdoses requires sedation and management of hyperpyrexia and cardiac arrhythmias. Most toxic symptoms, including paranoid psychoses, resolve quickly when the drug is stopped. An antipsychotic drug may be needed to control florid symptoms, but if this medication can be avoided the differential diagnosis from schizophrenia will be easier.

The treatment of amphetamine dependence is difficult because craving for the drug can be intense. **Abstinence** is the usual goal and to achieve this a full range of social and psychological interventions may be needed (see above). Benzodiazepines may be helpful for managing acute distress occasioned by a severe withdrawal syndrome. Antidepressants do not appear to be effective in promoting abstinence though may be appropriate for treatment of a persistent depressive disorder. Abstinence-based programmes are not suitable for all misusers and in view of the considerable harm that is associated with severe intravenous misuse, some specialist centres undertake maintenance treatment with oral amphetamine. There is no clear evidence base for this practice, but it may achieve the goal of harm reduction in carefully selected situations (see Bruce, 2000), and randomized controlled trials are needed. For a review of pharmacological treatments, see Srisurapont *et al.* (2004).

Cocaine

Cocaine is a central nervous stimulant with effects similar to those of amphetamines (described above). It a particularly powerful positive reinforcer in animals and causes strong dependence in humans. These latter effects probably stem from the ability of cocaine to block the re-uptake of dopamine into presynaptic dopamine terminals. This leads to substantial increases in extracellular levels of dopamine in the nucleus accumbens and consequent activation of the physiological 'reward system' (Robbins and Everitt, 1999).

Cocaine is administered by injection, by smoking, and by sniffing into the nostrils. The latter practice sometimes causes perforation of the nasal septum. In 'freebasing', chemically pure cocaine is extracted from the 'street' drug to produce 'crack', which has a very rapid onset of action, particularly when inhaled.

Epidemiology In 2003 about 15 per cent of Americans reported lifetime use of cocaine with an additional 3 per cent acknowledging use of the crack derivative. Usage of these dugs in the past month were 6 per cent and 1 per cent respectively (SAMHSA, 2004). Cocaine use in the USA has been associated with high levels of violent crime. The incidence of cocaine use in the UK and Europe has increased over the last decade, but to a lesser extent than that seen in the USA. Lifetime use for cocaine in the UK is about 6 per cent with the highest prevalence in young people in the 'dance' scene, the socially marginalized and people with opiate dependence (Ramsay *et al.*, 2001). It is likely that the great majority of cocaine users do not present to services.

Clinical effects The psychological effects of cocaine include excitement, increased energy, and euphoria. This can be associated with grandiose thinking, impaired judgement, and sexual disinhibition. Higher doses can result in visual and auditory hallucinations. **Paranoid ideation** may lead to **aggressive behaviour**. More prolonged use of high doses of cocaine can result in a paranoid psychosis with violent behaviour. This state is usually short-lived but may be more enduring in those with a pre-existing vulnerability to psychotic disorder. Formication ('cocaine bugs'), a feeling as if insects are crawling under the skin, is sometimes experienced by cocaine misusers.

The physical effects of cocaine include increases in pulse rate and blood pressure. Dilatation of the pupils is often prominent. Severe adverse effects of cocaine use include **cardiac arrhythmias, myocardial infarction, myocarditis**, and **cardiomyopathy**. Cocaine use has also been associated with cerebrovascular disease, including cerebral infarction, subarachnoid haemorrhage, and transient ischaemic attacks. Seizures and respiratory arrest have been reported. **Obstetric complications** include miscarriage, placental abruption, and premature labour.

Tolerance and dependence In persistent users, tolerance to the effects of cocaine develops and a withdrawal syndrome similar to that seen following withdrawal of amphetamines can occur. After acute cocaine use, the 'crash' consists of dysphoria, anhedonia, anxiety, irritability, fatigue, and hypersomnolence. If the preceding cocaine use has been relatively mild, such symptoms resolve within about 24 hours. After more prolonged use, the symptoms are more severe and extended, and are associated with intense craving, depression, and occasionally severe suicidal ideation. Craving for cocaine can re-emerge after months of abstinence, particularly if the subject is exposed to psychological or social cues previously associated with its use.

Treatment Acute intoxication may require sedation with benzodiazepines or, in severe cases, an antipsychotic agent. Concurrent medical crises such as seizures or hypertension should be managed in the usual way.

As with amphetamines, the treatment of cocaine dependence is difficult because of the intense craving associated with abstinence from the drug. For moderate cocaine users it may be sufficient to provide psychological and social support on an outpatient basis. Heavy and chaotic users with strong dependence will need more intensive management, perhaps as inpatients. There is little evidence to support pharmacological treatments to date, though several approaches have been evaluated. The evidence base does not support the use of antidepressant drugs, carbamazepine or dopamine agonists such as bromocriptine or amantadine (see Lima *et al.*, 2003a, b). There are some hints that disulfiram may be of benefit, probably not through any effect on concomitant alcohol use (Carroll *et al.*, 2004). Various psychotherapeutic programmes may be helpful in subjects with cocaine dependence. These include cognitive–behavioural approaches, contingency management and programmes incorporating twelve step approaches (Higgins *et al.* 2003). As far as individual treatment programmes are concerned, it is worth noting that subjects who misuse cocaine often misuse other drugs such as opioids and alcohol.

MDMA (ecstasy)

The recreational use of **3,4 methylenedioxymethamphetamine (MDMA)** or 'ecstasy' increased rapidly in the last decade and is still increasing but more slowly. In 1998 about 5 per cent of 16–24 year olds reported using ecstasy in the last year and in 2002 the number had risen to about 7 per cent (Aust *et al.*, 2002). In the US in 2003, lifetime risk for ecstasy use was about 5 per cent and in the last year about 0.9 per cent rather less than that seen in the UK (SAMHSA, 2003). Ecstasy is a synthetic drug classified in the DSM-IV substance list as a hallucinogen. However, it has stimulant as well as mild hallucinogenic properties. It is usually taken in tablet or capsule form in a dose of about 50–150 mg. Given in this way, its effects last for about 4–6 hours. Like amphetamines, ecstasy increases the release of dopamine but it also releases 5-hydroxytryptamine (5-HT), which may account for its hallucinogenic properties.

Clinical effects Ecstasy produces a positive mood state with feelings of euphoria, sociability, and intimacy. It also produces sensations of newly discovered insights and heightened perceptions. The physical effects of ecstasy include loss of appetite, tachycardia, bruxism, and sweating. Tolerance to successive doses of ecstasy develops quickly. Weekend users describe a midweek 'crash' in mood which may represent withdrawal effects (Curran and Travill, 1997).

Adverse reactions Rarely, ecstasy can cause severe adverse reactions, and deaths due to hyperthermia and its complications have been reported in healthy young adults. Hyperthermia probably results from the effect of ecstasy in increasing brain 5-HT release, together with the social setting in which the drug is customarily taken (crowded parties with prolonged and strenuous dancing). Deaths have also been reported through cardiac arrhythmias, though pre-existing cardiac disease may have played a role. Intracerebral haemorrhage has occurred in ecstasy users, probably as a consequence of hypertensive crises. Cases of toxic hepatitis could reflect impurities in manufacture or an idiosyncrasy in metabolism (Winstock, 2000).

The use of ecstasy has been associated with acute and chronic paranoid psychoses but, as with other drug-induced psychotic states, it is not clear how far such disorders represent idiosyncratic reactions of vulnerable individuals. There are also reports of 'flashbacks', which are the recurrence of abnormal experiences weeks or months following drug ingestion. Such effects have been reported with other hallucinogens (see below).

In experimental animals, including primates, repeated treatment with ecstasy produces **degeneration of 5-HT nerve terminals** in cortex and forebrain. Therefore it is possible that such effects could occur in humans, and brain-imaging studies show changes in serotonin transporter binding consistent with 5-HT neuronal damage (McCann *et al.*, 1998). Whether such a change could be associated with long-term neuropsychological or psychiatric sequelae is not known.

Prevention and harm reduction Although the risk of serious harm following acute ecstasy use appears to be low, it is important to inform potential users about the acute risks and the potential long-term hazard of neurotoxicity. Consumption of large doses and pre-existing psychiatric disorder are likely to be associated with increased risk of adverse reactions. Education may also help users to avoid heatstroke by encouraging breaks from dancing and the consumption of sufficient isotonic replacement fluid during vigorous exercise.

Hallucinogens

Hallucinogens are sometimes known as psychedelics, but we do not recommend this term because it does not have a single clear meaning. The term psychotomimetic is also used because the drugs produce changes that bear some resemblance to those of the functional psychoses. However, the resemblance is not close, and so we do not recommend this term.

The synthetic hallucinogens include lysergic acid diethylamide (LSD), dimethyltryptamine, and methyldimethoxyamphetamine. Of these drugs, LSD is encountered most often in the UK. Hallucinogens also occur naturally in some species of mushroom, and varieties containing **psilocybin** are consumed for their hallucinogenic effects. The mode of action of hallucinogenic drugs is unclear, but most act as partial agonists at brain 5-HT_{2A} receptors.

Epidemiology Trends in both the USA and Europe suggest that misuse of hallucinogens has increased over the last fifteen years. For example, between 1988 and 1997 the proportion of US high school students reporting lifetime hallucinogen use rose from 7.7 to 13.6 per cent. Life time risk in 2003 was estimated at 14.5 per cent (SAMHSA, 2004). In the UK 29 per cent of people aged 16–29 reported having used hallucinogens at least once in their lifetime, with 5 per cent acknowledging use in the last month (Ramsay *et al.*, 2001).

Clinical effects The effects of LSD have been most studied and will be described here. The physical actions of LSD are variable. There are initial sympathomimetic effects: heart rate and blood pressure may increase and pupils dilate. However, overdosage does not seem to result in severe physiological reactions.

In predisposed subjects, the hypertensive effects of hallucinogens can cause adverse myocardial and cerebrovascular effects. The psychological effects develop during a period of 2 hours after LSD consumption and generally last from 8 to 14 hours. The most remarkable experiences are distortions or intensifications of sensory perception. There may be confusion between sensory modalities (synaesthesia), with sounds being perceived as visual or movements experienced as if heard. Objects may be seen to merge with one another or move rhythmically. The passage of time appears to be slowed and experiences seem to have a profound meaning.

A distressing experience may be distortion of the body image, with the person sometimes feeling that they are outside their own body. These experiences may lead to panic with fears of insanity. The mood may be exhilaration, distress, or acute anxiety. According to early reports, behaviour could be unpredictable and extremely dangerous, with the users sometimes injuring or even killing themselves through behaving as if they were invulnerable. Since then there may have been some reduction in such adverse reactions, possibly because users are more aware of the dangers and take precautions to ensure support from other people during a 'trip'.

Whenever possible, adverse reactions should be managed by 'talking down' the user, explaining that the alarming experiences are due to the drug. If there is not time for this, an anxiolytic such as diazepam should be given and is usually effective. Tolerance to the psychological effects of LSD can occur, but a withdrawal syndrome has not been described. Whether dependence occus is uncertain but it is likely to be rare (Nichols, 2004).

It has been argued that use of LSD can cause long-term abnormalities in thinking and behaviour or even schizophrenia but the evidence for this is weak. However, flashback, i.e. the recurrence of psychedelic experience weeks or months after the drug was last taken, is a recognized event. A number of medications, including benzodiazepines and anticonvulsants, have been reported as helpful in the management of flashback but there are no controlled trials (Halpern and Pope, 2003).

Phencyclidine

Phencyclidine is sufficiently different from the hallucinogens in its actions to require a separate description. It can be synthesized easily, and is taken by mouth, smoked, or injected. Phencyclidine was developed as a disassociative anaesthetic, but its use was abandoned because of adverse effects such as delirium and hallucinations. It is related to the currently used anaesthetic agent ketamine.

Both phencyclidine and ketamine antagonize neurotransmission at **N-methyl-D-aspartate (NMDA) receptors**, which may account for their hallucinogenic effects. The psychological effects of ketamine in healthy volunteers have been used to model some of the clinical symptoms and cognitive changes seen in patients with schizophrenia (Krystal *et al.*, 1999) and are discussed on p. 289.

Phencyclidine is widely available in the USA but is little used in the UK. Most users of phencyclidine also use other drugs, particularly alcohol and cannabis. Ingestion of phencylcidine may be inadvertent because it is often added to other 'street' drugs to boost their effects.

Clinical effects Small doses of this drug produce drunkenness, with analgesia of fingers and toes, and even anaesthesia. Intoxication with the drug is prolonged, with the common features being agitation, depressed consciousness, aggressiveness and psychotic-like symptoms, nystagmus, and raised blood pressure. With high doses there may be ataxia, muscle rigidity, convulsions, and absence of response to the environment even though the eyes are wide open. Phencyclidine can be detected in the urine for 72 hours after it was last taken.

With serious overdoses, an adrenergic crisis may occur with hypertensive heart failure, cerebrovascular accident, or malignant hyperthermia. Status epilepticus may appear. Fatalities have been reported, due mainly to hypertensive crisis but also to respiratory failure or suicide. Other people may be attacked and injured. Chronic use of phencyclidine may lead to aggressive behaviour accompanied by memory loss. Tolerance to the effects of phencyclidine occurs, though withdrawal symptoms are rare in humans. Animal studies suggest that dependence could occur in heavy users (Abraham, 2000).

Treatment of phencyclidine intoxication Treatment of acute intoxication is symptomatic, according to the features listed above. Haloperidol, or diazepam, or both, may be given. Caution should be employed if using benzodiazepines alone because of the risk of further behavioural disinhibition. Chlorpromazine should be avoided because it may increase the anticholinergic effects of phencyclidine and worsen mental state. Hypertensive crisis should be treated with antihypertensive agents such as phentolamine. Respiratory function needs to be carefully monitored because excessive secretions may compromise the airway in an unconscious patient.

Volatile substances (solvents, inhalants)

The misuse of **volatile substances (also known as solvents)** is not new but public concern about widespread misuse was first apparent in the USA in the 1950s. Similar concerns emerged in the UK in the early 1970s. Although public interest has waned since then, there is a continuing high level of volatile substance misuse, particularly amongst adolescents.

The pharmacological actions of volatile substances in the central nervous system are not clear but, like alcohol, they may increase the fluidity of neuronal cell membranes and could also increase brain GABA function (Beckstead *et al.*, 2000).

Epidemiology Volatile substance misuse is a worldwide problem. In the NSDUH survey in 2003, about 10 per cent of the American population had used volatile substances at least once in their lives, but only about 0.2 per cent in the past month (National Institute on Drug Abuse, 1991). In the UK, up to a fifth of young people have tried sniffing volatile substances (Miller and Plant, 1996). Volatile substance misuse is very prevalent among the young homeless populations in South American countries.

Volatile substance use occurs mainly in **young men**. Use is more common in those from lower socioeconomic backgrounds. Most of the young people known to use volatile substances do so as a group activity, and only about 5 per cent are solitary users. There is some evidence that a subgroup of volatile substance users have antisocial personalities and are likely to use and misuse multiple substances. However, the epidemiological data suggest that most who use volatile substances do so only a few times and then abandon the practice (Ives, 2000).

Substances used and methods of use The volatile substances used are mainly solvents and adhesives (hence the name 'glue sniffing'), but also include many other substances such as petrol, cleaning fluid, aerosols of all kinds, agents used in fire extinguishers, and butane. Toluene and acetone are frequently used. In this chapter the term 'volatile substance' will be used to describe all these various substances. The methods of ingestion depend on the substance; they include inhalation from tops of bottles, beer cans, cloths held over the mouth, plastic bags, and sprays. Volatile substance use may be associated with taking other illicit drugs or with tobacco or alcohol consumption, which can be heavy.

Clinical effects The clinical effects of volatile substances are similar to those of alcohol consumption. The central nervous system is first stimulated and then depressed. The stages of intoxication are similar to those of alcohol: euphoria, blurring of vision, slurring of speech, incoordination, staggering gait, nausea, vomiting, and coma. Compared with alcohol intoxication, volatile substance intoxication develops and wanes rapidly (within a few minutes, or up to 2 hours). There is early disorientation and two-fifths of cases may develop hallucinations, which are mainly visual and often frightening. This combination of symptoms may lead to serious accidents.

Adverse effects Volatile substance misuse has many severe adverse effects, of which the most serious is **sudden death**. These fatalities occur during acute intoxication, and about 100 such deaths occurred annually in the UK in the 1990s (Ives, 2000). About half the deaths are due to the direct toxic effects of the volatile substance, particularly cardiac arrhythmias and respiratory depression. The rest are due to trauma, asphyxia (plastic bag over head), or inhalation of stomach contents.

Chronic users may show evidence of **neurotoxic effects** and severe and disabling peripheral neuropathy has been described in teenager misusers. Other neurological adverse effects, particularly associated with toluene, include impaired cerebellar function, encephalitis, and dementia. Volatile substance misuse can also damage other organs including liver, kidney, heart, and lungs. Gastrointestinal symptoms include nausea, vomiting, and haematemesis.

Tolerance and dependence Dependence can develop if use is regular, but physical withdrawal symptoms are unusual. When such symptoms occur they usually consist of sleep disturbance, irritability, nausea, tachycardia, and, rarely, hallucinations and delusions. With sustained use over 6–12 months, tolerance can develop.

Diagnosis The diagnosis of acute volatile substance intoxication is suggested by several features: glue on the hands, face, or clothes; chemical smell on the breath; rapid onset and waning of intoxication; disorientation in time and space. Chronic misuse is diagnosed mainly on an admitted history of habitual consumption, increasing tolerance, and dependence. A suggestive feature is a facial rash ('glue-sniffers rash') caused by repeated inhalation from a bag.

Treatment As noted above, for many users experimentation with volatile substances is a temporary phase which does not appear to lead to persistent misuse or dependence. Advice and support may be sufficient for such subjects. However, a significant subgroup of those who misuse volatile substances also misuse other substances such as alcohol and opioids. Such subjects are more likely to have an antisocial personality disorder and to have experienced a chaotic and abusive family life. Treatment of this group is difficult, and a full range of psychological and social treatments is likely to be needed (see above). There is no specific pharmacotherapy for volatile substance misuse, but associated psychiatric disorders such as depression may require treatment in their own right.

Prevention Prevention of volatile substance misuse may best be directed at the large numbers of young people who experiment with volatile substances through curiosity or peer pressure. Policies include the restriction of sales of volatile substances to children and adolescents. Education, particularly concerning the risk of severe injury and death (which can, of course, occur in occasional or first-time users), seems worthwhile. Wider social measures such as the provision of improved recreational facilities have also been advocated. For a review of volatile substance misuse see Ives (2000).

Further reading

Department of Health (1999) *Drug misuse and dependence – Guidelines of clinical management*. HMSO, London. (Current practice guidelines for assessment and treatment of drug misuse.)

Lingford-Hughes, AR, Welch S and Nutt D (2004) Evidence-based guidelines for the treatment of substance misuse, addiction and comorbidity: recommendations from the British Association for Psychopharmacology. *Journal of Psychopharmacology* **18**(3) 293–335. (Excellent summary of the pharmacological management of alcohol and substance misuse.)

Miller, WR and Rollnick, S (1991) *Motivational interviewing: preparing people to change addictive behaviour*. Guilford Press, London. (Account of how best to motivate drug misusers to change their drug habit.)

Robson, P (1999) *Forbidden drugs*. Oxford University Press, Oxford. (Readable account of illicit drugs, reasons for use and treatment of misuse.)

CHAPTER 19

Problems related to sexuality and gender identity

Chapter contents

This chapter is concerned with four topics related to sexuality and gender: sexual orientation, sexual dysfunction, abnormalities of sexual preference, and disorders of gender identity.

1. **Sexual orientation** refers to the various aspects of sexual attraction towards members of the opposite or the same sex.
2. **Sexual dysfunction** denotes impaired or dissatisfying sexual enjoyment or performance. Such conditions are common.
3. **Abnormalities of sexual preference** are uncommon, but they take many forms and therefore require relatively more space than the more common sexual dysfunctions.
4. **Gender identity** is a person's sense of being male or female. When this sense of identity is at variance with the anatomical sex, the person is said to have a gender identity disorder.

To decide what sexual activities are abnormal requires an understanding of the wide variations that exist in normal sexual functioning. The chapter begins with an account of these variations. No account is given of sexual physiology; readers seeking information on this subject are referred to Levin (2000).

Variations in sexual behaviour

Human sexual behaviour is very varied. It is not known what determines this variation but it is likely that it has biological and social determinants. Compared with the behaviour of other primates, human sexual behaviour is less tied to biological factors; for example, it is not limited to a periods of oestrus. Also the biologically determined sexual signals related to the breasts, pubic hair, buttocks, and lips are augmented in many cultures by the use of make-up, perfumes, and clothing. In other cultures, clothing is used to hide these innate sexual signals by covering the arms, legs, and, in some societies, the women's faces. Moreover, man's artistic abilities are used to produce erotic images and writing that increase sexual arousal.

Social rules control the range of sexual behaviours that may be expressed. Sexual relations between family members are widely prohibited by social rules and also in law. Sexual relations with unrelated minors are also widely forbidden, though ages of consent vary in different societies. Some sexual behaviours that were generally condemned in the past are now widely accepted. For example, in the late nineteenth century, masturbation was condemned in many countries as sinful and also harmful to health; now it is widely accepted as normal. In ancient Greece, homosexual relations were widely accepted; in the more recent past they have been condemned; now they are generally accepted though condemned by some religions groups. Clinicians need to be aware of these variations in sexual behaviour and attitudes, and refrain from imposing their own values and attitudes on their patients.

Surveys of sexual behaviour

One way to discover what sexual behaviours are common is to ask people. The first major investigation was carried out by the group led by American biologist Alfred Kinsey (Kinsey *et al.*, 1948, 1953). The surveys were large (12 000 males and 8000 females), but the subjects were not representative of the general population. Thus, although the results were valuable in showing the range of sexual behaviour, the estimates of frequency could not be generalized. This is even more the case now since the surveys were carried out in the 1950s and sexual attitudes and behaviour have changed in many ways since then.

More recent surveys have collected reports from more representative samples of US and UK populations. Whilst similar findings might be expected in countries with comparable cultures, the results should not be generalized too widely.

In the **US survey** (Michael *et al.*, 1994), 3194 English-speaking adults were interviewed. About 20 per cent of those approached refused to be interviewed and although this is a generally satisfactory response rate for this kind of study, it is possible that those who refused had sexual attitudes and behaviour different from those of the rest. The main findings were:

- Men thought about sex more often than did women. Half the men reported sexual thoughts several times a day; most women reported sexual thoughts a few times a week or less.
- The percentages of men and women reporting various frequencies of sexual intercourse were: none in the last year, 14 per cent; a few times in the last year, 16 per cent; a few times a month, 40 per cent; 2–3 times a week, 26 per cent; more than this, 8 per cent.
- A third of females aged 18–60 said they were uninterested in sex.
- The most appealing sexual activity was vaginal intercourse (80 per cent), followed by watching the partner undress (50 per cent of males; but 30 per cent of females).
- Oral sex was common: 68 per cent of women had given it and 73 per cent had received it at some time.
- Anal sex was said to be unappealing by 73 per cent of men and 87 per cent of women.
- Frequency of intercourse was related inversely to age, and to the length of time that the couple had been together. It was not related to race, education, or religion. However, reported sexual practices did vary with race and social class.

The **UK survey** concerned 18 876 adults (Wellings *et al.*, 1994). Although the findings were similar to those of the US survey, they should be interpreted cautiously since, of those approached, nearly 30 per cent refused to be interviewed. The mean frequency of intercourse of those in their twenties was about 5 per month falling to 2 per month in those aged 55–59. Oral sex was the most common sexual activity after vaginal intercourse. Anal intercourse was infrequent: only 14 per cent of males and 13 per cent of females said that they had practised it. In another UK survey 30 per cent of males and 26 per cent of females reported that their first experience of intercourse was before the age of 16 (Wellings *et al.*, 2001).

Homosexual intercourse has been less studied than heterosexual intercourse but it is probably no less variable. With the obvious exception of vaginal intercourse, it includes all the sexual activities described by heterosexual people, including oral-genital contact and mutual masturbation. For males, it may include anal intercourse, and for women the use of an artificial phallus. Sexual partners may exchange roles in these acts, or one partner may be always passive and the other always active.

Apart from these survey results, it is widely accepted that many sexual activities that are regarded as abnormal when they are the preferred form of sexual behaviour, are practised widely as a minor component of both heterosexual and homosexual activity, for example, painful stimulation, or wearing certain clothes to increase arousal.

Sexual orientation

Kinsey *et al.* (1948) found that people cannot be divided sharply into those with homosexual and those with heterosexual orientation. Between people who are exclusively heterosexual and those who are exclusively homosexual is a continuum of people who experience in varying degrees both homosexual and heterosexual attraction and fantasies, who engage in varying mixtures of homosexual and heterosexual behaviour and relationships, and who adopt various degrees of homosexual and heterosexual lifestyles. For this and other reasons, Klein *et al.* (1985) suggested that sexual orientation should be assessed against six criteria: sexual attraction, sexual fantasies, sexual behaviour, affectional relationship preference, lifestyle, and self-identification. The expression of homosexual and heterosexual behaviour varies in the same person with age and with circumstances. The potential for bisexual attraction and behaviour seems to be greater in adolescence than in adult life. Also, homosexual behaviour is more likely to be expressed when heterosexual behaviour is unavailable, for example in prisons; and more likely to be suppressed when religious beliefs or the attitudes in the society are strongly disapproving.

In the study referred to above, Kinsey *et al.* (1948) estimated that 10 per cent of men were 'more or less exclusively homosexual' for at least 3 years, and that 4 per cent of men were exclusively homosexual throughout their lives. Kinsey *et al.* (1953) reported that 4 per cent of single women were continuously homosexual from the ages of 20 to 35. Neither study was of a representative sample of the population, and subsequent estimates suggest that the true figure may be nearer 3 per cent of men and 1 per cent of women (Gagnon and Simon, 1973; Laumann *et al.*, 1994).

Lifestyle is an aspect of sexual orientation that varies according to cultural factors. Nevertheless, in most societies the majority of homosexual people have lifestyles similar to those of heterosexual people. Other homosexual people prefer work and leisure activities that are more often chosen by members of the opposite sex. A small minority of homosexual people adopt the mannerisms and dress resembling, sometimes in an exaggerated way, those of the opposite sex. (Unlike transsexual people, they do this while recognizing that their gender corresponds to their anatomical sex.) Most people of either sexual orientation seek lasting relationships, but in both groups a promiscuous minority seek a series of brief sexual experiences.

Self-identification also varies considerably among people of the same sexual orientation. Some exclusively homosexual people experience strong feelings of identity with other homosexual people and seek their company in preference to that of heterosexuals.

Determinants of sexual orientation

The determinants of sexual orientation are not known. Several theories have been proposed, concerned with: genetic factors, birth order, hormonal influences, neuroanatomical differences, and psychological factors. For a review see Mutanski *et al.*, 2002.

Genetic determinants

Twin and adoption studies

Several investigators have reported that MZ twins are more often alike in respect of homosexuality than are DZ twins (Kallmann, 1952; Eckhert *et al.*, 1986; Bailey and Pillard, 1991; King and McDonald, 1992). These findings are compatible with a genetic aetiology, but could also reflect early environment which is in some ways is more similar for MZ twins than for DZ twins. Adoption studies may relevant to this latter possibility but there has been no conclusive investigation.

Molecular genetic and chromosome studies have not produced convincing evidence of a difference between either male or female homosexual people and heterosexuals.

Birth order

Having an older brother increases the chance of homosexuality. The reason is unknown but it has been suggested that the maternal immune system becomes sensitized to some aspect of the male fetus (see Quinsey, 2003).

Hormonal theories

Research with animals indicates that the intrinsic pattern of the mammalian brain is female, and that the development of male brain characteristics depends on androgen production by the fetus. In animals, male or female brain characteristics are inferred from differences in reproductive behaviour, such as mounting by the male and the lordosis of the sexually receptive female. It is uncertain whether information about the neural control of these mating behaviours is relevant to human sexual orientation. Moreover, although male animals engage at times in sexual behaviour with other males, exclusively homosexual behaviour probably occurs only in humans.

If prenatal androgen activity is a determinant of sexual orientation, there should be an excess of people with homosexual orientation among males with syndromes of prenatal androgen deficiency or insensitivity, and among females with syndromes involving androgen excess. No such increase has been observed among men with androgen deficiency or insensitivity (Byrne and Parsons, 1993). However, an increased rate of homosexual orientation has been reported among women with congenital virilizing adrenal hyperplasia (Money *et al.*, 1984; Byrne and Parsons, 1993). The interpretation of this finding is uncertain because these females are born with masculinized external genitalia, and it is possible that sexual orientation in adult life was affected by this feature rather than by a direct effect of hormones on the brain.

Neuroanatomical differences

Reports of differences between homosexual and heterosexual men, in the structure of the several hypothalamic nuclei (LeVay, 1991; Swaab and Hoffman, 1990), have been criticized on technical grounds (Byrne and Parsons, 1993).

Psychological causes

Theories about psychological causes of sexual orientation derive mainly from psychoanalytical studies of single cases or of highly selected groups of homosexual people. They rely on the unconfirmed recollections by adults of events in early childhood. The theories generally suppose that homosexual orientation among males is determined by poor relationships with the parents in early childhood: a distant relationship with, or prolonged absence of the father; or an overprotective mother. It is supposed that either can interfere with the development of a heterosexual orientation. Similarly, homosexual orientation among females is supposed to result from problems in early relationships with a mother who is rejecting or indifferent (Wolff, 1971). These theories have not been supported by scientific evidence.

Psychological problems related to sexual orientation

Most people of either sexual orientation are contented and have a stable relationship with a partner. However, people may consult doctors about four kinds of problem related to sexual orientation. Many of these problems are related to public attitudes, religious convictions, and personal beliefs that conflict with the person's sexual orientation.

Uncertainty about sexual orientation

Shy and sexually inexperienced young men may seek advice because they are uncertain of their sexual orientation. They can be helped by sympathetic discussion in which they are allowed time to reflect on their feelings and their situation.

Problems in adolescence

Young people who have realized that they are partly or predominantly homosexual may be uncertain about the implications for their lives, especially if they encounter intolerant attitudes. Some of these young people are bullied at school. A study of American school students showed a higher rate of suicide intent and suicide attempts among male homosexual students than heterosexuals. The corresponding rates among females were not increased (Remafedi *et al.*, 1998).

Some young people ask whether their sexual orientation is likely to change as they grow older. There are no reliable data, but it seems that a person who has reached adult life without experiencing heterosexual attraction or fantasies is unlikely to develop these later.

Problems in early adult life

People of either sexual orientation may ask for help with emotional disorders related to sexual or social relationships, or when their sexual urges conflict with religious or other beliefs. Some homosexual people ask for help with problems related to the unfavourable attitudes of other people. Some homosexual women marry and then seek advice, often at the suggestion of the spouse, about dysfunction in heterosexual intercourse.

Problems in middle age

People of either sexual orientation who have not formed a stable sexual relationship may become lonely and depressed if they do not have close friends and family. Men who have depended previously on casual sexual experiences may find these harder to arrange as they grow older.

Other problems

Other problems are often related to fears of sexually transmitted diseases, nowadays most often the possibility of having contracted AIDS, or a positive result of testing for HIV. People with these problems require appropriate medical treatment and counselling.

Problems of sex and gender identity

Classification of problems of sex and gender identity

In both DSM-IV and ICD-10 problems of sex and gender identity are classified in three groups:

1. sexual dysfunction;
2. disorders known as paraphilias in DSM-IV and disorders of sexual preference in ICD-10;
3. gender identity disorders.

In DSM-IV these conditions are grouped together under the heading of sexual and gender identity disorders. In ICD-10 they appear in two parts of the classification: sexual dysfunctions are in F5, 'physiological dysfunction associated with mental or behavioural factors'; disorders of sexual preference and of gender identity are in F6, 'abnormalities of adult personality and behaviour'. The two classifications are shown side by side in Table 19.1. In both systems each of the three main categories is classified further. **Sexual dysfunctions** are divided according to the stage of the sexual response that is mainly affected: disorders of sexual desire; disorders of sexual arousal; disorders of orgasm. There are also categories for the painful conditions vaginismus and dyspareunia. The slight differences in terminology between DSM-IV and ICD-10 are shown in Table 19.1.

Paraphilias (abnormalities of sexual preference) are subdivided in both classifications. The only substantial difference is that DSM-IV has a category for the uncommon disorder known as frotteurism, a condition which in ICD-10 would be classified under 'other abnormalities of sexual preference'.

Gender identity disorders are divided in DSM-IV, but not in ICD-10, into those in children and those in adolescents and adults.

TABLE 19.1 Classification of sexual and gender identity disorders

DSM-IV	ICD-10
Sexual dysfunction	*Sexual dysfunction not caused by organic disorders**
Sexual desire disorders	Lack or loss of sexual desire
Hypoactive sexual desire disorder	
Sexual aversion disorder	Sexual aversion and lack of sexual enjoyment
Sexual arousal disorder	
Female sexual arousal disorder	Failure of genital response
Male erectile disorder	
Orgasm disorders	Orgasmic dysfunction
Female orgasmic disorder	
Male orgasmic disorder	
Premature ejaculation	Premature ejaculation
Sexual pain disorders	
Dyspareunia	Non-organic dyspareunia
Vaginismus	Non-organic vaginismus
Sexual dysfunction due to a general medical condition	Excessive sexual drive
Paraphilias	*Disorders of sexual preference***
Exhibitionism	Exhibitionism
Fetishism	Fetishism
Frotteurism	–
Paedophilia	Paedophilia
Sexual masochism	Sadomasochism
Sexual sadism	
Voyeurism	Voyeurism
Transvestic fetishism	Fetishistic transvestism
Gender identity disorders	*Gender identity disorders****
In children	
In adolescents and adults	

* In ICD-10 sexual dysfunction is part of F5, behavioural syndromes associated with physiological disturbances and physical factors.

** In ICD-10 disorders of sexual preference are part of F6, disorders of adult personality and behaviour (to aid comparison with DSM- IV, the order in which the disorders appear has been changed from that in the text of ICD-10).

***In ICD-10 gender identity disorders are part of F6.

Sexual dysfunctions

In men sexual dysfunction refers to repeated impairment of normal sexual interest and/or performance. In women it refers more often to a repeated unsatisfactory quality to the experience; sexual intercourse can be completed, but without enjoyment. What is regarded as normal sexual intercourse, and therefore what is thought to be impaired or unsatisfactory, depends in part on the expectations of the two people concerned. For example, one couple may regard it as normal that the woman seldom achieves orgasm, whilst another may seek treatment.

As explained above, problems of sexual dysfunction are classified into those involving:

- Sexual desire and sexual enjoyment.
- The genital response (erectile impotence in men, lack of arousal in women).
- Orgasm (premature or retarded ejaculation in men, orgasmic dysfunction in women).

- Pain (vaginismus and dyspareunia in women; painful ejaculation in men).

It is important to remember that sexual dysfunction may not be disclosed directly but revealed during enquiries about another complaint, such as depression or poor sleep, or gynaecological symptoms.

Prevalence of sexual dysfunctions

In the UK a stratified probability sample of 11,161 people aged 16–44 were asked about sexual problems lasting more than one month and lasting more than 6 months (Mercer *et al.*, 2003). The response rate was 65 per cent. It is not known whether the self reported problems would have met diagnostic criteria for the corresponding sexual dysfunction. The reported rates are shown in Table 19.2. More women than men reported problems and among both the majority of problems lasted less than 6 months.

Two UK studies have surveyed general practice patients. Dunn *et al.* (1998) carried out a postal survey. A third of the men who responded and two-fifths of the women reported a current sexual problem. Erectile dysfunction and premature ejaculation were the most common problems among the men. Vaginal dryness and infrequent orgasm were the most common problems among the women. Half of those with a problem reported that they would have liked help, but only one in ten had received it. Nazareth *et al.* (2003) surveyed patients from 13 London general practices with a response rate of 70 per cent to the questionnaire. About 22 per cent of men and 40 per cent of women met criteria for an ICD diagnosis of a sexual problem. The most frequent were: inhibited female orgasm (19 per cent); lack or loss of sexual desire (17 per cent of women and 7 per cent of men); male erectile dysfunction (9 per cent); and female sexual arousal dysfunction (3.6 per cent).

In about a third of couples seen for treatment, both partners have a problem, usually low libido in the woman and premature ejaculation in the man. For a review of the prevalence – and also causes and treatment of sexual dysfunction – see Heiman (2002a).

TABLE 19.2 Reported frequency of problems related to sexual functions among people aged 16–44 with a sexual partner*

	Lasting 1 month (%)	Lasting 6 months (%)
Males		
Lack of sexual interest	17	2
Erectile difficulty	6	1
Premature orgasm	12	3
Anxiety about performance	9	2
Females		
Lack of sexual interest	40	10
Unable to reach orgasm	14	4
Pain on coitus	12	3
Anxiety about peformance	7	2

*Data from Mercer *et al.* (2003). Respondents could report more than one disorder.

General causes of sexual dysfunction

Sexual dysfunction arises from varying combinations of a poor general relationship with the partner, low sexual drive, ignorance about sexual technique, and anxiety about sexual performance. Other important factors are physical illness, depressive and anxiety disorders, medication, and alcohol or drug misuse. Some of these factors will now be considered. When assessing aetiology in an individual, it is important to recognize that both psychological and physical factors are often present.

Low sexual drive

Sexual drive varies between people but the reason for this is not known. In males, increasing sexual drive at puberty is related to increased output of androgens. Conversely, lowered androgen levels after castration, treatment with oestrogens, and the administration of anti-androgenic drugs are associated with reduced male sexual drive. However, no convincing association has been shown between low androgen levels and low sexual drive in men seeking help for this problem. Also, treatment with androgens does not usually increase sexual drive in men with normal endocrine function. Small doses of androgens do however increase sexual drive in women (Hawton, 1985).

Anxiety

Anxiety is an important cause of sexual dysfunction. Sometimes anxiety is an understandable consequence of an earlier frightening experience such as a man's failure in his first attempt at intercourse, or a woman's experience of sexual abuse or assault. Sometimes the anxiety relates to frightening accounts of sexual relationships received from parents or other people. Psychoanalysts suggest that anxiety about sexual relationships originates from even earlier experiences, namely failure to resolve the oedipal complex in boys or the corresponding attachment to the father in girls (see p. 91). There is no scientific support for these ideas.

Physical illness and surgical treatments

Sexual dysfunction sometimes dates from a period of abstinence associated with pregnancy or childbirth, or from the debilitating effects of physical illness (Table 19.3). Of the diseases that have a direct effect on sexual performance, **diabetes mellitus** is particularly important. In one study, 22 per cent of men and 27 per cent of women with type I diabetes reported lasting sexual dysfunction. The dysfunction is thought to be related to autonomic neuropathy, or vascular disorders; in women it was associated also with depression - as it was also in the control group (Enzlin *et al.*, 2002, 2003). For a review of the pathophysiology of diabetic sexual dysfunction, see Morano (2003).

TABLE 19.3 Medical and surgical conditions commonly associated with sexual dysfunction

Medical
Endocrine
◆ Diabetes, hyperthyroidism, myxoedema,
◆ Addison's disease, hyperprolactinaemia
Gynaecological
◆ Vaginitis, endometriosis, pelvic infections
Cardiovascular
◆ Angina pectoris, previous myocardial infarction
Respiratory
◆ Asthma, obstructive airways disease
Arthritic
◆ Arthritis from any cause
Renal
◆ Renal failure with or without dialysis
Neurological
◆ Pelvic autonomic neuropathy, spinal cord lesions, stroke
Surgical
◆ Mastectomy
◆ Colostomy, ileostomy
◆ Oophorectomy
◆ Episiotomy, operations for prolapse
◆ Amputation

Modified from Hawton and Oppenheimer (1983).

Sexual dysfunction after **myocardial infarction** may result from anxiety and medication side-effects rather than from physical causes (H. A. Taylor, 1999). Most of the associations between physical disease or its treatment and sexual dysfunction are obvious. Nevertheless, doctors often fail to think of the sexual consequences of disease and the (often unexpressed) problems that result.

Effects of medication

Several drugs have side-effects that involve sexual function (Table 19.4). The most important drugs are antihypertensives (especially adrenoceptor antagonists), antipsychotics (especially thioridazine), monoamine oxidase inhibitors, and specific serotonin re-uptake inhibitors. Anxiolytics, sedatives, and hormones have more effect on the sexual activity of men than of women. Apart from these prescribed drugs, the excessive use of alcohol and street drugs impairs sexual performance.

General approach to the assessment of patients with sexual dysfunction

History taking

Whenever possible, the sexual partner should be interviewed as well as the patient. The two should be seen separately, and then together. The following enquiries are important (see Table 19.5).

TABLE 19.4 Some drugs that may impair sexual function

Therapeutic agents
Antihypertensives
◆ Diuretics, spironolactone, sympatholytics,
◆ α-blockers, β-blockers
Antidepressants
◆ Tricyclics, monoamine oxidase inhibitors, specific serotonin re-uptake inhibitors
Mood regulators
◆ Lithium
Anxiolytics and hypnotics
◆ Benzodiazepines
Antipsychotics
◆ Especially thioridazine
Hormonal agents
◆ Anabolic steroids, corticosteroids, oestrogens
Misused substances
◆ Tobacco, alcohol, cocaine, marijuana

TABLE 19.5 Assessment of sexual dysfunction

Define the problem (ask both partners)
Origin and course
With other partners?
Sexual drive
Knowledge and fears
Social relationships generally
Social relations between the partners
Psychiatric disorder
Substance misuse
Medical illness; medical or surgical treatment
Why seek help now?
Physical examination
Laboratory tests -see text
(Special tests for erectile function)

- **Define the problem** as it appears to each partner. Details should not be omitted because the interviewer feels embarrassed.
- **Origin and course** Has the problem always been present or did it start after a period of normal functioning?
- **Has the problem occurred with more than one partner?** Each partner should be asked this question separately.
- **Strength of sexual drive** is assessed by asking each partner separately about frequency of intercourse and masturbation, about sexual thoughts, and about feelings of sexual arousal.
- **Knowledge of sexual technique and anxiety about sex** Possible sources of misinformation and anxiety are considered by asking about the family's attitude to sex, and the extent of sex education and sexual experience. Each partner should be asked about the sexual technique of the other.
- **Social relationships with the opposite sex** Is either partner shy or socially inhibited?
- **The couple's social relationship** Some couples ask for help with sexual problems which are the result and not (as they suggest) the cause of marital conflict.
- **Psychiatric disorder** Is either partner suffering from a psychiatric disorder, especially a depressive disorder, which might account for the sexual problem, directly or through the drugs used to treat it (see Table 19.4)?
- Misuse of alcohol or drugs (see above).
- **Physical illness and medical or surgical treatment** - particular attention should be given to the factors listed in Tables 19.3 and 19.4.
- **Why have they sought help now?** The sexual problem may have increased, and/or one partner may have threatened to end the relationship.

Physical examination and special investigations

Physical examination If the general practitioner or another specialist has not already done so, a physical examination should be carried out (see Table 19.6).

Laboratory tests should be arranged in appropriate cases; for example, fasting blood sugar, testosterone, sex-hormone-binding globulin, luteinizing hormone, and prolactin in men with erectile dysfunction.

For further information about the examination of people with sexual dysfunction Tomlinson (2005).

General approaches to the treatment of sexual dysfunction

Before directing treatment to the sexual problem, it is important to consider whether **couple therapy** is more appropriate because the sexual problem is secondary to a problem in the relationship. If it is appropriate to focus treatment on the sexual problem, **advice and education** may be all that is needed.

If **sex therapy** is appropriate, it should be directed to both partners whenever possible. The usual approach,

TABLE 19.6 Important points in the physical examination of men presenting with sexual dysfunctions

General examination (directed especially to evidence of diabetes mellitus, thyroid disorder, and adrenal disorder)
Hair distribution
Gynaecomastia
Blood pressure
Peripheral pulses
Ocular fundi
Reflexes
Peripheral sensation
General examination
Penis: congenital abnormalities, foreskin, pulses, tenderness, plaques, infection, urethral discharge
Testicles: size, symmetry, texture, sensation
Prostate – in men aged over about 50 years

Adapted from Hawton (1985).

which owes much to the original work of Masters and Johnson (1970), has four characteristic features:

1. the partners are treated together;
2. they are helped to communicate better about their sexual relationship;
3. they receive education about the anatomy and physiology of sexual intercourse;
4. they take part in a series of 'graded tasks'.

Masters and Johnson held that two other factors were important. The first was that treatment should be intensive, for example, seeing both partners every day for up to 3 weeks. The second was that treatment should be carried out by a man and a woman working as co-therapists. It has been shown that neither of these additional factors is essential; good results can be obtained when treatment is given once a week and when only one therapist sees the couple.

Treatment as a couple Although better results are obtained when the couple are treated together, some help can be given to a patient who has no regular partner. Such patients can at least discuss their difficulties and possible ways of overcoming them. Discussion of this kind can sometimes help to overcome social inhibitions.

Communication Communication is not only the ability to talk freely about specific sexual problems; it is also concerned with increasing understanding of the other person's wishes and feelings. Each partner may believe that the other should know instinctively how to give pleasure during intercourse, so that failure to please is attributed to lack of concern or affection rather than to ignorance. Such failure can be overcome by helping the partners to express their own desires more frankly.

Education Education stresses the physiology of the sexual response. For example, if the problem is anorgasmia in the woman, the doctor may explain the longer time needed for a woman to reach sexual arousal, and may emphasize the importance of foreplay, including clitoral stimulation, in bringing about vaginal lubrication. Suitably chosen sex education books can reinforce the therapist's advice. Such counselling is often the most important part of the treatment of sexual dysfunctions.

Graded tasks These begin with tender physical contact. The couples are encouraged to caress any part of the other person's body except the genitalia in order to give enjoyment (Masters and Johnson call this the 'sensate focus'). Next, the couple may stimulate each other's genitalia, but not go on to penetrative sex. At both stages, each partner is encouraged to discover the experience most enjoyed by the other and to provide this experience. They are strongly discouraged from checking their own state of sexual arousal because this checking generally has an inhibiting effect. (Such checking is a common habit in people with sexual disorder, and has been called the 'spectator role'.) Graded tasks are not only directly beneficial; they also help to uncover any hidden fears or areas of ignorance that need to be discussed.

For further information about sexual therapy for couples, see Hawton (1995) and Crowe (1998).

Results of sex therapy

There have been few adequately controlled studies of sex therapy. Early studies suggested that the general methods described above are successful in about a third of cases, and lead to some worthwhile improvement in a further third (Heinman and LoPiccolo, 1983; Hawton *et al.*, 1986). Improvement at the end of treatment are maintained for months (Heinman and LoPiccolo, 1983), but may not be sustained 3 years after therapy (De Amicis *et al.*, 1985). The results seem to be as good in problems of long duration as in others (Hawton *et al.*, 1986).

Types of sexual dysfunction

Lack or loss of sexual desire (hypoactive sexual desire disorder)

Description and causes Complaints of diminished sexual desire are much more common among women than among men. The term *lack* of sexual desire indicates that the condition has been present since the start of sexual activity. The term *loss* of sexual desire indicates that the condition developed after a period when sexual desire was normal. Loss may be global or situational.

Global lack of desire suggests a biologically determined low level of sexual drive; or homosexual orientation when the complaint relates to heterosexual intercourse.

Global loss of desire suggests a medical or psychiatric cause. Medical causes include low testosterone, high prolactin, systemic disease, gynaecological disease, and the side-effects of medication such as antipsychotics and SSRIs. Psychiatric causes include depressive disorder, the consequences of sexual trauma, and severe intrapsychic conflict leading to inhibition. Loss of desire after a depressive disorder usually returns to the previous level as the disorder resolves, but occasionally it persists. Among women, sexual desire may diminish premenstrually, during and immediately – and for some women for longer – after pregnancy, and after hysterectomy or breast removal. Women who experience loss of desire in these circumstances should be reassured that this is common and likely to be short-lived.

Situational loss of desire often reflects general problems in the relationship between the sexual partners.

Assessment Problems of sexual desire and sexual arousal among women with psychiatric disorder are often overlooked and women should have the opportunity to discuss their sexual lives with a woman professional

Sexual desire is assessed by asking about:

- **imagery** the frequency and nature of sexual imagery and dreams;
- **desire** for and **frequency** of sexual behaviour, with a partner or alone.

Potential causes are assessed by asking about:

- relationship problems: loss of affection, anger, etc.;
- sexual orientation, sexual preferences;
- tiredness, anxiety, depression;
- past sexual experiences causing fear or disgust.
- medical causes: Those listed above should be considered, including testosterone and prolactin measurement in selected cases.

For a review of the assessment of sexual desire disorders see Rosen and Leiblum (1987).

Treatment Because there is little research evidence, treatment is based mainly on clinical experience. Any psychiatric or medical causes should be treated. Couple therapy, cognitive therapy or counselling may be tried, depending on the apparent causes and the person's preferences. Testosterone may increase desire in patients who have low levels of bioavailable testosterone but there is no evidence from controlled trials of sustained increase of sexual desire in patients with low sexual desire and normal testosterone levels. Daily apomorphine has been reported to benefit premenopausal women with hypoactive sexual desire disorder (Caruso *et al.*, 2004) but further trials are needed.

Sexual aversion disorder

Sexual enjoyment is sometimes replaced by a positive aversion to genital contact. When this aversion is persistent or severe and accompanied by avoidance of almost all genital sexual contact with a sexual partner, the condition is classified as sexual aversion disorder. The causes of the condition are not well understood; they seem to be similar to the psychological causes of hypoactive sexual desire disorder. Assessment and treatment is similar to that for hypoactive sexual desire disorder.

Specific sexual fears

A few women are made extremely anxious by specific aspects of the sexual act, such as being touched on the genitalia, the sight or smell of seminal fluid, or even kissing. Despite these specific fears, they may still enjoy other parts of sexual intercourse. Assessment and treatment follows the general approach described on pp. 477–9.

Female sexual arousal disorder

Lack of sexual arousal in the female appears as reduced vaginal lubrication. This reduction may be due to:

- inadequate sexual foreplay by the partner;
- lack of sexual interest; or
- anxiety about intercourse.

After the menopause, hormonal changes may lead to reduced vaginal secretions. Assessment and treatment follow the general approach described on pp. 477–9. There are reports of beneficial effects of sildenafil citrate but a controlled clinical trial (Basson *et al.*, 2002) did not find significant diffrences from placebo and more research is needed. In any case, medication should be prescribed only after full consideration of psychological and other potential causes (see Bancroft, 2002).

Male erectile disorder

This condition is the inability to reach an erection or to sustain it long enough for satisfactory coitus. It may be present from the first attempt at intercourse (primary) or develop after a period of normal function (secondary). It is more common among older than younger men (in contrast with premature ejaculation, see below).

Causes: Primary cases may occur through a combination of low sexual drive and anxiety about sexual performance. **Secondary cases** may arise from diminishing sexual drive in the middle-aged or elderly, loss of interest in the sexual partner, anxiety, depressive disorder, and organic disease and its treatment. It is thought that abnormalities of the vascular supply to the penile erectile tissue are important factors in erectile failure associated with some physical diseases including diabetes, and peripheral vascular disease.

Assessment The following aspects of the general assessment are particularly important:

- Has there been a previous period of normal function? Erectile failure may be a transient disorder arising at times of stress, or may reflect loss of interest in the sexual partner.

- Has the failure occurred with more that one partner?
- Does erection occur during foreplay?
- Does erection occur on waking or in response to masturbation? Erection in these circumstances suggests psychological causes for the failure of erection at other times.
- Is there evidence of alcohol or drug abuse (ask the partner as well as the patient)?
- Are there possible effects of any medication?

Special tests for erectile dysfunction When aetiology is uncertain after history taking, physical examination, and blood tests, several special investigations may be considered. The **Rigiscan** helps to assess penile tumescence and rigidity. Measurements can be made during exposure to visual sexual stimuli, in response to a vibrator, or during sleep. These tests help to differentiate between psychogenic and neurological impairment. If vascular impairment is suspected, **Doppler ultrasound** and/or **duplex ultrasonography** may help to identify arterial or venous dysfunction. **Intracavernosal prostaglandin** produces a penile response if there is vascular capability. More specialized investigations may be indicated when vascular surgery appears to be indicated. For a review see Althof and Seftel (1995).

Treatment Any reversible causes should be treated. Psychological causes may respond to appropriate **cognitive or psychodynamic therapy**, although temporary relapses may occur

Oral medication The phosphodiesterase type 5 inhibitors sidenafil, vardenafil and tadalafil inhibit the breakdown of cyclic GMP by a phosphodiesterase situated in the vascular smooth muscle of the penis. They do not initiate arousal but enhance the effects of sexual stimulation. Care should be taken to observe the manufacturer's advice about contraindications, side-effects, and interactions with other drugs. The most common side-effects are headache, flushing, dyspepsia and nasal congestion. These effects are generally reversible and diminish during continued treatment. Of the three, tadalafil has the longest half life and period of responsiveness. For further information about sildenafil see Kuthe (2003).

Treatment for vascular or neurogenic causes Several treatments are available for patients with impotence due to vascular or neurogenic abnormalities, including those secondary to diabetes. These methods include drugs, vacuum devices, the surgical correction of vascular abnormalities, and penile prostheses.

- **Intracavernosal injections** of the smooth muscle relaxant papaverine, or the α-receptor blocker phenoxybenzamine, produce erection and have been used to treat impotence (Virag, 1982; Padma-Nathan *et al.*, 1987), as have injections of prostaglandins (Lee *et al.*, 1988). Alprostadil is a newer drug available for intracavernosal injection (Linet and Ogrinc, 1996). Small doses of the chosen drug are given at first, and increased gradually. When an appropriate dose has been determined, patients are taught to inject themselves. (Doses are not given here because the treatment should be learned from a doctor experienced in its use.) Overdose can lead to prolonged erection, which may require the aspiration of blood and the injection of an α1-agonist such as phenylephrine (Kirby, 1994).
- **Intraurethral treatment** Alprostadil can be administered by the intraurethral route (see Padma-Nathan *et al.*, 1997) as well as by the intracavernosal route described above.
- **Vacuum devices** can be tried for patients who do not respond to intracavernosal drug injections (Wylie *et al.*, 2003). The penis is placed in a surrounding cylinder in which the pressure is reduced; an erection follows, and is maintained by applying a restricting band to the base of the penis before the cylinder is removed. Although this procedure is generally effective in producing an erection, it is disliked by many patients.
- **Surgical methods** have been used to treat erectile disorder resulting from proven vascular abnormalities. Microsurgery can be used to revascularize the corpora cavernosa when there are stenoses or occlusions in the arteries. Short-term improvement rates of about 50 per cent have been reported in selected cases (Goldstein, 1986). An alternative approach is to insert a penile prosthesis, which may be semi-rigid or capable of being inflated before intercourse

For a review of erectile dysfunction and its treatment see Ralph and McNicolas (2000).

Female orgasmic dysfunction

Many women do not regularly reach orgasm during vaginal intercourse but do so in response to clitoral stimulation. Whether failure to reach orgasm regularly should be regarded as a disorder has been questioned (e.g. Heiman, 2002b). Nevertheless some women regard it as a problem and ask for advice and help.

Causes This disorder arises from normal variations in sexual drive, poor sexual technique by the partner, lack of affection for the partner, tiredness, depressive disorder, physical illness including gynaecological disorders, long term effects of sexual abuse, and the effects of medication.

Assessment In addition to the general assessment, the following questions are important:

- Has the woman ever achieved orgasm?
- If so, during intercourse with another partner, or masturbation, or in response to a particular fantasy?

Medication such as SSRIs, other antidepressants, and antihypertensives are possible causes.

Treatment The partner is encouraged to use the sensate focus technique (see above). Also the woman can use graduated self stimulation, manually or with a vibrator, or increased engorgement of the clitoris can be brought about by a vacuum device (Billups, 2002). Whichever approach is chosen, help should be given for any relationships or other problems.

Male orgasmic disorder

This term refers to serious delay in, or absence of, ejaculation. Usually the problem occurs only during coitus, but it may also occur during masturbation. It is usually associated with a general psychological inhibition about sexual relations, but it may be caused by drugs including antipsychotics, monoamine oxidase inhibitors, and specific serotonin uptake inhibitors.

Premature ejaculation

This term refers to habitual ejaculation before penetration or so soon afterwards that the women has not gained pleasure. It is more common among younger than older men, especially during their first sexual relationships.

Causes This disorder is so common in sexually inexperienced young men that it can be regarded as a normal variation. When it persists, it is often because of fear of failure.

Treatment Psychological causes should be treated with the general approach described on p. 478. If the partner is willing, this disorder can be treated with the 'squeeze technique'. When the man indicates that he will soon have an orgasm, the woman grips the penis for a few seconds and then releases it suddenly. Intercourse is then continued. An alternative 'start-stop' method has been described in which the woman attempts to regulate the amount of sexual stimulation during intercourse. Similar techniques can be used during masturbation. In the 'quiet vagina' technique, the penis is contained within the vagina for increasing periods without any movement, before the man ejaculates. It is important to understand the woman's point of view thoroughly before asking her to assist in such treatment.

SSRIs and some other antidepressants such as clomipramine delay ejaculation, whether this is normal or premature. However, the effect is generally lost when the medication stops. If used at all, medication should not be the first line of treatment, and should be combined with psychological measures.

Sexual pain disorders

Dyspareunia This term refers to pain on intercourse. Such pain has many causes. Pain experienced after partial penetration may result from impaired lubrication of the vagina, from scars or other painful lesions, or from the muscle spasm of vaginismus. Pain on deep penetration strongly suggests pelvic pathology such as endometriosis, ovarian cysts and tumours, or pelvic infection, though it can be caused by impaired lubrication associated with low sexual arousal.

Vaginismus Vaginismus is spasm of the vaginal muscles which causes pain when intercourse is attempted, in the absence of a physical lesion causing pain. The spasm is usually part of a phobic response to penetration, and may be made worse by an inexperienced partner. Spasms often begin as soon as the man attempts to enter the vagina; in severe cases it occurs even when the woman attempts to introduce her own finger. Severe vaginismus may prevent consummation of marriage. So called 'virgin wives' may have a generalized fear and guilt about sexual relationships rather than a specific fear of penetration. Some women with vaginismus are married to passive men who have low libido and are able to accept their wives' refusal to permit full sexual relations (Dawkins, 1961). Low libido in the man then becomes evident when the treatment has reduced the woman's problem.

Points of special relevance in the sexual history include:

- the circumstances that provoke spasm (intercourse, tampon, partner's finger, patient's own finger);
- the partner's sexual technique;
- any history of traumatic sexual experience.

Treatment There have been very few trials of treatment for dyspareunia (see McGuire and Hawton (2003) for a Cochrane review), so that therapy has to be based on clinical experience. Treatment employs the general sex therapy techniques described above with emphasis on a ban on vaginal intercourse. Fears are treated with cognitive or psychodynamic approaches, and the woman is helped to desensitize herself gradually by inserting first her finger and then dilators of increasing size.

Pain on ejaculation This problem is uncommon. The usual causes are urethritis or prostatitis. Sometimes no cause is found.

Sexual dysfunction among the physically handicapped

Physically handicapped people have sexual problems arising from several sources:

- **specific effects** of the physical handicap on sexual function, for example, disease of the nervous system affecting the autonomic nerve supply;
- **general effects** such as tiredness, and pain;
- **fears** about the effects of intercourse on the handicapping condition;
- **lack of information** about the sexual behaviour of other people with the same disability.

Much can be done to help disabled people by overcoming fears and discussing the forms of sexual activity that are possible despite their disability, and, if appropriate, using appropriate parts of the methods described above for treating sexual dysfunction.

Abnormalities of sexual preference (paraphilias)

The study of these disorders in the past

For centuries, abnormalities of sexual preference were regarded as offences against the laws of religion rather than conditions that doctors should study and treat. The systematic investigation of these disorders began in the 1870s. Krafft-Ebing (1840–1902), a professor of psychiatry in Vienna, wrote a systematic account of paraphilias in his book *Psychopathia sexualis*, first published in 1886. Soon afterwards, Schrenck-Notzing (1895) reported successful treatment with therapeutic suggestion. In England, Havelock Ellis (1859–1939) wrote extensively about these and other sexual disorders.

The concept of abnormal sexual preference

This concept has three aspects:

1. **Social** the behaviour does not conform to some generally accepted view of what is normal. The accepted view is not the same in every society or at every period of history; for example, regular masturbation was regarded as abnormal by many medical writers in Victorian England.
2. **Harm** that might be done to another person involved in the sexual behaviour. Intercourse with young children or extreme forms of sexual sadism are examples.
3. **Suffering** experienced by the person himself. This suffering is related to the attitudes of the society in which the patient lives (for example, attitudes to cross-dressing), to conflict between the person's sexual urges and his moral standards, and to the person's awareness of harm or distress caused to others.

General considerations

Mode of presentation

Abnormalities of sexual preference may come to medical attention in several ways, and the doctor should be aware of the different modes of presentation.

Direct requests for help

A doctor may be consulted directly by the person with the abnormalities. He may be asked to help by the spouse or other sexual partner, sometimes because the behaviour has just been discovered, and sometimes because known behaviour has become more frequent and can be tolerated no longer.

Indirect presentations

Sometimes the problem is presented as sexual dysfunction, and the abnormality of sexual preference is discovered only in the course of history taking.

As a forensic problem

A doctor may be asked for an opinion about a patient charged with an offence arising from an abnormality of sexual preference. Offences of this kind include the stealing of clothes by fetishists, indecent exposure, the behaviour of a 'peeping Tom', appearing in public in clothes of the opposite sex, sexual assaults upon children, and rape. With one exception, these offences are discussed below in relation to the corresponding abnormality of sexual preference. The exception is rape, with is considered with other sexual offences on p. 742.

The role of psychiatrists

There are different opinions about the extent to which doctors should attempt to alter abnormal sexual preferences. There seems to be no reason why doctors should not try to help people who wish to alter unusual patterns of sexual behaviour, but they should not try to impose treatment on people who do not want it. How to decide who really wants psychiatric help is a difficult point that is taken up later in this chapter.

Pornography

The reading of pornography is not a sexual disorder but it is considered here because doctors may be asked about the effects of such publications. Since some of the publications are designed for people with unusual sexual preferences, this is a convenient point at which to consider the topic. In a study of men and women in Norway in 2002 (Traeen *et al.*, 2004), 90 per cent of respondents had seen pornography at least once, usually in a magazine (76 per cent) or a film (67 per cent), but also on the Internet (24 per cent). Far fewer watched it regularly. It is not known whether these sources of pornography provide a harmless outlet for sexual impulses, including those that might otherwise be inflicted on another person, or whether they increase such impulses and make people more likely to act on them. The question has been approached in several ways.

Epidemiological studies have attempted to relate the numbers of sexual offences to changes in the law on pornography but the results are inconclusive.

Clinical experience with the paraphilias suggests that the use of pornographic material can increase the related content of fantasies during sexual arousal. However, it is not known whether an increase in fantasies leads to an increase of the corresponding behaviour.

Public policy on these important matters, like many others, has to be decided on limited scientific information. Without more definite evidence, it seems appropriate that pornographic material relating sexual activity to violence or to children should not be available, especially to young people whose sexual development is incomplete. Such material is, however, widely available on the Internet and it is difficult to regulate the output. Other arguments for restricting pornography are that it debases women and exploits and harms children in the making of the material and in other ways; and that it has not been proved that the material is harmless.

Advice to individuals

Doctors may be asked what effect pornographic material, discovered by a wife or parent, may have on a husband or adolescent son. Doctors should explain the different points of view and the uncertainty of the scientific evidence. They should indicate that the effects are likely to differ in different people and according to the nature of the material and the frequency of use. They should offer to interview the person. If the person's sexual life is reviewed thoroughly, some useful advice can generally be given. Such advice should extend to broader aspects of personal relationships and not merely to the effects of the pornographic material.

Types of abnormality of sexual preference

Abnormalities of sexual preference can be divided into two groups: abnormalities of the 'object' of the person's sexual interest, and abnormalities in the preference of the sexual act. Abnormalities of the sexual 'object' include fetishism, paedophilia, transvestic fetishism, zoophilia, and necrophilia. Abnormalities of preference of the sexual act include exhibitionism, voyeurism, sadism, masochism, and autoerotic asphyxia.

General aspects of the assessment of abnormalities of sexual preference

Assessment is often in the context of possible or actual legal proceedings. It is important therefore to explain the relation of the interview to any proceedings, explain confidentiality and its limits, and obtain necessary consent to the interview. Leading questions may be needed to help the patient reveal some problems, but any information obtained in this way should be checked by asking for examples of the behaviour in question. People seen for the assessment of abnormality of sexual preference often have more that one kind of abnormal preference (Abel and Osborn, 2000), though they may not volunteer this information when first interviewed. It may need more than one interview before the patient feels able to confide the full extent of the sexual behaviour. Whenever possible, consent should be obtained for an interview with any regular sexual partner, and with other informants who may be able assist with, for example, the assessment of personality.

Assessment includes a psychiatric history and should include the following steps:

- **exclude mental disorder**, especially when the abnormal sexual preference comes to notice for the first time in middle age or later. Abnormal sexual preference is sometimes secondary to dementia, alcoholism, depressive disorder, or mania. These conditions probably release the behaviour in a person who has previously experienced the corresponding sexual fantasies but controlled them.
- **detail the sexual behaviour**. Obtain details of the normal and of the abnormal sexual behaviour, currently and in the past. Remember that, as noted above, it is not uncommon for people to have more than one form of abnormal sexual preference.
- **describe the wider significance of the behaviour**. Find out what part the abnormal sexual preference is playing in the patient's life other than as a source of sexual arousal. It may be a comforting activity that helps to ward off feelings of loneliness, anxiety, or depression. If so, unless other means are found to deal with such feelings, treatment that reduces the abnormal sexual preference may worsen the patient's emotional state.
- **assess motivation**. Motives for seeking treatment are often mixed. People who have little wish to change

their sexual behaviour may consult a doctor because of pressure from a sexual partner, a relative, or the police. Such people may hope to be told that no treatment will help, so as to justify the continuation of their paraphilia. Others seek help when they are depressed and feel guilty about their behaviour. Strong wishes for change, expressed during a period of depression, may fade quickly as normal mood returns. Strong motivation is important whatever the proposed mode of treatment, so its assessment is important.

- **psychophysiological assessment**. Some specialists use penile plethysmography or polygraphy to assess sexual interests (see Abel and Osborn, 2000). In the former, changes in penile circumference are measured while the patient views visual material or listens to audiotapes. Positive responses can be discussed with the patient. However, the method is of limited value because people can produce false-negative responses by directing their attention away from the stimuli. Polygraphy, measuring several physiological variables, can also reflect sexual arousal to stimuli. Its limitations resemble those of penile plethysmography. These methods are not part of routine assessment.

General aspects of the management of abnormalities of sexual preference

Some aspects of management apply to all kinds of abnormality of sexual preference. These aspects are described here. Management specific to a particular disorder is described below with the other aspects of the disorder.

Agreeing the aims

The aim of treatment should be discussed with the patient: whether it is to control, or if possible give up, the behaviour, or to adapt better to the behaviour so that less guilt and distress are felt. In considering these aims, the doctor will have to take into account whether any psychological or physical harm is being caused to other people. At this early stage it is important to make clear that, whatever the aim, treatment will require considerable effort on the part of the patient.

Aiding adjustment

If the agreed aim is better adjustment, treatment will be by counselling designed to explore the person's feelings and to help him to identify the problems caused by his sexual practices and to find ways of reducing them. If the agreed aim is change, the first step is to seek ways of improving ordinary heterosexual relationships. Treatment is directed to any anxieties that are impeding social relationships with the opposite sex. Attention is then directed to any sexual inadequacy using the methods outlined earlier in this chapter. Usually, these two steps are the most important part of treatment.

Anticipating problems from abstinence

Some people occupy much of their time in preparing for the sexual act (for example, fetishists may spend many hours searching for a particular kind of women's underclothes). As already noted, such behaviour may become a way or warding off feelings of loneliness or despair. To safeguard against these feelings, the person should be helped to develop leisure activities, seek new friends, and find other ways of coping with unpleasant emotions.

Reducing the paraphilia

Only when these steps have been taken should attention be directed to ways of suppressing the unwanted sexual behaviour. Sometimes the preceding steps are enough to strengthen the person's capacity to control himself, but additional help is often needed.

Masturbation fantasies about the paraphilia often maintain the abnormal sexual behaviour. Therefore the person should be encouraged to keep any such fantasies out of mind while masturbating, and to try to imagine normal heterosexual intercourse instead. If he cannot dismiss the abnormal fantasies, he should try to modify them progressively so that the sexual themes become less abnormal and increasingly concerned with ordinary heterosexual intercourse.

Hormonal treatment

Most patients with paraphilias are men, and for some, treatment to reduce androgen levels is a helpful adjunct to psychological treatment. Generally, cyproterone acetate, a testosterone antagonist, is used Europe for this purpose, and medroxyprogesterone acetate is used in the USA. Both have been reported to benefit some exhibitionists and paedophiles (see Murray, 1998). Long acting agonists of luteinizing hormone-releasing hormone have been reported to benefit several kinds of paraphilia but there is insufficient evidence to decide the place of these agents in therapy (see Briken *et al.*, 2003).

Behavioural treatment

Behavioural treatment has been used to reduce the paraphilia directly, and also to help indirectly by treating any sexual inadequacy. Several direct methods have been tried including advice about changing masturbation fantasies (see above). **Covert sensitization** makes an immediate link in imagination between paraphiliac thoughts and urges, and humiliating adverse consequences that are normally delayed such as discovery by family or arrest. In smell or taste aversion, an unpleasant odour or taste is associated with the paraphilic fantasies. The long-term efficacy of these techniques has not been demonstrated convincingly.

Relapse prevention focuses on the situations in which paraphilic urges are likely to be experienced. Patients are encouraged to identify these situations and to avoid them. Particular attention is paid to the earliest stages of the chain of behaviour leading up to the paraphilias, for example an action by the patient which regularly makes his wife angry, and thus provides an excuse to go to a place where the paraphilia may be stimulated. For a review of psychological treatments for paraphilias, see Wylie (1994).

Legal considerations

Many people with abnormal sexual preferences appear before the courts. Sanctions such as a suspended sentence or probation order can sometimes help the patient to gain control of his own behaviour. However, doctors should not agree to treat patients who are referred against their wishes. Sexual offences are considered further on pp. 740–4.

Types of abnormality of preference for the sexual object

These abnormalities involve preferences for an 'object' other than another adult in the achievement of sexual excitement. The alternative 'object' may be inanimate, as in fetishism and transvestic fetishism, or may be a child (paedophilia) or an animal (zoophilia).

Fetishism

In sexual fetishism, the preferred or only means of achieving sexual excitement are inanimate objects or parts of the human body that do not have direct sexual associations. The disorder shades into normal sexual behaviour; it is not uncommon for men to be aroused by particular items of clothing, such as stockings, or by parts of the female body that do not have direct sexual associations, such as the hair. The condition is abnormal when the behaviour takes precedence over the usual patterns of sexual intercourse.

Prevalence Sexual fetishism as the sole or preferred means of sexual arousal is uncommon, but no exact figures are available for the rate in the community.

Description Fetishism usually begins in adolescence. It occurs almost exclusively among men, although a few cases have been described among women. Most fetishists are heterosexual but some are homosexual – 20 per cent according to Chalkley and Powell (1983). The objects that can evoke sexual arousal are many and varied, but for each person there is usually a small number of objects or classes of objects. Among the more frequent are rubber garments, women's underclothes and high-heeled shoes, and, for homosexual fetishists, men's shoes (Weinberg *et al.*, 1994). Sometimes the object is an attribute of a person (partialism), for example, lameness or deformity, or a part of the human body, such as the hair or foot, or the absence of a part through amputation (apotemnophilia). The texture and smell of objects is often as important as their appearance, for example furs, velvet, rubber garments, and polished leather. Contact with the object causes sexual excitement, which may be followed by solitary masturbation or by sexual intercourse incorporating the fetish if a willing partner or paid prostitute is available.

Fetishists may spend much time seeking desired objects. Some buy them, some steal – for example, underclothes from a washing line. When the 'object' is an attribute of a person, many hours may be spent in searching for and following someone with the attribute, for example, a woman with a limp. Fetishists often hoard fetish objects such as women's shoes or underclothes, or pictures of such objects.

Aetiology The cause is unknown but several theories have been proposed:

- **Conditioning** Fetishism was the first sexual disorder for which a theory of association learning was put forward. Binet (1877) suggested that the condition arose by a chance coming together of sexual excitation and the object that becomes the fetish object.
- **Psychoanalytical theories** These suggest that sexual fetishism arises when castration anxiety is not resolved in childhood, and the man attempts to ward off this anxiety by maintaining in his unconscious mind the idea that women have a penis (Freud, 1927). In this view, each fetish is a symbolic representation of a phallus. Although some fetishes can be interpreted in this way, others require tortuous interpretations if the general hypothesis is to be sustained (see for example Stekel, 1953). There is no objective evidence to support the theory.
- **Brain dysfunction** Over the years, occasional cases have been reported in which fetishism is associated with EEG evidence of temporal lobe dysfunction (e.g. Epstein, 1961) or with frank epilepsy (e.g. Mitchell *et al.*, 1954). However, there is no evidence of such associations in most cases, and the reported cases may be chance associations.
- **Maintaining factors** However fetishism arises, clinical experience suggests that it is maintained, in part,

by inhibited expression of normal sexual behaviour, for example, by shyness or fears, and by the reinforcing effects of sexual release during actual or imagined contact with the fetish object.

Prognosis There are no reliable follow-up data. Clinical experience suggests that fetishism in adolescents and young adults often diminishes or ceases when satisfying heterosexual relationships have been established. The prognosis appears to be worse for solitary single men who are shy with women and without a sexual partner than for those who are younger and socially better adjusted. The prognosis is generally worse when the behaviour is frequent and has persistently broken social conventions and legal barriers. Legal proceedings instituted for the first time may increase motivation to control the behaviour.

Treatment There are case reports of successful treatment by **psychoanalysis** and by **behaviour therapy** but no controlled trials. Clinical experience indicates that the **general measures** earlier in the chapter are generally as effective as either of these special techniques. Medication is considered in the general section, above.

Transvestic fetishism

In ICD-10 this condition is known as fetishistic transvestism. The term transvestic fetishism is used here because it indicates a similarity to the cases of sexual fetishism in which the object is an article of clothing. Transvestic fetishism varies from the occasional wearing of a few articles of clothing of the opposite sex to complete cross-dressing. Transvestic fetishism is rare among women (almost all women who cross-dress are transsexual or lesbian) and the description below applies to men.

Prevalence Estimates of the percentage of the population who have ever cross-dressed vary from 1.5 per cent to 10 per cent.

Description The person usually begins to put on articles of women's clothing at about the time of puberty. He usually starts by putting on only a few garments, but as time goes by he adds more until eventually he may dress entirely in clothes of the other sex. Transvestic fetishists generally experience sexual arousal when cross-dressing and the behaviour often terminates with masturbation. Sexual arousal is more frequent in younger people. It may diminish as they grow older, so that the person dresses mainly to feel feminine. Sometimes the clothes are worn in public, either underneath male outer garments or in some cases without such precautions against discovery.

Unlike the transsexuals described later, transvestic fetishists have no doubt that their gender conforms with their external sexual characteristics. Most are heterosexual and many have sexual partners though most of those seen by psychiatrists hide the behaviour from the partner. If the partner has discovered the behaviour, most express distress and disgust but a few assist in obtaining the clothing.

Aetiology The cause is unknown. There are several theories, all unsupported by evidence:

- **Genetic factors** There is no convincing evidence that the chromosomal sex or hormonal make-up of transvestic fetishists is abnormal. Transvestic fetishism is not familial and there is no evidence that it is inherited.
- **Brain dysfunction** Although occasional associations with temporal lobe dysfunction have been reported (Davies and Morgenstern, 1960; Epstein, 1960), there is no evidence for such an association in the majority.
- **Conditioning** has been suggested as a cause – see fetishism above.
- **Psychoanalytical theories** resemble those concerning fetishism – see above. They are not supported by objective evidence.

Prognosis There are no reliable follow-up studies. Clinical experience suggests that most cases persist for years, becoming less severe as sexual drives decline in middle age or later. However, there are wide variations in outcome, and the comments made earlier about the prognosis of fetishism apply here as well. A minority of transvestic fetishists gradually develop the idea that they are women: they continue to cross-dress but without sexual arousal, so that they resemble transsexual people (see p. 491).

Treatment There is no specific treatment for transvestic fetishism. Management is with the general procedures described on p. 485.

Paedophilia

Paedophilia is repeated sexual activity (or fantasy of such activity) with prepubertal children as a preferred or exclusive method of obtaining sexual excitement. It is almost exclusively a disorder of men. Paedophilia has to be distinguished from intercourse with young people who have passed puberty but not yet reached the legal age of consent (which differs between legislations). Paedophilia is not concerned with the borderline of legal consent but with intercourse between an adult and a prepubertal child.

Prevalence There is no reliable information about the prevalence of paedophilia. From the existence of child prostitution in some countries, the ready sale of pornographic material depicting sex with children, and the number of Internet sites it is evident that interest in sexual relationships with children is not rare. However, paedophilia as an exclusive form of sexual behaviour is probably uncommon.

Description Paedophiles usually choose a child aged between 6 years and puberty, but some seek a very young child. The child may be of the opposite sex (heterosexual paedophilia) or the same sex (homosexual paedophilia). Some paedophiles approach children within their extended family, or in their professional care; others befriend unrelated children. Although most paedophiles seen by doctors are men of middle age, the condition is established early in life. There is no evidence that an established interest in adult sexual partners changes to an interest in child partners. With younger children, fondling or masturbation is more likely than full coitus, but sometimes young children are injured by forcible attempts at penetration. There are rare and tragic cases of paedophilia associated with sexual sadism. (Sexual abuse of children is described on p. 699.)

Differential diagnosis Paedophilia has to be distinguished from exhibitionism towards young girls (in which no attempt is made to engage in direct sexual contact). Occasionally sexual contact with children may be sought by people with subnormal intelligence, dementia, and alcoholism.

The child Most of the females involved in paedophilia are aged between 6 and 12 years, most of the male children involved in homosexual paedophilia are somewhat older. Of the children involved in cases of paedophilia coming to the attention of the law, many have cooperated in sexual activity more than once with the same or another adult. Most of these children have been involved through fear rather than interest but a small minority are promiscuous and delinquent.

The **effects on the child** of sexual abuse are considered on p. 699.

Aetiology This is unknown. Paedophiles often have a marked incapacity for relationships with adults and fears of relationships with women.

Prognosis In the absence of reliable information from follow-up studies, prognosis has to be judged in individual patients by the length of the history, the frequency of the behaviour, the absence of other social and sexual relationships, and the strengths and weaknesses of the personality. Behaviour that has been frequently repeated is likely to persist despite efforts at treatment.

Treatment There is no evidence that any treatment is effective. Paedophiles who are genuinely motivated to control their impulses may be helped by support and problem-solving counselling. Attempts to treat those convicted of sex offences are considered on p. 742.

For a review of paedophilia, see McConaghy (1998).

Other abnormalities in the preference of sexual object

Zoophilia Zoophilia, otherwise called bestiality or bestiosexuality, is the use of an animal as a repeated and preferred or exclusive method of achieving sexual excitement. It is uncommon and rarely encountered by doctors.

Necrophilia In this extremely rare condition sexual arousal is obtained through intercourse with a dead body. Occasionally there are legal trials of men who murder and then attempt intercourse with the victim. No reliable information is available about the causes or prognosis of this extreme form of abnormal sexual preference.

Abnormalities in the preference for the sexual act

The second group of abnormalities of sexual preference involves variations in the behaviour that is carried out to obtain sexual arousal. Generally, the acts are directed towards other adults, but sometimes children are involved (for example, by some exhibitionists).

Exhibitionism

Exhibitionism is the repeated exposing of the genitals to unprepared strangers for the purpose of achieving sexual excitement but without any attempts at further sexual activity with the other person. The name exhibitionism was suggested by Lasègue (1877). (This technical use of the term is clearly different from its everyday sense of self-display.)

Prevalence This is not known. Almost all are men, except for a very few women exhibitionists who repeatedly expose the breasts and an even smaller number who expose the genitalia.

Description Amongst exhibitionists seen by doctors, most are aged 20–40 years and two-thirds are married (Gayford, 1981). In some, the urge to exhibitionism is persistent; in others it is episodic. The act of exposure is usually preceded by a feeling of mounting tension. Most exhibitionists choose places from which escape is easy. The exhibitionist may step out from a hiding place and exposes his penis; or suddenly reveal the penis which was hidden, for example, behind a newspaper. Occasionally the exhibitionist appears nude.

Some masturbate during exposure; others do this afterwards. The exhibitionist seeks to evoke a strong emotional reaction from the other person. Whatever this reaction may be, it is interpreted by the exhibitionist as sexual interest, though it is in fact shock, fear, or even laughter. This distorted interpretation is accompanied by a state of intense excitement.

As a broad generalization, two groups of exhibitionists can be described. The first group includes men of inhibited temperament who struggle against their urges and feel much guilt after the act; they sometimes expose a flaccid penis. The second group includes men who have aggressive traits, sometimes accompanied by features of antisocial personality disorder. They usually expose an erect penis, often while masturbating. They gain pleasure from any distress they cause and often feel little guilt.

In the UK, if a man is brought to court because of exhibitionism, he is charged with the offence of indecent exposure (see Chapter 26, p. 742). About four-fifths of men charged with indecent exposure are exhibitionists.

Exhibitionism and the making of obscene phone calls There is uncertainty about the relationship between exhibitionism and the making of obscene phone calls by men who talk to women about sexual activities while masturbating. It has been suggested (Tollison and Adams, 1979) that these obscene callers are also exhibitionists, but it is not easy to identify them in order to study their psychopathology.

Aetiology The cause of exhibitionism is unknown. Psychoanalytical theories suggest failure to resolve Oedipal conflict or a general inhibition of relationships with women. In an influential paper, Rickles (1950) suggested some exhibitionists describe unduly close relationships with their mothers and a poor relationship with ineffectual fathers. However, these accounts are retrospective, and may not reflect the actual circumstances of the patient's upbringing. Also, many people describe similar experiences in childhood, but do not become exhibitionists.

Exhibitionism that starts in middle or old age is occasionally associated with organic disease of the brain or alcoholism. It is possible that these conditions reduce previously effective control of urges to exhibitionism.

Prognosis There is no reliable follow-up information. Men who exhibit only once do not fall within the definition of the disorder. Clinical experience suggests a variable outcome for the rest. Among men who exhibit repeatedly but only at times of stress, the prognosis depends on the likelihood of the stressors returning. Exhibitionists who repeat often, and not solely at times of stress, are likely to persist with the behaviour for years despite treatment by psychiatrists or punishment by the courts. In keeping with these clinical impressions, the evidence from the courts is that the reconviction rate for indecent exposure is low after a first conviction but high after a second conviction. Although a history of exhibitionism is given by some men who commit rape, it seems that most exhibitionists do not go on to commit violent sexual acts nor do they interfere with children (Rooth, 1973).

Treatment Any associated psychiatric disorder such as depressive disorder, alcoholism, or dementia should be sought and treated appropriately if found. Many treatments have been tried specifically for exhibitionism, including psychoanalysis, individual and group psychotherapy, and covert sensitization. There is no satisfactory evidence that any of these treatments is generally effective. A practical approach combines counselling and behavioural techniques. Counselling deals with the effects of exhibitionistic behaviour and with problems in personal relationships. Behavioural techniques are concerned with self-monitoring to identify circumstances that trigger the behaviour and to help the person avoid them. Cyproterone acetate and related drugs have been used to reduce the sex drive, but are not recommended because of uncertain results and problems of gynaecomestia and depression with long-term use. The general measures described on p. 485 can be tried, though without high expectation of success. For further information about exhibitionism, see Abel and Osborn (2000).

Sexual sadism

Sadism is named after the Marquis de Sade (1740–1814) who inflicted extreme cruelty on women for sexual purposes. Sexual sadism is achieving sexual arousal, habitually and in preference to heterosexual intercourse, by inflicting pain on another person, by bondage, or by humiliation.

Prevalence Inflicting pain in fantasy or practice is a not uncommon accompaniment of other forms of sexual behaviour. Sex shops sell chains, whips, and shackles, whilst some pornographic magazines and web sites provide pictures and descriptions of sadistic sexual practices. Sexual sadism as the predominant sexual practice is probably uncommon, but its frequency is not known.

Description Beating, whipping, and tying are common forms of sadistic activity. Repeated acts may be with a partner who is a masochist or a prostitute who is paid to take part. Sadism may be a component of homosexual as well as heterosexual acts. The acts may be symbolic, with little actual damage, and some involve humiliation rather than injury. However, at times, serious and permanent injuries are caused. Extreme examples are the rare 'lust murders', in which the killer inflicts serious repeated injuries – usually stabbings and mutilations – on the genitalia of his victim. In these rare cases, ejaculation may occur during the sadistic act or later by intercourse with the dead body (necrophilia). An historically significant description is given by Hirschfeld (1944).

Aetiology This is not known. Psychoanalytical explanations draw attention to the association between love and aggressive feelings that is supposed to exist in the young child's early relationship with his parents. Behavioural formulations rely on association learning. Neither explanation is supported by objective evidence.

Prognosis There is no reliable follow-up information. Clinical experience suggests that, once established, the behaviour is likely to persist for many years.

Treatment No treatment has been shown to be effective in clinical trials. Men who have committed serious injury are dealt with by legal means. The risks must not be underestimated when potentially dangerous behaviour has been planned or has taken place.

Sexual masochism

Sexual masochism is achieving sexual excitement, as a preferred or exclusive practice, through the experience of suffering or humiliation. As a predominant activity it differs from the common use of minor painful practices as an accompaniment to sexual intercourse. The condition is named after Leopold von Sacher-Masoch (1836–1905), an Austrian novelist, who described sexual gratification from the experience of pain.

Prevalence Fantasies of being beaten or humiliated are sufficiently common among males to create a demand for pornographic publications on this theme, and for prostitutes who enable the person to act out the fantasies. Established sexual masochism is probably uncommon, though no exact information is available.

Description The suffering may take the form of being beaten, trodden upon, bound, or chained, or the enactment of various symbolic forms of humiliation, for example, dressing as a child and being punished. Masochism, unlike most other sexual deviations, occurs in women as well as in men. It may occur in homosexual as well as heterosexual relationships. Some masochists desire dangerous behaviours such as strangulation, a practice that can increase sexual excitation through the resulting partial anoxia (see also auto-erotic asphyxia, below).

Aetiology This is not known. Conditioning theory suggests that it arises as a result of association between sexual arousal and beatings received as punishment around puberty. Psychoanalytical theory suggests that masochism is sadism turned inwards, and therefore is explicable in the same way as sadism (see above). Neither theory is supported by evidence.

Prognosis There is no reliable follow-up information. Clinical experience suggests that, once established as a preferred form of sexual behaviour, masochism is likely to persist for many years.

Treatment Psychoanalysis and behavioural treatments have been proposed but neither has been shown to be effective. General measures (see p. 485) can be tried, without high expectation of success.

Voyeurism

Many men are sexually excited by observing others engaged in intercourse. Voyeurism is observing the sexual activity of others repeatedly as a preferred means of sexual arousal. The voyeur also spies on women who are undressing or without clothes, but does not attempt sexual activity with them. Voyeurism is usually accompanied or followed by masturbation. Some voyeurs use video cameras to record women undressing or engaging in sexual activities (Simon, 1997).

Voyeurism is a disorder of heterosexual men whose heterosexual activities are usually inadequate. Although the voyeur usually takes great care to hide from the women he is watching, he often takes considerable risks of discovery by other people. Hence most voyeurs are reported by passers-by, and not by the victim.

Aetiology Among adolescents voyeuristic activities are not uncommon as an expression of sexual curiosity, but they are usually replaced by direct sexual experience. The voyeur continues to watch because he is shy, socially awkward with girls, or prevented from normal sexual expression by some other obstacle. Psychoanalytical explanations follow the general lines described above for other sexual disorders. Behavioural theories seek an explanation in terms of chance associations between a first experience of peeping and sexual arousal. Neither theory is supported by evidence.

Prognosis No reliable information is available.

Treatment No treatment has been shown to be effective in clinical trials. It is reasonable to try the general measures described earlier in this chapter.

Other abnormalities of preference of the sexual act

Auto-erotic asphyxia Auto-erotic asphyxia is the practice of inducing cerebral anoxia to heighten sexual arousal while masturbating. Asphyxia is usually induced by partial strangulation with cords or by plastic bags placed over the head. The practice occurs almost exclusively in men. It is hazardous and may lead to death. The act may be accompanied by the use of objects to produce anal stimulation, by the use of fetish objects, or by cross-dressing. The person may look at himself in a mirror or photograph himself, or he may apply bondage, for example by tying the ankles. Few people who practise auto-erotic asphyxia seek help from doctors. Most information about the condition comes from forensic studies of persons who have died during the act although occasional cases have been studied in life (e.g. Quinn and Twomey, 1998). For further information see Blanchard and Hucker (1991) or Hucker (1990).

Frotteurism In frotteurism, the preferred form of sexual excitement is by rubbing the male genitalia against another person, or by fondling the breasts of an unwilling participant, who is usually a stranger, generally in a crowded place such as an underground train.

Coprophilia, coprophagia, sexual urethism, and urophilia In coprophilia, sexual arousal is induced by thinking about or watching the act of defecation and this is the preferred sexual activity; in coprophagia arousal follows the eating of faeces. In sexual urethism, which occurs mainly in women, erotic arousal is obtained by stimulation of the urethra. Urophilia refers to sexual arousal obtained by watching the act of urination, being urinated upon, or drinking urine.

The prevalence of these disorders is not known, but some are sufficiently common to demand provision from prostitutes. Further information can be found in Tollison and Adams (1979).

Abnormalities of gender identity

Transsexualism

Transsexual people are convinced that they are of the gender opposite to that indicated by their chromosomes. They have an overpowering wish to live as a member of the gender group opposite to their anatomical sex, and seek to alter their bodily appearance and genitalia.

In the past, the condition was called eonism because it was exemplified by the Chevalier d'Eon de Beaumont. In psychiatric literature, the condition was mentioned by Esquirol in 1838 and described in more detail by Krafft-Ebing in 1886 (see Krafft-Ebing, 1924). In the 1960s, the attention of doctors and the public was directed to the condition by a number of striking reports and by a book by Benjamin (1966).

Terminology

The terms transsexual male and transsexual female are used in different ways. Transsexual people generally prefer the usage in which transsexual female refers to people identified at birth as male, but experiencing themselves as female; transsexual males are people who were identified at birth as female but experience themselves as male. In the past medical literature transsexual male has more often been used to denote people identified at birth as males but experiencing themselves as female. In the following account, we generally use the terms male to female transsexual, and female to male transsexual as they describe the sequence of events in the person's life. Thus male to female transsexuals are people who were identified at birth as male, but who later experience themselves as female. Some transsexual people object to the use of the word transsexual as a noun. When the word transsexual is used in this way in the following account, it denotes a transsexual person, just as heterosexual is widely used as a noun to denote a heterosexual person.

Many transsexual people consider that their condition should not be listed as a psychiatric disorder. However, it is listed in both ICD and DSM, and this listing may assist transsexual people who request treatment since in many countries treatment under a state health scheme or private insurance is restricted to disorders listed in one of the classifications of diseases.

Prevalence

Epidemiological data are difficult to obtain. A survey in the Netherlands gave the prevalence of gender identity disorder in adults as about 1 per 10 000 born male and 1 per 30 000 born female (Kesteren *et al.*, 1996). Among those seeking help at clinical centres, male to female transsexual people exceed female to males by about 4 to 1 (Green, 2000a).

Description

Transsexual people have a strong conviction, usually starting before puberty, of belonging to the sex opposite to that to which they were assigned. Parents sometimes report that, as children, these people preferred the company and pursuits of children of the opposite anatomical sex, although such a history is not invariable. However, follow-up studies of effeminate boys have found that they more often grow up as homosexual than as transsexual adults (see Green, 1974).

By the time that medical help is requested, most transsexual people have started to cross-dress at times. In contrast with transvestic fetishists, male to female transsexuals cross-dress to feel more like a woman, not to produce sexual arousal. (Contrast also homosexual men who dress as women to attract other male homosexuals.) Make-up may be worn and the hair is arranged in a feminine style; facial and body hair may be gradually removed by electrolysis. These physical changes may be added to by cultivating feminine gestures, raising the pitch of voice, and seeking changes in social role.

Male to female transsexual people often ask for help in altering the appearance of the breasts and external genitalia. Usually the first requests are for oestrogens to enlarge the breasts. Later requests may be for surgery to the breasts, castration and removal of the penis, and operations to create an artificial vagina. Many transsexual people are greatly distressed by their predicament. Depression is common, and some make suicide attempts, and some some threaten self-castration if they cannot have surgery. These threats should be taken seriously because they indicate extreme distress and are sometimes carried out.

Female to male transsexual people adopt masculine dress, voice, gestures, and social behaviour. They wish to have intercourse in the role of male with a heterosexual woman (and not with a female homosexual). Some ask for mastectomy or hysterectomy, and a few for plastic surgery to create an artificial penis.

Aetiology The causes of this condition are unknown. The following factors have been investigated:

Genetic causes Transsexual people have normal sex chromosomes, and there is no convincing evidence of a genetic cause.

Early upbringing There is no convincing evidence that transsexual people have been brought up in the gender role opposite to their anatomical sex. As noted above, most boys with gender identity disorder grow up as homosexual rather than transsexual adults.

Endocrine causes No definite endocrine abnormality has been found in adult transsexual people. It has been suggested that the condition might result from hormonal abnormalities during intrauterine development. When pregnant rhesus monkeys are given large doses of androgens, their female infants behave more like males during play (Young *et al.*, 1964). Also, female children with adrenogenital syndrome, who are exposed to large amounts of androgen before and after birth, have been reported to show boyish behaviour in childhood (Ehrhardt *et al.*, 1968) although they do not grow up as transsexual. A high rate of polycystic ovarian disease has been reported in female to male transsexual people (Bosinski *et al.*, 1997) very few with this ovarian condition have gender identity disorder (Green, 2000a).

Differences in brain structure The volume of the central subdivision of the bed nucleus of the stria terminalis is larger in men than in women. One study of six post-mortem brains from male to female transsexual people found the size of the nucleus similar to that in described in women (Zhou *et al.*, 1995). However the results have been criticized on technical grounds (Green, 2000a).

Transition from transvestism In a minority of male to female transsexual people, the condition begins after many years of transvestic fetishism. These people start by cross-dressing to obtain sexual excitement, but the resultant arousal gradually diminishes. At the same time, they gradually become convinced that they are women.

Course There is no reliable information about the course of untreated transsexual people. One influential report (Harry Benjamin International Gender Dysphoria Association, 2001) concluded that some carefully diagnosed transsexual people change their aspirations; some adapt to their desired gender indentities without medical help; and others give up their wish to change during the early stages of treatment. It is not known what proportion of transsexual people fall into each of these groups.

Treatment First stages Treatment generally follows the standards of care document of the Harry Benjamin International Gender Dysphoria Association (2001). The following account summarizes the steps; for further information see the original publication or Green (2000a).

- **Agreeing a plan** Transsexual people have often decided what treatment they require and may be impatient to obtain it. They may regard psychiatric assessment as an unnecessary obstacle in the path to hormonal treatment and surgery. Some threaten suicide or self-mutilation if their own timetable is not met. Such threats should always be taken very seriously as an indication of great distress, and a need for immediate help. Nevertheless, it should be explained that certain stages have to be gone through. The first is to demonstrate the psychological stability that is essential if the person is to succeed in the transition that is sought. To help establish this stability, the person needs to pass through the 'real life experience' (see below).
- **Counselling** should deal with the range of options including those not considered previously by the person seeking help. It emphasizes the need to set realistic goals and to consider the full consequences of any changes that are contemplated, both on the person concerned and on family including any children. The counsellor should also discuss the likelihood that no therapy can permanently eradicate all vestiges of the person's original sex asignment (Harry Benjamin International Gender Dysphoria Association, 2001)

The 'real life experience' A male to female transsexual person has to become accustomed to appearing, speaking, and behaving as a woman. Facial hair is often removed by electrolysis or laser treatment and voice training may be required. The experience requires the person to live in the new gender role continuously for at least 1 year, and preferably for two. During this time the person has to be employed full time in work or as a student. (The criterion of full-time employment may be difficult to meet at times of high unemployment.) Appropriate hormone treatment (see below) is prescribed during this year. To be eligible for hormone treatment, the person must (i) be over the age of 18 years, (ii) understand what hormones can and cannot do, including their adverse effects, and (iii) have completed successfully either 3 months of the real life experience or an agreed period of counselling. At the end of the year, people who can demonstrate to an assessment panel that they are better adjusted in the new gender role than in the old, may be considered for surgery.

Hormonal treatment: Oestrogens may be prescribed to produce breast enlargement. The effects of oestrogen on breast development are as variable in genetic males as they are in genetic females, but in most cases fat increases around the hips and buttocks, giving a more female appearance. Prolonged oestrogen treatment carries the risk of deep vein thrombosis (van Kesteren *et al.*, 1997). Malignant breast tumours have been reported (e.g. Symmers, 1968), but there were no cases in a more recent series of 816 male to female transsexual people (van Kesteren *et al.*, 1997).

Androgens may be prescribed to female to male transsexual people. The voice deepens, hair increases on the face and body, menstruation ceases, the clitoris enlarges, and the sex drive increases. These changes are generally more pronounced than the changes in male to female transsexual patients taking oestrogen. Prolonged use of androgens carries the risk of liver damage.

Surgery People who have successfully passed the previous stages of treatment may be considered for surgery. Because there is still some uncertainty about the long-term outcome of surgical treatment (see below), opinions differ about this treatment. Decisions should be taken jointly by psychiatrist and a surgeon, in consultation with the primary care physician, each with special experience of the treatment of this condition. Surgery should be followed by intensive and long term support.

For a male to female transsexual person, possible surgical procedures include mammoplasty, penectomy, orchidectomy, and the creation of vagina-like structure. The latter is constructed from penile skin, with the addition of other skin or large intestine.

For a female to male transsexual person, surgical procedures include mastectomy, ovariectomy, and phalloplasty. In the latter, a 'microphallus' is formed from the clitoris (already enlarged by androgens), or from skin taken from another part of the body (see Green, 2000a).

Help for the family Many transsexual people are married and some have children. Spouses, and especially children, require help in coming to terms with the effects on their own lives of the changes in the transsexual person. Concerns may be expressed about the possibility of gender role problems in the children. Green (1998) studied 34 children with a transsexual parent and found no instances of gender identity disorder.

Outcome More than a dozen follow-up studies have been reported, but none has been able to compare patients allocated randomly to surgery or no surgery. A review of the English language literature over a 10-year period found that 90 per cent of male to female transsexual people were reported to have had a successful outcome of sex reassignment surgery (Green and Fleming, 1991). However, this figure must be viewed cautiously because of possible bias in selection and loss from follow-up (see Green, 2000a). In one study (Mate-Kole *et al.*, 1990), 40 patients were selected for surgery, and then allocated alternately to treatment within 3 months, or treatment after 2 years. Two years after their operation the first group had lower scores for neurotic symptoms and somewhat better work adjustment than the group that was still waiting for the operation. Meyer and Reter (1979) compared operated patients with unoperated ones and found a similar rate of improvement in the two groups. However, this finding cannot be generalized since the groups were not randomly assigned, only half the patients were assessed at follow-up, and the follow-up period was longer for those who had recived an operation.

Dual-role transvestism

This term is used in ICD-10 to describe people who wear clothes of the opposite sex but are neither transvestic fetishists (seeking sexual excitement) nor transsexuals (wishing a change of gender and sexual role). Instead they enjoy cross-dressing in order to gain temporary membership of the opposite sex.

Gender identity disorder of adolescence and adulthood – non-transsexual type

This term is used in DSM-IV to denote people who have passed puberty and feel a persistent or recurrent discomfort or sense of inappropriateness about their assigned gender identity. They cross-dress persistently or repeatedly, or imagine themselves doing this, but are not sexually excited by these actions or fantasies nor preoccupied with change in their primary or secondary sex characteristics.

Gender identity disorders in children

Parents more often seek advice about effeminate behaviour in boys than about masculine behaviour in small girls (it is not clear whether such behaviour in girls is less frequent or more socially acceptable). Effeminate boys prefer girlish games and enjoy wearing female clothing. The outcome amongst these boys is variable; some develop normal male interests and activities. Most boys with gender disorder in childhood become homosexual men. Further information is given by Green (2000b).

Other aspects of sexual behaviour

Rape and incest are discussed in Chapter 26 on forensic psychiatry.

Ethical problems in the diagnosis and treatment of disorders of sexuality and gender

Any of the ethical problems associated with the practice of psychiatry can arise when sexual disorders are treated but the following are especially likely to cause difficulty.

The professional relationship

When sexual problems are the main topic of the interviews, there is an increased risk that the relationship between patient and therapist will become sexualized. Medical codes of practice contain an absolute prohibition against a sexual relationship with a patient because this exploits the patient and undermines the general trust in doctors.

Confidentiality

Problems may arise when one sexual partner reveals information to the therapist and refuses to allow it to be passed to the other partner, even though it is relevant. The problem can usually be avoided if a full history is taken from both partners before deciding whether sex therapy is an appropriate treatment, and if the therapist does not see the partners separately after therapy has started.

Diagnosis, stigmatization, and responsibility

It has been objected that to give a psychiatric diagnosis to a pattern of sexual behaviour has two undesirable consequences. First, it can stigmatize the person; second, it can excuse behaviour that is morally wrong. Both problems are a reminder that the concept of diagnosis was developed mainly to assist with questions about treatment. It cannot be applied uncritically to other problems including those of responsibility.

Many people with the behaviour diagnosed as gender identity disorder argue that the diagnosis stigmatizes them because it implies that the behaviour is pathological rather than a normal variation. A similar objection was made in the past about homosexual behaviour at a time when it was viewed as a disorder (which is no longer the case). The question about transsexual people is still the subject of some debate. In debates on this or related topics, a clear distinction has to be made between medical evidence and religious prohibitions – even though the two may, at times, coincide. For example, in the late nineteenth century, masturbation was regarded as morally wrong, and also medically harmful. The practice was condemned by the church and treated by doctors.

Some people argue that to diagnose certain kinds of sexual behaviour as a disorder excuses the person from responsibility for the effects of his behaviour. However, whilst the diagnosis of a disorder allows the person to adopt the sick role (see p. 165), this role does not absolve the person from all responsibilities. Indeed, it adds the responsibility to seek help, and does not remove the responsibility of not doing harm to other people.

Further reading

Gelder, MG, López-Ibor, JJ Jr and Andreasen, NC (eds) (2000) *The new Oxford textbook of psychiatry*, Section 4.11: Sexuality, gender identity, and their disorders. Oxford University Press, Oxford. (The four chapters in this section include an account of normal sexual function.)

Golombek, S and Fivush, R (1998) Gender development. In H Freeman, I Pullen, G Stein and G Wilkinson (eds), *Psychosexual disorders*, Chapter 2. Gaskell, London.

Tomlinson, J (ed.) (2005) *ABC of sexual health*. BMJ Books, London. (A series of concise, practical reviews of the assessment and treatment of sexual dysfunctions and other aspects of sexual health.)

CHAPTER 20

Psychiatry of the elderly

Chapter contents

Older people with mental health problems present particular challenges to the practice of old age psychiatry and the organization of its services. They are often physically as well as mentally frail and this affects presentation and course. On the other hand, they have the advantage of a rich history to tell and a lifetime's experience of responding to fortune and adversity. Dementia comprises a substantial part of the clinical practice.

When considering psychiatric disorder in the elderly, the clinician must be able to collect and integrate information from a variety of sources, and produce a management plan which takes account of physical and social needs, as well as the psychological. This plan is likely to involve the cooperation of several professionals. It is in this clinical complexity that much of the challenge and fascination of old age psychiatry lies.

This chapter deals with the psychiatry of old age, with two important exceptions, both of which were covered in Chapter 14:

- Delirium (pp. 329–30).
- The clinical features and aetiology of dementia (pp. 330–46).

Normal ageing

Demography

In 1993, 6 per cent of the world's population was over 65 years of age. However, in the more developed countries the proportion was about 14 per cent, whilst in less developed countries it was 4 per cent. Less developed countries have higher birth rates, but the life expectancy at birth is substantially lower than in developed countries: 60 years compared to 73. In the UK, life expectancy at birth has increased from 41 in 1840 to 46 in 1900, 69 in 1950, and 76 in 2004.

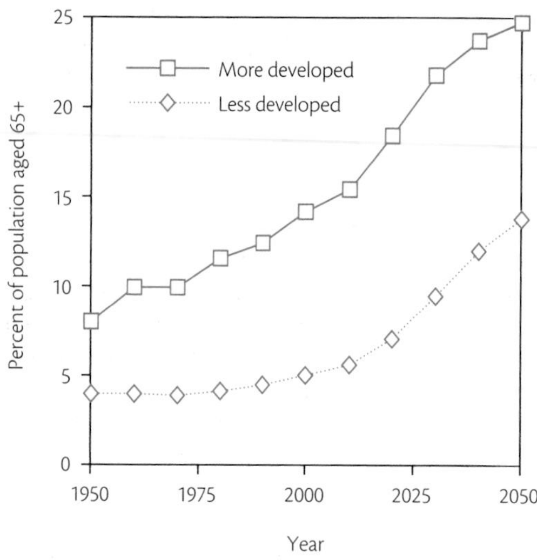

Fig. 20.1 Percentage of the population aged 65+ for more developed and less developed countries. Data from 1996 United Nations population estimates and projections. From AF Jorm (2000).

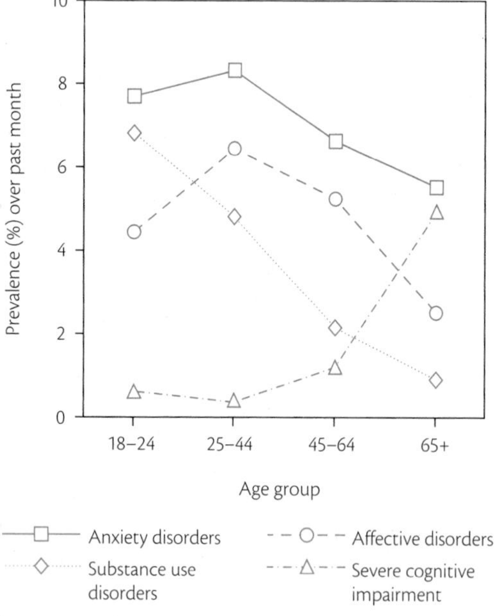

Fig. 20.2 Prevalence of mental disorders across age groups: data are 1-month prevalence rates from the Epidemiologic Catchment Area Study using DSM-III criteria. From AF Jorm (2000).

TABLE 20.1 Percentage change in population of the world, 1975–2000

Age	Total	% Change 1975–2000	
		Developed	Less developed
<15	57.6	20.2	72.6
15–24	41.8	8.6	50.0
25–34	56.5	4.2	75.0
35–44	72.2	16.9	95.0
45–54	74.5	33.2	104.2
55–64	64.5	30.5	86.7
65–74	68.9	33.2	104.2
75–79	84.3	53.4	121.2
>80	91.7	64.7	138.0

Source United Nations (1988).

Table 20.1 and Figure 20.1 show that the difference in age structure of the population is changing; the proportion of older people in less developed countries is increasing much faster than it is in developed countries. Although some psychiatric disorders become less common (Figure 20.2), the prevalence of dementia increases rapidly with age (see below), and all countries face the increasing problem of managing large numbers of cognitively impaired older people.

The effects of ageing

Physical changes in the brain

The weight of the human brain decreases by approximately 5 per cent between the ages of 30 and 70 years, by a further 5 per cent by the age of 80, and by another 10–20 per cent by the age of 90. As well as these changes, the ventricles enlarge and the meninges thicken. MRI studies show a complex temporal and spatial profile of changes affecting both grey and white matter, with volume reductions prominent in hippocampus, association cortex, and cerebellum (Raz *et al.*, 2005).

There is some loss of neurons, though this is regionally selective and much less marked than formerly believed, and reductions in synapses and dendrites appear more important. The cytoplasm of some neurons contain a pigment, **lipofuscin**. The ageing brain also tends to accumulate senile plaques and neurofibrillary tangles, but with a more restricted distribution and smaller numbers than in Alzheimer's disease. Neurofibrillary tangles are usually limited to neurons in hippocampus and entorhinal cortex; while senile plaques can also occur in neocortex and amygdala. Similarly, a small proportion of brains from healthy old people contain

Lewy bodies. For a review of the neuropathology of normal ageing, see Hof and Morrison (2004).

At a biochemical level, brain ageing is thought to reflect changes in calcium regulation and mitochondrial function (Toescu *et al.*, 2004), driven in part by oxidative damage due to free radicals (Barja, 2004) and alterations in certain growth factor and neurotransmitter signalling pathways (Hof and Morrison, 2004; Mattson *et al.*, 2004).

The neuropsychology of ageing

Assessment of cognitive function in the elderly is complicated by the frequent presence of physical ill health, notably sensory deficits, and by the need to carefully distinguish normality from the earliest phase of dementia.

Longitudinal studies suggest that intellectual function, as measured by standard intelligence tests, shows a significant decline only in later old age. A characteristic pattern of change occurs with psychomotor slowing and impairment in the manipulation of new information. By contrast, tests of well-rehearsed skills such as verbal comprehension show little or no age-related decline.

Short-term memory, as measured by the digit span test, for example, does not change in the normal elderly. Tests of working memory show a gradual decrease in capacity, so that the elderly perform significantly less well than the young if attention has to be divided between two tasks or if the material has to be processed additionally in some way. The elderly can usually recall remote events of personal significance with great clarity. Despite this, their long-term memory for other remote events shows a decline; for a review see Morris (1997). Overall, there appears to be a balance between losses in flexible problem-solving, and the benefits of accumulated wisdom derived from experience.

As well as these cognitive and motor changes, there are important alterations in personality and attitudes, such as increasing cautiousness and rigidity.

Physical health

In addition to a general decline in functional capacity and adaptability with ageing, chronic degenerative conditions are common. As a result, the elderly consult their family doctors frequently and occupy half of all hospital beds. These demands are particularly large in those aged over 75. Medical management is made more difficult by the presence of more than one disorder, the consequent increased risk of side-effects of treatment, and by psychiatric and social problems (Kane, 1985).

Sensory and motor disabilities are frequent among elderly people. In a study of over 80-year-olds in Jerusalem, 50–60 per cent reported problems with vision, hearing or walking, and 22 per cent had difficulties talking (Davies and Fleishchman, 1981). These figures are representative of those reported in other countries.

Social circumstances

For most people, ageing brings with it profound changes in social circumstances. Retirement affects not only income but also social status, time available for leisure, and social contacts. Loss of income is a serious problem facing many elderly people, and financial problems were the commonest worry reported in a large European survey of over 65-year-olds.

Social isolation is a fact of life for many older people, especially in developed countries. In the UK and USA, about a third of those over 65 lived alone in 1993, compared with 7 per cent in Chile and 3 per cent in China. The figure in the UK increased markedly in the second half of the last century: in 1851 it was 7 per cent, and in 1921, 11 per cent. However, for many older people, living alone is not seen as a problem and is aided by slowly increasing pensioner incomes and greater availability of suitable housing. Many see family, friends, and neighbours regularly and provide as much support as they receive. In a 1993 European Commission survey, 44 per cent of older Europeans saw a relative every day. This figure was highest in southern Europe and lowest in northern Europe, but, interestingly, reported loneliness showed the same pattern, being highest in countries with the highest levels of family contact.

Table 20.2 summarizes data from the 2001 Great Britain Census (www.statistics.gov.uk/cci/) regarding the proportion of elderly people who live at home alone, or who live in a 'communal establishment', i.e. residential care or long-stay hospital bed. In both statistics, women predominate, reflecting the greater number of widows than widowers (and thus women who lack a spouse to care for them), and the higher level of disability reported by women than men at any given age. Note also that the lower row indicates that 93 per cent of elderly people, including 67 per cent of over 85-year-olds, live at home rather than in residential care.

TABLE 20.2 Percentages of people living alone, or in residential care, in England and Wales, 2001

Place of dwelling	Aged 65 and over		Aged 85 and over	
	Men	Women	Men	Women
At home, alone	21	43	42	70
In residential care	2	5	11	21

Other factors

Not only does the number of elderly people change with time, but there are marked changes in experiences and expectations with successive cohorts. In Europe, the generation born in the early decades of the twentieth century mostly received only basic education, had large families, worked long hours in unprosperous conditions, and experienced two world wars. Those who survived had considerable resilience and powers of endurance. By comparison, those born 50 years later grew up mostly in more affluent circumstances, with more education, and with higher expectations. In the UK and most parts of Europe there have been rapid recent changes in ethnic composition and in household structure. All these factors will affect demands on both health and social services in the future (Royal Commission on Long Term Care, 1999).

Epidemiology of psychiatric disorder in the elderly

Kay *et al.* (1964) carried out the first systematic prevalence study of psychiatric disorder amongst elderly people in the general population, including those living at home as well as those living in institutions, in an area of Newcastle-upon-Tyne, in northern England. The findings (Table 20.3) have been broadly replicated in subsequent surveys, taking into account changes in diagnostic criteria (e.g. inclusion of depression in their category of neurosis), and the problems of case finding. For example, a recent large French population study of people aged 65 or over found a point prevalence of 14 per cent for anxiety disorder, 11 per cent for phobia, 3 per cent for major depression, and 1.7 per cent for psychosis, using an interview to make DSM-IV diagnoses (Ritchie *et al.*, 2004). These figures mask the significant changes in prevalence and proportions of disorders at different stages of old age, as shown by a large Swedish study (Skoog, 2004), summarized in Table 20.4.

TABLE 20.3 Prevalence of psychiatric disorder in over 65 year olds

Disorder	Prevalence (%)
Dementia (severe)	5.6
Dementia (mild)	5.7
Neurosis and personality disorder	12.5
Manic depression	1.4
Schizophrenia	1.1
Any disorder	26.3

Kay *et al.* (1964).

TABLE 20.4 Changing prevalence of psychiatric disorders with age amongst the elderly

Age	Dementia*	Depression	Anxiety disorders	Psychotic disorders
70 (n = 392)	2	6	6	1
75 (n = 303)	5	6	4	2
79 (n = 206)	11	11	3	3
85 (n = 494)	31	13	10	5

*Moderate or severe

Figures are percentages. Adapted from Skoog (2004).

Other surveys have shown a high prevalence of psychiatric disorder among elderly people in sheltered accommodation and in hospital. A third of the residents in old people's homes have significant cognitive impairment. In general hospital wards, a third to a half of the patients aged 65 or over suffer from some form of psychiatric illness.

It has frequently been reported that general practitioners are unaware of many of the psychiatric problems amongst elderly people living in the community. Moreover, the presentation of such disorders to general practitioners and psychiatrists is determined as much by social factors as by a change in the patient's mental state. For example, there may be a sudden alteration in the patient's environment, such as illness of a relative, or a bereavement. Sometimes an increasingly exhausted or frustrated family decide that they can no longer continue to care for an old person. At other times there is an element of manipulation by relatives who are trying to rid themselves of an unwanted responsibility.

As in younger subjects, there are gender differences in the prevalence, presentation and course of some psychiatric disorders, and in treatment needs (Lehmann, 2003).

Dementia

Although there are references in classical literature, dementia in the elderly has been recognized by modern medicine since the French psychiatrist Esquirol described **démence senile** in 1838. Esquirol's description was in general terms, but it can be recognized as similar to the present-day concept (Alexander, 1972). Kraepelin distinguished dementia from psychoses due to other organic causes such as neurosyphilis, and he

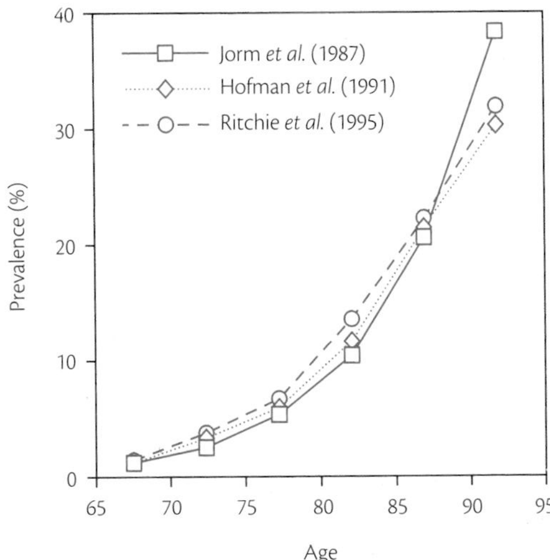

Fig. 20.3 Prevalence rates for dementia across age groups: data from three meta-analyses. From AF Jorm (2000).

divided it into presenile, senile, and arteriosclerotic forms. In an important study, Roth (1955) showed that dementia in the elderly differed from affective disorders and paranoid disorders in its poorer prognosis.

Following Roth (1955), there has been extensive research on the prevalence of dementia, and several meta-analyses (Figure 20.3). Prevalence rises steeply with age, up to the age of 90; thereafter the increase slows, and about a quarter of centenarians remain cognitively intact (Perls, 2004). As discussed in Chapter 14, the commonest causes are Alzheimer's disease, vascular dementia, and dementia with Lewy bodies, with frequent coexistence of features of more than one disorder.

Mood disorder

Despite the focus on dementia in the elderly, depressive disorders are considerably commoner. A systematic review of community-based studies found an average prevalence of clinically relevant depression of 13.5 per cent for those aged 55 or over, of which 9.8 per cent was classed as minor and 1.8 per cent as major. Prevalence was higher in women and among older people living in adverse circumstances (Beekman *et al.*, 1999). The figures show that a high proportion of depressed elderly people do not meet criteria for major depression, but are instead variously labelled as having minor depression, dysthymia, or subthreshold depression. However, this does not diminish its clinical significance, since these cases have similar morbidity and course as do patients meeting criteria for major depression (Beekman *et al.*, 1997, 2002).

Rates of depression depend on the setting. Koenig and Blazer (1992) reported the following rates: 0.4–1.4 per cent in the community, 5–10 per cent among medical outpatients, 10–15 per cent among medical inpatients, and 15–20 per cent among nursing home patients. These variations likely reflect the frequent comorbidity of depression in the elderly with other psychiatric (Devanand, 2002) and physical (Krishnan *et al.*, 2002) disorders, notably those with a vascular basis (see p. 512). For example, rates of depression are higher in those with cardiac problems and neurodegenerative disorders, and a third of patients have an alcohol misuse disorder. These comorbidities may also contribute to the increased disabilities and mortality rate, especially from cardiac events (Penninx *et al.*, 1999), experienced by elderly people with depression. Elderly prisoners have particularly high rates of depression (Fazel *et al.*, 2001).

The high prevalence of depressive disorder masks the fact that first episodes become less common after the age of 60, and rare after the age of 80. There is current debate as to whether late-onset depression has a different biological basis than depression starting earlier in life (see p. 511).

The incidence of suicide increases steadily with age (Chapter 17), and suicide in the elderly is usually associated with depressive disorder (Waern *et al.*, 2002). Unlike depressive disorder, bipolar disorder and mania appear to become less common in old age (Depp and Jeste, 2004).

Anxiety and stress-related disorders

In general practice, Shepherd *et al.* (1966) found that, after the age of 55, the incidence of new cases of neurosis (i.e. anxiety disorder) declined; however, the frequency of consultations with the general practitioner for neurosis did not fall – presumably as a result of chronic or recurrent cases. Surveys in the general population indicate that after the age of 65 some new cases of emotional disorder appear, with a prevalence of cases of at least moderate severity of about 12 per cent (Kay and Bergmann,1980). Post-traumatic stress disorder has a prevalence of about 1 per cent in the elderly (van Zeist *et al.*, 2003).

For review of anxiety disorders in the elderly see Alwahhabi (2003).

Schizophrenia-like disorders and paranoid states

Schizophrenia-like and paranoid disorders in the elderly have been a long-standing source of debate and terminological confusion (see Box 13.2), with the terms

paraphrenia and **late paraphrenia** still commonly if loosely used. In future versions of ICD and DSM, the term **'very-late-onset-schizophrenia-like-psychosis'** will cover psychoses of this kind arising after 60 years of age. The delineation of this group, and its separation from the **'late-onset schizophrenia'** which will apply to those with onset between ages 40 and 59 years, is based on differences in its symptom profile and associated risk factors (Howard *et al.*, 2000).

Patients with 'very-late-onset-schizophrenia-like-psychosis' form approximately 10 per cent of admissions to psychiatric wards for the elderly. There are no good data on the prevalence in the community because it is difficult to identify all cases of a condition in which many sufferers keep their experience to themselves and are unlikely to cooperate with 'doorstep' interviews. Also, in this setting, it may be difficult to distinguish cases from those with psychotic symptoms occurring in dementia or in severe depression.

Principles and practice of old age psychiatry

Having surveyed the epidemiological landscape, in this section we outline the principles and practice of old age psychiatry, in terms of assessment, management, and service organization, and how this reflects the characteristics and needs of its patients and their disorders. The remainder of the chapter proceeds to describe the specific features and treatments of the individual psychiatric disorders of old age.

Organization of services

An international consensus statement has defined the essential elements of a mental health service for elderly people (Wertheimer, 1997):

- Primary healthcare team
- Specialist old age psychiatry team
- Inpatient unit
- Rehabilitation
- Day care
- Availability of respite care
- Range of residential care facilities
- Family and social supports
- Liaison with geriatric medicine
- Education of health care providers to the needs of elderly people with psychiatric problems
- Research, especially into epidemiological issues, and evaluation of services.

The 'team' concept is highlighted as being the key to effective provision of care (Collighan *et al.*, 1993), with multidisciplinary involvement the norm. However, beyond these broad points of consensus, national policies have differed considerably in terms of the development of services and how they are implemented (Johnston and Reifler, 2000). In the USA, emphasis has been placed on care in hospitals and nursing homes. In Europe, Canada, and Australasia, there has been varying emphasis on social policies to provide sheltered accommodation and care in the community. In this section, services in the UK will be described as an example. Health, social, and voluntary services will be described separately, although good care depends on close collaboration at all levels, from strategic planning to the coordinated provision of care for each individual patient. Reflecting this need, health and social services, and their budgets, are now being integrated in the UK.

Health services

Primary care

The general practitioner has a central role in assessment and management of the problems of mentally ill older people. In the UK, all patients over the age of 75 are offered an annual health check, providing an opportunity for regular screening for psychiatric disorders. In many instances, the general practitioner, together with other health professionals in primary care, assesses and manages patients without referring them to a specialist. Even in the case of disorders for which referral will usually follow, such as dementia, the general practitioner is still responsible for the initial assessment and diagnosis (Turner *et al.*, 2004). However, as already mentioned, general practitioners do not detect all the psychiatric problems of the elderly at an early stage, nor do they always provide all the necessary long-term medical supervision. These problems are partly due to lack of awareness of the significance of psychiatric illness among the elderly, and partly to the provision of a service in which doctors respond to requests from patients rather than seeking out their problems. Some old age psychiatry services will only accept referrals from a general practitioner, but increasingly referrals may be accepted directly from any source, though liaison with the general practitioner will always be important. In some areas, community psychiatric nurses (CPNs) work in primary care, though it is more usual for them to be part of old age psychiatry teams in secondary care.

Old age psychiatry services

The organization of psychiatric services varies in different localities, since it reflects the local styles of service providers, local needs, and the extent of provision for this age group by general psychiatric services, as well as national policies. Nevertheless, there are some general principles of planning. The aims should be to maintain the elderly person at home for as long as possible, to respond quickly to medical and social problems as they arise, to ensure coordination of the work of those providing continuing care, and to support relatives and others who care for the elderly person at home. There should be close liaison with primary care, other hospital specialists who may be involved, social services, and voluntary agencies. A multidisciplinary approach should be adopted with a clinical team that may include psychiatrists, psychologists, community psychiatric nurses, occupational therapists, and social workers. Some members of the team should spend more of their working day in patients' homes and in general practices than in the hospital. It is important that the care provided by these different agencies is coordinated, and in the UK, the Care Programme Approach is intended to improve coordination by making a single person, the key worker, responsible for ensuring that appropriate assessment, care planning, and review takes place (p. 637). The contributions of the various parts of an old age psychiatry service will now be considered.

Domiciliary psychiatric care. Increasingly, assessment and treatment take place in the patient's own home, which is both more convenient for the patient and offers a more relevant and realistic assessment of the difficulties facing the patient and carers. Community psychiatric nurses act as a bridge between primary care and specialist services. The nurses may assess referrals from general practitioners, monitor treatment in collaboration with general practitioners and the psychiatric services, and take part in the organization of home support for the demented elderly.

Outpatient clinics have a smaller part to play in providing care for the elderly than for younger patients because assessment at home is particularly important for old people. However, such clinics are convenient for the assessment and follow-up of mobile patients. There are advantages when these clinics are staffed jointly by medical geriatricians and old age psychiatrists. In recent years, **memory clinics** have been developed in many areas for the specialist assessment of patients with early memory problems (Phipps and O'Brien, 2002); in the UK, these clinics also serve as the focus for prescription of drugs used to treat Alzheimer's disease, since their availability is limited (p. 509).

Day hospitals and day centres. Although some treatments can be provided at home, others may require the patient to attend a day hospital, where a high level of stimulation and social interaction can also be provided. In the 1950s, day care began in geriatric hospitals. A few years later the first psychiatric day hospitals for the elderly were opened. Psychiatric day hospitals should provide a full range of diagnostic services and offer both short-term and continuing care for patients with functional or organic disorders, together with support for relatives. Currently, day care is more often provided by day centres rather than in day hospitals; these centres combine health and social care elements, and often also involve financial and practical involvement from voluntary organisations, such as the Alzheimer's Society. Day centres provide an important and cost-effective component of the services available for the elderly with psychiatric problems. In particular, day care has become a mainstay of care for those with mild to moderate dementia. All day-based arrangements depend crucially on adequate transport facilities.

Inpatient units. Inpatient teams should be able to provide multidisciplinary assessment and treatment of patients with severe mental health problems. In addition to psychiatrists and psychiatric nurses, teams may include occupational therapists, psychologists, speech and language therapists, physiotherapists, social workers, health care assistants, and others. There is substantial variation in different areas as to the composition of the team and as to whether patients with functional illnesses are cared for separate from or together with those with organic disorders.

Geriatric medicine. There is inevitably some overlap in the characteristics of patients treated by units for geriatric medicine and those treated in psychiatry units. Both are likely to treat patients with dementia, although old age psychiatry units are more likely than geriatric units to treat patients with functional psychiatric disorders. In the past there was considerable concern that many patients were 'misplaced' and therefore received poor treatment, stayed too long in hospital, and had an unsatisfactory outcome. Research has generally not confirmed these concerns. For example, Copeland *et al.* (1975) found that although 64 per cent of patients admitted to geriatric hospitals were psychiatrically ill, only 12 per cent appeared to be wrongly placed. Moreover, the outcome of these misplaced patients did not appear to be affected adversely: it seems that many patients can be cared for equally well in either type of hospital. The optimal placement of the rest depends on the relative predominance of behavioural and physical problems. Medical and psychiatric teams need to cooperate closely if all patients are to receive appropriate treatment.

Long-term hospital care. In some countries, most elderly psychiatric patients are still treated in the wards of psychiatric hospitals. However, the nature of the care provided is more important than the type of institution in which it is given. The basic requirements are opportunities for privacy and the use of personal possessions, together with occupational and social therapy. Provided that these criteria are met, long-term hospital care can be the best provision for very disabled patients. In the UK, hospital provision of long-term care has been drastically reduced (with some increase in the level of community care), and long-term care is now largely provided outside hospital in residential and nursing homes. There is an active debate on how long-term care should be funded, since care provided by the NHS is free whilst care provided through the social services is means tested (Royal Commission on Long Term Care, 1999).

Social services

Domiciliary services

In addition to medical services, domiciliary services include home helps, meals at home, laundry, telephone, and emergency call systems. In the UK, local authorities both provide and commission these services; they also support voluntary organizations and encourage local initiatives such as good neighbour schemes and self-help groups. In a random sample of nearly 500 people aged 65 and over living at home, Foster *et al.* (1976) found that 12 per cent were receiving domiciliary services but a further 20 per cent needed them. Although these provisions are increasing, so are the numbers of those requiring them. Bergmann *et al.* (1978) have argued that if resources are limited, more should be directed to patients living with their families than to those living alone. This is because the former can often remain at home if they receive such help, whereas many of the latter require admission before long, even when extra help is given.

Residential and nursing care

Older people may need a variety of social service accommodation, ranging from entirely independent housing through sheltered housing schemes, where there may be some communal provision, often including access to a warden, to residential or nursing homes where there are staff available at all times. There is a need for special housing for the elderly, conveniently sited and easy to run. Ideally, the elderly should be able to transfer to more sheltered accommodation if they become more disabled, without losing all independence or moving away from familiar places. In many communities in the UK, there is still not enough variety of accommodation offering a range of independence. Provision of this kind is better in many parts of Europe, the USA, and Australasia (Grundy, 1987).

'Continuing care' refers to the provision of homes where staff are available on site at all times. In residential homes, the needs of residents for help with personal care can be met by care assistants with relatively little training, whereas in nursing homes residents will have need for regular nursing care, and therefore the staff will include a substantial number of trained nurses. Some, but not all, nursing homes specialize in the care of older people with mental health problems.

In the UK, local social services are responsible for providing residential homes and other sheltered accommodation, although many independent organizations and charities also provide residential homes for older people. The growth of continuing care provision in the private sector has had some advantages in encouraging a greater variety of facilities, but in some places undue emphasis on the cost rather than the standard of care, together with a lack of coordinated planning, has made it difficult to develop integrated local services to meet the needs of the elderly. Over the past two decades there has been a steady rise in the level of disability of residents in residential homes.

Voluntary services

Voluntary agencies play a large and increasing role in the provision of facilities and support to patients, their families, and carers. It is essential that their contributions are integrated with health and social service provisions. In addition, any discussion of service provision for the elderly mentally ill must acknowledge the major part played by informal carers.

Informal carers

Informal carers are unpaid relatives, neighbours, or friends who look after disabled (usually demented) elderly persons at home. The term differentiates these people from formal carers such as paid home helps and district or community psychiatric nurses. Informal carers provide substantially more care to older people than do the statutory services, and their role in the overall provision of care should not be underestimated. Most informal carers of older people are (in descending order of frequency) spouses, daughters, or sons. About twice as many women as men are informal carers. About half of all informal carers are themselves elderly.

Several studies have shown that patients suffering from dementia place the greatest stress on carers (Baumgarten *et al.*, 1994). In general, the more severe the dementia, the greater the strain. Incontinence, behavioural disturbance at night, and aggression are the most distressing problems for carers. As assessed by the General Health Questionnaire, many carers have symptoms as severe as those of a psychiatric case. Symptoms diminish when the patient has moved to permanent residential care (Morris *et al.*, 1988; Henderson, 1990).

Accurate assessment of carers' needs is important, and in the UK, social services now have a statutory responsibility to provide this, where requested. Table 20.5 summarizes the key recommendations made by Levin (1997). Time should be spent with family carers in giving advice about the care of patients and discussing their problems. Such support can help families avoid some of the frustration and anxiety of caring for elderly relatives. Published guides, increasingly available on the internet, are useful. Other practical help may include day-care or holiday admissions, and laundry and meal services to the home. With such assistance many patients can remain in their own homes without imposing an unreasonable burden on their families. The assessment of need and carer support may often need to be multidisciplinary; both community psychiatric nurses and care managers (social workers) play essential roles in coordinating these services, supporting relatives, and providing direct nursing care.

TABLE 20.5 Support for carers of elderly patients with dementia

1. Early identification of dementia
2. Comprehensive medical and social assessment of identified cases
3. Timely referrals between agencies, for example, from general practitioner to old age psychiatrist
4. Continuing reviews of each patient's needs, and back-up for carers
5. Active medical treatment for any intercurrent illness
6. The provision of information, advice, and counselling for carers
7. Regular help with household and personal care tasks
8. Regular breaks for carers, for example, by providing day care and respite care for the patient
9. Appropriate financial support
10. Permanent residential care when this becomes necessary.

Despite the increasing focus on carers' needs, there is little evidence that any interventions are effective upon their psychosocial wellbeing (Thompson and Briggs, 2000). However, there is some support for problem-solving and behavioural management strategies (Pusey and Richards, 2001).

Psychiatric assessment in the elderly

The principles and basic purpose of assessment of older people are not substantially different from that of all patients: it is intended to establish a diagnosis, to develop the best possible plan of care, and inform prognosis. However, there are differences of emphasis and process:

- The assessment is likely to take longer, requiring more than one interview and with a greater reliance on informants. For example, in assessment of suspected dementia, an informant is essential to complete the history, and to verify the extent to which the impairments are affecting the patient's capabilities and safety. In the evaluation of cognitive impairment, time will also be required to administer rating scales.
- The assessment is likely to extend beyond a strictly medical understanding of the patient's conditions and its treatment to include assessment of the wider psychosocial situation, taking account not only of the patient's needs but also those of carers and other involved people. This is particularly relevant for the patient with moderate or severe dementia.
- The physical examination and laboratory investigations play a larger role, because of the greater prevalence of organic disorders as a cause of psychiatric symptoms in the elderly. The psychiatric assessment may also bring coincidental medical problems to light.

For review of assessment of psychiatric disorder in the elderly, see Jacoby (2000b).

The referral

It is important to establish at the outset what prompted the referral, and what is hoped to be gained from it. This may well require information to be collected even before the patient is seen, not least in order to establish the most useful way to approach the assessment. In any one case, each person involved in care may have different, and possibly conflicting, needs.

Informants

Many old people seen by psychiatrists are unable to give complete or reliable information about themselves. Frequently there is a partner or other close relative living with the patient, but in other cases it may be necessary to talk to neighbours or friends. It may be useful to spend considerable time telephoning relatives or others who may be able to give information about family history or previous personality. Many patients seen for the first time will already be well known to their general practitioner or to other health professionals, and it is always worth consulting them.

Where to assess the patient

In the UK, most old age psychiatrists prefer to assess patients in their own homes, in keeping with international recommendations (Wertheimer, 1997). This enables much essential 'real life' information about the patient's ability to function at home to be gained (for example, making a cup of tea, or recognizing relatives in family photographs); it also avoids the patient appearing excessively disorientated simply because of the disturbing effect of having to travel to a hospital for assessment in an unfamiliar environment. It is also likely to make it easier to interview other members of the family, and to assess the level of support from neighbours or outside carers, who may be prepared to be available at the patient's home during the assessment.

Old age psychiatrists may also be asked to assess patients on general hospital wards. Although this will normally provide much less information about the patients' circumstances, it has the advantage of making close liaison with the hospital team possible. Conditions on hospital wards are often unfavourable for a quiet, private interview, but it is important to spend time reading the notes carefully, talking to nursing and other staff, and then requesting the use of an office or side room in which to see the patient. Even if the family or other carers cannot be present, it may be possible to telephone them. Similar principles apply to assessment in residential and nursing homes.

Increasingly, patients with early cognitive impairments are being offered assessments in a memory clinic (p. 501), usually in a hospital outpatient setting. For some patients this offers advantages of a systematic and detailed assessment, and enables relevant further investigations and follow-up to be arranged as efficiently as possible.

The assessment

The information required about the medical and psychiatric history is the same as in younger patients. However, it may be necessary to piece it together from accounts given by the patient and by other informants. It is of particular importance to obtain a clear medical history and to determine past and present medication.

During the mental state examination, assessment of cognitive function has a particular significance, especially for those in whom memory impairment is apparent or suspected; this assessment requires a range of clinical questions and observations, supplemented by one or more of the questionnaires available for this purpose (Table 14.9, p. 334), such as the Mini-Mental State Examination, p. 67).

Since physical problems are extremely common, the psychiatrist will often need to examine the patient thoroughly (especially if this has not been done recently by the general practitioner) including a neurological examination. Laboratory investigations are important for patients on admission, and in all others with significant psychiatric disorder (for investigation of dementia, see p. 333).

Finally, the assessment process includes assessments of risk, and of the needs of the carer(s), discussed above, since most elderly people with mental disorders live in their own homes and are cared for by family or, occasionally, by good neighbours or friends.

Psychiatric treatment in the elderly

As with assessment, the principles of psychiatric treatment in the elderly resemble that of other adults, but their greater age does require three issues which impact upon treatment to be borne in mind (Oppenheimer, 2000):

- Patients are likely to have multiple problems. Psychiatric, physical and social difficulties usually coexist to some extent. 'Treatment' may thus include a broad range of interventions beyond those normally associated with psychiatry, such as antibiotics for a urinary tract infection, or liaision with a district nurse or dietitian. These complex treatment needs are reflected in the multidisciplinary nature of services, described above, and require careful planning and integration of treatment provision.
- Clear boundaries between normality and disease are rare. This poses challenges for treatment thresholds and service provision.
- Lack of competence is common, because of cognitive impairment. There is an increasing focus on how (lack of) competence should be assessed, and responded to. The question of competence underlies a range of ethical and legal issues in which old age psychiatrists become involved (see below).

Physical treatments

The efficacy of psychotropic drugs is generally not affected by age, and elderly patients should not be denied effective drug treatment, especially for depressive disorders. However, as noted in Chapter 21 (p. 523), prescribing in the elderly requires particular caution, for two main reasons:

- The rate of unpleasant or dangerous side-effects is high, and can produce delirium and other psychiatric disorders. Most problems arise with drugs used to treat cardiovascular disorders (hypotensives, diuretics, and digoxin) and those acting on the central nervous system (antidepressants, hypnotics, anxiolytics, antipsychotics, and antiparkinsonian drugs). These problems arise because of differences in pharmacokinetics with ageing, and the greater number of drugs which elderly people are prescribed, increasing the chances for harmful interactions. There is particular concern regarding antipsychotics in dementia (p. 508).
- Compliance with treatment may be compromised in those who live alone, have poor vision, or who are forgetful or confused.

Given these factors, the following points should be borne in mind when prescribing for the elderly person with a psychiatric disorder:

- Always start with a low dose, increase slowly, and expect the final dose to be considerably lower than in younger patients. The main exception to this is SSRIs, for which comparable doses are used.
- All medication should be reviewed regularly, and kept to a minimum. Before starting a drug in the elderly, it is good practice to state clearly in the notes the reason for the decision (including, for example, the score on a depression rating scale), and the criteria by which the effects of the treatment will be assessed. If good evidence of efficacy is not achieved, medication should be gradually withdrawn.
- The drug regimen should be as simple as possible. Medicine bottles should be labelled clearly, and memory aids, such as packs containing the drugs to be taken on a single day with daily dose requirements, should be provided. If possible, drug taking should be supervised.

Electroconvulsive therapy

ECT remains one of the most effective and valuable treatments for serious depressive disorder in the elderly (p. 513). Advanced age is not a contraindication for ECT. However, attention should be paid to the physical health of all elderly patients undergoing this treatment, and frail patients should be assessed by an experienced anaesthetist before receiving ECT.

Psychological treatment

In all patients, supportive therapy with clearly defined aims can be helpful, including joint sessions with the spouse or carer.

In patients with no cognitive impairment, the specific psychological therapies used in younger subjects remain appropriate, for the same range of disorders and with similar expectations of success. In particular, cognitive and behavioural interventions for mood and anxiety disorders are effective and often preferred by the patient. Family or systems therapy, although not widely available, is advocated as it explicitly recognizes the patient in his or her social context (Jacoby, 2000b). Psychodynamic psychotherapy is less appropriate for the elderly and seldom used.

Even mild cognitive impairment militates against use of most of the common psychological therapies, since it is likely to prevent the patient understanding or implementing the treatment (Oppenheimer, 2000). However, a range of specialized psychological and behavioural interventions (e.g. reminiscence therapy) are becoming widely used in this group, with the benefits targeted as much at the carer as at the patient, as described below (p. 507).

See Woods and Charlesworth (2002) for a review of psychological assessment and treatment in the elderly.

Psychosocial treatments

Some patients can achieve independence through measures to encourage self-care, and domestic skills, and to increase social contacts. For those living at home, a domiciliary occupational therapist may be helpful in advising on environmental or other modifications which will help the patient to live in a more independent way. More severely impaired patients living in institutional care can benefit from an environment in which individual needs and dignity are respected and each person retains some personal possessions. Further psychosocial interventions of this kind are discussed in the section on treatment of dementia.

Legal, financial, and ethical issues

Both the law and ethical principles apply equally to the elderly as to younger people, and these issues are discussed elsewhere in this book. However, certain legal and ethical issues relevant in psychiatry have particular relevance to the elderly (Table 20.6), for several reasons:

- The nature of the common illnesses from which they suffer, especially dementia, which compromises their competence to make decisions and give consent.
- Problems arising from increasing age and frailty, for example, driving.
- The greater likelihood and proximity of death, giving a greater urgency to issues such as testamentary capacity (see Posener and Jacoby, 2002 for a review) and advance directives.

In the UK, these issues will be affected by forthcoming legislation (the Mental Capacity Bill) which is currently before Parliament.

Financial affairs

Older people, particularly those with mental health problems, may have difficulty in managing their financial affairs. In the UK, if the issues are relatively simple, for example, involving only a state pension and benefits, the person can request that someone else, known as an appointee, collects these benefits on his behalf. Alternatively, while the person still has mental capacity to understand what is involved, he can make an Enduring Power of Attorney in favour of one or more others. The attorney then has authority to carry out any financial transaction on behalf of that person. If the donor of the power subsequently becomes mentally unable to manage his own affairs, the attorney may continue to do so on his behalf (in the UK, provided the arrangement is registered with the Court of Protection). Sometimes a person becomes mentally incapable of managing his affairs without having made any formal arrangement for someone else to act on his behalf; under these circumstances, an application supported by medical evidence of incapacity may be made to the Court of Protection for a receiver to be appointed to manage his affairs. It is important to note that all these provisions apply only to financial affairs, and do not carry any authority to make treatment decisions on behalf of the patient.

Driving

A common practical problem is the inability of older patients to drive safely, especially those with mild dementia (p. 333) and Parkinson's disease (p. 341). As with other disorders, doctors generally have an obligation, which overrides confidentiality, to inform authorities responsible for the provision of driving licences. In practice, elderly people often make the decision to stop driving anyway, or are persuaded to do so by relatives.

TABLE 20.6 Ethical and legal issues in the elderly
Confidentiality in relation to information from carers
Confidentiality of information about financial circumstances
Consent to treatment
◆ Capacity to consent to physical and psychological treatment
◆ Advance directives
◆ Decisions 'not to treat'
Damaging behaviour
Management of financial affairs
◆ Nominating another to take responsibility (Power of Attorney)
◆ Procedures to enable others to take responsibility
Entitlement to drive a vehicle
Consent to participate in research

Abuse and neglect of the elderly

Abuse and neglect of the elderly by family members or other carers is an issue of increasing concern for all healthcare professionals working with the elderly. Its psychiatric relevance arises in part from the finding that people with dementia are particularly likely to be abused.

Elder abuse refers to actions by a carer or other trusted person that cause harm or create a serious risk of harm to an elderly person (whether or not harm is intended), or to failure by a caregiver to satisfy the elder's basic needs or protect them from harm. Five forms of 'elder abuse' are recognized: physical, psychological, sexual, financial, and neglect. Prevalence rates of 2–10 per cent are reported, with a higher risk associated with several circumstances:

- the abused person has dementia
- the carer and abused person live together
- social isolation of the abused person, e.g. lack of close friends
- the carer has a psychiatric disorder or misuses alcohol
- the carer is heavily dependent (e.g. financially) on the person being abused.

Elder abuse has a threefold increased mortality rate compared to matched elderly people (Lachs *et al.*, 1998), as well as with other adverse outcomes ranging from depression to placement in a nursing home.

Although there is now widespread awareness of the problem and the need to identify elder abuse and respond to it, there is no evidence about the effectiveness of interventions. At present, a range of measures are used, such as increased social support, respite care, marital counselling, and carer education programs. Legal approaches (e.g. guardianship, law enforcement agencies) may also be necessary.

Elder abuse is reviewed by Lachs and Pillemer (2004).

Dementia

The clinical, epidemiological and aetiological features of dementia were covered in Chapter 14. Here, the management of dementia is covered, in two sections. First, the treatment of psychiatric and behavioural disturbances of dementia, for which non-pharmacological and pharmacological strategies are used. Second, the treatment of Alzheimer's disease and some other specific dementias for which drugs are becoming available.

Treatment of behavioural and psychological symptoms of dementia

A spectrum of behavioural changes and psychological symptoms occur during the course of dementia, as described in Chapter 14 and summarized in Table 20.7. These features affect about 60 per cent of sufferers at some stage of the illness, although the overall prevalence and frequency of individual features varies according to the type of dementia (Lyketsos *et al.*, 2000). The behavioural and psychological symptoms cause considerable difficulties for carers, and their management can be difficult; there is increasing concern about the inappropriate use of medication, yet a shortage of evidence-based non-pharmacological alternatives.

TABLE 20.7 Behavioural and psychological symptoms of dementia

Behaviours
◆ Agitation
◆ Shouting
◆ Wandering
◆ Apathy
◆ Inappropriate sexual behaviour
◆ Impaired sleep
Symptoms
◆ Delusions
◆ Hallucinations
◆ Depression
◆ Anxiety
Contributory factors
◆ Constipation
◆ Pain
◆ Superimposed delirium
◆ Sensory deficits

Before any treatment is considered, careful assessment is required, with attention paid to several points:

- The nature of the problem behaviour(s) should be clearly identified, including duration, severity, and any suspected causative or modifying factors. Rating scales may be useful (Table 14.9, p. 334). Examples of remediable causal factors include urinary tract infections, constipation, and pain. The latter is often overlooked and adequate analgesia therefore not provided (Scherder *et al.*, 2005). Pain in dementia may be due to concurrent physical problems (e.g. leg ulcers, arthritis), or part of the disease process.
- A mental state examination is needed to determine if the behaviour can be explained in terms of an underlying psychopathology. For example, whether there is evidence of psychotic symptoms, low mood or anxiety. If this examination, together with the history and other observations, supports a diagnosis (e.g. of psychosis, depression, or delirium), it will likely influence the treatment plan. On other occasions, however, no such diagnostic evidence may be forthcoming, in which case the behaviour is dealt with on its merits.
- The natural history is that behavioural and psychological symptoms of dementia tend to fluctuate and often last less than three months (Hope *et al.*, 1999). Any treatment, especially if drugs are used, should reflect this fact. Regular reassessment, and trials of medication withdrawal, should be an integral part of the management plan.
- Behavioural changes in dementia are usually problems for the carer rather than for the patient. This reality should be borne in mind when treatment decisions are made, especially as informed consent is often not possible because of the patient's cognitive impairment.

Non-pharmacological treatment of behavioural and psychological symptoms

If a behaviour or symptom is deemed, following assessment, to be sufficient to require treatment, a hierarchical approach should be employed. First, to treat any

TABLE 20.8 Non-pharmacological interventions for behavioural and psychological symptoms in dementia

Sensory stimulation
◆ Music therapy ◆ Aromatherapy (e.g. lavender oil) ◆ Bright light therapy ◆ Massage/touch ◆ White noise
Behavioural management
◆ Differential reinforcement ◆ Stimulus control
Social contact
◆ One on one interaction ◆ Pet therapy ◆ Simulated contact, e.g. videos
Exercise
Structured activity programs
Environmental modifications
◆ Reduced stimulation ◆ Wandering areas
Carer education and support
Combination therapies

underlying remediable cause, as outlined above. If the problem persists, the next approach should be based on modification of the person's environment, or a behavioural or psychological intervention, the choice of which will be influenced by the nature of the problem, the severity of the dementia, the setting, and the resources and expertise available (Table 20.8). Medication should be reserved for those in whom such approaches prove unsuccessful.

Most of the interventions in Table 20.8 have some evidence of effectiveness, with the largest number of studies being carried out on sensory stimulation and behavioural management (Cohen-Mansfield, 2001). However, in virtually no case is there substantial randomized controlled evidence. One exception is a study showing that an intervention comprising exercise and a carer training programme improved depression and physical health in 153 Alzheimer's disease patients, with a trend towards less institutionalization for behavioural problems two years later (Teri *et al.*, 2003). For review of non-pharmacological interventions in dementia, see Cohen-Mansfield (2001) and Livingston *et al.* (2005).

TABLE 20.9 Drugs used to treat behavioural and psychological symptoms in dementia

Typical antipsychotics
Atypical antipsychotics
Cholinesterase inhibitors
Antidepressants, e.g. trazodone
Carbamazepine
Valproic acid
Anxiolytics
Memantine

Drug treatment of behavioural and psychological symptoms

High rates of prescribing of psychotropic drugs in dementia, largely to control behavioural problems, have been reported in nursing homes and other institutions. For example, in a 1996 study, up to 30 per cent of residents in Glasgow nursing homes were receiving antipsychotics (McGrath and Jackson, 1996), as were 18 per cent of those with dementia in a large American survey (Liperoti *et al.*, 2003). A range of drug classes are in use (Table 20.9). However, the evidence shows that medication has at most a modest effect and, in the case of antipsychotics, may be associated with considerable morbidity and even mortality, as noted below. Reflecting these increasing concerns, medication for behavioural problems and psychological symptoms in dementia should not be contemplated until:

- A full assessment has been carried out.
- Aggravating physical and environmental factors have been addressed.
- Non-pharmacological strategies have been attempted.

For review, including a medication algorithm, see Sink *et al.* (2005).

Antipsychotics

Two meta-analyses have shown that typical antipsychotics given over 3–16 weeks are modestly better than placebo for managing difficult behaviours in dementia, but a larger meta-analysis limited to haloperidol found that only aggression might be reduced (Anonymous, 2003a). These benefits must be set against the significant risk of extrapyramidal side-effects, postural hypotension, tardive dyskinesia, and the many other side-effects of typical antipsychotics to which the elderly are prone.

Atypical antipsychotics are now more widely used than typical antipsychotics in this population (Liperoti *et al.*, 2003), with the expectation of a better tolerability and perhaps greater efficacy. There are no meta-analyses, but randomized trials suggest both risperidone and olanzapine have benefits against aggression and psychosis that are comparable to those seen for typical antipsychotics (Sink *et al.*, 2005).

The increasing concern about the use of antipsychotics in dementia is enhanced by three other serious potential risks.

1. They may increase the risk of stroke. This has led to warnings specifically about the use of olanzapine and risperidone, but the evidence suggests that any such risk is shared by all antipsychotics (Gill *et al.*, 2005).
2. Antipsychotics can precipitate an irreversible and sometimes fatal syndrome of parkinsonism, inpaired consciousness and autonomic disturbance, notably in patients with dementia with Lewy bodies (McKeith *et al.*, 2004).
3. Antipsychotics may hasten cognitive decline (McShane *et al.*, 1997), an observation confirmed in a randomized trial of quetiapine (Ballard *et al.*, 2005). The mechanism is unknown, but may relate to antimuscarinic actions. The latter study also found that the drug was ineffective in treatment of agitation.

Current British guidelines recommend that antipsychotics should not be used in dementia unless the patient's problems are severe, associated either with psychotic symptoms or serious distresss, or if the behaviour poses a danger of physical harm. Restrictions are also in force in the USA to limit antipsychotic use in nursing homes. Antipsychotics should be used rarely, if ever, in dementia with Lewy bodies. Assessment for vascular risk factors is advised because of the risk of stroke. Treatment should start with a low dose, which is increased slowly, and the effects monitored regularly. As there is no evidence of differential efficacy, the choice of antipsychotic should be based on the side-effect risk profile, with particular attention to extrapyramidal and anticholinergic effects and sedation.

Cholinesterase inhibitors

Cholinesterase inhibitors were developed to treat the cognitive symptoms of Alzheimer's disease. They have become widely used to treat behavioural problems and psychological symptoms too, in part because of the increasing concern surrounding antipsychotics. However, it is unclear whether they are effective against these aspects of dementia. A meta-analysis showed statistically significant but very small benefits (Trinh *et al.*, 2003), and subsequent trials (Ballard *et al.*, 2005) and reviews (Anonymous, 2003a) have drawn negative conclusions.

Other drugs

One randomized trial has shown efficacy for carbamazepine against agitation and aggression (Tariot *et al.*, 1998). Antidepressants are effective against depression in dementia, with SSRIs and trazodone being commonly used. Anxiolytics should not normally be used in dementia because of the risks of sedation, falls, and tolerance. There is no good evidence regarding valproic acid or memantine.

Drug treatment of Alzheimer's disease

Treatment of behavioural and cognitive symptoms continues to be the most important element of therapy of dementia. However, in recent years, the first drugs intended to treat dementia itself have emerged, with the advent of cholinesterase inhibitors for Alzheimer's disease. Other treatments for this disease, and for other dementias, are also being developed. For review, see Cummings (2004).

Cholinesterase inhibitors

A loss of acetyl choline was the first substantial neurochemical feature of Alzheimer's disease to be discovered (p. 339) and led to the development of cholinesterase inhibitors as the first effective treatments for the disease. Although their efficacy is limited and they do not alter the disease process, they have an important role in clinical practice and their discovery was responsible for bringing a new therapeutic optimism to the field. They work by increasing the survival and thence availability of acetyl choline at the synapse; some may also enhance activity at nicotinic cholinergic receptors.

The first cholinesterase inhibitor was tacrine, but its use was limited by hepatotoxicity. The currently available drugs are donepezil, rivastigmine, and galantamine. All received regulatory approval, for use in mild to moderate Alzheimer's disease, based upon trial data showing benefits, relative to placebo, on cognitive function (usually measured on the cognitive portion of the Alzheimer's Disease Assessment Scale (ADAS-Cog) and upon global functioning (assessed with the Clinician Interview-Based Impression of Change scale with carer input; CIBIC-Plus). The efficacy of the three drugs is similar, but there are no head-to-head comparisons. The size of effect is relatively modest. For example, benefits of about 3 points on the ADAS-Cog (range of scores, 0–70), and 0.4 on CIBIC-Plus (range of scores, 1–7). As disease progression averages about 7 points on the ADAS-Cog per year, cholinesterase inhibitors may be viewed as delaying progression by about six months. Expressed another way, the drugs roughly double the chances of a patient improving by four ADAS-Cog points. Whether these effects translate into better functioning in daily living activities is unclear.

Side-effects are relatively common and can be troublesome. They include nausea, vomiting, diarrhoea, muscle cramps, insomnia, bradycardia, syncope, and fatigue. Their occurrence can be reduced by starting with a low dose, taking the drug with meals, and increasing dose slowly.

Treatment should be instituted by a specialist (usually old age psychiatrist, or neurologist or geriatrician), following a formal assessment of the patient, from which the diagnosis of Alzheimer's disease is made, and its severity established, with a minimum MMSE score of 12. The response should be assessed 2–4 months later, and the drug continued only if the MMSE score has not declined, together with evidence of global or behavioural improvement. In those who show this initial response, the drug should continue as long as the MMSE score remains above 12, taking into account the patient's overall condition and global functioning. Decisions to stop medication are complicated by the possibility that this is followed by an accelerated cognitive decline, such that within months the patient returns to the expected level of functioning had treatment never occurred.

The current status of cholinesterase inhibitors in the treatment of Alzheimer's disease remains controversial. Advocates emphasize the unequivocal evidence of efficacy, the anecdotal evidence for more substantial benefits in some patients, and carers and charities are vocal in their support. Reflecting these positive views, use of cholinesterase inhibitors is considered a standard of care in American practice guidelines (Doody *et al.*, 2001), and supported in the UK (National Institute for Clinical Excellence, 2001). Trials showing efficacy at earlier stages of the illness (Seltzer *et al.*, 2004) strengthen this view. However, others are much more cautious, noting that the size of effect of cholinesterase inhibitors is small to moderate (Rockwood, 2004), and their practical effectiveness and cost-effectiveness remain under debate (AD2000 Collaborative Group, 2004). At the time of writing, the concern about cost-effectiveness has led to renewed debate in the UK as to whether cholinesterase inhibitors will continue to funded on the National Health Service.

Memantine

The only other drug currently licensed for treatment of Alzheimer's disease is memantine, which is a NMDA glutamate receptor antagonist. The rationale is that neurotoxicity caused by excess glutamate transmission through the NMDA receptor might contribute to the disease process.

In a 28-week randomized controlled trial of 252 patients, Reisberg *et al.* (2003) showed that memantine has modest cognitive benefits, as rated by clinician and carer, compared to placebo in moderate to severe Alzheimer's disease (MMSE score at entry of 3–14). Memantine may therefore have a role at a more advanced stage of the illness than cholinesterase inhibitors. However, the effectiveness and cost-effectiveness of memantine in clinical practice remain to be established (Anonymous, 2003b), and it cannot be prescribed on the British NHS.

Ginkgo biloba

Extracts from the leaves of the maidenhair tree, *Gingko biloba*, have long been used in China as a remedy for various diseases. The herb has also been advocated for, and trialled in, Alzheimer's disease and other dementias. Current data show that its effects are minimal, and the evidence is less consistent than for cholinesterase inhibitors; the herb is, however, well tolerated (Kurz and Van Baelen, 2004).

Novel treatment approaches

Treatments under development are intended to modify the disease process, and thus produce greater and more persistent benefits than current drugs (Citron, 2004).

Targeting β-amyloid

The increasing evidence that β-amyloid is central to the Alzheimer's disease process (p. 338) has led to this molecule and its biochemical pathways becoming the key treatment targets (Hardy and Selkoe, 2002). Three main approaches are being used:

- Drugs to inhibit the enzymes ('secretases') by which β-amyloid is formed from its precursor molecule.
- Drugs to prevent aggregation of β-amyloid.
- Immunization strategies in which either β-amyloid, or antibodies against it, are used to vaccinate patients with – or, potentially, those at risk of – Alzheimer's disease (Dodel *et al.*, 2003). This approach arose from unexpected findings in a mouse model of the disease, discussed in Box 14.1, p. 337 (Schenk *et al.*, 1999). There is preliminary evidence of efficacy from a clinical trial and neuropathological case reports, but the trial had to be halted because encephalitis developed in some subjects (Bennett and Holtzmann, 2005). Further studies using different vaccines are underway. If successful, the ramifications will be considerable not just for the psychiatry of old age, but for society.

Other strategies

As discussed in Chapter 14, exposure to hormone replacement therapy, non-steroidal anti-inflammatories, and statins, has been associated with lower rates of Alzheimer's disease (p. 338). Each of these drugs has therefore been used to treat the condition, but without benefit (Launer, 2003; Citron, 2004). Based on the evidence that homocysteine is a risk factor for Alzheimer's disease, trials of folate supplementation are also underway. Other targets include tau and its phosphorylation (p. 337).

Drug treatment of other dementias

There are no drugs currently licensed for any other common dementia. However, several of the approaches being used in Alzheimer's disease are also being applied in these disorders.

Vascular dementia

Few randomized trials exist for treatment or prevention of vascular dementia. Existing data suggest some efficacy of cholinesterase inhibitors; this is probably due to ischaemic damage to cholinergic neurons rather than the unintentional inclusion of patients with Alzheimer's disease or mixed dementia (Erkinjuntti *et al.*, 2004). Non-cholinergic drugs, notably vasodilators and anti-hypertensives, have a strong theoretical rationale in vascular dementia, but there is no good evidence of efficacy in treatment or prevention (Pantoni, 2004).

Dementia with Lewy bodies

Cholinergic deficits are at least as pronounced in this dementia as in Alzheimer's disease, and there is considerable, albeit largely anecdotal, evidence that cholinesterase inhibitors are correspondingly effective (Simard and van Reekum, 2004). Their efficacy may extend to some of the behavioural and psychological symptoms (Wild *et al.*, 2003), and to the dementia of Parkinson's disease (Emre *et al.*, 2004).

Frontotemporal dementia

There have been no fully published drug trials of frontotemporal dementia. Preliminary data suggest the antidepressant trazodone, which blocks 5-HT2 receptors, may have some benefits for the behavioural disturbance (Pasquier *et al.*, 2003). Cholinesterase inhibitors are unlikely to be useful as cholinergic deficits are not a prominent feature.

Prion disease

Various drugs and immunization strategies are under investigation (Mallucci and Collinge, 2005), stimulated by the emergence of variant CJD (p. 344). The antimalarial drug quinacrine is currently being trialled, and some patients are receiving intraventricular injections of the anticoagulant pentosan polyphosphate; at present there is no evidence that either is effective.

Huntington's disease

Treatments under investigation include minocycline (a tetracyline with neuroprotective properties), antibodies, cell grafting, and gene therapy (Hersch, 2003).

Mood disorder in the elderly

Depressive disorder

Clinical features

There is no clear distinction between the clinical features of depressive disorders in the elderly and those in younger people, but some symptoms are more striking in the elderly. Post (1972) reported that a third of depressed elderly patients had severe retardation and agitation. Depressive delusions concerning poverty and physical illness are common, and occasionally there are nihilistic delusions such as beliefs that the body is empty, non-existent, or not functioning (see Cotard's syndrome, p. 221). Hallucinations of an accusing or obscene kind may occur. Depression itself is sometimes not conspicuous and may be masked by other symptoms, particularly hypochondriacal complaints. Depressive disorder in the elderly should always be considered when the patient presents with anxiety, hypochondriasis, or confusion. For a review, see Alexopoulos (2005).

Depressive pseudodementia

Some retarded depressed patients present with pseudodementia, i.e. they have conspicuous difficulty in concentration and remembering, but careful clinical testing shows that there is no major defect of memory. Differentiation of these patients from those with early dementia (in whom depression may occur) is important and can be difficult. Pointers suggestive of depressive pseudodementia include:

- The patient's complaint of memory disturbance tends to be greater than the informant's account of memory problems in everyday life.
- Depressive symptoms that predated the memory difficulties.
- 'Don't know' responses and poor involvement with neuropsychological tests are characteristic.
- A personal or family history of mood disorder.

Aetiology

In general, the aetiology of depressive disorders of first onset in late life almost certainly resembles the aetiology of similar disorders at younger ages, with biological

(Krishnan, 2002) psychological and social influences (Blazer and Hybels, 2005).

Twin studies show a moderate heritability in both men and women, comparable to but somewhat lower than that for depression of early onset, suggesting a slightly smaller genetic contribution (Johnson *et al.*, 2002), and consistent with less familial aggregation (Maier *et al.*, 1991).

It might be expected that the loneliness and hardship of old age would be important predisposing factors for depressive disorder. Surprisingly, there is no convincing evidence for such an association (Murphy, 1982). Indeed, Parkes *et al.* (1969) even found that the association between bereavement and mental illness no longer held in the aged.

Vascular depression

A role for vascular factors in depression in the elderly was noted by Post (1972) and has become the prominent hypothesis since Alexopoulos *et al.* (1997) coined the term 'vascular depression'. There is now strong and diverse evidence for a multifaceted and bidirectional relationship between late-life depression and vascular disease and its risk factors (Thomas *et al.*, 2004). The evidence is both epidemiological and biological. The latter includes findings that the neuropathological basis of the white matter hyperintensities seen frequently in late-life depression on MRI scans reflects focal areas of ischaemia and infarction.

It is unclear whether 'vascular depression' is a discrete subgroup, or whether vascular factors are part of the biological contribution to depression in the elderly in general (Baldwin, 2005). There is some suggestion that the presence of vascular risk factors is associated with poorer treatment response, more cognitive impairment, and poorer outcome (Baldwin *et al.*, 2004).

Differential diagnosis

As noted above, it is sometimes difficult to distinguish between depressive pseudodementia and dementia, a problem compounded by the fact that depression may occur during the course of dementia. It is essential to obtain a detailed history from other informants and to make careful observations of mental state and behaviour using the differentiating features listed on p. 511. Psychological testing can be a useful adjunct, but it requires experienced interpretation and it usually adds little to skilful clinical assessment. At times, dementia and depressive illness coexist. If there is real doubt, a trial of antidepressant treatment may be appropriate.

The possibility that a mood disorder is secondary to physical disease or drugs must always be considered in the elderly, given the frequent coexistence of such conditions and widespread use of medication.

Less frequently, depressive disorder has to be differentiated from a non-affective psychotic disorder, such as a delusional disorder. When persecutory ideas occur in a depressive disorder, the patient usually believes that the supposed persecution is justified by his wickedness.

Course and prognosis

In a classic study, Post (1972) described that depression in the elderly follows the rule of threes: a third recover, a third remain the same, a third deteriorate and become 'chronic invalids'. More recent studies have generally found a similar, if not poorer, outcome (Cole *et al.*, 1999). For example, in a 6 year longitudinal study of 277 elderly depressed people, Beekman *et al.* (2002) found that 32 per cent had a severe, chronic course, 44 per cent had a fluctuating course, and only 23 per cent achieved substantial remissions. Even the 'subthreshold' group, noted above, tended to have a poor outcome. The natural history of depression in old age has implications for its management (see below).

Factors said to predict a good prognosis for depression in old age are:

- Onset before the age of 70.
- Short duration of illness.
- Good previous adjustment.
- Absence of disabling physical illness.
- Good recovery from previous episodes.
- Religiosity (self-reported faith, or belonging to religious group).

Poor outcome is associated with the severity of the initial illness, presence of organic cerebral pathology, poor compliance with treatment, and severe life events in the follow-up period. As discussed in Chapter 17, the risk of suicide remains high in elderly people with depression, especially men (Jacoby, 2000a).

Despite the evidence that a history of depression is a risk factor for dementia, there is no evidence that late-life depression is a prodrome of dementia (Schweitzer *et al.*, 2002), and there is no shared genetic predisposition (Heun *et al.*, 2001).

Treatment

The principles of the treatment of depressive disorder are the same as for younger adults, as described in Chapter 11. Effective treatments thus exist, but they are often not implemented, both because cases are not diagnosed and because the interventions are not provided (Chew-Graham *et al.*, 2004). Guidelines for the management of late-life depression in primary care have been produced (Baldwin *et al.*, 2003). With elderly patients it is especially important to be aware of the risk of suicide. Any intercurrent physical disorder should be thoroughly treated.

Antidepressants appear to be as effective as in younger people (Katona and Livingston, 2002), although there are few data (Taylor and Doraiswamy, 2004). The drugs should be used cautiously, perhaps starting with half the normal dosage and increasing this slowly in relation to side-effects and response. SSRIs are generally preferred to tricyclics because of their lower propensity for side-effects and cardiotoxicity. Potential interactions with other drugs being taken by the patient must also be noted, and may influence the choice of antidepressant (Spina and Scordo, 2002). For patients who do not respond to the maximum tolerated dose of an antidepressant, it may be necessary to use a combination of drugs as in younger patients, or to combine medication with psychological treatment.

As with medication, psychological interventions show similar efficacy in the elderly, and are often preferred by patients, but are of very limited availability in primary care, where over 90 per cent of cases are managed (Thompson *et al.*, 1987). There is increasing evidence that, within this setting, outcome is improved by models of collaborative care in which specialists provide some input, and care is supplemented by education about depression and medication (Unützer *et al.*, 2002).

ECT is appropriate for depressive disorder with severe and distressing agitation, suicidal ideas and behaviour, life-threatening stupor, or failure to respond to drugs. Concerns that ECT is dangerous, or ineffective, in elderly subjects are unwarranted, and it should be used with a similar threshold as in younger patients (p. 565), albeit sometimes at a lower frequency. If a patient has previously responded to antidepressants or ECT, but does not respond in the present episode, undetected physical illness should be sought as a cause.

After recovery, full-dosage antidepressant medication should be continued for at least several months, as in younger patients, although the evidence suggests that in older people treatment should continue for considerably longer, and possibly permanently (Old Age Depression Interest Group, 1993).

Bipolar disorder

Broadhead and Jacoby (1990), in the first prospective study of mania in old age, found that the clinical picture was the same as in younger patients but that a depressive episode, immediately after the manic episode occurs more frequently. Mixed affective episodes may be somewhat commoner than in younger subjects, and organic factors play a greater role (Depp and Jeste, 2004). Aetiological factors have been reviewed by Krishhan (2002).

Management of bipolar disorder in the elderly follows the principles described in Chapter 11. Lithium prophylaxis is valuable, but the blood levels should be monitored with special care and kept at the lower end of the therapeutic range (0.4–0.6 mmol/l). See Shulman (2002) for a review.

Anxiety disorders in the elderly

In later life, anxiety and emotional disorders are seldom causes for referral to a psychiatrist, although this may be largely because of non-presentation by patients and lack of recognition or referral by general practitioners. It does not reflect their rarity in the population, as shown by the high rates seen in the study of Ritchie *et al.* (2004), and it is now recognized that anxiety disorders in the elderly are clinically more important than previously acknowledged. On the other hand, the possibility that anxiety symptoms are secondary to an underlying depressive episode should always be actively considered before the diagnosis is made.

Symptoms of anxiety disorders among the elderly are often non-specific, with features of both anxiety and depression. Hypochondriacal symptoms may be prominent (Lindesay, 2000).

Personality disorder is a predisposing factor, whilst physical illness and life events such as retirement or change of accommodation may act as precipitants. A first onset of panic attacks in an elderly person should always prompt a search for an underlying physical or depressive disorder (Flint and Gagnon, 2003).

The approach to treatment is similar to that of anxiety disorders in younger adults (Alwahhabi, 2003; Flint and Gagnon, 2003), with a preference for psychological and behavioural interventions, and with cautious use of medication.

Schizophrenia-like disorders in the elderly

Schizophrenia usually begins in early adulthood or middle age (Chapter 12), but new onset cases after age 60, though rare, are well recognized. This section concentrates on the features that characterize such cases compared to schizophrenia of younger onset. It also highlights some issues affecting the management of all patients with schizophrenia as they become elderly.

The complicated terminology in this area has been covered previously, and its existence reflects the long-standing view that these cases are, to some extent, clinically different from earlier onset cases (Box 13.2, and p. 499). However, there is no evidence that age of onset separates schizophrenia into categorically distinct subtypes.

For review of late-onset schizophrenia, see Howard *et al.* (2000) and Tune and Salzman (2003).

Clinical features

Although the core symptoms and overall clinical profile is very similar to those of younger onset cases, the relative prominence of some features does differ (Table 20.10); of these, the extreme rarity of thought disorder and negative symptoms is the most striking.

Neuropsychologically, a similar generalized cognitive impairment is seen regardless of age of onset, but late-onset cases show somewhat milder deficits, especially in working and verbal memory. This profile contrasts with the marked decline in intellectual performance and development of moderate to severe dementia which occurs in a significant minority of elderly patients whose illness began earlier in life (Harvey, 2001; see p. 272).

TABLE 20.10 Features characteristic of late-onset compared to early-onset schizophrenia

Symptoms which are commoner
◆ Visual, tactile and olfactory hallucinations
◆ Third person, running commentary, and derogatory auditory hallucinations
◆ Persecutory delusions
◆ Partition delusions
Symptoms which are less common
◆ Formal thought disorder
◆ Affective flattening
◆ Affective blunting
◆ Negative symptoms
Other features
◆ Female predominance
◆ No clear genetic loading
◆ Association with sensory deficits and social isolation
◆ Less premorbid educational and psychosocial impairment
◆ Less working memory and verbal learning impairment
◆ Much lower antipsychotic doses required

Adapted from Howard *et al.* (2000).

Course and prognosis

There are no contemporary data on the course or outcome of schizophrenia with onset in old age. There is no good evidence that it heralds or progresses to dementia.

Differential diagnosis

Compared to younger-onset schizophrenia, there is a greater likelihood that an elderly patient presenting with psychotic symptoms has an organic psychosis of some kind. Thus, all elderly patients presenting with a first onset of schizophrenia-like features should be assessed carefully to exclude a delirium, dementia, or organic psychosis due to a neurological or medical disorder such as neurosyphilis, HIV, or neoplasm. As in younger patients, schizophrenia must also be distinguished from other psychiatric disorders in which psychotic symptoms occur, notably delusional disorder or affective psychosis. Such distinctions may be particularly difficult if the patient presents with persecutory beliefs but no other clear symptoms, and if there is a history suggestive of paranoid personality traits. For those in whom visual hallucinations are an isolated symptom, consider Charles Bonnet syndrome (p. 515).

Aetiology

Familial aggregation is much less common than in earlier onset schizophrenia, suggestive of a smaller genetic predisposition. There is no familial association with neurodegenerative or cerebrovascular disorders. Brain imaging changes are similar in nature and magnitude to those described in younger onset schizophrenia. Unlike late-life depression, rates of white matter hyperintensities are not increased. A role for sex hormones in the aetiology of late-onset schizophrenia has been proposed (Seeman, 1997), based upon the female predominance, but there is little direct evidence. Schizoid or paranoid personality traits are common in elderly people who develop late-onset psychotic disorders (Kay *et al.*, 1976).

Treatment

Antipsychotic medication is the mainstay of treatment of late onset schizophrenia, as in younger cases. However, much lower doses (10–20 per cent of a 'normal' dose) are often sufficient; this is not just a reflection of age of the patient, since higher doses are typically needed for earlier onset cases when they reach the same age. Another reason for cautious use of antipsychotic medication is that the risk of tardive dyskinesia appears to be considerably greater than in younger patients (Jeste *et al.*, 1995), though this may be independent of age at onset of illness. Atypical antipsychotics probably have a lower tardive dyskinesia risk than do typical antispsychotics in this age group, but recent concerns that they may increase cerebrovascular events in the elderly must be taken into account (p. 509). Cognitive and other psychological interventions may reduce disability, as in earlier-onset cases, although there is little direct evidence (Schimming and Harvey, 2004).

Management of schizophrenia in the elderly must also pay due attention to the complex medical and social needs of many patients; services are often fragmentary and inadequate, in part because of the emphasis on younger subjects (Cohen *et al.*, 2000).

Personality disorder in the elderly

As discussed in Chapter 7, some personality traits and disorders attenuate with age, whilst others remain or become exaggerated. A meta-analysis found that the prevalence of personality disorder in the over 50s was 7–10 per cent (Abrams and Horowitz, 1996), somewhat lower than in younger adults. The decline is mostly attributable to a decline in cluster B personality disorders (Cohen *et al.*, 1994), whereas obsessive-compulsive and schizoid characteristics may become more prominent (Engels *et al.*, 2003). Schizoid or paranoid traits may become accentuated by the social isolation of old age, sometimes to the extent of being mistaken for a delusional disorder or schizophrenia. Criminal behaviour is unusual, with only 1.7 per cent of men in England and Wales who are found guilty of indictable offences being aged 60 or older (Fazel *et al.* 2001).

Personality disorder is often comorbid in elderly subjects with depression and other psychiatric disorders (Devenand, 2002) and, as in younger patients, likely to be associated with a poorer prognosis. Personality disorder may also be a risk factor for late-life depression (Abrams *et al.*, 1987).

For review of personality disorder in the elderly, see Holroyd (2000).

Other psychiatric syndromes of the elderly

Senile squalor syndrome

The **senile squalor syndrome** is also known as **Diogenes' syndrome** (Clark *et al.*, 1975). It is characterized by severe neglect of self and surroundings, domestic squalor and social withdrawal and isolation. **Syllogomania** (the hoarding of rubbish) also occurs. It may be precipitated by stressful life events, and is associated with a high mortality after hospital admission. Other causes of self-neglect must be excluded, notably dementia, psychosis or severe depression. The person usually stubbornly refuses all offers of help, and it is difficult to decide when to intervene using compulsory powers.

For review, see Reyes-Ortiz (2001).

Charles Bonnet syndrome

Charles Bonnet syndrome refers to the occurrence of visual hallucinations without any other features of psychosis, dementia, or delirium. The syndrome is important, since misdiagnoses, especially of psychosis, resulting in inappropriate treatments, have been reported. It is named after a Swiss philosopher who described the case of his own grandfather in 1760.

The syndrome is particularly common in elderly people with failing eyesight, in whom there is a prevalence of 10–15 per cent. It is said to occur in up to 3.5 per cent of referrals to old age psychiatrists.

The visual hallucinations are well formed, elaborate, vivid, and perceived in external space. They may be transient or persistent, and either variable in content or stereotyped. They have no personal meaning for the patient. Although they meet most of the criteria for true hallucinations (pp. 6–7), the patient usually retains some insight into their unreality, and can often make the image disappear by closing their eyes.

The condition tends to improve if vision is restored, or when total blindness occurs. There is no specific treatment. It has been suggested that the syndrome may be an early indication of dementia, but this is unproven.

For review, see Jacob *et al.* (2004).

Further reading

Gelder MG, Lopez-Ibor JJ, Andreasen NC (eds) (2000) *The new Oxford textbook of psychiatry*, Section 8: The psychiatry of old age. Oxford, Oxford University Press.

Jacoby R, Oppenheimer C (2002) *Psychiatry in the elderly*, 3rd edn. Oxford, Oxford University Press. (Definitive textbook.)

CHAPTER 21

Drugs and other physical treatments

Chapter contents

This chapter is concerned with the use of drugs and other physical treatments such as electroconvulsive therapy and neurosurgical procedures. Psychological treatments are the subject of Chapter 22. This separation, although convenient when treatments are described, does not imply that the two kinds of therapy are to be thought of as exclusive alternatives when an individual patient is considered; on the contrary, many patients require both. In this book, the ways of combining treatments are considered in other chapters where the treatment of individual syndromes is discussed. It is important to keep this point in mind when reading this chapter and the next.

Our concern is with clinical therapeutics rather than basic psychopharmacology, which the reader is assumed to have studied already. An adequate knowledge of the mechanisms of drug action is essential if drugs are to be used in a rational way, but a word of caution is appropriate. The clinician should not assume that the therapeutic effects of psychotropic drugs are necessarily explained by the pharmacological actions that have been discovered so far. For example, substantial delay in the effects of antidepressant and antipsychotic drugs suggests that their actions on transmitters, which occur rapidly, are only the first steps in a chain of biochemical changes.

This caution does not imply that a knowledge of pharmacological mechanisms has no bearing on psychiatric therapeutics. On the contrary, there have been substantial advances in pharmacological knowledge since the first psychotropic drugs were introduced in the 1950s, and it is increasingly important for the clinician to relate this knowledge to his use of drugs.

History of physical treatments

Physical treatments have been applied to patients with psychiatric disorders since antiquity, though, in retrospect, the most that could be claimed for the best of these interventions is that they were relatively harmless. Of course, the same holds for the management of patients with general medical disorders, for which similar treatments, such as bleeding and purging, were often used regardless of diagnosis. It is wise not to be too censorious about the treatment of disorders of which the aetiology is still largely unknown, but to bear in mind that 'it may well be that in a hundred years current therapies, psychotherapies as well as physical therapies, will be looked upon as similarly uncouth and improbable' (Kiloh *et al.*, 1988).

Historically, physical treatments can be divided into two main classes:

- those that were aimed at producing a direct change in a pathophysiological process, usually by some alteration in brain function;
- those that were aimed at producing symptomatic improvement through a dramatic psychological impact.

The latter interventions were often based on philosophical theories about the moral basis of madness. For example, many physicians appear to have followed the proposal of Heinroth (1773–1843) that insanity was the product of evil and personal wrongdoing. Accordingly, restraint with chains and corporal punishment were seen as appropriate remedies. Other physical treatments, such as the spinning chair introduced by Erasmus Darwin (1731–1802), seemed designed to produce a general 'shock to the system', and perhaps thereby interrupt the morbid preoccupations of the patient. A less arduous regimen was the use of continuous warm baths, often given in combination with cold packs. This treatment was recommended by clinicians as distinguished as Connolly (1794–1866) and Kraepelin (1856–1926), and was still in use at the Bethlem Hospital in the 1950s.

Drugs that produce changes in the function of the central nervous system, such as opiates and anticholinergic agents, have been used in the treatment of mental disorders for hundreds of years. Whilst some of these drugs may sometimes have had calming effects, they were of no specific value in the treatment of psychiatric disorders. Often a physical treatment was used, not because of proven efficacy, but because it was recommended by an eminent and vigorous physician. Also, the assessment of efficacy depended almost entirely on uncontrolled clinical observation.

In 1933, about 10 years after the isolation of insulin by Banting and Best, Sakel introduced **insulin coma treatment** for psychosis (Sakel, 1938). A suitable dose of insulin was used to produce a coma, which was terminated by either tube feeding or intravenous glucose. A course of treatment could include up to 60 comas. Not surprisingly, serious side-effects were common, and a mortality of at least 1 per cent could be expected depending on the standard of the clinic and on the physical state of the patient. Insulin coma treatment was rapidly taken up throughout Europe and many specialized treatment units were built. There was a great improvement in the morale of patients and staff because of the belief that this dramatic treatment could cure symptoms of some of the most serious psychiatric disorders.

There were always some practitioners who doubted the efficacy of insulin coma treatment. Their doubts were reinforced by a controlled trial by Ackner and Oldham (1962), who found that, in patients with schizophrenia, insulin coma was no more effective than a similar period of unconsciousness induced by barbiturates. This study was published about the time when chlorpromazine was introduced, and both factors led to a rapid decline in the use of insulin coma treatment. It should be noted that the controlled studies did not exclude the efficacy of insulin treatment in some circumstances, and a number of workers continued to maintain that it was effective. Therefore it is interesting that recent experimental studies have shown that insulin administration causes striking changes in the release of monoamine neurotransmitters in the brain. Perhaps the main lesson to be learned from insulin coma treatment is that the introduction of a new medical treatment should be preceded by adequate controlled trials to determine whether it is therapeutically more effective or safer than current therapies (see Chapter 6). This lesson is particularly important in psychiatry because the aetiology of some disorders may be obscure and outcome may vary widely, even amongst patients with the same clinical syndrome.

Electroconvulsive therapy (ECT) was introduced about the same time as insulin coma treatment. Unlike the latter, ECT has retained a place in current clinical practice. The rationale for convulsive therapy was a postulated antagonism between schizophrenia and convulsions such that the one would exclude the other. This view is erroneous in so far as schizophrenia-like illnesses are actually more common in patients with temporal lobe epilepsy than would be expected by chance (see p. 349). Astute clinical observation, in combination with controlled trials, has shown that ECT is effective

BOX 21.1 INTRODUCTION OF SOME PHYSICAL TREATMENTS IN PSYCHIATRY

1934	Insulin coma treatment (Sakel)
1936	Frontal leucotomy (Moniz)
1936	Metrazole convulsive therapy (Meduna)
1938	Electroconvulsive therapy (Cerletti and Bini)
1949	Lithium (Cade)
1952	Chlorpromazine (Delay and Deniker)
1954	Benzodiazepines (Sternbach)
1957	Iproniazid (Crane and Kline)
1957	Imipramine (Kuhn)
1966	Valpromide (valproate) in bipolar disorder (Lambert *et al.*)
1967	Clomipramine in obsessive–compulsive disorder (Fernandez and Lopez-Ibor)
1971	Carbamazepine in bipolar disorder (Takezaki and Hanaoka)
1988	Clozapine in treatment-resistant schizophrenia (Kane *et al.*)
1999	Lamotrigine in bipolar depression (Calabrese *et al.*)

in the acute treatment of severe mood disorders. Thus, even though the rationale for the introduction of ECT was incorrect and its mode of action remains unclear, controlled trials have confirmed that, in carefully defined clinical situations, ECT is a safe and effective treatment (see p. 565).

The action of **lithium** in reducing mania was a chance finding by Cade (1949) who had been investigating the effects of urates in animals and had decided to use the lithium salt because of its solubility. Lithium is a toxic agent, and so Cade's important observations did not make a significant impact on clinical practice until the following decade, when controlled trials showed that lithium was effective in both the acute treatment of mania and the prophylaxis of recurrent mood disorders.

Other agents that revolutionized psychopharmacology were introduced about this time (Box 21.1). Their efficacy and their indications were first recognized through clinical observation, and were subsequently confirmed by controlled clinical trials. None of these agents was introduced on the basis of an aetiological hypothesis. Indeed, such aetiological hypotheses as there are in biological psychiatry have been largely derived from knowledge of the mode of action of effective drugs. Thus the dopamine receptor antagonist properties of antipsychotic drugs have given rise to the dopamine hypothesis of schizophrenia, whilst the action of tricyclic antidepressants and monoamine oxidase inhibitors (MAOIs) in facilitating the effects of noradrenaline and 5-hydroxytryptamine (5-HT) has led to the various monoamine hypotheses of mood disorders.

The last 30 years have brought a period of consolidation in psychopharmacology. Clinical trials have been widely used to refine the indications of particular drug treatments and to maximize their risk:benefit ratios. New compounds have continuously become available but because most have been derived from previously described agents their range of activity is not strikingly different from that of their predecessors. In general, however, the newer agents are better tolerated and sometimes safer – developments which are important for clinical practice.

There may now be grounds for more optimism about the prospects for advances in psychopharmacology. For example, there is rapidly increasing knowledge about chemical signalling in the brain. Numerous neurotransmitters and neuromodulators interact with specific families of receptors, many of which exist in a number of different subtypes. Several of these receptors have been cloned, and selective ligands for them are becoming available. There is increasing knowledge as to how these chemical messengers may modify behaviour through their interactions with specific brain regions and distributed neuronal circuits.

Future compounds developed as consequence of these scientific advances are likely to differ from current drugs in their range of behavioural effects and could lead to important new developments in psychopharmacology. Given the complex causes of psychiatric disorders, it seems likely that detailed knowledge of aetiology and pathophysiology may lag behind advances in therapeutics. Of course, this disparity is not uncommon in general medicine. It serves to reinforce the importance of **randomized clinical trials** in the assessment of new psychopharmacological treatments.

General considerations

The pharmacokinetics of psychotropic drugs

Before psychotropic drugs can produce their therapeutic effects, they must reach the brain in adequate amounts. How far they do so depends on their absorption, metabolism, excretion, and passage across the blood–brain barrier. A short review of these processes is given here. The reader who has not studied them before is referred to the chapter on pharmacokinetics in Grahame-Smith and Aronson (2002). The following processes are important:

- absorption
- distribution
- metabolism
- excretion.

Absorption

In general, psychotropic drugs are easily absorbed from the gut because most are **lipophilic** and are not highly ionized at physiological pH values. Like other drugs, they are absorbed faster from an empty stomach, and in reduced amounts by patients suffering from intestinal hurry or malabsorption syndrome.

Distribution

Psychotropic drugs are distributed in the plasma where most are largely bound to proteins; thus diazepam, and amitriptyline are about 95 per cent bound. They pass easily from the plasma to the brain because they are highly lipophilic. For the same reason, they enter fat stores, from which they are released slowly long after the patient has ceased to take the drug. This means that psychotropic drugs tend to have **large volumes of distribution**.

Metabolism

Most psychotropic drugs are **metabolized in the liver**. This process begins as the drugs pass through the liver in the portal circulation on their way from the gut. This 'first-pass' metabolism reduces the amount of available drug, and is one of the reasons why larger doses are needed when a drug such as chlorpromazine is given by mouth than when it is given intramuscularly. The extent of this liver metabolism differs from one person to another. It is altered by certain other drugs which, if taken at the same time, induce liver enzymes (for example, carbamazepine) or inhibit them (for example, selective serotonin re-uptake inhibitors [SSRIs]).

Some drugs, such as carbamazepine, induce their own metabolism, especially after being taken for a long time. Not all drug metabolites are inactive; for example, fluoxetine is metabolized to a hydroxy derivative, norfluoxetine, which is also a potent 5-HT re-uptake inhibitor. Where drugs give rise to active metabolites, measurements of plasma concentrations of the parent drug alone are a poor guide to therapeutic activity.

Excretion

Psychotropic drugs and their metabolites are excreted mainly through the **kidney**. When kidney function is impaired, excretion is reduced and a lower dose of drug should be given. Lithium is filtered passively and then partly reabsorbed by the same mechanism that absorbs sodium. The two ions compete for this mechanism; hence reabsorption of lithium increases when that of sodium is reduced. Certain fractions of lipophilic drugs such as chlorpromazine are partly excreted in the bile, enter the intestine for the second time, and are then partly reabsorbed, i.e. a proportion of the drug is recycled between intestine and liver.

Measurement of circulating drug concentrations

As a result of individual variations in the mechanisms described above, plasma concentrations after standard doses of psychotropic drugs vary substantially from one patient to another. Tenfold differences have been observed with the antidepressant drug nortriptyline. Therefore it might be expected that measurements of the plasma concentration of circulating drugs would help the clinician. With the exception of lithium, however, this practice is rarely helpful because the plasma drug levels that predict therapeutic response or toxicity within individuals vary so much. Clearly for any drug to work it must be present in plasma above a certain minimum concentration and for some medications 'target' levels have been suggested. However, it is still not unusual for some individuals to show a therapeutic response where plasma levels are lower than recommended.

Pharmacodynamic measures

As an alternative to these assays, it may be possible to measure the pharmacological property, which is thought to be responsible for the therapeutic effect of a particular drug. For example, positron emission tomography can be used to measure directly the degree of brain dopamine receptor blockade produced by antipsychotic drugs during treatment. Such information has proved valuable in designing appropriate dosage regimens of antipsychotic drugs (see Table 21.6). However, these pharmacodynamic measures have not yet been able to identify why some patients do not respond to medication. For example, the degree of dopamine receptor blockade is the same in patients who respond to antipsychotic drugs as in those who do not (Geaney *et al.*, 1992). Pharmacogenetic approaches to prediction of treatment response (Box 21.2) are a topic of current interest (for a review see Staddon *et al.*, 2002).

Plasma half-life

Plasma concentrations of drugs vary throughout the day, rising immediately after the dose and falling at a rate that differs between individual drugs and individual people. The rate at which a drug level declines after a single dose varies from hours with lithium carbonate to weeks with slow-release preparations of

BOX 21.2 PHARMACOGENETICS IN PSYCHIATRY

- Polymorphic (allelic) variation in DNA may result in the production of proteins that interact in different ways with psychotropic drugs
- These polymorphic variations may modify the likelihood of therapeutic response or the development of adverse effects
- Genetic variation in CYP metabolizing enzymes can affect blood levels of drugs and thereby brain exposure. Mutations in the gene for CYP2D6 may be associated with antipsychotic drug-induced tardive dyskinesia
- Alleles associated with decreased expression of 5-HT transporter are associated with poorer response to SSRIs
- Therapeutic response to clozapine may be associated with specific alleles of the 5-HT_{2A} receptor
- Weight gain with antipsychotic drugs is associated with an allele of the 5-HT_{2C} receptor

injectable antipsychotic agents. Knowledge of these differences allows more rational decisions to be made about appropriate intervals between doses.

The concept of **plasma half-life** is useful here. The half-life of a drug in plasma is the time taken for its concentration to fall by a half, once dosing has ceased. With most psychotropic drugs, the amount eliminated over time is proportional to plasma concentration and in this case it will take approximately five times the half-life for the drug to be eliminated from plasma. Equally, when dosing with a drug begins, it will take five times the half-life for the concentration in plasma to reach steady state. This can be important when planning treatment. For example, MAOIs should not be given with SSRIs. Therefore if a patient is taking sertraline, which has an elimination half-life of about 26 hours, it will be important to leave at least five times the half-life (a week is recommended) before starting MAOI treatment. When sertraline treatment begins, the plasma concentrations will continue to rise for about a week before reaching a steady state.

Drug interactions

When two psychotropic drugs are given together, one may interfere with or enhance the actions of the other. Interference may arise through alterations in absorption, binding, metabolism, or excretion (**pharmacokinetic interactions**), or by interaction between the pharmacological mechanisms of action (**pharmacodynamic interactions**).

Pharmacokinetic interactions

Interactions affecting **drug absorption** are seldom important for psychotropic drugs, although it is worth noting that absorption of chlorpromazine is reduced by antacids. Interactions due to **protein binding** are also uncommon, although the chloral metabolite trichloroacetic acid may displace warfarin from albumin. Interactions affecting **drug metabolism** are of considerable importance. Examples include the inhibition of the metabolism of antipsychotic drugs by SSRIs and the stimulation of the metabolism of tricyclic antidepressants by carbamazepine, which induces the relevant **cytochrome P450 enzymes** (see below). Interactions affecting **renal excretion** are mainly important for lithium, the elimination of which is decreased by thiazide diuretics.

Cytochrome P450 enzymes There have been significant developments in the understanding of the microsomal cytochrome P450 enzyme system. These enzymes are located mainly in the liver but also in other tissues including gut wall and brain. Their role is to detoxify exogenous substances such as drugs and their activity can be increased or decreased by concomitant drug administration. This can give rise to clinically important drug interactions (Grahame-Smith and Aronson, 2002). Importantly, several new antidepressants, particularly selective SSRIs, potently inhibit P450 enzymes (see Table 21.11).

Pharmacodynamic interactions

Pharmacodynamic interactions are exemplified by the serotonin syndrome in which drugs that potentiate brain 5-HT function by different mechanisms (for example, SSRIs and MAOIs) can combine to produce dangerous 5-HT toxicity (see p. 550).

As a rule, a single drug can be used to produce all the effects required of a combination; for example, many antidepressant drugs have useful anti-anxiety effects. It is desirable to avoid combinations of psychotropic drugs whenever possible; if a combination is to be used, it is essential to know about possible interactions. The *British National Formulary* provides a useful guide.

Drug withdrawal

Many psychotropic drugs do not achieve useful therapeutic effects for several days or even weeks. After drugs have been stopped, there is often a comparable delay before their effects are lost. Psychotropic and, indeed, many other classes of drugs produce neuroadaptive changes during repeated administration. Tissues therefore have to readjust when drug treatment is stopped; this readjustment may appear clinically as a **withdrawal or abstinence syndrome**. Characteristic abstinence syndromes have been described for antidepressants, antipsychotics and anxiolytics while sudden discontinuation of lithium can provoke a 'rebound' mania. It is important to be able to distinguish withdrawal syndromes from relapse of the disorder being treated. In addition, the risk of abstinence symptoms makes it prudent to withdraw psychotropic drugs slowly wherever possible.

General advice about prescribing

Use well-tried drugs

It is good practice to use well-tried drugs with therapeutic actions and side-effects that are thoroughly understood. The clinician should become familiar with a small number of drugs from each of the main classes. In this way he can become used to adjusting the dosage and recognizing side-effects. Well-tried drugs are usually less expensive than new preparations.

Give an adequate dose

Having chosen a suitable drug, the doctor should prescribe it in **adequate doses**. He should not change the drug or add others without a good reason. In general, if there is no therapeutic response to one established drug, there is no likelihood of a better response to another that has very similar pharmacological properties (provided that the first drug has been taken in adequate amounts). However, since the main obstacle to adequate dosage is usually side-effects, it may be appropriate to change to a drug with a different pattern of side-effects – for example, from a tricyclic antidepressant to an SSRI or vice versa.

Use drug combinations cautiously

Occasionally, combinations of psychotropic drugs are given deliberately in the hope of producing interactions that will be more potent than the effects of either drug taken alone in full dosage (for example, a tricyclic antidepressant with a MAOI). This practice, if it is to be used, is best carried out by experienced psychiatrists (or under their guidance) because the adverse effects of combinations are less easy to predict than those of single drugs.

Dosing and treatment duration

When a drug is prescribed, it is necessary to determine the dose, the interval between doses, and the likely duration of treatment. The dose ranges for commonly used drugs are indicated later in this chapter. Ranges for others will be found in the manufacturers' literature, the *British National Formulary*, or a comparable work of reference. Within the therapeutic range, the correct dose for an individual patient should be decided after considering the severity of symptoms, the patient's age, and weight, and any factors that may affect drug metabolism (for example, other drugs being taken or renal disease).

Next, the interval between doses must be decided. Psychotropic drugs have often been given three times a day, even though their duration of action is such that most can be taken once or twice a day without any undesirable fall in plasma concentrations between doses. Less frequent administration has the advantage that outpatients are more likely to be reliable in taking drugs. In hospital, less frequent drug rounds mean that nurses have more time for psychological aspects of treatment. Some drugs, such as anxiolytics, are required for immediate effect rather than continuous action; they should not be given at regular intervals but shortly before occasions on which symptoms are expected to be at their worse. The duration of treatment depends on the disorder under treatment; it is considered in the chapter dealing with the clinical syndrome.

What patients want to know

Psychotropic drugs have the aim of changing what people think and feel; not surprisingly many patients have misgivings about taking them. It is therefore important to make clear what the drug is being used for, what therapeutic effects are expected and when they should start to appear. Other key questions that must be dealt with are:

- What effects will I experience on first taking the drug?
- What side-effects can I expect?
- What serious side-effects should I report immediately?
- For how long should I take the drug?
- Is the drug addictive?
- What will I notice when I stop the drug?

Compliance, concordance, and collaboration

Many patients do not take the drugs prescribed for them. This problem is greater when treating outpatients, but also occurs in hospital where some patients find ways of avoiding drugs administered by nurses.

If patients are to take medication reliably, they must be convinced of the need to take it, free from unfounded fears about its dangers, and be aware of how to take it. Each of these requirements presents particular problems when the patient has a psychiatric disorder. Thus patients with schizophrenia or seriously depressed patients may not be convinced that they are ill or they may not wish to recover. Deluded patients may distrust clinical staff, and hypochondriacal patients may fear dangerous side-effects. Anxious patients often forget the prescribed dosage and frequency of their drugs. Therefore it is not surprising that many psychiatric patients do not take their drugs in the prescribed way. It is important for the clinician to pay attention to this problem. Time spent in discussing the patient's concerns is time well spent, for it often increases compliance with treatment. Written instructions can be a valuable adjunct and are now often included with drug packaging.

The successful and safe use of medication requires an essentially **collaborative** relationship between patient and doctor. Some have proposed that the term **concordance** should therefore be preferred to **compliance**, which carries the implicit assumption that the patient's job is to obey instructions (Mullen, 1997). Whatever the term used, it is clearly important to recognize that the use of drug treatment, particularly in psychiatry, requires a thorough understanding of the **patient's attitude** to both their illness as its treatment.

Ethical aspects of drug prescription

The ethical issues in this complex area have been reviewed by Brown and Pantelis (1999):

1. The basis of ethical prescribing is the practitioner's comprehensive knowledge of risk and benefits of drug therapies. This will be derived from evidence-based approaches where possible.
2. The doctor-patient relationship is the appropriate framework through which this knowledge is communicated to the patient
3. The therapeutic partnership between patient and doctor must lead to true informed consent, which includes the right of competent patients to refuse treatment.

Difficulties arise where the evidence base of treatment is lacking and where there is uncertainty as to what approach to pursue. Here the clinician has the responsibility to advise treatments that would be supported by peer opinion and to use clinical guidelines. The clinician should also support the right of patients to genuinely effective treatment where this is being hindered by cost constraint and other economic factors.

Prescribing for special groups

Children and the elderly

Psychotropic drugs usually lack specific licenses for use in young people and relevant controlled trials are sparse. However, recent advice from the UK Committee on safety of Medicines is that the efficacy of some SSRIs and venlafaxine treatment in depressed adolescents does not outweigh their disadvantages in terms of agitation and suicidal behaviour (see also Whittington *et al.*, 2004). Practitioners need to make themselves aware of local guidelines concerning the use of psychotropic medication in young people and seek specialist advice when in doubt.

Clinical trials of most psychotropic medications often exclude older patients even though conditions such as depression are more common in the elderly. Elderly patients are often sensitive to side-effects of medication and may have impaired renal or hepatic function; for these reasons it is important to start treatment with low doses.

Pregnant women

There are special problems about prescribing psychotropic drugs in pregnancy because of the risk of **teratogenesis**. Information about the teratogenic risk of individual drugs can be obtained from the relevant manufacturer and the *British National Formulary*, although available evidence is often scanty or difficult to interpret. The practitioner and patient have the difficult task of weighing this information against the risk of managing the illness without medication. In addition, a substantial number of pregnancies are unplanned. For this reason, it is prudent where possible to advise women of child-bearing age who require psychotropics specifically to avoid pregnancy until the need for the drug treatment is over (for a review of the use of psychotropic drugs in pregnancy, see Wieck, 2004).

Anxiolytics and antidepressants

Anxiolytic drugs are seldom essential in early pregnancy, and psychological treatments can usually be used. If medication is needed, in general, **benzodiazepines** have not been shown to be teratogenic although one meta-analysis has shown an increased risk of oral clefts after first trimester exposure. If an **antidepressant drug** is required, it is probably better to use long-established preparations such as **imipramine** or **amitriptyline** for which there is no consistent evidence of a teratogenic effect after many years of use. There is also reasonable experience with **fluoxetine**, which does not appear to be associated with an increased risk of major malformations.

Antipsychotic drugs and mood stabilizers

It is seldom necessary to start **antipsychotic drugs** in early pregnancy. There is little evidence that high potency agents such as **haloperidol** carry an increased teratogenic risk. However, there may be a higher rate of congenital malformations in babies exposed to lower potency agents such as **chlorpromazine**. There is little information on the teratogenic risk of newer antipsychotic agents.

Lithium treatment early in pregnancy has been associated with cardiac abnormalities in the fetus, particularly **Ebstein's anomaly**; therefore, women considering pregnancy have been recommended to discontinue lithium before conceiving. Similarly, women who become pregnant whilst taking lithium have usually been advised to stop the treatment. However, recent epidemiological studies have suggested that whilst the relative risk of Ebstein's anomaly is increased at least tenfold in infants exposed to lithium in the first trimester, the absolute risk is still fairly low, **between 0.05–0.1 per cent**. Withdrawal of lithium carries a high risk of relapse in people with bipolar illness and the balance of risk to mother and baby may therefore suggest continuation of lithium treatment during pregnancy in some cases.

Anticonvulsant drugs such as **carbamazepine** and **valproate** are increasingly used as mood stabilizers. However, both these agents are clearly associated with an increased risk of neural tube defects as well as other fetal abnormalities. The neural tube defects associated with anticonvulsant use may be associated with changes in folate metabolism. However, a role for folate treatment in their prevention has not been established.

Neonatal toxicity

Exposure to psychotropic drugs in the later stages of pregnancy can give rise to **neonatal toxicity** either through the presence of the drug or a withdrawal syndrome. For example, it has been reported that among babies born to mothers who have been receiving **tricyclic antidepressants** there may be withdrawal reactions including tremulousness, vomiting, poor feeding, and seizures. Direct anticholinergic effects such as gastrointestinal stasis and bladder distension have also been reported. These reactions, whilst clearly problematic, appear to settle quickly without causing lasting sequelae.

There are also reports that late exposure to SSRIs may be associated with an increased risk of neonatal complications including jitteriness, hypoglycaemia, poor muscle tone, and respiratory difficulties (Sanz *et al.*, 2005). The perinatal toxicity associated with **lithium** use includes 'floppy baby syndrome' with cyanosis and hypotonicity whereas **benzodiazepine** treatment can result in impaired temperature regulation together with breathing and feeding difficulties.

Animal studies suggest that fetal exposure to psychotropic medication can cause **longer-term abnormalities in brain development and behaviour**. Thus far, however, a limited number of human studies have not detected such effects in children followed up for the first few years of life.

Breast-feeding

Psychotropic drugs should be prescribed cautiously to women who are **breast-feeding**. **Diazepam** and other **benzodiazepines** pass readily into breast milk and may cause sedation and hypotonicity in the infant. Antipsychotic drugs and antidepressants also enter breast milk, although rather less readily than diazepam. **Sulpiride**, however, is excreted in significant amounts and should be avoided. **Fluoxetine** and its metabolites could also accumulate, but other SSRIs are present in small amounts and breast-feeding can be permitted while the baby is observed for sedation or feeding difficulties (see Weissman *et al.*, 2004). It is usually advised that mothers should express and discard breast milk that has been exposed to peak plasma plasma levels of the drug concerned.

Lithium salts enter the milk freely, and serum concentrations in the infant can approach those of the mother so that breast-feeding requires great caution. However, the amounts of **carbamazepine** and **valproate** in breast milk are considered too low to be harmful. A general issue is that, even when the concentration of a particular drug in breast milk is low and no detectable clinical effect upon the infant can be discerned, it is nevertheless possible that subtle longer-term effects on brain development and behaviour could occur. For this reason, some authorities recommend that women receiving psychotropic medication should not breastfeed at all. A more pragmatic view is provided by the *British National Formulary*.

What to do if there is no therapeutic response

1. Is the drug being taken as recommended? The first step is to find out whether the patient has been taking the drug in the correct dose. He may not have understood the original instructions, or may be worried that a full dose will produce unpleasant side-effects. Some patients fear that they will become dependent if they take the drug regularly. Other patients may have little wish to take drugs for the reasons discussed above.

2. Is the patient is taking any other drug which could affect the metabolism or pharmacological action of the psychotropic agent? Misuse of licit or illicit sub-

stances might interfere with the therapeutic actions of psychotropic drugs.

3. Is the diagnosis correct? Review the diagnosis to make sure that the treatment is appropriate before deciding whether to increase the dose.

Failure to respond adequately to psychotropic medication is a common reason for psychiatric referral. Specific pharmacological approaches for individual disorders are discussed in the relevant chapters.

The classification of drugs used in psychiatry

Drugs that have effects mainly on mental symptoms are called **psychotropic**. Psychiatrists also use **antiparkinsonian agents**, which are employed to control the side-effects of some psychotropic drugs. Anticonvulsant drugs have a growing role if the treatment of mood disorders.

Psychotropic drugs are conventionally divided into different classes, as shown in Table 21.1, but the therapeutic actions of particular compounds are not confined to one diagnostic category. For example, SSRIs are classified as antidepressants and are effective in the treatment of major depression, but they also produce useful therapeutic effects in anxiety states, obsessive-compulsive disorders, and eating disorders. Of course, this breadth of effect does not mean that the latter syndromes are forms of depression. It merely emphasizes that the neuropsychological consequences of facilitating brain 5-HT function may provide beneficial effects in a variety of psychiatric disorders.

Whilst there is considerable understanding of the pharmacological actions of psychotropic drugs, little is known about the neuropsychological consequences of these pharmacological actions and about the ways in which neuropsychological changes are translated into clinical benefit in different diagnostic syndromes. At present, therefore, the best plan is to classify drugs according to their major therapeutic use but to bear in mind that the therapeutic effects of different classes of drugs **may overlap considerably**.

The main groups of drugs will now be reviewed in turn. For each group, an account will be given of therapeutic effects, pharmacology, principal compounds available, pharmacokinetics, unwanted effects (both those appearing with ordinary doses and the toxic effects of unduly high doses), and contraindications. General advice will also be given about the use of each group in everyday clinical practice, but specific applications to the treatment of individual disorders will be found in the chapters dealing with those conditions. Drugs that have a limited use in the treatment of a single disorder, for example, **disulfiram** for alcohol problems or ***cholinesterase inhibitors*** for dementia, are discussed in the chapters dealing with the relevant clinical syndromes.

TABLE 21.1 Classification of clinical psychotropic drugs

Class of drug	Examples	Indications of classes
Antipsychotic	Phenothiazines	Acute treatment of schizophrenia and mania, prophylaxis of schizophrenia
	Butyrophenones	
	Substituted benzamides	
Antidepressant	Tricyclic antidepressants	Major depression (acute treatment and prophylaxis),
	MAOIs	anxiety disorders, obsessive-compulsive disorder
	SSRIs	(SSRIs)
Mood stabilizer	Lithium	Acute treatment of mania
	Carbamazepine	Prophylaxis of recurrent mood disorder
Anxiolytic	Benzodiazepines	Generalized anxiety disorder
	Azapirones (buspirone)	
Hypnotic	Benzodiazepines	Insomnia
	Cyclopyrrolones ('z drugs')	
Psychostimulant	Amphetamine	Hyperkinetic syndrome of childhood
	Modafinil	Narcolepsy

Anxiolytic drugs

Anxiolytic drugs such as **benzodiazepines**, have been prescribed widely and often inappropriately. Before prescribing anxiolytic drugs it is always important to seek the causes of anxiety and to try to modify them. It is also essential to recognize that a degree of anxiety can motivate patients to take steps to reduce the problems that are causing it. Hence removing all anxiety in the short term is not always beneficial to the patient in the long run. Anxiolytics such as benzodiazepines are most useful when given for a short time, either to tide the patient over a crisis or to help them tackle a specific problem.

Tolerance is a particular problem with barbiturates and benzodiazepine-like anxiolytic drugs, and drug dependence can develop. Because the benzodiazepines are still widely used anxiolytics, they will be considered first. **Antidepressants** are increasingly used to treat specific anxiety syndromes but their therapeutic actions differ in important ways from benzodiazepine-like drugs. Their indications in the treatment of anxiety disorders will be considered here but their detailed pharmacology is discussed in the section on antidepressant drugs. When reading this section, it is important to keep in mind that psychological treatments are effective in the management of anxiety disorders and have certain advantages over drug treatment, including more sustained efficacy after treatment cessation as well as fewer adverse effects.

Benzodiazepines

Pharmacology

Benzodiazepines have several actions:

- anxiolytic
- sedative and hypnotic
- muscle relaxant
- anticonvulsant.

Their pharmacological actions are mediated through specific receptor sites located in a supramolecular complex with gamma-aminobutyric acid (GABA) receptors. Benzodiazepines enhance GABA neurotransmission, thereby altering indirectly the activity of other neurotransmitter systems such as those involving noradrenaline and 5-HT.

Compounds available

Many different benzodiazepines are available. They differ both in the potency with which they interact with benzodiazepine receptors and in their plasma half-life (Box 21.2). In general, **high-potency benzodiazepines** and those with **short half-lives** are more likely to be associated with dependence and withdrawal. Benzodiazepines with short half-lives (less than 12 hours) include lorazepam, temazepam, and lormetazepam.

Because of problems with dependence, long-acting benzodiazepines are preferable for the management of anxiety, even if such treatment is to be given intemittently on an 'as required basis'. Long-acting benzodiazepines include drugs such as diazepam, chlordiazepoxide, alprazolam, and clonazepam. **Diazepam** is rapidly absorbed and can be used both for the continuous treatment of anxiety and for treatment 'as required'. **Alprazolam**, a high-potency benzodiazepine, is effective in the treatment of panic disorder. This therapeutic efficacy is not confined to alprazolam because equivalent doses of other high-potency agents such as **clonazepam are** also effective.

Flumazenil is a benzodiazepine receptor antagonist that produces little pharmacological effect by itself but blocks the actions of other benzodiazepines. Therefore it may be useful in reversing acute toxicity produced by benzodiazepines but carries a risk of provoking acute benzodiazepine withdrawal. Flumazenil is available for intravenous use only.

Pharmacokinetics

Benzodiazepines are rapidly absorbed. They are strongly bound to plasma proteins but, because they are lipophilic, pass readily into the brain. They are metabolized to a large number of compounds, many of which have therapeutic effects of their own; temazepam and oxazepam are among the metabolic products of diazepam. Excretion is mainly as conjugates in the urine.

BOX 21.3 HALF-LIVES OF SOME DRUGS ACTING AT ABA/BENZODIAZEPINE RECEPTOR COMPLEX

Diazepam	20–100 h*
Chlordiazepoxide	5–30 h*
Lorazepam	8–24 h
Temazepam	5–11 h
Zaleplon	1–1.5 h
Zopiclone	4–6 h
Zolpidem	1.5–2 h
Chlormethiazole	4–6 h (4–12 h in elderly)
Chloral	6–8 h

*Active metabolite

Benzodiazepines with short half-lives, such as temazepam and lorazepam, have a 3-hydroxyl grouping, which allows a one-step metabolism to inactive glucuronides. Other benzodiazepines, such as diazepam and clorazepate, are metabolized to long-acting derivatives, such as desmethyldiazepam, which are themselves therapeutically active.

It is now common practice to give benzodiazepines (often in combination with low-dose antipsychotic drugs) to produce a rapid calming effect in psychosis. In this situation, benzodiazepines may be given parenterally and it is worth noting that the absorption of diazepam following intramuscular injection is poor, and lorazepam should be preferred if this route of administration is used.

Unwanted effects

Benzodiazepines are well tolerated. When they are given as anxiolytics, their main side-effects are due to the sedative properties of large doses, which can lead to **ataxia and drowsiness** (especially in the elderly) and occasionally to **confused thinking and amnesia**. Minor degrees of drowsiness and of impaired coordination and judgement **can affect driving skills** and the operation of potentially dangerous machinery; moreover, people affected in this way are not always aware of it. For this reason, when benzodiazepines are prescribed, especially those with a longer action, patients should be advised about these dangers and about the potentiating effects of alcohol. The prescriber should remember that these effects are more common among elderly patients and those with impaired renal or liver function.

Although in some circumstances benzodiazepines reduce tension and aggression, they can also lead to a **release of aggression** by reducing inhibitions in people with a tendency to aggressive behaviour. In this they resemble alcohol. This possible effect should be remembered when prescribing to those judged to be at risk of child abuse or to any person with a previous history of impulsive aggressive behaviour.

Toxic effects

Benzodiazepines have few toxic effects. Patients usually recover from large overdoses because these drugs do not depress respiration and blood pressure as barbiturates do. Even so, fatal overdoses of benzodiazepines have occasionally been reported.

Drug interactions

Benzodiazepines, like other sedative anxiolytics, potentiate the effects of alcohol and of drugs that depress the central nervous system. Significant respiratory depression has been reported in some patients receiving combined treatment with benzodiazepines and clozapine.

Dependence and withdrawal

It is now generally agreed that **dependence** develops after prolonged use of benzodiazepines. The frequency depends on the drug and the dosage, and has been estimated as up to 50 per cent of patients who are long-term users. Benzodiazepines are associated with a withdrawal syndrome and tolerance. While drug seeking behaviour is less common, it certainly can occur and benzodiazepines are not uncommonly involved in polydrug misuse and dependence (see Ashton, 2004).

The **withdrawal syndrome** associated with benzodiazepines is characterized by several different kinds of symptoms:

- apprehension, anxiety, insomnia
- tremor
- nausea
- heightened sensitivity to perceptual stimuli and perceptual disturbances
- depression and suicidal thinking
- epileptic seizures (rarely).

Since many of these symptoms resemble those of anxiety disorder, it can sometimes be difficult to decide whether the patient is experiencing a benzodiazepine withdrawal syndrome or a recrudescence of the anxiety disorder for which the drug was prescribed originally. Perceptual disturbances are more likely to indicate benzodiazepine withdrawal.

Withdrawal symptoms generally begin within 2–3 days of stopping a short-acting benzodiazepine and within 7 days of stopping a long-acting one. The symptoms generally last for 3–10 days. Withdrawal symptoms seem to be more frequent after drugs with a short half-life than after those with a long half-life. If benzodiazepines have been taken for a long time, it is best to withdraw them gradually over several weeks (Schweizer and Rickels, 1998). If this is done, withdrawal symptoms can be minimized or avoided.

Azapirones (buspirone)

Indications and pharmacology

The only drug in the azapirone class currently marketed for the treatment of anxiety is **buspirone**. Buspirone is effective in the treatment of generalized anxiety disorder but is not helpful in the treatment of panic disorder. Unlike the benzodiazepines, the anxiolytic effects of buspirone take several days to develop. It is also important to note that buspirone cannot be used to treat benzodiazepine withdrawal.

Pharmacologically, buspirone has no affinity for benzodiazepine receptors but stimulates a subtype of 5-HT receptor called the **5-HT$_{1A}$ receptor**. This receptor is found in high concentration in the raphe nuclei in the brainstem where it regulates the firing of 5-HT cell bodies. Administration of buspirone lowers the firing rate of 5-HT neurons and thereby decreases 5-HT neurotransmission in certain brain regions. This action may be the basis of its anxiolytic effect.

Pharmacokinetics and unwanted effects

Buspirone has poor systemic availability because it has an extensive first-pass metabolism. The side-effect profile differs from that of benzodiazepines. For example, buspirone treatment does not cause sedation but instead is often associated with **lightheadedness, nervousness**, and **headache** early in treatment. There is little evidence that tolerance and dependence occur during buspirone use, although such a judgement must always be made with circumspection.

Drug interactions

Buspirone is relatively free from significant drug interactions, but combination with MAOIs has been reported to cause raised blood pressure.

Antidepressant drugs used for anxiety

Antidepressant drugs usually ameliorate the anxiety that accompanies depressive disorders. Tricyclic antidepressants have also been shown to be as effective as benzodiazepines in the management of both **generalized anxiety** and **panic disorder** whether or not significant depressive symptoms are present. Similarly, both SSRIs and MAOIs are effective in the treatment of panic disorder, but the selective noradrenaline uptake inhibitor maprotiline is not. Recent studies have also shown that SSRIs are effective in the treatment of **social phobia** and **obsessive-compulsive disorder** (see Bandelow *et al.*, 2002).

The therapeutic profile of antidepressant drugs in the treatment of anxiety differs significantly from that of benzodiazepines. The time of onset of effect is much slower with antidepressants and, particularly in panic disorder, there may be an **exacerbation of symptoms** early in treatment. However, the ultimate therapeutic effect of antidepressants is as least as great and they are less likely to produce cognitive impairment (Nutt and Bell, 1997). In addition, the use of antidepressants is not associated with tolerance and dependence though, as noted above, sudden cessation of treatment can cause abstinence symptoms.

Antipsychotic drugs used for anxiety

These drugs are sometimes prescribed for their anxiolytic effects. In low doses that do not lead to side-effects (for example, flupenthixol, 1.0 mg), they are generally no more effective than benzodiazepines. Nevertheless, antipsychotic drugs have a small place as anxiolytics in the treatment of two groups of patients – those with persistent anxiety who have become dependent on other drugs, and those with aggressive personalities who respond badly to the disinhibiting effects of other anxiolytics. However, even low-dose antipsychotic treatment, if maintained, is not free from the risk of **tardive dyskinesia**.

Beta-adrenoceptor antagonists used for anxiety

These drugs relieve some of the autonomic symptoms of anxiety, such as tachycardia, almost certainly by a peripheral effect. They are best reserved for anxious patients whose main symptom is palpitation or tremor, particularly in social situations. An appropriate drug is **propranolol** in a dose of 20–40 mg three times a day. Contraindications are heart block, systolic blood pressure below 90 mmHg or a pulse rate of less than 60/minute, and a history of bronchospasm. Beta-adrenoceptor antagonists precipitate heart failure in a few patients and should not be given to those with atrioventricular node block as they decrease conduction in the atrioventricular node and bundle of His. They can exacerbate Raynaud's phenomenon and hypoglycaemia in diabetics.

Advice on management

Before an anxiolytic drug is prescribed, the cause of the anxiety should always be sought. In addition, it is helpful to classify the nature of the anxiety disorder because this can have implications for drug treatment. It is worth remembering that whilst medication is undoubtedly helpful in the treatment of anxiety syndromes, **psychological treatments** are also effective and are often preferred by patients. In practice, medication tends to be used when psychological treatments are not readily available or have not been successful.

For most patients with **generalized anxiety symptoms**, attention to life problems, an opportunity to talk about their feelings, and reassurance from the doctor are enough to reduce anxiety to tolerable levels. If an anxiolytic is needed, a benzodiazepine should be given for a short time – not more than 3 weeks – and withdrawn gradually. It is important to remember that dependency is particularly likely to develop among people with alcohol problems. If the drug has been taken for several weeks, the patient should be warned that he may feel tense for a few days when it is stopped.

A compound such as **diazepam** is suitable for both the intermittent treatment of anxiety and continuous treatment throughout the day. The use of diazepam on an 'as needed' basis usually means that lower total doses are consumed and the risk of tolerance and dependence is diminished. For longer-term treatment of severe generalized anxiety disorder, **antidepressant medication** is more appropriate.

Antidepressants are often helpful in the treatment of **panic disorder**, although the risk of early symptomatic worsening must be remembered and explained to the patient. The use of small doses early in treatment (for example, 10 mg imipramine, 5 mg citalopram) can be helpful. High-potency benzodiazepines such as **alprazolam** and **clonazepam** are effective in panic disorder but can cause cognitive impairment and withdrawal problems. They may be helpful, however, in patients who do not respond to other treatments. **MAOIs** can also be used in treatment-resistant patients (Bandelow *et al.*, 2002).

Other anxiolytic drugs should be kept for the specific purposes outlined above: beta-adreno-ceptor antagonists for control of palpitations and tremor caused by anxiety, low-dose antipsychotic drugs for patients who respond badly to the disinhibiting effects of sedative anxiolytics (for example, abnormally aggressive patients) or patients who have become dependent upon them.

Hypnotics

Hypnotics are drugs used to improve sleep. Many anxiolytic drugs also act as hypnotics, and they have been reviewed in the previous section. Hypnotic drugs are prescribed widely and often continued for too long. This reflects the frequency of insomnia as a symptom (Ohayon and Lemoine, 2004). Insomnia is reported more often by women and the elderly. Effective psychological treatments are available for the management of insomnia and they appear to have a more sustained duration of action than hypnotics (Morin *et al.*, 1999).

Pharmacology

The ideal hypnotic would increase the length and quality of sleep without residual effects the next morning. It would do so without altering the pattern of sleep and without any withdrawal effects when the patient ceased to take it. Unfortunately, no drug meets these exacting criteria. It is not easy to produce drugs that affect the whole night's sleep and yet are sufficiently eliminated by morning to leave behind no sedative effects.

Most prescribed hypnotics **enhance the action of GABA** either through interaction with the benzodiazepine receptor or other adjacent sites located on the GABA macromolecular complex. Antihistamines and low doses of sedating antidepressants such as amitriptyline and trazodone are also used to facilitate sleep.

Compounds available

The most commonly used hypnotics are **benzodiazepines** or non-benzodiazepine ligands which act at or close to the benzodiazepine receptor site. The latter include **zopiclone, zolpidem** and **zaleplon (the 'Z drugs')**. The actions of these drugs can be reversed by the benzodiazepine receptor antagonist, flumazenil. Among other available hypnotic agents are **chloral hydrate** (or its derivatives), **chlormethiazole**, and **sedating antihistamines** (the latter are often present in 'over the counter' preparations).

Of the benzodiazepines, the shorter-acting compounds such as temazepam and lormetazepam are appropriate as hypnotics because of their relative lack of hangover effects (see Box 21.3). Other benzodiazepines that have been marketed as hypnotics, such as flurazepam and nitrazepam, have a long duration of action and produce significant impairments in tests of cognitive function on the day following treatment.

Zopiclone is a cyclopyrrolone. Zopiclone produces fewer changes in sleep architecture than benzodiazepine hypnotics. The most common side-effect is a **bitter after-taste** following ingestion, but behavioural disturbances including **confusion, amnesia**, and **depressed mood** have been reported. **Zolpidem and zaleplon** are similar agents with shorter half lives. Zaleplon has the shortest duration of action of all currently marketed hypnotics (about 1 hour). It has been recommended for 'as needed' use in patients who wake in the middle of the night and cannot fall asleep again.

Other hypnotic drugs that facilitate GABA include **chloral hydrate**, which is sometimes prescribed for children and old people. It is a gastric irritant and should be diluted adequately. **Chloral** is also available in tablet form. **Clomethiazole edisylate** is a hypnotic drug with anticonvulsant properties. It has often used to prevent withdrawal symptoms in patients dependent on alcohol. For this reason, it is sometimes thought, mistakenly, to be a suitable hypnotic for alcoholic patients. This belief is wrong because the drug is as likely as any other hypnotic drug to cause dependency and can cause **respiratory depression** when combined with alcohol. It retains a place in the treatment of insomnia in the elderly because of its short duration of action. Unwanted effects include **sneezing, conjunctival irritation**, and **nausea**.

Unwanted effects

As well as specific side-effects of individual compounds noted above, all hypnotics have a number of general problems associated with their use. One of the most important is the presence of **residual effects**, which are experienced by the patient on the next day as feelings of being **slow** and **drowsy**. This is accompanied by deficits in daytime performance. Such effects are less apparent with the shorter-acting compounds noted above. Other problems include the **development of tolerance** in which the original dose of the drug has progressively less efficacy and **'rebound' insomnia** on withdrawal, which makes preparations difficult to stop. **Tolerance** is less of a problem with sedating antidepressants, but such drugs have long half-lives accompanied by residual psychomotor effects the next day.

Interactions

The most important interaction of hypnotic drugs is with **alcohol** where a potentiated effect can be seen. The interaction between **clomethiazole and alcohol** is particularly dangerous and can result in death from respiratory failure. For this reason there must be adequate supervision if the drug is used during withdrawal of alcohol. It should not be prescribed for alcoholics who continue to drink. Hypnotics will also potentiate the effect of other drugs with sedating actions such as some antidepressant and antipsychotic agents.

Advice on management

Before prescribing hypnotic drugs, it is important to find out whether the patient is really sleeping badly and, if so, why. Many people have unrealistic ideas about the number of hours they should sleep. For example, they may not know that length of sleep often becomes shorter in middle and late life. Others take 'cat naps' in the daytime, perhaps through boredom, and still expect to sleep as long at night. Some people ask for sleeping tablets in anticipation of poor sleep for one or two nights, for example when travelling. Such temporary loss of sleep is soon compensated by increased sleep on subsequent nights, and any supposed advantage in alertness after a full night's sleep is likely to be offset by the residual effects of the drugs.

Among the common causes of disturbed sleep are excessive caffeine or alcohol, pain, cough, pruritus, and dyspnoea, and anxiety and depression. When any primary cause is present, this should be treated, not the insomnia. Often simple 'sleep hygiene' measures may be helpful (see p. 372). If, after careful enquiry, a hypnotic appears to be essential, it should be prescribed for a few days only. The clinician should explain this to the patient, and should warn him that a few nights of restless sleep may occur when the drugs are stopped, but this restlessness will not be a reason for prolonging the prescription.

The prescription of hypnotics for children is not justified, except for the occasional treatment of night terrors and somnambulism. Hypnotics should also be prescribed with particular care for the elderly, who may become confused and get out of bed in the night, perhaps injuring themselves. Many patients are started on long periods of dependency on hypnotics by the prescribing of 'routine night sedation' in hospital. Prescription of these drugs should not be routine; it should be a response only to a real need, and should be stopped before the patient goes home.

Recent guidance from the UK National Institute for Clinical Excellence (2004e) has re-inforced advice to use hypnotic medicines only for **short periods in disabling insomnia**. In addition, the use of zopiclone, zolpidem and zaleplon was not recommended because of the lack of evidence for their superiority over benzodiazepine medications and their higher cost.

Antipsychotic drugs

This term is applied to drugs that reduce psychomotor excitement and control symptoms of psychosis. Alternative terms for these agents are **neuroleptic** and **major tranquillizer**. None of these names is wholly satisfactory. Neuroleptic refers to the side-effects rather than to the therapeutic effects of the drugs and major tranquillizers does not refer to the most important clinical action. The term antipsychotic is used here because it appears in the *British National Formulary*.

The main therapeutic uses of antipsychotic drugs are to reduce **hallucinations, delusions, agitation,** and **psychomotor excitement** in schizophrenia, mania, or psychosis secondary to a medical condition. The drugs are also used prophylactically **to prevent relapses** of schizophrenia. The introduction of chlorpromazine in 1952 led to substantial improvements in the treatment of schizophrenia and paved the way to the discovery of the many psychotropic drugs now available.

Pharmacology

Antipsychotic drugs (Table 21.2) share the property of **blocking dopamine receptors**. This may account for their therapeutic action, a suggestion supported by the close relationship between their potency in blocking

TABLE 21.2 A list of antipsychotic drugs

Phenothiazines
◆ Chlorpromazine
◆ Thioridazine
◆ Pipothiazine
◆ Trifluoperazine
◆ Fluphenazine
Thioxanthines
◆ Flupenthixol
◆ Clopenthixol
Butyrophenones
◆ Haloperidol
Dibenzodiazepines
◆ Clozapine
◆ Olanzapine
Dibenzothiazepine
◆ Quetiapine
Substituted benzamides
◆ Sulpiride
◆ Amisulpride
Benzisoxazole
◆ Risperidone

dopaminergic receptors *in vitro*, and their therapeutic strength.

Dopamine receptors are of several biochemical and morphological subtypes. Most antipsychotic drugs bind strongly to dopamine D_2 receptors, and this action appears to account for both their antipsychotic activity and their propensity to cause movement disorders. Positron emission tomography (PET) studies suggest that an antipsychotic effect is obtained when D_2 receptor occupancy lies between 60–70 per cent. Higher levels are associated with extrapyramidal movement disorders and hyperprolactinaemia (see Kapur *et al.*, 1999).

Distinction between typical and atypical antipsychotic drugs

The term **atypical** antipsychotic agent has been introduced to distinguish newer antipsychotic drugs from conventional agents such as chlorpromazine and haloperidol. Whilst the definition of the term 'atypical' varies in the literature, a fundamental property of an atypical antipsychotic is the ability to produce an antipsychotic effect **without causing extrapyramidal side-effects**. This definition is not free of difficulty; for example, haloperidol prescribed in sufficiently low doses may also have this effect. However, it is true to say that atypical antipsychotic agents have a lower likelihood of producing extrapyramidal side effects through their usual therapeutic range.

Another property sometimes attributed to atypical antipsychotic drugs is improved efficacy against **positive** and **negative** symptoms of psychosis relative to typical agents. Whilst this is true of the prototypic atypical antipsychotic, clozapine, it is not clear how far more recently developed compounds meet this exacting criterion. The evidence this respect is stronger for amisulpiride, risperidone and olanzapine (see Davis *et al.*, 2003). Whether atypical antipsychotic drugs may **improve cognitive performance** more than conventional agents in patients with schizophrenia is a topic of active investigation (Mortimer, 2004).

Pharmacology of typical (conventional) antipsychotics

All these drugs are effective dopamine receptor antagonists but many possess additional pharmacological properties which influence their **adverse effect profile**.

Phenothiazines Phenothiazines fall into three groups:

1. **Aminoalkyl compounds** such as chlorpromazine antagonize α_1-adrenoceptors, histamine H_1receptors and muscarinic cholinergic receptors. Blockade of α_1-adrenoceptors and histamine H_1-receptors gives chlorpromazine a sedating profile, while α_1-adrenoceptor blockade also causes hypotension. The anticholinergic activity may cause dry mouth, urinary difficulties, and constipation, while on the other hand offsetting the liability to produce extrapyramidal effects.
2. **Piperidine compounds** such as thioridazine and pipothiazine are similar to chlorpromazine but are very potent muscarinic antagonist with a correspondingly low incidence of movement disorders.
3. **Piperazine compounds** such as trifluoperazine or fluphenazine are the most selective dopamine receptor antagonists, the least sedating and the most likely to produce extrapyramidal effects.

Thioxanthenes and butyrophenones

Thioxanthines such as **flupenthixol** and **clopenthixol** are similar in structure to the phenothiazines. The therapeutic effects are similar to those of the piperazine group. Butyrophenones such as **haloperidol** have a different structure but are clinically similar to the thioxanthenes. They are potent dopamine receptor antagonists with few effects at other neurotransmitter

TABLE 21.3 Atypical antipsychotics

Drug	EPS*	Prolactin	Weight gain	Adverse effects
Amisulpride	+	+++	+	Insomnia, agitation, nausea, constipation, Q-T prolongation (rare)
Sulpiride	+	+++	+	Insomnia, agitation, abnormal liver function tests
Clozapine	0	0	+++	Agranulocytosis – white cell monitoring mandatory, myocarditis and myopathy (rare), fatigue, drowsiness, dry mouth, sweating, tachycardia, postural hypotension, nausea, constipation, ileus, urinary retention, seizures, diabetes
Olanzapine	+/0	+	+++	Somnolence, dizziness, oedema, hypotension, dry mouth, constipation, diabetes
Quetiapine	0	0	++	Somnolence, dizziness, postural hypotension, dry mouth, abnormal liver function tests, Q-T prolongation (transient)
Risperidone	+	+++	++	Insomnia, agitation, anxiety, headache, impaired concentration, nausea, abdominal pain
Zotepine	+	+++	+++	Constipation, dry mouth, insomnia, sleepiness, tiredness
Aripirazole	0	0	0	Agitation, insomnia, nausea, vomiting

*EPS, extrapyramidal symptoms: 0, not present; +, sometimes; ++, often; +++, can be excessive.

receptors. They are not sedating but have a high propensity to cause extrapyramidal side-effects.

Pharmacology of atypical antipsychotic drugs (see Table 21.3)

Selective D_2 receptor antagonists Atypical antipsychotic drugs have a diverse pharmacology but currently two main groupings can be discerned. On the one hand are substituted benza**mides** such as **sulpiride** and **amisulpride**. These drugs are highly selective D_2 receptor antagonists which, for reasons that are not well understood, seem less likely to produce extrapyramidal movement disorders. They also lack sedative and anticholinergic properties. They do, however, cause substantial increase in plasma prolactin.

5-HT_2-D_2 receptor antagonists The other major group of atypical antipsychotic drugs possess **5-HT_2 receptor antagonist propertie**s. In other aspects, for example, potency of dopamine D_2 receptor blockade, these drugs differ significantly from one another (Meltzer, 2004). **Risperidone** is a potent antagonist at both 5-HT_2 receptors and dopamine D_2 receptors. It also possess α_1-adrenoceptor blocking properties, which can cause mild sedation and hypotension. **Zotepine** has a similar pharmacological profile to risperidone but has a somewhat low selectivity for 5-HT_2 over D_2 receptors. It is also a stronger antihistamine, making it more likely to cause weight gain.

Olanzapine is a slightly weaker D_2 receptor antagonist than risperidone but has anticholinergic and histamine H_1 receptor blocking activity. This gives it strong sedating effects. **Quetiapine** has modest 5-HT_2 receptor antagonist effects with even weaker D_2 receptor antagonist effects. It has a very low propensity to produce movement disorders.

Sertindole is a potent 5-HT_2 receptor antagonist with weak D_2 receptor antagonist effects. Sertindole produces clinically significant effects of the QT interval in the electrocardiogram and its use is currently suspended. **Ziprasidone** is another 5-HT_2 and D_2 receptor antagonist currently in clinical development. It differs from the other 5-HT_2/D_2 receptor antagonists described here because its also binds to 5-HT_{1A} receptors and is a noradrenaline re-uptake inhibitor. Somnolence and dizziness are common side-effects of ziprasidone and it causes relatively little weight gain. It has a tendency to increase the QTc interval and has not been licensed in the UK. **Aripiprazole** is a partial dopamine agonist that also has 5-HT_2 receptor blocking properties. It has an activating profile and dopaminergic side-effects such as insomnia, nausea and vomiting. It is less likely to cause weight gain or significant EPS.

To some extent these latter drugs were designed to reproduce the pharmacological profile of **clozapine**, which was the first antipsychotic agent to show definite benefit in the treatment of patients whose psychotic symptoms had failed to respond to conventional agents. In addition, clozapine has a low liability to produce movement disorders and is therefore usually regarded as the prototypic atypical antipsychotic drug (Kane *et al.*, 1988). Clozapine is a **weak dopamine D_2**

receptor antagonist but has a high affinity for 5-HT$_2$receptors; it also binds to a variety of other neurotransmitter receptors including histamine H_1, 5-HT$_2$, α_1-adrenergic and muscarinic cholinergic receptors (Meltzer, 2004). Various studies have attempted to define a therapeutic plasma range for clozapine with inconsistent results. A reasonable compromise is 350–500 µg/l.

The pharmacological basis for the increased efficacy of clozapine is not well understood. It is clear, however, that the use of clozapine is associated with a high risk of **leucopenia**, which restricts its use to patients who do not respond to or who are intolerant of other antipsychotic drugs. The haematological monitoring of clozapine treatment is discussed below.

Depot antipsychotic drugs

Slow-release preparations are used for patients who need to take antipsychotic medication to prevent relapse but cannot be relied on to take it regularly. These 'depot' preparations include the esters **fluphenazine decanoate, flupenthixol decanoate, zuclopenthixol decanoate, haloperidol decanoate**, and **pipothiazine palmitate**. All are given intramuscularly in an oily medium. Zuclopenthixol acetate reaches peak plasma levels within 1–2 days and has a shorter duration of action than other depots. It is used for the immediate control of acute psychosis but its superiority to ordinary intramuscular injections is not established. A slow release injection of risperidone is now available.

Pharmacokinetics

Antipsychotic drugs are well absorbed, mainly from the jejunum. When they are taken by mouth, part of their hepatic metabolism is completed as they pass through the portal system on their way to the systemic circulation (first-pass metabolism). Antipsychotic drugs are **highly protein bound**.

With the exception of **amisulpride**, which is excreted unchanged by the kidney, antipsychotic drugs are extensively metabolized by the liver to produce a range of active and inactive metabolites. Following administration of chlorpromazine, for example, about 75 metabolites have been detected in the blood or urine. This complex metabolism has made it difficult to interpret the clinical significance of plasma concentrations of most antipsychotics; hence the plasma measures are seldom used in everyday clinical work. The half-life of most antipsychotic drugs (around 20 hours) is sufficient to allow once-daily dosing. **Quetiapine**, however, has a half-life of about 7 hours, and twice-daily dosing is recommended.

The pharmacokinetic profile of **depot preparations** differs substantially from standard preparations. For all compounds except zuclopenthixol acetate, several weeks is needed for steady-state drug levels to be reached in plasma (Table 21.4). This means that relapse after treatment discontinuation is likely to be similarly delayed.

Drug interactions

Antipsychotic drugs potentiate the effects of other **central sedatives**. They may delay the hepatic metabolism of tricyclic antidepressants and antiepileptic drugs, leading to increased plasma levels of these latter agents. The **hypotensive** properties of chlorpromazine may enhance the effects of **antihypertensive drugs** including ACE inhibitors.

Antipsychotic drugs, particularly **pimozide** and **thioridazine, can increase the QT interval** and should not be given with other drugs likely to potentiate this effect, such as anti-arrhythmics, astemizole and terfenadine, cisapride and tricyclic antidepressants. There are also reports of increased risk of cardiac arrhythmias when pimozide has been combined with clarithro-

TABLE 21.4 Some pharmacokinetic properties of depot antipsychotic drugs

Depot	Time to peak plasma level (days)	Time to steady state (weeks)	Usual frequency of administration (weeks)	Equivalent dose (mg)
Flupenthixol decanoate	7–10	8	2	40
Fluphenazine decanoate	1–2	8	2	25
Haloperidol decanoate	3–9	1	2	100
Pipothiazine palmitate	9–10	8–12	4	5
Zuclopenthixol decanoate	4–7	8	2	200
Risperidone slow release injection	28	6	2	25

Adapted from D. Taylor (1999).

mycin and erthyromycin. **Clozapine** should not be given with any agent likely **to potentiate its depressant effect on white cell count** such as carbamazepine, co-trimoxazole, and penicillamine. **SSRIs** slow the hepatic metabolism and increase blood levels of several antipsychotic drugs including haloperidol, risperidone, and clozapine.

Unwanted effects

The many different antipsychotic drugs share a broad pattern of unwanted effects that are mainly related to their **antidopaminergic, antiadrenergic**, and **anticholinergic** properties (see Table 21.5). Details of the effects of individual drugs will be found in the *British National Formulary* or a similar work of reference. Here we give an account of the general pattern, with examples of the side-effects associated with a few commonly used drugs.

TABLE 21.5 Some unwanted effects of antipsychotic drugs

Antidopaminergic movement effects
◆ Acute dystonia
◆ Akathisia
◆ Parkinsonism
◆ Tardive dyskinesia
Antiadrenergic effects
◆ Sedation
◆ Postural hypotension
◆ Inhibition of ejaculation
Anticholinergic effects
◆ Dry mouth
◆ Reduced sweating
◆ Urinary hesitancy and retention
◆ Constipation
◆ Blurred vision
◆ Precipitation of glaucoma
Other effects
◆ Cardiac arrhythmias
◆ Weight gain and diabetes
◆ Amenorrhoea
◆ Galactorrhoea
◆ Hypothermia

Extrapyramidal effects

These are related to the antidopaminergic action of the drugs on the **basal ganglia**. As already noted, the therapeutic effects may also derive from the antidopaminergic action, though at mesolimbic and mesocortical sites. Atypical agents produce a more effective dopamine receptor blockade at the latter sites than at the basal ganglia and fewer movement disorders. The effects on the extrapyramidal system fall into four groups (see Barnes and Spence, 2000):

1. **Acute dystonia** Acute dystonia occurs soon after treatment begins, especially in young men. It is observed most often with butyrophenones and with the piperazine group of phenothiazines. The main features are torticollis, tongue protrusion, grimacing, and opisthotonos, an odd clinical picture which can easily be mistaken for histrionic behaviour. It can be controlled by an anticholinergic agent given carefully by intramuscular injection.

2. **Akathisia** Akathisia is an unpleasant feeling of physical restlessness and a need to move, leading to an inability to keep still. Agitation with suicidal ideation can also occur. Akathisia may wrongly be mistaken for a worsening of psychosis and more antipsychotic medication inappropriately prescribed. It usually occurs in the first 2 weeks of treatment with antipsychotic drugs, but may begin only after several months. Akathisia is not reliably controlled by antiparkinsonian drugs, β-adrenoceptor antagonists and short-term treatment with benzodiazepines may be helpful. The best strategy is to reduce the dose of antipsychotic drug, if possible.

3. **Parkinsonian syndrome** Antipsychotic-induced Parkinsonism is characterized by akinesia, an expressionless face, and lack of associated movements when walking, together with rigidity, coarse tremor, stooped posture, and, in severe cases, a festinant gait. This syndrome often does not appear until a few months after the drug has been taken, and then sometimes diminishes even though the dose has not been reduced. The symptoms can be controlled with antiparkinsonian drugs. However, it is not good practice to prescribe antiparkinsonian drugs prophylactically as a routine, because not all patients will need them. Moreover, these drugs themselves have undesirable effects in some patients; for example, they occasionally cause an acute organic syndrome, and may worsen or unmask concomitant tardive dyskinesia.

4. **Tardive dyskinesia** Tardive dyskinesia is particularly serious because, unlike the other extrapyramidal effects, it does not always recover when the drugs are stopped. It is characterized by chewing and sucking movements, grimacing, choreoathetoid movements,

and possibly akathisia. The movements usually affect the face, but the limbs and the muscles of respiration may also be involved. Whilst the syndrome is seen occasionally among patients who have not taken antipsychotic drugs, it is more common among those who have taken antipsychotic drugs for a number of years. It is also sometimes seen in patients taking dopamine receptor blockers for other indications, for example, metoclopramide for chronic gastrointestinal problems.

Epidemiology Tardive dyskinesia is more common among **women, the elderly**, and patients who have **diffuse brain pathology**. A diagnosis of **mood disorder** is also a risk factor. In about half the cases, tardive dyskinesia disappears when the antipsychotic drug is are stopped. Estimates of the frequency of the syndrome vary in different series, but it seems to develop in about 20 per cent of patients with schizophrenia treated with long-term conventional antipsychotic medication. Preliminary data suggest that the incidence of tardive dyskinesia is less with **atypical antipsychotic agents** such as clozapine, olanzapine, and risperidone than with haloperidol (Kane, 2004; Jeste, 2004). However, cases still occur, albeit at a lower level.

Pathophysiology The cause of tardive dyskinesia is uncertain, but it could be supersensitivity to dopamine as a result of prolonged dopaminergic blockade. This explanation is consistent with the observations that tardive dyskinesia may be aggravated by stopping antipsychotic drugs or by the administration of anticholinergic antiparkinsonian drugs (presumably by upsetting further the balance between cholinergic and dopaminergic systems in the basal ganglia).

Treatment Many treatments for tardive dyskinesia have been tried but none is universally effective. Therefore it is important to reduce its incidence as far as possible by limiting long-term antipsychotic drug treatment to patients who really need it. At the same time, a careful watch should be kept for abnormal movements in all patients who have taken antipsychotic drugs for a long time. If dyskinesia is observed, the antipsychotic drug should be stopped if the state of the mental illness allows this.

Although tardive dyskinesia may first worsen after stopping the drug, in many cases it will improve over several months. If the dyskinesia persists after this time or if the continuation of antipsychotic medication is essential, a trial can be made of an atypical agent such as olanzapine or quetiapine with weaker dopamine receptor antagonist properties. This can sometimes lead to remission of the disorder. Other agents that have been tried include vitamin E, although the evidence for its efficacy is conflicting.

Tardive dystonia

Although the two conditions can coexist, tardive dyskinesia needs to be distinguished from **tardive dystonia** which is the long-term persistence of a dystonic movement disorder. Clinically the condition is indistinguishable from the various idiopathic dystonias which present, for example, with blepherospasm or torticollis. The diagnosis of drug-induced tardive dystonia is made on the basis of exposure to dopamine receptor blocking agents and a negative family history for dystonia. Treatment is unsatisfactory. Anticholinergic drugs are ineffective and the condition often persists after withdrawal of the antipsychotic agent. However, clozapine has been reported to be useful as has local injection of botulinum toxin into the affected muscle group.

Anti-adrenergic effects

These include sedation, postural hypotension with reflex tachycardia, nasal congestion, and inhibition of ejaculation. The effects on blood pressure are particularly likely to appear after intramuscular administration, and may appear in the elderly whatever the route of administration.

Anticholinergic effects

These include dry mouth, urinary hesitancy and retention, constipation, reduced sweating, blurred vision, and, rarely, the precipitation of glaucoma.

Other effects

Cardiac conduction defects Cardiac arrhythmias are sometimes reported. ECG changes are more common in the form of **prolongation of the QTc interval** and T-wave changes. The use of **pimozide** has been associated with serious cardiac arrhythmias. Cautious dose adjustment with ECG monitoring is recommended. Studies have also suggested that thioridazine might be relatively more likely to produce QT prolongation which has resulted in the indications for thioridazine being greatly restricted in the UK.

Depression Depression of mood had been said to occur, but this is difficult to evaluate because untreated patients with schizophrenia may have periods of depression. It is certainly possible that excessive dopamine receptor blockade in the mesolimbic forebrain could be associated with anhedonia and loss of drive, which could then resemble depression or negative symptoms of schizophrenia.

Endocrine and metabolic changes Some patients **gain weight** when taking antipsychotic drugs, especially chlorpromazine and atypical agents such as olanzapine, zotepine, and clozapine (Table 21.3). Schizophrenia itself has been associated with an increased risk of diabetes and this risk is probably increased by antipsychotic drugs, partly but not completely through associated weight gain. Atypical antipsychotics are probably more likely to be associated with impaired glucose tolerance than conventional agents. Whether there are differences between different atypical agents is a matter of dispute but olanzapine and clozapine have been implicated most frequently (see Taylor, 2004).

Galactorrhoea and **amenorrhoea** are induced in some women by high prolactin levels and it is possible that low libido and sexual dysfunction may also result. There may also be an increased risk of osteoporosis. Some atypical agents do not increase prolactin levels significantly (Table 21.3). (For a review of the adverse effects of hyperprolactinaemia, see Wieck and Haddad, 2004)

Hypothermia, seizures and eye problems In the elderly, **hypothermia** is an important unwanted effect. Some antipsychotic drugs, particularly lower potency agents, such as chlorpromazine and clozapine, **lower seizure threshold** and can increase the frequency of seizures in epileptic patients. Prolonged **chlorpromazine** treatment can lead to **photosensitivity** and to accumulation of pigment in the skin, cornea, and lens. **Thioridazine** in high dose (more than 800 mg/day) has caused **retinal degeneration**.

Sensitivity reactions Phenothiazines, particularly **chlorpromazine**, have been associated with cholestatic jaundice, but the incidence is low (about 0.1 per cent). Blood cell dyscrasias also occur rarely with antipsychotic drugs, but are most common with clozapine. Skin rashes can also occur.

Adverse effects of clozapine

The use of clozapine is associated with a significant risk of **leucopenia** (about 2–3 per cent), which can progress to agranulocytosis. Weekly blood counts for the first 18 weeks of treatment and at 2-weekly intervals thereafter are mandatory. After a year, the frequency of blood sampling may be lowered to monthly. With this intensive monitoring, the early detection of leucopenia can be followed by immediate withdrawal of clozapine and by reversal of the low white cell count. This procedure greatly reduces, but does not eliminate, the risk of progression to agranulocytosis. It is usually recommended that clozapine be used as the sole antipsychotic agent in a treatment regimen. Clearly, it is wise to avoid concomitant use of drugs such as **carbamazepine**, which may also lower the white cell count.

Because of its relatively weak blockade of dopamine D_2 receptors, clozapine is unlikely to cause extrapyramidal movement disorders, including tardive dyskinesia. It does not increase plasma prolactin; hence galactorrhoea does not occur. However, its use is associated with **hypersalivation, drowsiness, postural hypotension, weight gain,** and **hyperthermia. Seizures** may occur at higher doses. Clozapine is a sedating compound, and cases of respiratory and circulatory embarrassment have been reported during combined treatment with clozapine and benzodiazepines. Rarely, fatal **myocarditis** and **myopathy** have been reported. The weight gain may be partly responsible for an increased risk of diabetes mellitus (American Diabetes Association, 2004).

The neuroleptic malignant syndrome

This rare but serious disorder occurs in a small minority of patients taking antipsychotic drugs, especially high-potency compounds. Most reported cases have followed the use of antipsychotic agents for schizophrenia, but in some cases the drugs were used for mania, depressive disorder, and psychosis secondary to a medical condition. **Combined lithium and antipsychotic** drug treatment may be a predisposing factor. The overall incidence is probably about 0.2 per cent of patients treated with antipsychotic drugs.

The onset is often, but not invariably, in the first 10 days of treatment. The clinical picture includes the rapid onset (usually over 24–72 hours) of severe motor, mental, and autonomic disorders together with **hyperpyrexia:**

- The prominent motor symptom is generalized muscular hypertonicity. Stiffness of the muscles in the throat and chest may cause dysphagia and dyspnoea.
- The mental symptoms include akinetic mutism, stupor, or impaired consciousness.
- Hyperpyrexia develops with evidence of autonomic disturbances in the form of unstable blood pressure, tachycardia, excessive sweating, salivation, and urinary incontinence.
- In the blood, **creatinine phosphokinase (CPK)** levels may be raised to very high levels, and the white cells increased.
- Secondary complications may include pneumonia, thromboembolism, cardiovascular collapse, and renal failure.

The mortality rate of neuroleptic syndrome appears to be declining over recent years but can still be of the order of 10 per cent. The syndrome lasts for 1–2 weeks after stopping an oral neuroleptic but may last two to three times longer after stopping long-acting preparations. Patients who survive are usually, but not invariably, without residual disability.

The differential diagnosis includes encephalitis, and in some countries heat stroke. Before the introduction of antipsychotic drugs, a similar disorder was reported as a form of catatonia sometimes called acute lethal catatonia. The condition can probably occur with any antipsychotic agent, but in many reported cases the drugs used have been haloperidol or fluphenazine. Cases have also been reported with atypical antipsychotic drugs, including clozapine. The cause could be related to excessive dopaminergic blockade, though why this should affect only a minority of patients cannot be explained.

Treatment is symptomatic; the main needs are to stop the drug, cool the patient, maintain fluid balance, and treat intercurrent infection. No drug treatment is certainly effective. **Diazepam** can be used for muscle stiffness. **Dantrolene**, a drug used to treat malignant hyperthermia, has also been tried. **Bromocriptine** a dopamine agonist is also recommended. Very ill patients require intensive care unit support with intubation and paralysis to maintain respiration and deal with renal failure.

Some patients who developed the syndrome on one occasion have been given the same drug again safely after the acute episode has resolved. Nevertheless, if an antipsychotic has to be used again, it is prudent to restart treatment cautiously with an atypical agent, used at first in low doses. At least 2 weeks should elapse before antipsychotic drug treatment is reinstated.

Contraindications to antipsychotic drugs

There are few absolute contraindications to antipsychotic medication and they vary with individual drugs. Before any of these drugs is used, it is important to consult the *British National Formulary* or a comparable work of reference. Contraindications include myasthenia gravis, Addison's disease, glaucoma (where compounds have significant anticholinergic activity), and, in the case of clozapine, any evidence of bone marrow depression. For patients with liver disease, chlorpromazine should be avoided and other drugs used with caution. Caution is also required when there is renal disease, cardiovascular disorder, epilepsy, or serious infection. Patients with Parkinson's disease sometimes require antipsychotic medication to deal with psychotic states induced by dopaminergic agents; an atypical agent is preferable in these circumstances. Antipsychotic drugs can produced severe movement disorders and changes in consciousness in some patients with dementia, particularly **Lewy body dementia**.

Antipsychotic drugs are associated with an increased risk of stroke so they should not be used in patients with cerebrovascular disease unless an underlying psychiatric disorder makes this essential. Recent advice from the UK Medicines and Healthcare Products Regulatory Agency (2004) has pointed to a three-fold increase in the risk of stroke when patients with dementia were treated with risperidone or olanzapine. This may, in fact, be similar to the risk seen with conventional antipsychotic drugs (Herrman *et al.*, 2004).

Dosage

Doses of antipsychotic drugs need to be adjusted for the individual patient and changes should be made gradually. Doses should be lower for the elderly, patients with brain damage or epilepsy, and the physically ill. The dosage of individual drugs can be found in the *British National Formulary* or a comparable work of reference or in the manufacturer's literature.

PET imaging studies

There has been an important trend for lower doses of antipsychotic drugs to be recommended. This is based in part on studies with PET which have demonstrated that adequate dopamine D_2 receptor blockade (in the basal ganglia at least) can be obtained with **low doses** of conventional antipsychotic drugs (about 5 mg haloperidol, for example) (Table 21.6) (Farde *et al.*, 1989; Kapur *et al.*, 1999). For newer drugs sufficient PET data is usually available to allow clear dosage recommendations.

Low recommended doses produce an adequate antipsychotic effect in the majority of patients. Higher doses may cause further calming but are likely to be associated with significant adverse effects, some of which may be serious (for example, cardiac arrhythmias). A prevailing view is that the combination of modest doses of antipsychotic drugs with a benzodiazepine is a safer and more effective means of producing rapid sedation than high doses of antipsychotic drugs.

Antipsychotic drugs and risk of sudden death

The association of **sudden unexplained death** with antipsychotic drug treatment is a matter of continuing debate. Patients with schizophrenia treated with antipsychotic drugs appear to have higher rates of cardiac arrest and ventricular arrythmias than controls. They are also more like to die through choking (Hennesy *et al.*, 2002, Ruschena *et al.*, 2003). This could be due to the illness or to treatment. However, antipsychotic drugs are known to alter **cardiac conduction**, and drugs such as chlorpromazine also produce hypotensive effects. Whilst the relationship between high doses of antipsychotic drug treatment and sudden death is not well established, it is clearly prudent to use as low a dose of an antipsychotic drug as the clinical circumstances permit. For a review of this area and the question of high-dose antipsychotic drug treatment see Royal College of Psychiatrists (1993).

An indication of the relative dosage of some commonly used drugs taken by mouth is given in Table 21.6. Some practical guidance on the most frequently used drugs is given in the next section.

Advice on management

Emergencies

Antipsychotic drugs and benzodiazepines are used to control psychomotor excitement, hostility, and other abnormal behaviour resulting from schizophrenia, mania, or organic psychosis. If the patient is very excited and is displaying abnormally aggressive behaviour, the aim should be to bring the behaviour under control as quickly and safely as possible. Current practice favours the use of low doses of drugs such as **haloperidol** (2–5 mg) or **lorazepam** (1–4 mg) singly or if necessary in combination. **Olanzapine** (2.5–10mg), which is now available as an intramuscular preparation for acute use, is an alternative. When using olanzapine intramuscularly it is important to be aware of the contraindications for its use, particularly patients with cardiovascular disease. **Intramuscular olanzapine should not be given with parenteral benzodiazepines**.

Haloperidol, olanzapine and lorazapam can be given orally or parenterally (diazepam is poorly absorbed intramuscularly). The intravenous route is possible for haloperidol and lorazapam but should be used only in exceptional circumstances. If haloperidol is used, an anticholinergic agent will reduce the risk of acute movement disorder. It is important to check for possible respiratory depression, particularly in the elderly or those with concomitant physical illness. The benzodiazepine antagonist **flumazenil** should also available (see Taylor *et al.*, 2003).

There are several other practical points in the management of the acutely disturbed patient that can be dealt with conveniently here. Although it may not be easy in the early stages to differentiate between mania and schizophrenia as causes of the disturbed behaviour, it is necessary to try to distinguish them from psychosis secondary to medical conditions and from outbursts of aggression in abnormal personalities. Among medical conditions it is important to consider post-epileptic states, the effects of head injury, transient global amnesia, and hypoglycaemia. If the patient has been drinking alcohol, the danger of potentiating the sedative effects of antipsychotic drugs and benzodiazepines should be remembered. Similarly, antipsychotic drugs that may provoke seizures should be used with caution in post-epileptic states.

For further information about the management of violence in healthcare settings and clinical guidelines see p. 751.

TABLE 21.6 Dosage and D_2 receptor blockade of some antipsychotic drugs

Drug	Relative dose (oral)	Maximum BNF dose (mg)	D_2 receptor occupancy *in vivo* (%) [daily dose (mg)]*
Chlorpromazine	100	1000	80 [200]
Trifluoperazine	5	NA	80 [10]
Haloperidol	2	30	80 [4]
Flupentixol	1	18	74 [10]
Sulpiride	200	2400	74 [800]
Clozapine	60	900	65 [600]
Risperidone	2	16	75 [4]
Olanzapine	8	20	75 [15]
Aripiprazole	5	30	80 [15]

NA, Not available.

* Farde *et al.* (1989); Nyberg and Farde (2000); Yokoi *et al.* (2002).

Drug treatment of the acute episode

When any necessary emergency measures have been taken, or from the beginning in less urgent cases, treatment with **moderate doses** of an oral antipsychotic drug should be started. An appropriate prescription would be haloperidol 4–12 mg daily in divided doses, chlopromazine 150–300 mg daily, riperidone 2–4 mg daily or olanzapine 10 mg daily.

In the early stages of treatment, the amount and timing of doses should be adjusted if necessary from one day to the next, until the most acute symptoms have been brought under control. Thereafter, regular once- or twice-daily dosage is usually appropriate. A careful watch should be kept for **acute dystonic reactions** in the early days of treatment. Watch should also be kept for **parkinsonian** side-effects as treatment progresses; if they appear, an antiparkinsonian drug should be given (see next section). For the elderly or physically ill, appropriate observations of temperature and blood pressure should be made to detect hypothermia or postural hypotension.

Whilst patients often become more settled a few days after starting antipsychotic drugs, improvement in psychotic symptoms is usually gradual, with resolution often taking a number of weeks. Again, current trends are to maintain the dose of antipsychotic drugs at a modest steady level and not to escalate the dose in the hope of speeding up the rate of improvement. For patients in whom agitation and distress continue to cause concern, it may be appropriate to add short-term intermittent treatment with a **benzodiazepine** rather than increase the dose of antipsychotic agent.

Current advice issued by the National Institute for Clinical Excellence is that atypical antipsychotic drugs should be preferred in patients:

- with a first episode of illness.
- patients demonstrating inadequate therapeutic response.
- patients experiencing adverse effects such as movement disorders or hyperprolactinaemia.
- clozapine is indicated for patients who are intolerant to or who do not respond to other atypical agents.

Drug treatment after the acute episode

Episodes of mania and acute psychosis secondary to medical conditions usually subside within weeks. However, patients with schizophrenia often require treatment for many months or years. Such maintenance treatment can be a continuation, often in a smaller dose, of the oral medication used to bring the condition under control.

Where patients do not take their drugs reliably, one of the intramuscular depot preparations may be useful. At the start of treatment a small test dose is given to find out whether serious side-effects are likely with the full dose (D. Taylor, 1999). The appropriate maintenance dose is then established by observation and careful follow-up. As noted earlier, depot preparations have long half-lives, and therefore it may take **several weeks** for maximum plasma concentrations to be reached. This has implications for the rate at which dose increases and decreases should be made, and also for the tapering of doses of oral antipsychotic medication once depot treatment has started.

It is important to find the **smallest dose** of medication that will control the symptoms; since this may diminish with time, regular reassessment of the remaining symptoms of illness and the extent of side-effects is needed. It is not necessary to give **antiparkinsonian drugs** routinely; if they are needed, it may be only for some days after the injection of the depot preparation (when the drug plasma concentrations are highest).

Antiparkinsonian drugs

Although these drugs have no direct therapeutic use in psychiatry, they are often required to control the **extrapyramidal side-effects** of typical antipsychotic drugs.

Pharmacology

Of the drugs used to treat idiopathic parkinsonism, currently only the **anticholinergic compounds** are used for drug-induced extrapyramidal syndromes. These drugs are antagonists of **muscarinic cholinergic receptors** both centrally and in the periphery. Some also possess **antihistaminic** properties.

Preparations available

Many anticholinergic drugs are available and there is little to choose between the compounds. However, some authorities suggest that the use of agents more selective for the **M_1 subtype** of the muscarinic receptor, for example, **biperiden**, may be associated with fewer peripheral anticholinergic effects. Other preparations employed include **procyclidine** and **benzhexol**. **Orphenadrine** and **benztropine** have combined antihistaminic and anticholinergic properties.

Pharmacokinetics

Limited data are available. Anticholinergic drugs appear to be well absorbed and are extensively metabolized in the liver. They are highly protein bound. Their half-lives are generally between 15–20 hours.

Unwanted effects

In large doses these drugs may cause an **acute organic syndrome**, especially in the elderly. Their anticholinergic activity can summate with those of antipsychotic drugs so that glaucoma or retention of urine in men with enlarged prostates may be precipitated. Drowsiness, dry mouth, and constipation also occur. These effects tend to diminish as the drug is continued.

Orphenadrine may be more toxic than other anticholinergic drugs in overdose whereas **benztropine** has been associated with heat stroke. All anticholinergic drugs can exacerbate tardive dyskinesia but are probably not a predisposing factor in its development (see Barnes and Spence, 2000).

Drug interactions

Antiparkinsonian drugs can induce **drug metabolizing enzymes** in the liver, so that plasma concentrations of antipsychotic drugs are sometimes reduced. As noted above, anticholinergic agents can potentiate the effects of other drugs with anticholinergic activity such as chlorpromazine and amitriptyline.

Advice on management

As noted already, anticholinergic drugs should not be given routinely because they may increase the manifestation of tardive dyskinesia. Patients receiving injectable long-acting antipsychotic preparations usually require anticholinergic drugs for only a few days after injection, if at all. There have been reports of misuse and dependence on anticholinergic drugs, possibly resulting from a mood-elevating effect.

If anticholinergic drugs are required, **biperiden** (2–12 mg daily) or **procyclidine** (5–30 mg daily) are appropriate for routine use. These drugs are usually given thrice daily, although their half-lives would suggest that less frequent dosing should be possible. It is best not to give anticholinergic drugs in the evening because of the possibility of excitement and **sleep disruption**.

Antidepressant drugs

Currently used antidepressant drugs can be divided into three main classes, depending on their acute pharmacological properties:

- **Monoamine re-uptake inhibitors:** Compounds that inhibit the re-uptake of noradrenaline and/or 5-HT (tricyclic antidepressants, SSRIs, selective noradrenaline and serotonin re-uptake inhibitors (SNRIs), and selective noradrenaline re-uptake inhibitors (NARIs).
- **Monoamine oxidase inhibitors (MAOIs):** Compounds that deactivate monoamine oxidase irreversibly (phenelzine and tranylcypromine) or reversibly (moclobemide)
- **5-HT$_2$ receptor antagonists:** These drugs (mianserin, mirtazepine, trazodone) have complex effects on monoamine mechanisms but share the ability to block 5-HT$_2$ receptors.

In the broad range of major depression, these drugs are of equivalent efficacy. The main distinctions between them are in their **adverse effects, toxicity,** and **cost** (Table 21.7). These three classes of drugs will be considered in turn after some comments on the possible mechanism of action of antidepressants.

Mechanism of action

The acute effect of re-uptake inhibitors and of MAOIs is to enhance the functional activity of noradrenaline and/or 5-HT. These actions can be detected within hours of the start of treatment and yet the full antidepressant effects of drug treatment can be delayed for several weeks. For example, it has been suggested that at least 6 weeks should elapse before an assessment of the effects of an antidepressant drug can be made in an individual patient.

To some extent, this delay in the onset of therapeutic activity may be due to pharmacokinetic factors. For example, the half-life of most tricyclic antidepressants is around 24 hours, which means that steady state in plasma drug levels will be reached only after 5–7 days. However, it seems unlikely that this can account completely for the lag in antidepressant activity.

An important feature of both noradrenaline and 5-HT pathways is that the cell bodies in the midbrain possess **inhibitory autoreceptors**, stimulation of which decreases cell firing. Drugs that acutely increase synaptic neurotransmitter levels of noradrenaline and 5-HT (such as tricyclics and MAOIs) indirectly activate these autoreceptors through dendritic release of noradrenaline and 5-HT. This action diminishes cell body firing and attenuates the increase in neurotransmission caused by the antidepressant drug.

Biochemical and behavioural studies have indicated that, as antidepressant treatment is continued for several days, the autoreceptors on noradrenaline and 5-HT cell bodies become **subsensitive**. The effect of this is to free noradrenergic and 5-HT neurons from inhibitory feedback control, and to restore the firing rate of the cell bodies to normal levels despite the presence of increased synaptic concentrations of noradrenaline and 5-HT. This would be expected to increase further the ability of antidepressant drugs to augment noradrenaline and 5-HT function.

These findings suggest that the clinical effects of antidepressant treatment result from an increasing potentiation of noradrenaline and 5-HT neurotransmission over time. Recent experimental studies have suggested that increased monoamine function can lead to activation of **intracellular second messengers** such as cyclic AMP and this in turn results in increased elaboration of **neurotropic factors** required for neuronal function and survival. This model proposes that the effects of antidepressants are expressed ultimately at the level of synaptic plasticity and remodeling (for a review see Manji *et al.*, 2003)

TABLE 21.7 Groups of antidepressant drugs

Drug	Advantages	Disadvantages
Tricyclic antidepressants	Well studied	Cardiotoxic*, dangerous in overdose
	No serious long-term toxicity at therapeutic doses	Anticholinergic side-effects
	Useful sedative effect in selected patients	Cognitive impairment
	Inexpensive	Weight gain during longer-term treatment
SSRIs	Lack cardiotoxicity: relatively safe in overdose	Long-term toxicity not fully evaluated
SNRI	Not anticholinergic	Gastrointestinal disturbance, sexual dysfunction
	No cognitive impairment	
	Relatively easy to give effective dose	May worsen sleep and anxiety symptoms initially
		Greater risk of drug interaction
		Expensive‡
Trazodone	Lack cardiotoxicity†, relatively safe in overdose	Daytime drowsiness
Mianserin	Not anticholinergic	Cognitive impairment
Mirtazepine	Useful sedative effect in selected patients	Less well established efficacy in severe depression
		Expensive

* Lofepramine has important differences from conventional tricyclic antidepressants.

† Cardiac arrhythmias have rarely been reported with trazodone.

‡ Some generic SSRIs are now available.

Tricyclic antidepressants

Pharmacology

Tricyclic antidepressants have a three-ringed structure with an attached side chain. A useful distinction is between compounds that have a terminal methyl group on the side chain (**tertiary amines**) and those that do not (**secondary amines**). In general, compared with the secondary amines, tertiary amines (for example, amitriptyline, clomipramine, and imipramine) have a higher affinity for the 5-HT uptake site and are more potent antagonists of α_1-adrenoceptors and muscarinic cholinergic receptors. Therefore, in clinical use, tertiary amines are more sedating and cause more anticholinergic effects than secondary amines (for example, desipramine, lofepramine and nortriptyline).

Tricyclic antidepressants inhibit the re-uptake of both 5-HT and noradrenaline. They also have **antagonist activities at a variety of neurotransmitter receptors**. In general, these receptor-blocking actions have been thought to cause adverse effects (Table 21.8), though some investigators have argued that the ability of some tricyclics to antagonize brain 5-HT_2 receptors may also mediate some of their therapeutic effects. Tricyclics have quinidine-like **membrane-stabilizing effects**, and this may explain why they impair cardiac conduction and cause high toxicity in overdose.

Pharmacokinetics

Tricyclic antidepressants are well absorbed from the gastrointestinal tract, and peak plasma levels occur 2–4 hours after ingestion. Tricyclics are subject to significant first-pass metabolism in the liver and are highly protein bound. The free fraction is widely distributed in body tissues. In general, the elimination half-life of tricyclics is such that it is unnecessary to give them more than once daily.

Tricyclics are metabolized in the liver by hydroxylation and demethylation; it is noteworthy that demethylation of tricyclics with a tertiary amine structure gives rise to significant plasma concentrations of the corresponding secondary amine. There can be substantial (10–40-fold) differences in plasma tricyclic antidepressant levels between individual subjects when fixed-dose regimens are employed.

Despite a considerable research effort, the role of plasma level monitoring in the use of tricyclics is not

TABLE 21.8 Some adverse effects of tricyclic antidepressants

Pharmacological action	Adverse effect
Muscarinic receptor blockade (anticholinergic)	Dry mouth, tachycardia, blurred vision, glaucoma,
	Constipation, urinary retention, sexual dysfunction,
	Cognitive impairment
α_1-Adrenoceptor blockade	Drowsiness, postural hypotension, sexual dysfunction,
	Cognitive impairment
Histamine H_1 receptor blockade	Drowsiness, weight gain
Membrane-stabilizing properties	Cardiac conduction defects, cardiac arrhythmias, epileptic seizures
Other	Rash, oedema, leucopenia, elevated liver enzymes

well established. In general, it has been difficult to show a consistent relationship between plasma level and therapeutic response. However, there is some agreement that plasma levels of **nortriptyline** demonstrate a curvilinear relationship with clinical outcome. The highest response rates occur with plasma concentrations in the range of 50–150 ng/ml, and above this level the response rate may actually decline.

However, the relationship between clinical response during amitriptyline treatment and total plasma levels of amitriptyline and nortriptyline is not clear, with different studies reporting variously a linear relationship, a curvilinear relationship, and no relationship at all.

There is some evidence that high levels of tricyclic antidepressants are more likely to be associated with toxic side-effects such as **delirium, seizures**, and **cardiac arrhythmias**. The risk of such side-effects is minimized if total plasma levels of tricyclic antidepressants are **lower than 300 ng/ml** (Burke and Preskorn, 1999). In this context it is worth noting that a small proportion of patients who metabolize drugs slowly may develop significantly increased plasma levels of tricyclics while taking routine clinical doses.

Overall, plasma-level monitoring has a useful but rather limited role in the management of tricyclic antidepressant treatment (Table 21.9). Plasma monitoring may be useful to assess concordance and is often helpful in patients who have not responded to what are usually adequate tricyclic doses, particularly if increases in dose above 200 mg daily are contemplated.

TABLE 21.9 Indications for plasma monitoring of tricyclic antidepressants

To check compliance
Toxic side-effects at low dose
Lack of therapeutic response and doses > 200mg
Coexisting medical disorder (e.g. epilepsy)
Possibility of drug interaction

Finally, plasma level monitoring is useful in patients with coexisting medical disorders, especially if there is a possibility of drug interaction. For example, in patients with seizure disorders, it is prudent to maintain plasma tricyclic levels within the usual range for the particular compound being used because tricyclics lower the seizure threshold. An additional level of complexity is added by the effects of coadministered anti-epileptic drugs which can increase or lower plasma tricyclic levels through pharmacokinetic interactions.

Compounds available

These include amitriptyline, amoxapine, clomipramine, desipramine, dosulepin (dothiepin), doxepin, imipramine, lofepramine, nortriptyline, and trimipramine. Some of these are sufficiently distinct from amitriptyline and imipramine to be worth separate mention.

Amoxapine is a fairly selective inhibitor of noradrenaline uptake but, unusually for a tricyclic antidepressant, produces significant **blockade of dopamine D_2 receptors**. The combined effect of amoxapine to increase noradrenaline neurotransmission and antagonize D_2 receptors has led to suggestions that this compound may be particularly useful in the treatment of depressive psychosis when combined treatment with antidepressant and antipsychotic drugs is often required. However, the use of a single preparation to produce a combined pharmacological effect limits prescribing flexibility. Furthermore, as might be expected, the D_2 receptor blocking properties of amoxapine may result in extrapyramidal disorders and hyperprolactinaemia.

Clomipramine is the most potent of the tricyclic antidepressants in inhibiting the re-uptake of 5-HT; however, its secondary amine metabolite, desmethylclomipramine, is an effective noradrenaline re-uptake inhibitor. In studies of depressed inpatients, the antidepressant effect of clomipramine was found to be superior to that of the SSRIs citalopram and paroxetine (Danish University Antidepressant Group, 1990). Unlike other tricyclic antidepressants, clomipramine is also useful in ameliorating the symptoms of **obsessive-**

compulsive disorder (whether or not there is a co-existing major depressive disorder).

Lofepramine is a tertiary amine which is metabolized to desipramine; however, during lofepramine treatment, desipramine levels are probably too low to contribute significantly to the therapeutic effect. Lofepramine is a fairly selective inhibitor of noradrenaline re-uptake, and has fewer anticholinergic and antihistaminic properties than amitriptyline. Lofepramine has been widely compared with other tricyclic antidepressants and in general its antidepressant efficacy appears equivalent (Anderson 1999).

The most important feature of lofepramine is that, unlike conventional tricyclics, it is not **cardiotoxic in overdose**. This means that lofepramine is likely to be safer than other tricyclics for patients with cardiovascular disease, though caution is still recommended. There have been reports of **hepatitis** in association with lofepramine, but it is not clear whether the incidence is greater than with other tricyclic antidepressants.

Maprotiline is often referred to as a quadricyclic antidepressant because the tricyclic nucleus is supplemented by an ethylene bridge across the middle ring. It is the most selective noradrenaline uptake inhibitor of the tricyclic antidepressants currently available, and has moderate antihistaminic properties but rather less anticholinergic effects than imipramine. It is not well established whether maprotiline is more effective than placebo for depression, but in comparative studies with reference tricyclics its therapeutic activity appears equivalent.

The use of maprotiline at doses above 200 mg has been associated with a **higher incidence of seizures** than is usual during tricyclic treatment. Therefore a dose range of 75–150 mg daily has been recommended, and the co-prescription of other drugs that may lower the seizure threshold, such as phenothiazines, should be approached with caution. Maprotiline has effects on the heart that are similar to those of conventional tricyclics, and in overdose it is at least as toxic.

Unwanted effects of tricyclic antidepressants

These are numerous and important (see Table 21.8).

- **Autonomic:** Dry mouth, disturbance of accommodation, difficulty in micturition leading to retention, constipation leading rarely to ileus, postural hypotension, tachycardia, and increased sweating. Retention of urine, especially in elderly men with enlarged prostates, and worsening of glaucoma are the most serious of these effects; dry mouth and accommodation difficulties are the most common. Nortriptyline and lofepramine have relatively fewer anticholinergic side-effects.
- **Psychiatric** Tiredness and drowsiness with amitriptyline and other sedative compounds; insomnia with desipramine and lofepramine; acute organic syndromes; mania may be provoked in patients with bipolar disorders.
- **Cardiovascular effects** Tachycardia and hypotension occur commonly. The electrocardiogram frequently shows prolongation of PR and QT intervals, depressed ST segments, and flattened T-waves. Ventricular arrhythmias and heart block develop occasionally, more often in patients with pre-existing heart disease.
- **Neurological** Fine tremor (commonly), incoordination, headache, muscle twitching, epileptic seizures in predisposed patients, and, rarely, peripheral neuropathy.
- **Other** Allergic skin rashes, cholestatic jaundice, and, rarely, agranulocytosis; weight gain and sexual dysfunction are also common.
- **Withdrawal effects** Tricyclic antidepressants should be withdrawn slowly if at all possible. Sudden cessation may be followed by nausea, anxiety, sweating, gastrointestinal symptoms, and insomnia.

Toxic effects

In overdosage, tricyclic antidepressants produce a large number of effects, some of which are extremely serious. Therefore urgent expert treatment in a general hospital is required, but the psychiatrist should know the main signs of overdosage. These can be listed as follows. The cardiovascular effects include **ventricular fibrillation, conduction disturbances, and low blood pressure**. Heart rate may be increased or decreased depending partly on the degree of conduction disturbance. The respiratory effects lead to **respiratory depression**. The resulting hypoxia increases the likelihood of cardiac complications. Aspiration pneumonia may develop.

The **central nervous system complications** include agitation, twitching, convulsions, hallucinations, delirium, and coma. Parasympathetic effects include dry mouth, dilated pupils, blurred vision, retention of urine, and pyrexia. Most patients need only supportive care, but cardiac monitoring is important and arrhythmias require urgent treatment by a physician in an intensive care unit. Tricyclic antidepressants delay gastric emptying, and so gastric lavage is valuable for several hours after the overdose. Lavage must be carried out with particular care to prevent aspiration of gastric contents; if necessary, a cuffed endotracheal tube should be inserted before lavage is attempted.

Antidepressants and heart disease

The cardiovascular side-effects of tricyclic drugs, noted above, coupled with their toxic effects on the heart when these drugs are taken in overdose, have led to the suggestion that tricyclic antidepressant drugs may be dangerous in patients with heart disease. Indeed, patients with abnormal cardiac function do seem to be more at risk of orthostatic hypotension and heart block during treatment.

Some of the newer antidepressants, particularly the SSRIs, appear safer in patients with cardiac disease. With the availability of safer drugs it is probably wise not to use tricyclic antidepressants for patients with clinical or electrocardiographic evidence of cardiac disease. A recent epidemiological study found a higher risk of myocardial infarction in patients maintained on tricyclics than those on SSRIs with an increase in relative risk of 2.2 (95% CI 1.2–3.8) (Cohen *et al.*, 2000), although interpretation of this effects is complicated by the observation that SSRIs may actually produce cardioprotective effects possibly by impairing platelet activity (Sauer *et al.*, 2003).

Antidepressants and epilepsy

Most classes of antidepressants lower seizure threshold to some extent. This can lead to an increased risk of seizures in patients who have epilepsy or are predisposed to it. In general, SSRIs and trazodone are believed less likely to lower the seizure threshold than tricyclics. MAOIs are also said not to lower seizure threshold.

Another complication is that antidepressant drugs can cause pharmacokinetic interactions with anticonvulsants in various ways. For example, SSRIs can increase carbamazepine levels whereas valproate can elevate tricyclic concentrations. Before prescribing an antidepressant with an anticonvulsant, it is prudent to check possible interactions in the *British National Formulary* (see also Table 21.11).

Interactions with other drugs

- Tricyclic antidepressants antagonize the hypotensive effects of α_2-adrenoceptor agonists such as clonidine but can be safely combined with thiazides and angiotensin-converting enzyme (ACE) inhibitors.
- The ability of tricyclics to block noradrenaline reuptake can lead to hypertension with systemically administered noradrenaline and adrenaline.
- Tricyclics should not be used in conjunction with anti-arrhythmic drugs, particularly amiodarone.
- Plasma levels of tricyclics can be increased by numerous other drugs including cimetidine, sodium valproate, calcium channel blockers and SSRIs. Tricyclics may increase the action of warfarin. Interactions of tricyclic drugs with MAOIs are considered later.

Contraindications

Contraindications include agranulocytosis, severe liver damage, glaucoma, prostatic hypertrophy and significant cardiovascular disease. The drugs must be used cautiously in epileptic patients and in the elderly.

Clinical use of tricyclic antidepressants

In the use of tricyclics the old adage is recommended that it is best to get to know one or two drugs well and stick to them. It is probably sufficient to be familiar with one sedating compound (for example, amitriptyline) and one less sedating drug (for example, nortriptyline). Other tricyclics can then be reserved for special purposes; for example, lofepramine can be used for patients who present the risk of overdose, whilst clomipramine can be reserved for patients in whom a depressive disorder is related to an obsessional illness.

The prescribing of amitriptyline can be taken as an example. At the outset it is important to explain to patients that, whilst side-effects may be noticed early in treatment, any significant improvement in mood may be delayed for a week or more, and therefore it is important to persist. Early signs of improvement may include better sleep and a lessening of tension. Common side-effects should be mentioned because a forewarned patient is more likely to continue with medication.

The usual practice of starting with a **low dose** of amitriptyline and building up is probably wise, because side-effects are generally milder and patients are more likely to develop tolerance to them. The starting dose will depend to some extent on the patient's age, weight, physical condition, and history of previous exposure to tricyclics; daily doses of 25–50 mg for an outpatient and 50–75 mg for an inpatient would be reasonable. The whole dose can be given at night about 1–2 hours before bedtime because the sedative effects of the drug will help sleep.

Patients should be **reviewed frequently** in the first few weeks of treatment when support and advice are helpful both to maintain morale and to ensure compliance with medication. Often the clinician can detect improvements in rapport and initiative early in treatment. It can then be useful to discuss these changes with the patient. The dose of amitriptyline to be aimed is about 125 mg daily or above. With careful monitoring and encouragement, this dose can usually be reached over 2–4 weeks. Whether lower doses of tricyclics are effective in less severe depressive states in primary care is still debated (Furukawa *et al.*, 2002).

In some patients, **side-effects** limit the rate of dosage increase, but if there is clinical improvement it is reasonable to settle for lower doses. In general, side-effects should not be greater than the patient can comfortably tolerate. For patients who show little or no improvement, it is usually advisable to continue amitriptyline for 4 weeks at the maximum tolerated dose before deciding that the drug is ineffective.

Some patients respond only to **higher doses** (up to 300 mg daily), and cautious increases towards this level are warranted provided that side-effects are tolerable. In doses above 225 mg daily, it is wise to **monitor plasma tricyclic levels** and the **electrocardiogram** before each further dosage increase.

Plasma tricyclic concentrations have to be interpreted in the context of a patient's clinical condition, but generally **levels above 450 ng/ml** are more likely to be associated with severe toxic reactions. In patients with concomitant medical disorders, a limit of **300 ng/ml** may be more appropriate (Burke and Preskorn, 1999).

In the ECG it is important to note any evidence of impaired cardiac conduction, for example, **lengthening of the QT interval** and the appearance of bundle branch block or arrhythmias. Because of the half-life of amitriptyline, each dose increase will take about a week to reach steady state. If the patient has not improved, and if they cannot tolerate an increase in dose or fails to respond to higher doses, then other treatments should be considered. Some possible strategies are outlined in Chapter 11 on mood disorders (see p. 259).

Maintenance and prophylaxis

If patients respond to amitriptyline, they should be maintained on treatment for **at least 6 months** because continuation therapy greatly reduces the risk of early relapse. The same dose of amitriptyline should be maintained if possible, but if side-effects become a problem the dose can be lowered until tolerance is again satisfactory.

It is often not clear when antidepressant drug treatment should be withdrawn, because in some patients depression is a recurrent disorder. Long-term prophylactic treatment may then be justified. Obviously the risk of recurrence increases with the number of episodes that the patient suffers, but other clinical and biochemical predictors of relapse are not well established.

Selective serotonin reuptake inhibitors (SSRIs)

Pharmacological properties

Six SSRIs - citalopram, escitalopram, fluoxetine, fluvoxamine, paroxetine, and sertraline - are available at present for clinical use in the UK. SSRIs are a structurally diverse group, but they all **inhibit the re-uptake of 5-HT** with high potency and selectivity. None of them has an appreciable affinity for the noradrenaline uptake site, and present data suggest that they have a low affinity for other monoamine neurotransmitter receptors.

Pharmacokinetics

In general, SSRIs are absorbed slowly and reach peak plasma levels after about 4–8 hours, although citalopram and escitalopram are absorbed more quickly. The half-lives of citalopram, escitalopram. fluvoxamine, paroxetine, and sertraline are between 20 and 30 hours, whereas the half-life of fluoxetine is 48–72 hours. The SSRIs are primarily eliminated by hepatic metabolism. Fluoxetine is metabolized to norfluoxetine, which is also a potent 5-HT uptake blocker and has a half-life of 7–9 days. Sertraline is converted to desmethylsertraline, which has a half-life of 2–3 days and is 5–10 times less potent than the parent compound in inhibiting the reuptake of 5-HT. The contribution of desmethylsertraline to the antidepressant effect of sertraline during treatment is unclear.

Efficacy of SSRIs in depression

The SSRIs have been extensively compared with placebo and with reference tricyclic antidepressants. The SSRIs are all clearly **superior to placebo** and are **generally as effective as tricyclics** in the treatment of major depression (see Anderson, 1999). Most comparative studies have been of moderately depressed outpatients and there has been concern that SSRIs may be less effective than conventional tricyclic antidepressants for more severely depressed patients, particularly inpatients (Anderson, 1999).

Unwanted effects of SSRIs

The **adverse effects** of SSRIs differ significantly from those of tricyclic antidepressants. A major difference is that SSRIs are **less cardiotoxic than tricyclic antidepressants** and are generally much **safer in overdose**, though concerns have been raised about the safety of citalopram in this respect. SSRIs also **lack anticholinergic effects** and are not sedating. Side-effects can be grouped as follows (Table 21.10):

- **Gastrointestinal** Nausea occurs in about 20 per cent of patients, though it may resolve with continued administration, dyspepsia, bloating, flatulence, and diarrhoea. With the exception of paroxetine, SSRIs are not usually associated with weight gain.

- **Neuropsychiatric** Insomnia, daytime somnolence, agitation, tremor, restlessness, irritability and headache. SSRIs have also been associated with seizures and mania, although they are probably less likely than tricyclics to produce the latter effects. By contrast, extrapyramidal side-effects such as parkinsonism and akathisia are more common during treatment with SSRIs than with tricyclics. In particular, paroxetine has been associated with acute dystonias in the first few days of treatment.
- **Other** Sexual dysfunction including ejaculatory delay and anorgasmia are common during SSRI treatment. Sweating and dry mouth are also reported. Cardiovascular side effects are rare with SSRIs, but some reduction in pulse rate may occur and postural hypotension has been reported. Fluoxetine has been associated with skin rashes and, rarely, a more generalized allergic reaction with arthritis. SSRIs have been associated with low sodium states secondary to inappropriate ADH secretion, especially in the elderly. As with tricyclic antidepressants, elevation of liver enzymes can occur but is generally reversible on treatment withdrawal. SSRIs may increase the risk of upper gastrointestinal bleeding, particularly when combined with non-steroidal anti-inflammatory drugs.
- **Suicidal behaviour** There have been anecdotal reports that SSRI treatment may be associated with hostile and suicidal behaviour. Meta-analyses of controlled trials of SSRIs have found no significant increase in suicidal ideation or suicidal acts, as compared with placebo or tricyclic antidepressants (Khan *et al.*, 2003; see also http://www.mhra.gov.uk/news/2004/SSRIfinal.pdf). However, like some other antidepressants, SSRIs can cause agitation and restlessness early in treatment and it is possible that in predisposed individuals this might trigger dangerous behaviour. A recent epidemiological study of depressed patients in primary care who received a first prescription for an antidepressant found no difference in rates of suicidal behaviour or completed suicide in patients taking SSRIs relative to TCAs (Jick *et al.*, 2004). Noteworthy, however, was the fourfold increase in risk of attempted suicide seen with all antidepressants in the first nine days of treatment, relative to the risk of longer-term treatment (greater than 90 days). In the small number of completed suicides, the relative risk in the first nine days of treatment was increased almost forty-fold (Jick *et al.*, 2004)

BOX 21.4 SUICIDE RATES AMONG PARTICIPANTS IN FDA TRIALS OF INVESTIGATIONAL ANTIDEPRESSANTS

Treatment	Placebo	SSRI	Other*
Number of patients	4,895	26,109	17, 272
Suicides	5	38	34
Per cent of suicides	0.10	0.15	0.20
95% CI interval	0.01–0.19	0.10–0.20	0.09–0.27

- TCAs together with a range of other antidepressants including bupropion, mianserin, mirtazapine, nefazodone, trazodone and venlafaxine.

From Khan *et al.* (2003)

There are a number of possible of reasons for this important phenomenon. For example, depressed people may visit their doctor and start treatment when they are at a particularly low ebb. Alternatively this observation may be a reflection of the traditional view that the greatest risk of suicidal behaviour occurs during the early stages of antidepressant treatment because improvement in motor retardation precedes resolution of depressed mood. Whatever the explanation it reinforces advice that patients should be closely monitored when starting antidepressant medication. It should also be noted that in adolescents there is evidence that some SSRIs can increase suicidal behaviour relative to placebo (see p. 688 and Ryan, 2005).

Interactions with other drugs

Pharmacodynamic interactions The most serious interaction reported is where simultaneous administration of SSRIs and MAOIs has provoked a **5-HT toxicity syndrome** ('the serotonin syndrome') with agitation,

TABLE 21.10 Side-effects of SSRIs

Gastrointestinal	*Common* nausea, appetite loss, dry mouth, diarrhoea, constipation, dyspepsia *Uncommon* vomiting, weight loss
Central nervous system	*Common* headache, insomnia, dizziness, anxiety, fatigue, tremor, somnolence *Uncommon* extrapyramidal reaction, seizures, mania
Other	*Common* sweating, delayed orgasm, anorgasmia *Uncommon* rash, pharyngitis, dyspnoea, serum sickness, hyponatraemia, alopecia

TABLE 21.11 Inhibition of P450 enzyme by SSRIs

	CYP 1A2	CYP 2D6	CYP 2C9	CYP 2C19	CYP 3A/4
Inhibitors	Fluvoxamine (+++)	Fluoxetine (+++)	Fluoxetine (+++)	Fluvoxamine (+++)	Fluvoxamine (++)
	Duloxetine (+)	Paroxetine (+++)	Fluvoxamine (+++)	Fluoxetine (++)	Fluoxetine (+)
		Duloxetine (++)		Venlafaxine (+)	
		Sertraline (+)			
Some substrates (plasma level (increased)	Olanzapine	Tricyclic anti-depressants	Warfarin	Tricyclic anti-depressants	Benzodiazepine
	Clozapine		Tolbutamide		Carbamazepine
	Haloperidol	Venlafaxine	Phenytoin	Diazepam	Quetiapine
	Tricyclic anti-depressants	Haloperidol		Propranolol	Clozapine
		Thioridazine		Omeprazole	
	Theophylline	Risperidone			
		Clozapine			
		Olanzapine			

Inhibition: +++, strong; ++, modest; +, mild.

hyperpyrexia, rigidity, myoclonus, coma, and death (for further details see the section on MAOIs). Other drugs that increase brain 5-HT function must be used with caution in combination with SSRIs; they include lithium and tryptophan, which have been reported to be associated with mental state changes, myoclonus, and seizures. Serotonin toxicity can also occur if SSRIs are combined with 5-HT receptor agonists such as sumatriptan.

SSRIs may potentiate the induction of extrapyramidal movement disorders by antipsychotic drugs, although this effect could be partly due to a pharmacokinetic interaction whereby SSRIs increase plasma levels of certain antipsychotic drugs (see below).

Pharmacokinetic interactions SSRIs can produce substantial inhibition of some hepatic cytochrome P450 enzymes and can decrease the metabolism of several other drugs, thereby elevating their plasma levels (Table 21.11). Examples where clinically important reactions have been reported include tricyclic antidepressants, antipsychotic agents, including clozapine and risperidone, anticonvulsants, and warfarin. Citalopram, escitalopram, and sertraline cause fewer reactions of this nature.

The clinical use of SSRIs in depression

Particularly in primary care SSRIs have supplanted tricyclics because of their better tolerability and greater ease of dosing. In clinical trials, the rate of drop-out due to adverse effects is modestly but significantly lower with SSRIs than tricylics; this difference may be greater in routine clinical practice (see Anderson, 1999). Economic analyses of the cost-benefit of SSRIs compared to tricyclics have given conflicting results but with the availability of generic forms of SSRI, costs of medication become less important in such calculations. However, tricyclics retain an important role in the treatment of patients who do not respond to newer agents. Meta-analysis suggests that, at appropriate dosage, *amitriptyline* is still the most efficacious of currently available antidepressants (Barbui and Hotopf, 2001). There are some clinical situations where SSRI treatment is more strongly indicated. These are listed in Box 21.5.

Although the overall efficacy of individual SSRIs does not differ significantly, there are a few clinical distinctions which are worth considering (Edwards and

BOX 21.5 INDICATIONS FOR SSRI TREATMENT IN DEPRESSION

- Concomitant cardiac disease*
- Intolerance of anticholinergic effects
- Significant risk of deliberate overdose
- Likelihood of excessive weight gain
- Sedation undesirable
- Depression and obsessive-compulsive disorder.

TABLE 21.12 Contrasts between SSRIs

Drug	Risk of pharmacokinetic interaction*	Discontinuation syndrome	Other
Citalopram	Low	Not commonly reported	May be less safe in overdose
Escitalopram	Low	Little data	Isomer of citalopram
Fluoxetine	High	Rare	Increased risk of agitation, slower onset of action
Fluvoxamine	High	Common	Less well tolerated
Paroxetine	High	Common	Acute dystonia early in treatment
Sertraline	Moderate	Common	May have dopaminergic effects

*Based on inhibition of cytochrome P450 enzymes. See Table 21.11.

Anderson, 1999) (Table 21.12). **Fluvoxamine** appears to have **higher drop-out rates** from trials and may be somewhat less well tolerated. **Fluoxetine** has the most **activating effect** and also has a distinctive pharmacokinetic profile in relation to its **long-acting metabolite** which has a half-life of about a week. On the one hand, this results in a potential for troublesome **drug interactions** several weeks after fluoxetine has been stopped. For example, at least 5 weeks should elapse between stopping fluoxetine and starting an MAOI. On the other hand, this slow tapering of plasma concentration results in fluoxetine being the least likely of the SSRIs to cause a **withdrawal syndrome**. **Escitalopram** is the active isomer of citalopram and is marketed as being more effective than the parent compound. At the moment the evidence for this claim is not compelling.

In treating depressive disorder, dosing is easier with SSRIs than with tricyclic antidepressants because most SSRIs can be started at a standard dose that can often be maintained throughout treatment. For example, although fluoxetine has been given in doses of up to 80 mg daily, there is little evidence of increasing therapeutic efficacy above the 20 mg dose.

As with tricyclic antidepressant treatment, patients starting SSRIs should be warned about likely **side-effects**, including nausea and some restlessness during sleep. A number of patients become more anxious and agitated during SSRI treatment; therefore it is important to explain that such effects are sometimes experienced during treatment but do not mean that the underlying depression is worsening. If patients persist with treatment, anxiety and agitation usually diminish, **but short-term treatment with a benzodiazepine** may be helpful, particularly if sleep disturbance is a problem. Small doses of **trazodone** (50–150 mg) may also help sleep, although there are occasional reports of serotonin toxicity with this combination (Mir and Taylor, 1999).

As with tricyclic antidepressants, when patients respond to SSRIs there is good evidence that **continuing treatment** for several months lowers the rate of relapse. In addition, placebo-controlled studies have shown that SSRIs are effective in the prophylaxis of recurrent depressive episodes. SSRIs should not be stopped suddenly as there have been reports of withdrawal reactions (insomnia, nausea, agitation, dizziness) after the cessation of treatment, particularly with paroxetine (for a review of antidepressant discontinuation syndromes see Haddad *et al.*, 2004). Liquid preparations of SSRIs can facilitate a slow withdrawal.

Monoamine oxidase inhibitors (MAOIs)

MAOIs were introduced just before the tricyclic antidepressants but their use has been less widespread because of both troublesome **interactions with foods and drugs** and uncertainty about their **therapeutic efficacy**. However, in adequate doses MAOIs are useful antidepressants, often producing clinical benefit in depressed patients who have **not responded** to other medication or ECT. In addition, MAOIs can be useful in **refractory anxiety states** (Thase *et al.*, 1995).

These beneficial effects have to be weighed against the need to adhere to **strict dietary and drug restrictions** in order to avoid reactions with tyramine and other sympathomimetic agents. In practice this means that conventional MAOIs are very rarely used as first line treatment.

Pharmacological properties

MAOIs inactivate enzymes that oxidize noradrenaline, 5-HT, dopamine, and tyramine, and other amines that are widely distributed in the body as transmitters, or are taken in food and drink or as drugs. Monoamine oxidase (MAO) exists in a number of forms that differ in their substrate and inhibitor specificities.

From the point of view of psychotropic drug treatment, it is important to recognize that there are two forms of MAO (type A and type B), which are encoded by separate genes. In general, **MAO-A** metabolizes intraneuronal **noradrenaline and 5-HT**, whereas both **MAO-A** and **MAO-B** metabolize **dopamine and tyramine**.

Compounds available

Phenelzine is the most widely used and widely studied compound. **Isocarboxazid** is reported to have fewer side-effects than phenelzine, and can be useful for patients who respond to the latter drug but suffer from side-effects of hypotension or sleep disorder. **Tranylcypromine** differs from the other compounds in combining the ability to inhibit MAO with an **amphetamine-like stimulating effect** which may be helpful in patients with anergia and retardation. Some patients, however, have become dependent on the stimulant effect of tranylcypromine. Moreover, compared with phenelzine, tranylcypromine is more likely to give rise to hypertensive crises, though less likely to damage the liver. For these reasons, tranylcypromine should be prescribed with particular caution.

Moclobemide is the most recently developed MAOI to be marketed. It differs from the other compounds in **selectively binding** to MAO-A, which it inhibits in a **reversible** way. This results in a lack of significant interactions with foodstuffs and a quick offset of action (Bonnet, 2003) (see below).

Pharmacokinetics

Phenelzine, isocarboxazid, and tranylcypromine are rapidly absorbed and widely distributed. They have short half-lives (about 2–4 hours), as they are quickly metabolized in the liver by acetylation, oxidation, and deamination. People differ in their capacity to acetylate drugs; for example, in the UK, approximately 60 per cent of the population are 'fast acetylators' who would be expected to metabolize hydrazine MAOIs more quickly than 'slow acetylators'. Some studies have shown a better clinical response to phenelzine in 'slow acetylators', but this finding has not been consistently replicated. However, it may underlie the observation that the best response rate with MAOIs occurs in studies that have used **higher dose ranges**, presumably because even patients who metabolize MAOIs quickly will receive an adequate dose.

Phenelzine, isocarboxazid, and tranylcypromine bind irreversibly to MAO-A and MAO-B by means of a covalent linkage. Hence, the enzyme is permanently deactivated and MAO activity can be restored only when new enzyme is synthesized. Thus, despite their short half-lives, irreversible MAOIs cause a **long-lasting inhibition of MAO**.

In contrast with these compounds, moclobemide binds reversibly to MAO-A. This compound has a short half-life (about 2 hours), and therefore its inhibition of MAO-A is brief, declining to some extent even during the latter periods of a thrice daily dosing regimen. Full MAO activity is restored **within 24 hours of stopping moclobemide**; with the irreversible MAOIs, 2 weeks or more may be needed for synthesis of new MAO.

Efficacy of MAOIs in depression

For many years MAOIs were in relative disuse because several studies, in particular a large controlled trial by the Medical Research Council (Clinical Psychiatry Committee, 1965), found phenelzine no better than placebo in the treatment of depressive disorders. It seems likely that the doses of MAOIs were too low in these early investigations; in the Medical Research Council study the maximum dose of phenelzine was 45 mg daily as against the current practice of doses up to 90 mg daily if side-effects permit. Subsequent studies have shown that in this wider dose range MAOIs are **superior to placebo** and are **generally equivalent to tricyclic antidepressants** in their therapeutic activity (see Thase *et al.*, 1995).

Investigations in the USA have confirmed early clinical impressions that MAOIs may be of particular value in the treatment of **atypical depression**. It also seems that MAOIs are more effective than tricyclic antidepressants for patients with **bipolar depression** if the clinical features include hypersomnia and anergia. Finally there is also good evidence that they may be beneficial for depressed patients who **do not respond to tricyclics and other re-uptake inhibitors**, whether or not the depression has endogenous features (see Thase *et al.*, 1995).

Unwanted effects

These include dry mouth, difficulty in micturition, postural hypotension, confusion, mania, headache, dizziness, tremor, paraesthesia of the hands and feet, constipation, and oedema of the ankle. Hydrazine compounds can give rise to hepatocellular jaundice (Box 21.6).

Interactions with foodstuffs

Some foods contain **tyramine**, a substance that is normally inactivated by MAO in the liver and gut wall. When MAO is inhibited, tyramine is not broken down and is free to exert its **hypertensive effects**. These effects are due to release of noradrenaline from sympathetic nerve terminals with a consequent elevation in

BOX 21.6 ADVERSE EFFECTS OF MAOIS

Central nervous system Insomnia, drowsiness, agitation, headache, fatigue, weakness, tremor, mania, confusion

Autonomic Blurred vision, difficulty in micturition, sweating, dry mouth, postural hypotension, constipation

Other Sexual dysfunction, weight gain, peripheral neuropathy (pyridoxine deficiency), oedema, rashes, hepatocellular toxicity (rare), leucopenia (rare)

blood pressure. This may reach dangerous levels and may occasionally result in **subarachnoid haemorrhage**. Important early symptoms of such a crisis include a severe and usually throbbing headache.

The incidence of hypertensive reactions is about 10 per cent in patients taking MAOIs, even in those who have received dietary counselling. Therefore regular reminders about dietary restrictions may be helpful, particularly in patients on longer-term treatment (Box 21.6). There have been reports of many foods being implicated in hypertensive reactions with MAOIs, but many of these have cited single cases and hence are of uncertain validity. Another complication is that the tyramine content of a particular food item may vary, as may the susceptibility of an individual patient to a hypertensive reaction. If a forbidden food has been consumed on one occasion without adverse effects, this does not preclude a future reaction.

It is notable that about four-fifths of all reported reactions between foodstuffs and MAOIs, and nearly all the deaths, have followed the **consumption of cheese**. Hypertensive reactions should be treated with parenteral administration of an α_1-adrenoceptor antagonist, such as **phentolamine**. If this drug is not available, **chlorpromazine** can be used. Recently, the use of oral **nifedipine** has been advocated. Whatever treatment is given, blood pressure must be monitored carefully.

Moclobemide and tyramine reactions

Tyramine is metabolized by both MAO-A and MAO-B. Experimental studies have shown that the hypertensive effect of oral tyramine is potentiated **much less by moclobemide** than by non-selective MAOIs (Bonnet, 2003). In patients taking moclobemide in doses up to 900 mg daily, the dose of tyramine required to produce a significant pressor response is above 100 mg. Even a five-course meal with wine would be unlikely to result in a tyramine intake of more than 40 mg.

BOX 21.7 FOODS TO BE AVOIDED DURING MAOI USE

- All cheeses except cream, cottage, and ricotta cheeses
- Red wine, sherry, beer, and liquors
- Pickled or smoked fish
- Brewer's yeast products (for example Marmite, Bovril, and some packet soups)
- Broad bean pods (such as Italian green beans)
- Beef or chicken liver
- Fermented sausage (for example, bologna, pepperoni, salami)
- Unfresh, overripe, or aged food (for example pheasant, venison, unfresh dairy products)

Tyramine has relatively little effect in patients receiving moclobemide because MAO-B (present in the gut wall and liver) is still available to metabolize much of the tyramine ingested. Another factor may be that the interaction between moclobemide and MAO-A is reversible, thus allowing displacement of moclobemide from MAO when tyramine is present in excess.

Interactions with drugs

Patients taking MAOIs must not be given drugs whose metabolism depends on enzymes that are affected by the MAOI. These drugs include **sympathomimetic amines** such as **adrenaline, noradrenaline,** and **amphetamine,** as well as **phenylpropanolamine** and **ephedrine** (which may be present in proprietary cold cures). **L-Dopa** and **dopamine** may also cause hypertensive reactions. Local anaesthetics often contain a sympathomimetic amine, which should also be avoided. **Opiates, cocaine,** and **insulin** can also be involved in dangerous interactions. Sensitivity to **oral antidiabetic** drugs is increased, with consequent risk of hypoglycaemia. The ability of MAOIs to cause postural hypotension can increase the **hypotensive effects** of other agents. Finally, the metabolism of carbamazepine, phenytoin, and other drugs broken down in the liver **may be slowed**.

The serotonin syndrome A number of drugs that potentiate brain 5-HT function can produce a severe **neurotoxicity syndrome** when combined with MAOIs. The main features of this syndrome are shown in Box 21.7. It is worth noting that some of these symptoms resemble the neuroleptic malignant syndrome (see p. 536) with which 5-HT neurotoxicity is occasion-

BOX 21.8 CLINICAL FEATURES OF THE SEROTONIN SYNDROME

Neurological Myoclonus, nystagmus, headache, tremor, rigidity, seizures

Mental state Irritability, confusion, agitation, hypomania, coma

Other Hyperpyrexia, sweating, diarrhoea, cardiac arrhythmias, death

ally confused. In view of the interactions between dopamine and 5-HT pathways, it is possible that similar mechanisms may be involved.

Current clinical data indicate that combination of **MAOIs** with **SSRIs, venlafaxine, and clomipramine** is contraindicated. The combination of MAOIs with **L-tryptophan** has also been reported to cause 5-HT toxicity. Adverse reactions have been reported between the 5-HT_{1A} receptor agonist, **buspirone,** and MAOIs. The use of 5-HT_1 receptor agonists, such as **sumatriptan,** should be avoided. Used with caution the combination of **lithium** with MAOIs seems safe and can be effective in patients with resistant depression.

If a 5-HT syndrome develops, all medication should be stopped and supportive measures instituted. In theory, drugs with 5-HT receptor antagonist properties such as cypropeptadine or propranolol may be helpful, but controlled studies have not been carried out (for a review of the serotonin syndrome, see Gillman and Whyte, 2004).

Combination of MAOIs with tricyclic antidepressants The combined use of MAOIs and tricyclic antidepressants fell into disuse because of the severe reactions associated with the 5-HT syndrome. Current views are that combination therapy is safe provided that the following rules are followed:

- Clomipramine and imipramine are not used. The most favoured tricyclics in combination with MAOIs are amitriptyline and trimipramine.
- The MAOI and tricyclic are started together at low dosage, or the MAOI is added to the tricyclic (adding tricyclics to MAOIs is more likely to provoke dizziness and postural hypotension).

The advantages and disadvantages of combined tricyclic and MAOI therapy have not been fully established. On the one hand, patients taking tricyclics with MAOIs are less likely to suffer from **MAOI-induced insomnia**; on the other hand, they are more likely to experience **postural hypotension** and troublesome **weight gain**. The combination is said to be useful in patients with **resistant depression**. Although formal studies have not been carried out in this patient group, there are case reports of patients for whom combined MAOI-tricyclic treatment was successful when either treatment alone had not been helpful. Low doses of **trazodone** (50–150 mg) are also used to ameliorate MAOI-induced insomnia; present experience suggests that this combination is generally well tolerated, although there are occasional reports of adverse effects that could represent serotonin toxicity (Mir and Taylor, 1999).

Contraindications

These include liver disease, phaeochromocytoma, congestive cardiac failure, and conditions that require the patient to take any of the drugs that react with MAOI.

Clinical use of MAOIs in depression

Because of the potential danger of drug interactions and the need for a tyramine-free diet, irreversible MAOIs are rarely used as first-line antidepressant agents. The exception may be when patients have previously shown a favourable response to these drugs as against other classes of antidepressants. Even in atypical depression, for which MAOIs may well be superior to tricyclic antidepressants, it is probably better to try an SSRI first because many patients will respond to this approach.

The clinical use of phenelzine can be taken as an example. Treatment should start with 15 mg daily increasing to 30 mg daily in divided doses (with the final dose not later than 3.00 p.m.) in the first week. Patients should be given **clear written instructions about foods to be avoided** (see below) and should be warned to take no other medication unless it has been specifically checked with a pharmacist or doctor who knows that the patient is taking MAOIs. As always, patients should be warned about the delay in therapeutic response (up to 6 weeks) and about common side-effects (sleep disturbance, dizziness).

In the second week, the dose of phenelzine can be increased to 45 mg daily. At this stage a greater increase to 60 mg may produce a quicker response, but it is also associated with more adverse effects. Accordingly, if feasible, it is better to find out whether an individual patient will respond to lower doses (about 45 mg) before increments are made (up to 90 mg daily). If patients do not respond to 45 mg, the dose can be increased by 15 mg weekly if side-effects permit.

The response to MAOIs can often be sudden; over the course of a day or two the patient suddenly feels better.

If there are signs of **overactivity** or **excessive buoyancy** in mood, the dose can be reduced and the patient monitored for signs of developing hypomania. Side-effects likely to be particularly troublesome are insomnia and postural hypotension. Insomnia is best managed by lowering the dose of MAOI if feasible. Otherwise, the addition of a benzodiazepine or trazodone (50–150 mg at night) can be helpful, although the latter drug can sometimes increase problems of dizziness and postural hypotension.

Postural hypotension can be a disabling problem with MAOIs. Again, dose reduction is worth considering. Various measures have been suggested, for example, the use of support stockings, an increase in salt intake, or even the use of a mineralocorticoid. Of course, the latter two measures have their own adverse effects.

Withdrawal from MAOIs

Patients who respond to MAOIs have often suffered from disabling depression for many months or even years. For such patients the usual practice is to continue therapy for at least 6 months to a year. With MAOIs, it is wise to lower the dose if the patient can tolerate the reduction without relapsing. Sudden cessation of MAOIs can lead to **anxiety** and **dysphoria**. Even gradual withdrawal can be associated with increasing anxiety and depression.

Clinical experience indicates that it is more difficult to stop MAOI than tricyclic antidepressant treatment. An explanation for this difference may be that MAOIs may produce a more severe discontinuation syndrome than other antidepressants; another possible explanation is that MAOIs are given to patients with chronic disabling disorders who frequently relapse. It is emphasized that, because of the time taken to synthesize new MAO, at least two **weeks should elapse** between the cessation of irreversible MAOI treatment and the easing of dietary and drug restrictions.

Moclobemide

In their freedom from tyramine reactions and their quick offset of activity, reversible type A MAOIs, such as **moclobemide**, have clear advantages over conventional MAOIs. As with other newer antidepressants, however, the therapeutic efficacy of moclobemide, particularly in more severely depressed patients, is not as well established and may be questionable (Anderson, 1999). Also, it is not yet known whether moclobemide will prove effective for patients with the various forms of atypical depression and tricyclic-resistant depression for which conventional MAOIs can be useful. A recent case series suggested that moclobemide may have a place in the treatment of patients with resistant depression when used in combination with other agents such as lithium and tricyclic antidepressants (Kennedy and Paykel, 2004).

The starting dose of moclobemide is 150–300 mg daily, which can be increased to 600 mg over a number of weeks. Treatment-resistant patients may require higher doses but above levels of 900 mg daily it is prudent to institute the usual MAOI dietary restrictions. Moclobemide is better tolerated than tricyclic antidepressants or irreversible MAOIs, but side-effects such as nausea and insomnia occur in about 20–30 per cent of patients.

Drug interactions of moclobemide

Moclobemide should not be combined with **SSRIs, venlafaxine** or **clomipramine** because a serotonin syndrome may result. Caution is needed with **sumatriptan**. Like the irreversible MAOIs, moclobemide may react adversely with **opiates**. Similarly, moclobemide may potentiate the pressor effects of **sympathomimetic amines**; therefore combined use should be avoided. Moclobemide should not be combined with **L-dopa** because of the risk of hypertensive crisis. **Cimetidine** delays the metabolism of moclobemide.

Other antidepressant drugs

Other antidepressant drugs are available for use in the UK and other countries. Their mechanism of action is such that they cannot easily be grouped with tricyclic antidepressants, SSRIs, or with MAOIs. These drugs also have differing adverse-event profiles. Therefore they are discussed individually below.

Mianserin

Mianserin is a quadricyclic compound with complex pharmacological actions. It has weak noradrenaline reuptake inhibiting effects, and is a fairly potent antagonist at several 5-HT receptor subtypes, particularly 5-HT_2 receptors. Mianserin is also a competitive antagonist at histamine H_1 receptors and α_1- and α_2-adrenoceptors. The latter action leads to an increase in noradrenaline cell firing and release. It is not a muscarinic cholinergic antagonist and is not cardiotoxic. Because of these various actions, mianserin has a **sedating profile**, but it is not anticholinergic and is relatively **safe in overdose**.

Pharmacokinetics Mianserin is rapidly absorbed, and the peak plasma concentration occurs after 2–3 hours. Its half-life is 10–20 hours, and the entire daily dose can be given in a single administration at night.

Efficacy Controlled trials have shown that mianserin is **superior to placebo** in the management of depression, and comparative studies against imipramine and clomipramine have shown no difference in effect. These studies are difficult to assess because of the wide range of doses that have been used. Many early studies of mianserin used doses of 30–60 mg daily, whereas much higher doses of up to 200 mg daily have sometimes been advocated for inpatients.

Unwanted effects The main adverse effects of mianserin are **drowsiness** and **dizziness**, though these effects can be lessened by starting at a modest dosage and then increasing gradually. **Weight gain** is a common problem. Dyspepsia and nausea have also been reported. Like tricyclics, mianserin appears to lower seizure threshold to some extent. Postural hypotension occurs occasionally.

The most serious adverse effect of mianserin is lowering of the white cell count, and **fatal agranulocytosis** has been reported. These adverse reactions occur more commonly in elderly patients. It is recommended that a blood count be obtained before starting mianserin treatment, and that the white cell count be monitored monthly for 3 months after treatment has started. Rare side effects of mianserin include arthritis and hepatitis.

Drug interactions Mianserin can potentiate the effect of other central sedatives. There is a theoretical risk that mianserin could reverse the effects of α_2-adrenoceptor agonists such as clonidine.

Mirtazapine

Mirtazapine is an analogue of mianserin with a generally similar pharmacological profile but a weaker affinity for α_1-adrenoceptors. It is said that this permits mirtazapine to activate 5-HT as well as noradrenaline neurons, though whether this occurs during clinical use is unclear. Like mianserin, mirtazepine has a **sedating profile**. Mirtazepine is known as a noradrenaline- and serotonin-specific antidepressant (NASSA).

Pharmacokinetics Mirtazapine is well absorbed with peak plasma levels being reached between 1 and 2 hours. The half-life is about 16 hours and the daily dose can be given at night. Mirtazapine is extensively metabolized by the liver and has only minor inhibitory effects on cytochrome P450 isoenzymes.

Efficacy Mirtazapine has demonstrated clinical efficacy in both **placebo-controlled and comparator trials** with SSRIs and tricyclic antidepressants in moderate to severely depressed patients. The effective dose is usually between 30 mg and 45 mg daily. Some have advocated that mirtazapine treatment should be instituted directly at a dose of 30 mg at night rather than a lower intermediate dose because at the higher dose excessive sedation may be actually less common. The theoretical reason given for this is that at the higher dose the powerful antihistaminic action of mirtazapine should be mitigated by activation of noradrenaline pathways.

Unwanted effects The common adverse effects of mirtazapine are attributable to its potent antihistaminic actions and include **drowsiness** and **dry mouth**. **Increased appetite** and **body weight** are also common. Thus far leucopenia does not appear more common with mirtazapine than with other antidepressants. The data sheet, however, recommends that physicians be vigilant for possible signs that might reflect low white cell count.

Drug interactions Mirtazapine may potentiate other centrally acting sedatives. As with mianserin, there is a theoretical risk that mirtazapine could reverse the effect of α_2-adrenoceptor agonists.

Trazodone

Trazodone is a triazolopyridine derivative with complex actions on 5-HT pathways. Studies *in vitro* suggest that trazodone has some weak 5-HT reuptake inhibiting properties which are probably not manifest during clinical use; for example, repeated administration of trazodone does not lower platelet 5-HT content.

Trazodone has antagonist actions at 5-HT_2 receptors but its active metabolite, *m*-chloro-phenylpiperazine (*m*-CPP), is a 5-HT receptor agonist. Therefore the precise balance of effects on 5-HT receptors during trazodone treatment is difficult to determine and may depend on relative blood levels of the parent compound and metabolite. Trazodone also blocks postsynaptic α_1-adrenoceptors. Overall it has a distinct **sedating profile**.

Pharmacokinetics Trazodone has a short half-life (about 4–14 hours). It is metabolized by hydroxylation and oxidation, with the formation of a number of metabolites including *m*-CPP. During treatment, plasma levels of *m*-CPP may exceed those of trazodone itself.

Efficacy Several controlled studies have shown that trazodone in doses of 150–600 mg is **superior to placebo** in the treatment of depressed patients. Trazodone also appears to have equivalent antidepressant activity to reference compounds such as imipramine. Many of these studies were carried out in moderately depressed outpatients, and the efficacy of trazodone relative to other antidepressants is not well established (see Anderson, 1999).

Some have maintained that the efficacy of trazodone is improved if treatment is started at low doses (50 mg) and increased slowly to 300 mg over 2–3 weeks. Despite the short half-life of trazodone, once-daily administration of the drug is often sufficient. The drug is usually given in the evening to take advantage of its sedative properties. Doses above 300 mg daily are usually better given in divided amounts. Lower doses (50–150 mg) are sometimes used in combination with SSRIs and MAOIs to ameliorate the sleep-disrupting effects of the latter agents.

Unwanted effects The major unwanted effect of trazodone is **excessive sedation**, which can result in significant cognitive impairment. **Nausea** and **dizziness** are also reported, particularly if the drug is taken on an empty stomach. The α_1-adrenoceptor antagonist properties of trazodone may **lower blood pressure** to some extent, and postural hypotension has been reported. Trazodone is less cardiotoxic than conventional tricyclics, but there are reports that **cardiac arrhythmias** may be worsened in patients with cardiac disease. Nevertheless, trazodone is less toxic in overdose than tricyclic antidepressants.

The most serious side-effect of trazodone is **priapism**. This reaction is seen rarely (about 1 in 6000 male patients). It can cause considerable problems, requiring the local injection of noradrenaline agonists such as adrenaline or even surgical decompression. Long-term sexual dysfunction has sometimes resulted. It is recommended that male patients be warned of this potential side effect and advised to seek medical help urgently if persistent erection occurs.

Drug interactions As with all sedative antidepressants, trazodone may potentiate the sedating effects of alcohol and other central tranquillizing drugs. Studies in animals have raised the possibility that trazodone could attenuate the hypotensive effect of clonidine, but it is not known whether such an interaction occurs in humans.

Reboxetine

Reboxetine is a morpholine and is structurally related to fluoxetine. It is a **selective noradrenaline re-uptake inhibitor (NARI)** with no clinically significant effects on other neurotransmitter receptors.

Pharmacokinetics After oral administration reboxetine reaches peak plasma levels after about 2 hours. Its half-life is around 13 hours and twice-daily administration is recommended. Reboxetine is metabolized by the liver where it is a substrate for cytochrome P450 CYP3A.

Efficacy Reboxetine has shown efficacy in **placebo controlled trials** and against active comparators including tricyclic antidepressants and SSRIs (Burrows *et al.*, 1998). It is claimed that reboxetine produces better improvement in social function in depressed patients than fluoxetine but this possibility requires further study. The usual dose of reboxetine is 4 mg twice daily with a maximum dose of 12 mg daily.

Unwanted effects Despite its low affinity for muscarinic receptors, reboxetine produces adverse effects characteristic of cholinergic receptor blockade, presumably through interactions of noradrenergic and cholinergic pathways. The most common side effects are **dry mouth, constipation, sweating**, and **insomnia. Urinary hesitancy, impotence, tachycardia**, and **vertigo** are also occasionally described.

Drug interactions Limited information is available. It is recommended that reboxetine should not be given with other agents that might **potentiate noradrenaline function**, such as MAOIs, or increase blood pressure, such as ergot derivatives. Plasma reboxetine levels might be increased by drugs that inhibit cytochrome P450 3A4, such as some antifungal agents, fluvoxamine, and macrolide antibiotics.

Venlafaxine

Venlafaxine is a phenylethylamine derivative which produces a **potent blockade of 5-HT re-uptake** with somewhat lesser effects on noradrenaline. In this respect the pharmacological properties of venlafaxine resemble those of clomipramine to some extent; however, unlike clomipramine and other tricyclic antidepressants, venlafaxine has a negligible affinity for other neurotransmitter receptor sites and so lacks sedative and anticholinergic effects. Because of these pharmacological properties, venlafaxine has been classified as a **selective serotonin and noradrenaline reuptake inhibitor (SNRI)**.

Pharmacokinetics Venlafaxine is well absorbed, achieving peak plasma levels about 1.5–2 hours after oral administration. The half-life of venlafaxine is 3–7 hours but it is metabolized to desmethylvenlafaxine which has essentially the same pharmacodynamic properties as the parent compound and a half-life of 8–13 hours. The extended release formulation of venlafaxine (venlafaxine XL) reaches a peak plasma level after about about 6 hours. This gives a long apparent half-life (about 15 hours) but the drug is still quickly eliminated. Once-daily dosing is possible with this preparation.

Efficacy Venlafaxine has been studied in both inpatients and outpatients with major depression and compared with placebo and active comparators. Current studies suggest that it **is more effective than placebo** and at least of equal efficacy to other available antidepressant drugs including tricyclic antidepressants (see

Anderson, 1999). Some and meta-analyses suggest that venlafaxine is more effective than SSRIs particularly for more severely depressed patients (Smith *et al.* 2002).

Venlafaxine has a wider dosage range than SSRIs, from 75–375 mg daily in two divided doses or up to 225 mg of the extended release preparation given as a single dose. The usual starting dose of venlafaxine is 75 mg daily, which may be sufficient for many patients. Upward titration can be considered where there is insufficient response.

Unwanted effects The adverse effect profile of venlafaxine resembles that of SSRIs, with the most common adverse effects being **nausea, headache, somnolence, dry mouth, dizziness**, and **insomnia**. **Anxiety** and **sexual dysfunction** may also occur. Venlafaxine occasionally causes **postural hypotension**, but in addition, dose-related **increases in blood pressure** can occur. Blood pressure monitoring is advisable in patients receiving more than 150 mg venlafaxine daily. Like SSRIs, venlafaxine can lower plasma sodium levels. Generally the extended release preparation of venlafaxine is better tolerated than the immediate release tablets but venlafaxine may be somewhat less well tolerated than SSRIs (National Institute for Clinical Excellence, 2004d).

Venlafaxine appear to be **more toxic than SSRIs** in acute overdose (Cheeta *et al.*, 2004). In the UK this has led the Committee on Safety of Medicines to advise that:

- venlafaxine should be used only in patients who have failed to respond to two adequate trials of other antidepressants
- venlafaxine is not recommended in patients with cardiovascular disease, hypertension or electrolyte imbalance
- Treatment with venlafaxine should be preceded by an ECG.

Similarly to SSRIs, sudden discontinuation of venlafaxine has been associated with symptoms of **fatigue, nausea, abdominal pain**, and **dizziness**. It is recommended that patients who received venlafaxine for 6 weeks or more should have the dose reduced gradually over at least a 1-week period and longer if possible. Preliminary evidence suggest that venlafaxine is less toxic in overdose than tricyclic antidepressants.

Drug interactions Unlike the SSRIs, venlafaxine appears to produce little effect on hepatic drug metabolizing enzymes and therefore should be less likely to inhibit the metabolism of coadministered drugs. Like other drugs that potently inhibit the uptake of 5-HT, venlafaxine should not be given concomitantly with **MAOIs** because of the danger of a toxic serotonin syndrome. It is also recommended that 14 days should elapse after the end of MAOI treatment before venlafaxine is started and that at least 7 days should elapse after venlafaxine cessation before MAOIs are given.

Duloxetine

Like venlafaxine, duloxetine is classified as an SNRI. It is about five times more potent in inhibiting the reuptake of 5-HT than that of noradrenaline. It has little effect on other neurotransmitter receptors (see Cowen *et al.*, 2005).

Pharmacokinetics Duloxetine is well absorbed with maximum blood levels occurring about 6 hours post ingestion. It has a half life of about 12 hours. It is extensively metabolized to therapeutically inactive compounds.

Efficacy Duloxetine given in a single dose of 60 mg daily has greater antidepressant efficacy than placebo and is equivalent in therapeutic activity to SSRIs. Whether, like venlafaxine, more extensive study will show a somewhat greater efficacy than SSRIs and utility in treatment-resistant patients, remains to be determined.

Unwanted effects The adverse effect profile of duloxetine is similar to that seen with other 5-HT promoting antidepressants and includes nausea, dry mouth, dizziness, gastrointestinal disturbances, insomnia and somnolence. Effects on sexual dysfunction are not well characterized. At therapeutic doses, duloxetine does not seem to increase blood pressure; there is little data on toxicity in overdose. As would be expected, abrupt cessation of duloxetine is associated with dizziness, insomnia, anxiety and headache (see Cowen *et al.*, 2005).

Drug interactions Duloxetine produces a moderate inhibition of CYP2D6 and to a lesser extent CYP1A2. It is therefore likely to increase blood levels of other drugs metabolized by these enzymes (Table 21.11). From its pharmacology, duloxetine should not be given concomitantly with **MAOIs** because of the danger of a toxic serotonin syndrome. For the same reason it seems advisable that 14 days should elapse after the end of MAOI treatment before duloxetine is started and that at least 7 days should elapse after duloxetine cessation before MAOIs are given.

L-Tryptophan

L-Tryptophan is a naturally occurring amino acid, present in the normal diet; about 500 mg of tryptophan is consumed daily in the typical Western diet. Most ingested tryptophan is used for protein synthesis and the formation of nicotinamide nucleotides; only a small proportion (about 1 per cent) is synthesized to 5-HT via 5-hydroxtryptophan (5-HTP). Tryptophan hydroxylase, the enzyme that catalyses the formation of 5-HTP from L-tryp-tophan, is normally unsaturated with tryptophan. Accordingly, increasing tryptophan availability to the brain increases 5-HT synthesis.

Pharmacokinetics L-Tryptophan is rapidly absorbed, with plasma levels peaking about 1–2 hours after ingestion. It is extensively bound to plasma albumin. The amount of L-tryptophan available for brain 5-HT synthesis depends on several factors, including the proportion of L-tryptophan free in plasma, the activity of tryptophan pyrrolase, and the concentration of other plasma amino acids that compete with L-tryptophan for brain entry

Efficacy There is only weak evidence that L-tryptophan has antidepressant activity when given alone, though it may be superior to placebo in moderately depressed outpatients. There is rather better evidence that L-tryptophan combined with MAOI treatment can enhance the antidepressant effects of MAOIs. Similar synergistic effects have been reported in some studies of L-tryptophan combined with tricyclics, though overall the therapeutic benefit of this combination is inconsistent.

Unwanted effects L-Tryptophan is generally well tolerated, although **nausea** and **drowsiness** soon after dosing are not unusual. In recent years, however, the prescription of L-tryptophan has been associated with the development of a severe scleroderma-like illness, the **eosinophilia-myalgia syndrome (EMS)**, in which there is a very high circulating eosinophil count (about 20 per cent of peripheral leucocytes) with severe muscle pain, oedema, skin sclerosis, and peripheral neuropathy. Fatalities have been reported.

It is now reasonably well established that EMS is not caused by L-tryptophan itself but rather by a **contaminant** formed in the manufacturing process used by a particular manufacturer (Kilbourne *et al.*, 1996). L-Tryptophan remains available for the treatment of **severe refractory depression**, when it can be used as an **adjunct** to other antidepressant medication (see for example, Barker *et al.*, 1987). Patients receiving L-tryptophan require regular monitoring for possible symptoms of EMS. L-Tryptophan should be withdrawn if there is any evidence that EMS may be developing and an urgent blood eosinophil count obtained.

Drug interactions The only significant drug interactions of L-tryptophan are with drugs that also increase brain 5-HT function. Thus, while administration of L-tryptophan with MAOIs may produce clinical benefit, there are also reports that this combination may lead to 5-HT neurotoxicity as described above. Similarly, the combination of L-tryptophan with **SSRIs** has been reported to cause myoclonus, shivering, and mental state changes (Gillman and Whyte, 2004).

St Johns Wort

St Johns Wort is an extract from the plant, *Hypericum perforatum*. It has been used in medicine for centuries for numerous indications including burns, arthritis, snakebite, and depression. The active principles are probably derived from six major product groups including **hypericins** and **hyperforins**. The pharmacology of St John's Wort is complex but animal experimental and some human studies indicate that it potentiates aspects of monoamine neurotransmission (see Nathan, 1999).

Efficacy There have been numerous trials of St Johns Wort, although these are difficult to interpret because the preparations and dosages have been difficult to standardize. In addition, the trials have been carried out in mild to moderately depressed subjects. A meta-analysis indicated that daily doses of total hypericum of 0.4–2.7 mg were **more effective than placebo** in this patient group (Linde *et al.*, 1996). However, more recent studies in patients with clearly diagnosed major depression have not shown substantial antidepressant effects (Werneke *et al.*, 2004).

Adverse effects and drug interactions St John's Wort is well tolerated with the most common side-effects being **gastrointestinal disturbance, dizziness**, and **tiredness**. Cases of mania during treatment have been described. Photosensitivity is also rarely reported. Hypericum extracts may **induce hepatic enzymes** and there are reports that St John's Wort treatment was associated with lowered levels of theophylline, cyclosporin, digoxin, and ethinyloestradiol. Finally, St Johns Wort may cause **serotonin neurotoxicity** when combined with SSRIs and other 5-HT potentiating drugs (see Ernst, 1999).

Bupropion

Bupropion is not marketed in the United Kingdom or Europe but has significant use as an antidepressant in the United States. In the UK it is licensed as an adjunct to smoking withdrawal. It is structurally and pharmacologically distinct from other antidepressants being a unicyclic aminoketone derivative. Bupropion enhances both dopamine and noradrenaline function in the brain, probably via re-uptake blockade.

Efficacy and adverse effects Numerous controlled trials have shown that the antidepressant effect of bupropion is superior to that of placebo and equivalent to SSRIs. In some respects the adverse effect profile of bupropion is similar to that of the SSRIs with insomnia, agitation, tremor and nausea most frequently reported. Unlike SSRIs, however, bupropion does not cause sexual dysfunction, which gives it an important advantage in some patients.

The main concern with the use of bupropion has been the increased risk of seizures. In its original formulation the risk of seizures at higher doses (0.4 per cent) was about four times greater than that associated with SSRIs (about 0.1 per cent). The risk appears less with the slow release formulation (bupropion SR) which has been marketed for smoking cessation; at doses of 300 mg and less the risk of seizures with bupropion SR appears to be about 0.1 per cent. This is the maximum dose recommended for smoking cessation and is the standard dose used when treating depression. Bupropion should not be used in patients with a history of seizures or eating disorder.

Drug interactions Bupropion should not be given with other drugs that might lower seizure threshold such as TCAs, antipsychotic drugs and anti-malarials. Administration with MAOIs is also contraindicated. Bupropion has been combined safely with lithium and in the United States is used by specialists to augment ineffective SSRI treatment.

Mood-stabilizing drugs

Several agents are grouped under this heading such as **lithium** and a number of anticonvulsant drugs including **carbamazepine** and **sodium valproate**. These three drugs are effective in the **prevention** of recurrent affective illness and also in the **acute treatment of mania**. Lithium also has useful antidepressant effects in some circumstances, but the antidepressant activity of carbamazepine and sodium valproate is less well established. Another, anticonvulsant, **lamotrigine**, shows promise in the treatment of bipolar depression but does not appear to be effective against manic states.

Lithium

Placebo-controlled trials have shown that lithium is effective in a number of conditions:

- the acute treatment of mania;
- the prophylaxis of unipolar and bipolar mood disorder;
- augmentation therapy in resistant depression;
- the prevention of aggressive behaviour in patients with learning disabilities.

Mechanism of action Animal studies have shown that lithium has important effects on the intracellular signalling molecules or 'second messengers' that are activated when a neurotransmitter or agonist binds to a specific receptor. At clinically relevant doses, lithium inhibits the formation of **cyclic adenosine monophosphate (cAMP)** and also attenuates the formation of various **inositol lipid-derived mediators**. Through these actions lithium could exert profound effects on a wide range of neurotransmitter pathways, many of which use the above messenger systems. More recent interest has focused on the ability of lithium to promote cell survival and increase synaptic plasticity perhaps through inhibition of the activity of the enzyme glycogen synthase kinase-3 (Pilcher, 2003).

Pharmacokinetics Lithium is rapidly absorbed from the gut and diffuses quickly throughout the body fluids and cells. Lithium moves out of cells more slowly than sodium. It is removed from plasma by **renal excretion** and by entering cells and other body compartments. Therefore there is a rapid excretion of lithium from the plasma, and a slower phase reflecting its removal from the whole-body pool.

Like sodium, lithium is filtered and partly reabsorbed in the kidney. When the proximal tubule absorbs more water, lithium absorption increases. Therefore **dehydration** causes plasma lithium concentrations to rise. Because lithium is transported in competition with sodium, more is reabsorbed by the kidney when sodium concentrations fall. This is the mechanism whereby **thiazide diuretics** can lead to toxic concentrations of lithium in the blood.

Dosage and plasma concentrations Because the therapeutic and toxic doses are close together, it is essential to measure plasma concentrations of lithium during treatment. Measurements should first be made after 4–7 days, then weekly for 3 weeks, and then, provided that a satisfactory steady state has been achieved, once every 6 weeks. Subsequently, lithium levels are often very stable, and plasma monitoring can be carried out at intervals of 2–3 months unless there are clinical indications for more frequent monitoring.

After an oral dose, plasma lithium levels rise by a factor of two or three within about 4 hours. For this reason, concentrations are normally measured approximately **12 hours after the last dose**, usually that given at night. It is important to follow this routine because published information about lithium concentrations refers to the level 12 hours after the last dose, and not to the 'peak' reached in the 4 hours after that dose. If an unexpectedly high concentration is found, it is important to establish whether the patient has inadvertently taken a morning dose before the blood sample was taken.

Previously, the accepted range for prophylaxis was 0.7–1.2 mmol/l measured 12 hours after the last dose. However, current trends are to maintain lithium at **lower plasma levels** (0.5–0.8 mmol/l), because this decreases the burden of side-effects. Some studies suggest that patients with lower lithium levels (0.4–0.7 mmol/l) experience more affective illness during maintenance treatment than patients with higher levels (0.8–1.0 mmol/l). However, this is not a consistent finding (see Ferrier *et al.*, 1999).

In practice, it seems that many patients can be managed satisfactorily if their lithium levels are kept in the 0.4–0.7 mmol/l range. However, if a patient's course is unstable, it may be worthwhile maintaining slightly higher lithium levels if side-effects permit. In the treatment of acute mania, plasma concentrations below 0.8 mmol/l appear to be ineffective and a range of 0.8–1.0 mmol/l is probably required. Serious toxic effects appear with concentrations above 2.0 mmol/l, though early symptoms may appear above 1.2 mmol/l (see Macritchie and Young, 2004).

A number of delayed-release preparations of lithium are now available, but their pharmacokinetics *in vivo* do not differ significantly from those of standard lithium carbonate preparations. Liquid formulations of lithium citrate are available for patients who have difficulty in taking tablets. Lithium may be administered once or twice daily. Frequency of administration does not appear to affect urine volume. In general, it is more convenient to take lithium as a single dose at night, but patients who experience gastric irritation on this regimen may be helped by divided daily dosage.

Unwanted effects (Table 21.13) A mild **diuresis** due to sodium excretion occurs soon after the drug is started. Other common effects include **tremor** of the hands, **dry mouth**, a **metallic taste**, feelings of **muscular weakness**, and **fatigue**.

Some degree of mild **thirst and polyuria** is common in patients taking lithium, probably because lithium blocks the effect of antidiuretic hormone (ADH) on the renal tubule. This is rarely of clinical significance, but up to a third of patients show progression to a **diabetes insipidus-like syndrome** with pronounced polyuria and polydipsia. This may necessitate withdrawal of lithium treatment although the use of lower plasma lithium levels may cause the syndrome to remit.

Some patients, especially women, gain some **weight** when taking the drug. Persistent fine tremor, mainly affecting the hands, is common, but coarse tremor suggests that the plasma concentration of lithium has reached toxic levels. Most patients adapt to the fine tremor; for those who do not, propanolol up to 40 mg three times daily may reduce the symptom. Both **hair loss** and coarsening of hair texture can occur.

TABLE 21.13 Some adverse effects of lithium, carbamazepine and valproate

	Lithium	**Carbamazepine**	**Valproate**
Neurological	Tremor, weakness, dysarthria, ataxia, impaired memory, Seizures (rare)	Dizziness, weakness, drowsiness, ataxia, headache, visual disturbance	Tremor, sedation
Renal/fluid balance	Increased urine output with decreased urine concentrating ability. Thirst, diabetes insipidus (rare), oedema	Acts to increase urine concentrating ability. Low sodium states, oedema	Increased plasma ammonia
Gastrointestinal/ hepatic	Altered taste, anorexia, nausea, vomiting, diarrhoea, weight gain	Anorexia, nausea, constipation, hepatitis	Anorexia, nausea, vomiting, diarrhoea, weight gain, hepatitis (rare) pancreatitis (rare)
Endocrine	Decreased thyroxine with increased TSH. Goitre, hyperparathyroidism (rare)	Decreased thyroxine with normal TSH	Menstrual disturbances
Haematological	Leucocytosis	Leucopenia, agranulocytosis (rare)	Low platelet count. Abnormal platelet aggregation
Dermatological	Acne, exacerbation of psoriasis, hair loss	Erythematous rash	Hair loss
Cardiovascular	ECG changes (usually clinically benign)	Cardiac conduction disturbances	

Thyroid gland enlargement occurs in about 5 per cent of patients taking lithium. The thyroid shrinks again if thyroxine is given while lithium is continued and it generally returns to normal a month or two after lithium has been stopped. Lithium interferes with thyroid production, and **hypothyroidism** occurs in up to 20 per cent of women patients with a compensatory rise in thyroid-stimulating hormone.

Tests of thyroid function should be performed every 6 months to help to detect these changes, but these intermittent tests are no substitute for a continuous watch for suggestive clinical signs, particularly **lethargy** and substantial **weight gain**. If hypothyroidism develops and the reasons for lithium treatment are still strong, thyroxine treatment should be added. Lithium has also been associated with elevated serum calcium levels in the context of **hyperparathyroidism**. This is occasionally associated with severe depression, making distinction from the underlying mood disorder difficult.

Reversible ECG changes also occur. These may be due to displacement of potassium in the myocardium by lithium for they resemble those of hypokalaemia, with T-wave flattening and inversion or widening of the QRS. They are rarely of clinical significance. Other changes include a reversible **leucocytosis** and occasional papular or maculopapular rashes.

Effects on **memory** are sometimes reported by patients, who complain particularly of everyday lapses of memory such as forgetting well-known names. It is possible that this impairment of memory is caused by the mood disorder rather than by the drug itself, but there is also evidence that lithium can be associated with impaired performance on certain cognitive tests.

Long-term effects on the kidney As noted above, lithium treatment decreases **tubular concentrating ability** and can occasionally cause diabetes inspidus. In addition, there have been reports that over many years of treatment lithium can sometimes cause an increasing and in some cases **irreversible decline** in tubular function. This may be more likely in patients with higher plasma concentrations of lithium and where concomitant psychotropic medication has been employed (Bendz *et al.*, 1994).

Several follow-up studies have examined the effect of longer-term lithium maintenance treatment on **glomerular function**. In general, any decline in glomerular function is usually mild and related to lithium intoxication. However, there are occasional case reports of substantial glomerular decline and even frank **renal failure** in lithium-treated patients when other causes of nephrotoxicity appear to be absent. With the current trends towards long-term prophylaxis of mood disorders, it is clearly wise to monitor plasma **creatinine** levels regularly. It seems likely that the risk of nephrotoxicity will be minimized by maintaining plasma lithium levels at the **lower end** of the therapeutic range provided that they are therapeutically effective for the individual patient (see Macritchie and Young, 2004).

Toxic effects These are related to dose. They include **ataxia, poor coordination of limb movements, muscle twitching, slurred speech**, and **confusion**. They constitute a serious medical emergency for they can progress through **coma** and **fits** to **death**.

If these symptoms appear, lithium must be stopped at once and a high intake of fluid provided. In severe cases, renal dialysis may be needed. Lithium is rapidly cleared if renal function is normal so that most cases either recover completely or die. However, cases of permanent neurological damage despite haemodialysis have been reported.

As noted earlier (p. 524), lithium can increase **fetal abnormalities**, particularly of the heart, although the magnitude of the individual risk is low. The decision whether or not to continue with lithium treatment during pregnancy must therefore be carefully weighed. Important factors include the likelihood of affective relapse if lithium is withheld and the difficulty that could be experienced in managing an episode of affective illness in the individual woman.

If pregnant patients continue with lithium, plasma levels should be monitored closely. Ultrasound examination and fetal echocardiography are valuable screening tests as the pregnancy progresses. Patients with a history of **bipolar disorder** have a substantially **increased risk** of psychotic relapse in the post-partum period. In such patients it may be worth considering the introduction of lithium shortly after delivery to provide a prophylactic effect. However, significant concentrations of lithium can be measured in the plasma of breast-fed infants which may make bottle-feeding is advisable (see p. 524).

Drug interactions (Box 21.9) Because of the narrow therapeutic index of lithium, **pharmacokinetic** drug interactions are of major clinical importance. **Pharmacodynamic** interactions may involve potentiation of **5-HT promoting agents**, leading to a serotonin syndrome. In addition, therapeutic plasma levels of lithium can be associated with **neurotoxicity** in the presence of certain other centrally acting agents.

ECT and surgery It is possible that the continuation of lithium during **ECT** may lead to neurotoxicity. If feasible, lithium treatment should be suspended or

BOX 21.9 SOME DRUG INTERACTIONS OF LITHIUM

Pharmacokinetic

Increased lithium levels

- Diuretics (frusemide safest)
- Non-steroidal anti-inflammatory drugs
- (aspirin/sulindac safest)
- ACE Inhibitors
- Angiotensin-II receptor antagonists
- Antibiotics (spectinomycin/metronidazole)

Decreased lithium levels

- Theophylline
- Sodium bicarbonate

Pharmacodynamic

5-HT neurotoxicity

- SSRIs (can be used safely with care)
- 5-HT_1 agonists

Extrapyramidal side-effects enhanced

- Antipsychotic agents, metoclopramide, domperidone

Enhanced neurotoxicity

- Carbamazepine, phenytoin, calcium channel blockers, methyldopa

plasma levels reduced during ECT because the customary overnight fast beforehand may leave patients relatively dehydrated the following morning. If possible, lithium treatment should be discontinued before **major surgery** because the effects of **muscle relaxants** may be potentiated. However, the risk of acute withdrawal and 'rebound' mania must be considered (see below).

Lithium withdrawal In some studies, abrupt **lithium withdrawal** has been associated with the rapid onset of mania. Undoubtedly there is an increased risk of recurrent mood disorder after lithium discontinuation, probably because lithium is an effective prophylactic agent and because it is used for disorders with a high risk of recurrence. However, there is probably also a lithium withdrawal syndrome with 'rebound' mania, although this may be restricted to patients with bipolar disorder.

The risk of rapid relapse is lessened if lithium is **discontinued slowly** over a period of several weeks. Even patients who have remained entirely well for many years may experience a further episode of affective disorder after lithium discontinuation. Most of these subjects will respond to the reintroduction of lithium (Tondo *et al.*, 1997).

Contraindications These include renal failure or recent renal disease, current cardiac failure or recent myocardial infarction, and chronic diarrhoea sufficient to alter electrolytes. Lithium should not be prescribed if the patient is judged unlikely to observe the precautions required for its safe use. This includes a propensity to discontinue it suddenly against advice.

The management of patients on lithium

Preparation A careful routine of management is essential because of the effects of therapeutic doses of lithium on the thyroid and kidney, and the toxic effects of excessive dosage. The following routine is one of several that have been proposed and can be adopted safely. Successful treatment requires attention to detail, and so the steps are set out below at some length.

Before starting lithium, a **physical examination** should be carried out, including the measurement of blood pressure. It is also useful to **weigh** the patient.

Blood should be taken for estimation of **electrolytes**, serum **creatinine**, and a **full blood count**. When a particularly thorough evaluation is indicated, **creatinine clearance** is carried out, with an 18-hour collection usually being adequate. **Thyroid function tests** are also necessary. If indicated, an ECG and pregnancy tests should be performed as well.

If these tests show no contraindication to lithium treatment, the doctor should check that the patient is not taking any drugs that might interact with lithium. A careful explanation should then be given to the patient. They should understand the possible early toxic effects of an unduly high blood level, and also the circumstances in which this can arise, for example, during intercurrent gastroenteritis, renal infection, or the dehydration secondary to fever. They should be advised that if any of these arise, they should stop the drug and seek medical advice.

It is usually appropriate to include another member of the family in these discussions. Providing **printed guidelines** on these points is often helpful (either written by the doctor, or in one of the forms provided by pharmaceutical firms). In these discussions a sensible balance must be struck between alarming the patient by overemphasizing the risks and failing to give him the information that he needs to take a collaborative part in the treatment.

Starting treatment Lithium should normally be prescribed as the carbonate, and treatment should begin and continue with a **single daily dose** unless there is gastric intolerance, in which case divided doses can be given. If the drug is being used for prophylaxis, it is appropriate to begin with 200–400 mg mg daily in a single dose. The lower is appropriate where patients are taking concomitant medication such as SSRIs that might interact with lithium.

Blood should be taken for lithium estimations every week and adjusting the dose until an appropriate concentration is achieved. A lithium level of 0.4–0.7 mmol/l (in a sample taken 12 hours after the last dose) may be adequate for prophylaxis, as explained above; if this is not effective, the previously accepted higher range of 0.8–1.0 mmol/l should be used if side-effects permit. In judging response, it should be remembered that several months may elapse before lithium achieves its full effect.

Continuation treatment As treatment continues, lithium estimations should be carried out every **6–12 weeks**. It is important to have some means of reminding patients and doctors about the times at which repeat investigations are required. Computerized databases may be helpful in this respect. **Every 6 months**, blood samples should be taken for electrolytes, urea, and creatinine, a full blood count, and the thyroid function tests listed above. If two consecutive thyroid function tests a month apart show evidence of **hypothyroidism**, lithium should be stopped or L-thyroxine prescribed. Troublesome **polyuria** is a reason for attempting a reduction in dose, whilst severe persistent polyuria is an indication for specialist renal investigation including tests of concentrating ability. A persistent **leucocytosis** is not uncommon and is apparently harmless. It reverses soon after the drug is stopped.

When lithium is given, the doctor must keep in mind the **interactions** that have been reported with psychotropic and other drugs (see above). It is also prudent to watch for toxic effects with extra care if ECT is being given. If the patient requires an anaesthetic for any reason, the anaesthetist should be told that the patient is taking lithium; this is because, as noted above, there is some evidence that the effects of muscle relaxant may be potentiated.

Lithium is usually continued for at least a year, and often for much longer. The need for the drug should be reviewed once a year, taking into account any persistence of mild mood fluctuations, which suggest the possibility of relapse if treatment is stopped. Continuing medication is more likely to be needed if the patient has previously had several episodes of mood disorder within a short time, or if previous episodes were so severe that even a small risk of recurrence should be avoided.

Some patients have taken lithium continuously for 15 years or more, but there should always be compelling reasons for continuing treatment for more than 5 years. As noted above, lithium should be withdrawn slowly, over a number of months if possible. Patients should be advised not to **discontinue lithium suddenly** on their own initiative.

Carbamazepine

Carbamazepine was originally introduced as an **anticonvulsant** and was found to have useful effects on mood in certain patients. Subsequently it was found to be beneficial in many bipolar patients, including those who had proved **refractory to lithium**. There is reasonable evidence that carbamazepine is effective in the management of **acute mania** and also in the **prophylaxis** of **bipolar disorder** though overall its efficacy is probably a little less than that of lithium. Carbamazepine may also have some benefit in the treatment of **drug-resistant bipolar depression**, but it does not have an established role in the prophylaxis of recurrent unipolar depression (see Goodwin, 2003).

Mode of action Like certain other anticonvulsants, carbamazepine blocks **neuronal sodium channels**. It is unclear whether this action plays a role in the mood-stabilizing effects. In both humans and animals carbamazepine facilitates 5-HT neurotransmission, an action it shares with lithium.

Pharmacokinetics Carbamazepine is slowly but completely absorbed and widely distributed. It is extensively metabolized, with at least one metabolite, carbamazepine epoxide, being therapeutically active. The half-life during long-term treatment is about 20 hours. Carbamazepine is a strong **inducer of hepatic microsomal enzymes** and can lower the plasma concentrations of other drugs.

Dosage and plasma concentrations The dosage of carbamazepine in the treatment of mood disorders is similar to that used in the treatment of epilepsy, within the range of 400–1600 mg daily. Treatment is usually given in divided doses twice daily, because this practice may improve tolerance. No clear relationship has been established between plasma carbamazepine concentrations and therapeutic response, but it seems prudent to monitor levels (about 12 hours after the last dose) and to maintain them in the usual anticonvulsant range as a guard against toxicity.

Unwanted effects (Table 21.13) Side-effects are common at the beginning of treatment. They include **drowsiness, dizziness, ataxia, diplopia, and nausea.** Tolerance to these effects usually develops quickly. A potentially serious side-effect of carbamazepine is **agranulocytosis**, though this complication is very rare (variously estimated from 1 in 10 000 to 1 in 125 000 patients).

A **relative leucopenia** is more common, with the white cell count often falling in the first few weeks of treatment, though usually remaining within normal levels. Rashes occur in about 5 per cent of patients. Elevations in **liver enzymes** may also occur and, rarely, **hepatitis** has been reported. Carbamazepine can cause disturbances of **cardiac conduction** and therefore is contraindicated in patients with preexisting abnormalities of cardiac conduction.

Carbamazepine lowers plasma **thyroxine concentrations**, but thyroid-stimulating hormone levels are not elevated and clinical hypothyroidism is unusual. Carbamazepine has also been associated with low sodium states. The unwanted effects of carbamazepine are compared with those of lithium and valproate in Table 21.13.

Drug interactions Carbamazepine **increases the metabolism** of many other drugs including tricyclic antidepressants, benzodiazepines, haloperidol, oral contraceptive agents, thyroxine, warfarin, other anticonvulsants, and some antibiotics. A similar mechanism may underlie the **decline in plasma carbamazepine** levels that occur after the first few weeks of treatment.

Carbamazepine levels may be **increased** by SSRIs and erythromycin. The pharmacodynamic effects and plasma levels of carbamazepine may be increased by some calcium-channel blockers such as diltiazem and verapamil. Conversely, carbamazepine may decrease the effect of certain other calcium-channel antagonists such as felodipine and nicardipine. **Neurotoxicity** has been reported when **carbamazepine and lithium** have been combined even in the presence of normal lithium levels. The manufacturers of carbamazepine recommend that combination of carbamazepine with **MAOIs** be avoided. However, there are case reports of these drugs being used safely together. It is possible that some MAOIs may increase plasma carbamazepine levels.

Clinical use of carbamazepine

The usual indications for carbamazepine are:

- the prophylactic management of bipolar illness in patients for whom lithium treatment is ineffective or poorly tolerated;
- in the treatment of patients with frequent mood swings and mixed affective states for which carbamazepine may be more effective than lithium;
- added to lithium treatment in patients who have shown a partial response to the latter drug; in these circumstances it is important to remember that this combination can cause neurotoxicity;
- in the acute treatment of mania, again usually as an alternative or addition to lithium.

If clinical circumstances permit, it is preferable to start treatment with carbamazepine slowly at a dose of 100–200 mg daily, increasing in steps of 100–200 mg twice weekly. Patients show wide variability in the blood levels at which they experience adverse effects; accordingly, it is best to titrate the dose against the side-effects and the clinical response.

Because of the risk of a **lowered white cell count**, it is prudent to monitor the count in the first 3 months of treatment. Patients should be instructed to seek help urgently if they develop a fever or other sign of infection. When patients have responded to the addition of carbamazepine to lithium, it is possible subsequently to attempt a cautious lithium withdrawal. However, the current clinical impression is that for many patients, the maintenance of mood stability requires continuing treatment with both drugs.

Sodium valproate

Like carbamazepine, sodium valproate was first introduced as an anticonvulsant. In recent years there has been increasing interest in using the drug in the management of mood disorders.

There have been several controlled studies indicating that valproate is effective in the **acute management of mania**. As yet there is less clear evidence that valproate is effective in **longer-term prophylaxis** of bipolar disorder. However, in a randomized trial Bowden *et al.* (2000) showed a marginal benefit for valproate over lithium and placebo in bipolar patients over a 1-year follow-up. There have been numerous case studies and open studies that have reported useful prophylactic effects of valproate in patients **unresponsive to lithium and carbamazepine**, including those with rapid cycling mood disorders (see Ferrier, 2001).

Mode of action Valproate is a simple branch-chain fatty acid with a mode of action that is unclear. However, there is some evidence that it can slow the breakdown of the **inhibitory neurotransmitter GABA.** This action could account for the anticonvulsant properties of valproate, but whether it also underlies the psychotropic effects is unclear.

Pharmacokinetics Valproate is rapidly absorbed, with the peak plasma concentrations occurring about 2 hours after ingestion. It is widely and rapidly distributed and has a half-life of 8–18 hours. Valproate is metabolized in the liver to produce a wide variety of metabolites, some of which have anticonvulsant activity. Unlike carbamazepine, valproate does not induce hepatic microsomal enzymes and, if anything, tends to delay the metabolism of other drugs.

Dosing and plasma concentrations Valproate can be started at a dose of 200–400 mg daily, which may be increased once or twice weekly to a range of 1–2 g daily. Plasma levels of valproate do not correlate well with either the anticonvulsant or the mood-stabilizing effects, but it has been suggested that efficacy in the treatment of acute mania is usually apparent when plasma levels are **greater than 50 μg/ml**.

Unwanted effects (Table 21.13) Common side-effects with valproate include **gastrointestinal disturbances, tremor, sedation, and tiredness**. Other troublesome side-effects include **weight gain** and **transient hair loss** with changes in texture on regrowth.

Patients taking valproate may have some elevation in **hepatic transaminase enzymes**; provided that this increase is not associated with hepatic dysfunction, the drug can be continued while enzyme levels and liver function are carefully monitored. However, there have been several reports of fatal **hepatic toxicity** associated with the use of valproate; most of these cases have occurred in children taking multiple anticonvulsant drugs. Valproate must be withdrawn immediately if vomiting, anorexia, jaundice, or sudden drowsiness occur.

Valproate may also cause **thrombocytopenia** and may inhibit platelet aggregation. **Acute pancreatitis** is another rare but serious side-effect, and increases in plasma **ammonia** have also been reported. Other possible side-effects include **oedema, amenorrhoea**, and **rashes**.

Drug interactions Valproate potentiates the effects of central sedatives. It has been reported to increase the side effects of other anticonvulsants (without necessarily improving anticonvulsant control). It may **increase plasma levels** of phenytoin and tricyclic antidepressants.

Clinical use

The efficacy of valproate in the acute and continuation treatment of mania has been established by several controlled trials (see Goodwin, 2003) and it is licensed for this indication in the UK in the form of the semisodium preparation. In the treatment of acute mania it produces a quicker onset of action than lithium and carbamazepine because it can be dosed at high levels initially. For example, a therapeutic effect can be apparent with a day or two employing a loading dose of valproate of 20 mg/kg. Valproate may also be more effective than lithium in the management of patients with **mixed affective states**.

In terms of prophylaxis, valproate seems more effective in the prevention of manic than depressive episodes. It has often been used in combination with lithium in bipolar patients who have shown a partial response to lithium, and this combination appears to be safe. Valproate has also been used in combination with carbamazepine. For patients who continue to show episodes of mood disturbance, valproate can be combined with antidepressant or antipsychotic drugs (Ferrier, 2001).

Lamotrigine

Lamotrigine is a triazine derivative which blocks voltage-dependent **sodium channels** and reduces excitatory neurotransmitter release, particularly that of **glutamate**. Lamotrigine is licensed in the UK as a monotherapy and adjunctive treatment for epilepsy.

Lamotrigine is not licensed for the treatment of mood disorders in the UK but there are open studies showing therapeutic benefit when it has been added to the medication of patients with **bipolar illness refractory to standard treatments**. In addition, placebo-controlled trials have shown that lamotrigine is effective as monotherapy in the acute treatment of **bipolar depression** (Calabrese *et al.*, 1999) and also in the longer-term prevention of this disorder (Bowden *et al.*, 2003). Used alone lamotrigine does not seem to have significant acute or prophylactic anti-manic actions.

Pharmacokinetics Following oral administration, lamotrigine is rapidly absorbed with peak plasma levels occurring after about 1.5 hours. The drug is extensively metabolized by the liver but does not induce cytochrome P450 enzymes. Its half-life is about 30 hours. A plasma therapeutic range has not been identified.

Adverse effects Skin eruptions, usually maculopapular in nature, occur in about 3 per cent of patients and may be associated with fever. They are most common in the first few weeks of treatment and their incidence can be reduced by careful initial dosing (see below). Other side-effects include **nausea, headache, diplopia, blurred vision, dizziness, ataxia, and tremor**. Very serious adverse effects such as **angioedema, Stevens- Johnson syndrome** and **toxic epidermal necrolysis** have been reported rarely.

Drug interactions Plasma levels of lamotrigine can be lowered by drugs that induce hepatic-metabolizing enzymes such as **carbamazepine**. Combination of carbamazepine and lamotrigine can also cause neurotoxicity. Lamotrigine levels are increased by concomitant administration of **valproate**.

Clinical use

Until more data are available, lamotrigine should be used in bipolar disorder only when more familiar agents have proved unsuccessful. Lamotrigine may then be helpful as an **adjunctive therapy**, paying due attention to the drug interactions noted above. Lamotrigine may also be useful in the treatment of **bipolar depression**, again when standard agents are poorly tolerated or unsuccessful. It is presumed that lamotrigine will be less likely to produce mania or rapid cycling in bipolar patients than conventional antidepressants, but this has yet to be clearly established.

When initiating lamotrigine treatment, to minimize the risk of rash, it is important to follow the **dosage recommendations in the *British National Formulary*** (25 mg daily for the first 2 weeks, followed by 50 mg daily for the next 2 weeks). The usual therapeutic dose in bipolar disorder is between 50–300 mg daily.

Gabapentin

Gabapentin was developed as a structural analogue of GABA. Despite its structural relationship to GABA, its anticonvulsant mechanism of action is uncertain, although it does increase **GABA turnover** in the brain.

Gabapentin is licensed as an adjunctive treatment for seizure disorders and is not licensed for the treatment of mood disorders. There are published case series showing benefit when gabapentin has been used as an adjunctive therapy in patients with **bipolar disorder resistant to standard medication regimens** (Young *et al.*, 1999). However, controlled trials in mania and refractory bipolar depression have yielded disappointing results (Yatham, 2004), Gabapentin has a **sedating** profile and may also have **anxiolytic** properties.

Pharmacokinetics After oral absorption peak, plasma levels of gabapentin are reached after 2–3 hours. Gabapentin is not metabolized by the liver and is excreted entirely by the kidney. Its half-life is about 5–7 hours and thrice-daily dosing is recommended.

Unwanted effects The most common side-effects of gabapentin are **somnolence, dizziness, fatigue, and nystagmus**. No serious adverse effects have been reported.

Drug interactions Probably because of its lack of hepatic metabolism, thus far no significant pharmacokinetic interactions of gabapentin with other medications have been described. It may potentiate the effects of other central sedatives.

Clinical use

As with lamotrigine, gabapentin can be considered in patients with bipolar disorder who have **not responded** to standard therapies. Gabapentin has a wide dosage range but the usual dose in bipolar illness is between 600 mg and 2400 mg daily. Sedative and anxiolytic effects are often apparent at lower doses. While effects of this nature might be useful in patients with refractory bipolar illness, there is currently no evidence from controlled trials that gabapentin has a place in the treatment of bipolar disorder.

Psychostimulants

This class of drugs includes mild stimulants, of which the best known is **caffeine**, and more powerful stimulants such as **amphetamine** and **methylphenidate**. Pemoline has intermediate effects. **Cocaine** is a powerful psychostimulant with a particularly high potential for inducing dependence (see p. 464). It is useful as a local anaesthetic but has no other clinical indications. All these psychostimulants **increase the release** and **block the re-uptake** of dopamine and noradrenaline. A new compound, **modafinil**, produces increases in alertness and decreases sleepiness, apparently through non-catecholaminergic mechanisms (Saper and Scammel, 2004), Modafinil is licensed for the treatment of narcolepsy.

Indications

Amphetamines were used for numerous conditions in the past, but they are now prescribed much less frequently because of the high risk of dependence. They are not appropriate for the treatment of obesity. In adults the agreed indication for amphetamines is **narcolepsy**. Methylphenidate is approved for the treat of attention deficit disorder in children. It is also effective in adults who have continued to display symptoms of attention deficit but the diagnosis and treatment of adult attention deficit disorder is controversial (see Zwi and York, 2004).

In the past, amphetamines were widely prescribed for the treatment of depression, but have been superseded by the antidepressant drugs. Some specialists, mainly in the USA, believe that psychostimulants may have a role either as sole agent or in combination with other antidepressant drugs for patients with **refractory depressive disorder**. Also, there is some interest in using psychostimulants for **elderly depressed patients**

with concomitant medical illness. A blanket proscription of psychostimulant treatment in depression therefore seems unjustified. However, psychostimulants should be used only by practitioners with special experience in the psychopharmacological management of resistant depression. Modafinil has been used with apparent benefit in open case series to treat sleepiness and fatigue in depressed patients receiving SSRIs (Menza *et al.*, 2000).

The main preparations are dexamphetamine sulphate, given for narcolepsy in divided doses of 10 mg daily increasing to a maximum of 50 mg daily in steps of 10 mg each week, and methylphenidate, which has similar effects. In narcolepsy, modafinil is used in doses of 200–400mg.

Unwanted effects These include restlessness, insomnia, poor appetite, dizziness, tremor, palpitations, and cardiac arrhythmias. Toxic effects from large doses include disorientation and aggressive behaviour, hallucinations, convulsions, and coma. Persistent abuse can lead to a paranoid state similar to paranoid schizophrenia. Amphetamines can cause severe hypertension in combination with MAOIs and to a lesser extent with tricyclic antidepressants. They are contraindicated in cardiovascular disease and thyrotoxicosis. Modafinil has been associated with dry mouth, nausea, abdominal pain, headache, tachycardia, anxiety and insomnia.

Other physical treatments

Electroconvulsive therapy (ECT)

History

Convulsive therapy was introduced in the late 1930s on the basis of the mistaken idea that epilepsy and schizophrenia do not occur together. It seemed to follow that induced fits should lead to improvement in schizophrenia. However, when the treatment was tried it became apparent that the most striking changes occurred not in schizophrenia but in **severe depressive disorders**, in which it brought about a substantial reduction in chronicity and mortality (Slater, 1951).

At first, fits were produced either by using cardiazol (Meduna, 1938) or by passing an electric current through the brain (Cerletti and Bini, 1938). As time went by, electrical stimulation became the rule. The subsequent addition of brief anaesthesia and muscle relaxants made the treatment safe and acceptable.

Indications

This section summarizes the indications for ECT. Further information about the efficiency of the proced-

BOX 21.10 INDICATIONS FOR ECT

It is recommended that electroconvulsive therapy is used only to achieve rapid and short-term improvement of severe symptoms after an adequate trial of other treatment options has proven ineffective and/or when the condition is considered to be potentially life-threatening in individuals with:

1. severe depressive illness
2. catatonia
3. a prolonged or severe manic episode.

National Committee for Clinical Excellence (2003)

BOX 21.11 INDICATIONS FOR ECT

In severe depressive illness, ECT may be the treatment of choice when the illness is associated with:

- Life-threatening illness because of refusal of foods and fluids
- High suicide risk

ECT may be considered for the treatment of severe depressive illness associated with:

- Stupor
- Marked psychomotor retardation
- Depressive delusions and hallucinations

ECT may be considered as second or third line treatment of depressive illness not responsive to antidepressant drugs

ECT may be considered for the treatment of mania associated with:

- Life-threatening physical exhaustion
- Mania that has not responded to appropriate drug treatment

ECT may be considered for the treatment of acute schizophrenia as a fourth line option for treatment resistant schizophrenia after treatment with two antipsychotic drugs and then clozapine has proved ineffective.

ECT may be indicated in patients with catatonia where treatment with a benzodiazepine (usually lorazapam) has proved ineffective.

Royal College of Psychiatrists (2005)
Source Scott (2005)

ure will be found in the chapters dealing with the individual psychiatric syndromes.

ECT is a rapid and effective treatment for **severe depressive disorders**. In the Medical Research Council trial (Clinical Psychiatry Committee, 1965) it acted faster than imipramine or phenelzine, and was more effective than imipramine in women and more effective than phenelzine in both sexes. The indications for ECT have recently been reviewed by the National Committee for Clinical Excellence (Box 21.10). Indications suggested by the Royal College of Psychiatrists (2005) are given in Box 21.11.

Both sets of guidelines accord with the impression of many clinicians, and with the recommendations of this book, that ECT should be used mainly when it is essential to bring about improvement quickly. Therefore, the strongest indications are an immediate **high risk of suicide, depressive stupor, or danger to physical health** because the patient is not drinking enough to maintain adequate renal function.

ECT can lead a rapid resolution of **mania** (Mukherjee *et al.*, 1994) but is generally reserved for patients who do not respond to drug treatment or for those whose manic illness is severe, requiring high doses of antipsychotic drugs.

On the basis of clinical case studies, it has long been held that ECT is useful in the treatment of **acute catatonic states**. Controlled studies have also shown that ECT is effective in patients with acute schizophrenia with predominantly positive symptoms. In these studies ECT is effective not only for affective symptoms but also for positive symptoms such as **delusions** and **thought disorder** (Brandon *et al.*, 1985). In general, however, ECT adds little to the effects of adequate doses of antipsychotic drugs, though it probably produces a greater rate of symptomatic improvement in the short term. It is unclear whether ECT has a role in the treatment of patients with schizophrenia whose positive symptoms do not respond to antipsychotic medication. There is greater evidence for the use of atypical antipsychotic drugs in this situation and ECT is not generally recommended (National Committee for Clinical Excellence, 2003), although the Royal College of Psychiatrists suggests it can be considered as a fourth line option.

Mode of action

Role of the seizure Presumably, the specific therapeutic effects of ECT must be brought about through physiological and biochemical changes in the brain. The first step in identifying the mode of action must be to find out whether the therapeutic effect depends on the seizure, or whether other features of the treatment are sufficient, such as the passage of the current through the brain and the use of anaesthesia and muscle relaxants.

Clinicians have generally been convinced that the patient does not improve unless a convulsion is produced during ECT procedure. This impression has been confirmed by several double-blind trials which, taken

Trial	Number of participants	Standardized effect size (95% CI)
Wilson 196310	12	−1.078 (−2.289 to 0.133)
West 198111	25	−1.255 (−2.170 to −0.341)
Lambourn 197815	40	−0.170 (−0.940 to 0.600)
Freeman 197812	40	−0.629 (−1.2647 to 0.006)
Gregory 198513	69	−1.418 (−2.012 to −0.824)
Johnstone 198014	70	−0.739 (−1.253 to −0.224)
Pooled fixed effects		−0.911 (−1.180 to −0.645)
Pooled random effects		−0.908 (−1.270 to −0.537)

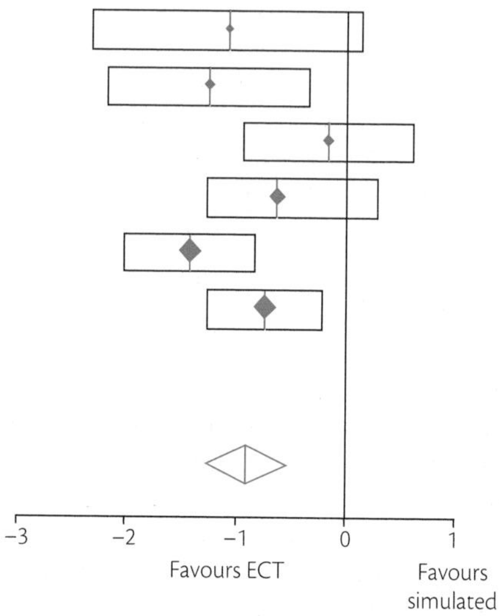

−3 −2 −1 0 1

Favours ECT

Favours simulated

Fig 21.1 Meta-analysis of randomized, placebo-controlled studies of ECT in depression. UK ECT Review Group (2003).

together, show that ECT is strikingly more effective than a full placebo procedure that includes anaesthetic and muscle relaxant (see UK ECT Review Group, 2003) (Figure 21.1).

This evidence does not necessarily support the notion that a full seizure is the sufficient and necessary therapeutic component of ECT, and recent studies have shown that this notion is incorrect. Modern ECT machines deliver brief pulses of electrical current that enable a seizure to be induced by administration of relatively low doses of electrical energy. With this mode of administration, both **electrode placement** and **electrical dosage** can have profound effects on the therapeutic efficacy of ECT. In particular, it appears that the **amount by which the applied electrical dose exceeds the seizure threshold of the individual patient** is an important determinant of both efficacy and cognitive side-effects of ECT. Furthermore, the seizure threshold varies greatly (about 15-fold) between individuals.

This situation has important implications for the practical management of ECT when the clinician's aim is to find the best balance between **therapeutic efficacy** and **cognitive side-effects** (see below). From a theoretical viewpoint, however, it can be concluded that an important determinant of ECT efficacy is how far the applied electrical energy **exceeds the seizure threshold** of the individual patient.

Neurochemical effects of ECT Electrical seizures in animals produce many biochemical and electrophysiological changes, and therefore it is difficult to identify the processes that are important in the antidepressant effect of ECT. It is of interest that some of the changes in brain monoamine pathways found in rodents after ECT (for example, **downregulation of noradrenaline β-adrenoceptors**) resemble those found after antidepressant drug treatment. In addition, both ECT and antidepressants increase the expression of **dopamine D_2 receptors** in the nucleus accumbens, which could be associated with improvements in motivational behaviour. In the case of ECT, this may involve interaction with **glutamatergic pathways**.

Physiological changes during ECT

If ECT is given without atropine premedication, the pulse first slows and then rises quickly to 130–190 beats/min, falling to the original resting rate or beyond towards the end of the seizure before a final less marked tachycardia lasting several minutes. Marked increases in blood pressure are also common and the systolic pressure can rise to 200 mmHg. Cerebral blood flow also increases by up to 200 per cent.

Unilateral or bilateral ECT

Overall bilateral ECT has a superior efficacy to unilateral ECT; however, bilateral ECT is associated with more cognitive impairment (UK ECT Review Group, 2003).

More recent studies of this issue have concluded that:

- high-dose right unilateral ECT (titrated to a dose five times greater than seizure threshold) is as effective as low-dose bilateral ECT and causes less cognitive impairment;
- high fixed-dose right unilateral ECT (about 400 millicoulombs) is more effective than moderately (2.5 times) suprathreshold right unilateral ECT;
- cognitive impairment with right unilateral ECT increases as dose exceeds seizure threshold but is less than any form of bilateral ECT.

These data suggest that that the most appropriate electrode placement for ECT is right unilateral with dose titrated to about five times above initial seizure threshold. This is likely to give the best overall combination of efficacy and lower cognitive impairment (Sackheim *et al.*, 2000). However, if the need for improvement is a particularly urgent, bilateral ECT should be considered. (For a meta-analytic review of treatment factors affecting the efficacy of ECT see UK ECT Review Group, 2003) (Box 21.12).

Unwanted effects after ECT

Subconvulsive shock may be followed by anxiety and headache. ECT can cause a brief **retrograde amnesia** as well as loss of memory for up to 30 minutes after the fit. **Brief disorientation** can occur, particularly with

BOX 21.12 EFFICACY OF ECT IN DEPRESSION IN RELATION TO ANTIDEPRESSANT TREATMENT AND DIFFERENT STIMULUS PARAMETERS

Treatment Comparison	Ham-D Difference (with 95% CI)	Effect size
ECT superior to antidepressant medication	5.2 (1.4–8.9)	0.46
Bilateral ECT superior to unilateral	3.6 (2.2–5.2)	0.32
Higher ECT dose superior	4.1 (2.4–5.9)	0.57

From the UK ECT review Group (2003).
HAM-D is Hamilton Rating Scale for Depression.

bilateral electrode placement. **Headache** can also occur. Some patients complain of confusion, nausea, and vertigo for a few hours after the treatment, but with modern methods these unwanted effects are mild and brief.

A few patients complain of **muscle pain**, especially in the jaws, which is probably attributable to the relaxant. There have been a few reports of sporadic major seizures in the months after ECT, but these may have had other causes. Occasional damage to the teeth, tongue, or lips can occur if there have been problems in positioning the gag or airway. Poor application of the electrodes can lead to **small electrical burns**. **Fractures**, including crush fractures of the vertebrae, have occurred occasionally when ECT was given without muscle relaxants.

All these physical consequences are rare provided that a good technique of anaesthesia is used and the fit is modified adequately. Other complications of ECT are rare and mainly occur in people suffering from physical illness. They include **cardiac arrhythmia, pulmonary embolism, aspiration pneumonia, and cerebrovascular accident**. Prolonged apnoea is a rare complication of the use of muscle relaxants. Rarely, **status epilepticus** may occur in predisposed subjects or in those taking medication that prolongs seizure duration.

Since the introduction of ECT, there has always been concern as to whether it may cause **brain damage**. When ECT is given to animals in the usual clinical regimen, there is no evidence that brain damage occurs. Also, structural imaging studies in patients have been reassuring on this point (UK ECT Review Group, 2003).

Memory disorder after ECT

As already mentioned, the immediate effects of ECT include loss of memory for events shortly before the treatment (**retrograde amnesia**), and impaired retention of information acquired soon after the treatment (**anterograde amnesia**). These effects depend on both electrode placement (unilateral versus bilateral) and electrical dose; electrode placement appears to be the more important factor.

Controlled studies indicate that the **anterograde amnesia** produced by ECT is **temporary**. Sackheim *et al.* (1993) found either no differences in memory tests or some improvements in the weeks after ECT. Depressive disorders substantially impair cognitive function, and many patients report their memory as subjectively improved after ECT (Sackheim *et al.*, 1993).

Possible long-term effects of ECT on memory take two forms. First, some patients describe loss of **memories for personal and impersonal remote events** (retrograde amnesia for remote events). For example, Squire *et al.* (1981) found that after bilateral ECT, in particular, there was a patchy loss of memory for some personal events, television programmes or major news items. More recently, Lisanby *et al.* (2000) found that 2 months after ECT there was some persistent loss of remote memories for impersonal events, which were more marked than those for personal events. Bilateral ECT caused more deficts in this respect than unilateral ECT.

The other possible complication is decreased ability to **learn new information** (long-term anterograde amnesia). For example, in a study of former patients who were complaining that they had suffered permanent harm to memory from ECT given in the past, Freeman *et al.* (1980) found that these patients did worse than controls on some tests in a battery designed to test memory. However, they also had residual depressive symptoms, and so it is possible that continuing depressive disorder accounted for the memory problems.

It seems reasonable to conclude that, when used in the usual way, **ECT is not usually followed by persisting anterograde memory disorder** and where this does occur it is mild and may be accounted for by concurrent depressive symptomatology (Cohen *et al.*, 2000). However, there may be some persisting retrograde amnesia for personal and impersonal memories, particularly with bilateral ECT. While this is not a significant problem for most patients, some people for reasons that are unclear have greater ECT-induced memory loss and are understandably distressed by it.

The mortality of ECT

The death rate attributable to ECT was estimated to be **3–4 per 100 000 treatments** by Barker and Barker (1959). This is similar to that seen with general anaesthesia in general medical conditions. The risks are related to the anaesthetic procedure and are greatest in patients with cardiovascular disease. When death occurs it is usually due to **ventricular fibrillation** or **myocardial infarction**.

Contraindications The contraindications to ECT are any medical illnesses that increase the risk of anaesthetic procedure by an unacceptable amount, for example, respiratory infections, serious heart disease, and serious pyrexial illness. Other contraindications are diseases likely to be made worse by the **changes in blood pressure and cardiac rhythm** that occur even in a well-modified fit; these include serious heart diseases, recent myocardial infarction, cerebral or aortic aneurysm, and raised intracranial pressure.

Mediterranean and Afro-Caribbean patients who might have **sickle cell trait** need additional care that oxygen tension does not fall. Extra care is also required with diabetic patients who take insulin. Although risks rise somewhat in old age, so do the risks of untreated depression and drug treatment.

Adverse effects, including increased cognitive impairment, have been reported when ECT has been given with **lithium**. **SSRIs** have been associated with prolonged seizures during ECT. Some anaesthetists prefer not to anaesthetize patients taking **MAOIs**, but ECT can, in fact, be given safely to patients receiving MAOI treatment.

Technique of administration

In this section we outline the technical procedures used at the time of treatment. Although the information in this account should be known, it is important to remember that ECT is a **practical procedure** that must be learned by apprenticeship as well as by reading.

ECT clinic ECT should be given in pleasant safe surroundings. Patients should not have to wait where they can see or hear treatment given to others. There should be waiting and recovery areas separate from the room in which treatment is given, and adequate emergency equipment should be available including a sucker, endotracheal tubes, adequate supplies of oxygen, and facilities to carry out full resuscitation. The nursing and medical staff who give ECT should receive **special training and accreditation**.

Arrival of patient The first step in giving ECT is to put the patient at ease and to check their identity. The case notes should then be seen to make sure that there is a valid consent form. The drug sheet should be checked to ensure that the patient is not receiving any drugs that might complicate anaesthetic procedures. It is also important to check for evidence of drug allergy or adverse effects of previous general anaesthetics. The drug sheet should be available for the anaesthetist to see. A full physical evaluation should have been carried out by the patient's treating doctor. Specialist advice should be sought when there may be medical contra-indications to ECT.

Electrode placement A decision about electrode placement should have been made by the treating doctor prior to treatment. In using unilateral treatment, it is important to apply the electrodes to the **non-dominant hemisphere**. In right-handed people, the left hemisphere is nearly always dominant; in left-handed people, either hemisphere may be dominant. Hence, if there is evidence that the patient is not right-handed, it is usually better to use bilateral electrode placements.

Anaesthetic procedures Prior to anaesthetic it is necessary to make sure that the patient has taken nothing by mouth for at least 5 hours, and then, with the anaesthetist, to remove dentures and check for loose or broken teeth. Finally, the record of any previous ECTs should be examined for evidence of delayed recovery from the relaxant (due to deficiency in pseudocholinesterase) or other complications.

The anaesthetic should be given by a trained anaesthetist (though this cannot always be achieved in developing countries). Suction apparatus, a positive-pressure oxygen supply, and emergency drugs should always be available. A tilting trolley is also valuable. As well as the psychiatrist and anaesthetist, at least one nurse should be present.

There is some debate as to whether atropine pretreatment helps to prevent vagal arrhythmias and dry excess bronchial secretion. There is little evidence that atropine in usual dosage is useful for these purposes. If an anticholinergic agent is required to dry secretions, glycopyrrolate should be used because it does not cross the blood–brain barrier.

Anaesthesia for ECT is best induced with **methohexitone**, a short-acting barbiturate. However, this agent is becoming increasingly difficult to obtain. Alternatives are **propofol, etomidate** or **thiopentone** but all have some drawbacks (Freeman 1999). **Propofol** is probably the most widely used in day-case anaesthesia but it can **decrease seizure length** during ECT and has also been associated with **delayed convulsions, delayed recovery**, and **anaphylaxis**.

The induction agent is followed immediately by a **muscle relaxant** (often suxamethonium chloride) from a separate syringe, although the same needle can be used. The anaesthetist is responsible for the choice of drugs and should also ensure that the lungs are well oxygenated before a mouth gag is inserted.

Application of ECT While the anaesthetic is being given, the psychiatrist checks both the **dose of electricity** and the **electrode placement** that has been prescribed for the patient. The skin is cleaned in the appropriate areas and moistened electrodes are applied. (If good electrical contact is to be obtained, it is also important that grease and hair lacquer are removed by ward staff before the patient is sent for ECT.) While dry electrodes can cause skin burns, it is also important to remember that excessive moisture causes shorting and may prevent a seizure response.

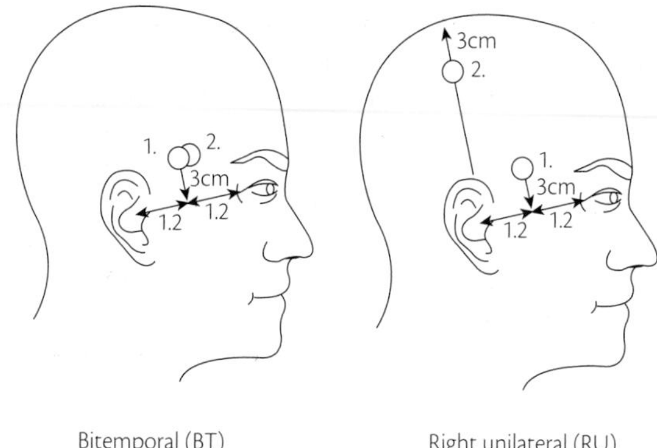

Fig 21.2 Electrode placements for ECT.

Although enough muscle relaxant should have been given to ensure that convulsive movements are minimal, a nurse or other assistant should be ready to restrain the patient gently if necessary. The electrodes are now secured firmly. For unilateral ECT, the first electrode is placed on the non-dominant side, 3 cm above the midpoint between the external angle of the orbit and the external auditory meatus. The second is **at least 10 cm** away from the first, vertically above the meatus of the same side (see Figure 21.2). A wide separation of the electrodes increases the efficacy of unilateral ECT (see Lock, 1999). The stimulus is then given.

For **fixed-dose right unilateral ECT** the initial dose should be set at 400 millicoulombs and subsequently adjusted according to clinical efficacy and cognitive side-effects. However dose-titration offers advantages in terms of individualizing the dose for each patient. In dose titration the seizure threshold for the individual patient is determined during the first ECT session by starting with a very low dose and increasing until a fit occurs (see Lock, 1999).

For **bilateral ECT**, electrodes are on opposite sides of the head, each 3 cm above the midpoint of the line joining the eternal angle of the orbit to the external auditory meatus – usually just above the hairline (Figure 21.2). When using bilateral electrode placement, the present practice is to administer a dose of electricity that is only modestly (about 50 per cent) above the seizure threshold for the individual. The seizure threshold for ECT is best determined by dose titration as described above. Otherwise an appropriate dose can be estimated from the fact that two-thirds of the population have seizure thresholds between 100 and 200 millicoulombs. In addition, seizure thresholds are higher in men than in women, and increase with age. For example, a reasonable starting dose for a male patient under 40 who is to receive bilateral ECT, would be 150 millicoulombs.

Subsequently this dose could be adjusted depending on the length of seizure, the cognitive side-effects, and clinical response. The dose might be increased if the seizure were short or absent, or if there were no improvement after several treatments. Conversely, troublesome post-ECT cognitive disturbance would indicate that the dose of electricity should be reduced or bilateral placement of the electrodes used.

It is important to note that seizure duration may **decrease** during a course of ECT because repeated treatment tends to increase seizure threshold. Thus, if a dose of electricity initially produced a seizure of satisfactory duration, it may subsequently need to be increased.

The seizure It is essential to observe carefully for evidence of seizure. If satisfactory muscle relaxation has been achieved, the seizure takes the following form. First the muscles of the face begin to twitch and the mouth drops open; then the upper eyelids, thumbs, and big toes jerk rhythmically for about half a minute. It is important not to confuse these convulsive movements with muscle twitches due to the depolarization produced by suxamethonium.

EEG monitoring has been used to check whether a seizure has been induced, but the records can be difficult to interpret because of the muscle artefact produced by direct stimulation of the frontalis muscle. An alternative is to **isolate one forearm from the effects of the muscle relaxant**. This can be done by blowing up a blood pressure cuff to above systolic pressure before the relaxant is injected; this pressure is maintained during the period in which the seizure should occur and then released. Seizure activity can then be observed in the muscles of the isolated part of the arm. When judging the appropriate cuff pressure, it is important to remember that systolic pressure rises during the seizure; if the cuff is not at sufficient pressure the relaxant will pass into the forearm at this stage.

There is no direct correlation between treatment outcome and duration of seizure activity, but it is recommended that the dose of electricity be adjusted to achieve a seizure duration of **between 20 and 50 seconds**. This duration is recommended because short seizures are likely to be therapeutically ineffective whereas long seizures are more likely to be associated with cognitive disturbance.

Psychotropic drugs may alter seizure threshold and seizure duration. For example, most antidepressant and antipsychotic drugs lower seizure threshold, whilst benzodiazepines valproate and lamotrigine have the reverse effect.

Recovery phase After the seizure, the lungs are oxygenated thoroughly with an airway in place. The patient remains in the care of the anaesthetist and under close nursing observation until breathing resumes and consciousness is restored. During recovery, the patient should be turned on their side and cared for in the usual way for anyone recovering from an anaesthetic after a minor surgical procedure. A qualified nurse should be in attendance to supervise the patient and reassure them. Meanwhile the psychiatrist makes a note of the date, type of electrode placement, drugs used, and amount of current, together with a brief description of the fit and any problems that have arisen. When the patient is awake and orientated, they should rest for an hour or so on a bed or in a chair.

If ECT is given to a day patient, it is especially important to make certain that no food or drink has been taken before they arrive at the hospital. They should rest for several hours and should not leave until it is certain that their recovery is complete; they should leave in the company of a responsible adult and certainly not riding a bicycle or driving a car.

Failed stimulations The most important problem, apart from those relating to the anaesthetic procedure, is failure to produce a clonic convulsion (a tonic jerk produced by the current must not be mistaken for a seizure). If it is certain that no seizure has appeared, checks should be made of the machine, electrodes, and contact with the skin. The possibility of shorting due to excess moisture on the scalp should also be considered. If all these are excluded, the patient may have either an unusually high resistance to the passage of current through the extracranial tissues and skull, or a high convulsive threshold. The charge can then be increased by 50% and a further stimulus given.

Frequency and number of treatments

ECT is usually given twice a week. In general, thrice-weekly ECT has **little therapeutic advantage** over a twice weekly regimen, and may produce more cognitive impairment (UK ECT Review Group, 2003).

Decisions about the length of a course of ECT have to depend on clinical experience since relevant information is not available from clinical trials. **A course of ECT is usually from six to a maximum of 12 treatments**. Progress should be reviewed after each treatment; there is usually little response until two or three treatments have been given, after which increasing improvement takes place. If the response is more rapid than this, fewer treatments may be given. If there has been no response after six to eight treatments, the course should usually be abandoned since it is unlikely that more ECT will produce useful change. Memory should also be assessed after each treatment. Significant cognitive impairment should lead to a reappraisal of the electrical dose and electrode placement.

Prevention of relapse

It is important that, whereas ECT may produce striking benefit in depressed patients, there is a **high relapse rate** unless continuation therapy with antidepressant medication is undertaken. Sometimes the choice of antidepressant drug can be difficult because if a patient does not respond to an adequate dose of an antidepressant drug prior to ECT, continuing the same drug after the course of ECT is completed **may not provide a useful prophylactic effect** (Sackheim *et al.*, 1990). Thus, if a patient has required ECT because of non-response to antidepressant medication, it is good practice to consider a different class of antidepressant drug or else lithium carbonate in the continuation and prophylactic phases of drug treatment.

A few patients respond well to ECT but continually relapse even when maintained on multiple drug therapy. In these circumstances some practitioners have given **maintenance ECT** at a reduced frequency, such as fortnightly or monthly. However, this practice was not recommended by the National Committee for Clinical Excellence.

Consent to ECT

Before a patient is asked to agree to ECT, it is essential provide a full **explanation of the procedure** and indicate its **expected benefits** and **possible risks**, especially the effects on memory. Appropriately written informations sheets should be a standard part of the consent procedure (see National Institute for Clinical Excellence, 2003).

Many patients expect severe and permanent memory impairment after treatment and some even expect to receive unmodified fits. Once the doctor is sure that the patient understands what he has been told, the latter is asked to sign a standard form of consent. The patient should understand that consent is being sought for the whole course of ECT and not just for one treatment, although it is essential to make clear that consent can be withdrawn at any time.

If a patient refuses consent or is unable to give it because he is in a stupor or for other reasons, and if the procedure is essential, further steps must be considered in the UK. The first is to decide whether there are grounds for involving the appropriate section of the Mental Health Act (see Appendix). The section does not allow anyone to give consent on behalf of the patient, but it does establish formally that he is mentally ill and in need of treatment. In England and Wales, the opinion of a second independent consultant is required by the Mental Health Act 1983. Readers working elsewhere should find out the relevant legal requirements.

If the decision is made in this careful way and fully explained, it is rare for patients to question the need for treatment once they have recovered. Instead, most acknowledge that treatment has helped, and they understand why it was necessary to give it without their expressed consent. In general, audits suggest that most patients feel that they have been helped by ECT; in terms of unpleasantness ECT tends to be rated in the same order as a visit to the dentist. The most common side effects complained of are memory problems, headache, dizziness and confusion (see Benbow and Crentsil, 2004).

Ethical aspects of ECT

As for drug treatment, the key issue for a competent patient is the concept of **full informed consent**. Generally ECT is widely regarded as a safe and effective treatment, a view supported by randomized controlled trials. However, it is important that patients be warned about the possibility of loss of remote memories outlined above. In addition, with medication-resistant patients, the issue of relapse should be discussed.

ECT in the case of non-competent patients raises difficult issues. Usually, in these circumstances ECT is needed to treat a patient whose life is placed at risk through their illness. The legal safeguards for patients are outlined above but the clinician has the duty to explain to the patient and their family the reasons for the action taken. Merskey (1999) emphasizes the value of 'a scrupulous fiduciary approach'.

Bright light treatment

The use of **phototherapy**, or **artificial bright light**, as a psychiatric treatment was first studied systematically by Rosenthal *et al.* (1984). These workers used bright light to treat patients with the newly identified syndrome of **seasonal affective disorder**. Since then, phototherapy has become the mainstay of treatment of **winter depression**, particularly in patients with **atypical depressive features** such as hyperphagia and hypersomnia (Eagles, 2004).

Mechanism of action

The light-dark cycle is believed to be one of the most important 'Zeitgebers' regulating circadian and seasonal rhythmicity in mammals. Initially, phototherapy was believed to ameliorate the symptoms of winter depression by extending the photoperiod. This was based on the view that patients with winter depression were particularly sensitive to the effects of short winter days and that bright light treatment produced a day length equivalent to that of summer.

More recent formulations have suggested that the antidepressant effect of bright light may be attributable to a **phase advance in circadian rhythm**. This is supported by the fact that controlled trials show that in most patients morning phototherapy is more effective than evening phototherapy. However, other studies have shown that bright light given at midday is also therapeutically effective. It is difficult to devise a truly plausible placebo condition for bright light treatment and some have argued that the antidepressant effects of bright light may be mediated in large measure by placebo effects, particularly patient expectation. (For a systematic review see Golden *et al.*, 2005.)

Equipment

A conventional light box contains fluorescent tubes mounted behind a translucent plastic diffusing screen. The tubes provide an output that can vary between 2500 and 10,000 lux. Light sources producing 10 000 lux are more expensive but may allow a **reduced duration of exposure** (30 minutes compared with 120 minutes) to secure a therapeutic effect.

Phototherapy has also been administered using **head-mounted units** or **light visors**. These instruments are attached to the head and project light into the eyes, allowing subjects to remain mobile while receiving treatment. Whilst light visors are more convenient to use than light boxes, results from placebo-controlled trials of light visors have proved disappointing and their use is not currently recommended.

Therapeutic efficacy and indications

The major indication for light therapy is seasonal affective disorder where patients experience winter depressions. Numerous controlled trials have shown that bright light treatment is more effective than placebo in patients with winter depression, particularly if they experience:

- increased sleep

- carbohydrate craving
- afternoon slump in energy.

Patients with more typical melancholic symptoms, for example, weight loss and insomnia, do less well with phototherapy as a sole treatment even where the disorder is seasonal in nature. Phototherapy may also be of benefit in other disorders characterized by depressed mood and appetite changes, for example, premenstrual syndrome and bulimia nervosa. The literature contains a number of controlled trials in such disorders where light treatment has improved ratings of depression. However, the difficulty of distinguishing specific and placebo effects of bright light makes the current data difficult to interpret.

Adverse effects

Generally, phototherapy is well tolerated although mild side-effects occur in up to 45 per cent of patients early in treatment. These include **headache, eye strain, blurred vision, eye irritation, and increased tension**. Insomnia can also occur, particularly with late evening treatment. Rare adverse events that have been reported include **manic mood swings** and **suicide** attempts, the latter putatively through light-induced alerting and energizing effects prior to mood improvement. Whether these rare events are actually adverse reactions to light is uncertain. There is no evidence that phototherapy employed in recommended treatment schedules causes ocular or retinal damage.

Clinical use of phototherapy

Since the best established indication for phototherapy is seasonal affective disorder, the following account will describe the use of bright light treatment in winter depression. One of the major practical difficulties in phototherapy is the time needed to administer the treatment. For this reason, a 10,000 lux light box may be preferred because the daily duration of therapy can be reduced to 30–45 minutes. It seems likely that cool-white light and full-spectrum light have equivalent clinical efficacy but because cool-white light is free of ultraviolet light it is theoretically safer.

The evidence suggests that bright light treatment of winter depression is most effective when administered in the early morning. However, treatments given at other times of day including the evening may prove beneficial and can be more convenient for individual patients. In an initial trial, therefore, it is best to recommend early morning treatment but to advise the patient that the exact timing of therapy can eventually represent a balance of therapeutic efficacy and practical convenience. Treatment should not be given late in the evening because of the possibility of **sleep disruption**.

Early morning phototherapy should start within a few minutes of awakening. Subjects should allow an initial duration of treatment of 30 minutes with a 10,000 lux light box or two hours with 2,500 lux equipment. They should seat themselves about 30–40 cm away from the light-box screen. They should not gaze at the screen directly but face it at an angle of about 45 degrees and glance across it once or twice each minute.

The antidepressant effect of light treatment can appear within **a few days** but in controlled trials longer periods – up to 3 weeks – can be needed before the therapeutic effects of bright light exceed those of placebo treatment. As noted above, mild side-effects are common in the early stages of treatment but usually settle without specific intervention. If they are persistent and troublesome, the patient can sit a little further away from the light source or reduce the duration of exposure. Exposure should also be reduced if elevated mood occurs.

Once a therapeutic response has occurred, it is necessary to **continue phototherapy** up to the point of natural remission, otherwise relapse will occur. It may be possible, however, to lower the daily duration of treatment. Phototherapy may also be started in advance of the anticipated episode of depression as this appears to have a **prophylactic effect**.

Neurosurgery for psychiatric disorders (psychosurgery)

History of procedure

Psychosurgery refers to the use of **neurosurgical procedures** to modify the symptoms of psychiatric illness by operating on either the nuclei of the brain or the white matter. Psychosurgery began in 1936 with the work of Moniz whose operation consisted of an extensive cut in the white matter of the frontal lobes (**frontal leucotomy**). This extensive operation was modified by Freeman and Watts (1942) who made smaller coronal incisions in the frontal lobes through lateral burr holes.

Although their so-called standard leucotomy was far from standardized anatomically, and although it produced unacceptable **side-effects** (see below), the procedure was widely used in the UK and other countries. There was enthusiasm for the initial improvements observed in patients, but this was followed by growing evidence of **adverse effects including intellectual**

impairment, emotional lability, disinhibition, apathy, incontinence, obesity, and epilepsy.

These problems led to a search for more restricted lesions capable of producing the same therapeutic benefits without these adverse consequences. Some progress was made, particularly with the incorporation of **stereotactic techniques** (see Christmas, 2004) but at the same time advances in pharmacology made it possible to use drugs to treat the disorders for which surgery was intended.

Current approaches

The term for psychosurgery is now often replaced with the phrase 'neurosurgery for mental disorders'. This change in terminology is intended to emphasize:

- the techniques involved now involve placement of localized lesions in specific cerebral sites;
- the treatment is for specific psychiatric conditions (treatment-resistant major depression and obsessive–compulsive disorder) and not for primary behavioural disturbance.

Indications

In the UK the indications for neurosurgery for mental disorders are restricted to major depression and obsessive–compulsive disorder that is chronic, treatment refractory and disabling. Neurosurgery is not indicated where these conditions arise as a consequence of organic brain disease or a pervasive developmental disorder.

Types of operation

Nowadays the older 'blind' operations have been replaced by stereotactic procedures that allow the lesions to be placed more accurately (Box 21.13). In the UK current procedures are limited to anterior capsulotomy and anterior cingulotomy. The lesions are produced either by radio-frequency thermo-coagulation or gamma radiation (the 'gamma knife'). Lesions are made bilaterally.

Effectiveness

In the absence of controlled trials, assessment has been in the form of long-term **follow-up studies**. A report by the Royal College of Psychiatrists (2000) found a 'marked improvement' rate 63 per cent of patients with major depression and 58 per cent of patients with obsessive–compulsive disorder (Box 21.14).

Adverse effects

With modern procedures severe adverse effects are rare. After the operation, headache and nausea are common and confusion occurs in about ten per cent of patients. These adverse effects last typically a few days but can persist for up to a month. Long-term cognitive impairment does not seem to occur (Table 21.14).

Clinical use

Neurosurgical procedures for mental disorders should not be carried out until the effects of several years of vigorous multi-modal treatment have been observed. If this rule is followed, the operation will hardly be used. In fact, less than 20 psychosurgical operations a year are currently carried out in the UK, about one-quarter the annual rate in the early 1980s. If the surgery is to be

BOX 21.14 OUTCOME OF PSYCHOSURGERY IN THE UK 1961–1997

	Depression (n = 727)	OCD (n = 478)
Marked improvement	63%	58%
Lesser improvement	22%	27%
No response	14%	14%
Worse	1%	1%

From the Royal College of Psychiatrists (2000)

BOX 21.13 STEREOTACTIC PROCEDURE USED IN PSYCHOSURGERY

Subcaudate tractotomy Lesion made beneath the head of each caudate nucleus, in the rostral part of the orbital cortex

Anterior cingulotomy Bilateral lesions within the cingulate bundles

Limbic leucotomy Subcaudate tractotomy combined with cingulotomy

Anterior capsulotomy Bilateral lesions in anterior limb of internal capsule

TABLE 21.14 Adverse effects of stereotactic psychosurgery

Acute
Operative mortality (less than 0.1%)
Haemorrhage, hemiplegia (less than 0.3%)
Transient confusion, lethargy
Long-term
Epilepsy (1–2%)
Weight gain (10%)
Frontal lobe syndrome (very rare)
Personality changes (usually mild)

considered at all, it should only be for chronic intractable obsessional disorder and severe chronic depressive disorders in older patients. There is no clear justification for neurosurgery for anxiety disorders or schizophrenia. For a review see Christmas *et al.* (2004).

Ethical issues

The ethical issues concerning the use of psychosurgery have been discussed by Merskey (1999). The brain is the organ of judgement and decision-making but it is regarded ethically permissible to operate, for example, on a brain tumour, if a patient gives consent. The situation with regard to psychosurgery is different because the tissue which is lesioned is not overtly diseased. However, surgeons do sometimes operate on tissue which is not diseased. The practical problems for psychosurgery (which distinguish it from ECT) are as follows:

- the lack of randomized studies to show that it is effective;
- the irreversibility of the procedure;
- the potentially serious nature of some of the adverse effects.

For these reasons it seems ethically appropriate that psychosurgery should be offered only to competent patients who are able to give full informed consent. Determining competence may, of course, be difficult in a patient with chronic severe mood disorder. In the UK, this has led to the development of safeguards under Section 57 of the 1983 Mental Health Act which require that:

1. the patient gives full informed consent
2. a multidisciplinary panel appointed by the Mental Health Act Commission confirms that the patient's consent is valid
3. the doctor on the multidisciplinary panel certifies that the treatment should be given. Before doing so, the doctor must consult two people, one a nurse and the other neither a nurse nor a doctor, who have been concerned with the patient's treatment.

Brain stimulation techniques

Transcranial magnetic stimulation

The use of transcranial magnetic stimulation (TMS) rests on the principle that if a conducting medium such as the brain is adjacent to a magnetic field, a current will be induced in the conducting medium. In TMS, an electromagnetic coil is placed on the scalp. Passage of high-intensity pulses of current in the coil produces a powerful magnetic field [typically about 2 tesla (T)], which results in current flow in neural tissue and neuronal depolarization. Neuropsychological effects of TMS are particularly likely when pulse of current are delivered rapidly, so-called **repetitive TMS or rTMS**. If the stimulation occurs more quickly than once per second (1 Hz), it is called **fast rTMS**. The use of appropriately-shaped coils allows reasonably localized stimulation of the main specific cortical areas.

Uses of TMS TMS has been used for many years in clinical neurophysiology to explore, for example, the integrity of motor cortex after stroke. In research settings, TMS is used to localize the cortical substrates of specific neuropsychological functions. For example, short-term verbal recall can be disrupted by rTMS administered over left temporal cortex.

Clinically rTMS has been used to relieve **depressive states**. Initially, studies used fast rTMS applied to left prefrontal cortex. In some, but not all studies, rTMS applied daily for 1–2 weeks was more effective than sham control treatment. However, other investigations have employed different kinds of electromagnetic coil, stimulation parameters, and site of coil application. A meta-analysis found only weak and transient effects of rTMS to improve depression ratings but overall the quality of the studies was low (Martin *et al.*, 2002).

TMS has also been employed in treatment studies of other disorders such as mania and obsessive–compulsive disorder. Findings in these conditions are still preliminary (Lisanby and Sackheim, 2002).

Adverse effects of TMS The use of single-pulse TMS in neurophysiological studies has not raised significant safety concerns. The major hazard with rTMS is the risk of inducing **seizures**. This is greater with fast rTMS than slow rTMS. Current safety protocols, which adjust the amount of magnetic stimulation in relation to the motor threshold of the individual, appear to have greatly reduced the likelihood of fits although subjects with risk factors (for example, family history of epilepsy) are generally excluded from TMS studies of healthy volunteers.

Minor side-effects are more common and include **muscle tension headaches**, and sufficient noise generated by the equipment to cause short-term changes in **hearing threshold**. This can be prevented by the use of earplugs (by both subjects and investigators). rTMS appropriately localized also has the potential to disrupt cognitive function but thus far changes have been temporary, and have not persisted after the stimulation is terminated. There are insufficient data to know whether there might be any long-term sequelae to the brain or other organs from the high-intensity magnetic field generated during TMS. No specific hazard has been revealed by current follow-up studies.

Vagal nerve stimulation

Vagal nerve stimulation (VNS) is an established treatment for patients with refractory epilepsy in whom it was noted to improve mood. It is currently undergoing trials in patients with treatment-resistant depression.

As well as providing an efferent parasympathetic outflow from the brain, the vagus nerve conveys afferent sensory fibres that synapse in the nucleus tractus solitarius and subsequently project to the forebrain. Stimulating the vagus nerve therapeutically involves an operative procedure during which a pulse-generator is implanted subcutaneously in the left anterior chest wall. Bipolar electrodes, connected to the generator, are placed around the left vagus nerve in the cervical region. These electrodes are intermittently stimulated by the generator, with the stimulation parameters being regulated by a telemetric 'wand' which is connected to a personal computer. Modification of stimulus parameters is used to balance adverse effects (see below) with therapeutic effects

Use in depression The main indication being explored for VNS is treatment resistant depression. Open studies have suggested that over 12 months about 50 per cent of subjects show a good clinical response. Currently the best antidepressant effects have occurred in patients who have a moderate degree of treatment resistance but who have not proved refractory to multiple trials of antidepressant and augmentation therapies (Marangell *et al.*, 2002).

Adverse effects of VNS During periods of vagal nerve stimulation hoarseness is common and throat pain, cough and dsypnoea can occur. These adverse effects decline with time and withdrawal from treatment is uncommon. Hypomania has rarely been reported but its relationship to VNS treatment is uncertain (see Christmas *et al.*, 2004).

Furthe r reading

Haddad P, Dursan S, Deakin JFW (2004) *Adverse syndromes and psychiatric drugs: a clinical guide*. Oxford University Press, Oxford. (Useful coverage of common adverse events associated with psychotropic drug use.)

Stahl, SM (2000) *Essential psychopharmacology*. Cambridge University Press, Cambridge. (Well illustrated account of basic pharmacology and clinical use of psychotropic drugs.)

Taylor, D, Paton C, Kerwin D (2003) The Maudsley Prescribing Guidelines. Martin Dunitz, London. (Excellent handbook of good prescribing practice.)

CHAPTER 22

Psychological treatment

Chapter contents

This chapter is concerned with various kinds of counselling, psychotherapy, behavioural and cognitive therapies, and some related techniques. The subject is large, and the chapter will be easier to follow if the reader's attention is drawn at this stage to certain aspects of the organization of the chapter:

- Psychological treatment is not given in isolation and the account in this chapter should be read in conjunction with the general advice about treatment in the chapters on physical treatment and on services.
- This chapter contains advice on the general value of various treatments. Advice about the value of these treatments for specific disorders is given in the chapters concerned with the relevant disorders.
- Psychological treatments are often combined with medication. Appropriate ways of doing this are considered in the chapters concerned with the relevant disorders.
- Because many different techniques of treatment are considered here, none can be described in detail and

TABLE 22.1 Psychological treatments considered in this chapter

suggestions for further reading are given in several places in the chapter.

- Although outline descriptions of technique are given in several places, supervised experience is essential before any of these treatments can be used with patients.
- Psychological treatments for sexual disorders are described in Chapter 19.

Terminology The word psychotherapy is used in two ways. In the first usage, psychotherapy denotes all forms of psychological treatment, including counselling and cognitive-behaviour therapy treatments. In the second usage, psychotherapy excludes counselling and cognitive-behaviour therapy. We have generally used the term psychological treatment to denote the broad sense. When we use the word psychotherapy, we usually qualify it to indicate a more precise meaning, for example, brief dynamic psychotherapy.

The treatments considered in this chapter are listed in Table 22.1, which also shows the general structure of the chapter.

How psychological treatments developed

The use of psychological healing is as old as the practice of medicine. Parallels have been drawn between aspects of modern techniques and the ceremonial healing carried out in some of the temples of ancient Greece. However, in the history of psychiatry, psychological treatment can be said to start in the nineteenth century with developments in hypnosis. These developments begin with the activities of Anton Mesmer (1734–1815), a Viennese physician who believed that magnetic forces could be used to alter the functions of the body. These forces could, he believed, arise not only from actual magnets but also from 'animal magnetism' present in the body of the therapist. He believed, moreover that the two sources could be combined to increase the therapeutic effect (see Block, 1980). Mesmer's theories were not generally accepted by the medical profession, but a Manchester doctor, James Braid, thought the phenomenum real but showed that it could be induced without magnets. He also suggested a more physiologically plausible explanation, namely that the state produced by 'mesmerism' was in some way related to sleep, and for this reason suggested the name hypnosis (Braid, 1843).

Treatment with hypnosis became popular in France, where a disagreement arose about its nature. In Nancy, A. A. Liebeault (1823–1904) and Hippolyte Bernheim (1837– 1919) followed Braid's idea that hypnosis was a normal state, allied to sleep, that could be induced in most people, and that its effects were brought about through suggestion. Bernheim's book *Suggestive therapeutics* (Bernheim, 1890) described the use of suggestion to treat hysteria and other neurotic conditions, as well as painful afflictions and gastrointestinal problems. The contrary view was championed by Jean Martin Charcot (1825–1893), a neurologist at the Salpetriere hospital in Paris. Charcot maintained that hypnosis was a pathological state which occurred only in patients with hysteria.

At that time, the main alternative to hypnosis was 'persuasion', a method in which symptoms and other problems were explained and discussed without any attempt to increase suggestibility. An important proponent of this approach was Paul Dubois, a Swiss professor of neuropathology, whose book *The psychic treatment of nervous disorders*, published in 1904 (and translated into English as Dubois, 1909) was widely influential. Dubois taught that although hypnosis had some limited value for hysteria, persuasive treatment was more appropriate for other neuroses.

In the late nineteenth century, most neuroses were treated by neurologists and when Freud began practice as a neurologist he saw many neurotic patients. To improve his therapeutic skills, he visited Bernheim and Charcot in France to study hypnosis (see Freud, 1892). When he returned to Vienna, Freud tried hypnosis with some of his neurotic patients and at first was pleased by its results. However, he could not maintain these early successes and he decided to use hypnosis not to change symptoms directly, but to release the emotion associated with the repressed ideas that he believed to be the cause of the symptoms. In 1889, he described his first use of this new technique in the case of Emmy von N.

Freud then remembered that Bernheim had shown that patients could recall forgotten events without hypnosis. To encourage his patients to do the same, he asked them to shut their eyes while he placed his hands on their forehead (Breuer and Freud, 1893–5, pp. 109, 279). Next Freud discovered that recall was as effective when the patient simply lay on a couch while the therapist kept out of sight. In this way the method of **free association** developed. Soon after this Freud began to encourage free associations and to comment on their significance, and he learned that it was necessary to control the intensity of the relationship with his patients. These discoveries formed the basic technique of psychoanalysis and subsequently of the larger group of dynamic psychotherapies. The interested reader is recommended to read one of the accounts written by Freud of the development of his techniques (Freud, 1895a, 1923). Freud's theories of mental functioning are summarized in this book on pp. 599–603.

Gradually, psychoanalytical and related techniques became more widely used than hypnosis or persuasion. Freud published striking accounts of his new treatment and elaborated his theories in increasingly complex ways. He attracted a group of followers, some of whom disagreed with Freud's further development of his ideas, and formed their own 'schools' of dynamic psychotherapy. These developments will be described briefly; more information will be found in the chapter by Holmes (2000) or the book by Munroe (1955).

Pierre Janet (1859–1947). In the same period that Freud was developing his ideas, Pierre Janet was also seeking the cause of the neuroses. Like Freud, Janet began his studies by investigating the use of hypnosis for hysteria, but his conclusions differed. Janet supposed that neuroses were caused by a loss of the normal integration of mental activities, a process he called dissociation. This dissociation related to a general weekness of nervous function which he called neurasthenia. Janet did not describe any technical innovations comparable to Freud's psychoanalysis and partly for this reason, his extensive writings have been less influential that those of Freud. A second reason is that Janet did not establish a school of followers, unlike Freud, who would develop his ideas.

Early departures from Freud's original group

Alfred Adler left Freud in 1910. He rejected the libido theory (see p. 90) and pointed instead to the influence of social factors in development. In his therapeutic technique, called individual analysis, he tried to understand how the patient's lifestyle had developed, and he focused on current problems. Adler's theories lacked the ingenuity and interest of Freud's ideas, and his treatment was not used widely. However, his ideas can be seen as the basis for the influential dynamic-cultural school of American analysts (see below). For more information about Adler's contributions see Ansbacher and Ansbacher (1964).

Carl Jung While Adler emphasized the real problems in the patient's life, Jung emphasized the inner world of fantasy, though he did not neglect contemporary issues. In his psychotherapy, Jung laid stress on the interpretation of unconscious material, deduced from dreams, paintings, and other artistic productions. Jung believed that part of the content of the unconscious mind was common to all people (the 'collective' unconscious) and was expressed in universal images which he called archetypes. Despite this emphasis on fantasy and the unconscious, the relationship between therapist and patient in Jungian analysis is less one-sided than in psychoanalysis in that the therapist is more active and reveals more about himself. For further information about Jung's ideas see Storr (2000).

The neo-Freudians

The **neo-Freudian** school of analysis developed in the USA in the 1930s. Its members accepted that the origins of character and of neurosis are in childhood but they did not accept Freud's idea that libido development in childhood was of crucial importance for subse-

BOX 22.1 THE NEO-FREUDIANS

Karen Horney took issue with Freud's view of the psychological development of women, especially the concept of 'penis envy'. For Horney, anxiety in childhood arose from the experience of being insignificant, helpless, and threatened. This anxiety was normally overcome by the experience of being brought up by loving parents. When children lack this experience, anxiety persists and defences develop against it. These defences include striving for affection, striving for power, and excessive submissiveness. Horney summarized the difference between her treatment and Freud's methods as follows: 'I differ from Freud in that after the recognition of the neurotic trends, while he primarily investigates their genesis, I primarily investigate their actual functions and their consequences' (Horney, 1939, p. 282).

Erich Fromm also rejected Freud's theory of instinctual development as a cause of neurosis. He accepted the importance of family influences in shaping character, and drew attention to wider cultural influences. Fromm was generally concerned more with social than with clinical issues, and his ideas did not greatly influence therapy.

Harry Stack Sullivan, unlike Fromm, was more interested in therapy than in theory. His treatment centred on the relationship between analyst and patient, and the discussion of everyday social encounters. Patient and therapist were more equal than in Freudian analysis, and Sullivan preferred pointed questions and provocative statements to interpretations based on theory (see Sullivan, 1953).

quent psychological health. Instead, family and wider social factors were considered more important. Three important figures in this school were Karen Horney and Erich Fromm, both refugees from Nazi Germany who settled in the USA in 1930s; and Harry Stack Sullivan an America. Their contributions are summarized in Box 22.1.

Melanie Klein developed Freud's theories about early infant development. She believed that psychoanalytical techniques could be adapted for use with very young children by interpreting their play as if it were the equivalent of the statements of adults. One of Klein's influential ideas concerned the 'object', a term that can refer both to an emotionally significant person (for example, the mother), to parts of that person (for example the mother's breast) and to the internal psychological representation of that person or part. Klein believed that for infants the experience of these 'objects' is linked to strong instinctual feelings of love and hate. Since the child is not at first able to experience mixed feeling, objects are either loved or hated. Therefore if an 'object' such as the mother evokes both kinds of feeling, the object is 'split' into good and bad parts. Later, children become able to experience mixed feeling, and can therefore can bring together the previously split objects (in other words, they can have both good and bad feelings about the same person). When this happens they feel remorse for the exclusively bad, past feelings. Klein referred to this sequence as the change from the paranoid-schizoid 'position' (her word for a developmental stage) to the depressive 'position'. The details of Klein's theory are difficult to summarize or to accept uncritically, but her general approach to therapy with children and the concept of 'objects' have been widely influential. For an outline of Klein's theories see Segal (1963), and for an account of Klein's technique of analysis of children see Klein (1963).

The object relations school began in Britain in the 1930s and 1940s as a development of Klein's ideas. **W. R. D. Fairburn** accepted Klein's theories of the importance of very early experiences with the mother, of objects, and of splitting. He supposed that both objects and the self could become split into three parts: (i) the ideal that never causes frustration, (ii) the 'libidinal' that can satisfy drives, and (iii) the 'antilibidinal' which causes frustration. Conflict between these last two leads usually to repression, but sometimes to sudden swings between opposite feelings. Fairburn's ideas were developed further and applied to therapy by **Harry Guntrip** and later by **Joseph Sandler**. For a review of objects relations theory see Gomez (1997).

Attachment theory originated in the work of **John Bowlby**, a British analyst. The theory is based not on drives, instincts and object relations but on the idea that infants need a secure relationship with their parents, and that insecure attachments can lead to difficulty in making relationships and to emotional problems. At the time, Bowlby's ideas had a considerable effect on the care of children, for example, by drawing attention to the need to maintain contact with the parents when a child is admitted to hospital. For a review of the historical development of attachment theory see Holmes (2000). For more recent developmentsin the theory see and Fonagy *et al.* (1996).

Brief psychodynamic psychotherapy This development of Freud's techniques can be said to have started from the work of Ferenczi, who saw the need to develop treatments shorter than psychoanalysis. He did this by setting time limits, making the role of the therapist less passive, and planning the main themes of treatment. These innovations have found their way into the brief dynamic psychotherapy used today (see p. 599).

Later developments Recent developments have continued the trend towards briefer treatment and have attended more to the patient's current problems , and less to those in the past. There are three main types:

1. **Interpersonal therapy** (see p. 587), developed by Klerman and Weissman, is directed to current interpersonal problems.
2. **Cognitive analytic therapy** (see p. 60), developed by Ryle, uses cognitive therapy techniques within a framework of psychodynamic understanding (see Llewellyn, 2003).
3. **Psychodynamic interpersonal therapy** (see p. 601) was developed by Hobson as a simpler 'conversational' form of treatment See Hobson (1985).

The development of cognitive–behaviour therapy

Behaviour therapy Interest in a treatment based on scientific psychology can be traced to Janet's (1925) methods of treatment which included re-education; to Watson and Rayner's (1920) use of learning principles in the treatment of children's fears; and to the use in the 1930s of aversion therapy for alcoholism. However, there was little progress until the 1950s when psychologists working at the Maudsley Hospital in London became disillusioned with the extravagant claims then made for psychoanalysis, and by its unscientific approach. They began to use learning principles to devise treatment for patients with phobic disorders, with the hope that the lessons learned with these conditions would be a guide to their wider use. At about the same time, Joseph Wolpe, a psychiatrist working in South Africa, was thinking along similar lines which he decribed in an influential book, *Psychotherapy by reciprocal inhibition* (Wolpe, 1958). In this book, Wolpe described a widely applicable treatment for neurotic disorders, based on learning theory and making use of existing methods of relaxation. Meanwhile, in the USA, Skinner (1953) suggested that the principles of operant conditioning could be used in the treatment of psychiatric disorders and for a while these ideas were influential.

Wolpe's ideas were adopted in the UK where they fitted well with the initiatives at the Maudsley Hospital, but in the USA there was more interest, at least among clinical psychologists, in Skinner's ideas. Later the two approaches converged, and the methods used in these two countries are now similar.

From the beginning there was a strong emphasis on the evaluation of the new treatment methods. The first clinical trial, to compare desensitization with individual and group dynamic psychotherapy, was reported in 1978 (Gelder *et al.*, 1978). By current standards, the trial had many shortcomings but it was followed by many more, carried out with increasing sophistication, so that there is now a strong evidence base for most of the behavioural methods in current use, whilst those without such a base have mostly fallen out of use.

Cognitive therapy began with the work of A. T. Beck, a US psychiatrist who had become dissatisfied with the results of psychoanalytical psychotherapy for depressive disorders, and sought an alternative. Beck was struck by certain recurring themes in the thinking of depressed patients, for example personal failure, and he suggested that these themes were an essential part of the disorder and had to be changed. Beck devised an ingenious way of changing the ideas by challenging them in special ways (see p. 596).

A second source of ideas leading to cognitive therapy was the work of a group of US psychologists who had become dissatisfied with operant conditioning methods in which the mind was regarded as a 'black box' and thoughts and feelings were ignored. For example, Meichenbaum (1977) proposed that the recurrent thoughts of people with emotional disorders played a part in maintaining their distress, and suggested how they might be controlled.

Cognitive-behaviour therapy These cognitive approaches were taken up by other psychologists and psychiatrists, and integrated with work on behaviour therapy to produce what eventually became the current methods of cognitive-behaviour therapy (described below). The strong evidence base, the clearly described procedures, and the relatively brief treatment time of cognitive-behaviour therapies have made them the preferred psychological treatment for many disorders.

Classification of psychological treatments

There are so many kinds of psychological treatment that it is useful to group them in a simple classification. Various classifications have been proposed, of which three will be considered here, followed by a simple scheme used here to help readers relate the treatments to their use in most healthcare systems.

I Classification by technique

- Eclectic
- Psychodynamic
- Cognitive behavioural
- Other, for example systems theory.

II Classication by number of patients taking part:

- **individual therapy** (one patient) may be chosen when the treatment needs to be tailored to the particular problems of the patient, or when group discussion would cause distress, either because of the nature of the problem (for example, a sexual deviation) or because of social anxiety
- **couple therapy** may be chosen when relationship problems are an important contributory cause of psychiatric disorder
- **family therapy** may be chosen when the difficulties of a child or adolescent are part of a wider problem in the family
- **small and large group therapy** may be chosen when several patients require similar treatment (for example, exposure treatment for agoraphobia), or when the contributions of other group members will be helpful (for example, to help alcohol abusers view their problems more objectively).

These first two types of classifications can be combined: for example, individual cognitive-behavioural; psychodynamic group therapy.

Uses of psychotherapy within a health service. Psychological treatment is the principal treatment for some psychiatric disorders, used alone or with medication. Counselling, crisis intervention and cognitive-behaviour therapies are used in this way when they have been shown to be effective in clinical trials. Dynamic psychotherapy is now used mainly to modify factors that are thought to increase the risk of relapse or recurrence of a disorder, for example, to help overcome low self esteem. In the past, dynamic psychotherapy was used to treat many conditions that would now be called 'subthreshold', that is, emotional problems that are distressing but are not severe or lasting enough to meet diagnostic criteria for a psychiatric disorder. Within a health service these problems are now treated with counselling, and the use of psychodynamic methods for this purpose is now mainly in private practice.

Consideration of these uses within a health service leads to a third classification:

- **Least complex and part of all healthcare** These are methods of counselling used for the less severe emotional problems, and to help people adjust to stressful situations or make difficult decisions (for example, whether to terminate a pregnancy). These methods merge into the every day use of the doctor-patient relationship in all medical practice.
- **Moderately complex and provided by most mental health professionals** This group includes the simpler forms of cognitive-behaviour therapy and some brief dynamic psychotherapies. These treatments are used to treat anxiety disorders and eating disorders, and some of the less severe mood disorders, often as part of a plan that includes medication and social measures.
- **Complex and provided by specialy trained therapists** This group includes the more complex psychodynamic and cognitive-behaviour therapies. The treatments are used to treat the more severe or complex disorders, alone or as part of a wider plan of management.

Common factors in psychological treatment

Research on psychological treatment has shown that, for many conditions, different methods achieve results which are similar and greater than those of no treatment. This finding suggests that in these cases the features that the psychotherapies share are more important than their differences. This conclusion was reached many years ago by Jerome Frank (1967) who suggested that the important common features are: the therapeutic relationship, listening sympathetically, allowing the release of emotion, providing informa-

BOX 22.2 COMMON FACTORS IN PSYCHOTHERAPY

The therapeutic relationship This is generally thought to be the most important of the common factors in psychotherapy. However, it may become too intense with resulting problems (see text).

Listening By listening attentively, the therapist shows concern for the patient's problems and begins to develop the helping relationship in which the patient feels understood.

Release of emotion Emotional release can be helpful at the beginning of treatment, but repeated release is seldom useful. Intense and rapid emotional release is called **abreaction**.

Restoration of morale Many patients have suffered repeated failures, and no longer believe that they can help themselves. By improving morale, the therapist helps the patient begin to help himself.

Providing information Distressed patients may remember little of what they have been told about their condition because their concentration is poor. Information should be as simple as possible and expressed clearly. It may be necessary to explain important points more than once, or write them down.

Providing a rationale All forms of psychological treatment provide reasons for the patient's condition, and this adds to the patient's confidence. The reasons may be stated directly by the therapist (as in short-term psychotherapy), or suggested indirectly through questions and interpretations (as in much long-term psychotherapy).

Advice and guidance These are part of all psychotherapy. In brief therapies, the advice and guidance is given directly; in long-term treatments the patient is made to seek the answers, but may still be guided - less obviously - in deciding which are right.

Suggestion Although, with the exception of hypnosis, suggestion is not deliberately increased in psychological treatments, all psychological treatment contains an element of suggestion. This suggestive element contributes to improvement in the early stages of treatment but it does not usually last long.

tion, providing a rationale for the patient's condition, restoring morale, using prestige suggestion, and forming a relationship. These features are shown in Box 22.2.

Transference and counter-transference

When the therapeutic relationship becomes intense it develops in ways that are called transference and counter-transference. Although more pronounced in dynamic approaches, transference and counter-transference develop to some extent during all psychological treatments. Therapists overlook this fact at their peril.

Transference is an element of the therapeutic relationship which becomes increasingly intense as treatment progresses. Transference is especially strong when the patient reveals to the therapist, personal problems that a person would normally reveal only to someone in an intimate relationship. This revelation increases the intimacy of the relationship with the therapist. Since the psychotherapist does not reciprocate by revealing any personal details, the patient responds to the feeling of intimacy by constructing a picture of the therapist by drawing (without realizing it) on memories of someone else with whom he has felt as intimate, and usually this person is a parent. When this happens, patients are said to have transferred to the therapist, feelings and attitudes from the relationship with the parents. This process is called transference. When the transferred feelings are good, transference is said to be positive; when the transferred feelings are bad, the transference is said to be negative. Just as feelings toward a parent are mixed, so transference has both positive and negative components, which may involve a complex mixture of love, hate, envy, and jealousy.

Countertransference In psychotherapy, therapists have to be genuinely concerned about their patients' most intimate problems and yet remain impartial and professional. Even with special training, therapists cannot always achieve this ideal combination of concern and detachment. They may then respond in ways that are not simply a reflection of their patients' personal qualities but also a displacement onto their patients of ideas and feelings related to other figures in the therapist's own life. This process is called **countertransference**. (Note that some writers include in countertransference realistic as well as unrealistic feelings and attitudes towards the patient.)

Transference problems Transference may lead to excessive dependency expressed in attempts to prolong interviews, requests for extra appointments, and behaviour demanding additional care, such as threats of suicide. Such dependency may make it difficult to end treatment because of a recrudescence of symptoms, and demands for further treatment. If dependency is noticed early and discussed appropriately with the patient, these further difficulties can usually be prevented. At the same time, patients can learn more about themselves by understanding the true origins of their feelings and behaviour not only to the therapist, but more widely.

Counter-transference problems arise when therapists become inappropriately involved in their patients' problems or inappropriately angry with them. These problems will be recognized earlier, when therapists scrutinize their feelings and recognize their origins in their personal experience. It is partly for this reason that training for intensive psychotherapy often includes a period of psychotherapy in which the future therapists are helped to understand the links between their past experiences and their current emotional reactions.

Counselling and crisis intervention

Counselling

In everyday usage, the word counselling denotes the giving of advice. As a technical term, it denotes a wider procedure concerned with emotions as well as with knowledge. There are many techniques of counselling, each used for a variety of problems, and in a variety of settings (for example, general medical practice, as part of psychiatric care, and in a student health service).

Counselling incorporates the non-specific factors shared by all kinds of psychotherapy (see Box 22.2). In all techniques, the relationship between the counsellor and the person counselled is important. The relative importance of giving information, allowing the release of emotion, and thinking afresh about the situation, vary according to the purpose of counselling. In the past much counselling used the **client-centred approach** in which counsellors take a passive role. They give little information and largely restrict their interventions to comments on the emotional content of the client's utterances; for example, instead of asking for clarification of facts, they might say 'that seems to make you angry' (reflection of feelings). The technique has been largely replaced, in healthcare systems, by the more structured and focused procedures (reviewed below), since these are generally agreed to be more rapidly effective. Non-directive approaches are, however, still used by some counsellors working independently.

Approaches to counselling

Problem-solving counselling is a highly structured form of counselling, suitable for patients whose problems are clearly related to stressful circumstances. It is mentioned first in this section because it is widely applicable to conditions in which life problems are exacerbating or maintaining a disorder. The basic counselling techniques are combined with a systematic approach to the resolution of problems. The patient is helped to:

- **identify and list** problems that are causing distress;
- **consider courses of action** that might solve or reduce each problem;
- **select** a problem and course of action that appear feasible and likely to succeed;
- **review** the results of the attempt to solve the problem and then either choose another problem for solution if the first action has succeeded, or choose another course of action if the first has not succeeded.

This approach has been shown to be effective for the less severe forms of mood disorder. For a review of problem-solving counselling see Mynors-Wallace (2001).

Interpersonal counselling was developed by Klerman *et al.* (1987) from interpersonal therapy (described on p. 587). It has many similarities to the problem-solving approach. Attention is focused on current problems in personal relationships within the family, at work, and elsewhere. These problems are considered under four headings: **loss, interpersonal disputes, role transitions, and interpersonal deficits**. Using a problem-solving approach similar to that described above, the therapist encourages patients to consider alternative ways of coping with their difficulties, and to try these out between sessions of treatment. The method has been shown to be effective for patients in primary care presenting with minor mood disorders (Klerman *et al.*, 1987).

Psychodynamic counselling places more emphasis on the influence of past experience on the development of current behaviour, an influence mediated in part through unconscious processes. The method is influenced by object relations theory, that is, by the idea that previous relationships leave lasting traces which affect self-esteem, and influence current relationships. The patient's emotional reactions to the counsellor are considered to be a source of information about problems in other relationships. This form of counselling is used, for example, in student health centres where the developmental approach fits well with problems that although manifest at university, often originated in experiences before the student entered university. Psychodynamic counselling has been described by Jacobs (1988). It has not been evaluated as thoroughly as the other two approaches.

Counselling for specific purposes

Debriefing

This approach is used for survivors of disasters, who are encouraged to recall the distressing events. The emphasis is on emotional release, and to ways of coping with the immediate problems. Evidence from clinical trials indicates that debriefing does not improve the outcome of survivors of disasters, and that methods using cognitive techniques may be more helpful (see p. 157).

Counselling for relationship problems

Counselling for relationship problems helps couples to talk constructively about problems in their relationship. The focus is on the need for each partner to understand the point of view, needs, and feelings of the other, and to identify positive aspects of the relationship as well as those causing conflict.

Grief counselling

Grief counselling focuses on working through the stages of grief (see p. 169). It combines an opportunity for emotional release (including in appropriate cases, the expression of anger); information about the normal course of grieving; encouragement to engage in final acts such as viewing the body and disposing of clothing; and advice about the practical problems of living without the deceased person. (Grief counselling is considered further on p. 170.)

Counselling for the late effects of trauma

Clinical experience strongly suggests that non-directive and unstructured approaches should not be used since they may result in the recollection of distressing experience without enabling the person to deal adequately with the resulting emotions or to do the necessary cognitive processing. Cognitive or psychodynamic methods appear to be more suitable, but they, too, require careful planning and skilful management.

Counselling about risks

Counselling about risks is exemplified by counselling about genetic risks and about the risks of sexually transmitted disease. The essential steps are to give information about the risks, provide an opportunity for reflection on the impact of the various outcomes, and to help the person decide how best to respond.

Counselling for students

Universities have counselling services for students who are usually experiencing adjustment disorders, or other stress-related disorders related to pressures of university life, often against a background of family or other interpersonal problems outside the university setting. Special skills are needed to phase the treatment to take account of the length of the university terms and the students' absence in the vacations.

Counselling in primary care

In primary care, many patients with minor psychiatric disorders are treated by practice counsellors who have received training but are not members of the medical, nursing, or social work professions. These counsellors use various methods of brief treatment with an average number of sessions - about seven, and the average length of each session of about 50 minutes (Sibbald *et al.*, 1996a). Although patients generally welcome this help, evidence for its effectiveness is conflicting (Bower at al., 2003; Chilvers *et al.*, 2001) and there are further uncertainties about its cost-effectiveness (Friedli *et al.*, 2000). Most of the counselling in these studies was non-directive, and it is possible that better results would be obtained with problem-solving techniques (see above).

Crisis intervention

This treatment helps patients cope with a crisis in their lives, and to learn effective ways of dealing with future difficulties. The approach is used, for example, after the break-up of a relationship. It can be used also in the aftermath of natural disasters such as floods and earthquakes, but cognitive methods (see below) are now often preferred in these circumstances. Crisis intervention, which originated in the work of Lindemann (1944) and Caplan (1961), is based on Caplan's description of four stages of coping:

1. emotional arousal with efforts to solve the problem;
2. if these fail, greater arousal leading to a disorganization of behaviour;
3. trials of alternative ways of coping;
4. if there is still no resolution, exhaustion and decompensation.

Crisis intervention seeks to limit the reaction to the first stage, or if this has been passed before the person seeks help, to avoid the fourth stage.

Problems leading to crisis

These can be divided usefully into:

- **loss problems** such as the loss of a person through death or separation, or the loss of a body part or the function of an organ;
- **role changes** such as entering marriage, parenthood, or a new job with added responsibilities;
- **relationship problems** such as those between sexual partners, or between parent and child;
- **conflict problems**, which are usually difficulties in choosing between two undesirable alternatives.

TABLE 22.2 Crisis intervention

Treatment is immediate, brief and collaborative
Stage I
◆ Reduce arousal
◆ Focus on current problems
◆ Encourage self-help
Stage II
◆ Assess problems
◆ Consider solutions
◆ Test solutions
Stage III
◆ Consider future coping methods

Crisis intervention methods

The methods generally resemble interpersonal counselling (p. 585) and problem-solving counselling (p. 585), though with a greater emphasis on reducing arousal. Treatment starts as soon as possible after the crisis and is brief, usually a few sessions over days or a few weeks. The approach is collaborative, involving the patient fully, and often including family or close friends. The focus is on current problems, although relevant past events are also considered. Patients in crisis have a high level of emotional arousal, which interferes with problem-solving, and the first aim of treatment is to reduce this level. Usually this can be achieved with reassurance and an opportunity to express emotions, but occasionally anxiolytic medication is required for a few days. Although the general approach is that patients should help themselves, in this first stage some arrangements may have to be made for them, for example, arrangements for the care of children.

The second stage of crisis intervention resembles the problem-solving counselling described above. The patient's problems and assets are assessed carefully. The patient is encouraged to suggest alternative solutions and to choose the most promising. The therapist's role is to encourage, prompt, and question. He does not formulate problems or suggest solutions directly but helps the patient to do so himself. The patient should discover general methods of coping that will be useful for solving future problems.

Indications

Clinical experience suggests that crisis intervention is most valuable for well-motivated people with stable personalities who are facing major but transitory difficulties; in other words, those who are most likely eventually to cope on their own. Crisis intervention is used, especially, after deliberate self-harm arising in response to a social crisis.

For a review of the application of crisis theory to crisis services, see Bridget and Polak (2003).

Supportive psychotherapy

Supportive psychotherapy is used to relieve distress or to help a person cope with difficulties, when problem-solving approaches are unlikely to succeed. It is used, for example, for some patients with chronic mental or physical illness and as part of the care of the dying (see p. 167). As a general rule, supportive treatment should not be used unless more active forms of intervention have failed or are highly unlikely to succeed.

Supportive therapy is based on the common factors of psychological treatment (see Box 22.2). Its basic elements are a therapeutic relationship, listening, allowing the release of emotions, explaining, encouraging hope, and persuasion. The various components will be considered briefly.

- **The therapeutic relationship** is used to sustain patients. It is important to avoid dependence since the treatment often has to be long lasting; but if patients are severely handicapped or have dependent personalities, it may be difficult to achieve this aim. If dependence cannot be avoided, it should be directed as far as possible to the group of staff caring for the patient and not to any individual. The risk of dependence will be less if, from the beginning, it is agreed with patients how much time can be allocated for the support.
- **Listening** As in all forms of psychological treatment, patients should feel that they have their doctor's full attention and sympathy while he is with them, and that their concerns are being taken seriously.
- **Information and advice** are important but their timing should be considered carefully. Information should always be accurate, but it is not necessary to explain everything at the first session. Indeed, patients with serious and incurable illness may need to receive information gradually, coping with parts before they face the whole extent of their problems. Most patients indicate, directly or indirectly, how much they wish to be told on each occasion.
- **Emotional release** can be helpful in the early stages of supportive treatment. However, repeated release of emotions is unlikely to be beneficial, except when a new problem has arisen, for example, in a progressive physical illness.
- **Encouraging hope** is important but premature or unrealistic reassurance can destroy a patient's confidence in the carers. Reassurance should be offered only when the patient's concerns have been fully understood. Reassurance must, of course, be truthful and patients who find that they have been deceived lose the basic trust on which supportive therapy depends. When a patient asks about prognosis, the therapist can give a range of outcomes, including the most optimistic that can be foreseen. Even with the most difficult problems, a positive approach can often be maintained by encouraging patients to build on their remaining assets and opportunities.
- **Persuasion** In supportive treatment, patients should generally decide to take actions themselves as a result of their understanding the situation. Nevertheless, it is sometimes appropriate for doctors to use their powers of persuasion to help patients to take some necessary step, for example, to continue to cope despite a temporary exacerbation of their condition.

Supportive treatment need not always be provided by a health professional. Self-help groups give valuable support to some patients and to relatives. Indeed, this form of support is sometimes more effective than support from a doctor since it is given by people who have struggled with the same problems as the patient. An account of supportive treatment is given by Bloch (1986).

Interpersonal psychotherapy

Interpersonal psychotherapy was developed as a structured psychological treatment for the interpersonal problems of depressed patients (Klerman *et al.*, 1984).

TABLE 22.3 Basic procedures of supportive treatment
◆ Develop a therapeutic relationship
◆ Listen to patients' concerns
◆ Inform, explain, and advise
◆ Allow the expression of emotion
◆ Encourage hope
◆ Review and develop assets
◆ Encourage self-help

The method has a wider application to other disorders in which similar problems are maintaining behaviour, for example, eating disorders. It is characterized by its approach rather than its techniques, which overlap with those of other kinds of psychotherapy.

The treatment is highly structured. The number and content of treatment sessions are planned carefully. The initial assessment period lasts one to three sessions. Interpersonal problems are considered under four headings:

1. bereavement and other loss
2. role disputes
3. role transitions
4. 'interpersonal deficits' such as loneliness.

Problems are considered by reference to specific situations and alternative ways of coping are evaluated. Clear goals are set and progress towards them is monitored. New coping strategies are tried out in homework assignments. In the middle phase of treatment, specific methods are used for each of the four kinds of problem listed above. For grief and other problems of loss, the methods resemble those described under grief counselling (p. 585). For interpersonal disputes, patients are helped to identify clearly the issues in the dispute, as well as any differences between their own values and those of the other person. They are helped to negotiate with the other person and to recognize their own contributions to problems that they ascribe to that person. Problems of role transition are dealt with in a similar way. Interpersonal deficits are discussed by analysing present relationship problems and the patient's previous attempts to overcome them, and by discussing alternatives. In the final two or three sessions, patients are helped to anticipate future problems and consider how they might overcome them.

Several clinical trials have shown that interpersonal therapy is effective for depressive disorders in adults and adolescents (Mufson 2004), dysthymia (Markowitz, 2003) and bulimia nervosa. For an account of interpersonal therapy, see Blanco and Weissman (2005).

Cognitive–behaviour therapy

All psychiatric disorders have cognitive and behavioural components and these features have to change if the patient is to recover. With other treatments, change comes about indirectly, for example as mood improves with antidepressant therapy or as the origins of the disorder are understood better with psychotherapy. In contrast, cognitive-behaviour therapy is designed to change cognitions and behaviour directly. Unlike dynamic psychotherapy, cognitive–behavioural therapy is not concerned with the ways in which the disorder developed in the past. Instead the focus is on the factors that are maintaining the disorder at the time of treatment.

Behaviour therapy is also concerned with factors that provoke symptoms or abnormal behaviour. These factors are most obvious in the phobic disorders, but they are important, though less obvious, in other disorders. For example, in bulimia nervosa, episodes of excessive eating may be provoked by situations which cause the patient to feel inadequate. One of the most frequent maintaining factors is **avoidance**, which is particularly important in phobic and other anxiety disorders in which it prevents the extinction of anxiety response.. Many behaviours are **maintained by their consequences**. For example, escape from an anxiety-provoking situation is followed by a fall in anxiety, and this fall reinforces the phobic avoidance. **Increased attention** is another powerful reinforcer of behaviour. For example, a child's noisy and unruly behaviour will be reinforced if the parents pay more attention when the child behaves in this way than when he is quiet and well behaved.

Cognitive therapy generally focuses on two kinds of abnormal thinking: **intrusive thoughts** ('automatic thoughts') and **dysfunctional beliefs and attitudes** ('dysfunctional assumptions'). Intrusive thoughts provoke an immediate emotional reaction, usually of anxiety or depression. Dysfunctional beliefs and attitudes determine the way in which situations are perceived and interpreted.

Three factors are thought to maintain dysfunctional beliefs and attitudes.

1. **Attending selectively** to evidence that confirms these beliefs and attitudes, and ignoring or discounting evidence that contradicts them. For example, patients with social phobias attend more to the critical behaviour of others, than to signs of approval.

2. **Thinking illogically** in several ways, of which three common ones are shown in Box 22.3.

3. **Safety-seeking behaviour.** This is behaviour carried out because the person believes that it reduces an immediate threat but which in the long-term perpetuates the person's concerns. For example, a patient who fears that she will faint during a panic attack, may tense her muscles every time she feels anxious, in the belief that this action prevents fainting. Although she has not fainted in hundreds of panic attacks, she believes that this is only because

BOX 22.3 EXAMPLES OF ILLOGICAL THINKING

Over-generalization Patients draw general conclusions from single instances (for example, he does not love me so no one will ever love me).

Selective abstraction Patients focus on a single unfavourable aspect of a situation and ignore favourable aspects.

Personalization Patients blame themselves for the consequences of the actions of other people.

All or nothing thinking Patients view people or situations in 'black or white' terms -e.g. a person is wholly good or wholly bad instead of mixture of good and bad qualities.

she has tensed her muscles on every occasion, and therefore continues to fear that she may faint in the future.

General features of cognitive–behaviour therapy

Certain features characterize cognitive behavioural treatments:

- **The patient as an active partner** The patient takes an active part in treatment, with the therapist acting as an expert advisor who asks questions, and offers information and guidance.
- **Attention to provoking and maintaining factors** Patients keep daily records to identify factors which precede or follow the disorder and may be provoking or maintaining it. This kind of assessment is sometimes called the **ABC approach**, the initials referring to antecedents, behaviour, and consequences.
- **Attention to ways of thinking** revealed by recording thoughts associated with the behavioral or emotional disturbance, the situations in which these thoughts appear, and the accompanying mood.
- **Treatment as investigation** Therapeutic procedures are usually presented as experiments which, even if they fail to produce Improvement, will help the patient find out more about the condition.
- **Homework assignments and behavioural experiments** Patients practise new behaviours between sessions with the therapist, or carry out experiments to test explanations suggested by the therapist. Box 22.4 contains an example of a behavioural experiment. Advice about the design of behavioural experiements is given by Bennet-Levy *et al.* (2004).

BOX 22.4 AN AGORAPHOBIC PATIENT'S RECORD OF A BEHAVIOURAL EXPERIMENT

Situation Shopping in a crowded supermarket

My predictions I shall panic and feel dizzy.
Unless I tense my stomach muscles and breath deeply, I shall faint.

Experiment When anxious, do not tense stomach muscles or breathe deeply.

Outcome I did panic quite badly. I felt dizzy but less so than usual.
I did not faint.

What I learnt I did not faint even though I had a severe panic and I did nothing to prevent fainting. I seem to be wrong in thinking I shall faint whenever I panic. Also tensing and deep breathing may not be having the effect I supposed. My therapist could be right in thinking that deep breathing makes me more dizzy.

What I should do next Repeat the experiment next time I go shopping.

- **Highly structured sessions** At each session, an agenda is agreed, and progress since the last session is reviewed, including any homework. New topics are considered, the following week's homework is planned, and the main points of the session are summarized.
- **Monitoring of progress** Assessment of progress does not rely solely on the patient's verbal account but typically includes the checking of daily records kept by the patient, and sometimes of formal rating scales.
- **Treatment manuals** are often available describing the procedures and the way in which they are to be applied. Manuals ensure that different therapists use procedures that are closely similar to those shown to be effective in clinical trials.

Assessment for cognitive–behaviour therapy

Topics to be covered

As well as a full psychiatric history, certain additional topics are addressed (see Table 22.4). For each of the presenting problems, the interviewer obtains an account of the antecedents, the behaviour, and the con-

TABLE 22.4 Topics to be considered in assessment for cognitive-behaviour therapy

1. Description of each problem including behaviour, thoughts and emotions ◆ Where it occurs most often ◆ Common prior events ◆ The patient's response to these events ◆ What follows the problem
2. Factors making the problem better or worse
3. Maintaining factors ◆ Avoidance ◆ Safety behaviours (see text) ◆ Selective attention ◆ Ways of thinking ◆ The responses of others

sequences (the ABC approach described above). Note that the term behaviour is used here in a wide sense to include thinking and emotion, as well as actions. By considering the sequence ABC on several occasions, regular patterns of thinking and responding are identified. The assessor is particularly concerned with patients' reasons for holding their beliefs, since this knowledge is essential in planning how arrange experiences that will negate and change the beliefs.

Sources of information for the assessment

Self-monitoring Patients record thoughts, behaviours and associated factors over days or weeks. The record is made as soon as possible after the events, so that important details are not forgotten. The record usually has columns for symptoms, thoughts, emotions, and actions; and the day and time at which they occurred. Events immediately preceding the problem are noted as well as those at the time, and afterwards.

Observations during treatment sessions Patients may be asked to imagine situations in which problems arise, and report the accompanying thoughts and emotions. Also, symptoms resembling those of the disorder may be induced (for example, panic-like symptoms produced by hyperventilation), and the accompanying thoughts and emotions noted. This technique can be used when treating panic disorder (see p. 595).

Special interviewing Although some patients are aware of their maladaptive beliefs and can describe them, other patients need help to do so. **Laddering** is one way of doing this: a series of questions is asked, each about the answer to the previous question. For example, a patient with an eating disorder might be asked what would happen if she were to gain weight; she might answer that she would lose her friends. To the question 'why?' she might reply that she would be unlikeable. To a further question 'why?' she might say that only thin people are attractive and popular.

The formulation

The information obtained in these several ways is combined with the usual psychiatric history in a formulation of:

- the type of **events that provoke** symptoms (for example, opening a conversation);
- any **special features of these events** (for example, speaking to a man of the same age);
- **background factors** (for example, an excessively critical parent); and
- **maintaining factors** including avoidance, safety behaviours, and ways of thinking.

The formulation is guided by the cognitive model of the disorder (for example the cognitive model of panic disorder - see p. 594. The therapist discussed the formulation with the patient and may build it up, step by step, as a diagram on paper or on a whiteboard. The formulation is modified as necessary as a result of this discussion.

Behavioural techniques

There are many behavioural techniques, some for a single disorder (for example, the enuresis alarm, p. 593), others used for a variety of disorders (for example, exposure, see below). Here we describe the more commonly used methods; evidence for the efficacy of each method as a treatment for a particular disorder, is considered in the chapter dealing with that disorder.

Relaxation training

This is the simplest behavioural technique. It is useful mainly for subthreshold states of anxiety, for stress-related disorders such as initial insomnia (Vienes *et al.*, 2003), and for mild hypertension (Yung and Keltner, 2000). In the original method, known as progressive relaxation, patients are trained to relax individual muscle groups one by one, and to regulate breathing (Jacobson, 1938). Because progressive relaxation is a lengthy procedure, simpler ones have been developed by, for example, Bernstein and Borkovec 1973) and by Öst (1987b). This latter - applied relaxation - is a rapid but intensive method, developed for the treatment of anxiety disorders for which it has worthwhile effects (Ost and Breitholz, 2000). All methods of relaxation can be learnt in part from tape-recorded instructions or in a group, and either reduces the time spent in training by the therapist. Relaxation has to be practised regularly between the training sessions and many patients lack the motivation to sustain this for long enough.

Exposure

Exposure is used to reduce avoidance behaviour, especially in the treatment of phobic disorders. For simple phobias, it is often sufficient to use exposure alone but for other phobic disorders exposure is usually combined with cognitive procedures (see p. 594). Exposure can be carried out **in practice**, that is in the actual situations that provoke anxiety; or **in imagination**, that is while imagining the phobic situations vividly enough to induce anxiety. Exposure can be gradual, starting with situations that provoke little anxiety and progressing through a series of increasingly more difficult ones (**desensitization**); or it can be intensive from the start (**flooding**). In practice, exposure is usually carried out with a speed and intensity between these two extremes and, whenever possible, in practice rather than in imagination.

Desensitization

In desensitization patients are helped to:

1. **Construct a hierarchy:** that is, a list is made of situations that provoke increasing degrees of anxiety. The list usually has about 10 items, chosen so that there is an equal increment of anxiety between each pair of items. If this aim is difficult to achieve, the severity of anxiety induced by certain items can be adjusted by introducing modifying factors. For example, the anxiety response to a situation may be less when the person is accompanied. Sometimes the anxiety-provoking situations seem so diverse that they cannot form a single hierarchy; for example, an agoraphobic patient may fear visiting the hairdresser, going to the cinema, and attending a teacher-parent evening. In such cases, a unifying fear should be sought, for example, the fear of being unable to leave a situation without embarrassment. When no common theme exists, two hierarchies are constructed.
2. **Enter or imagine entering the situations** on the hierarchy until they can do this without anxiety.
3. **Use relaxation** while entering or imagining the situation so as to reduce the anxiety response, and make imagery more vivid.
4. Repeat with each item on the hierarchy.

When exposure to the actual situation is impractical, for example with phobia of flying, desenstization in imagination is used. Otherwise exposure in practice is used because it is generally more effective.

Flooding

In flooding, patients enter situations near the top of the hierarchy from the start of treatment and remain there until the anxiety has diminished. The process is repeated with other near-maximal stimuli. Because many patients find the experience distressing and the results have not been shown to be better than desensitization, flooding is seldom used.

Exposure in everyday practice

Most exposure treatment is carried out in a way that is intermediate in speed and intensity between those used in desensitization and in flooding. Sessions last about 45 minutes. The patient enters a feared situation every day, either alone or with a relative or friend. Usually anxiety diminishes with each exposure. If it does not, it may be because treatment started with items too high on the hierarchy so that treatment should start again from an item lower on the hierarchy. Some patients fail to progress because they disengage from anxiety-provoking situations by thinking of other things. If patients can reduce this defensive behaviour progress can usually be made.

Exposure with response prevention

This is a treatment for obsessional rituals. The procedure is based on the observation that the urge to carry out rituals diminishes if the rituals can be restrained for a long period (usually about an hour). The steps in the procedure are:

1. The therapist **explains the rationale of treatment and agrees targets** for exposure with the patient. A target might be to touch a 'contaminated' object such as a door handle, and not to wash the hands during the next hour. A more advanced target might be to do all the household cleaning without washing the hands until the task is completed. Patients need to feel confident that every task will be agreed in advance and that they will never be faced with the unexpected.
2. The therapist may demonstrate the necessary exposure himself, a procedure known as **modelling**.
3. At first, therapists accompany and support patients while they strive to prevent the rituals; later they do this on their own.
4. When the necessary restraint has been achieved, the urge to carry out rituals is made greater by persuading the patient to enter situations that provoke this urge. Since these situations have previously been avoided, the procedure is called **exposure**.

The obsessional thoughts that accompany rituals usually improve as the rituals are brought under control. Obsessional thoughts occuring without rituals are more difficult to treat. **Habituation training** is a form of mental exposure treatment: patients dwell on the obsessional thoughts for long periods or listen repeatedly to a tape-recording of the thoughts spoken aloud for an hour or more. (A second technique for obsessional thoughts, **thought stopping**, is described below under distraction techniques (p. 594).

Social sklls training

Some aspects of social behaviour can be regarded as skills that can be learned, for example, making eye contact, or starting a conversation. These skills can improved through modelling, guided practice, role play and video-feedback. The training is useful mainly for socially inadequate people, and as part of a wider programme of rehabilitation for people with chronic mental disorder.

Assertiveness training

Assertiveness training is a form of social skills training used to treat people who have difficulty in being appropriately assertive. Patients enact social encounters in which moderate self assertion would be appropriate, for example, being ignored by a gossiping shop assistant. By a combination of coaching, modelling, and role reversal, patients are encouraged to practise appropriate verbal and non-verbal behaviour, and to judge the level of self-assertion appropriate to various situations. The techniques are described further by Paterson (2000).

Anger management

In this form of social skills training, patients are helped to:

- identify the situations that lead to anger.
- identify attitudes that lead to anger that is out of proportion to an facts of the situation.
- identify any factors that reduce restraints on anger, especially the use of alcohol.
- discover and practise alternative ways of dealing with situations that provoke anger: for example delaying their response until anger can be brought under control.

Self-control techniques

All behavioural treatments aim to increase patients' control over their own behaviour. Self-control techniques attempt to do this directly without the intermediate step of changing thoughts or emotions as would be done in cognitive therapy. Self-control techniques are based on operant conditioning principles, and on Bandura's (1969) studies of the role of self-reward in the control of social behaviour. The techniques are useful when the behaviour is potentially controllable but the patient has found it difficult to achieve this. Overeating and excessive smoking are examples of such behaviours. Since cognitive and emotional factors are importantdeterminants of behaviour, self-control methods are usually part of a wider cognitive–behaviour programme, for example in the treatment of eating disorders (see p. 597).

Self-control treatment has three stages:

1. **Self-monitoring**, that is, the keeping of daily records of the problem behaviour and the circumstances in which it appears. For example, patients who overeat record what they eat, when they eat, and any associations between eating, stressful events, and mood states. Keeping such a record is in itself a powerful stimulus to self-control for patients who have previously avoided facing the true extent of their problem, or are unaware of the factors that control it. Later, the daily records of the behaviour are used to assess progress.
2. ***Self-evaluation***: Achievements to be rewarded are agreed with the patient and progress is monitored by the patient.
3. **Self-reward** It is often useful to devise a system of reward points that can be accumulated to earn a material reward. Thus a woman might award herself a point for each day that she keeps to her diet, and buy herself new shoes when she reaches a pre-agreed number of points.

Contingency management

Contingency management, like self-control techniques, is concerned with providing rewards for desired behaviour and removing reinforcement from undesired behaviour. However, instead of relying on self-monitoring and self-reinforcement, in contingency management another person monitors the behaviour, and provides the reinforcers. The latter are usually social reinforcers such as indications of approval or disapproval, or enjoyable activities earned by accumulating points. Contingency management is used mainly in the treatment of children and people with learning dsiability.

Contingency management has four stages:

1. **Define and record the behaviour** The behaviour to be changed is defined and another person (usually a nurse, or parent) is trained to record it; for example, a mother might count the number of times a child with learning difficulties shouts loudly.

2. **Identify the stimuli and reinforcements** Stimuli for the behaviour are identified by recording the events that regularly precede it. Sometimes the abnormal behaviour is provoked by the actions of another person: aggressive behaviour often starts in this way. **Reinforcers** are identified by recording the events that immediately follow the behaviour. Often the reinforcing effect of these events is not obvious to the people involved; for example, parents may be unaware that by paying more attention to their child when he shouts than at other times, they are reinforcing the shouting.
3. **Change the reinforcement** Reinforcement is directed away from the problem behaviours and to desired behaviours; for example, parents are helped to attend less when their child shouts and more when he is quiet.
4. **Monitor progress** As treatment progresses, records are kept of the frequency of the problem behaviours and of the desired behaviours.

Contingency management is used alone and also as part of a wider programme, for example in the treatment of substance abuse (see Petry and Simcic, 2002) . The principles of contingency managementhave been applied to a group of patients living together in a ward or hostel, an arrangement called a **token economy**. However, token economies are seldom used now because the beneficial changes are limited and do not generalize to other situations.

The account of contingency management by Rimm and Masters (1979) is still useful.

Enuresis alarms

This behavioural treatment was developed specifically for nocturnal enuresis (see p. 689). In the original 'pad and bell' method, two metal plates forming part of a circuit with a battery and a bell, were separated by a pad and placed under the sheets of the bed. If the child passed urine while asleep, the pad became moist and its resistance fell, allowing current to flow between the plates, and to activate the bell (or buzzer). Nowadays a small sensor attached to the pyjamas replaces the plates and pad. The noise of the alarm wakes the child, who must then rise to empty his bladder and if necessary, change the bed sheet. After this procedure has been repeated on several nights, the child begins to wake before his bladder empties involuntarily. Eventually he sleeps through the night without being enuretic. The waking from sleep before passing urine can be understood as the result of classical conditioning. It is less easy to understand how the treatment leads to an uninterrupted dry night. The procedure is considered further on p. 689.

Complex behavioural techniques

Habit reversal

Habit reversal is a complex procedure used generally to treat tics, Tourette's syndrome and stuttering. The treatment has five components: (i) training in becoming aware of the onset of the behaviour (ii) monitoring the behaviour, (iii) training in initiating competing responses, that are incompatible with the behaviour (iv) relaxation and (v) social support. Positive effects have been reported (e.g. by Verdellen Keijers *et al.*, 2004) but at the time of writing, there is insufficient evidence to decide the effectiveness of the treatment.

Eye movement desensitization and reprocessing

This treatment was developed for post-traumatic stress disorder. There are three components:

- **exposure** using imagined scenes of the traumatic events;
- **a cognitive component** in which patients attempt to replace negative thoughts associated with the images, with positive ones; and
- **saccadic eye movements** induced by asking the patient to follow rapid side-to-side movements of the therapist's finger.

At the time of writing, there is insufficient high quality evidence to reach a firm conclusion about the value of the method (see Hertlein and Ricci, 2004). However, evidence has not so far supported the claim (e.g. Shapiro, 1995) that the third of these components is important. When the procedure was compared with exposure therapy it was not more effective (Devilly and Spence, 1999; Taylor *et al.*, 2003).

Behavioural techniques no longer in general use

Biofeedback

This technique assists patients to be aware of changes in a bodily function, such as blood pressure, over which they otherwise have little or no control. Information about the function is presented in an easily understood form such as a tone of varying pitch or a visual display. The person then tries to alter the function, usually in an indirect way such as relaxing. Biofeedback is not in general use because it has not been proved that it adds to the effects of relaxation alone. The technique may be of some value when normal sensory information has been lost, for example, after spinal injury (Brudny *et al.*, 1974). For further information see Basmajian (1983) or Stroebel (1985).

Aversion therapy

Aversion therapy was one of the earliest behavioural techniques, having been developed in the 1930s as a treatment for alcohol dependence. Negative reinforcement was used to suppress unwanted behaviour, but the method fell out of use because of two problems. First, negative reinforcement has only temporary effects on behaviour. Second, the use of negative reinforcement causes ethical problems. Although patients consent to the use of the negative stimuli, the therapist is nevertheless using something which, in other circumstances, might be used for punishment. The problem of separating treatment from punishment is particularly difficult with disorders which are, or could be, the subject of legal proceedings.

Cognitive techniques

Four methods are commonly used to bring about cognitive restructuring, that is change in cognitions:

1. **Distraction**, that is, focusing attention away from distressing thoughts. This is done by attending to something in the immediate environment (for example, the objects in a shop window); by engaging in a demanding mental activity (such as mental arithmetic); or by producing a sudden sensory stimulus (for example, snapping a rubber band on the wrist). The last technique is called 'thought stopping'.
2. **Neutralizing** The emotional impact of anxiety provoking thoughts can be reduced by rehearsing a reassuring response, for example, 'my heart is beating fast because I feel anxious, not because I have heart disease'. To make it easier to focus on reassuring thoughts, patients may carry a 'prompt card' on which the reassuring thoughts are written.
3. **Challenging beliefs** The therapist produces evidence that contradicts the beliefs. It is, however, generally insufficient to challenge the beliefs in this logical way because (as noted above) such beliefs often persist because people think in illogical ways. They over-generalize from single instances, and they pay more attention to evidence that supports their beliefs than evidence that contradicts them (see Beck, 1976). Therefore the therapist not only provides information but also attempts to reveal and change the illogical ways of thinking. He does this in two ways by asking questions such as those shown in Box 22.5; and by arranging behavioral experiments of the kind shown in Box 22.4 (p. 599). For further practical information about behavioural experiments see Bennett-Levy *et al.* (2004).
4. **Reassessing the patient's responsibility** Some beliefs persist because patients overestimate the extent of their responsibility for events that have multiple determinants. Patients can be helped to reassess their responsibility by constructing a **pie chart** that shows all the determinants. For example, a mother who feels responsible for ensuring that every member of her family is happy and successful, would make a 'pie chart' showing the contribution of all the factors that determine their state of mind (events at school or at work, relationships with friends, even the weather). By allocating appropriately sized sectors to each of these other factors before entering their own contribution, patients discover that there is less room for the latter than they had supposed.

Cognitive –behavioural treatments

Treatments for anxiety disorders

In the treatment of anxiety dosorders, cognitive techniques are combined with exposure (see above, p. 591). The importance of exposure is proportional to the amount of avoidance behaviour, being greater in the phobic disorders and less important in generalized anxiety disorders.

Three kinds of cognition are considered in treatment:

1. **fear of fear:** general concerns about the effects of being anxious, for example losing control
2. **fear of symptoms** concerns about specific symptoms, for example, fears that palpitations are a sign of heart disease,
3. **fear of negative evaluation:** concerns that other people will react unfavourably to the patient.

The balance of these cognitions varies in the different anxiety disorders. In generalized anxiety disorder, fear of fear and general worry pedominate (see p. 180). In social phobia, fears of negative evaluation are particularly important, as are concerns about blushing and trembling. In agoraphobia, fear of fear (especially thoughts that the person will faint, die, or lose control) and fears about the symptoms of a panic attack are important. Such cognitions are modified using the techniques outlined above, that is, by giving information, by questioning the logical basis of the fears, and by arranging behavioural experiments.

Information about the physiology of anxiety helps patients to attribute symptoms such as dizziness and palpitations to the correct cause, instead of to physical illness such as heart disease (a common concern of these patients). The **illogical basis of the fears** is discovered by questioning the patient's own evidence for her beliefs. **Behavioral experiments** are devised to the patient's beliefs and the alternative explanation suggested by the therapist.

Anxiety management is a general treatment for anxiety disorders.It has the following stages:

1. **Assessment** Patients keep a diary record of:
   - the frequency and severity of symptoms
   - the situations in which they occur
   - avoidance behaviour
2. **Information** about the physiology of anxiety and any other matters that will correct misconceptions
3. **Explanation** of the various vicious circles of anxiety (see above and Chapter 9)
4. **Relaxation** training as a means of controlling anxiety
5. **Exposure** to situations that provoke anxiety (see above p. 591)
6. **Distraction** to reduce the impact of anxiety provoking thoughts (see p. 591)

BOX 22.5 USEFU.L QUESTIONS FOR CHALLENGING BELIEFS

What is your evidence for this belief?

Is there an alternative way of looking at the situation?

How might other people think if in the same situation?

Are you focusing on what you felt rather than on what happened?

Are you forgetting relevant facts? Are you focusing on irrelevant matters?

Are you overestimating how likely this is?

Are you applying to yourself, higher standards than you would apply to others?

Are you thinking in black and white terms when you should consider shades of grey?

Are you overestimating your responsibility for the outcome?

What is the worst that could happen, and how bad would this be?

What if the worst should happen? How bad would it be? Could you cope?

Are you underestimating what you can do to deal with the situation?

Adapted from Clark (2000)

Treatment for panic disorder is focused on the characteristic beliefs, namely that physical symptoms of anxiety are evidence of a serious physical condition, usually heart disease (see p. 194). These beliefs create a vicious circle in which anxiety symptoms such as tachycardia generate additional anxiety, and this further increases the physical symptoms. Treatment has the following stages.

1. **Explanation** The therapist explains that physical symptoms are part of the normal response to stress, and how fear of these symptoms sets up a vicious circle of anxiety.
2. **Record keeping** Patients record the anxious cognitions that precede and accompany their panic attacks
3. **Demonstration** The therapist demonstrates that:
   (i) physical symptoms can provoke anxious cognitions, for example by asking the patient to induce such symptoms by over-breathing or strenuous exercise and noting the accompanying thoughts and fears.

   (i) these cognitions can induce anxiety for example by asking patients to concentrate their minds on the cognitions and observe the effect.

   This demonstration that physical symptoms lead to anxious thoughts, which in turn lead to anxiety, helps to **validate the vicious circle account** of the aetiology of panic attacks.
4. **Safety seeking behaviours** Attention is given to safety behaviours, and to any dysfunctional beliefs which make ordinary situations stressful (see p. 588).
5. **Behavioural experiments** are used to test the patient's ideas against those proposed by the therapist. For useful detail about the devising of these experiments, see Hackmann (2004).
6. **Cognitive restructuring** when they experience symptoms, and they observe the effect of this change on the severity of the panic attacks. By repeating this sequence many times they gradually gain control of the panic attacks.

Treatment for post-traumatic stress disorder includes attention to the intrusive visual images that characterize the condition. Patients imagine repeatedly the situations depicted in these images, as they would do in systematic desensitization (see above). They try to change the content of the images progressively and in small steps to images that are less distressing. Patients are also helped to integrate and process the fragmentary and distressing recollections of the traumatic events. Treatment for post-traumatic stress disorder is considered further on p. 161). For further information about the techniques used, see Mueller *et al.* (2004).

For further information about cognitive treatment of anxiety disorders see Clark (2000).

Cognitive–behaviour therapy for depressive disorders

Cognitive therapy for depressive disorders was developed by A. T. Beck (1976) as the first effective form of cognitive therapy. It is a complex procedure intended to alter three aspects of the thinking of depressed patients: negative intrusive thoughts, beliefs and assumptions that render ordinary situations stressful, and errors of logic that allow these beliefs and assumptions to persist despite evidence to the contrary.

Monitoring: is of three kinds:

1. Patients identify intrusive thoughts (for example, 'I am a failure') by writing down their thoughts when their mood is low.
2. Therapists uncover dysfunctional beliefs and assumptions by asking questions such as those in Box 22.5. A typical belief of a depressed patient is 'unless I always try to please other people, they will not like me'.
3. Patients record their activities and mark each one P if it was pleasurable and a M if it was accompanied by a sense of mastery and achievement.

If the patient is severely depressed the monitoring of thoughts is deferred and attention focussed on activities. The resulting 'activity schedule' is used to encourage activities that have been identified as leading to pleasure and mastery. The schedule also helps to bring a sense of order and purpose into the patient's life. At this stage the therapist helps the patient to reduce the need to make decisions, which are difficult for someone who is severely depressed.

If the patient is less severely depressed, treatment begins with an explanation of the cognitive model of depression and an attempt is made to reduce intrusive thoughts. This is done through distraction (see p. 594) and by rehearsing reassuring alternatives (for example, 'even though I think my work is bad, my boss praised me yesterday'). To help the patient concentrate on the positive statement, the alternative can be written on a prompt card. As treatment proceeds, more time is spent in challenging depressive cognitions using the techniques outlined in Box 22.5 combined with behavioural experiments For further information about the devising of these experiments see Fennell *et al.* (2004).

The following points are important in relation to cognitive therapy for depression

- **Reviewing evidence** Depressed patients are particularly prone to focus on evidence that supports their negative ideas and overlook evidence that contradicts them. The therapist should help patients give appropriate weight to the positive evidence.
- **Considering alternatives** Depressed patients often reject postive alternatives to their thoughts and beliefs. The therapist can help the patient consider alternatives by asking questions such as: What do you think that another person would think about this situation? What would you think if another person had done what you have done? (See Box 22.5 for additional questions.) Behavioural experiments are used as another way of challenging beliefs and assumptions.
- **Considering consequences** Patients should be helped to see the consequences of thinking negative thoughts; for example, the thought that everything is hopeless may prevent them from attempting even small changes that could accumulate beneficially.
- **Considering errors of logic** (Box 22.6) The patient should be helped to by ask himself questions such as: 'Am I thinking in black and white terms?' 'Am I drawing too wide conclusions from this single event?' 'Am I blaming myself for something for which I am not responsible?' 'Am I exaggerating the importance of events?' These questions are asked in relation to specific ideas, beliefs and situations.
- **Considering beliefs** As depression improves, more attention is given to the patient's beliefs since abnormal beliefs can lead to relapse. The technique of laddering (p. 590) can be used to uncover these beliefs. Useful questions include:
  'In what ways is this idea helpful?'
  'In what ways is it unhelpful?'
  'What alternatives are there?'
- **'Mindfulness'** Teasdale has suggested that people who are prone to depression have a cognitive set whereby thoughts and feelings are experienced as events rather than as aspects of the self, and that

BOX 22.6 LOGICAL ERRORS IN DEPRESSIVE DISORDERS

Exaggeration magnifying small mistakes and thinking of them as major failures.

Catastrophizing expecting serious consequences of minor problems (e.g. thinking that a relative who is late home has been involved in an accident).

Overgeneralizing thinking that the bad outcome of one event will be repeated in every similar event in future (e.g. that having lost one partner, the person will never find a lasting relationship).

Ignoring the positive dwelling on personal shortcomings or on the unfavourable aspects of a situation while overlooking favourable aspects.

modifying this set reduces the risk of relapse. At the time of writing, the evience for this idea is incomplete (see Teesdale *et al.*, 2002).

For a more detailed account of cognitive therapy for the depressed patient, see Fennell (2000).

Cognitive–behaviour therapy for bulimia nervosa

The treatment of bulimia nervosa by cognitive–behaviour therapy is based on the idea that the central problems are excessive concern about shape and weight, and low self-esteem. This concern leads to extreme dieting, which makes the control of eating more difficult and leads to binge-eating. Self-induced vomiting, sometimes combined with abuse of laxatives and diuretics, prevents weight gain and also reduces restraint on overeating, leading to more binges and a greater tendency to diet. In this way a vicious circle is set up which can be interrupted by:

- restoring a regular pattern of eating three meals a day,
- increasing restraint on binge-eating, and
- discussing ideas about shape, weight, and self-esteem.

The therapist attends first to the disordered pattern of eating before attempting to modify cognitions. He **explains the cognitive model** and relates it to the patient's experience. He emphasizes the importance of regular meals, the causal role of long periods of fasting, and the ill-effects of repeated vomiting, and of repeatedly taking laxatives and diuretics. **Patients keep records** of what they eat, when they eat, and when they induce vomiting or take laxatives and diuretics. The situations that provoke binge-eating are recorded. With this information, patients are more able to control the urge to overeat and, subsequently, the bouts of vomiting. **Patients take precautions** to help them control their eating:

- meals are eaten in a place separate from that in which food is prepared or stored;
- a limited amount of food is available at each meal, for example two slices of bread are put on the table but not a whole loaf;
- a small amount of food is left on the plate and then thrown away, in order to mark the end of the meal; and
- when shopping for food, a list is made in advance and purchases are limited strictly to the items and quantities on the list.

The therapist strongly discourages frequent checking of weight and of appearance, since both habits maintain the disorder.

Because patients often binge when they are unhappy, lonely, or bored, they are helped to **find other ways of dealing with unpleasant emotions**. For example, they might seek out friends or listen to music. Vomiting usually stops when binges are under control. The dangers of abuse of laxatives and diuretics are emphasized once more, and patients are encouraged strongly to throw away all such drugs.

When eating is under better control, **attention turns to cognitions**. Patients record these together with the eating behaviour. Relevant cognitions are concerned not only with body shape and weight but also with self-esteem. Examples of these cognitions are:

- to be fat is to be a failure;
- dieting is a sign of strong will and self-control;
- it is necessary to be thin to be happy and successful.

Such beliefs persist because of the **illogical ways of thinking** see Box 22.3 (p. 589), namely selective use of evidence, overgeneralization from limited instances, all or none reasoning, and overestimation of the person's contribution to events with multiple causes. The questioning used to identify cognitions and illogical thinking resembles that described in Box 22.5. Behavioural experiments are used, as in other forms of cognitive therapy (for an account, see Cooper *et al.*, 2004). Some patients with bulimia nervosa may have a distorted body image, and this cannot usually be changed directly by cognitive procedures. However, the distortion often diminishes as the other symptoms are brought under control.

Treatment also exists in a self help format that can be effective with well motivated patients - see Box 22.7.

For further information about cognitive–behaviour therapy for bulimia nervosa see Fairburn *et al.* (1993) and Wilson, Fairburn and Agrass (1996). For a review of its efficacy see Wilson and Fairburn (2002).

Cognitive–behaviour therapy has not been shown to be effective in **anorexia nervosa**. However, some of the underlying principles can be applied in management (see p. 366).

Cognitive–behaviour therapy for hypochondriasis

The approach is twofold: to identify behaviours that maintain the disorder, and to change hypochondriacal ideas directly. The relevant behaviours are

- repeatedly seeking reassurance, which relieves anxiety briefly but reinforces the concerns in the longer term,
- checking bodily functions (for example, counting the pulse rate),
- checking bodily structure (for example, palpating for lumps).

BOX 22.7 SELF-HELP FOR BULIMIA NERVOSA

Monitoring
  a daily record of eating, binges, and vomiting
  weighing no more than once a week

Regular planned meals
  three normal-sized meals a day
  with three small between-meal snacks

Stop binges
  eat only the planned amount
  keep other food out of sight
  keep limited stocks
  take just enough money when buying food

Control vomiting
  urge to vomit declines as binges stop

Control purging
  reduce laxatives/diuretics, if necessary, in stages

Find alternatives to binge eating
  list distracting activities
  try them

Reduce life problems
  see problem-solving counselling (Table 18.2)

For further information see Fairburn (1995).

Hypochondriacal ideas are approached along the lines described above in relation to cognitive-behaviour therapy for anxiety and depressive disorders, using questioning and behavioural experiments. For further information see Salkovskis and Bass (1997).

Cognitive–behaviour therapy for schizophrenia

There are two approaches. The first aims to help the patient **reduce and cope better with stressors** that may be exacerbating the disorder; and to **cope better with hallucinations**. The techniques for dealing with stressors are similar to those described above, namely identifying and finding ways of dealing with stressful situations. Patients are helped to cope with hallucinations by distancing themselves and repeating statements that neutralize their effects.

The aim of the second approach is to **challenge delusions**. This approach is directed to secondary delusions, especially those that seem to have developed to explain hallucinations. The therapist encourages the patient to regard the delusions as beliefs rather than facts, and to discuss alternatives. To do this effectively requires a detailed formulation of each patient's delusions and other beliefs. In questioning the basis of the delusions, the therapist has to be careful not to appear to be challenging them directly. Instead he tries to persuade the patient to consider the consequences of holding the delusion and what would be the consequences of thinking in another way. The therapist then tries to reformulate the delusion as a way of making sense of certain experiences, which can be understood in terms of the knowledge the patient had at the time, but should now be reconsidered. Patients selected for their willingness to reconsider their delusions are likely to differ in other ways from the majority of people with schizophrenia and it is not known how much the changes reported with this treatment are brought about by it rather than resulting from the method of selection. Positive effects have been reported but more evidence is needed before the effectiveness of the treatment can be decided (see Cormac *et al.* [2004] and the further discussion on p. 300).

For further information about the treatment see Turkington *et al.* (2005).

Cognitive therapy for personality disorder

A. T. Beck suggested that the techniques he had developed for the treatment of depressive disorders could be adapted for personality. He described beliefs and ways of thinking that characterize each type of personality disorder. Each disorder can be considered in terms of the person's self-view, the views of others, general beliefs, perceived threats, main strategies for coping, and primary affective responses. Beck also suggested a 'schema' characteristic of each type of personality disorder and consisting of statements that can be challenged in treatment. For example, the schema for histrionic personality disorder includes the following statements:

- 'Unless I captivate people, I am nothing';
- 'To be happy, I need other people to admire me';
- 'I must show people that they have hurt me'.

Schemas are challenged using the general techniques of cognitive therapy (see p. 594 and Box 22.5). As yet the treatment has not been evaluated as fully as the other cognitive treatments described in this section. For more information about the general use of cognitive therapy for personality disorders, see the book by Beck and Freeman (1990), or Beck (1998).

Dialectic behaviour therapy for borderline personality disorder

Linehan *et al.* (1994) developed this treatment for patients with borderline personality disorder who repeatedly harmed themselves. Despite the name, treatment uses cognitive as well as behavioural techniques. The treatment, which is highly structured, is described in a manual. Therapy is intensive with individual sessions, skills training in a group, and access by telephone to the therapist between sessions. It is delivered by a small team of therapists and lasts for up to a year.

Individual sessions have four elements:

1. **Cognitive-behavioural** techniques (see p. 589) including self-monitoring, and a collaborative style of working with the patient
2. **Dialectical** ways of thinking about problems such as seeing causality in terms of both/and rather than either/or and the possibility of reconciling opposites. This approach helps to avoid confrontations with the patient.
3. **'Mindfulness'**, that is, the practice of detachment from experience.
4. **Aphorisms**, that is, phrases that encapsulate the approach: for example, although people may not have caused all their problems, they have to solve them anyway.

During the sessions, treatment goals are prioritized: deal first with life-threatening situations; then with matters that could reduce collaboration with treatment; and after that with behaviours that impair qaulity of life.

Skills training sessions are usually provided in a weekly group lasting 2 hours or more. Patients learn (i) the control of anger and other strong emotions; (ii) toleration of distress; (iii) interpersonal skills; (iv) mindfulness. The procedures for teaching these skills are described in a manual

Telephone contact is designed to help patients get through crises by using the skills learnt in the sessions. The hours at which contact will be available are agreed in advance between patient and therapist.

Dialectic behaviour therapy has been claimed to give good results with borderline personality disorder, but at the time of writing, further evaluation is needed. For further information see Palmer (2002).

Individual dynamic psychotherapies

Brief insight-oriented psychotherapy

This kind of psychotherapy seeks to uncover the origins of a psychiatric disorder in early life experience, and seeks for unconscious factors that account for abnormal thinking, emotions, and behaviour. In its usual form, it aims to produce limited but worthwhile changes through weekly sessions for 6–9 months (brief in contrast to full psychoanalytic treatment - see p. 602). The treatment is focused upon specific problems; hence the alternative term **focal psychotherapy**. The procedures can be summarized as follows.

Starting treatment

The initial assessment is important and should not be hurried. As well as assessing suitability for brief treatment (see below), the aim is select the problems that are to be the focus of treatment. This focus and the length of treatment are agreed with the patient. Usually, some problems remain at the end of treatment, and this possibility is explained at the start. The therapist also explains the general aim of linking past and present behaviour patterns. He indicates that the therapist's role is to help patients find their own solutions to their problems, not to do it for them. From the start, an atmosphere is created in which patients feel involved, listened to, and safe to speak about ideas and fantasies that they have not previously revealed to anyone.

Subsequent sessions

In subsequent sessions patients are encouraged to:

- give specific examples of the selected problems, and consider how they thought, felt, and acted at the time;
- talk freely about emotionally painful subjects, within limits of topics agreed with the therapist;

- express ideas and feelings even if they seem illogical or shameful;
- review their own part in any difficulties that they ascribe to other people;
- look for common themes in their problems and their responses to situations;
- consider how present patterns of behaviour began, what function they served in the past, and why they may be continuing;
- consider alternative ways of thinking and behaving in the situations that cause difficulties;
- try out new and more adaptive ways of behaving and responding to emotions.

The therapist's role is to respond to the emotional as well as to the intellectual content of the patient's utterances (for example, 'it sounds as though you felt angry when this happened'). He helps the patient to examine feelings that previously have been denied, and to think about past situations in which similar feelings were experienced. The therapist pays as much attention to patients' non-verbal behaviour as to their words, because discrepancies between the two often point to problems that have not been expressed directly. He maintains the focus, that is, he avoids problem areas which are too complex to deal with in the agreed time.

Interpretations by the therapist may be (i) hypotheses linking present or past events and behaviours; (ii) comments about defence mechanisms, for example, blocks in recall during the sessions, or ways in which the patient unconsciously protects himself from unpleasant feelings in his daily life.

Transference and counter-transference The therapist is alert to the development of transference and counter-transference (see p. 584). **Transference** may reveal how the patient responds to other people at the present time, or how he responded to his parents in childhood. In brief therapy, **counter-transference** is usually taken to include both appropriate and inappropriate responses by the therapist to the patient's emotional state. A therapist who has insight into his own reactions will be more objective and understand the patient's situation better. Because such insight is difficult to achieve, therapists often work with a supervisor who can help to identify the counter-transference. Some therapists undergo a period of personal psychotherapy to understand better how events in their past determine their responses to their patients.

Ending treatment

To ensure that treatment ends on time, realistic goals should be chosen and the focus should remain on these goals. Also, potential problems related to termination should be discussed from an early stage. As the end of treatment approaches, patients should feel that they have a better understanding of the chosen problems and should be more confident about dealing with them. It is often useful to ease the termination of treatment by arranging a few follow-up appointments spaced over 2 or 3 months.

Indications

Because there is no satisfactory, adequate evidence from randomized clinical trials, the indications for short-term dynamic psychotherapy have to be based on clinical experience which suggests that. treatment is more useful

I When the problem:

(i) can be conceptualized in psychodynamic terms

(ii) is emotional or interpersonal (rather than a specific psychiatric disorder)

(iii) involves low self-esteem, and recurrent problems in forming intimate relationships.

II When the person

(i) has adequate social support while treatment continues

(ii) is willing to bring about change though their own efforts,

(iii) can look honestly at their own motives,

(iv) is capable of ceasing self-exploration when the sessions end.

Contraindications

Clinical experience suggests that contraindications include obsessional or hypochondriacal disorders, severe mood disorder, schizophrenia in which exploration of past emotional problems may increase present distress; and some personality disorders, especially those leading to acting out of problems.

See Ursano and Ursano (2000) for a concise account of the theories and methods of brief individual dynamic psychotherapy, or the review by Hobbs (2005).

Very brief treatment.

Recently, attempts have been made to reduce the length (and cost) of dynamic therapy still further by focusing on a small number of recurrent interpersonal problems and on the patient's own contribution to these problems. Patients are expected to take an active part in overcoming their problems and a follow-up session may be offered at which their efforts to do this are discussed. For a review of very brief treatment see Aveline (2001).

Cognitive-analytical therapy

Cognitive analytic therapy was developed by Ryle (1990) as a brief form of therapy. Treatment is based on a procedural sequence model that supposes that purposeful behaviour activity follows a sequence of: aim generation, evaluation of the environment, planning, action, evaluation of the consequences and, if necessary, revision. Procedural sequences can be faulty in three ways:

- **Traps** that is repetitive cycles of behaviour in which the consequences of behaviour perpetuate it. For example, depressed people think in ways that make for failure and further depression more likely (see p. 596).
- **Dilemmas** which are false choices or unduly narrowed options. For example, people who fear angry feelings may think they have to choose between placation and aggression: they choose to placate others who then take advantage of them, thus making them even more angry.
- **Snags** which are the anticipation of highly negative consequences of actions such that the action is never carried out and therefore never subject to a reality check.

The **theory of reciprocal roles** was developed when cognitive analytic therapy was appled to borderline personality disorder. Ryle supposed that, starting from childhood, people develop internalized 'templates' of social roles. These templates consist of a role for the self, a role for the other person, and a paradigm of the relationship. Examples of such roles include teacher/pupil, bully/victim, and abuser/abused. When one person adopts one of the reciprocal roles, the other feels under pressure to adopt the other. According to Ryle, these 'templates' can become abnormal in three ways:

1. The repertoire of different roles is restricted or distorted
2. Roles cannot be switched easily
3. Roles are inflexible and cannot be adapted to new situations.

Scaffolding is important: it is the provision of just enough support to enable patients to discover their own solutions. Scaffolding has to be flexible and appropriate to the different needs of each patient.

Outline of the procedures

Following assessment and an explanation of the treatment, the patient is helped to construct a list of problems, moods and behaviours and asked to record their occurrence in a daily diary. From the history and the diary, recurrent maladadaptive behaviours, role problems and faulty procedural sequences are identified and formulated, often using diagrams to explain the procedural sequences. For example, a faulty sequence might begin with the idea that one must try to please everyone, leading to giving way to others, and thence to frustration and feelings of failure and anger. Specific examples of the general procedures are sought in the diaries, and homework is arranged whereby alternative procedures are tried out, for example asserting oneself appropriately. The origins of maladaptive procedures are considered also from a psychodynamic viewpoint. For example, present maladaptive behaviour is viewed as arising from behaviour that was adaptive when the person was younger.

The formulation is summarized in the form of a letter to the patient. With help from the therapist, the patient tries to become aware of these behaviours, procedural sequences and role problems, and attempts gradually to change them. From the start, transference and countertransference problems are anticipated, identified and discussed. Treatment usually lasts for 16–24 sessions. When it ends, the therapist writes another letter to the patient summarizing progress, prognosis and future action. Patients with borderline personality usually need additional help before they can become aware of their problems ('develop an observing I'). This help is often in the form of modelling of ways in which the maladaptive elements can be evaluated and analysed, often with the aid of diagrams. Object relations (see above) and social interaction concepts are used to understand the genesis of the problems, but defence mechnisms are not viewed as important.

In the absence of high quality evidence from randomized clinical trials, the use of cognitive-analytical therapy is based mainly on clinical experience; it does not have the strong evidence base of cognitive therapy.

For further information about cognitive analytic therapy see Ryle and Kerr (2002) or the review see by Denman (2001).

Psychodynamic interpersonal therapy

This form of brief treatment was developed by Hobson (1985). It is similar to interpersonal therapy (see p. 587) but with more use of the patient–therapist relationship as a tool for understanding and changing interpersonal problems (but less interpretation of transference than in other kinds of psychodynamic therapy). Important features are:

- the assumption that the presenting problems arise from or are made worse by disurbed interpersonal relationships
- the therapist is supportive and encouraging
- the therapist tries to understand the patient through exploring feelings and through the therapist–patient relationship
- the therapist uses metaphor to communicate with the patient
- the patient's distress is linked to particular problems in relationships
- the patient tests out solutions in his daily life.

The treatment has been tested in clinical trials with, for example, high utilizers of psychiatric services (Guthrie *et al.*, 1999), chronic functional dyspepsia (Hamilton *et al.*, 2000), and deliberate self-harm (Guthrie *et al.*, 2001).

Long-term individual dynamic psychotherapy

Long-term individual dynamic psychotherapy is a general term referring to many kinds of individual psychotherapy lasting for longer that the 9 months that is often taken as the upper limit of brief dynamic psychotherapy. The longest, most intensive, and best known form is psychoanalysis, and most methods are derived from it. Long-term dynamic psychotherapy is costly, and because its results have not been shown to be better than those of shorter forms of treatment, it is not generally available as part of the health services of most countries. When it is used, it is usually for patients judged unsuitable for short-term psychotherapy, even though it is in these cases that its effects are least certain.

The primary aim of long-term dynamic psychotherapy is to increase insight, defined as 'the conscious recognition of the role of unconscious factors on current experience and behaviour' (Fonagy, 2000). Insight requires more than an awareness of these factors; it involves the integration of this knowledge into ways of thinking, feeling and behaving, a process that is called 'working through'. Insight is achieved by bringing to conscious awareness mental contents that were previously outside consciousness, by interpreting their significance, and by linking past experiences with present modes of functioning.

Unconscious material is brought to conscious awareness through free association, and by examining the content of fantasies and dreams. Analysis of the patient's unrealistic responses to the therapist (the transference) provides further information about unconscious processes. Therapists vary in the extent to which they work with the transference. Analysis of the counter-transference provides further relevant information since it reflects not only the therapist's psychological make-up but also aspects of the patient to which the therapist is responding. The need to understand the counter-transference is one reason why therapists generally undergo personal psychotherapy as part of their training to undertake long-term dynamic psychotherapy.

Attempts to access unconscious material and to increase insight activate **resistance** of three kinds.

1. Resistance by repression which blocks access to unconscious material.
2. Transference resistance which restricts the intensity of the relationship with the therapist.
3. A negative therapeutic reaction which is expressed in new symptoms that retard progress.

Although resistance impedes progress, analysis of resistance can increase insight.

Interpretations are generally regarded as one of the main techniques of this kind of treatment. However, the use of interpretations varies considerably between the various types of long-term dynamic psychotherapy. Interpretations may be concerned with defences, unconscious processes, transference, or the links between past experience and present patterns. Transference interpretations are often used, in keeping with the greater importance of transference in long-term, compared with short-term therapy.

Other ways in which long-term psychodynamic psychotherapy differs from brief dynamic psychotherapy are that:

- *It is less structured*; patients are encouraged to talk and associate ideas freely without a specific focus.
- *The therapist is less active* and guides the patient less. He tries to make the material clearer by asking questions, pointing out contradictions, commenting on evasions and resistance, and making interpretations.
- *Patients are seen more frequently* (up to five times a week). This is one of the factors leading to the more intense transference noted above. In psychoanalysis, transference may be increased further by arranging

that the therapist sits out of direct vision of the patient who lies on a couch.

For a fuller account of psychoanalysis and other long-term dynamic psychotherapies, see Gabbard (2005).

Results of and indications for long-term dynamic psychotherapy

In general, the research literature does not contradict the impression of experienced clinicians that most patients can be helped as effectively with short-term dynamic therapy as with longer methods. Clinical experience suggests that if long-term therapy is ever appropriate, it is for patients who have long-lasting and complicated emotional difficulties, or significant maturational problems in their personal development. Specific psychiatric disorders respond less well than do problems of personality and relationships. Long-term psychotherapy should not be used with patients with schizophrenia, manic-depressive disorder, or marked paranoid personality traits. Histrionic and schizoid personality disorders, whilst not contraindications, are particularly difficult to treat.

Treatment in groups

Small-group psychotherapy

This section is concerned with psychotherapy carried out with a group of usually about eight patients. Treatment in larger groups is considered later. Small-group psychotherapy is used most often to modify interpersonal problems; as a form of supportive treatment; or to encourage adjustment to the effects physical or mental illness.

How group psychotherapy developed

Group therapy is often said to have originated from the work of Joseph Pratt, an American physician who used groups to assist patients with pulmonary tuberculosis (Pratt, 1908). Pratt's groups were supportive and educational and more obvious precursors of modern group psychotherapy were J. L. Moreno, a Romanian who migrated to the USA, and Trigant Burrow, an American (Burrow, 1927). The main roots of group therapy were, however, in the experience of treating war neuroses in the 1940s in the UK.

In the Northfield Military Hospital in England, S. H. Foulkes developed group analysis (Foulkes and Lewis, 1944). He based his approach on psychoanalysis so that the group leader took a rather passive role, and used analytical interpretations (Foulkes 1948, p. 136). W. R. Bion, a Kleinian analyst who also worked at Northfield Hospital, developed a different approach (Bion, 1961). He focused specifically on the unconscious defences of the group as a whole rather than on the problems of individual members.

Further developments took place in the USA in the 1960s and early 1970s, where so-called action groups were used to provide a more intense form of group experience. Many variations of group technique have developed but it is now generally accepted that the features that the different methods have in common are more important than the differences.

Classification of small-group therapies

Pines and Schlapobersky (2000) have suggested a useful classification based on the goals of the group (specific versus non-specific) and the activity of the leader (high versus low). The resulting four categories are therefore:

1. **Specific goals - high leader activity:** includes structured programmes for alcohol and drug dependence, as well as cognitive–behaviour therapy carried out in a group;
2. **Specific goals - low leader activity:** includes problem solving groups;
3. **Non-specific goals - high leader activity:** includes the many kinds of short-term group therapy, as well as psychodrama;
4. **Non-specific goals - low leader activity:** includes the various kinds of psychodynamic group such as the Tavistock, eclectic, and interpersonal approaches, and group analytical therapy.

Several of these methods will be discussed below.

Terminology

Groups are often described in terms of their structure, process, and content:

- **Structure** describes the enduring reciprocal relationships between each member of the group and the therapist, and between the members.
- **Process** describes the short-term changes in emotions, behaviours, relationships, and other experiences of the group.
- **Content** refers to the observable events in the group meetings: the themes, responses, and discussions, and the silences.

Therapeutic factors in group therapy

Group treatments share the therapeutic factors common to all kinds of psychological treatment, namely restoring hope, releasing emotion, giving information, providing a rationale, and prestige suggestion (see Box 22.2). In group treatment, there are additional factors not present in individual therapies but common to all kinds of group psychotherapy. These factors are shared experience, support to and from group members, socialization, imitation, and interpersonal learning (see Yalom, 1985). These factors are summarized in Box 22.7.

BOX 22.7 THERAPEUTIC FACTORS IN GROUP THERAPY

Universality (shared experience) Helps patients to realize that they are not isolated and that others have similar experiences and problems. Hearing about experiences is often more convincing and helpful than reassurance from a therapist.

Altruism Supporting others increases the self-esteem of the person giving the support, as well as helping the receiver. Mutual support is one of the factors leading to a sense of belonging to the group.

Group cohesion The feeling of belonging to the group is especially valuable for patients who previously have felt isolated. Group cohesion can sustain the group when problems threaten to destroy it

Socialization The acquisition of social skills within a group as a result of the comments and reactions members provide about one another's behaviour. Members can try out new social behaviours within the safety of the group.

Imitation is learning from observing and adopting the behaviours of other group members. If the group is run well, patients imitate adaptive behaviours; if it is not run well, they may imitate maladaptive behaviours such as extravagant displays of emotion, or talking in a way that deflects attention from their own emotional problems.

Interpersonal learning is learning from the interactions within the group and from practising new ways of interacting. Interpersonal learning is an important component of group therapy.

Recapitulation of the family group As the group proceeds, interactions are increasingly unrealistic and based on past relations between patients and their parents and siblings. This group transference develops eventually in all groups; it is encouraged and used in some treatments, mainly those using a psychoanalytical approach.

General indications for group therapy

Group or individual therapy?

There is no evidence that the results of group therapy differ in general from those of individual psychotherapy of the same duration and used for the same problem, or that the results of any one form of group therapy differ from those of the rest. In particular, there is no evidence that encounter groups or action techniques are superior to other methods, and there is some evidence that they can increase symptoms in some patients (Yalom *et al.* 1973).

What problems are suitable?

Group therapy appears to be useful for patients whose problems are mainly in relationships. As in individual psychotherapy, results are generally thought to be better in patients who are **young, well-motivated, able to express themselves fluently, and free from severe personality disorder**. Groups are often suitable for patients with moderate degrees of social anxiety, presumably because such patients benefit from the opportunity to rehearse social behaviour. (Severe social anxiety is a contraindication.)

General contraindications for group therapy

These are similar to the contraindications for individual psychotherapy (see above), with the addition of severe social anxiety. Also, a group should never include a member whose problems are so unlike those of the others that he may become an outsider or a scapegoat.

Types of small group psychotherapy

Supportive groups

Many of the therapeutic factors present in a group (see Box 22.7) are at work in supportive treatment. In a supportive group, the therapist should encourage self-help and ensure that the experiences of the group members are used positively. He should ensure that relationships do not become too intense, protect vulnerable patients when necessary, and ensure that each member is supported and gives support to other members. The problems that can arise in therapeutic groups (see below) may develop also in supportive groups. The leader of a supportive group should be alert to these potential problems and be capable of dealing with them along the lines described below (p. 606).

Self-help groups

Self-help groups are organized and led by patients or ex-patients who have learned ways of overcoming or adjusting to their difficulties. The other group members benefit from this experience, from the opportunity to talk about their own problems and express their feelings, and from mutual support. Group processes develop as much in these groups as in any other, so it is important that those who lead them have appropriate training and support. Some groups, such as Alcoholics Anonymous, have strict rules of procedure; others have a professional advisor.

There are self-help groups for people who suffer from many kinds of problems, for example, Alcoholics Anonymous (see p. 448), groups to help people lose weight (Weight Watchers), groups for patients with chronic physical conditions such as colostomy, groups for people facing special problems such as parents with a handicapped child, and groups for the bereaved (CRUSE Clubs). Only a few self-help groups have been evaluated. One study found that a self-help group for recently bereaved women was as effective as brief dynamic psychotherapy (Marmar *et al.*, 1988).

For a review of self-help groups see Lieberman (1990).

Therapeutic groups

Interpersonal group therapy

Interpersonal group therapy developed particularly from the work of Yalom (1985). Treatment is focused on problems in current relationships and examines the ways in which these problems are reflected in the group. The past is discussed only in so far as it helps to make sense of the present problems.

Stages of treatment

The first stage The group members try to depend on the therapist, seeking expert advice about their problems and about the way they should behave in the group. Before long, some members become disillusioned by the therapist's refusal to solve their problems and miss meetings or come late. Other members leave because they are anxious about talking in the group.

The second stage The remaining members begin to know each other better, they become used to discussing each other's problems, and they begin to seek answers. This is the stage in which most change can be expected. The therapist encourages the examination of current problems and relationships, and comments on the dynamics of the group.

The last stage The group can become dominated by the residual problems of the members who have made least progress and who still show the most dependency. This development should be anticipated by starting to discuss these and other problems of termination several months before the group is due to end.

Preparation for the group

It is useful to prepare patients for their experience in a group by emphasizing the following points:

- **Confidentiality:** the proceedings of the group are confidential.
- **Reliability:** members must attend regularly and on time, and not leave early.
- **Disclosure:** members are required to disclose their problems.
- **Concern:** members must show concern for the problems of others.
- **Disappointment:** at first members may be disappointed at the lack of rapid change, or frustrated at the need to share the time available for speaking.
- **Keeping apart:** The group members must not meet outside the group; if this rule is ever broken, it must be reported to the next meeting of the group.
- **Duration:** the length of the group is explained, together with need to remain until the end.

Setting up the group

General considerations About eight members are chosen. They should have some problems in common, and no member should have problems that set him aside from the rest. Members should be able to empathize with each other's difficulties and willing to assist each other. Meetings should be held in a room of adequate size, with the chairs arranged in a circle so that all members can see one another.

Meetings usually last for 60–90 minutes to allow adequate time for every member to take part; they are usually held once a week and generally continue for 12–18 months. Most groups are **closed**, that is, no new members join after the first few weeks. (Groups that accepts new members are called **open**; such groups are usually supportive or educational.)

One or two therapists? Some groups are run by one therapist, some by co-therapists. The advantage of employing two therapists is that one can help the other to recognize and deal with counter-transference problems (which are as important in group as in individual psychotherapy). The potential disadvantages are that the two therapists may develop different views about the running of the group, or may behave defensively with one another. However, when the therapists trust each other's judgements and if any differences are discussed as they arise, they can provide further insight into the group process. At the start, differences between co-therapists may be discussed outside the group. However, when the group is well integrated, such differences can be discussed within the group, as a way of increasing the members' understanding of interpersonal processes.

Managing the group

The therapist should be aware of **five basic issues** that are likely to require attention:

1. the conflict between each member's wish to be helped and the requirement to help others;
2. the conflict between a wish to gain the therapist's approval and the desire to be approved by the other members of the group;
3. the process by which members of a group establish a hierarchy of dominance, and the rivalries that this produces;
4. the risk that one person may become a scapegoat when the group is dissatisfied;
5. the risk that members may be excessively passive and dependent on the therapist instead of working out solutions themselves.

The group therapist's role has been compared to that of the conductor of an orchestra. He helps the members to work in harmony, prevents any one member from dominating the group, and regulates the speed and emotional intensity of the discourse. He also helps the members to understand one another, to accept suggestions, and to see aspects of themselves in other people. If a therapeutic group is working well, members are active, they give and take, and they support each other. They discuss problems constructively and do not blame or scapegoat other members.

Some problems in group therapy

However skilful the therapist, certain problems commonly arise in the course of group therapy:

Formation of subgroups Some members may form a coalition based on age, social class, shared values, or other characteristics. Because subgroups disrupt the therapeutic process, the therapist should be alert for early signs of such alliances. He should discourage them by asking the group to discuss the reasons for their formation.

Members who talk too much In its early stages the group may welcome a talkative member who relieves the others of the need to speak about themselves. As meetings continue, the group is likely to become dissatisfied with this member for monopolizing time that would be better shared. The therapist should draw attention to this problem at an early stage, before the group rejects the talkative member. He can do so by asking the group why they allow one person to absolve the rest from the need to speak about themselves.

Members who talk too little The therapist should assist silent members to speak and should therefore understand the reasons for silence. Some patients are generally awkward in company; some are afraid to reveal a specific problem to the group and fear that this problem will be uncovered if they speak; and some are silent because they are angry and dissatisfied with the progress of the group.

Conflict between members The therapist should not take sides in conflicts but should encourage the whole group to discuss the issue in a way that leads them to understand why the conflict has arisen, for example, because a hostile transference has developed.

Avoidance of the focus The usual focus of a group is on the current problems of the members and on the reflection of these problems in the interactions of the group. The past experience of the members is considered in so far as it assists understanding present problems. Sometimes the group members talk excessively about the past as a way of avoiding their present difficulties. When this happens, the therapist can ask questions or use interpretations as an indirect way of bringing the discussion back to the present problems of the members. For example, a woman who dwells inappropriately on past difficulties with her overpowering father, may be asked whether she does this because she feels that one of the men in the group is behaving in a similar way.

Potentially embarrassing revelations A group member may say, for example, that he has been unfairly criticized by a member of the group. The therapist should then help the group to examine the remark constructively to understand whether the feelings relate to past or present experiences outside the group as well as to experiences within it. Such discussions are more useful when they are specific. For example, it is more useful to discuss why a woman feels angry when a particular man in the group offers her advice than to discuss why she has a general problem of anger with men. Consideration of the specific instances will lead to understanding of the wider problem.

To supplement this outline of interpersonal group therapy, the reader is referred to Bloch and Aveline (1996).

Group analysis

This technique, which was pioneered by Foulkes (see above) is one of the most widely used within the UK health Service. It differs from the interpersonal method described above (i) in the greater use of interpretations about transference and unconscious mechanisms; and (ii) in the use of 'free-floating discussion' instead of a focus. The therapist ('conductor') points out conflicts, preoccupations, and evasions, and makes interpretations. Particular attention is given to transferences to the therapist and between members, which are interpreted as reflecting relations in earlier life with parents and siblings. The resulting hypotheses about previous relationships are used to understand current problems. This process leads to questioning of long-held assumptions, and to greater self-understanding. As the group progresses, the leader becomes less active, and exerts his influence more by example than as an expert, thereby encouraging and allowing the members to take more responsibility for the proceedings.

For a fuller account of group analysis, see Pines and Schlapobersky (2000) or Montgomery (2002).

Encounter groups and psychodrama (action techniques)

In **encounter groups** the interaction between members is made more intense and rapid in the hope that this will lead to greater change. The encounter can be entirely verbal, using challenging language, or it can include touching or hugging between the participants. Sometimes the experience is intensified further by prolonging the group session for a whole day or even longer (**marathon groups**). Although some participants are helped by encounter groups, many are not, and an early study showed that a few are made worse (Lieberman et al., 1973). Adverse effects are more likely in people with substantial emotional disorders, and in groups using the most confrontational methods.

Psychodrama is another form of intensive group experience. The group enacts events from the life of one member, in scenes reflecting either current relationships or those of the family in which the person grew up. The enactment usually provokes strong feelings in the person represented, and often reflects the problems experienced by other members of the group. Members sometimes exchange roles so as to understand better the other person's point of view. The drama is followed by a group discussion. Instead of building a drama round the personal experiences of one member, the action may be concerned with problems that the participants share, for example, how to deal with authority. This method is called **sociodrama**. For an account of psychodrama see Holmes and Karp (1991).

Action techniques are now used mainly as an adjunct to other group methods. A session of psychodrama can provide topics for discussion when a group using other methods is failing to make progress. Role reversal can help some patients to view their problems more objectively and perhaps for the first time from the standpoint of other people.

Large-group therapy

Ward groups

This form of group therapy is part of the daily programme of many psychiatric wards. It is also a characteristic component of the programme of a therapeutic community. Large groups usually include all the patients in a treatment unit together with some or all of the staff. At the simplest level, large groups allow patients to express problems of living together. At a more ambitious level, such groups can attempt to change their members, presenting to each member examples of his disordered behaviour or irrational responses. At the same time, support is provided by other members who share similar problems and opportunities for social learning. The group is sometimes used as a kind of governing body that formulates rules and seeks to enforce them. Because large groups can evoke much anxiety, in patients and also in staff, great care should be taken in conducting them. The general principles resemble those of small group therapy (see above). Special care is needed to prepare new members for the experience, regulate the emotional level of the sessions, protect vulnerable people, and excuse those too unwell to take part.

Therapeutic communities

In a therapeutic community, every shared activity is viewed as a potential source of change. Members live, work and play together and learn about themselves through the reactions of other members in the course of these activities. Within the safe environment of the community, they are encouraged to practise new behaviours and appreciate points of view other than their own. Members take part in frequent group meetings. Maxwell Jones, one of the founders of this form of treatment, referred to it as a living-learning situation (Jones, 1968) others have called it a culture of enquiry. There are usually 20–30 members of the community and they stay for between 9 and 18 months. The underlying principles of the regimen have been summarized as **democracy, reality confrontation, permissiveness, and communality** (Rapoport, 1960).These translate into the features shown in Box 22.8.

The role of the staff is to ensure a basic structure within which members of the community can interact. The amount of staff activity is greater when there are conflicts and other problems within the unit, and less when the members are able to function effectively. Staff help members to understand their interactions,

BOX 22.8 PRINCIPAL FEATURES OF A THERAPEUTIC COMMUNITY

Informality There are few rules, and staff dress and behave informally.

Mutual help The members support each other and help others to change.

Permissiveness Members tolerate behaviour that they might not accept elsewhere.

Directness and honesty Members respond directly to distortions of reality and other kinds of self-deception.

Shared decisions Members and staff join in the day-to-day decisions about the running of the unit, and the behaviour of its members, and usually about the admission of new candidates.

Shared activities Members provide some of the 'hotel' services in the community in order that each has a job with responsibilities to other people.

and ensure that problems are discussed constructively. Conflicts commonly arise between the need to allow patients to behave in ways that will lead to greater self-awareness and the need to prepare them for return to the outside world; and the need to help individuals versus the need to deal with processes in the group. The staff have to ensure a balance within the unit, protecting the vulnerable and ensuring safety. The staff also arrange that there is a sufficient variety of activities to allow members to find something in which they can work cooperatively, and for which they can take responsibility.

Therapeutic community day units have been developed in some centres for the treatment of personality disorder (see Bateman and Fonagy 1999, 2001). They provide a system of additional support during the hours when the community is closed, for example through a network of telephone contacts.

Indications and contraindications

It is difficult to assess the value of the therapeutic community method and there is no satisfactory body of evidence from clinical trials. Indications are also uncertain but are thought to include personality disorders of the dyssocial and unstable types, including those associated with previous drug dependence (all communities have a rule of abstinence). Contraindications include severe depression, hypomania, schizophrenia, paranoid personality, and persistent violence. Potential members need to be highly motivated to change, and willing to spend a long time in treatment. These last two requirements make it difficult to compare results of those who remain in treatment with those who remain in treatments that demand less of the patients.

Preparation

Patients in all forms of psychotherapy seem to be less likely to drop out if they understand what to expect. Membership of a therapeutic community is especially demanding and many communities provide written informatioms and audio- or videotapes to supplement the explanation given during the assessment interview. Some have a trial period before the patient commits to the full programme.

For further information about therapeutic communities see Kennard (1998) or Campling (2001).

Psychotherapy with couples and families

Couple therapy

Couple therapy is usually given either because conflict in a relationship appears to be the cause of emotional disorder in one of the partners, or because the relationship is unsatisfactory or likely to break up, and both partners wish to save it. In the apparently simple step from treating an individual to treating a couple, there is an important conceptual change in that the problem is not thought of as confined to one person but shared between two. The problem is conceived as resulting from the way in which the couple interact and treatment is directed to this interaction. In assessing the interaction, it is useful to examine issues that are important in all relationships for example the sharing of values, concern for the welfare and personal development of the partner, tolerance of differences, and an agreed balance of dominance and decision-making. It is useful also to bear in mind the three stages of most marriages or other long-term relationships: living together, bringing up children, and readjusting when the children leave home. To avoid imposing values, the therapist adopts a 'target problem' approach, whereby couples are required to identify the difficulties that they would like to put right.

Several techniques of therapy have developed, based on psychodynamic, behavioural, and systems theory approaches, and on a combination of techniques drawn from the last two approaches.

Psychodynamic couple therapy

The central idea is that the behaviour of a married couple is importantly determined, from the moment that they choose each other, by unconscious forces. Each person selects a partner who is perceived as completing unfulfilled parts of him or herself. When the selection is successful, the couple complement one another, but sometimes one partner fails to live up to the (unconscious) expectations of the other. For example, a wife may criticize her husband for failing to show the independence and self-reliance that she lacks herself. Also, each partner may project on the other unwanted aspects of the self which are split off and denied. For example, a husband may project on to his wife the vulnerability that he feels but cannot accept as part of himself.

The aim of this kind of treatment is to help each partner to understand his own emotional needs and how they relate to those of the other. This may be done in several ways. One therapist may see the couple together, two therapists may see them together (each therapist having a primary concern with one of them), or two therapists may see the patients separately but meet regularly to coordinate their treatments. Therapists take a more active part than they would in the analytical treatment of a single patient. Also, interpretations are concerned more with the relationship between the partners than with transference involving the therapist.

For a review of psychodynamic approaches to couple therapy see Scharff and Scharff (2005).

Systems approaches to couple therapy

The focus of treatment is on the hidden rules that govern the behaviour of the couple towards one another, on disagreements about who makes these rules, and on inconsistencies between these two 'levels' of interaction. Important concepts include enmeshment, that is, excessive involvement with the other person, and the idea of a cycle of cause and effect such that neither person is wholly to blame. These ideas are discussed around conflicts arising in the everyday life of the couple, for example, who decides where to go on holiday, and how the couple decide who is to decide this. In this way it is hoped to arrive at a more balanced and more cooperative relationship. Some therapists use '**paradoxical injunctions**', that is, provocative statements designed to elicit a (beneficial) counter-response that the couple have previously resisted. One or two therapists may take part but the partners are always seen together. The account of the method given by Haley (1963) is still valuable.

Cognitive behavioural couple therapy

This form of couple therapy is brief and highly structured. It is based on the principles of operant conditioning. The therapist tries to identify ways in which undesired behaviour between the couple is being reinforced unwittingly by one of its consequences. Each partner is asked to say what alternative behaviours they desire in the other. These behaviours must be described in specific terms, for example 'talk to me for half an hour when you come in from work' rather than 'take more notice of me'. Each partner agrees a way of rewarding the other when the desired behaviour is carried out. The reward could be the expression of approval and affection, or doing something that the partner desires. This exchange is called 'reciprocity negotiating'. In addition, the couple is helped to communicate more directly, to listen to one another, and to express individual wishes more clearly. Described briefly, the treatment may seem a crude form of bargaining that is remote from a loving relationship. In practice it can enable a couple to cooperate and give up habits of criticism and nagging, with consequent improvement in their feelings for one another. The method has been described by Stuart (1980). Some therapists add cognitive approaches based on the ideas of Beck (1988). For a review of cognitive-behaviour therapy with couples see Dattilio (2005).

The behavioural-systems couple therapy

The approach described here was developed by Crowe for use with problems of couples encountered in psychiatric practice. It is described in detail by Crowe and Ridley (1990). As the name implies, it has two sets of components. The behavioural components are 'reciprocity negotiating' (see above) and training in communication. The systems components are 'structural moves' (see below), timetables and tasks, and the use of paradox. These components are drawn together progressively, starting with the simplest and adding complexity only when it is clearly necessary. Figure 22.1 shows the order in which the procedures are combined. Behavioural methods are used for simpler cases and the more complex systems procedures are added for couples with more symptoms, less willingness to accept the relationship as the focus of treatment, and more rigid patterns of interaction. The various procedures have been described above.

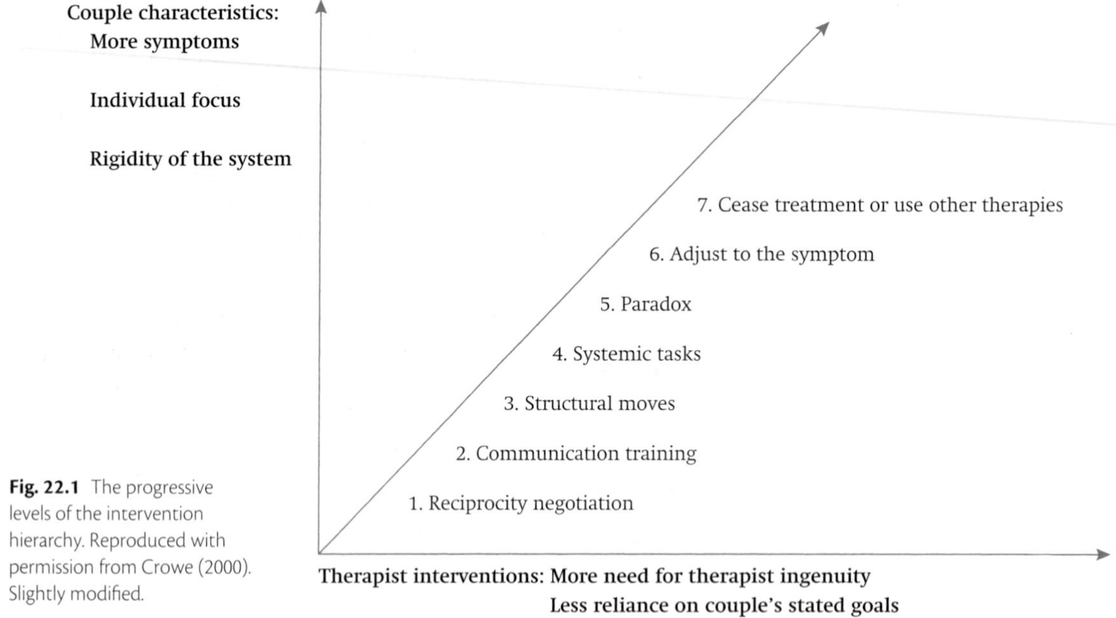

Fig. 22.1 The progressive levels of the intervention hierarchy. Reproduced with permission from Crowe (2000). Slightly modified.

Treatments last usually for 5–10 sessions over 3–6 months. The therapist has to develop a relationship with both partners without favouring either or taking sides. He maintains a focus on mutual interactions, and helps them to make changes in the way they interact. The therapist's role is more like that of the director of a play than a negotiator. He encourages the couple to speak to each other, not to the therapist, and comments on what they say and do in the sessions. Difficulties may arise with couples who communicate well about intellectual matters but not about their feelings. In such cases, instead of questioning one person, it is often better to ask the other partner to put the question. For example, 'Could you ask John what he thinks about what you said?' Sessions usually end with a summary message for the couple to consider together when they return home.

Special techniques

Structural moves include requiring disagreement, reversed role play, and sculpting. Couples may be **asked to disagree** about something when one partner dominates the other who habitually gives in to avoid disagreement. The topic does not matter, the aim is to help the passive partner express an opinion forcefully and to help the other to value it. **Role reversal** helps one partner to understand the point of view and experience of the other. In **sculpting**, the partners take up positions, silently, to express some aspect of the relationship without words; for example, one partner may depict the depth of her dissatisfaction with the relationship through a tableau in which the two sit side by side, looking away from one other.

Systemic tasks concern interactions that occur either too seldom or too often. A timetable is made in which specific times are allocated for the interaction. For example, if the couple do not spend undivided time together, times are agreed at which they will spend time together without any distractions. If one partner returns repeatedly to the same complaint, it is agreed that complaints will be made only at specific times, and that the other will agree to listen at these times.

Paradox The use of paradox has been described above. Paradoxical injunctions should be given only after consideration of possible consequences other than the intended one, and in the context of a caring relationship. Often the paradox is to 'prescribe the symptom'. The therapist tells the couple to continue with the problem behaviour, and give a reason that is unacceptable to the couple. Crowe (2000) gives an example in which the therapist tells a chronically depressed and passive wife that she should go in this way because otherwise she and her husband would argue all the time. The intervention was intended to stir the wife into greater activity and assertiveness, which in this case was achieved. The example shows the importance of understanding the personality of each partner before venturing a paradox, which could have an opposite and unfortunate effect in another case. For further information about behavioural-systems couple therapy, see Crowe and Ridley (1990).

Informal approaches

In practice, many couples are helped in more informal ways using the general principles outlined above and restricting interventions to those at the bottom of the hierarchy depicted in Figure 22.1.

Evaluation of couple therapy

The use of couple therapy has to be based mainly on clinical impressions since few clinical trials have been reported. A reviews by Baucom (1998) indicated that marital therapy is better than no treatment: behavioural and insight-orientated couple therapy had about equal effects; and the behavioural form of marital therapy was followed by improvement in up to two-thirds of reported cases. Leff *et al.* (2000) found that an ecletic form of couple therapy was as effective as antidepressant treatment for people with depression who were living with a partner who criticized them.

For a historical review of couple therapy see Gurman and Fraenkel (2002)

Family therapy

Several or sometimes all members of a family members take part in this treatment. Usually both parents are involved, often together with the child whose problems have led the family to seek help. They may be joined by other children, grandparents, or others members of the extended family. The aim of treatment is to improve family functioning, and so to help the identified patient. Since success depends on the collaboration of several people, drop-out rates are high. Whatever their method, family therapists have the following goals for the family:

- improved communication,
- improved autonomy for each member,
- improved agreement about roles,
- reduced conflict, and
- reduced distress in the member who is the patient.

Family therapy dates from the 1950s. It can be traced to two sources: an influential book by Ackerman (1958) called *The psychodynamics of family life*, and the work on communication by Bateson and his colleagues mentioned above. Ackerman's work led to psychodynamic methods of treatment, whilst Bateson's treatments led to the systems approach. The latter approach was developed further in the USA by Salvador Minuchin who advocated a practical approach to resolving problems in his structural family therapy; and in Italy by the Milan school who used hypotheses about the family system to suggest ways of promoting change. These approaches are described briefly below, together with an eclectic approach. The reader will find fuller accounts in the chapter by Bloch and Harari (2005) and the book edited by Gurman (2003).

Indications and contraindications for family therapy

Family therapy is used mainly in the treatment of problems presented by young people living with their parents. These problems are often related to difficulties in communication between members of the family, or to role problems. In the practice of adult psychiatry, family therapy is often combined with other treatment, for example, antidepressant medication for a depressive disorder, Family therapy is used in treating some young people with anorexia nervosa after weight has been restored by other means (see p. 364). Special kinds of family treatment have been developed to reduce relapses in schizophrenia (see p. 299).

Psychodynamic family therapy

This method is based on the idea that current problems in the family originate in the separate past experiences of its individual members, particularly those of the parents. Present problems arise in part from unconscious conflicts within individual members who need to gain insight into these conflicts if they are to change their behaviour. The therapist's task is to help members gain this insight and to understand how their own problems and those of other family members interact. The therapist does this by examining his own relationship with each of the family members. The therapist uses the non-directive method described under individual dynamic psychotherapy (p. 600).

A related approach has been developed by Skynner (1991) using **object relations theory** (see p. 581). Skynner emphasized ways in which the childhood experience of a parent affects the ways that they relate to their own children; for example, a mother who received no adequate mothering may develop a 'projective system', i.e. expectations shaped by her childhood experiences rather than current reality. Projective systems affect the parents' ways of relating to one another as well as to the children. Sometimes a conflict between the projective systems of the parents is resolved by diverting the projections onto the child. By identifying these systems, the therapist helps the family resolve their conflicts.

Structural family therapy

The term family structure refers to a set of unspoken rules that organize the ways in which family members relate to one another. Some rules determine the hierarchy in the family, for example, that parents have more authority and responsibility than children. Some rules determine cooperation in the family, for example, that father and mother share certain tasks and responsibilities, and take on others individually. In some families, both parents set rules for behaviour and admonish children when the rules are broken; in other families, the father is the strict parent. Rules also determine boundaries; sometimes these are broken, for example, when an unhappy wife involves her son in her problems with her husband. In structural family therapy, hypotheses about these rules are often presented to the family in a paradoxical way; for example, 'You seem to be very dependent on your wife; what does she do to make you feel less competent?' Such interventions, which increase family tension in the short term, are intended to bring about change.

Systemic family therapy

Systemic family therapy is concerned with the present functioning of the family, rather than with the past experiences of its members. The therapist's task is to identify the family's unspoken rules, their disagreements about who makes these rules, and their distorted ways of communicating. The therapist helps the family to understand and modify the rules, and to improve communication.

In the **Milan approach** (Palazzoli *et al.*, 1978) there are usually 5–10 sessions, spaced at intervals of a month or more ('long brief therapy'). **Circular questioning** is often used to assess the family. In this technique, one person is asked to comment on the relationships of others, for example, the mother may be asked how her husband relates to their son, and others are asked to comment on her response. The purpose is to discover and clarify confused or conflicting views. A hypothesis is then constructed about the family functioning. For example, the boundary between the parent and child subsystems may have been breached, in that one parent has an inappropriately strong alliance with one of the children. Such hypotheses are presented to the family, who are asked to consider them in and between sessions. The family may be asked to try to behave in new ways. Sometimes the therapist provokes change with paradoxical injunctions designed to provoke the family into making changes that they cannot make in other ways. For example, if the patient fears that the parents will separate, the injunction may be designed to make them prove the therapist wrong and so bring them closer.

Criticisms of the systems approach are that they ignore on the one hand the effects of past experience and unconscious motives, and on the other the effects of realistic problems such as unemployment and poverty. A review of ten outcome studies of Milan systemic family therapy (five of which included comparison groups) found it as effective as other kinds of family therapy. There was symptomatic improvement in about two-thirds of patients, and improved functioning in about half the families. Generally, these results were obtained in less than ten sessions (Carr, 1991).

Eclectic family therapy

In everyday clinical work, especially with adolescents, it is practicable to use a simple short-term method designed to bring about limited changes in the family. For this purpose, it is appropriate to concentrate on the present situation of the family and to examine how the members communicate with one another. The number of family members taking part is decided on practical grounds; for example, some children may be too young, whilst others may be away from home. The interval between sessions is varied to allow time for the family to work together on the problems raised in treatment.

Assessment

Assessment begins with the family structure which can be summarized as a genogram using conventional symbols (see Figure 22.2). Further questions concern the current and past state of family life, and the roles of the members. Several kinds of questioning may be used: circular questioning (see above); questions about the roles of the members (who takes care of others, who worries most, who decides, etc.); about triadic relationships (for example, what does A do when B criticizes C); and about responses to a previous change (for example, the death of a grandparent).

The therapist tries to answer two questions: how does the family function, and are family factors involved in the patient's problems? Bloch and Harari (2005) have proposed a useful framework in which to consider these questions.

1. How does the family function?
    - **structure** recorded in the genogram: for example, single parent, a step parent, size and age spread of the sibship;
    - **changes and events** such as births, deaths, departures, and financial problems;

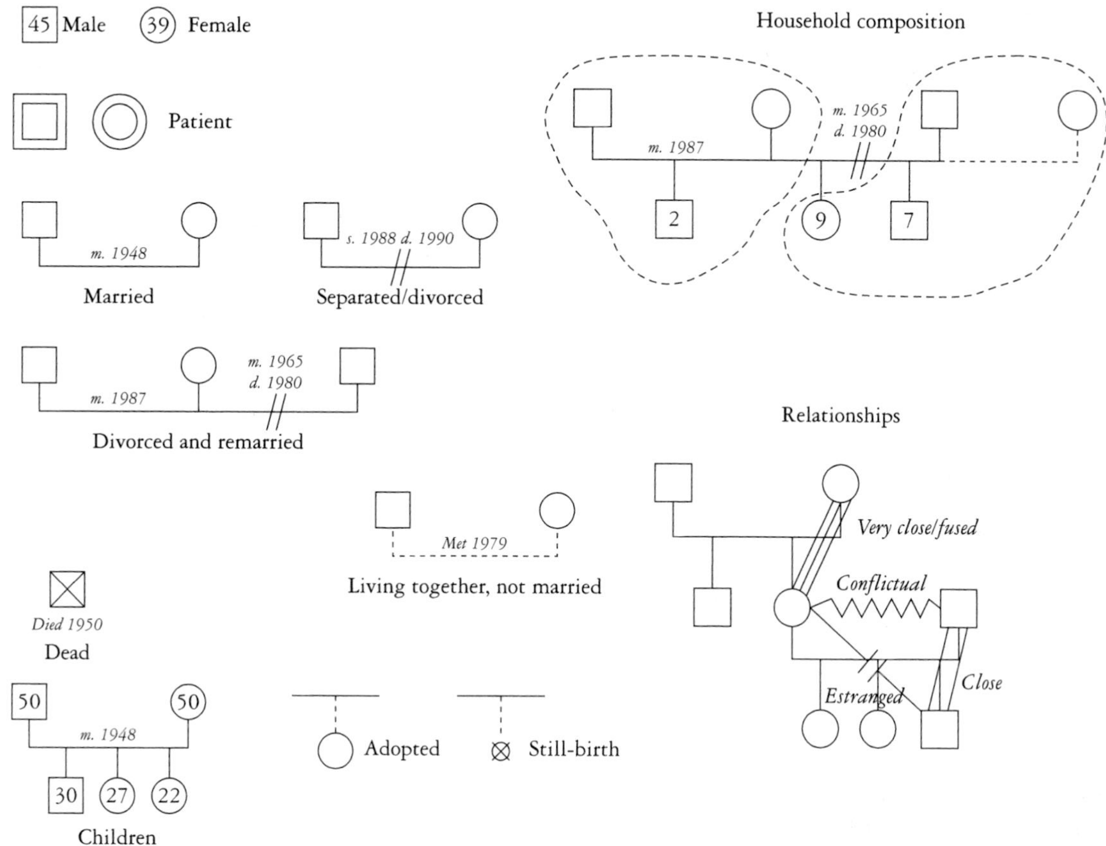

Fig. 22.2 Symbols used in the construction of a genogram. Reproduced with permission from Bloch and Harari (2000).

- **relationships** close, distant, loving, conflictual, etc;
- **patterns of interaction** involving two or more people, for example, a child who sides with one parent against the other.

2. Are family factors involved in the patient's problems? The family may be:

- **reacting** to the patient's problems – but there may be unrelated problems as well;
- **supporting** the patient;
- **contributing** to the patient's problems, for example, the problems of a daughter who cannot leave her lonely mother.

The answers to these questions lead to a hypothesis about what should and can change.

Intervention

Specific goals for change are agreed with the members of the family, who are asked to consider how any changes will affect themselves and others, and what has prevented the family from making the changes. Paradoxical injunctions may be included but should be made only after the most careful consideration of the range of possible responses. The therapist should remember that interchanges in the sessions are likely to continue when the family return home, and try to ensure that this does not lead to further problems.

Results of family therapy

In a meta-analysis of the results of 19 studies of family therapy, the effect was found to be comparable to that of other forms of psychotherapy. About 75 per cent of patients receiving family therapy had a better outcome than similar patients receiving minimal or no treatment (Markus *et al.*, 1990). For children and adolescents, family therapy appears to be an effective treatment for eating disorders, substance abuse, and conduct disorder, though the patients treated were not necessarily representative of the groups as a whole (see Cottrell and Boston, 2002).

For further information about family therapy in psychiatry see Bloch and Harari (2000).

Psychotherapy for children

The kinds of psychotherapy discussed so far do not lend themselves to the treatment of young children who lack the necessary verbal skills. In practice there are fewer difficulties than might be expected, because many emotional problems of younger children are secondary to those of their parents and it is often appropriate to direct psychotherapy mainly to the parents.

Some psychotherapists believe that it is possible to use the child's play as equivalent to the words of the adult in psychotherapy. Klein developed this approach extensively by making frequent analytical interpretations of the symbolic meaning of the child's actions during play, and by attempting to relate these actions to the child's feelings towards his parents. Although ingenious, this approach is highly speculative since there is almost no evidence against which the interpretations can be checked. Anna Freud developed child psychotherapy by a less extreme adaptation of her father's techniques to the needs of the child. She recognized the particular difficulty for child analysis of the child's inability or unwillingness to produce free associations in words. However, she considered that neither play with toys, nor drawing and painting, nor fantasy games could be an adequate substitute. Moreover, she cautioned against the use of uncontrolled play, which may lead to the acting out of aggressive urges in a destructive way. Anna Freud accepted that non-analytical techniques could be helpful for many disorders of development. These techniques include reassurance, suggestion, the giving of advice, and acting as role model (an 'auxiliary ego'). However, for neurotic disorders in childhood, and for the many mixed disorders, she advocated analytical techniques to identify the unconscious content of the disorder and to interpret it in a way that strengthens ego functions. A concise account of Anna Freud's views on child analysis is contained in Freud (1966, Chapters 2 and 6).

In the UK, most psychotherapy for children is eclectic; the therapist tries to establish a good relationship with the child and to learn about his feelings and thoughts, partly through talking and listening, and partly through play. Older children can communicate verbally with adults but younger children can communicate better through actions, including play. The therapist can help children to find words that express thoughts and feelings, and thus can make it easier for them to control and change these thoughts and feelings. However, it is important to ensure that the therapist's interpretations are reflecting the child's own thoughts and not implanting new ideas. Child psychotherapy is discussed further in Chapter 24 on child psychiatry (p. 662). For a more detailed account see Target *et al.* (2005).

Psychotherapy for older people

Increasing emphasis is being placed on the provision of psychological treatments as part of the care plan for elderly patients. Provided they do not have cognitive impairment, elderly patients can take part in any of the treatments descibed for younger adults. When using cognitive therapy, it is important to search for minor degrees of cognitive impairment insufficient to affect general functioning but enough to impair the patient's grasp and retention of the details of the therapy. For a review of psychotherapy for the elderly see Garner (2003) and for a fuller account see Cook *et al.* (2005).

Other psychological treatments

Treatments of mainly historical interest

Hypnosis

Hypnosis is a state in which the person is relaxed and drowsy, and more suggestible than usual. Enhanced suggestibility leads to diminished sensitivity to painful stimuli, vivid mental imagery, hallucinations, failures of memory, and 'age regression' (behaving as would a much younger person). Although enhanced suggestibility is characteristic of hypnosis, it is not confined to it. Some people respond in a similar way to suggestion when in a state of full alertness (Barber, 1962), and there seem to be no phenomena peculiar to the hypnotic state.

Hypnosis can be induced in many ways. The main requirements are that the subject should be willing to be hypnotized and convinced that hypnosis will occur. Most hypnotic procedures contain some combination of a task to focus attention (such as watching a moving object), rhythmic monotonous instructions, and the use of a graduated series of suggestions, for example, that the person's arm will rise. The therapist uses the suggestible state either to implant direct suggestions of improvement or to encourage recall of previously repressed memories.

Indications for hypnosis

Hypnosis is used infrequently in psychiatry. A light trance is used occasionally as a form of relaxation. For this purpose hypnosis has not been shown to be generally superior to relaxation. A deeper trance is used occasionally to enhance suggestion in order to relieve symptoms, especially those of conversion disorder. Although sometimes effective in the short term, this method has not been shown to be superior to suggestion without hypnosis. Also, the sudden removal of symptoms by suggestion under hypnosis can be followed by an increase of anxiety or depression. Hypnosis has been used to aid the recall of memories in psychotherapy, but there is no evidence that this procedure improves outcome. For these reasons the authors do not recommend the use of hypnosis in clinical psychiatry. Readers seeking more information about hypnosis are referred to Burrows *et al.* (2002).

Autogenic training

This technique was described by Schultz in 1905 and was in use mainly in continental Europe as a treatment for physical symptoms caused by emotional disorder (Schultz, 1932). Patients practise exercises in which they learn to induce feelings of heaviness, warmth, or cooling in various parts of the body, and to slow their respiration. Repeated use of these exercises is supposed to induce changes in autonomic nervous activity and thereby to benefit patients with physical symptoms arising in stress-related and anxiety disorders. It has not been established that autonomic changes after autogenic training differ substantially from those after simple relaxation, nor is there any good evidence that it has a specific therapeutic effect. Interested readers are referred to Schultz and Luthe (1959).

Abreaction

Abreaction (the unrestrained expression of emotion) has long been used to relieve mental distress and some psychiatric symptoms. Although is seldom used today, it is considered here because of its historical interest. Abreaction is part of many forms of religious healing (see below). It was used in psychiatry during the Second World War to bring rapid relief from acute war neuroses (probably acute stress disorders and the early stages of post traumatic stress disorder), notably by Sargant and Slater (1940). In civilian practice, abreaction is less effective, perhaps because fewer disorders are the result of overwhelming stress (those that are so caused – the post-traumatic stress disorders – are considered on p. 157). Abreaction can be brought about simply by strong encouragement to relive the traumatic events; but in wartime the procedure was sometimes facilitated by giving a small dose of sedative drug intravenously. For more information about the latter procedure see Sargant and Slater (1963).

Meditation and traditional healing

Meditation

Although not in regular use in psychiatry, meditation is increasingly used by people with minor psychiatric problems as an alternative to psychiatric treatment. There are many methods of meditation, each associated with a different system of belief, but sharing several features. The first is instruction in relaxation and the regulation of breathing. The second is a way of directing attention away from the external world and from the stream of thoughts that would otherwise occupy the mind. Often the person achieves this by repeating a word or phrase (a mantra). The third common feature is the setting aside, from the day's other activities, periods when calm can be restored. Finally, the person joins a group of people who are convinced that the methods work, and encourage each other to practise it. Such group pressure, which is often lacking from hospital-based programmes of relaxation, may explain some of the reported successes of the methods.

There is insufficient evidence to decide the value of meditation. Clinical experience indicates that many of the patients who find them helpful have problems related to a style of life that is too stressful and hurried. For a review of the various forms of meditation and their effects see West (1990).

Traditional healing

There are many kinds of traditional healer but they can be divided into four groups (Jilek 2000):

- **Herbalists** are concerned mainly with plant remedies, some of which are known to contain active ingredients while others appear to be placebos.
- **Medicine men** and women use verbal or ritual methods of healing, sometimes combined with plant remedies. They are believed to have special powers, often of supernatural origin.
- **Shamans** use methods like those of medicine men but also enter into altered states of consciousness in which they are believed to communicate with spirits or ancestors, and to recover the abducted souls of people made ill by this supposed loss.
- **Diviners** discover and name the cause of illness by interpreting oracles (in clear or in altered consciousness), from the content of dreams, or through some form of communication with ancestors or spirits.

All kinds of traditional healers use methods which are likely to activate the non-specific processes identified as common to many kinds of western psychological treatment (see Box 22.1). In addition, they are aware of the value of naming a condition and answering the questions – 'Why am I afflicted?' and 'Why is this member of our family afflicted?' – thus ending uncertainty and relieving blame and guilt. Some traditional healers use therapeutic suggestion, and many involve the family both in the diagnostic process and in the rituals of treatment. Some employ cleansing or purification rituals to eliminate supposed polluting agents. A few healers use sacrificial rites to appease supernatural beings, sometimes combining these with confession and a promise of changed behaviour. These rituals may be conducted in a group ceremonial involving the wider community as well as the patient and the family. These practices are likely to activate the common factors of group therapy, described in Box 22.7.

Many traditional healers distinguish between 'western' diseases that respond to specific medication, and others in which their procedures help the patient and support the family. There is some scientific evidence that traditional healing is effective for substance abusers (see Jilek, 2000) and much anecdotal evidence that it is helpful in minor mental disorders.

For more information about traditional healing and its relevance to psychiatry, see Jilek (2000).

Ethical problems in psychological treatment

Autonomy

The need for informed consent is as great in psychological treatment as in other treatment and to give such consent the patient must understand the nature of the treatment and its likely consequences. This requirement is easily met in cognitive-behaviour therapies which are clearly defined and have been subjected to clinical trial. The course of dynamic psychotherapy and group psychotherapy is less easy to specify at the start, but a broad description should be provided. Such preparation is not only ethically desirable but also likely to improve the therapeutic alliance. A further problem arises when one of the aims of a dynamic psychotherapy is to free the patient from psychological constraints and thereby increase autonomy. In such treatment, it is necessary to review the situation with the patient to ensure that he is fully aware of, and consents to, the new aims and consequences of treatment.

Confidentiality

Group psychotherapy presents special problems of confidentiality. Patients should understand fully the requirement to talk of personal matters in the group but they need to understand equally clearly the requirement to treat as confidential the revelations of other patients. Family therapy presents similar problems, especially if the therapist agrees to see one member outside the family session, and is told of a family secret (relating, for example, to an extramarital affair). When possible, the therapist should refuse to meet individual members in this way but arrange for a colleague to do so when such a meeting seems indicated (for example, if one member is seriously depressed). Similar problems arise in couple therapy.

The problem of when a therapist should reveal confidential material to a third party is the same as in other treatment situations, namely that it is justified when there is a substantial risk to a third party.

Exploitation

Patients receiving psychological treatment are vulnerable to exploitation, sometimes because of the experiences that caused them to seek psychotherapy, but also because of the relationship with the therapist. As in other branches of medicine, exploitation may be financial or sexual. Financial exploitation is a potential problem in private practice in which treatment may be prolonged for longer than is necessary to achieve the patient's goals. Occasionally the exploitation is sexual. In the medical and other caring professions, such exploitation is prohibited in professional codes of conduct; it is not a matter for utilitarian arguments.

Another form of exploitation is the imposition on the patient of the therapist's values. This may be open and direct, for example, when a therapist imposes his view that termination of pregnancy is morally wrong. Or it may be concealed and indirect, for example, when a therapist expresses no opinion but nevertheless gives more attention to the arguments against termination than to those for it. Similar problems may arise, for example, in couple therapy when the therapist's values may affect his approach to the question whether the couple should separate.

In group psychotherapy, one patient may be exploited by another. One patient may bully or scapegoat another within the sessions of treatment, or may seek a sexual relationship between the sessions. The therapist should protect vulnerable patients within the sessions, and make a rule that patients should not meet between the sessions. If they do meet, they should report this to the group at the next session and the matter should be discussed.

Further reading

Bloch, S (2005) *An introduction to the psychotherapies*, 4th edn. Oxford University Press, Oxford. (An introduction to the commonly used psychological treatments with a chapter on ethics.)

Bateman, A, Brown, D and Pedder, J (2000) *Introduction to psychotherapy: an outline of psycho-dynamic principles and practice,* 3rd edn. Tavistock/Routledge, London. (An account of dynamic theory, and practice in individual, couple, family and group formats.)

Frank, JD and Frank JB (1993) *Persuasion and healing*, 3rd edn. Johns Hopkins Press, Baltimore, MD. (A revised version of a landmark account of the non-specific factors in psychotherapy.)

Gabbard, G, Beck, JS and Holmes, J (2005) *Oxford textbook of psychotherapy*. Oxford, Oxford University Press. (A comprehensive set of reviews of the major forms of psychotherapy and their use in clinical practice.)

Gurman, AS (ed.) (2003) *Family therapy: theory practice and research*. Brunner-Routledge. (A comprehensive work of reference.)

Hawton, K, Salkovskis, PM, Kirk, JW and Clark, DM (2000) *Cognitive behavioural approaches for adult psychiatric disorders: a practical guide*, 2nd edn. Oxford University Press, Oxford. (An introduction with many valuable practical examples.)

CHAPTER 23

Psychiatric services

Chapter contents

The last two chapters dealt with the treatment of individual patients. This chapter is concerned with the provision of psychiatric care for populations. It deals mainly with the needs of and provisions for people aged 18–65.

Services for children are described on p. 661; services for the elderly are described on p. 500; and services for patients with learning difficulties are described on p. 722. The organization of psychiatric services in any country inevitably depends on the organization of general medical services in that country. This chapter will refer specifically to services in the UK, but the principles embodied in these services apply widely.

The chapter begins with an account of the historical development of psychiatric services. This is followed by descriptions of the commonly available psychiatric services and of the problems encountered with these provisions. The chapter ends with a consideration of some innovations designed to overcome these problems.

The history of psychiatric services

Until the middle of the eighteenth century, there were hardly any special provisions for the mentally ill in Europe. In England, for example, the only hospital for these patients was the Bethlem Hospital, founded in 1247. In most of continental Europe, there was a similar lack of hospital provision except in Spain where some hospitals were present from the Middle Ages (Chamberlain, 1966). This provision reflects the Islamic influence in Spain, for mental illness was viewed differently within Islam and Christianity. Both faiths regarded mental illness as the result of supernatural intervention: within Judeo-Christian teaching, it indicated demonic possession and/or the effects of sin; within Islamic teaching the intervention was not necessarily malign nor necessarily the result of wrongdoing. In keeping with this more positive approach, Islamic medicine was more concerned for mental disorder and the Arab physician Rhazes cared for mental patients in Baghdad in the tenth century.

In Britain until the middle of the eighteenth century, most mentally ill people lived in the community, often with help from Poor Law provisions, or were in prison. In England, the Vagrancy Act of 1744 made the first legal distinction between paupers and lunatics, and made provision for the treatment of the latter. In response, private provisions for the mentally ill ('madhouses' – later to be called private asylums) were developed mainly for those who could pay for care, but also for some paupers supported by their parishes (Parry-Jones, 1972). At about the same time, a few hospitals or wards were established through private benefaction and public subscription. The Bethel Hospital in Norwich was founded in 1713. In London, the lunatic ward at Guy's Hospital was established in 1728, and in 1751, St Luke's Hospital was founded as an alternative to the overcrowded Bethlem Hospital. Then, as now, the value of psychiatric wards in general hospitals was debated (Allderidge, 1979).

Moral management

At the end of the eighteenth century, public concern in many countries about the poor standards of private and public institutions led to renewed efforts to improve the care of the mentally ill. In Paris in 1793, Pinel gave an important lead by releasing patients from the chains that were used for restraint. Subsequently he introduced other changes to make the care of patients more humane. In England, similar reforming ideas were proposed by William Tuke, a Quaker philanthropist who founded the Retreat in York in 1792. The Retreat provided pleasant surroundings and adequate facilities for occupation and recreation. Treatment was based on 'moral' (i.e. psychological) management and respect for patients' wishes, in contrast with the physical treatments (usually bleeding and purging) and the authoritarian approach favoured by most doctors at that time. This enlightened form of care was described several years later by William Tuke's grandson, Samuel, in *A description of the Retreat*, published in 1813. These humane methods were adopted in other hospitals as it became clear that many mentally ill patients could exert self-control and did not require physical restraint and drastic medical treatment.

The asylum movement

Despite such pioneering efforts, in the early years of the nineteenth century many mentally ill people received no care and lived as vagrants or as inmates of workhouses and gaols. Also, there was public concern in England about the welfare of those in care, following reports of scandalously low standards in some private madhouses. This concern led to the County Asylum Act of 1808, which provided for the building of mental hospitals in each of the English counties. Unfortunately, little was done by the county authorities, and in 1845 it was necessary to enact the Lunatics Act, which required the building of an asylum in every county. At first the new asylums provided good treatment in spacious surroundings. Moral management was championed, especially by members of the Nonrestraint Movement, which had started with the work of Gardiner Hill at the Lincoln Asylum in 1837 and was developed further by John Conolly at the Middlesex County Asylum, Hanwell. In 1856, Conolly published a significant book, *The treatment of the insane without mechanical restraints*.

Unfortunately, these liberal steps were soon followed by a new restrictive approach. Increasing public intolerance led to the transfer of more and more patients from the community and prisons to the new asylums. Initial optimism about the curability of psychiatric disorder dissipated, as the limitations of moral treatment became apparent. More gloomy views about organic and hereditary causes prevailed. By the 1850s, the problems of overcrowded asylums were evident. Attempts were made to house patients with chronic illness in less restrictive and more domestic surroundings in detached annexes or houses in the grounds of the asylum. Other hospitals returned patients to the community either by boarding them out with a family (a form of care which was practised most successfully at Gheel in Belgium) or by returning them to workhouses. The Lunacy Commissioners, whose role was to oversee the care of the mentally ill, were concerned that these arrangements could lead to abuse, and were opposed to them. Nevertheless, nineteenth-century asylums, even when overcrowded, provided a standard of care for the mentally ill that was lacking elsewhere. Thus the mentally ill were protected from exploitation, and were provided with shelter, food, and general healthcare. These benefits were counterbalanced by the disadvantages of loss of personal choice and autonomy, and of a monotonous and overprotective regimen that could lead to institutionalism.

Under the increasing pressures of overcrowding and staff shortages, there was less and less time for moral management. Again, a custodial approach was adopted. This change to custodial care was endorsed by the Lunacy Act 1890, which imposed restrictions on discharge from hospital. These custodial arrangements continued into the twentieth century, and their legacy is still seen in the size and structure of the large Victorian hospitals in which most psychiatry was practised until recently. See Jones (1972) and Rothman (1971) for accounts of psychiatric hospitals in the UK and the USA in the nineteenth century.

Arrangements for early treatment

In the UK, the start of a return to more liberal policies was signalled shortly before the First World War, by a substantial gift of money by Henry Maudsley, a wealthy psychiatrist, to provide for a hospital devoted to early treatment. Unfortunately, the war interfered with the project, and the opening of the Maudsley Hospital was delayed until 1923. The hospital provided an outpatient service and voluntary inpatient treatment in surroundings in which teaching and research were carried out.

In the years between the wars, the impetus for change increased. The Mental Treatment Act 1930 repealed many of the restrictions on discharge of patients imposed by the Lunacy Act 1890, and allowed county asylums to accept patients for voluntary treatment. The 1930 Act also encouraged local authorities to set up outpatient clinics and to establish facilities for aftercare. Therapeutic optimism increased further as two new treatments were discovered: insulin coma (later abandoned) and electroconvulsive therapy. At the same time, efforts were made to improve conditions in hospitals, to unlock previously locked wards, and to encourage occupational activities. Similar changes took place in other countries.

In most countries, these reforms were halted by the Second World War. Psychiatric hospitals became understaffed as doctors and nurses were recruited to the war effort. They also became overcrowded as some were allocated to the care of the war injured, with the result that their patients had to be relocated among the rest. The effects of the war on an English county asylum have been described by Crammer (1990). In Germany, many psychiatric patients died in a eugenics programme - a shameful period in the history of a country that had been in the forefront of psychiatric progress in the nineteenth and early twentieth centuries. For an account of the Nazi eugenics programme, see Burleigh (2000).

Social psychiatry and the beginning of community care

After the Second World War, several influences led to further changes in psychiatric hospitals. Social attitudes had become more sympathetic towards disadvantaged people. Among psychiatrists, wartime experience of treating 'battle neuroses' had encouraged interest in the early treatment of mental disorder and in the use of group treatment and social rehabilitation. In the UK, the advent of the National Health Service led to a general reorganization of medical services including psychiatry. The introduction of chlorpromazine in 1952 made it easier to manage disturbed behaviour of patients with psychosis, and therefore easier to open wards that had been locked, to engage patients in social activities, and to discharge some of them into the community.

Despite these changes, services continued to be concentrated on a single site, often remote from centres of population. In the USA, Goffman (1961) argued that state hospitals were 'total institutions', i.e. segregated communities isolated from everyday life. He described such institutions as impersonal, inflexible, and authoritarian. In the UK, Wing and Brown (1970) found that some of the large mental hospitals were characterized by 'clinical poverty' and 'social poverty'. Vigorous methods of social rehabilitation were used to improve conditions in hospital and to reduce the effects of long years of institutional living. Occupational and industrial therapies were used to prepare chronically disabled patients for the move from hospital to sheltered accommodation or to ordinary housing (Bennett, 1983). Many long-stay patients were responsive to these vigorous new methods. There was optimism that newly admitted patients could also be helped in these ways.

For patients in the community, day hospitals were set up to provide continuing treatment and rehabilitation, and hostels were opened to provide sheltered accommodation. As a result of all these changes, the numbers of patients in psychiatric hospitals fell substantially in the UK and in other countries. The changes were particularly rapid in the USA. Despite these changes, services were still based in large mental hospitals that were often far from patients' homes. Unfortunately, in many places the provision of community facilities was insufficient for the needs of all newly discharged patients.

Hospital closure

After the initial success of discharging many institutionalized patients, it was optimistically proposed that large asylums could be closed and replaced by small psychiatric units in general hospitals, with support from community facilities. In most countries, the programme of hospital closure took place gradually. A notable exception was Italy, which at first lagged behind most other countries but later made rapid changes. In 1978, the Italian Parliament passed Law

180, which aimed to abolish the mental hospitals and replace them by a comprehensive system of community care. Admission to psychiatric hospitals was prohibited, and there were requirements that psychiatric units be set up in general hospitals and that community services be developed in defined areas. The scheme was based on the work of Franco Basaglia in hospitals in north-east Italy, and on the proposals of the professional and political movement he founded. This movement - Psichiatria Democratica - combined an extreme left-wing political view that patients in psychiatric hospitals were the victims of oppression by the capitalist system with the conviction that severe mental illness was induced by social conditions and not by biological causes. Basaglia's forceful personality and qualities of leadership helped him to succeed in finding new ways of caring for patients in the community. Other workers found it difficult to repeat his successes. At first the effects of this sudden change were varied. In those parts of Italy where the reforms were financed adequately and were implemented by enthusiastic staff, the new provisions were successful. In areas where the provision of new facilities was inadequate, there were problems (Bollini and Mollica, 1989). With more time, these initial difficulties were largely overcome and the state mental hospital system came to an end in 1989 (Burti, 2001).

In the UK and elsewhere, the pace of change was slower, but similar problems arose. Some patients could not manage in the community without intensive support, and even then required repeated readmission to hospital so that the arrangements became known as the 'revolving door policy'. The rehabilitation services had been expected to discharge patients in an improved state, but they found it necessary to provide continuing care for so many that it was difficult to take on new patients. Some discharged patients attended day hospitals for years without further improvement (Gath *et al.*, 1973). It became clear that earlier views of the benefits of 'de-institutionalization' had been over optimistic, and that services outside hospital were inadequate to provide the help needed by discharged patients and their families. Attempts were made to develop more adequate community facilities, a policy known as community care.

The rise of community care

As hospitals closed, psychiatric services had to perform three functions. The first was to treat, in the community, people with severe mental illness who would previously have remained in hospital for many years. The second was to assist primary care services with the detection, prevention, and early treatment of the less severe psychiatric disorders. The third was to treat severe acute psychiatric disorder as far as possible without lengthy admission to hospital and as near as possible to the person's home. These functions were to be carried out for a defined population. Services were to be comprehensive and deliver continuity of care, and be provided by multidisciplinary teams. These general principles were applied rather differently in the UK and in the USA.

In the UK, emphasis was placed initially on the providing for those who had benn discharged from long-term hospital care. In the USA, more emphasis was given to the prevention and early treatment of mental disorder as a way of avoiding admission to hospital. In the USA, the Joint Commission on Mental Illness and Health issued a report in 1961 recommending community treatment, delivered from community mental health centres (CMHCs) staffed from several disciplines. The centres offered psychological and social care and generally placed more emphasis on crisis intervention and treatment of acute psychiatric disorders than on the care of patients with chronic and severe mental illness. This emphasis led to dissatisfaction with the centres as people discharged from long-term hospital care found their way into private hospitals or prisons, or joined the homeless population of large cities (Goldman and Morrisey, 1985).

In the UK and elsewhere, some commonly agreed principles about community services developed from these early experiences:

- **Minimizing inpatient care** Hospital admissions were to be brief, and as far as possible to psychiatric units in general hospitals rather than to psychiatric hospitals. Whenever practicable, people were to be treated as outpatients or day patients.
- **Providing rehabilitation** originally with the hope that most people would progress to independent living, but subsequently with the more modest aim of preventing further deterioration.
- **Multidisciplinary teams** Care was to be provided by teams, usually of psychiatrists, community nurses, clinical psychologists, and social workers, working in collaboration with members of voluntary groups.
- **Legal reform** new laws were introduced to limit the uses of compulsory treatment and to encourage alternatives to inpatient care and to give greater emphasis to the rights of the individual.

As experience increased after the reforms had begun, additional features were introduced:

- **Care packages** based on an assessment of each person's needs.
- **Case management** by a named care worker who coordinated the work of others involved in care.
- **User involvement** Service users were increasingly involved in planning both their own treatment and the services for the population.
- **Outreach** to take services to vulnerable people who may otherwise find it difficult to engage with the care that is offered, and to arrange follow up.
- **Risk assessment** carried out regularly and leading if necessary to changes in the care plan.

These developments led to the current pattern of services which is described below.

TABLE 23.1 Approximate one-year prevalence of psychiatric disorder in the community

	US survey* (%)	UK survey† (%)
All disorders	20.0	–
Non-specific neurotic disorder	–	7.7 to 12.4
Anxiety disorders	13.5	4.7
Substance misuse	8.8	6.9
Affective disorders	4.3	2.1
Obsessive–compulsive disorders	1.7	1.2
Schizophrenia	1.0	0.4‡
Somatization	0.1	–

* Data based on Robins and Regier (1991). All rates are for one-year prevalence.

† Data from Jenkins *et al.* (1997). Rates are for one-week prevalence except for functional psychosis for which one-year prevalence is shown.

‡ Functional psychosis'.

– Indicates not assessed.

Rates of psychiatric disorder in the community

To determine what psychiatric services are required for a community, it is necessary to know the frequency of mental disorder in the population and the needs for treatment of the people with the disorders identified in this way. Policy decisions have then to be made about the division of care between primary and specialist medical services, between medical and social services, and between people with different kinds of mental disorder. In recent years within the NHS the tendency has been to concentrate resources on people who are severely mentally ill, whilst to treating as many as possible of the less severely ill in primary care.

It is difficult to determine the exact frequency of mental disorders in a community (for methods of epidemiological research, see p. 92), but approximate estimates are usually sufficient for service planning. Table 23.1 shows two sets of figures, one from a large population survey in the USA, the other from a household survey in Great Britain. The higher figure for anxiety disorders in the US survey is balanced by the figure for non-specific neurotic disorder in the UK survey. The other differences may relate to variations in the methods used in the two surveys rather than any major differences in the true population rates.

These and other surveys indicate that psychiatric disorders are common with about one in five experiencing one of these disorders in the course of one year. However, many of the conditions are brief anxiety and depressive disorders arising in reaction to stressful circumstances. Anxiety disorders are most frequent, followed by misuse of drugs or alcohol. Mood disorders come next in frequency. Obsessional disorders and schizophrenia are much less frequent.

Rates of psychiatric disorder among primary care attenders

How many affected persons seek help?

Table 23.2 shows that among the adult population of the UK, between 260 and 315 per thousand persons are found, in community surveys, to have a psychiatric disorder. Not all these people seek medical advice. Some cope on their own, others are supported by family, friends, clergy, or non-medical counsellors. People with substance misuse are particularly likely to consider that they do not need medical help.

Table 23.2 also shows that, in the UK where primary care services are well developed, about nine in ten people with a psychiatric disorder attend a general practitioner. The factors which determine whether a person seeks medical help for a psychiatric disorder include:

- the **severity and duration** of the disorder;
- the person's **attitude to psychiatric disorder**; some people feel ashamed and embarrassed to ask for help;

TABLE 23.2 Pathways to care with rates of psychiatric disorder among adults at each level of care*

	Cases per 1000 per annum
In the community	260–315
Attending primary care	230
Detected in primary care†	102
Attending psychiatric services	24
Inpatient	6

* Modified from Goldberg and Huxley (1992).

† Conspicuous psychiatric morbidity' (see opposite).

- **knowledge about possible help**; if people do not know what help can be provided, they are less likely to seek help;
- the person's **perception of the doctor's attitude** to psychiatric disorder; if the doctor is viewed as unsympathetic, the person is less likely to ask for help;
- the **attitudes and knowledge of family and friends**; if these people are unsympathetic, the affected person may be less likely to seek help.

How many affected persons attend primary care?

Table 23.2 shows that about 230 per thousand of the adult population attend primary care each year with a psychiatric disorder. Put in another way, Shepherd *et al.* (1966) in a seminal paper, estimated that in one year about 10 per cent of adults registered with a general practitioner consult for a condition that is wholly psychiatric, and 5 per cent consult with a disorder with a both psychiatric and physical components. More recently, Üstün and Sartorius (1995) estimated that about a quarter of attenders in primary care have at least one psychiatric disorder diagnosed by ICD-10 criteria, most being anxiety and depressive disorders.

Strathdee and Jenkins (1996) looked more closely at the frequency of various disorders in primary care and estimated that, for a practitioner with a list of 2000, there would be among the adult attenders:

- 60–100 with depression;
- 70–80 with anxiety;
- 50–60 with situational reactions;
- 2–4 with schizophrenia;
- 6–7 with affective psychosis;
- 4–5 with alcohol or drug dependence

- Similar findings have been reported for children. Among those aged 7–12 years attending primary care, almost a quarter had psychiatric disorder, divided about equally into emotional, conduct, and mixed conduct and emotional disorders (Garralda and Bailey, 1986). Among adolescents attending general practice, about a third have a psychiatric disorder (Garralda, 1994). As with adults, many of the children and adolescents with psychiatric disorder complain of physical symptoms, and in some of these cases the psychiatric disorder is not detected.

How long do the disorders last?

Many disorders seen in primary care are short lived reponses to temporary stressors but Goldberg *et al.* (2000) estimated that about 20 per cent of psychiatric disorders in general practice run a protracted course.

Hidden and conspicuous morbidity

Table 23.2 shows that rather less than half of the disorders present among attenders are likely to be detected. This is because patients do not always reveal the psychiatric symptoms because they are ashamed, or uncertain whether the doctor will be sympathetic, or reveal only physical symptoms of th mental disorder. Factors that affect the doctor's success in detecting these hidden disorders are discussed below (p. 629).

Assessing need

Need, demand, supply, and utilization

In the simplest terms, need is what people benefit from; demand is what people ask for; supply is what is provided; and utilization is what is used (Thornicroft and Tansella, 2000). Some of these simple definitions have to be expanded.

Need Breakey (2000) has suggested two definitions of need:

1. **For individuals** the services which professionals, service users and relatives believe ought to be provided over a relevant time period in order that the patient remains as healthy as is permitted by current knowledge;
2. **For populations** the services that a consensus of professionals, users, and the informed public believe to be required by a population over a relevant time period for its members to remain or become as healthy as permitted by current knowledge, and measured by objective epidemiological outcomes.

Psychiatrists, other health professionals, service users, and relatives may have different opinions about the benefits of various measures and the priority to be assigned to each (see for example Slade *et al.*, 1998). Service users commonly say that their most important aims are financial security, friendships, satisfying work, a sexual partner, and freedom from the side-effects of medication. Psychiatrists on the other hand might give more priority to symptom relief and the reduction of risk.

Unmet need In considering individuals, psychiatrists use this term to denote problems for which a sevice user has not received an adequate trial of a potentially effective intervention (see Marshall, 1994).

Demand is affected by the extent to which people know what services could be provided and by their assessment of the relevance and efficacy of those services. Some service users may wish to receive alternative medicine remedies, while professionals favour evidence-based conventional methods. Following media reports of rare cases of extremely violent behaviour the public may demand that priority is given to secure services.

Utilization: while need is unrelated to cost, utilization is affected by it. Where patients incur no direct cost (as in the National Health Service), utilization is affected by indirect costs such as the requirement to take time from work or pay for childcare while receiving the service. Utilization depends also on the accessibility and acceptability of services provided.

The assessment of the needs of individuals

Clinical assessment

Every psychiatric evaluation includes an assessment of the needs for treatment, often expressed as a care plan. Primm (1996) has suggested a useful mnemonic for the areas of need (see Table 23.3).

Standardized assessment

The following are examples of methods for assessing need. They are used principally for research: for ordinary clinical purposes, the use of standardized methods does not make care planning more effective (Marshall *et al.*, 2005a; Ashaye *et al.* 2003).

- **The Camberwell Assessment of Need**, which is directed especially to the needs of the seriously mentally ill (Phelan *et al.*, 1995). Twenty-two domains of need are assessed including accommodation, self-care, psychotic symptoms, physical health, safety, substance use, childcare, and finances.
- **The Cardinal Needs Assessment** (Marshall *et al.*, 1995), which assesses unmet need (see above).
- **The Needs for Care Assessment**, which was developed principally for research (Brewin *et al.*, 1987).
- **Level of care** An alternative approach is to assign patients to a level of care. Wing (1994) suggested six levels: the lowest for those who need no professional help; the second for those who can be treated (Marshall *et al.*, 2005). In primary care; the remaining levels for those who need specialist care, ranging from outpatient care (level 3) to long-term care, whether in the community or in hospital (level 6).

TABLE 23.3 SHARES: a mnemonic for the areas of need of disabled mentally ill patients

Symptoms
Housing – provision and supervision
Activities of daily living – includes nutrition, self-care and leisure
Recreation, training, and occupation
Employment
Significant others

Adapted from Primm (1996).

Assessment of the needs of a population

First, the number of people with each of the various psychiatric disorders is determined by extrapolating from epidemiological studies of similar populations, correcting for any special characteristics of the local population such as a greater number of elderly people or of people from ethnic minorities. Estimates of the needs for services for people in each diagnostic group are then applied to these population estimates. In practice, it is seldom possible to provide for all these needs and priorities have to be set; in the UK, people with serious mental illness have high priority.

Planning a psychiatric service

Locality planning

In most counties, the planning of psychiatric services is centred on a geographical area, often called a **sector or a catchment area**. In Europe, sectors vary in size considerably from about 15 000–50 000 in Sweden to 250 000 in Germany (see Thornicroft and Tansella, 2000).

Locality planning has **advantages** since it:

- allows for local variations in the make-up of the population, for example, an unusually large proportion of elderly people;
- integrates otherwise separate parts of the psychiatric services, for example, services for adolescents and adults;

- integrates psychiatric and medical services, for example, services for child psychiatry and paediatrics;
- integrates medical, social and voluntary services.

Locality planning also has some **disadvantages**:

- it may not be cost-effective to provide services for conditions which require specialist care but are of low prevalence, for example, patients needing medium or high security;
- the quality of services may differ between sectors though this can be reduced by setting of national minimal standards;
- health service and social service sectors may not be co-terminous, though this can be reduced by collaboration between the service providers.

The planning process

There is no universally accepted method of planning psychiatric services. Approaches differ between countries, and within countries they are frequently revised as professional and political ideas change. It is, nevertheless, possible to outline several parameters that influence planning. In this section, we describe these parameters and show how they have influenced the planning in the National Health Service in England. We use this example of a planning strategy to illustrate how principles can be translated into practice, and do not suggest that it is better than others.

Sources of finance A psychiatric service, may be funded through: direct charging, medical insurance, taxation, charitable donations or a combination of these sources. Insurance-based and self-payment services tend to be more flexible and efficient for those who use them, but risk neglecting those who are least able to pay. Services funded directly by the state are generally more equitable, but risk being underfunded, bureaucratic, and unresponsive to the needs of the users. The English NHS which is funded through taxation, has attempted to increase responsiveness and efficiency by creating a pseudo-market in which state funding is given to local Primary Care Trusts who buy (commission) care from Trusts providing secondary care.

Central control versus local autonomy. A nation's psychiatric services should be of uniform quality across the country and yet responsive to local need. The English NHS has attempted to achieve this difficult balance by delegating to local Primary Care Trusts (PCTs) the detailed purchasing of services for the local population, whilst specifying what kind of services these Trusts must buy. This specification is contained in a National Service Framework for Mental Health and in the NHS Plan, and set out in more detail in Policy Implementation Guides. Targets have been derived from these policy documents, and these targets have to be achieved by every PCT in England within a certain time. Examples of these targets include the setting up of assertive outreach teams, crisis teams, and early intervention services. The progress of PCTs and provider Trusts towards meeting these targets is monitored by Strategic Health Authorities and is reflected in a national system of hospital 'star ratings' which are made available to the public.

In addition to these targets for services, the National Institute of Clinical Excellence (NICE) has produced evidence-based guidelines for specific treatments that should be provided. These guidelines specify the treatment that people with different disorders can expect from the NHS (for example guidelines on the treatment of schizophrenia). Each provider Trust is expected to implement these guidelines, and audit progress in doing so, and their success is subject to evaluation by the national Health Care Commission.

Adapting services to local conditions. Local factors must always be taken into account when planning psychiatric services. Of particular importance are:

- **degree of urbanization** (which determines, amongst other things, the rates of psychosis),
- **ethnic make-up** of the population,
- **its dispersal** (for example over a large rural area),
- **age** structure,
- level of **deprivation**,
- **availability** of facilities and staff.

Integrating psychiatric, social and voluntary care. People with mental illness require a broad range of services and to provide them often requires the involvement of more than one agency. For example, a person with schizophrenia may receive medication from a psychiatrist, day care from social services, and accommodation from a voluntary organisation. Effective care planning requires collaboration between these and other organizations. The English NHS attempts to achieve this through Local Implementation Teams (or LITs) made up of representatives of primary care trusts, psychiatric providers, social services, voluntary organizations, service users and carers. LITs are charged with assisting Primary Care Trusts in the implementation of national targets, as set out in the National Service Framework.

Within the NHS there is a growing tendency to integrate the work of medical and social services in providing care for people with mental illness. For example, community mental health teams, which include social workers, are required to have an integrated management structure, and social services departments increasingly delegate the management of mental health social workers to the NHS, while they amalgamate their commissioning with that of Primary Care Trusts. In some places, certain services are commissioned jointly by NHS and voluntary providers, an arrangement that can be particularly successful in meeting the needs of marginalized groups such as refugees or the homeless.

Agreeing boundaries between primary and secondary care Since up to one in four consultations with a general practitioner concerns psychiatric illness (see above) the potential demand for specialist psychiatric care is very great. It is important therefore to agree the division of responsibilities between primary and specialist providers, otherwise the number of referrals to secondary care could exceed the capacity available. This division of responsibilities should be flexible, otherwise some people could be denied the specialist care they need, and others who are ready to leave hospital may not receive the aftercare that they require. The English NHS has addressed this problem in several ways. First, by encouraging investment in Primary Care Mental Health Workers to increase the capacity of primary care to treat milder psychiatric illness. Second, by encouraging a single channel of access to specialist care, with agreed referral protocols which are monitored and enforced. Third, through experiments in integrating psychiatric services entirely into Primary Care Trusts.

Specialist versus generic services A choice has to be made between generic community mental health teams and specialized teams such assertive outreach teams for people with severe mental illness, or early intervention teams for people with first episode psychosis. Within the English NHS the current trend is towards specialized teams with a mandate that all service users who require them will have access to an Assertive Outreach Team, a Crisis/Home Treatment Team, and an Early Intervention Service. There are also some moves towards specialized services for women and for people with personality disorders.

Boundaries between psychiatric subspecialities. It is difficult to specify precisely the point of transition between the various psychiatric subspecialities. The transitions between child and adolescent psychiatric services and general adult services, and between general adult services and services for the elderly are especially difficult to define. A cut-off point by age is clear but is not necessarily good for service users – for example, an older person with schizophrenia is not well served if she loses access to her well known psychiatrist, key worker and day care on her sixty-fifth birthday. On the other hand, more flexible arrangements tend to lack the clarity that is needed to avoid boundary disputes. The English NHS has incorporated the need for agreed transitional protocols into its national targets for Primary Care Trusts and Psychiatric Trusts.

Involvement of service users and carers When users of services and carers are involved in planning, the quality of the services usually improves and people have more confidence in them. Service users and carers can contribute usefully to local, regional and national planning. To achieve this level of engagement of users and carers requires a determined and sustained effort from professionals. In recent years the English NHS has achieved a high degree of service user and carer involvement, for example, service users and carers have been involved in drafting the guidelines for the National Institute for Clinical Excellence. All NHS Psychiatric Trusts have service user and carer committees and some have service user or carer representatives at board level.

Recognizing the needs of women Psychiatric services should take account of the needs of women such as: childcare; the choice of seeing a woman health worker; and areas for women only within inpatient units (including secure units), day-patient services, and residential accommodation. There should be provisions for women with perinatal psychiatric disorders, and attention to the needs of women within services such as those for eating disorders, substance misuse, personality disorder, and self-harm. Women from black and ethnic minority groups have special needs, as do women who have suffered violence or abuse. Women often report dissatisfaction with the available services and may not benefit from them (J. Williams *et al.*, 2001). Therefore women should be involved in service planning. The NHS Plan and the Mental Health National Service Framework both draw attention to the needs of women.

Quality control and performance improvement The planning of services needs to ensure that their performance can be monitored and improved continuously. This aim can be achieved with a variety of internal and external controls. Within the English NHS the key internal control is **clinical governance** which is essen-

BOX 23.1 NINE PRINCIPLES OF SERVICE PLANNING: THE THREE ACES*

1. *Autonomy* patients should be able to make choices
2. *Continuty:* over time and between different parts of the service
3. *Effectiveness* evidence that the intended benefits are achieved
4. *Accessibility* care should be provided where and when it is needed
5. *Comprehensiveness* in relation to the various needs and users
6. *Equity* the distribution of resources, and the way this is decided should be fair and explicit
7. *Accountability* to the users and funders of the Service
8. *Coordination* within the mental health service, and between it and other services
9. *Efficiency* the maximum reduction of need from the available resources

Adapted from Thornicroft and Tansella (2000)

tially a continuous process of improving quality and controlling risk. Key elements of clinical governance include: evidence-based practice, access to knowledge and clinical information, research and development, and assessment of clinical quality and effectiveness (including audit and checks on adherence to guidelines). The NHS also has several external control mechanisms, including inspections by the Health Care Commission, monitoring of attainment of national targets, external audit and external inquiries into untoward events. A delicate balance needs to be struck between the need to demonstrate good performance and the dangers of over-regulation.

Thornicroft and Tansella (2000) described a slightly different way of considering the principle underlying service planning and developed a useful nemonic (see Box 23.1).

The components of a mental health service

If they are to meet the needs of people with mental illness, mental health services need many components.

1. **Primary mental healthcare teams** supporting primary care, carrying out initial assessments;
2. **Outpatient care;**
3. **Specialist psychological treatments** often integrated into the specialist or primary mental healthcare teams;
4. **Crisis/home-based treatment teams** treating acute mental disorder at home;
5. **A&E liaison services** – often part of the crisis service – assessing and treating people who present to A&E departments;
6. **General hospital liaison services** for medically ill people who have mental health problems;
7. **Assertive community treatment teams** for severely mentally ill people who are difficult to engage or high users of services;
8. **Early Intervention Services** for people in their first episode of psychosis and the 3 years thereafter;
9. **Employment services**, including supported employment which helps people find paid employment and supports them in it through job coaching, services that link to training and education;
10. **Vocational rehabilitation** which includes sheltered workshops, transitional employment and the Clubhouse model;
11. **Day hospitals, day care services** including drop-in centres;
12. **Self-help and service user groups and advocacy services;**
13. **Inpatient services**;
14. **Forensic services** with accomodation for high, medium and low levels of security, and court-diversion schemes;
15. **Other residential services** including short-term accommodation outside hospital for acutely ill people or those in other forms of crisis;
16. **Services for special groups** such as people with eating disorders and Mother and Baby Units;
17. **Social and welfare services:** help with obtaining benefits, advocacy, community support workers, home help/meals;
18. **Services for special groups** outreach services to marginalized groups, such as the homeless and refugees.

Services for psychiatric disorder in primary care

Classification of psychiatric disorders in primary care

ICD-10 and DSM-IV were developed for use in psychiatry. They are too detailed for routine use in primary care, and their fine distinctions are seldom helpful in selecting treatment in this setting. The World Health Organization has therefore developed a simpler classification for use in primary care. Each diagnosis is linked to a plan of management.

Identification of psychiatric disorders in primary care

The first stage of providing services for psychiatric disorders in primary care is to detect them. This is not a simple matter because, as explained above, some people with a psychiatric disorder do not present with psychiatric symptoms but complain instead of physical symptoms. The latter may be those of a coincidental minor physical illness or part of the symptoms of the psychiatric disorder, for example, palpitations in an anxiety disorder or tiredness in a depressive disorder. Some patients are aware that they have an emotional problem but describe physical rather than psychiatric symptoms because they fear that the doctor may not respond sympathetically to psychiatric illness. Other patients are unaware that their physical symptoms have a psychological origin. The term **conspicuous morbidity** refers to the cases that are detected, **hidden morbidity** refers to the rest. Hidden morbidity is generally less severe than conspicuous morbidity.

As explained above, how effectively general practitioners identify undeclared psychiatric disorder depends on:

- their ability to gain the patients' confidence, thus enabling them to disclose the psychiatric problems of which they are aware;
- skill in assessing whether physical symptoms are caused by physical or psychiatric illness. This requires a good knowledge of physical medicine as well as psychiatry.

Disorders treated in primary care

Most psychiatric disorders in primary care attenders can be treated successfully by the general practitioner or another member of the practice team. Examples are most adjustment disorders, the less severe anxiety and depressive disorders, somatization (see below), and some cases of alcohol misuse. The following additional points should be noted; for a fuller account see (Goldberg *et al.*, 2000).

Patients presenting physical symptoms In primary care, many patients with psychiatric disorder present with physical symptoms. Such patients are often called **somatizers**. Many of these patients will reveal associated psychiatric symptoms and accept a psychiatric diagnosis when interviewed appropriately – **facultative somatizers**. Others deny psychiatric symptoms and reject a psychiatric diagnosis, however skilfully they are examined – **pure somatizers**.

Distressed high users attend frequently with a variety of complaints. Most are female and middle-aged. About 80 per cent have a present or past psychiatric disorder, usually depression, somatization, or generalized anxiety; and about 60 per cent have a concurrent physical illness (Katon *et al.*, 1990). Since most refuse to be referred to a psychiatric team, the general practitioner has to manage them. One approach is help patients to make links between physical symptoms and stressful life events, leaving out reference to any intervening psychological processes; and to discuss how life stresses might be reduced.

Disorders referred from primary care to the psychiatric services

Table 23.2 shows that on average about one in four of the patients with psychiatric disorder, identified by general practitioners, is treated by the psychiatric services. This referred group includes patients with severe depressive disorders, bipolar disorders, schizophrenia, and dementia. General practitioners are more likely to refer patients with other disorders when:

- the diagnosis is uncertain;
- the condition is severe;
- there is a significant suicide risk,
- the condition is chronic;
- necessary treatment cannot be provided by a member of the primary care team;
- previous treatment in primary care has been unsuccessful;
- psychiatric services are accessible and responsive;
- the patient is willing to attend.

Treatments provided by the primary care team

For acute disorders

Acute problems are generally treated with counselling, used alone or combined with medication. Some practices also provide simple behavioural treatments. Since general practitioners seldom have time to provide counselling for all those who would benefit from it, the primary care team often includes a counsellor. With additional training, practice nurses can take on this role effectively (Wilkinson *et al.*, 1993). The availability of a counsellor has not been shown to reduce the prescribing of psychotropic drugs in the practice (Mynors-Wallis *et al.*, 1995; Sibbald *et al.*, 1996b); however, medication and counselling often have complementary roles.

For chronic disorders

The respective roles of the general practitioner and the community team should be defined clearly in relation to any patient with chronic mental disorder, and reviewed regularly. For example, in the care of some patients with chronic schizophrenia, the general practitioner might care for physical health, assess general progress, administer and encourage compliance with medication, and support the family. Kendrick *et al.* (1995) found that even with additional training, general practitioners are not very effective in making structured assessments of patients with long-term psychiatric illness. It is generally better that the psychiatric team assess those patients, and agree a plan with the general practitioner. This plan will include elements provided by the psychiatric team, and elements provided by the primary care team, as in the example above.

Work in primary care by the psychiatric team

There are four ways in which a psychiatric team can work with the primary care team.

Advise and train general practitioners and their staff

In this style of working, the psychiatrist and other members of the team do not see patients but give advice based on the general practitioner's assessment of patients. The psychiatrist may also hold seminars or case discussions with the primary care staff. This arrangement increases the skills of the members of the primary care team, thus making them more effective in treating similar patients in future. The psychiatric nurse may work similarly with the practice nurses who can play an important part in treating psychiatric disorder.

Assess and refer

The psychiatrist assesses patients when the general practitioner is uncertain about diagnosis or treatment. He may do this on his own or jointly with the general practitioner. Patients identified as needing specialist treatment are then referred to a psychiatric outpatient clinic in the usual way.

Assess and treat

The psychiatrist works mainly in primary care, seeing most patients at the primary care centre or at home, rather than in the hospital outpatient clinic. Clinical psychologists and psychiatric nurses also work in primary care, providing assessment, counselling, or behavioural treatment. Patients no longer need to visit a psychiatric clinic, but there may be little contact between the psychiatric and primary care teams.

Share care

This approach fits with the care plan approach used for patients with severe mental illness, but it is not restricted to this group of patients. The general practitioner and the leader of the psychiatric team agree how each team will contribute to an overall plan of management, and a key worker is appointed.

The most appropriate of these ararrangements depends on the resources of the general practitioners, the accessibility of hospital outpatient clinics (generally greater in urban than in rural areas), and the number of primary care centres in which the psychiatrist works (the more centres, the less time for work in each).

Agreeing priorities in primary care

There is debate whether members of the community psychiatry team should accept referrals direct from the general practitioner, or whether referrals should be screened and prioritized by the leader of the psychiatric team leader in order to maintain the team's focus on patients with serious mental disorder. Without screening, community psychiatric nurses may take on large numbers of patients with minor disorders (Warner *et al.*, 1993) for whom their work may not be cost-effective (Gournay and Brooking, 1994). To avoid conflict, priorities and referral procedures should be agreed at the start of the collaboration between the primary care providers and the community psychiatric team.

Specialist services for acute psychiatric disorder

The patients referred to specialist care

Patients treated by the psychiatric services are a subgroup of people with mental disorder. In some countries patients can go directly to a specialist so that patients treated by the psychiatric services may not be very different from those treated in primary care. In countries such as the UK where the general practitioner acts as the 'gatekeeper' to specialist services, the number and types of patient reaching the psychiatric services depend on:

- the willingness of general practitioners to treat psychiatric disorder;
- the treatment skills and resources of the primary care team;
- patients' willingness to attend for specialist psychiatric advice;
- the general practitioner's criteria for referral to the psychiatric services;
- the psychiatric services' criteria for accepting referrals.

Studies of the behavioural training of parents have now firmly established the effectiveness of this approach in improving parenting skills and parent-child relationships, and reducing antisocial behaviour in children. Research is now focusing on which families can benefit, and long-term effects (for example Scott *et al.*, 2001). For a review of parent training programmes, see Scott (2002).

Family therapy

This is a specific form of treatment to be distinguished from the general family approach to treatment, described above. In family therapy, the symptoms of the child or adolescent are considered as an expression of malfunctioning of the family, which is the primary focus of treatment. Several approaches have been used based on behavioural or psychoanalytical, interpersonal or structural theories. These kinds of therapy are described on pp. 611–14. In practice, most therapists adopt an eclectic approach (see p. 612).

The **indications** for family therapy are still debated, but there is general agreement that it can be used appropriately when:

- the child's symptoms are judged to be part of a disturbance of the whole family;
- individual therapy is not proving effective;
- family difficulties have arisen during another kind of treatment.

The **contraindications** for family therapy are that the parents' marriage is breaking up, or the child's problems do not seem to be closely related to family function. It is important that a therapist's interest in family therapy should not prevent a thorough evaluation of the case and the use of other treatments when indicated.

Uncontrolled **evaluations** of family therapy have led to claims that it has substantial effects. Controlled evaluations suggest more modest benefits for children with a wide range of emotional and behavioural disorders. For example, in a study of children with emotional and behavioural disorders, the benefits of Milan Family Therapy were no greater than those of eclectic treatment (Simpson, 1990). The main exception is in the treatment of anorexia nervosa in adolescents for which dynamic family therapy has effects greater than those of a control treatment (Russell *et al.*, 1987; Robin *et al.*, 1999).

For further information on family therapy, and its evaluation, see Jacobs and Pearse (2002).

Group therapy

Group therapy may be carried out with parents, or with older children and adolescents. Parents may be helped by the opportunity to discuss shared problems of child management or other difficulties. Children may benefit from the support, discussion, and opportunities for modelling adaptive behaviour that form part of group therapy. Group therapy is described on pp. 603–606. The general effectiveness of group therapy for children and adolescents is reviewed by Jacobs (2002).

Social work

Social workers play an important role in the care of children with psychiatric disorders and of their families. In the UK, they have statutory duties for the protection of children who are at risk within the family, and who require special care or special supervision. They help parents to improve their skills in caring for their children and to solve problems with finances or accommodation. Social workers carry out family assessments and family therapy, and may also provide individual counselling for the child and members of the family.

Occupational therapy

Occupational therapists can play a valuable part in assessment of the child's development, in psychological treatment, and in devising measures to improve parent-child interaction. They work both in day- and inpatient units, and in the community. They work closely with teachers both in assessing and providing therapeutic activities for children.

Special education

Children attending at outpatient clinics, and the smaller number who are day- or inpatients, often benefit from additional educational arrangements. Special teaching may be needed to restore confidence, and remedy backwardness in writing, reading, and arithmetic, which is common among children with conduct disorders as well as those with specific developmental disorders. For further information about special education see Howlin (2002).

Substitute care

Residential care

Residential care can be valuable for children with symptoms that result from or are maintained by a severely unstable home environment or extreme parental rejection. Children considered for residential placement often have conduct disorders and severe educational problems. Removal of a child from home should be considered only after every practical effort has been made to improve the circumstances of the family. Residential care may be provided in a foster home, a children's home (in which a group of about 10 children live in circumstances as close as possible to those of a large family), or a residential school.

Residential care, other than fostering, is seldom arranged for children under 5 years of age because they have a special need for attachment to parental figures. In general, children who have been in residential care have high rates of psychosocial problems in later childhood and in adult life. As men they most often have problems with the law, whilst as women they most often have unmarried pregnancy and parenting problems. It is not clear how far these problems relate to the experience of residential care or to previous adverse experiences that led to the residential placement. Reports of the abuse of children placed within care are reminders of the need to ensure good training and supervision of the staff of children's homes and residential schools.

For a review of residential care see Rushton and Minnis (2002).

Fostering

Foster care may be of three kinds:

1. **short-term emergency care**, for example, when a caregiver is ill or when the parents of an autistic child need respite;
2. **medium-term care**, which may be followed by return home, for example, if the caregiver is receiving treatment for problems that led to neglect or abuse of the child;
3. **long-term care**, in which the child remains until able to leave independently.

Children in long-term foster care have more problems than children who have been adopted, but it is difficult to determine how far these problems are related to experiences before fostering and how far they are due to the lesser security of fostering as against adoption. Problems seem to be greater when the fostered child is older and when children in the fostering family are of the same age as the fostered child. Children in foster care usually retain some contact with their biological parents but it is not helpful to the child to have sporadic and distressing contacts. For a review of fostering see Rushton and Minnis (2002).

Inpatient and day-patient care

Child psychiatric inpatient units require easy access to paediatric advice, adequate space for play, easy access to schooling, and an informal design that still allows close observation. There should be some provisions for mothers to stay with their children.

Admission for inpatient treatment is usually arranged for any of three reasons:

1. **severity:** the disorder is too severe to treat in any other way, for example, extreme hyperactivity, severe pervasive developmental disorder, life threatening anorexia nervosa, and school refusal resistant to outpatient treatment;
2. **observation** when the diagnosis is uncertain;
3. **separation:** inpatient treatment can provide a necessary period away from a severely disturbing home environment, for example, when there is child abuse or gross overprotection.

Sometimes the mother is admitted as well as the child, thus helping to maintain the bonds between the two. This arrangement also allows close observation of the ways in which the mother responds to the child, for example in cases of child abuse. It is also an opportunity for the mother to learn new parenting skills by taking an increasing part in the child's care while both remain in hospital.

Day-hospital treatment for children provides many of the advantages of inpatient care without removing them from home. Unless there is any danger that the child may be abused, remaining at home has the advantage that relationships with other family members are maintained. Day care can relieve the family from some of the stressful effects of managing an overactive or autistic child.

For a review of inpatient and day-patient care see Green (2002).

Intensive home-based care and outreach services

Increasingly, intensive community-based support is provided for children and adolescents with severe problems. Such support requires a well staffed and experienced team of professionals. Though valuable, such services do not remove the need for inpatient provision (Henggeler *et al.*, 1999). For a review of outreach services for children, see Green (2002).

Review of syndromes

The review of syndromes begins with the problems encountered in pre-school children. Specific and perva-

TABLE 24.4 Arrangement of sections on disorders of children in this and other chapters

Problems of pre-school children and their families	Mood disorders
Specific developmental disorders Specific reading disorder Mathematics disorder (specific arithmetic disorder) Communication disorders	(School refusal)
Motor skills disorder	Other childhood psychiatric disorders Functional enuresis Faecal soiling Elective mutism Stammering Dementia Schizophrenia
Pervasive developmental disorders Childhood autism Rett's disorder Overactive disorder with mental retardation and stereotyped movements Childhood disintegrative disorder Asperger's syndrome Atypical autism and pervasive developmental disorder	Gender identity disorders Effeminacy in boys Tomboyishness in girls
	Suicide and deliberate self-harm
Hyperkinetic disorder	Psychiatric aspects of physical illness in childhood
Conduct disorders Truancy	Psychiatric problems of adolescence
(Juvenile delinquency)	Child abuse Physical abuse (non-accidental injury) Emotional abuse Child neglect Non-organic failure to thrive and deprivation Dwarfism Sexual abuse
Anxiety disorders Separation anxiety disorder Phobic anxiety disorder Social anxiety disorder of childhood Sibling rivalry disorder Post-traumatic stress disorder Obsessive–compulsive disorders	Conditions considered in other chapters Tic disorders (p. 352) Suicide and deliberate self-harm (pp. 412 and 422) Factitious disorder by proxy (p. 390)
Somatoform disorders and other unexplained physical symptoms Conversion disorders	

sive developmental disorders are described next. An account is then given of the main psychiatric disorders of childhood, in the order in which they appear in the major systems of classification. Other psychiatric disorders of childhood appear next before a brief account of the disorders of adolescence (which are generally similar to those of either childhood or adult life). The chapter ends with the subject of child abuse. Table 24.4 shows the arrangement of the remaining sections of this chapter and shows where to find information about three additional conditions which occur in both childhood and adult life.

Problems of pre-school children and their families

It has already been noted that in the pre-school years children are learning several kinds of social behaviour. They are acquiring sphincter control. They are learning how to behave at mealtimes, to go to bed at an appropriate time, and to control angry feelings. They are also becoming less dependent. All these behaviours are learned within the family. The psychiatric problems of pre-school children centre around these behaviours and they often reflect factors in the family as well as factors in the child. Many psychological problems at this age are brief, and can be thought of as delays in normal development. Most of these problems are treated by general practitioners and paediatricians. The more serious problems may be referred to child psychiatrists.

Prevalence

In a much quoted study, Richman *et al.* (1982) studied 705 families with a 3-year-old child in a London borough. The most frequent abnormalities of behaviour in these children were bed-wetting at least three times a week (present in 37 per cent), wetting by day at least once a week (17 per cent), overactivity (14 per cent), soiling at least once a week (13 per cent), difficulty in settling at night (13 per cent), fears (13 per cent), disobedience (11 per cent), attention seeking (10 per cent), and temper tantrums (5 per cent).

Whether these behaviours are reported as problems depends on the attitudes of the parents as well as on the nature, severity, and frequency of the behaviour. Richman *et al.* overcame this difficulty by making their own ratings of the extent of problems. They based this assessment on the effects on the child's well-being and the consequences for the other members of the family. They used common-sense criteria to decide whether the problems were mild, moderate, or severe. Seven per cent of 3-year-olds in their survey had behaviour problems of marked severity and 15 per cent had mild problems. The behaviours most often rated as problems were temper tantrums, attention-seeking, and disobedience.

Prognosis

As explained above, many psychological problems of pre-school children are brief. However, Richman *et al.* (1982) found that certain problems detected in 3-year-old children were still present at the age of 8. These problems were overactivity, difficulty in controlling the child, speech difficulty, and autism.

Aetiology

Aetiological factors are related to the stage of development, the child's temperament, and influences in the family. There are wide individual variations in the rate at which normal development proceeds, particularly in sphincter control and language acquisition. As noted above (p. 652), a child's temperamental characteristics are evident from the earliest weeks. These characteristics are capable of affecting the mother's response – how much time she spends with her child, how often she picks up her child, and so on. These maternal responses may in turn affect the child's development. Behaviour problems at this age are also associated with poor marital relationships, maternal depression, rivalry with siblings, and inadequate parental behaviour. See Campbell (1995) for further information.

Some common problems of pre-school children

Temper tantrums

Occasional temper tantrums are normal in toddlers, and only persistent or very severe tantrums are abnormal. The immediate cause is often unwitting reinforcement by excessive attention and inconsistent discipline on the part of the parents. When this arises it is often because the parents have emotional problems of their own or because the relationship between them is unsatisfactory.

Temper tantrums usually respond to kind but firm and consistent setting of limits. In treatment it is first necessary to discover why the parents have been unable to set limits in this way. They should be helped with any problems of their own and advised how to respond to the tantrums.

Sleep problems

The most common sleep difficulty is wakefulness at night, which is most frequent between the ages of 1 and 4 years. About a fifth of children of this age take at least an hour to get to sleep or are wakeful for long periods during the night. When wakefulness is an isolated problem and not very distressing to the family, it is enough to reassure parents that it is likely to improve. When sleep disturbances are severe or persistent, two possible causes should be considered. First, the problems may have been made worse by physical illness or an emotional disorders. Second, they may have been exacerbated by the parents' excessive concern and inability to reassure the child. If no medical or psychiatric disorder is detected, the reasons for the parents' concerns should be sought and dealt with as far as possible. Some parents overstimulate their child in the evening, or unwittingly reinforce crying in the night by taking the child into their own bed. A behavioural approach to these problems is generally helpful. Hypnotic medication may be used very occasionally for special occasions but should not be used for long.

Other sleep problems such as nightmares and night terrors are common among healthy toddlers but they seldom persist for long. They are discussed on p. 374.

For a review of sleep problems see Stores (2001).

Feeding problems

Minor food fads or food refusal are common in pre-school children, but do not usually last long. In a minority the behaviour is severe or persistent, although not accompanied by signs of poor nourishment. When this happens it is often because the parents, who are often overattentive and perfectionistic, are unwittingly reinforcing the child's behaviour.

Treatment is directed to the parents' management of the problem. They should be encouraged to ignore the feeding problem and refrain from offering the child special foods or otherwise attempting to do anything unusual to persuade the child to eat. Instead, the child should be offered a normal meal and left to decide whether to eat it or not.

Pica

Pica is the eating of items generally regarded as inedible, for example soil, paint, and paper. It is often associated with other behaviour problems. Cases should be investigated carefully because some are due to brain damage, or autism, or mental retardation. Some are associated with emotional distress, which should be reduced if possible. Otherwise, treatment consists of common-sense precautions to keep the child away from the abnormal items of diet. Pica usually diminishes as the child grows older. For a review of the history of ideas about pica see Parry-Jones and Parry-Jones (1992).

Reactive attachment disorder of infancy and early childhood

As explained above, children's attachments to their parents vary in their security, and they may vary between caregivers, for example insecure with one parent but secure with the other. Attachment disorders are more extreme variations from the norm and they do not correspond exactly with any of the types of insecure attachment describe earlier (see p. 655). They are pervasive affecting all relationships; and they cause distress. They start before the age of 5 years and are associated with grossly abnormal caregiving. There are two subtypes, disinhibited and inhibited.

- **Disinhibited** These children seek comfort but do so indiscriminately, seeking it as much from strangers as from caregivers. As infants, they relate to these people with clinging behaviour, and in early childhood with attention-seeking. Such behaviour has been described most clearly in children raised in institutions, or experiencing repeated changes in foster care. In DSM-IV, the diagnosis requires that the disturbance of relationships appears to be a direct result of abnormal caregiving. ICD-10 does not use this criterion but requires that the behaviour is present in several situations.
- **Inhibited** This type is less clearly defined. The children show a combination of behavioural inhibition, vigilance, and fearfulness, which is sometimes called frozen watchfulness. They show a mixture of approach and avoidance behaviours. They are miserable and difficult to console, and sometimes aggressive. Some fail to thrive. This behaviour is seen among children who have been abused (see p. 697).

Aetiology It seems that these syndromes are related more to the type of caregiving (abusive or institutional) than to the child.

Prognosis Insecure attachment in infancy is often followed by conflicts with caregivers and behaviour problems later in childhood. It seems that, improvement can occur if the child experiences a secure attachment to a caregiver, for example, as a result of fostering or adoption. However most of this information has not been derived from studies using ICD-10 or DSM-IV criteria.

For a review of attachment disorders see O'Connor (2002).

Assessment and treatment of the problems of pre-school children

Assessment Usually the information is largely from the parents. The assessor seeks to discover whether the problem is primarily in the child or related difficulties in the mother or the entire family. The problem behaviour is assessed, together with the child's general level of development, and the functioning of the family.

Treatment Apart from particular points already mentioned under the specific disorders, treatment includes advice for the mother (and if necessary for other family members) about relevant aspects of child-rearing. There is little evidence about the value of treatment. Behavioural methods are probably useful, and language delay may benefit from special teaching. Occasionally medication is needed to reduce extreme overactivity (see p. 677). It is often helpful to arrange for the child to spend part of the day away from the family in a playgroup or nursery school. For further information about the assessment of pre-school children see American Academy of Child and Adolescent Psychiatry (1998a).

Specific developmental disorders

Both DSM-IV and ICD-10 contain categories for specific developmental disorders, which are circumscribed developmental delays that are not attributable to another disorder or to lack of opportunity to learn (Table 24.5). It is debatable whether these conditions should be classified as mental disorders at all, since many children meeting the criteria have no other signs of psychopathology. In ICD-10, these developmental disorders are divided into specific developmental disorders of scholastic skills, speech and language, and motor function. In DSM-IV, the same disorders are called learning disorder, communication disorders, and motor skill disorder, respectively.

Specific developmental disorders of scholastic skills are divided further into specific reading disorder, specific spelling disorder, and specific arithmetic disorder. In DSM-IV, these conditions are called reading disorder, disorder of written expression, and mathematics disorder, respectively.

Specific reading disorder

In DSM-IV, this condition is named reading disorder. It is defined by a reading age well below (usually defined as 2 standard deviations below) the level expected from the child's age and IQ. In a much quoted study, the disorder was found in about 4 per cent of 10–11-year-olds in the Isle of Wight, and about twice that percentage in London (Yule and Rutter, 1985) and subsequent investigations have confirmed these estimates.

TABLE 24.5 Specific disorders of psychological development

DSM-IV	ICD-10
Learning disorder	*Specific developmental disorders of scholastic skills*
Reading disorder	Specific reading disorder
Disorder of written expression	Specific spelling disorder
Mathematics disorder	Specific disorder of arithmetic skills
	Mixed disorder of scholastic skills
Communication disorders	*Specific developmental disorders of speech and language*
Phonological disorder	Specific speech articulation disorder
Expressive language disorder	Expressive language disorder
Mixed receptive–expressive language disorder	Receptive language disorder
–	Acquired aphasia with epilepsy*
Stuttering	(stuttering†)
Motor skills disorder	
Developmental coordination disorder	Specific developmental disorder of motor function

* In DSM-IV acquired aphasia with epilepsy is classified as an (acquired) receptive-expressive language disorder.

† Stuttering though common is not listed as a disorder.

Clinical features

Specific reading disorder is to be distinguished from general backwardness in scholastic achievement resulting from low intelligence, lack of opportunity to learn at home or at school, or poor visual acuity. The child has serious delay in learning to read, evident from the early years of schooling, and sometimes been preceded by delayed acquisition of speech and language. Writing and spelling are impaired, and in older children these problems may be more obvious than the reading problems. Errors in reading and spelling include omissions, substitutions, or distortions of words, slow reading, long hesitations, and reversals of words or letters. There may also be poor comprehension. There may be associated emotional problems, but development in other areas is not affected. Compared with children with general backwardness at school, those with specific reading retardation are much more often boys; they are also more likely to have minor neurological abnormalities, and are likely to come from socially disadvantaged homes.

Specific reading retardation is associated with conduct disorder more often than would be expected through chance (Rutter *et al.*, 1970a, b). The association may arise in part because the two conditions have common neurodevelopmental or temperamental origins; in part because reading retardation leads to conduct problems at school when the child is frustrated by failures; and in part because conduct disorder gives rise to problems in learning to read.

Aetiology

Reading is a complex skill which depends on more than one psychological process and is learned in several stages. It is not surprising,therefore, that no single cause has been identified for specific reading disorder. A widely held theory of the learning of reading is that children first use visual methods: they learn the appearance of whole words, and cannot decipher new words. The next stage of learning is alphabetical: children become able to decode new words from the sounds associated with the letters. In the final stage, reading becomes automatic and flexible in combining visual and alphabetical methods. (This model of reading, although not accepted by all, is useful in clinical practice.)

Dyslexia It has been suggested that there is a subgroup of 'dyslexics' with a neuropsychological syndrome of poor coordination, constructional difficulties, and left/right confusion. While many children with specific reading disorder have one or two of these problems, there is no convincing evidence for a separate subgroup with these features. Despite this lack of evidence, the concept of dyslexia is in common use and has some value in conveying to laymen the message that the reading problems are not due to laziness or stupidity, and that the child needs help.

Genetic causes The frequent occurrence of reading disorder in family members suggests a genetic cause, and the family patterning suggests that there is not a single mode of inheritance (Rutter *et al.*, 1990). Several quantitative trait loci have been reported to link to reading disorder, including loci on chromosomes 2, 3, 6, 7, 15 and 18 (see for example Kaminen *et al.* 2003). At the time of writing, the most consistent findings concern an area of chromosome 6p (see for example Francks *et al.* 2004).

Neurological causes Children with cerebral palsy and epilepsy have increased rates of specific reading disorder. It has been suggested that children who have specific reading disorder, but no obvious neurological disease, may have minor and less obvious neurological abnormalities. The evidence does not support this idea. Another suggestion is that there is a **disorder of brain maturation** affecting one or more of the skills required in reading. This explanation is consistent with the following findings: difficulty in visual scanning, confusion between right and left, and general improvement with age.

Social factors It seems likely that difficulties insufficient in themselves to cause reading retardation sufficient to be diagnosed as specific reading disorder, may do so when the child is brought up in an illiterate or otherwise disadvantaged family, receives little attention at school, or changes school frequently.

For a review of aetiology, see Vellutino *et al.* (2004).

Assessment and treatment

It is important to identify the disorder early. **Assessment** is carried out by an educational or clinical psychologist using an individually administered standardized test of reading accuracy and comprehension. **Treatment** is educational unless there are additional medical or behavioural problems requiring separate intervention. Treatment should be started as early as possible before the child has a sense of failure. Several educational approaches are used but it is most important to reawaken the interest of a child with a long experience of failure. Parental interest and continued extra teaching seem to be helpful, but there is no evidence that any one method of teaching is better than others. If there are behavioural problems secondary to frustration caused by the reading difficulty, they may lessen as reading improves; others may need separate attention.

Prognosis

Prognosis varies with the severity of the condition. Among children with a mild problem in the middle years of childhood, only about a quarter achieve normal reading skills by adolescence. Very few with severe problems in mid-childhood overcome them by adolescence. Whilst there is insufficient evidence to be certain what happens to these people as adults, those with substantial difficulties in adolescence seem likely to retain them (Maughan *et al.*, 1985).

For a review of reading disorders see Snowling (2002).

Mathematics disorder (specific arithmetic disorder)

The first of these terms is used in DSM-IV; the term in parentheses is used in ICD-10. Difficulty with arithmetic is probably the second most common specific disorder. Problems include failure to understand simple mathematical concepts, failure to recognize numerical symbols or mathematical signs, difficulty in carrying out arithmetic manipulations, and inability to learn mathematical tables. These problems are not due simply to lack of opportunities to learn and are evident from the time of the child's first attempts to learn mathematics. Although causing less severe handicap in everyday life than reading difficulties, mathematics disorder can lead to secondary emotional difficulties when the child is at school.

Epidemiology The incidence reported in several studies lies between 1.3–6 per cent and frequently co-occurs with specific reading difficulties (see Snowling 2002).

Aetiology This is uncertain but cognitive deficits involving working memory have been implicated. Dyscalculia occurs in some adults with parietal lobe lesions, but no brain damage has been found in children with specific arithmetic disorder.

The **assessment** is usually based on the arithmetic subtests of the Wechsler Intelligence Scale for Children (WISC) and the Wechsler Adult Intelligence Scale (WAIS) and on specific tests. **Treatment** is by remedial teaching but it is not known whether it is effective. The **prognosis** is not known. For a review see Snowling (2002).

Communication disorders (developmental disorders of speech and language)

Children vary widely in their achievement of speech and language. Half of all children use words with meanings by 12.5 months and 97 per cent do so by 21 months. Half form words into simple sentences by 23 months (Neligan and Prudham, 1969). Vocabulary and complexity of language develop rapidly during the preschool years. However, when children start school, 1 per cent are seriously retarded in speech and 5 per cent have difficulty in making themselves understood by strangers. The process by which language is acquired is complex and is still not fully understood. Language disorders are associated with psychiatric problems because (i) the two may be an expression of a common brain abnormality; and (ii) language disorder impairs social interaction and education.

Causes of speech and language disorder

No cause can be found in the majority of children with speech and language disorders. These cases are said to have specific developmental speech and language disorder. It is most important to detect the primary conditions that are present in the minority. The most common of these causes is **learning disability**. Other important causes are **deafness, cerebral palsy, autism, and autistic spectrum disorders**. **Social deprivation** can cause mild delays in speaking or add to the effects of the other causes.

Classification

The classification differs in some ways between ICD-10 and DSM-IV. ICD-10 uses the title 'specific developmental disorders of speech and language', whereas DSM-IV has the wider title 'communication disorders'. Three disorders appear in both classifications, though with some differences in nomenclature:

- phonological disorder (DSM-IV) or specific speech articulation disorder (ICD-10);
- specific developmental expressive language disorder (the term is used in both classifications);
- mixed receptive-expressive disorder (DSM-IV); here ICD-10 has the narrower term specific developmental receptive language disorder. (The reason for the difference is explained below.)

ICD-10 (but not DSM-IV) has a fourth category of acquired aphasia with epilepsy. In DSM-IV, the wider title of the group allows the inclusion of stuttering; The narrower title in ICD-10 does not cover stuttering, which is coded instead under behavioural disorders of childhood (see Table 24.4).

Phonological disorder (specific developmental speech articulation disorder)

In this condition, accuracy in the use of speech sound is below the level appropriate for the child's mental age but language skills are normal. Errors in making speech sounds are normal in children up to about the age of 4 years, but by age 7 most speech sounds should be normal. By age 12 years nearly all speech sounds should be made normally. Children with specific speech articulation disorder make errors of articulation so severe that it is difficult for others to understand their speech. Speech sounds may be omitted or distorted, or other sounds substituted. In assessing speech production, appropriate allowance should be made for regional accents and dialects. The sounds affected most often are those developing later in the normal sequence of development (l, r, s, z, th, and ch for English speakers).

Prevalence depends on the criteria used to determine when speech production is abnormal; a rate of 2–3 per cent has been cited among 6- to 7-year-olds (American Psychiatric Association, 1994a).

Specific developmental expressive language disorder

In this disorder, the ability to use expressive spoken language is markedly below the level appropriate for the child's mental age. Language comprehension is within normal limits but there may be abnormalities in articulation. Language development varies considerably among normal children, but the absence of single words by 2 years of age, and of two-word phrases by 3 years of age signifies abnormality. Signs at later ages include restricted vocabulary, difficulties in selecting appropriate words, and immature grammatical usage. Non-verbal communication, if impaired, is not affected as severely as spoken language, and the child makes efforts to communicate. Disorders of behaviour are often present.

Cluttering Some children speak rapidly and with an erratic rhythm such that the grouping of words does not reflect the grammatical structure of their speech. This abnormality, which is known as cluttering, is classified as an associated feature of expressive language disorder in DSM-IV but in ICD-10 it is classified (with stammering) among other behavioural disorders of childhood.

Prevalence of expressive language disorder depends on the method of assessment; a rate of 3–5 per cent of children has been proposed (American Psychiatric Association, 1994a).

Prognosis It is reported that about half of the children meeting DSM-IV criteria develop normal speech by adult life, while the rest have long-lasting difficulties (American Psychiatric Association, 1994a). Prognosis is worse when the language disorder is severe, and when there is a comorbid condition, such as conduct disorder.

Treatment Treatment is mainly through special education. Psychiatrists are likely to be involved when there is a comorbid disorder, and may need to advise the parents about the child's rights for special education.

For a review of expressive language disorder, see American Academy of Child and Adolescent Psychiatry (1998b).

Receptive-expressive (or receptive) developmental language disorder

In this disorder the understanding of language is below the level appropriate to the child's mental age. In almost all cases, expressive language is also disturbed (a fact recognized in DSM-IV by the term receptive-expressive language disorder).

The development of receptive language ability varies considerably among normal children. However, failure to respond to familiar names, in the absence of non-verbal cues, by the beginning of the second year of age, or failure to respond to simple instructions by the end of the second year, are significant signs suggesting receptive language disorder – provided that deafness, learning disability, and pervasive developmental disorder have been excluded. Associated social and behavioural problems are particularly frequent in this form of language disorder.

The **prevalence** depends on the criteria for diagnosis, but a frequency of up to 3 per cent of school-age children has been suggested (American Psychiatric Association, 1994a).

The **prognosis** is poor with around 75 per cent continuing throughout childhood. The prognosis is worse when the language disorder is severe, or there is a comorbid condition, such as conduct disorder.

Treatment is through special education. The psychiatrist's role is the same as in expressive language disorder (see above).

For a review of receptive language disorder see American Academy of Child and Adolescent Psychiatry (1998b).

Acquired epileptic aphasia (Landau–Kleffner syndrome)

In this rare disorder, a child whose language has so far developed normally loses both receptive and expressive language but retains general intelligence. There are associated EEG abnormalities, nearly always bilateral and temporal, and often with more widespread disturbances. Most of the affected children develop seizures either before or after the change in expressive language. The disorder starts usually between 3 and 9 years of age, usually over several months but sometimes more rapidly.

The **aetiology** is unknown. The **prognosis** is variable: about two-thirds of children are left with a receptive language deficit, but the other third recover completely. **Treatment** of the seizures does not always lead to improvement in language.

Assessment of speech and language disorders

Early investigation is essential both to determine the nature and severity of the speech and language disorder and to exclude mental retardation, deafness, cerebral palsy, and pervasive developmental disorder. The speech-producing organs should be examined. **It is particularly important to detect deafness at an early stage.**

Parents can give some indication of the child's speech and language skills, especially if they complete a standardized inventory. With younger children it may be necessary to rely on this information, but children from about the age of 3 years can be tested by a standard test of language appropriate to the child's age. If possible, such a test should be carried out by a speech therapist or a psychologist specializing in the subject.

Treatment

Treatment depends partly on the cause but usually includes a programme of speech training carried out through play and social interaction. In milder cases this help is best provided at home by the parents who are given information on what to do. More severe difficulties are likely to require specialized help in a remedial class or a special school. Treatment should start early.

For a review the development of speech and language disorders see Bishop (2002). For more information about investigation and management of these conditions, see Busari and Weggelar (2005).

Motor skills disorder

Some children have delayed motor development, which results in clumsiness in school work or play. In ICD-10, this condition is called specific developmental disorder of motor function. It is also known as clumsy child syndrome or specific motor dyspraxia. The children can carry out all normal movements, but their coordination is poor. They are late in developing skills such as dressing, walking, and feeding. They tend to break things and are poor at handicrafts and organized games. They may also have difficulty in writing, drawing, and copying. IQ testing usually shows good verbal but poor performance scores.

These children are sometimes referred to a psychiatrist because of secondary emotional disorder. An explanation of the nature of the problem should be given to the child, the family, and the teachers. Special teaching may improve confidence. It may be necessary to exempt the child from organized games or other school activities involving motor coordination. There is usually some improvement with time. For further information see Graham *et al.* (1999).

Pervasive developmental disorders

The term pervasive developmental disorder refers to a group of disorders characterized by abnormalities in communication and social interaction and by restricted repetitive activities and interests. These abnormalities occur in a wide range of situations. Usually, development is abnormal from infancy and most cases are manifest before the age of 5 years.

Six conditions are included under this rubric in ICD-10 (see Table 24.6); two of which do not appear in DSM-IV, namely atypical autism and overactive disorder with mental retardation and stereotyped movements. The incidence of all forms of pervasive developmental disorder was thought to be around 3/1000, although the most recent surveys suggest double this incidence (Fombonne, 2003). Changes in case definition and improved recognition may account for part of this increase trend.

Autistic spectrum disorder (ASD) This term is often used to denote the whole range of pervasive develop-

TABLE 24.6 Pervasive developmental disorders

DSM-IV	ICD-10
Autistic disorder	Childhood autism
Rett's syndrome	Rett's syndrome
Childhood disintegrative disorder	Other childhood disintegrative disorder
	Overactive disorder with mental retardation and stereotyped movements
Asperger's disorder	Asperger's syndrome
Pervasive developmental disorder not otherwise specified (including atypical autism)	Atypical autism Pervasive developmental disorder not otherwise specified

mental disorders including those that do not exactly meet formal diagnostic criteria. It recognizes that the boundaries between the different syndromes are difficult to decide and that it can be more helpful to parents to think of a continuum of disability.

Childhood autism (autistic disorder)

This condition was described by Kanner (1943) who suggested the name infantile autism. The term childhood autism is used in ICD-10 but autistic disorder is the term in DSM-IV.

Clinical features

In his original description, Kanner (1943) identified the main features, which are still used to make the diagnosis. In both DSM-IV and ICD-10, three kinds of abnormality are required to make the diagnosis of autism:

1. abnormalities of social development;
2. abnormalities of communication;
3. restriction of interests and behaviour.

Of these, the abnormalities of social development are the most specific to autism. The clinical picture is variable both between persons, and in the same person at different ages.

Abnormal development is usually apparent before the age of 3 years. There are reports that early signs of autism can be detected in infancy, for example absence of babbling and pointing by 12 months, lack of imitation and oversensitivity to sounds, and dislike of change (for more detail, see LeCouteur and Baird, 2003).

Abnormalities of social development The child is unable to make warm emotional relationships with people (autistic aloneness). Autistic children do not respond to their parents' affectionate behaviour by smiling or cuddling. Instead, they appear to dislike being picked up or kissed. They are no more responsive to their parents than to strangers and do not show interest in other children. There is little difference in their behaviour towards people and inanimate objects. A characteristic sign is **gaze avoidance**, that is, the absence of eye-to-eye contact.

Abnormalities of communication Speech may develop late or never appear. Occasionally, it develops normally until about the age of 2 years and then disappears in part or completely. This lack of speech is a manifestation of a severe cognitive defect. As autistic children grow up, about half acquire some useful speech, although serious impairments usually remain, such as the misuse of pronouns and the inappropriate repeating of words spoken by other people (echolalia). Some autistic children are talkative, but their speech is a repetitive monologue rather than a conversation with another person.

The cognitive defect also affects non-verbal communication and play; autistic children do not take part in the imitative games of the first year of life, and later they do not use toys in an appropriate way. They show little imagination or creative play.

Restriction of interests and behaviour Obsessive desire for sameness is a term applied to the autistic child's stereotyped behaviour and distress if there is a change in the environment. For example, some autistic children insist on the same food repeatedly, on wearing the same clothes, or on engaging in repetitive games. Some are fascinated by spinning toys.

Odd behaviour and mannerisms are common. Some autistic children carry out odd motor behaviours such as whirling round and round, twiddling their fingers repeatedly, flapping their hands, or rocking. Others do not differ obviously in motor behaviour from normal children.

Other features Autistic children may suddenly show anger or fear without apparent reason. They may be overactive and distractible, sleep badly, or soil or wet themselves. Some injure themselves deliberately. About 25 per cent of autistic children develop **seizures**, usually about the time of adolescence.

Intelligence level Kanner originally believed that the intelligence of autistic children was normal. Later research has shown that three-quarters have IQ scores in the 'retarded' range, and this finding appears to represent true intellectual impairment (Rutter and Lockyer, 1967). Some autistic children show areas of ability despite impairment of other intellectual functions, and in some cases they have exceptional but restricted powers of memory or mathematical skill (Hermelin and O'Connor, 1983).

Epidemiology

The **prevalence** of autism is probably about 1 per 1000 children. It is four times as common in boys as in girls (Fombonne, 2003). The prevalence of autistic spectrum disorders has been estimated as 5–6 per 1000 in younger children (LeCouteur and Baird, 2003). It has been reported that rates of autism are rising but this could be because of changes in definition and ascertainment (Barbaresi *et al.*, 2005).

Aetiology

The cause of childhood autism is unknown but the social, language and behavioural problems in autism suggest abnormalities in not one but several neural systems.

Genetic influences are of great importance, probably with the involvement of several genes. The condition is 50 times more frequent in the siblings of affected persons than in the general population (Rutter *et al.*, 1990). Several twin studies have shown a much higher concordance between monozygotic than between dizygotic twins (for example, Rutter *et al.*, 1993; Bailey *et al.*, 1995) with a hereditability of about 90 percent. Cognitive abnormalities are more frequent among the siblings of autistic probands than in the general population, suggesting that the phenotype may be wider than the syndrome of autism as currently defined (Bailey *et al.*, 1998). Autism has been linked especially to regions on chromosomes 2, 7 and 15 (Veenstra-VanderWeele and Cook, 2004).

Organic brain disorder Structural brain studies have established that autistic children have larger brain volumes than normal children. Functional MRI (fMRI) scanning is providing important information about brain abnormalities in autism. Hypoactivation of the amygdala, frontal and temporal areas has been found, suggesting malfunctioning of areas involved in social processing; and in the area of the fusiform nucleus which is involved in face processing.

Other evidence for biological causes A third of autistic children have high peripheral serotonin levels. Autism is associated with fragile X syndrome (see p. 718), Rett syndrome, and tuberose sclerosis, but in only a small proportion of cases. About 10 percent of autistic children have a concomitant medical condition of some kind (Rutter *et al.*, 1994a).

Unsupported theories

MMR vaccine Claims of an association with MMR vaccine have not been confirmed in careful epidemiological studies.

Abnormal parenting In a much quoted paper, Kanner (1943) suggested that autism was a response to abnormal parents who were characterized as cold, detached, and obsessive. Kanner's idea has not been substantiated (see Koegel *et al.*, 1983). It is now thought that any psychological abnormalities in the parents are likely to be either a response to the problems of bringing up the autistic child, or (more likely) a manifestation in the parents of the genes that have produced autism in the child. Although unsupported by evidence, persistent lay beliefs about the role of parenting still cause distress among the parents who hear of it.

Relation to schizophrenia There is no evidence for a relationship between childhood autism and schizophrenia.

For a review of aetiology see Volkmar *et al.* (2004).

Psychopathology

Theory of mind in autism This theory attempts to identify a basic psychological disorder in autism. By the age of 4 years, normal children are able to form an idea of what others are thinking. As an example, consider a normal child who watches while another normal child is first shown the location of a hidden object and then sent out of the room while the object is moved to a new hiding place. The child who has remained in the room will conclude that the child who left temporarily will expect the object to be in the original position when he returns to the room. An autistic child tends to lack this appreciation of what another child is likely to be thinking. In the example, an autistic child is likely to say that the child who left the room will think that the object has been moved to its new place. It is not certain how specific to autism is this difficulty in appreciating what others know and expect, nor how central it is to the psychopathology. In any case, its cause is not known. For a review of the evidence for the theory of mind in autism, see Baron-Cohen *et al.* (2000).

Other possible 'core' psychological disorders in autism include impairment of frontal lobe executive functions involved in planning and organization, resulting in perseveration and poor self-regulation; and impaired ability to extract high-level meaning from diverse sources of information. None of these proposed core psychopathologies can account for more than a part of the clinical picture of autism.

Differential diagnosis

It is more usual to encounter partial syndromes than the full syndrome of childhood autism. These partial syndromes must be distinguished from :

- **Deafness** – excluded by appropriate tests of hearing.
- **Communication disorder** (see p. 669) which differs from autism in that the child usually responds normally to people and has good non-verbal communication.

- **Learning disability** in which responses to other people are more normal than those of an autistic child. Also, an autistic child has more impairment of language relative to other skills than is found in a learning-disabled child of the same age.
- Asperger's syndrome (see p. 675).
- Childhood disintegrative disorder (see p. 674).

Prognosis

Between 10–20 per cent of children with childhood autism begin to improve between the ages of about 4–6 years, and are eventually able to attend an ordinary school and obtain work. A further 10–20 per cent can live at home but cannot work and need to attend a special school or training centre and remain very dependent on their families and/or support services. The remainder, at least 60 per cent, improve little and are unable to lead an independent life; many need long-term residential care. Those who improve may continue to show language problems, emotional coldness, and odd behaviour. As noted already, a substantial minority develop epilepsy in adolescence. Pointers to better prognosis are communicative speech by the age of about 6 years and higher IQ although outcome is highly variable even within the normal IQ range (Howlin *et al.*, 2004).

Assessment

Assessment should be concerned with more than the diagnosis of autism. The following additional factors need to be considered (Lord and Rutter, 1994):

- cognitive level;
- language ability;
- communication skills, social skills and play;
- repetitive or otherwise abnormal behaviour;
- stage of social development in relation to age, mental age, and stage of language development;
- associated medical or conditions;
- psychosocial factors including the needs of the family.

For a review of diagnosis and assessment see Baird *et al.* (2003).

Management

In the absence of any specific treatment, management has three main aspects: management of the abnormal behaviour, education and social services, and help for the family.

Management of abnormal behaviour Contingency management (see p. 592) may control some of the abnormal behaviour of autistic children. Such treatment is often carried out at home by the parents, instructed and supervised by a clinical psychologist. It is not known whether this treatment has any lasting benefit, but in autism even temporary changes are often worthwhile for the patient and the family.

Education and social services Most autistic children require special schooling. It is generally thought better for them to live at home and to attend special day schools. If the condition is so severe that the child cannot stay in the family, residential schooling is necessary. Special care is needed to avoid an institutional atmosphere, since this can increase social withdrawal. In some cases, the educational and residential needs of autistic children can be provided through the services for the learning disabled. Older adolescents may need vocational training.

For a review of psychological and educational treatments see Howlin (1998).

Help for the family The family of an autistic child needs considerable help to cope with the child's behaviour, which is often difficult ot understand and distressing. They need prompt assessment of their child's needs and easy access to appropriate eductional and other provisions. Although doctors may be able to do little specifically to help the patient, they must not withdraw from the family, who need continuing support as well as support for their efforts to help the child themselves, and obtain help from educational and social services. Some parents request genetic counselling and it seems that the risk of a further autistic child is about 3 per cent (Lord and Rutter, 1994). Many parents find it helpful to join a voluntary organization in which they can meet other parents of autistic children and discuss common problems.

Other suggested treatments Individual psychotherapy has been used in the hope of effecting more fundamental changes but there is no evidence that it succeeds. Nor is there evidence that any medication is effective except in the short term control of (i) behaviour problems, when an atypical antipsychotic drug may be effective; .(ii) anxiety, depression, or self-injury when an SSRI is sometimes helpful; (iii) hyperactivity when a stimulant may be of value – though with the possibility of an accompanying increase in repeitive behaviours.

For a general review of treatment see Volkmar *et al.* (2004).

Rett's disorder

Rett's disorder (or Rett's syndrome) is a rare X-linked condition which occurs almost exclusively in girls. The reported prevalence is 0.8 per 10 000 girls (Kerr and Stevenson, 1985). After a period of normal development in the first months of life, head growth slows and over the next 2 years there is arrest of cognitive development and loss of purposive skilled hand movements. Stereotyped movements develop with hand-clapping and hand-wringing movements. Ataxia of the legs and trunk may develop. Interest in the social environment diminishes in the first few years of the disorder, but may increase again later. Expressive and receptive language development is impaired severely and there is psychomotor retardation. Some patients develop severe learning disability. The disorder is associated with sporadic mutations in the MECP2 gene, located on the X chromosome; aberrant imprinting (p. 103) of the gene may also occur. MECP2 regulates expression of genes involved in brain development. For review, see Jellinger (2003).

Childhood disintegrative disorder

Childhood disintegrative disorder (also known as Heller's disease) begins after a period of normal development usually lasting for more than 2 years. It is unclear how far the childhood disintegrative disorder is distinct from childhood autism. It resembles childhood autism in the marked loss of cognitive functions, abnormalities of social behaviour and communication, and unfavourable outcome. It differs from childhood autism in the loss of motor skills and of bowel or bladder control. The condition may arrest after a time, or progress to a severe neurological condition. For a review see Harris (1996).

Asperger's syndrome

This condition was first described by Asperger (1944) and his original paper, in German, has been translated into English by Frith (1991). The condition has also been referred to as autistic psychopathy and is more common in boys than girls. The children develop normally at first but by the third year begin to lack warmth in their relationships. They go on to show marked abnormalities of social behaviour similar to those of childhood autism. There may be stereotyped and repetitive activities, often in the form of intense but narrow interests rather than motor mannerisms. The condition differs from autism in that there is no general delay or retardation of cognitive development or language, though speech may be stilted and intonation unusual. Conversation may consist more of repeated monologues than social interchange. They are eccentric, solitary, and may spend much time in narrow interests. Many of these children are clumsy. They are more interested in others than are children with autism but they do not share interests or pleasures with others, and are without friends.

Epidemiology The prevalence of the syndrome is uncertain and reported rates depend on the definition used in the research. Using ICD-10 criteria, Ehlers and Gillberg (1993) reported a rate of about 39 per 10 000 but only four cases were detected and the confidence limits of this estimate extend from 0.6 to 56 per 10 000 (see Fombonne, 1999, p. 781). Whatever the true frequency, the condition is increasingly recognized as important and the children are recognized as requiring educational and other help.

Aetiology The cause of Asperger's syndrome is unknown. It is uncertain whether the condition is a milder variant of childhood autism or a separate disorder.

Prognosis The abnormalities usually persist into adult life. Most people with the disorder can work, but few form successful relationships and marry.

For a review of Asperger's syndrome, see Volkmar and Klin (2000).

Atypical autism, and pervasive developmental disorder NOS

The terms atypical autism (ICD-10) and pervasive developmental disorder, not otherwise specified (NOS) (DSM-IV) denote a residual category for pervasive developmental disorders that resemble autism but do not meet the diagnostic criteria for any of the syndromes within this group. The prevalence of these cases varies according to the criteria adopted but most investigations show that they are at least as common as autism (see Fombonne, 1999). It is not known what is the relation between these cases and those which meet the criteria for the other syndromes within the group of pervasive developmental disorders.

Hyperkinetic disorder

About a third of children are described by their parents as overactive, and 5–20 per cent of school children are so described by teachers. These reports encompass a continuum of behaviour varying from normal high spirits to a severe and persistent disorder. This overactivity often varies in different situations. Hyperkinetic disorders are severe forms of overactivity associated with marked inattention; hence the widely used term attention-deficit hyperactivity disorder adopted in DSM-IV. In ICD-10, the term is hyperkinetic disorder and because of slight differences in the criteria for disgnosis (see below), cases diagnosed as hyperkinetic disorder are rather more severe than those meeting the criteria for attention-deficit hyperactivity disorder.

Clinical features

The cardinal features of this disorder are:

- extreme and persistent restlessness;
- sustained and prolonged motor activity;
- difficulty in maintaining attention;
- impulsiveness and difficulty in withholding responses.

These features are pervasive, occuring across situations though they can vary somewhat in different situations so that parents and teachers may give rather different accounts of the child's behaviour.

Children with the disorder are often reckless, and prone to accidents. They may have learning difficulties, which result in part from poor attention and lack of persistence with tasks. Many develop minor forms of antisocial behaviour as the condition continues, particularly disobedience, temper tantrums, and aggression. These children are often socially disinhibited and unpopular with other children. Mood fluctuates, but low self-esteem and depressive mood are common.

Restlessness, overactivity, and related symptoms often start before school age. Sometimes the child was overactive as a baby, but more often significant problems begin when the children begin to walk; they are constantly on the move, interfering with objects and exhausting their parents.

Diagnostic criteria

In both ICD-10 and DSM-IV the cardinal features for the diagnosis of the disorder are impaired attention, hyperactivity, and impulsiveness starting in childhood and lasting for at least six months to a degree that is maladaptive and inconsistent with the developmental level of the child. However, the two systems differ in the details of the criteria for diagnosis:

- ICD-10 requires that the symptoms started before 6 years of age; DSM-IV specifies before 7 years of age.
- ICD-10 requires both hyperactivity and impaired attention; DSM-IV requires either inattention, or hyperactivity with impulsiveness.
- ICD-10 requires that the criteria are met both at home and at school, whereas DSM-IV requires only that they be present in one situation with impairment (which does not have strict criteria) in the other.

The result of these differences is that children who meet ICD-10 criteria are more severely impaired than those who meet DSM-IV criteria.

In ICD-10 the disorder can be further classified as:

1. disturbance of activity and attention, and
2. hyperkinetic conduct disorder.

The latter term is used when criteria for both hyperkinetic disorder and conduct disorder are met. (The provision is made because the presence of associated aggression, delinquency, or antisocial behaviour is associated with a less good outcome - see below.)

Comorbidity About half of children with the disorder meet diagnostic criteria for other conditions as well, principally conduct disorder; depressive disorder or anxiety disorder. Learning disability and language impairment is also commonly present. Autistic children are often hyperactive and inattentive, but these features are regarded as part of the syndrome of childhood autism; hyperactivity disorder is not diagnosed in addition to autism.

Epidemiology

Estimates of the prevalence of hyperkinetic disorder vary according to the criteria for diagnosis. Using DSM-IV criteria, a prevalence of 3–5 per cent is proposed (American Psychiatric Association, 1994a). Using ICD-10 criteria, a prevalence of 1.7 per cent was found among primary school boys (Taylor *et al.*, 1991). Rates seem to be increasing, possibly due to increased recognition of the disorder. Rates are about three times higher in boys than in girls, and higher with younger age. The disorder is more frequent in areas of social deprivation and among children raised in institutions.

Aetiology

The aetiology is uncertain though much of the evidence suggests a disorder of higher cognitive executive function, related to abnormalities of neurotransmission in the prefrontal cortex and associated subcortical structures, and with genetic as well as environmental origins.

Neurological findings Signs suggesting neurodevelopmental impairment or delay are found in children with hyperkinetic disorder, for example, clumsiness, language delay, and abnormalities of speech (Schachar, 1991). Although these signs are generally associated with birth complications, they could result from factors acting at an earlier stage of development of the brain. The disorder occurs in a quarter of children following severe traumatic brain injury (Max *et al.*, 2004).

Neuroimaging studies show functional abnormalities in the prefrontal and other areas associated with executive function and the cerebellum (see Roth and Saykin, 2004).

Genetic studies: Investigations of family members, twins and adopted children, and monozygotic and dizygotic twins, all suggest that genetic factors are important with heritability estimates of 70 per cent or more. Compared with controls, probands with attention-deficit hyperactivity disorder have more first-degree relatives with the same disorder (Biederman *et al.* (1992). Also there is a much higher concordance among monozygotic than dizygotic pairs (Eaves *et al.*, 1997). Adoption studies show that the biological parents of children with the attention-deficit hyperactivity disorder are more likely to have had the same or a related disorder than are the adoptive parents (van den Oord *et al.*, 1994).

Linkage has been reported between attention deficit hyperactivity disorder and polymorphisms of genes involved in the dopaminergic transmitter system, including the dopamine D_4 receptor gene (Smalley *et al.*, 1998), and the dopamine transporter gene (see Heiser *et al.*, 2004).These findings are consistent with evidence that drugs affecting the dopamine system lead to improvement in the disorder (see below). It seems that there are multiple genes of small effect but further work is required before their significance can be understood. For a review of the genetic causes see Heiser *et al.* (2004).

Social factors Social factors increase the childs innate tendency to hyperactivity. Thus, as noted above, overactive behaviour is more frequent among young children living in poor social conditions and institutions. Also, studies of twins indicate that both shared and non-shared environmental effects contribute to aetiology (Eaves *et al.*, 1997).

Other suggested causes In the past, lead intoxication (Needleman *et al.*, 1979) has been suggested as causes of hyperkinetic syndrome, and more recently zinc deficiency has been suggested, but there is no convincing evidence that either of these is a common cause. Some parents report that certain food additives increase their child's overactivity but there is no evidence that this is a general cause (see Schachar and Ickowicz, 2000 for a review).

Prognosis

Overactivity usually lessens gradually as the child grows older, especially when it is mild and not present in every situation. It usually ceases by puberty. The prognosis for any associated learning difficulties is less good, whilst antisocial behaviour has the worst outcome. When the overactivity is severe, and is accompanied by learning failure or associated with low intelligence, the prognosis is poor and the conditions may persist into adult life, usually as antisocial disorder and drug misuse rather than continued hyperactivity. It is uncertain whether mood and anxiety disorders are increased in adult life. See Willoughby (2004) for further information about prognosis. For a review of attention-deficit hyperactivity disorder in adults see Wilens *et al.* (2002).

Treatment

Support and psychological treatment A hyperactive child exhausts his parents, who need support from the start of treatment, particularly as it may be difficult to reduce the child's behaviour. Teachers also need support, and special education may be needed. Psychosocial intervention is usually combined with stimulant medication except in the milder cases. Family, group or behaviour therapy are all used but are less generally effective than medication in treatment trials. Behavioural treatment is directed to any conduct problems, often by modifying the response of the carers or teachers to these problems.

Medication *Stimulant drugs* should be tried when there is severe restlessness and attention deficit. These drugs increase dopamine and noradrenaline activity and it is thought that these actions underlie their therapeutic effects. The most commonly prescribed medication is methylphenidate. Dexamphetamine is also used, and longer acting preparations are now available. Dosage should be related to body weight following the manufacturers' instructions and advice about contraindications. The potential short-term benefits are decreased restlessness, aggressiveness and, sometimes, improved attention. These effects do not usually diminish with time, but it has not been shown that they are associated with better long-term outcome. The **side-effects** include irritability, depression, insomnia, and poor appetite. High doses may provoke stereotyped behaviour, which disappears when the dose is reduced. With high doses, there may be some slowing of growth, but adult stature and weight do not seem to be affected (Taylor, 1994; Spencer *et al.*, 1996). Also, tics may be made worse.The drug may be needed for many months and some children take it for years; careful monitoring is essential. Some parents are understandably reluctant to agree to long-term drug treatment for their children. In such cases it can be helpful to give the drugs for a trial period so that the benefits and disadvantages can be assessed for the particular child. The drug may be stopped from time to time in an attempt to minimize side-effects and to confirm that medication is still needed.

The noradrenaline re-uptake inhibitor, *atomoxetine*, has also been licensed for the treatment of hyperkinetic syndrome. Common adverse effects of atomoxetine include nausea, abdominal pain, loss of appetite and sleep disturbance. Rarely (about 1 in 50,000 patients treated) severe liver damage can occur. While atomoxetine has the theoretical advantage of lacking psychostimulant properties, experience with its use is necessarily limited compared to methylphenidate

In clinical trials, short-term benefits of stimulants have been shown in about two-thirds of children with hyperkinetic syndrome (Ottenbacher and Cooper, 1983), but the long-term benefits are uncertain. It seems best to reserve drug treatment for more severe cases that have not responded to other treatment. Surprisingly, there is no report of children treated in this way becoming addicted to the medication. For guidance on the use of stimulants in treatment see American Academy of Child and Adolescent Psychiatry (2002) and National Institute for Clinical Excellence (2000).

For a review of the evidence about stimulants as a treatment for this disorder, see College Research Unit of the Royal College of Psychiatrists (1999).

For a general review of management of the disorder, see National Institute for Clinical Excellence (NICE 2005b).

Conduct disorders

Conduct disorders are characterized by severe and persistent antisocial behaviour. They form the largest single group of psychiatric disorders in older children and adolescents.

Clinical features

The essential feature of conduct disorder is persistent abnormal conduct which is more serious than ordinary childhood mischief. The abnormal behaviours centre round defiance, aggression and antisocial acts. In the pre-school period, the disorder usually manifests as defiant and aggressive behaviour in the home, often with overactivity. The behaviours include disobedience, temper tantrums, physical aggression to siblings or adults, and destructiveness. In later childhood, conduct disorder is manifest in the home as stealing, lying, and disobedience, together with verbal or physical aggression. Later, the disturbance often becomes evident outside as well as inside the home, especially at school, or as truanting, delinquency, vandalism, and reckless behaviour, or as alcohol or drug abuse. Antisocial behaviour among teenage girls includes spitefulness, emotional bullying of peers, sexual promiscuity, and running away.

In children older than 7 years, persistent stealing is abnormal. Below that age, children seldom have a real appreciation of other people's property. Many children steal occasionally, so that minor or isolated instances need not be taken seriously. A small proportion of children with conduct disorder present with sexual behaviour that incurs the disapproval of adults. In younger children, masturbation and sexual curiosity may be frequent and obtrusive. Promiscuity may be a particular problem in adolescent girls. Fire-setting is rare, but obviously dangerous.

To constitute conduct disorders, these behaviours have to be more persistent that a reaction to changing circumstances such as adjusting to the arrival in the family of a new step-parent. There is no sharp dividing line between conduct disorder and ordinary bad behaviour; instead there is a continuum on which diagnostic criteria define a cut-off point. The cut-off defines the most severe cases that have the worst outcome and are most in need of help. Much of this help is social or educational, but psychiatrists have an important role in identifying comorbid disorders and arranging multidisiplinary care.

Classification

Both ICD-10 and DSM-IV require the presence of three symptoms from a list of 15, and a duration of at least 6 months. The criteria are closely similar in the two systems of classification.

Because conduct disorders vary widely in their clinical features, both systems divide conduct disorders. In DSM-IV, they are divided into childhood-onset type (onset before 10 years of age) and adolescent-onset type (with onset at 10 years of age or later). DSM-IV has an additional category, '*oppositional defiant disorder*', for persistently hostile defiant provocative and disruptive behaviour outside the normal range but without aggressive or dyssocial behaviour. This disorder occurs mainly in children below 10 years of age. ICD-10 has four subdivisions of conduct disorder: socialized conduct disorder, unsocialized conduct disorder, conduct disorders confined to the family context, and oppositional defiant disorder.

Prevalence

The prevalence of conduct disorders is difficult to estimate because the dividing line between them and normal rebelliousness is imprecise. Approximate rates were established many years ago, and have not been revised by more recent evidence. Rutter *et al.* (1970a) found the prevalence of 'antisocial disorder' to be about 4 per cent among 10–11 year olds on the Isle of Wight. In a subsequent study in London about twice this rate was found (Rutter *et al.*, 1975a, 1976a). A subsequent study in a province of Canada found a rate of 5.5 per cent (Offord *et al.*, 1987). Higher rates have been reported in older adolescents (see Scott 2000). Studies in the community, in psychiatric practice, and in the juvenile courts all indicate that conduct disorders are about three times more common in boys than girls (Rutter *et al.*, 1970a; Gath *et al.*, 1977). Higher rates are associated with low socioeconomic status and large family size.

Aetiology

Environmental factors are important. Conduct disorders are commonly found in children from unstable, insecure, and rejecting families living in deprived areas. Antisocial behaviour is frequent among children from broken homes, those from homes in which family relationships are poor, and those who have been in residential care in their early childhood. Conduct disorders are also related to adverse factors in the wider social environment of the neighbourhood and school (Rutter *et al.*, 1975b).

Genetic factors Conduct disorder clusters in families but twin and adoption studies indicate shared environment is more important than genes. It seems that persistent cases originating in childhood have a stronger genetic aetiology than those starting in adolescence (Silberg *et al.*, 1996). Alcoholism and antisocial personality disorder in the father are reported to be strongly associated with conduct disorder in the children (Earls *et al.*, 1988); the association could be through genetic or environmental mechanisms. There is evidence that a variant of the monoamine oxidase-A gene predisposes to conduct disorder but only when combined with adverse factors in the child's environment (see Foley *et al.*, 2004). If genetic factors are involved, it is not known whether they exert their effect through influencing temperament, or in some other way.

Organic factors Children with brain damage and epilepsy are prone to conduct disorder, as they are to other psychiatric disorders.

Other associations An important finding in the Isle of Wight survey was a strong association between antisocial behaviour and specific reading disorder (see p. 668). It is not known whether antisocial behaviour and reading disorder result from common predisposing factors, or whether one causes the other and, if so, which is primary.

See Earls and Mezzacappa (2002) for a review of the aetiology of conduct disorder.

Prognosis

The long-term outcome of conduct varies considerably with the nature and extent of the disorder. In an important study, Robins (1966) found that almost half of people who had attended a child guidance clinic for conduct disorder in adolescence showed some form of antisocial behaviour in adult life. No cases of sociopathic disorder were found in adult life among those with diagnoses other than conduct disorder in adolescence. Follow-up of conduct-disordered children cared for in children's homes and of controls led to similar conclusions: about 40 per cent of the conduct-disordered children had antisocial personality disorder in their twenties, and many of the rest had persistent and widespread social difficulties below the threshold for diagnosis of a personality disorder. Pervasive social difficulty in adult life was also related to upbringing in a children's home, but conduct disorder had an additional effect when the effect of this variable was controlled (Zoccolillo *et al.*, 1992).

Among **males**, the symptoms and behaviours in adult life usually resemble those in childhood, with antisocial personality traits, aggression, alcohol and drug misuse, and criminality.

Among **females**, the picture in adult life corresponds less closely to that in earlier years, with a range of emotional and personality problems.

Factors predicting poor outcome (see Goodman and Scott, 2005, pp. 68–9) are:

In the young person:

- early onset;
- many and varied symptoms and behaviours;
- severe symptoms and behaviours;
- pervasiveness (at home, in school, and elsewhere);
- associated hyperactivity.

In the family:

- parental psychiatric disorder;
- parental criminality;
- high hostility/discord focused on the child.

Treatment

Mild conduct disorders often subside without treatment other than common-sense advice to the parents. For more severe disorders, treatment for the child is often combined with treatment and social support for the family. Any coexisting disorders (e.g. ADHD, depression) should be treated. There is no convincing evidence that any treatment affects the overall long-term prognosis. Nevertheless, some short-term benefits can often be achieved, and in some cases adverse family factors can be modified in a way that could improve prognosis. Some families are difficult to help by any means, especially where there is material deprivation, chaotic relationships, and poorly educated parents. See Earls and Mezzacappa (2002) and American Academy of Child and Adolescent Psychiatry (1997b) for practice guidelines.

Parent training programmes These programmes use behavioural principles (see p. 662). Parents are taught how the child's antisocial behaviour may be reinforced unintentionally by their attention to it, and how it may be provoked by interactions with members of the family. Parents are also taught how to reinforce normal behaviour by praise or rewards and how to set limits on abnormal behaviour, for example, by removing the child's privileges such as an hour less time to play a game. As aids to learning, parents are provided with written information and videotapes showing other parents applying behavioural procedures. For a review of parent training programmes see Scott (2002).

Anger management Young people who are habitually aggressive have been shown to misperceive hostile intentions in other people who are not in fact hostile. They also tend to underestimate the level of their own aggressive behaviour, and choose inappropriate behaviours rather than more appropriate verbal responses. Anger management programmes seek to correct these ideas by teaching how to inhibit sudden inappropriate responses to angry feelings: for example, the child says to himself 'Stop! What should I do?' They also learn how to reappraise the intentions of other people and use socially acceptable forms of self-assertion.

Other methods Remedial teaching should be arranged if there are associated reading difficulties. Group therapy is seldom helpful (Kazdin, 1997). Medication is of little value unless there is comorbid disorder which is appropriately treated in this way.

Residential care Occasionally, residential placement may be necessary in a foster home, group home, or special school. This should be done only for compelling reasons. There is no evidence that institutional care improves the prognosis for conduct disorder.

Truancy

The treatment of truancy requires separate consideration. A direct and energetic approach is called for. Pressure should be brought to bear upon the child to return to school and, if possible, the support of the family should be enlisted. At the same time, an attempt should be made to resolve any educational or other problems at school. In all this, it is essential to maintain good communications between clinician, parents, and teachers. If other steps fail, court proceedings may need to be initiated.

Juvenile delinquency

A juvenile delinquent is a young person who has been found guilty of an offence that would be categorized as a crime if committed by an adult. In most countries, the term applies only to a young person who has attained the age of criminal responsibility - at present 10 years in the UK, but ranging widely in other countries. Thus delinquency is not a psychiatric diagnosis but a legal category. However, juvenile delinquency may be associated with psychiatric disorder, especially conduct disorder. For this reason, it is appropriate to interrupt this review of the syndromes of child psychiatry to consider juvenile delinquency.

The majority of adolescent boys, when asked to report their own behaviour, admit to offences against the law and a fifth are convicted at some time (West and Farrington, 1973). Most offences are against property. Many fewer girls than boys are delinquent although the ratio has fallen from 11:1. to 4.:1 over the past 40 years. Similar rates have been reported in other countries (D. J. Smith, 1995). Amongst boys who are convicted, only about half are convicted again and few juvenile delinquents continue to offend in adult life. In one study, three-quarters of those with three or more convictions as juveniles went on to offend as adults (Farrington, 2002). In considering these figures, it has to be remembered that crime statistics may be misleading. Nevertheless, there seems to be a substantial similarity in the characteristics of self-reported offenders and of convicted offenders (West and Farrington, 1973).

Delinquency is sometimes equated with conduct disorder. This is wrong, for although the two categories overlap, they are not the same. Many delinquents do not have conduct disorder (or any other psychological disorder). Equally, many of those with conduct disorder do not offend. Nevertheless, in an important group, persistent law-breaking is preceded and accompanied by abnormalities of conduct, such as truancy, aggressiveness, and attention-seeking, and by poor concentration.

Causes

The causes of juvenile delinquency are complex and overlap with the causes of conduct disorder. The causes are reviewed briefly here; for a fuller account see Rutter *et al.* (1998).

Social factors Delinquency is related to low social class, poverty, poor housing, and poor education. There are marked differences in delinquency rates between adjacent neighbourhoods, which differ in these respects. Rates also differ between schools. Many social theories have been put forward to explain the origins of crime, but none offers a completely adequate explanation. For a review of social factors see Farrington (2000).

Family factors Many studies have found that crime runs in families (Farrington *et al.*, 1996). For example, about half of boys with criminal fathers are convicted, compared with a fifth of those with fathers who are not criminals (West and Farrington, 1977). The reasons for this are poorly understood but they may include poor parenting and shared attitudes to the law.

In a much quoted retrospective study, Bowlby (1944) examined the characteristics of 'juvenile thieves' and argued that prolonged separation from the mother during childhood was a major cause of their problems. More recent work has not confirmed such a precise link (see p. 654). Although delinquency is particularly common among those who come from broken homes, this seems to be largely because separation often reflects family discord in early and middle childhood (Rutter and Madge, 1976). Other family factors correlated with delinquency are large family size and child-rearing practices, including erratic discipline and harsh or neglecting care.

Factors in the child: Genetic factors appear to be less significant among the causes of delinquency than in the more serious criminal behaviour of adult life (see p. 732). (The possible role of genetic factors in conduct disorder is considered above.) There are important relationships between delinquency and somewhat below average **IQ** as well as **educational and reading difficulties** (Rutter *et al.*, 1976a). There are at least two possible explanations for the latter finding. Temperament or social factors may predispose to both delinquency and reading failure. Alternatively, reading difficulties may result in frustration and loss of self-esteem at school, and these may in turn predispose to antisocial behaviour. **Physical abnormalities** probably play only a minor role among the causes of delinquency, even though brain damage and epilepsy predispose to conduct disorder.

Assessment

When the child is seen as part of an ordinary psychiatric referral and the delinquency is accompanied by a psychiatric syndrome, the latter should be assessed in the usual way. Sometimes the child psychiatrist is asked to see a delinquent specifically to prepare a court report. In these circumstances, as well as making enquiries among the parents and teachers, it is essential to consult any social worker or probation officer who has been involved with the child.

TABLE 24.7 Assessment of young offenders*

The offence
◆ nature and seriousness
◆ characteristics of victim
◆ motive
◆ role in the group, if others involved
◆ attitude to the offence and the victim
Other problem behaviours
◆ other offences – number, nature, whether detected/convicted
◆ violence
◆ self-harm
◆ cruelty to children or animals
◆ fire-setting

* Modified from Goodman and Scott (2005) Table 7.1.

Psychological testing of intelligence and educational achievements can be useful. Other factors to be taken into account are shown in Table 24.7. The form of the report is similar to that described earlier (p. 660). It should include a summary of the history and present mental state together with recommendations about treatment.

Violence among adolescents

There is concern about increasing rates of violent offences by adolescents. The causes of violent behaviour among young people are not fully understood, and most violent offenders commit other kinds of offence. In the UK, Bailey and Aulich (1997) studied 50 cases of the most extreme form of violence among juveniles – homicide. Many had pre-existing conduct or emotional disorders, and adverse family and social circumstances. A smaller number had learning difficulties. However, none of the 76 features studied separated these young people from other young offenders. Similar findings have been reported from the USA (Meyers and Kemph, 1990). For further information see Bailey and Dolan (2004).

Management

In this section we consider measures intended to reduce the chances of further offending. Many of the children and adolescents who appear before juvenile courts have psychiatric disorders including conduct disorders, mood disorders, attention-deficit hyperactivity disorder, substance misbuse and dependence, learning disability, and epilepsy. These disorders are treated in ways described elsewhere in this chapter.

Psychiatrists who treat delinquent children and adolescents need to understand the legal system in the country in which they work. The legal responses include a warning not to offend again, a fine, the requirement that the parent or guardian take proper control, supervision by a social worker, a period at a special centre, or an order committing the child to the care of the local authority. The exact provisions vary from one country to another. Since delinquent behaviour is common, mainly not serious, and usually a passing phase, it is generally appropriate to treat first offences with minimal intervention coupled with firm disapproval. The same applies to minor offences that are repeated. A more vigorous response is required for more serious, recurrent delinquency. For this purpose a community-based programme is usually preferred, with the main emphasis on improving the family environment, reducing harmful peer group influences, helping the offender to develop better skills for solving problems, and improving educational and vocational accomplishments. In the UK, such a programme has been introduced by the setting up of Young Offender Teams. When this approach fails, custodial care may be considered.

The main aim of the law as it applies to children and young persons is treatment rather than punishment. There has been extensive criminological research to determine the effectiveness of the measures used. The general conclusions are not encouraging, though not surprising since, as explained above, delinquency is strongly related to factors external to the child, including family disorganization, antisocial behaviour among the parents, and poor living conditions. The risk of reconviction are greater among children who have had any court appearance or period of detention than among children who have committed similar offences without any official action having been taken (West and Farrington, 1977).

Of the many special approaches to the treatment of delinquency, three have been shown to have some benefit.

1. **Functional family therapy** (Alexander and Parsons, 1982). The therapist works with the family at home for about three months with the following aims: (i) to motivate the family (ii) to select a specific problem and find how to change it, and (iii) to learn to generalize the problem-solving skills acquired in the second stage.
2. **Multisystemic therapy** (Henggeler *et al.*, 1999) has six elements: (i) family therapy, (ii) helping the young person to find non-delinquent friends, (iii) personal development, including assertiveness training, (iv) improving family problem-solving skills (v) liaison with teachers, and (vi) coordination of other involved agencies.
3. **Multidimensional treatment foster care** (Chamberlain, 1990) The young person lives in a foster home, away from delinquent friends, for about six months and learns better life skills. At the same time, the family are taught skills needed to respond to the young person more effectively.

Studies of these and other approaches indicate the need to match the type of treatment to the needs of the particular offender. Some seem to respond better to authoritative supervision, others to more permissive counselling. However, it is not yet possible to provide any satisfactory guidelines for matching treatment and offender. See Bailey and Dolan (2004) for a review of forensic aspects of child and adolescent psychiatry.

Anxiety disorders

There is no clear dividing line between normal anxiety and anxiety disorders in childhood. In ICD-10, anxiety disorders in childhood are classified as emotional disorders with onset specific to childhood (Table 24.8). DSM-IV does not contain this category and with two exceptions classifies childhood anxiety disorders in the same way as anxiety disorders in adult life. The exceptions are separation anxiety disorder and reactive attachment disorder, which are listed under the heading 'other disorders of infancy, childhood or adolescence'. ICD-10 has a diagnosis of sibling rivalry disorder. DSM-IV does not have this diagnosis in the main classification, but sibling relationship problems can be coded under 'other conditions that may be the focus of clinical attention'. An individual child's disorder may fulfil the criteria for more than one disorder listed in ICD-10 or DSM-IV, for example, phobic disorder and separation anxiety disorder.

Prevalence

The prevalence of anxiety disorders in childhood is uncertain because epidemiological studies have usually employed the wider category of emotional disorder, or asked about symptoms rather than syndromes of anxiety. In their survey of the Isle of Wight, Rutter *et al.* (1970a) found a prevalence of emotional disorders of 2.5 per cent in both boys and girls. In a London suburb, the corresponding figure was doubled (Rutter *et al.*,

TABLE 24.8 Anxiety disorders in childhood

DSM-IV	ICD-10
	F93 Emotional disorders with specific onset in childhood
Separation anxiety disorder	Separation anxiety disorder of childhood
Phobic anxiety disorder*	Phobic anxiety disorder of childhood
Social phobia*	Social anxiety disorder of childhood
Sibling relationship problems†	Sibling rivalry disorder
	*Other anxiety disorders**
Post-traumatic stress disorder*	Post-traumatic stress disorder
Obsessive–compulsive disorder*	Obsessive–compulsive disorder

* There is no separate category for these disorders in childhood; the adult categories are used (see text).

† Listed under 'other conditions that may be the focus of clinical attention'.

1975a). (In both places, the rate of conduct disorder was about twice that of emotional disorder.) More recent surveys of the general population suggest rates of anxiety disorders of 6–9 per cent among 7–11-year-olds, of which about half was separation anxiety disorder (see below) (Anderson *et al.*, 1987; Bird, 1996).

Anxiety at different ages

Anxiety is common in childhood, but its nature changes as the child grows older: infants pass through a stage of fear of strangers; during pre-school years separation anxiety and fears of animals, imaginary creatures, and the dark are common; in early adolescence these fears are replaced by anxiety about social situations and personal adequacy. Anxiety disorders in childhood resemble these normal anxieties and follow the same developmental sequence though they are more severe and more prolonged. Phobias and separation anxiety disorder usually start in early childhood, and social anxiety disorder starts in adolescence.

Separation anxiety disorder

Separation anxiety disorder is a fear of separation from people to whom the child is attached which is clearly greater than normal separation anxiety of toddlers or pre-school children, or persists beyond the usual pre-school period, and is associated with significant problems of social functioning. The onset is before the age of 6 years. The diagnosis is not made when there is a generalized disturbance of personality development.

Clinical picture

Children with this disorder are excessively anxious when separated from parents or other attachment figures, and unrealistically concerned that harm may befall these persons or that they will leave the child. They may refuse to sleep away from these persons or, if they agree to separate, may have disturbed sleep with nightmares. They cling to their attachment figures by day, demanding attention. Anxiety is often manifested as physical symptoms of stomach ache, headache, nausea, and vomiting, and may be accompanied by crying, tantrums, or social withdrawal. Separation anxiety disorder is one cause of school refusal (see p. 689).

Epidemiology

Community surveys suggest that rates of separation anxiety disorder are about 3–4 per cent among 7–11-year-old boys and girls (Anderson *et al.*, 1987; Benjamin *et al.*, 1990).

Aetiology

Separation anxiety disorder is sometimes precipitated by a frightening experience. This may be brief, for example, admission to hospital, or prolonged, for example, conflict between the parents. In some cases separation anxiety disorder develops in children who react with excessive anxiety to a large number of everyday stressors and who are therefore said to have an anxiety-prone temperament. Sometimes the condition appears to be a response to anxious or overprotective parents.

Course

The disorder often improves with time, but may worsen again when there is a change in the child's routine, such as a move of school. Some cases progress to generalized or other anxiety disorders in adult life.

Treatment

Account should be taken of the whole range of possible aetiological factors including stressful events, previous actual separation, an anxiety-prone temperament, and the behaviour of the parents. Stressors should be reduced if possible, and the children should be helped to talk about their worries. It is more important to involve the family, helping them to understand how their own concerns or overprotection effect the child, and to find ways of making the child feel more secure. Anxiolytic drugs may be needed occasionally when anxiety is extremely severe, but they should be used for short periods only. When separation anxiety is worse in particular circumstances, the child may benefit from the behavioural techniques used for phobias as described in the next section.

Phobic anxiety disorder

This diagnosis for children corresponds to specific phobia for adults (see p. 185). Minor phobic symptoms are common in childhood. They usually concern animals, insects, the dark, school, and death. The prevalence of more severe phobias varies with age. Severe and persistent fears of animals usually begin before the age of 5, and nearly all have declined by the early teenage years. At age 11 a rate of only about 2 per cent has been found (Anderson *et al.*, 1987; Milne *et al.*, 1995).

Course

Most improve but a minority, probably 10–15 per cent, persist into adult life (Last *et al.*, 1997).

Treatment

Most childhood phobias improve without specific treatment provided the parents adopt a firm and reassuring approach. For phobias that do not improve, simple behavioural treatment can be combined with reassurance and support. The child is encouraged to encounter feared situations in a graded way, as in the treatment of phobias in adult life. Dynamic psychotherapy has also been used, but it is not obviously more effective than simple behavioural treatment. For a review see Compton *et al.* (2004).

Social anxiety disorder of childhood

This term is used in ICD-10 to describe disorders starting before the age of 6 years in which there is anxiety with strangers greater or more prolonged than the fear of strangers, which normally occurs in the second half of the first year of life. Children with this condition tend to have an inhibited temperament in infancy (Schwartz *et al.*, 1999). These children are markedly anxious in the presence of strangers and avoid them. The fear, which may be mainly of adults or of other children, interferes with social functioning. It is not accompanied by severe anxiety on separation from the parents.

Aetiology and treatment resemble those of other anxiety disorders of childhood.

Sibling rivalry disorder

This category is listed in ICD-10 for children who show extreme jealousy or other signs of rivalry of a sibling, starting during the months following the birth of that sibling. The signs are clearly greater than the emotional upset and rivalry which is common in such circumstances, and they are persistent and cause social problems. When the disorder is severe there may be hostility and even physical harm to the sibling. The child may regress in behaviour, for example, losing previously learned control of bladder or bowels, or act in a way appropriate for a younger child. There is usually opposition to the parents and behaviour intended to obtain their attention, often with temper tantrums. There may be sleep disturbance and problems at bedtime.

In treatment, parents should be helped to divide their attention appropriately between the two children, to set limits for the older child, and to help him or her feel valued.

Post-traumatic stress disorder

Although not included in ICD-10 among the anxiety disorders with onset usually in childhood, post-traumatic stress disorder (PTSD) can occur in childhood life. The clinical picture resembles that of the same disorder in adult life (see p. 157) with disturbed sleep, nightmares, flashbacks, and avoidance of reminders of the traumatic events. Children with PTSD often have irrational separation anxiety, and young children may show regressive behaviour.

Aetiology

As in adults, the cause is an encounter with exceptionally severe stressors, for example, those encountered by children caught up in war, civil unrest, or natural disasters. Physical and sexual abuse may also provoke PTSD in children (Goodwin, 1988). As with adults, cases after vehicle and other accidents are more common than those after the less frequent major disasters. One study found a rate of about 14 per cent of PTSD among children involved in road accidents (Keppel-Benson *et al.* (2002).

Prognosis

The prognosis of the disorder has not been studied systematically in childhood, but severe reactions have been reported to last for 6 months to a year or longer (Yule, 1994).

Treatment

Treatment resembles that for adults (see p. 157). As with adults, immediate counselling (debriefing) is often provided for all those involved in a disaster. At least for adults, the value of this procedure is doubtful, unless cognitive therapy procedures are incorporated to help the victim 'process' the memories of the events (see p. 585). It is likely that the same principles apply to the treatment of children.

Obsessive–compulsive disorders

Obsessive–compulsive disorders are rare in childhood. However, several related forms of repetitive behaviour are common, particularly between the ages of 4 and 10 years. These repetitive behaviours include preoccupation with numbers and counting, the repeated handling of certain objects, and hoarding. Normal children commonly adopt rituals such as avoiding cracks in the pavement or touching lamp posts. These behaviours cannot be called compulsive because the child does not struggle against them (see p. 13 for the definition of obsessive and compulsive symptoms). The preoccupations and rituals of obsessive–compulsive disorder are more extreme than these behaviours of healthy children and take up an increasing amount of the child's time, for example, rechecking schoolwork many times or frequently repeated handwashing.

Clinical picture

Obsessional disorder rarely appears in full form before late childhood, though the first symptoms may appear earlier. The onset may be rapid or gradual.

Obsessional disorders in childhood generally resemble those in adult life (see p. 13). The presenting symptoms are more often rituals than obsessional thoughts. Washing rituals are the most frequent, followed by repetitive actions and checking. Obsessional thoughts are most often concerned with contamination, accidents or illness affecting the patient or another person, and concerns about orderliness and symmetry. The content of symptoms often change as the child grows older. The obsessional symptoms may be provoked by external cues such as unclean objects. Children with obsessional symptoms usually try to conceal them, especially outside the family. Obsessional children often involve their parents by asking them to take part in the rituals or give repeated reassurance about the obsessional thoughts.

Aetiology

Genetic factors are suggested by the observation that obsessive–compulsive disorder is more frequent among the first-degree relatives of children and adolescents with obsessive–compulsive disorder than among the general population (Lenane *et al.*, 1990.) However, the probands in this study had been referred for treatment, and it is possible that this biased the sample since parents with obsessive–compulsive disorder may be more likely to seek treatment for their affected children. Familial aggregation of cases might indicate social learning rather than genetic inheritance but studies of the children of parents with obsessive–compulsive disorder have a variety of emotional disorders, rather than mainly obsessive-compulsive disorders (Black *et al.*, 2003). The association of obsessive compulsive disorder with Tourette syndrome (see below) suggests that they may share genetic causes. At the time of writing, no confirmed linkages have been identified.

Neurotransmitter disorders Studies with adults suggest the involvement of serotonin systems in the brain (see p. 198) and the response of children to SSRIs (see below) suggests that they may share this involvement.

Neurological factors Obsessive–compulsive disorder in childhood is associated with certain conditions thought to arise from dysfunction of the basal ganglia. Some children with obsessive–compulsive disorder have tics or choreiform movements. Conversely, children with Tourette syndrome have obsessional and compulsive symptoms, and these symptoms have also been described in children with Sydenham's chorea (see below).

Autoimmune factors The association with Sydenham's chorea, which is thought to be an autoimmune disorder following Group A beta-haemolytic streptococcal infection, has led to the description of a subtype of childhood-onset obsessive–compulsive disorder with similar aetiology. The condition is known as paediatric autoimmune neuropsychiatric disorder associated with streptococcal infection - PANDAS. See Snider and Swedo (2004) for a review.

See Rapoport and Swedo (2002) for a review of aetiology in general.

Epidemiology

The overall prevalence of obsessive–compulsive disorder in young people up to 18 years of age is between 1–4 per cent (see Flament and Chabane, 2000) with equal rates in males and females. Rates are much lower in young children and rise exponentially with age (Heyman *et al.*, 2001).

Associated disorders

Severe and persistent obsessional thoughts and compulsive rituals in childhood are often accompanied by anxiety and depressive symptoms. In some cases there is an associated anxiety or depressive disorder. As noted above, tics occur in between 17 and 40 per cent of children with obsessive–compulsive disorder (Geller *et al.*, 1996). Many of the children with Tourette syndrome have obsessional symptoms, and it is important to make the distinction between this condition and obsessive–compulsive disorder.

Prognosis

There have been no large long term follow-up studies but the available evidence indicates that obsessive–compulsive disorder in childhood has a generally poor prognosis, often persisting into adult life though sometimes with fluctations in severity (see Rappoport and Swedo, 2002).

Treatment

The first step is to inform the child, the parents and the teachers about the disorder and allow time for questions. When obsessional symptoms occur as part of an anxiety or depressive disorder, treatment is directed to the primary disorder. True obsessional disorders of later childhood are treated along similar lines to the same disorder in adults (see p. 199), with cognitive-behavioural methods, medication, or a combination of the two. Cognitive-behavioural methods have to be modified somewhat with younger children to take account of their stage of development (Piacentini and Langley, 2004). Whatever the treatment, it is important to involve the family.

Medication Both SSRIs and clomipramine are more effective that placebo. (In the UK both sertraline and fluvoxamine are licensed for the treatment of obsessive–compulsive disorder in people under 18). As in adults, the symptoms are reduced but not removed by this treatment: in one trial, with children and adolescents with obsessive- compulsive disorder, treatment with sertraline gave a remission rate of 20 per cent, modest but worthwhile when compared with the placebo rate of 4 per cent. In the same trial, the remission rate with cognitive-behavioural treatment was 40 per cent and of combined treatment 54 per cent (Pediatric OCD Treatment Study Team, 2004).

Immunological treatments have been tried for the PANDAS syndrome (see Snider and Swedo, 2003), but so far without convincing evidence of success.

Somatoform disorders and other unexplained physical symptoms

Children with a psychiatric disorder often complain of somatic symptoms which do not have a physical cause. These complaints include abdominal pain, headache, cough, and limb pains. Most of these children are treated by family doctors. The minority who are referred to specialists are more likely to be sent to paediatricians than to child psychiatrists.

Chronic fatigue syndrome

This condition, which is described on p. 386, occurs in children over the age of 11 years and in adolescents (Farmer *et al*,. 2004). The principles of treatment resemble those for the treatment of the disorder in adults (see p. 388). Cognitive-behaviour therapy, similar to that used for adults (see p. 388), has been found to be effective in adolescents (Stulemeijer *et al.* (2005). Often it is best for treatment to be carried out jointly by a paediatrician and a psychiatrist or clinical psychologist. Although the longer term prognosis for fatigue is probably quite good, the short-term effects on school performance can have serious consequences (Patel *et al.*, 2003).

Recurrent abdominal pain

Recurrent abdominal pain has been estimated to occur in between about 5–17 per cent of all children, and it is a common reason for referral to a paediatrician. In most cases abdominal pain is associated with headache, limb pains, and sickness. Physical causes for the abdominal pain are seldom found and psychological causes are often suspected. Some are related to anxiety, some to 'masked' depressive disorder (see p. 687), and some to stressful events. Treatment is similar to that for other emotional disorders. Follow-up suggests that a quarter of cases severe enough to require investigation by a paediatrician develop psychiatric problems or unexplained physical symptoms in adult life.

Conversion disorders

Conversion disorders (or conversion and dissociative disorder in ICD terminology) are described on p. 206. They are more common in adolescence than in childhood, both in individual patients and in the rare epidemic form of the disorders (see p. 208). In childhood, symptoms are usually mild and they seldom last long. The most frequent symptoms include paralyses, abnormalities of gait, and inability to see or hear normally. As in adults, conversion symptoms can occur in the course of organic illness as well as in a primary conversion disorder. As with adults, organically determined physical symptoms are sometimes misdiagnosed as conversion disorder when the causation physical pathology is difficult to detect and stressful events coincide with the onset of the symptom (Rivinus *et al.*, 1975). For this reason, the diagnosis of conversion disorder should be made only after the most careful search for organic disease.

Epidemiology

Conversion disorders are encountered rarely in community suveys, including the original Isle of Wight study (Rutter *et al.*, 1970a). Among children referred to paediatricians, these disorders have been reported in 3–13 per cent. In a survey of prepubertal children referred to a psychiatric hospital, Caplan (1970) found that conversion disorder was diagnosed in about 2 per cent. In almost half of this 2 per cent, organic illness was eventually detected either near the time or during the 4–11-year follow-up. Amblyopia was the symptom of organic disorder most likely to be originally diagnosed as psychogenic.

Treatment

Conversion and other somatoform disorders should be treated as early as possible before secondary gains (see p. 206) accumulate. The psychiatrist and paediatrician should work closely together. Thorough physical investigation is required before the psychiatric diagnosis is made but unnecessary physical investigation should be avoided. Treatment is directed mainly at reducing any stressful circumstances and encouraging the child to talk about the problem. Symptoms may subside with these measures, or may need management comparable to that used for conversion disorder in adults with physiotherapy and behavioural methods for motor symptoms.

For a review of child psychiatric syndromes with somatic presentation see Garralda (2000).

Mood disorders

Mania is generally thought to be extremely uncommon before puberty although there have been claims that it is more frequent than this (see Biederman, 1998). The following account is therefore concerned with depressive disorders.

It is normal for healthy children to feel depressed in response to distressing circumstances, for example when a parent is seriously ill or a grandparent has died. Some, including those experiencing grief, may also lose interest, concentrate poorly, and eat and sleep badly. This section is not concerned with these normal forms of unhappiness. Neither is it concerned with depressive symptoms that are part of another psychiatric disorder such as anxiety disorder or conduct disorder. **Mood disorders in adolescence are considered on p. 694.**

Clinical picture

The clinical picture of major depression in childhood is in most ways similar to that in adults. The differences are that young children do not express guilt in an adult way, and may have difficulty in describing feelings of sadness. Also their sleep may not be disturbed in the ways found amongst adults with depressive disorder (see p. 694). About a quarter of children with major depressive disorder have evening corticol hypersecretion, and this is especially likely to be present in chronic depressive disorders (see Goodyer *et al.*, 2001).

Masked depression Some pychiatrists have suggested that in children, depressive disorders can present with little or no depressed mood but instead with symptoms such unexplained abdominal pains, headache, anorexia, and enuresis (Kovacs, 1996). However, while these latter symptoms can be the first to be brought to medical attention, their investigation should include the possibility of a depressive disorder. When this is done, history taking and mental state examination will reveal sadness, anhedonia, irritability and other typical symptoms of depressive disorder that were not volunteered initially (Luby *et al.*, 2003).

Epidemiology

Depressive disorders are infrequent before puberty (they are more common thereafter, see p. 694). Estimates of major depressive disorder give figures of 1 per cent of children in middle childhood. Before puberty, rates of depressive disorders are higher among males. They are less likely than depression in adolescence to lead to adult depression, and are more often associated with family dysfunction (Harrington, 2002). Many children who meet diagnostic criteria for depressive disorder also meet the criteria for another diagnosis, especially an anxiety disorder (see Goodyer, 2000). For more information, see Harrington (2002).

Aetiology

The causes of depressive disorder in childhood appear to be similar to those of depressive disorder in adult life (see p. 231).

Genetic factors As noted above, bipolar disorders seem to be rare in childhood so the available information concerns depressive disorders. The rates of depressive disorder among first-degree relatives of children with depressive disorder are greater than the rates in the general population, suggesting genetic factors. Differences in method between studies prevents an accurate assessment of hereditability but it is likely that genetic factors are less important in depression in childhood than they are in adolescence (Rice *et al.*, 2002).

Genetic factors could be acting in several ways. They could: (i) influence directly the biological mechanisms of depression; (ii) increase vulnerability to adverse life events; (iii) and increase the likelihood of experiencing stressful events, for example by causing personality features that lead to the repeated breakdown of relationships (Silberg *et al.*, 1999).

Cortisol As noted above, evening cortisol secretion is increased in some children with major depressive disorder. At an older age, cortisol hypersecretion in non depressed adolescents predicts the onset of depression independently of psychosocial measures (see Goodyer *et al.*, 2003). Such a relationship has not been shown in children, but it suggests the general posssibility that hypersecretion of cortisol could have some direct or indirect causative role.

Other causes Negative **life events** often precede the onset of depressive disorder in children, as they do in adults (Goodyer *et al.*, 1985). **Temperament** also seems important, especially the tendency to react intensely to environmental stimuli (Goodyer *et al.*, 1993). Family environment plays an important part in causing depression in adolescents, especially when a parent has depression (Hammen *et al.*, 2004) and it is likely that the same is true in children.

Prognosis

There are continuities between depressive disorders in childhood and adult life. Harrington *et al.* (1990) followed up people who, when children, had been treated for a depressive disorder diagnosed by criteria similar to those in use today. Of the index group, 58 per cent had a depressive disorder in adult life compared with 31 per cent of a control group. However, members of the index group were no more likely than controls to have other kinds of psychiatric disorder in adult life.

Treatment

General measures Any distressing circumstances should be reduced as far as possible, while the child is helped to talk about feelings. The possibility of depression in the parents should be considered and treated if necessary. With a school-age child, the management plan should involve the teachers to help them understand the effect of depression on the child's performance, and to help to identify and reduce any stressors at school, including bullying. The nature of the disorder is explained to the parents and, in terms appropriate to age, to the child. This explanation, and the approach to possible stressors, should take full account of culture and ethnicity.

Psychological treatment If depression does not improve with the above measures, a specific psychological treatment should be considered. Cognitive therapy, interpersonal therapy, and brief family therapy can be used though most of the evidence for their efficacy is from trials with older children and adolescents.

Medication When a child has failed to respond to psychosocial measures, or the depressive disorder is severe at the outset, drug treatment can be considered. Clinical trials of tricyclic antidepressant drugs for depressed children, have not shown significant benefits but SSRIs, including fluoxetine, have been reported to be more effective than placebo. It has not been established, however, that the benefit is great enough, in relation to potential adverse effects, to justify the general use of SSRIs for childhood depression (Jureidini *et al.*, 2004). This conclusion is the stronger when unpublished trial data are considered as well as published findings (Whittington *et al.*, 2004).

In clinical practice, the decision about medication should be made by a specialist in child psychiatry. The potential benefits and adverse effects are examined for each child, and discussed with the carers and, in appropriate terms, with the child. The information should include the delay between starting medication and improvement, and common side-effects. If an antidepressant is prescribed, it should always be combined with some form of psychological treatment. Of the available drugs, most evidence is available about fluoxetine. At the time of writing, other SSRIs and venlafaxine are not recommended for the treatment of depression in those under 18 (see http://www.mhra.gov.uk/news/2003.htm).

In view of the possibility of relapse, the child's progress should be followed for up to a year after improvement. Very occasionally, when depression is particularly severe and unresponsive to care in the community, it may be necessary to treat the child in hospital.

For guidelines about the care of children with depressive disorders see NICE (2005a).

Suicide in childhood

Suicide in childhood is considered on pp. 412–13.

School refusal

School refusal is not a psychiatric disorder but a pattern of behaviour that can have many causes. It is convenient to consider it at this point in the chapter because of its association with anxiety and depressive disorder. School refusal is one of several reasons for repeated absence from school. Physical illness is the most common. A small number of children are deliberately and repeatedly kept at home by parents to help in the home or for other reasons. Some are truants who could go to school but choose not to, often as a form of rebellion. Finally, school refusers stay away from school because they are anxious or miserable when there. In an important study, Hersov (1960) compared 50 school refusers and 50 truants, all referred to a child psychiatric clinic. Compared with the truants, the school refusers came from more neurotic families, were more depressed, passive, and overprotected, and had better records of schoolwork and behaviour.

Prevalence

Temporary absences from school are extremely common, but the prevalence of school refusal is uncertain. In the Isle of Wight study school refusal was reported in rather less than 3 per cent of 10- and 11-year-olds with psychiatric disorder (Rutter *et al.*, 1970a). It is most common at three periods of school life, between 5 and

7 years, at 11 years with the change of school, and especially at 14 years and older.

Clinical picture

At times, the first sign to the parents that something is wrong is the child's sudden and complete refusal to attend school. More often there is an increasing reluctance to set out, with signs of unhappiness and anxiety when it is time to go. These children often complain of somatic symptoms of anxiety such as headache, abdominal pain, diarrhoea, sickness, or vague complaints of feeling ill. These complaints occur on school days but not at other times. Some children appear to want to go to school but become increasingly distressed as they approach it. The final refusal can arise in several ways. It may follow a period of gradually increasing difficulty of the kind just described. It may appear after an enforced absence for another reason, such as a respiratory tract infection. It may follow an event at school such as a change of class. It may occur when there is a problem in the family such as the illness of a grandparent to whom the child is attached. Whatever the sequence of events, the children are extremely resistant to efforts to return them to school and their evident distress makes it hard for the parents to insist that they go.

Aetiology

Several causes have been suggested. Separation anxiety is particularly important in younger children. In older children there may be a true school phobia, i.e. a specific fear of certain aspects of school life including travel to school. Some fear bullying, or failure to do well in class. Other children have no specific concerns but feel generally inadequate and depressed. Some older children have a depressive disorder.

Prognosis

Clinical experience suggests that most younger children eventually return to school. However, a proportion of the most severely affected adolescents do not return before the time when their compulsory school attendance ceases. There have been few studies of the longer prognosis of school refusal. It seems that of those with the more severe problems, between a third and a half have emotional problems over the next ten years (Berg and Jackson, 1985; Flakierska *et al.*, 1988) This prognosis of less severe cases may be better.

Treatment

Except in the most severe cases, arrangements should be made for an early return to school. There should be discussion with the schoolteachers, who should be asked about the child's problems, asked how they can help the child to catch up with missed education, and advised how to manage any difficulties that mat arise when the child returns. By the time that help is sought, parents often have difficulty in pressuring the child to go to school. It is then more satisfactory for someone other than the parent to accompany the child to school at first. Sometimes the parents need help with their own problems before they can help the child. In severe cases, a more formal graded behavioural programme is necessary. In the most severe cases admission to hospital may be required to reduce anxiety or depression before the child can return to school. Occasionally a change of school is appropriate.

Any depressive disorder should be treated. Otherwise, treatment is psychosocial. In all cases the child should be encouraged to talk about his feelings and the parents given support.

See King and Bernstein (2001) for a review of school refusal.

Other childhood psychiatric disorders

Functional enuresis

Functional enuresis is the repeated involuntary voiding of urine occurring after an age at which continence is usual (see below) in the absence of any identified physical disorder. Enuresis may be nocturnal (bed-wetting) or diurnal (daytime wetting) or both. Most children achieve daytime and night-time continence by 3 or 4 years of age. Nocturnal enuresis is often referred to as primary if there has been no preceding period of urinary continence. It is called secondary if there has been a preceding period of urinary continence.

Nocturnal enuresis can cause great unhappiness and distress, particularly if the parents blame or punish the child. This unhappiness may be made worse by limitations imposed by enuresis on activities such as staying with friends or going on holiday.

Epidemiology

Estimates of prevalence vary, depending on the definition and method of assessment.In the UK, the prevalence of nocturnal enuresis occuring once a week or more is about 10 per cent at 5 years of age, 4 per cent at 8 years, and 1 per cent at 14 years. Similar figures have been reported from the USA. Nocturnal enuresis occurs more frequently in boys. Daytime enuresis has a lower prevalence and is more common in girls than boys. More than half of daytime wetters also wet their beds at night.

Aetiology

Nocturnal enuresis occasionally results from physical conditions but more often appears to be caused by delay in the maturation of the nervous system, either alone or in combination with environmental stressors. There is some evidence for a genetic cause; about 70 per cent of children with enuresis have a first-degree relative who has been enuretic (Bakwin, 1961). Also, concordance rates for enuresis are twice as high in monozygotic as in dizygotic twins (Hallgren, 1960). Linkage has been reported to several different loci (see Super and Postlewaite, 1997), but further research is required before the significance of the findings can be assessed (see Von Gontard *et al.*, 1998 for a review).

Although most enuretic children are free from psychiatric disorder, the proportion with psychiatric disorder is greater than that of other children. Enuresis is more frequent in large families living in overcrowded conditions. Stressful events are associated with the onset of secondary enuresis. Rigid or other particular kinds of training have not been proved to be important.

Assessment

A careful history and appropriate physical examination is required to exclude undetected physical disorder, particularly urinary infection, diabetes, or epilepsy, and to assess possible precipitating factors and the child's motivation. A question should be asked about faecal soiling.

Psychiatric disorder should be sought. If none is found, an assessment should be made of any distressing circumstances affecting the child. The attitudes of the parents and siblings to the bed-wetting are evaluated. The parents are asked how they have tried to help the child, and their motivation to do more is assessed.

Treatment

Any physical disorder should be treated. If the enuresis is functional, an explanation should be given to the child and the parents that the condition is common and the child is not to blame. It should be explained to the parents that punishment and disapproval are inappropriate and unlikely to be effective. The parents should be encouraged to reward success without drawing attention to failure, and not to focus attention on the problem. Many younger enuretic children improve spontaneously soon after an explanation of this kind, but those over 6 years of age are likely to need more active measures.

The next step is usually advice about restricting fluid before bedtime, lifting the child during the night, and the use of star charts to reward success.

Enuresis alarms Children who do not improve with these simple measures may be treated with an **enuresis alarm**. Modern alarms consist of a detector pad attached to the night clothes, and an alarm buzzer carried in a pocket or on the wrist. When the child begins to pass urine the detector is activated and the alarm sounds. The child turns off the alarm, gets up to complete the emptying of the bladder, and changes pyjamas and sheets as necessary, with help from the parents if needed. The method requires about 6–8 weeks of treatment and some families break off before this has been completed.

The enuresis alarm seldom succeeds with children under the age of 6, or those who are uncooperative. For the rest, the alarm method, carried to completion, is effective within a month in about 70–80 per cent of cases, although about a third relapse within a year (Butler *et al.*, 1990). It seems that children with associated psychiatric disorder do less well than the rest.

Medication The synthetic antidiuretic hormone desamino-D-arginine vasopressin (desmopressin) has a more prolonged action than natural vasopressin. It is used in the treatment of nocturnal enuresis in children over five years of age. It can be given as a tablet or in a nasal spray. In one clinical trial about half the enuretic children treated with intranasal hormone became dry (Miller and Klauber, 1990), and good results have been reported for an oral preparation (Skoog *et al.*, 1997). However, patients relapse when treatment is stopped. Side-effects of the oral preparation include rhinitis and nasal pain; other side-effects are nausea and abdominal pain. For this reason it is often used for temporary relief at important times, for example during an overnight stay with friends.

Enuresis can be treated with imipramine in a dose related to the child's age in accordance with the manufacturer's instructions. Most bed-wetters improve initially, but most relapse when the drug is stopped. For this reason and because of their side-effects and the danger of accidental overdose, the tricyclics are seldom used to treat enuresis.

See Clayden *et al.* (2002) for a review of enuresis.

Faecal soiling

At the age of 3 years, 6 per cent of children are still soiling themselves with faeces at least once a week; at 7 years the figure is 1.5 per cent. By the age of 11 years, the figure is only 1 per cent once a month or more. Soiling is three times more frequent in boys than in girls.

The term **encopresis** is used but in two senses. In its wider sense it is a synonym for faecal soiling. In its narrower sense it denotes the repeated deposition of formed faeces in inappropriate places including the underclothes. Because of this ambiguity, the term faecal soiling is used here.

Children who soil their clothes for any reason may feel ashamed, deny what has happened, and try to hide the dirty clothing.

Aetiology

Faecal soiling has several causes:

- **Constipation with overflow** is a common cause. Constipation has many causes, but common ones are low-fibre diet, pain on defecation due, for example, to an anal fissure, or refusal to pass faeces as a form of rebellion. Hirschsprung's disease is an uncommon but important cause. Soiling results when, after prolonged constipation, liquid faeces leak round the plug of hard faeces in the rectum.
- **Fear of using the toilet** Occasionally children who have no pain on passing faeces fear sitting on the toilet for other reasons, for example, for fear that some harmful creature lives there. Shy or bullied children may fear going to the toilet at school.
- **Failure to learn bowel control** This can occur in children with learning disability or children of normal intelligence whose training has been inconsistent or inadequate.
- **Stress-induced regression** Children who have recently learned control may lose it as a result of a highly stressful experience such as sexual abuse.
- **Rebellion** Some children appear to defecate deliberately in inappropriate places and some children smear faeces on walls or elsewhere. Usually the family has many social problems, and often the child has other emotional or behavioural difficulties. The act appears to be a form of aggression towards the parents, though this intention is usually denied by the child.

Treatment

Treatment depends on the cause. The first step is to check for chronic constipation, and if it is present, to treat the cause. For this, joint assessment with a paediatrician may be needed. Even when constipation is not the main cause, it may require treatment as a secondary problem. A child who is fearful of the toilet should be reassured sympathetically. Inadequate toilet training may be improved using behavioural techniques including achievable targets, and star charts or other rewards, together with help for the parents. Stress-induced regression usually disappears when the child has been helped to overcome the trauma. Soiling as rebellion is more difficult to treat since it is generally part of wider social and psychological difficulties which may require intensive and prolonged help. If outpatient treatment fails in these cases, or in those due to inadequate or unsuitable training, the child may respond to behavioural management in hospital. If the child is admitted, the parents need to be closely involved in the treatment to avoid relapse when the child returns home.

Prognosis

Whatever the cause, it is unusual for encopresis to persist beyond the middle teenage years, although associated problems may continue. When treated, most cases improve within a year.

For a review of faecal soiling see Clayden *et al.* (2002) For clinical guidelines on the management of chronic constipation and soiling in children see Felt *et al.* (1999).

Selective mutism

In this condition, sometimes called elective mutism, a child refuses to speak in certain circumstances, although he does so normally in others. Usually speech is normal in the home but lacking in school. There is usually no defect of speech or language, though some children have one. Often there is other negative behaviour such as refusing to sit down or to play when invited to do so. These children often have a comorbid anxiety disorder. The condition usually begins between 3 and 5 years of age after normal speech has been acquired. Although reluctance to speak is not uncommon among children starting school, clinically significant elective mutism is rare, probably occurring in about 1 per 1000 children. Assessment is difficult because the child often refuses to speak to the psychiatrist so that diagnosis depends to a large extent on the parents' account. In questioning the parents, it is important to ask whether speech and comprehension are normal at home. Although psychotherapy, behaviour modification, and speech therapy have been tried, there is no evidence that any treatment is generally effective. In some cases, elective mutism lasts for months or years. A 5–10-year follow-up of a small group showed that only about half had improved (Kolvin and Fundudis, 1981).

For a review see Kolvin (2000).

Stammering

Stammering (or stuttering) is a disturbance of the rhythm and fluency of speech. It may take the form of repetitions of syllables or words, or of blocks in the production of speech. Stammering is four times more frequent in boys than in girls. It is usually a brief problem in the early stages of language development. However, 1 per cent of children suffer from stammering after they have entered school.

The cause of stammering is not known, although many theories exist. It seems unlikely that all cases have the same causes; genetic factors, brain damage, and anxiety may all play a part in certain cases but do not seem to be general causes. Stammering is not usually associated with a psychiatric disorder even though it can cause embarrassment and distress. Most children improve whether treated or not. Many kinds of psychiatric treatment have been tried, including psychotherapy and behaviour therapy, but none has been shown to be effective. The usual treatment is speech therapy.

Tic disorders

Tic disorders including Gilles de la Tourette syndrome are considered on p. 352.

Dementia

Dementing disorders are rare in childhood. They result from organic brain diseases such as lipidosis, leucodystrophy, or subacute sclerosing panencephalitis. Some of the causes are genetically determined and may affect other children in the family. The prognosis is variable. Many cases are fatal, others progress to profound mental retardation.

Schizophrenia

Schizophrenia is almost unknown before 7 years of age, and seldom begins before late adolescence. When it occurs in childhood, the onset may be acute or insidious. The whole range of symptoms that characterize schizophrenia in adult life may occur (see Chapter 12), and in both DSM-IV and ICD-10 the criteria for diagnosis in children are the same as those used with adults; there is no separate category of childhood schizophrenia. Before symptoms of schizophrenia appear, many of these children are odd, timid, or sensitive, and their speech development is delayed. Early diagnosis is difficult, particularly when these non-specific abnormalities precede the characteristic symptoms.

Treatment is with antipsychotic drugs as in the management of schizophrenia in adults, though with appropriate reductions in dosage. The child's educational needs should be met and support given to the family. See Hollis (2002) for a review of schizophrenia in childhood.

Gender identity disorders

Effeminacy in boys

Some boys prefer to dress in girls' clothes and to play with girls rather than boys. Some have an effeminate manner and say that they want to be girls. The cause of this condition is unknown and there is no evidence of any endocrine cause. Various family influences have been suggested, including the encouragement of feminine behaviour by the parents, a lack of boys as companions in play, a girlish appearance, and a lack of an older male with whom the child can identify. However, many children experience these influences without being effeminate.

In **treatment** it is difficult to know how far intervention is appropriate. Associated emotional disturbance in the child may require help, and it may be useful to investigate and discuss any family behaviours that seem to be contributing to or maintaining the child's behaviour. The prognosis is uncertain. Adult males with transvestism and transsexualism frequently recall enjoying feminine play as children, but follow-up studies of effeminate behaviour in early childhood show that the condition is more likely to be associated with homosexuality or bisexuality in adult life than with transsexualism or transvestism (Zuger, 1984; Green, 1985).

Tomboyishness in girls

In girls, the significance of marked tomboyishness for future sexual orientation is not known. It is usually possible to reassure the parents, and sometimes necessary to discuss their attitudes to the child and their responses to her behaviour.

For a review of gender identity disorders see Zucker (2002).

Suicide and deliberate self-harm

Both deliberate self-harm and suicide are rare amongst children less than 12 years of age (though more common in adolescence). These problems are discussed in the chapter on suicide and deliberate self-harm (pp. 412 and 422). For a full account see King and Apter (2003).

Psychiatric aspects of physical illness in childhood

The associations between physical and psychiatric disorders in children resemble those in adults (see Chapters 14 and 16). There are three main groups of association which are met at least as frequently in paediatric as in child psychiatric practice:

1. psychological and social consequences of physical illness;
2. psychiatric disorders presenting with physical symptoms without a physical cause, for example, abdominal pain;
3. physical complications of psychiatric disorders; for example, eating disorders and faecal soiling.

Most medical disorders that may affect children are discussed in the chapter on psychiatry and medicine (Chapter 16). In this section we consider only some problems special to childhood.

The consequences of childhood physical illness

Psychiatric disorder provoked by physical illness

Delirium When physically ill, children are more likely than adults (except the elderly) to develop delirium. A familiar example is delirium caused by febrile illness.

Other psychiatric disorder In the Isle of Wight study of children (Rutter *et al.*, 1970a), the prevalence of psychiatric disorder was only slightly increased with physical illnesses that do not affect the brain, but considerably increased with organic brain disorder or epilepsy.

Other effects Chronic illness may lead to poor reading ability and affect general intellectual development. It may affect self-esteem and the ability to form relationships. These consequences may persist into adult life.

Effect on parents

The effects on parents are greater when the child's physical illness is chronic or disabling. Their response depends on factors such as the nature of the physical disorder, the temperament of the child, the parents' emotional resources, and the circumstances of the family. The parents may experience a sequence of emotional reactions like those of bereavement, and their marital and social lives may be affected. Most parents eventually develop a warm, loving relationship with a handicapped child and cope successfully with the difficulties. A few manage less well: they may have unrealistic expectations, or they may be rejecting or overprotective.

Effect on siblings

The brothers and sisters of children with physical problems may feel neglected, irritated by restrictions on their social activities, or resentful of having to spend so much time helping in the case of the handicapped child. Although some studies have shown more emotional and behavioural disturbances in siblings than would be expected by chance (e.g. Breslau and Prabucki, 1987), most siblings manage well and some even benefit through increased abilities to cope with stress and to show compassion for others.

Management

Everyone involved in the care of physically disabled children should be aware of the psychological difficulties commonly experienced by these children and their families. When giving distressing information to families, it is particularly important to take time. It may be necessary to see the family several times, and to provide continuing advice and support. The paediatrician and the child psychiatrist should collaborate closely, and with each other and with with teachers and any social workers or others involved with the child. Short periods of relief care may be needed to enable the family to continue with the care of a handicapped child.

Advice on imparting to parents the diagnosis of life-threatening illness affecting their children is given by Wooley *et al.* (1989). For childhood cancer see p. 400.

Children in hospital

Bowlby (1951) identified successive stages of protest, despair, and detachment in children who were isolated from the parents during admission to hospital. To avoid these problems it is important to prepare children for admission by explaining in appropriate terms what will happen, and by introducing to them the members of staff who will care for them. Also, the family should be able to visit frequently and, if possible, take some take part in the care of the child. If the child is young, one of the parents should be able to sleep in the hospital if family circumstances allow this.

These arrangments are especially important when hospital admission is long or repeated.

Psychiatric problems of adolescence

There are no specific disorders of adolescence. Nevertheless, special experience and skill are required to apply the general principles of psychiatric diagnosis and treatment to patients at this time of transition between childhood and adult life. It is often particularly difficult to distinguish psychiatric disorder from the normal emotional reactions of the teenage years. For this reason, this section begins by discussing how far emotional disorder is an inevitable part of adolescence. For a general review of problems in adolescence and their treatment, the reader is referred to Goodman and Scott (2005, Chapter 22).

Psychological changes in adolescence

Considerable changes - physical, psychosexual, emotional, and social - take place in adolescence. During this time the young person becomes physically and sexually mature, and develops cognitive abilities comparable to those of adults, though they have still to acquire experience. Adolescents strive to find an identity that reflects their aspirations as well as those of their family, and which is compatible with their abilities and their circumstances. In this process, the influence of the peer group is important as well as that of parents and teachers.

In many less developed countries, the adolescent starts work and gradually takes on more responsibility. In developed countries education continues into mid- or late-adolescence and responsibilities come later. Adolescents are expected both to conform with the rules of society and to become more independent and develop restraints on their own behaviour. Many of the problems of adolescence relate to conflicts between these two expectations, or to the rejection of the rules of society. While such problems are sometimes conspicuous, they are not inevitable. Rutter *et al.* (1976a) concluded that rebellion and parental alienation are uncommon in mid-adolescence, however inner turmoil, as indicated by reports of misery, self-depreciation, and ideas of reference, is present in about half of all adolescents. This turmoil seldom lasts for long and often goes unnoticed by adults. There may also be problems in relationships and sexual difficulties. Among older adolescents, rebellious behaviour increases some become estranged from school during their final years of compulsory attendance. These problems may be expressed as excessive drinking of alcohol, the misuse of drugs and solvents (discussed in Chapter 18), and irresponsible behaviour in driving cars and motorcycles, and of other kinds.

Epidemiology of psychiatric disorder in adolescence

Although psychiatric disorders are only a little more common in adolescence than in the middle years of childhood, the pattern of disorder is markedly different, being closer to that of adults. In adolescence, anxiety is rather less common than in earlier years, and depression and school refusal are more frequent. An epidemiological study of adolescents in the USA (Whitaker *et al.*, 1990) found that the most common disorders were dysthymic disorder, major depression, and generalized anxiety disorder, followed by bulimia and anorexia nervosa, obsessive–compulsive disorder, and panic disorder.

Clinical features of psychiatric disorders of adolescence

Anxiety disorders

School refusal is common between 14 years of age and the end of compulsory schooling, and at this age is often associated with other psychiatric disorders. Generalized anxiety states are less common in adolescence than in childhood. Social phobias begin to appear in early adolescence; agoraphobia appears in the later teenage years.

Conduct disorders

About half the cases of conduct disorder seen in adolescents have started in childhood. Those that begin in adolescence differ in being less strongly associated with reading retardation and family pathology. Among younger children, aggressive behaviour is generally more evident in the home or at school. Among adolescents, it is more likely to appear outside these settings as offences against property. Truancy also forms part of the conduct disorders occurring at this age.

Mood disorders

In depressive disorder of adolescence, depressive mood may be less immediately obvious than anger, alienation from parents, withdrawal from social contact with peers, underachievement at school, substance abuse, and suicide attempts. Bipolar disorder occurs in adolescence and it too may appear first as abnormal behaviours.

Epidemiology Depressive symptoms are more common in adolescence than in childhood. In the Isle of Wight study they were 10 times more frequent among 14-year-olds than among 10-year-olds.

Aetiology The hereditability of major depression in adolescents is greater than in children. As in children genes could act indirectly for example through behaviours that increase negative life events (see p. 687). Independent life events, in the family or elsewhere, interact with the genetic predisposition (Hammen *et al.*, 2004).

Treatment

As with depressed children, a stepped care model is appropriate starting with the general measures described already for childhood depressive disorder (p. 687).

Psychological treatments are considered next. There is more evidence about their effectiveness for adolescents than there is for children, and cognitive-behaviour therapy has been shown to be effective for moderately severe depression (Harrington *et al.*, 1998a, b). There is also some evidence that interpersonal therapy is effective.

Medication For bipolar disorder, lithium usually reduces recurrence in adolescents as it does in adults. There is also some use of other mood-stabilizing drugs such as valproate (see p. 562) Particular care is required in deciding dosage.

For depressive disorders some SSRIs have shown to be effective (Emslie *et al.*, 1997; Keller *et al.*, 2001), but concerns have been expressed about the possibility that the drugs may provoke suicidal thought and behaviour in some people (see p. 546). In the UK, fluoxetine is the only antidepressant drug considered to have a favourable risk:benefit profile. The other SSRIs. Venlafaxine and mirtazapine are not recommended. Tricyclic antidepressant drugs have not shown significant benefits over placebo in depressed adolescents (National Institute for Clinical Excellence, 2005). Medication should be combined with psychological treatment and patients should be monitored for agitation and suicidal thoughts. In a large randomized trial in depressed adolesecents, the combination of fluoxetine and cognitive behaviour therapy was superior to fluoxetine alone which in turn was superior to cognitive behaviour therapy alone (March *et al.*, 2004).

ECT In rare cases, with extremely severe, life-threatening depression, unresponsive to medication, ECT may be considered for older adolescents (National Institute for Clinical Excellence, 2005).

Prognosis Depression in adolescence may recur and is often followed by depression in adult life, and by a long term increase in suicide rate (see Goodman and Scott, 2005, p. 95). Attempts to prevent recurrence of unipolar depressive disorders have not so far been proved effective (Merry *et al.*, 2004). For bipolar disorder, lithium prophylaxis appears to be effective, as in adults (see p. 557).

See Goodyer (2001) for fuller information about depressive disorder in adolescence.

Schizophrenia

Schizophrenia in adolescence is more common in boys than in girls. Usually the diagnosis presents little difficulty. When there is difficulty it is usually in detecting characteristic symptoms, especially in patients whose main features are gradual deterioration of personality, social withdrawal, and decline in social performance. The prognosis may be good for a single acute episode with florid symptoms, but is poor when the onset is insidious.

Eating disorders

Problems with eating and weight are common in adolescence. They are discussed in Chapter 15 since they resemble closely the same conditions in adult life. It is particularly important to involve the parents and perhaps other family members in the treatment of an adolescent patient with eating disorders. Formal family therapy has been shown to be of value for anorexia nervosa in adolescents. For a review see Steiner and Lock (1998).

Suicide and deliberate self-harm

In recent years there has been a marked increase in suicide and deliberate self-harm among adolescents. These subjects are discussed in Chapter 17 (pp. 412 and 422).

Alcohol and substance abuse

Problems of substance abuse in adolescence are similar to those in adults, as described in Chapter 18. Excessive drinking is common among adolescents, especially among those with conduct disorder. Most adolescent heavy drinkers seem to reduce their drinking as they grow older, but a few progress to more serious drinking problems in adult life. Prevention programmes have been developed but there is no evidence they are effective (Foxcroft *et al.*, 1997).

Occasional drug taking is common in adolescence and is often a group activity. The use of cannabis and ecstasy are especially frequent. Solvent abuse is largely confined to adolescence and is usually of short duration (see p. 467). Abuse of drugs such as amphetamines, barbiturates, opiates, and cocaine is less common but more serious, since most drug-dependent adults have experimented with these drugs during adolescence. There is a strong association between conduct disorder in childhood and drug-taking in adolescence (Robins, 1966).

Most adolescents experiment with drugs for short periods and do not become regular users. Those who persist in taking drugs are more likely to come from discordant families or broken homes, to have failed at school, and to be members of a group of persistent drug users. Feelings of alienation and low self-esteem may also be important.

Since regular drug-taking starts less often in adult life than in adolescence, the limitation of drug-taking among adolescents is an important aim, but there is no evidence that it can be achieved. Drug-dependency clinics specifically for adolescents have been provided in the USA, for example, but their effectiveness has not been demonstrated convincingly.

See American Academy of Child and Adolescent Psychiatry (1998c) for advice about the assessment and treatment of adolescents with substance abuse problems.

See Bonomo and Proimus (2005) for a brief account of substance misuse by adolescents.

Sexual problems

Concern about sexuality is normal in adolescence. Sexual abuse is increasingly a cause of referral to psychiatrists (see p. 699).

Teenage pregnancy is an important problem. Most are terminated and some of the remainder are unwanted. There is a raised incidence of prenatal complications as compared with older mothers. Teenage mothers may experience the same post-partum disorders as other mothers (described on p. 402). Very young mothers frequently have difficulties as parents and there is a poor outlook for many teenage marriages. Pregnant teenagers need access to continuing medical and social services during and after pregnancy.

Assessment of adolescents

There are special skills in interviewing adolescents. In general, young adolescents require an approach similar to that used for children, while with older adolescents it is more appropriate to employ that used with adults. It must always be remembered that a large proportion of adolescents attending a psychiatrist do so somewhat unwillingly and also that most have difficulty in expressing their feelings in adult terms. Therefore psychiatrists must be willing to spend considerable time establishing a relationship with their adolescent patients. To do this, they must show interest in the adolescents, respecting their point of view, and talking in terms that they can understand. As in adult psychiatry, it is important to collect systematic information and describe symptoms in detail, but with adolescents the interviewer must be prepared to adopt more flexible approach to the interview.

It is usually better to see the adolescent before interviewing the parents. In this way, it is made clear that the adolescent is seen as an independent person. Later, other members of the family may be interviewed and sometimes the family seen as a whole. As well as the usual psychiatric history, particular attention should be paid to information about the adolescent's functioning at home, in school, or at work, and about relationships with peers. Relevant physical examination should be carried out unless it has been performed by the doctor who made the referral.

Such an assessment should allow allocation of the problem to one of three classes. In the first, no psychiatric diagnosis can be made and reassurance is all that is required. In the second, there is no psychiatric diagnosis but the adolescent, anxious parents or disturbed family need help. In the third, there is a psychiatric disorder requiring treatment.

Treatment of adolescents

Treatment methods are intermediate between those employed in child and adult psychiatry. As in the former, it is important to work with relatives and teachers. It is necessary to help, reassure, and support the parents and sometimes extend this to other members of the family. This is especially important when the referral reflects the anxiety of the family about minor behavioural problems rather than the presence of a definite psychiatric disorder. However, it is also important to treat the adolescent as an individual who is gradually becoming independent of the family. In these circumstances, family therapy as practised in child psychiatry is usually inappropriate and may at times be harmful.

Services for adolescents

The proportion of adolescents in the population who are seen in psychiatric clinics is less than the proportion of other age groups. Of those referred, some of the less mature adolescents can be helped more in a child psychiatry clinic. Some of the older and more mature adolescents are better treated in a clinic for adults. Nevertheless, for the majority the care can be provided most appropriately by a specialized adolescent service provided that close links are maintained with child and adult psychiatry services and with paediatricians. There are variations in the organization of these units and the treatment they provide, but most combine individual and family psychological treatment with the possibility of drug treatment for severe disorders. Most units accept outpatient referrals not only from doctors but also from senior teachers, social workers, and the courts. When the referral is non-medical, the general practitioner should be informed and the case discussed. All adolescent units work with schools and social services. Inpatient facilities are usually limited in extent, so that it is important to agree with social services what kinds of problems need admission to a health service unit and which should be cared for in residential facilities provided (in the UK) by social services. Reasons for admission to a health service inpatient unit include the following:

- severe or very unusual mental symptoms requiring that the person's mental state be observed carefully, investigations carried out, or treatment monitored closely;
- behaviour that is dangerous to the self or others and that is due to psychiatric disorder. When dangerous behaviour relates to personality and circumstances and not to illness, a hospital unit is not more effective than secure residential accommodation, and the behaviour of such adolescents may be stressful for others with mental disorders.

Child abuse

In recent years, the concept of child abuse has been widened to include the overlapping categories of physical abuse (non-accidental injury), emotional abuse, sexual abuse, and neglect. Most of the literature on child abuse refers to developed countries, rather than to developing countries in which children may face poor nutrition, and other hardships such as severe physical punishment, abandonment, and employment as beggars and prostitutes.

The term **fetal abuse** is sometimes applied to behaviours detrimental to the fetus, including physical assault and the taking by the mother of substances likely to cause fetal damage. **Factitious disorder (or Munchausen syndrome) by proxy** is the name given to apparent illness in children, which has been fabricated by the parents, and to conditions induced by parents, for example, by partly smothering the child (see p. 390).

For a general review of child abuse and neglect see Jones (2000).

Physical abuse (non-accidental injury)

Estimates of the prevalence of physical abuse vary with the criteria used. In the United Kingdom about 3 young persons per 1000 of the range 0–18 are on the Child Protection Register (Goodman and Scott, 2005, p. 170). Higher rates have been reported in the US (see Jones, 2000). Less severe injury is probably much more frequent, but often does not come to professional attention.

Clinical features

Parents may bring an abused child to the doctor with an injury said to have been caused accidentally. Alternatively, relatives, neighbours, or other people may become concerned and report the problem to police, social workers, or voluntary agencies. The most common forms of injury are multiple bruising, burns, abrasions, bites, torn upper lip, bone fractures, subdural haemorrhage, and retinal haemorrhage. Some infants are smothered, usually with a pillow, and the parents report an apnoeic attack. Suspicion of physical abuse should be aroused by the pattern of the injuries, a previous history of suspicious injury, unconvincing explanations, delay in seeking help, and incongruous parental reactions. The psychological characteristics of abused children vary but include fearful responses to the parents, other evidence of anxiety or unhappiness, and social withdrawal. Such children often have low self-esteem, may avoid adults and children who make friendly approaches, and may be aggressive.

TABLE 24.9 Risk factors for child abuse

The parent(s)
◆ Youth
◆ Low intelligence
◆ Social isolation/no-one to give help
◆ Breakdown of relationship with partner
◆ Poor parenting skills: lack of awareness of child's needs/harsh punishment/little reward
◆ Experience as a child: abused or neglected
◆ Criminal record
◆ Psychiatric problems: depression/substance abuse/personality disorder
The child
◆ Factors leading to weak attachment to the parents:
◆ Premature/malformed
◆ Separation from mother during early life (e.g. neonatal unit)
◆ Difficult temperament/cries a lot
The environment
◆ Problem neighbourhood: high levels of family violence/problem schools/high unemployment
◆ Little feeling of community
◆ Assessment and management

Aetiology

There are many interacting causes, see Table 16.2.

The environment Child abuse is more frequent in neighbourhoods in which family violence is common, schools, housing, and employment are unsatisfactory, and there is little feeling of community.

The parents Factors associated with child abuse include youth, abnormal personality, psychiatric disorder, lower social class, social isolation, disharmony and breakdown in marriage, and a criminal record. When a parent has a psychiatric disorder, it is most often a personality disorder; only a few parents have disorders such as schizophrenia or affective disorder. Many parents give a history of having themselves suffered abuse or deprivation in childhood. In abusing families, relationships between the parents are harsher and colder than in matched controls (Jones and Alexander, 1978). Although child abuse is much more common in families with other forms of social pathology, it is certainly not limited to such families.

In the children, risk factors include premature birth, early separation, need for special care in the neonatal period, congenital malformations, chronic illness, and a difficult temperament.

Assessment and management

Doctors and others involved in the care of children should always be alert to the possibility of child abuse. They need to be particularly aware of the risks to children who have some of the characteristics described above, or are cared for by parents with the predisposing factors listed.

Points that may raise suspicion include:

- delay in seeking help
- a vague or inconsistent account of the way injuries came about
- an account inconsistent with the nature and extent of injury
- apparent lack of concern for child; defensive or suspicious response to questions.

Doctors who suspect abuse should refer the child to hospital and inform a paediatrician or casualty officer of their suspicions. The pediatrician will carry out a physical examination, noting any of the physical consequences described above. (For further information about the physical examination, see a textbook of pediatrics). In the hospital emergency department, inpatient admission should be arranged for all children in whom non-accidental injury is suspected. If possible, the doctor's concerns should be discussed with the parents, and in any case they should be told that admission is necessary to allow further investigations. If the parents refuse admission, it may be necessary in England and Wales to apply to a magistrate for a Place of Safety Order; similar action may be appropriate in other countries. During admission, assessment must be thorough and include photographs of injuries and skeletal radiography. Radiological examination may show evidence of previous injury or, occasionally, of bone abnormalities such as osteogenesis imperfecta. A CT scan may be needed if subdural haemorrhage is suspected. All findings must be fully documented.

Once it has been decided that non-accidental injury is probable, a senior doctor should talk to the parents. Other children in the family should be seen and examined. In assessing the parents, the following points should be considered (Skuse and Bentovim, 1994):

- Do they acknowledge their part in the abuse?
- Do they accept the need to change their behaviour?
- Do they show a willingness to try new approaches to the child?
- Will they accept help with their personal or relationship problems?

The subsequent procedure will vary according to the administrative arrangements in different countries. In the UK, the Social Services Department should be notified so that they can organize a case conference for the exchange of information and opinions between various representatives of hospital and community services. It may be decided to put the child's name on a child abuse register, thereby making the Social Services Department responsible for visiting the home and checking the problem regularly.

In some cases, the risk of returning the child to the parents is too great and separation is required. If the parents do not agree to separation, a care order can be sought by the Social Services Department. When abuse is severe, prolonged, or permanent, separation may be necessary and parents may face criminal charges. Because there are known cases of injury or death in children returned to their parents, it is vitally important that most careful assessment be made before physically abused children are returned. Countries vary in the requirements and procedures for reporting and monitoring possible physical abuse in children, and readers should inform themselves of the arrangements in the area in which they work.

For further information about the assessment of children who may have been abused, see American Academy of Child and Adolescent Psychiatry (1997a) or Jones (2000).

Prognosis

Children who have been subjected to physical abuse are at high risk of further problems. For example, the risk of further severe injury is probably between 10–30 per cent, and sometimes the injuries are fatal. Abused children are likely to have subsequent high rates of physical disorder, delayed development, and learning difficulties. There are also increased rates of behavioural and emotional problems in later childhood and adult life even when there has been earlier therapeutic intervention (Lynch and Roberts, 1982; Cohn and Daro, 1987). As adults, many former victims of abuse have difficulties in rearing their own children. The outcome is better for abused children who can establish a good relationship with an adult and can improve their self-esteem; and for those without brain damage (Lynch and Roberts, 1982; Rutter, 1985). Some of these outcomes may be related in part to the factors predisposing to abuse, such as poor environment (see above), as well as to the abuse itself.

Emotional abuse

The term emotional abuse usually refers to persistent neglect or rejection sufficient to impair a child's development. However, the term is sometimes applied to gross degrees of overprotection, verbal abuse, or scapegoating, which impair development. Emotional abuse often accompanies other forms of child abuse.

Emotional abuse has various effects on the child, including failure to thrive physically, impaired psychological development, and emotional and conduct disorders (Rutter, 1985). Diagnosis depends on observations of the parents' behaviour towards the child, which may include frequent belittling or sarcastic remarks about him during the interview. One or both parents may have a disorder of personality, or occasionally a psychiatric disorder. The parents should be interviewed separately and together to discover any reasons for the abuse of this particular child; for example, he may fail to live up to their expectations, or may remind them of another person who has been abusive to one of them. The parents' mental state should be assessed. For a review see Hart *et al.* (1998).

Treatment

In treatment, the parents should be offered help with their own emotional problems and with the day-to-day interactions with the child. It is often difficult to persuade parents to accept such help. If they reject help and if the effects of emotional abuse are serious, it may be necessary to involve the social services and to consider the steps described above for the care of children suffering physical abuse. The child is likely to need individual help.

Child neglect

Child neglect is the failure to provide necessary care. It can take several forms including emotional deprivation, neglect of education, physical neglect, lack of appropriate concern for physical safety, and denial of necessary medical or surgical treatment. These forms of neglect may lead to physical or psychological harm including poor academic performance, and disturbed behaviour (Hildyard and Wolfe, 2002).

Child neglect is more common than physical abuse, and it may be detected by various people, including relatives, neighbours, teachers, doctors, or social workers. Child neglect is associated with adverse social circumstances, and is a common reason for a child to need foster care.

Non-organic failure to thrive and deprivation dwarfism

Paediatricians recognize that some children fail to thrive for no apparent organic cause. In children under 3, this condition is called non-organic failure to thrive (NOFT); in older children it is called psychosocial short stature syndrome (PSSS) or deprivation dwarfism.

Clinical picture

Non-organic failure to thrive is caused by the deprivation of food and close affection. In the children seen in the psychiatric service, there is usually evidence of problems in the parent-child relationship since the child's early infancy; these include rejection and, in extreme cases, expressed hostility towards the child. There may be physical or sexual abuse as well. However, not all cases have such causes; in some the failure to thrive is related to abnormal chewing and swallowing mechanisms (Wilensky *et al.*, 1996). The infant who is failing to thrive may present either with recent weight loss, persistently low weight, or reduced height. There may be cognitive and developmental delay. The infant may be irritable and unhappy, or, in more severe cases, lethargic and resigned. There is a clinical spectrum ranging from infants with mild feeding problems to those with all the severe features described above. If food and care are provided, the infants usually grow and develop quickly (Kempe and Goldbloom, 1987).

Psychosocial short stature or 'deprivation dwarfism' These children have abnormally short stature, unusual eating patterns, retarded speech development, and temper tantrums. Although short in stature, the children may be of normal weight. Growth hormone secretion is abnormal (Stanhope *et al.*, 1988). Emotional and behavioural disorders occur and there may be cognitive and developmental delay with impairment of language skills. The children have low self-esteem and are commonly depressed. There is usually a history of deprivation or of psychological maltreatment. Away from the deprived environment, these children eat ravenously.

Treatment

In treating either syndrome, the first essential is to ensure the child's safety, which often requires admission to hospital. Subsequently, some children can be managed at home, but some need foster care. Some parents can be helped to understand their child's needs and to plan for them; other parents are too hostile to be helped. If help is feasible, it should be intensive and should probably focus on changing patterns of parenting. It is unusual for the parents to be psychiatrically ill, but some have severe post-partum depression or other psychiatric disorder.

Prognosis

With both syndromes, the prognosis for severe cases is poor for psychological development and physical growth. The mortality rate is significant (Oates *et al.*, 1985). Some of the less severe cases improve when removed from the abusing environment. Some children have to be placed permanently in foster care because family patterns are resistant to change. The abnormal behaviour is usually lost quickly and mental development follows physical growth (Skuse, 1989).

Factitious disorder by proxy

This condition, in which a parent brings a child for treatment of fabricated symptoms, is discussed on p. 390.

Sexual abuse

The term sexual abuse refers to the involvement of children in sexual activities which they do not fully comprehend and to which they cannot give informed consent, and which violate generally accepted cultural rules. The term covers various forms of sexual contact with or without varying degrees of violence. The term also covers some activities not involving physical contact, such as posing for pornographic photographs or films. The abuser is commonly known to the child and is often a member of the family (incest). A minority of children are abused by groups of paedophiles (sex rings).

Epidemiology

The annual incidence is about 2 per 1000 children per year (Jones, 2000). The prevalence of sexual abuse has been estimated from criminal statistics or from surveys, but differences in definition and thoroughness of reporting making it difficult to interpret published figures. It is agreed that children are more often female - probably about 2–3:1 (Finkelhor, 1986). The offender is usually male. Much sexual abuse takes place within the family, and stepfathers are over-represented among abusers (Russell, 1984). The extent of sexual abuse by women is not known. Faller (1987) reported that four-fifths of the women involved were the mothers of at least one of their victims, and McCarty (1986) found that many of the women abusers reported having been sexually abused themselves as children.

Retrospective studies suggest that between 20–50 per cent of women in populations surveyed recall some experience of abuse in childhood (Peters *et al.*, 1986). These figures include a wide range of experiences, ranging from minor touching to repeated intercourse. Effects on adults of abuse in childhood are described below.

Clinical features

The presentation of child sexual abuse depends on the type of sexual act and the relationship of the offender to the child. Children are more likely to report abuse when the offender is a stranger. Sexual abuse may be reported directly by the child or a relative, or it may present indirectly with unexplained problems in the child, such as physical symptoms in the urogenital or anal area, pregnancy, behavioural or emotional disturbance, or precocious or otherwise inappropriate sexual behaviour. In adolescent girls, running away from home or unexplained suicide attempts should raise the suspicion of sexual abuse. When abuse occurs within the family, marital and other family problems are common.

Effects of sexual abuse

Early emotional consequences of sexual abuse include anxiety, fear, depression, anger, and inappropriate sexual behaviour, as well as reactions to any unwanted pregnancy. A sense of guilt and responsibility is common. Some children show signs of post-traumatic stress disorder. It is not certain how common these reactions are, or how they relate to the nature and circumstances of the abuse.

Long-term consequences include depressed mood, low self-esteem, self-harm, difficulties in relationships, and sexual maladjustment in the form of either hypersensitivity or sexual inhibition. Effects of abuse are generally greater when the abuse has involved physical violence and penetrative intercourse. Some of the long-term effects may be related to the events surrounding the disclosure of the abuse, including any legal proceedings, and to other problems in the family such as neglect of the children and sexual deviance or substance abuse (Seghorn *et al.*, 1987). Nevertheless, even when these other factors are controlled for, sexual abuse in childhood seems to be associated with psychiatric disorder later in life, especially with depressive disorders, anxiety disorders and personality disorders (Spataro *et al.*, 2004).

Aetiology

Sexual abuse of children occurs in all socioeconomic groups though it is more frequent among socially deprived families. However there is not the strong association with low social class found with physical abuse. Finkelhor (1984) suggests that there are several preconditions which make sexual abuse more likely: in the abuser, deviant sexual motivation, impulsivity, a lack of conscience, and a lack of external restraints (for example, cultural tolerance); in the child, a lack of resistance (through insecurity, ignorance, or other causes of vulnerability).

Assessment

It is important to be ready to detect sexual abuse and to give serious attention to any complaint by a child of being abused in this way. When abuse has been established, it is important to assess whether it is likely to continue if the child remains at home and, if so, how dangerous it is likely to be. It is also important not to make the diagnosis without adequate evidence, which requires social investigation of the family as well as psychological and physical examination of the child.

The child should be interviewed sympathetically and encouraged to describe what has happened. Drawings or toys may help younger children to give a description, but great care must be taken to ensure that they are not used in a way that suggests to the child, events that have not taken place. Young children can recall events accurately, but they are more suggestible than adults. Interviewing is difficult and whenever possible it should be carried out by a child psychiatrist or social worker with special experience. See Jones (2003) for further advice on interviewing.

At an appropriate time it is often necessary to arrange a physical examination, including inspection of the genitalia and anal region and, if intercourse may have taken place within 72 hours, the collection of specimens from the genital and other regions. Usually this physical examination should be carried out by a paediatrician or police surgeon with special experience in the problem (see Royal College of Physicians, 1991 for advice about physical examination).

The final decision as to whether abuse has taken place should be made after collecting information from the child, the physical examination, and social enquiries about the family. The decision is followed by steps to protect the child. The arrangements vary in different countries, and readers should find out how they apply in the country in which they are working.

For further information about assessment see American Academy of Child and Adolescent Psychiatry (1997a).

Management

The initial management and the measures to protect the child are similar to those for physical abuse (see p. 697), including a decision about separating the child from the family. There are particular difficulties involved in intervening with families in which sexual abuse has occurred. These include a marked tendency to deny the seriousness of the abuse and of other family problems, and in some cases deviant sexual attitudes and behaviour of other family members, possibly including other children. Individual and group treatment has been used for the offenders with the general aim of enabling the person to reduce denial and consider the effects of the abuse on the child. If the mother has a history of abuse, this needs to be discussed to help her understand how this may have affected her response to her child's abuse.

Some sexually abused children have highly abnormal sexual development for which they require help. They also need counselling to help them to deal with the emotional impact of the abuse, to come to terms with it, and to improve low self-esteem. Help should be in the form of a staged programme of rehabilitation for the whole family rather than a brief intervention. Of the specific interventions, cognitive therapy has the best evidence for efficacy for sexually abused children who have psychiatric symptoms (Ramchandani and Jones, 2003).

For a review of the treatment of child sexual abuse see Jones (2000).

Ethical and legal problems in child and adolescent psychiatry

As well as the ethical and legal problems related to the treatment of adults and discussed in Chapter 3 and elsewhere, the following issues are particularly likely to arise in the care of children with psychiatric disorders.

Conflicts of interest

In general, the interests of the child take precedence over those of the parents. This principle is most obvious, and most easily followed, in cases of child abuse. In other cases, the decision is more difficult, for example, when a depressed mother is neglecting her child and is likely to become more depressed if substitute care is arranged. Such problems can usually be resolved by discussion with the parents, and between the professionals caring for the child and for the parent.

Confidentiality

The care of children often involves collaboration between medical and social services, and sometimes with teachers. Different agencies may have different policies about the confidentiality of records, and doctors should take account of these differences when deciding what information to disclose.

Consent

In each country, the law decides an age below which parents give consent on behalf of the child. Below this age, the child's agreement should be obtained, if possible, since this will aid treatment, but if the child refuses the parents can decide. This problem arises, for example, when an adolescent under the legal age of consent refuses treatment for anorexia nervosa. The parents can also refuse treatment; however, their right to do so is linked to their duty to protect the child. In cases in which the parents' refusal appears not to be in the interests of the child, countries generally have provisions for a decision by a court of law.

Some of the complexities of English law can be mentioned briefly to illustrate the problems that have to be resolved in all legal systems. A fuller account of these and other issues is given by Hope *et al.* (2003). Readers should find out how these issues are dealt with in the country in which they are working before they undertake the care of patients under the age at which adult rules of consent apply.

In English law, the age from which people are judged legally capable of giving or refusing consent is 18 years. However, English law recognizes that most of those aged between 16 and 18 years have the capacity to give consent to treatment and allows them to do so without the need for consent by a parent. The position is less clear when a 16- or 17-year-old does not consent to treatment but it is probably the case that the parents' consent is sufficient. The decision in each case is likely to depend on the consequences of refusal; the more severe these are, the more likely is it that a court would accept that the child's refusal can be overridden by the parents. Further complexities arise with children under 16, some of whom are competent to give consent to certain treatments. There is no general assumption of competence at this age, and it has to be established in the individual case, but if it is established, the minor can give consent. The question arose most notably in respect to the provision of contraception without the additional consent of a parent. In the Gillick case, it was ruled that, in English law, the minor could consent without the need to obtain the consent of the parent. It is probable, however, that with certain more invasive and risky treatments, the consent of a parent could be legally necessary - as well as clinically desirable. If a minor under the age of 16 years refuses treatment, this can be overruled by the parents if refusal is likely to result in harm. A final complexity concerns the definition of a parent. This problem arises, for example, when the person accompanying the child is not the person recognized by the law as having parental responsibility. For example, in English law, a father who is not married to the mother does not automatically have legal responsibility.

Consent for research poses similar problems for subjects below the legal age of consent. In most countries, parents consent on behalf of their children, and they may find it difficult to balance the risks to the child against the benefits, which are usually not to their child but to other children who might be treated for the same condition in the future. It is important that they are able to discuss the issues fully, and generally with a person additional to the person who is requesting the consent (for example, a nurse). Guidelines on British have been published, for example, British Paediatric Association (1992). For a brief account see Larcher (2005).

Further reading

Black, D, Hendriks, JH and Wolkind, S (eds) (1998) *Child psychiatry and the law*, 3rd edn. Gaskell, London. (Deals with all aspects of child psychiatry and the law, within the framework of English law. Directly relevant to those working in the UK, although the general issues apply more widely.)

Gelder, MG, López-Ibor, JJ Jr and Andreasen, NC (eds) (2000) *New Oxford textbook of psychiatry*, Part 9: Child and adolescent psychiatry. Oxford University Press, Oxford. (The 33 chapters in this part of the textbook provide a comprehensive account of the subject written for the general psychiatrist.)

Goodman, R and Scott, S (2005) *Child psychiatry*, 2nd edn. Blackwell Science, Oxford. (A concise introduction to the subject.)

Hopkins, B, Ronalg, RG, Michel, GF and Rochat, P (2004) *The Cambridge enclyclopaedia of child development*. Cambridge University Press, Cambridge. (A comprehensive source of information about child development.)

Rutter, M and Taylor, E (eds) (2002) *Child and adolescent psychiatry*, 4th edn. Blackwell, Oxford. (An established, comprehensive work of reference.)

APPENDIX History taking and examination in child psychiatry

The format and extent of an assessment will depend on the nature of the presenting problem. The following scheme is taken from the book by Graham (1991), which should be consulted for further information. Graham suggests that *clinicians with little time available should concentrate on the items in bold type*

1 **Nature and severity of presenting problem(s). Frequency. Situations in which it occurs. Provoking and ameliorating factors. Stresses thought by parents to be important.**

2 **Presence of other current problems or complaints.**
- (a) **Physical.** Headaches, stomach ache. Hearing, vision. Seizures, faints, or other types of attacks.
- (b) Eating, sleeping, or elimination problems.
- (c) **Relationship with parents and siblings. Affection, compliance.**
- (d) Relationships with other children. Special friends.
- (e) Level of activity, attention span, concentration.
- (f) Mood, energy level, sadness, misery, depression, suicidal feelings. General anxiety level, specific fears.
- (g) Response to frustration. Temper tantrums.
- (h) Antisocial behaviour. Aggression, stealing, truancy.
- (i) **Educational attainments, attitude to school attendance.**
- (j) Sexual interest and behaviour.
- (k) Any other symptoms, tics, etc.

3 Current level of development.
- (a) Language: comprehension, complexity of speech.
- (b) Spatial ability.
- (c) Motor coordination, clumsiness.

4 Family structure.
- (a) Parents. Ages, occupations. **Current physical and emotional state**. History of physical or psychiatric disorder. Whereabouts of grandparents.
- (b) Siblings. Ages, presence of problems.
- (c) Home circumstances: sleeping arrangements.

5 Family function.
- (a) **Quality of parental relationship. Mutual affection. Capacity to communicate about and resolve problems. Sharing of attitudes over child's problems.**
- (b) **Quality of parent-child relationship. Positive interaction: mutual enjoyment. Parental level of criticism, hostility, rejection.**
- (c) Sibling relationships.
- (d) Overall pattern of family relationships. Alliance, communication. Exclusion, scapegoating. Intergenerational confusion.

6 Personal history.
- (a) Pregnancy complications. Medication. Infectious fevers.
- (b) Delivery and state at birth. Birth weight and gestation. Need for special care after birth.
- (c) Early mother-child relationship. Post-partum maternal depression. Early feeding patterns.
- (d) Early temperamental characteristics. Easy or difficult, irregular, restless baby and toddler.
- (e) Milestones. Obtain exact details only if outside range of normal.
- (f) **Past illnesses and injuries. Hospitalizations.**
- (g) Separations lasting a week or more. Nature of substitute care.
- (h) Schooling history. Ease of attendance. Educational progress.

7 **Observation of a child's behaviour and emotional state.**
- (a) Appearance. Signs of dysmorphism. Nutritional state. Evidence of neglect, bruising, etc.
- (b) Activity level. Involuntary movements. Capacity to concentrate.
- (c) Mood. Expression of signs of sadness, misery, anxiety, tension.
- (d) Rapport, capacity to relate to clinician. Eye contact. Spontaneous talk. Inhibition and disinhibition.
- (e) Relationship with parents. Affection shown. Resentment. Ease of separation
- (f) Habits and mannerisms.
- (g) Presence of delusions, hallucinations, thought disorder.
- (h) Level of awareness. Evidence of minor epilepsy.

8 Observation of family relationships.
- (a) Patterns of interaction – alliances, scapegoating.
- (b) Clarity of boundaries between generations: enmeshment.
- (c) Ease of communication between family members.
- (d) Emotional atmosphere of family. Mutual warmth. Tension, criticism.

9 Physical examination of child.

10 Screening neurological examination.
- (a) Note any facial asymmetry
- (b) Eye movements. Ask the child to follow a moving finger and observe eye movement for jerkiness, incoordination.
- (c) Finger-thumb apposition. Ask the child to press the tip of each finger against the thumb in rapid succession. Observe clumsiness, weakness.
- (d) Copying patterns. Drawing a man.
- (e) Observe grip and dexterity in drawing.
- (g) Jumping up and down on the spot.
- (h) Hopping.
- (i) Hearing. Capacity of child to repeat numbers whispered two metres behind him.

CHAPTER 25

Learning disability (mental retardation)

Chapter contents

This chapter is concerned with a general outline of the features, epidemiology, and aetiology of learning disability (mental retardation), the organization of services and, more specifically, with the psychiatric disorders affecting these people. Many of the psychiatric problems of children with learning disability are similar to those of children of normal intelligence; an account of these problems is given in Chapter 24 on child psychiatry.

Terminology

Over the years, several terms have been applied to people with intellectual impairment from early life. In the nineteenth and early-twentieth centuries, the word idiot was used for people with severe intellectual impairment, and imbecile for those with moderate impairment. The special study and care of such people was known as the field of **mental deficiency**. When these words came to carry stigma, they were replaced by the terms **mental subnormality and mental retardation**. The term **mental handicap** has also been widely used, but now the term **learning disability** is generally preferred in the UK. However, the term mental retardation is still used in ICD-10 and DSM-IV, and is employed in many countries. Moreover, in the US the term learning disability is generally applied to dyslexia and similar forms of specific disability rather than to mental retardation. For this reason the term **intellectual disability** is gaining acceptance, but it is not yet used so widely that we judge it appropriate to adopt it in this chapter, where we continue to use the term learning disability unless the historical or other context requires otherwise.

The development of ideas about learning disability

A fundamental distinction has to be made between general intellectual impairment starting in early childhood (learning disability or mental retardation) and intellectual impairment developing later in life (dementia). In 1845, Esquirol made this distinction when he wrote:

> Idiocy is not a disease, but a condition in which the intellectual faculties are never manifested; or have never been developed sufficiently to enable the idiot to acquire such an amount of knowledge as persons of his own age and placed in similar circumstances with himself are capable of receiving.
>
> (Esquirol, 1845, pp. 446–7)

Early in the twentieth century, Binet's tests of intelligence provided quantitative criteria for ascertaining the condition. These tests also made it possible to identify lesser degrees of the condition that might not be obvious otherwise (Binet and Simon, 1905). Unfortunately, it was widely assumed at the time that people with such lesser degrees of intellectual impairment were socially incompetent and required institutional care.

Similar views were reflected in the legislation of the time. For example, in England and Wales the Idiots Act of 1886 made a simple distinction between idiocy (more severe) and imbecility (less severe). In 1913, the Mental Deficiency Act added a third category for people who 'from an early age display some permanent mental defect coupled with strong vicious or criminal propensities in which punishment has had little or no effect'. As a result of this legislation, people of normal or near normal intelligence were admitted to hospital for long periods simply because their behaviour offended against the values of society. Although some of these people had committed crimes, others had not: for example, girls whose repeated illegitimate pregnancies were interpreted as a sign of the 'criminal' propensities mentioned in the Act.

Although, in the past, the use of social criteria clearly led to abuse, it is unsatisfactory to define mental retardation in terms of intelligence alone. Social criteria must be included, since a distinction must be made between people who can lead a normal or near-normal life and those who cannot. DSM-IV defines mental retardation as:

> a significantly sub-average general intellectual functioning, that is accompanied by significant limitations in adaptive functioning in at least two of the following skill areas: communication, self-care, home living, social/interpersonal skills used for community resources, self direction, functional academic skills, work, leisure, health and safety

and having an onset before the age of 18. Having defined the disorder in this way, it is subdivided by level of intelligence. In both ICD-10 and DSM-IV the subtypes are: mild (IQ 50–70); moderate (IQ 35–49); severe (IQ 20–34); profound (IQ below 20).

The original WHO classification of impairment, disability, and handicap is useful when considering the problems of people with learning disability. (WHO now employs a more positive terminology with activity replacing disability, and participation replacing handicap.) The impairment is of the central nervous system; the disability (or limitation of activity) is in learning and acquiring new skills. The extent to which impairement leads to disability (limits activity) depends, in part, on experiences in the family and at school, and on the correction of associated problems such as deafness. The final stage, handicap (or limited participation), depends on the degree of disability and on other factors such as the support that is provided.

Educationalists use other terms and these differ between countries. In the UK, the term is **special needs**, whereas in the USA, three groups are recognized: educable mentally retarded (EMR), trainable mentally retarded (TMR), and severely mentally retarded (SMR).

Epidemiology

Epidemiology of learning disability

In 1929, in an important survey of schoolchildren in six areas of the UK, E. O. Lewis found that the total prevalence of mental retardation was 27 per 1000, and the prevalence of moderate and severe learning disability (IQ less than 50) was 3.7 per 1000. Subsequent studies in many countries have broadly confirmed these early findings. In the population aged 15–19, the prevalence of moderate and severe learning disabilities is between 3.0 and 4.0 per 1000. The prevalence of moderate and severe learning disability has changed little since the 1930s. However, **incidence** of severe learning disability has fallen substantially, because antenatal, natal, and neonatal care have improved. The reason that prevalence has not changed is because people with learning disability are living longer, particularly those with Down syndrome. This change has also affected the age distribution of people with severe learning disability, so that the number of adults has increased.).

Tizard (1964) drew attention to the distinction between **'administrative' prevalence** and 'true' prevalence. He defined administrative prevalence as 'the numbers for whom services would be required in a community which made provision for all who needed them'. (In practice, the term usually means the number with needs who are known to the service providers.) If the true prevalence of all levels of learning disabilities (IQ less than 70) is 20–30 per 1000 of the population of all ages (Broman *et al.*, 1987), then the administrative prevalence is about 10 per 1000 of all ages. In other words, less than half of all such people require special provision. Administrative prevalence is higher in lower socioeconomic groups and in childhood when more people need services. It falls after the age of 16 (Richardson, 1992) because there is continuing slow intellectual development and gradual social adjustment.

For a review of the epidemiology of learning disability see Fryers (2000).

Epidemiology of psychiatric disorder among people with learning disability

The published rates of psychiatric disorder among people with learning disability vary widely because of difficulties with the case ascertainment, detection and definition. Old studies primarily had the selection bias of including mainly people from institutions. Although more recent studies have included people from the community, it is difficult if not impossible to detect all adults with learning disabilities – particularly those with mild disability. Different studies have used different methods of case detection, varying from from the study of case notes to direct interviews with subjects. The diagnostic criteria used in different studies have also varied: some used screening instruments, others used structured diagnostic instruments. Also studies have varied in whether they included behaviour disorders in the count of psychiatric disorders.

In an important early survey of all children aged 9–11 years with an IQ under 70, Rutter *et al.* (1970a) found that almost a third were rated as 'disturbed' by their parents, whilst about 40 per cent were so rated by their teachers. These rates were three to four times higher than the rates among intellectually normal children. Among children with severe learning disabilities, most surveys using standardized instruments have found that about half have psychiatric disorder, with the highest rates among those with the most profound learning disabilities (see Scott, 1994).

There is no statistically significant difference in the point prevalence of schizophrenia, mood disorders or anxiety disorders between adults with mild to moderate learning disability and adults in the general population (Deb *et al.*, 2001a). If, however, diagnoses such as behaviour disorder and personality disorder are added, the rates among the learning disabled rise quite considerably (Deb *et al.*, 2001b). Some childhood-onset disorders such as autism and attention deficit hyperactivity disorder may also be more frequent among adults with learning disability compared with the genera adult population, though there is uncertainty because these disorders are not generally included in surveys of the adult population. Among people with severe learning disability, certain kinds of behaviour disorder are especially frequent, notably hyperactivity, stereotypies, and self-injury (Deb *et al.*, 2001c).

Clinical features of learning disability

General description

The most frequent manifestation of learning disability is uniformly low performance on all kinds of intellectual tasks including learning, short-term memory, the use of concepts, and problem-solving. Specific abnormalities may lead to particular difficulties. For example, lack of visuospatial skills may cause practical difficulties, such as inability to dress, or there may be disproportionate difficulties with language or social interaction, both of which are strongly associated with behaviour disorder. Among children with learning disability, the common behaviour problems of childhood tend to occur when they are older and more physically developed than children in the general population, and the problems last longer. Such behaviour problems usually improve slowly as the child grows older but may be replaced by problems that start in adult life.

Mild learning disability (IQ 50–70)

People with mild learning disability account for **about 85 per cent** of people with learning disability. Usually their appearance is unremarkable and any sensory or motor deficits are slight. Most people in this group develop more or less normal language abilities and social behaviour during the pre-school years, and their learning disability may never be formally identified. In adult life, most people with learning disability can live independently in ordinary surroundings, though they may need help in coping with family responsibilities, housing and employment, or when under unusual stress.

Moderate learning disability (IQ 35–49)

People in this group account for **about 10 per cent** of those with learning disability. Many have better receptive than expressive language skills, which is a potent cause of frustration and behaviour problems. Speech is usually relatively simple and often better understood by people who know the patient well. Many make use of simplified signing systems such as Makaton sign language. Activities of daily living such as dressing, feeding, and attention to hygiene are usually acquired over time but other activities of daily living such as the use of money and road sense generally require support. Similarly, supported employment and residential provision are the rule.

Severe learning disability (IQ 20–34)

It is difficult to estimate IQ accurately when the score is below 34 because of the difficulty in administering the tests in a valid manner to people in this group. Estimates suggest that people with severe learning disability account for **about 3–4 per cent** of the learning disabled. In the pre-school years their development is usually greatly slowed. Eventually many of them can be helped to look after themselves under close supervision and to communicate in a simple way, for example, by using objects of reference. As adults they can undertake simple tasks and engage in limited social activities, but they need supervision and a clear structure to their lives.

Profound learning disability (IQ below 20)

People in this group account for **1–2 per cent** of people with learning disability. Development across a range of domains tends to be around the level expected of a 12-month-old infant. Accordingly, people with profound learning disability are a vulnerable and highly needy group who require support and supervision, even for simple activities of daily living.

TABLE 25.1 Features of mild, moderate, severe and profound learning disability

	Mild	Moderate	Severe/profound
IQ range	69–50	49–35	<35
Percentage of cases	85%	10%	5%
Ability to self-care	Independent	Need some help	Limited
Language	Reasonable	Limited	Basic or none
Reading and writing	Reasonable	Basic	Minimal or none
Ability to work	Semi-skilled	Unskilled, supervised	Supervised basic tasks
Social skills	Normal	Moderate	Few
Physical problems	Rare	Sometimes	Common
Aetiology discovered	Sometimes	Often	Usually

Physical disorders among people with learning disability

Physical disorders are common among people with learning disability but they are not always identified. A person with learning disability may not complain of feeling ill, and conditions may be noticed only because of changes in behaviour. Relatives should be told of the possible significance of such changes and encouraged to seek help. Clinicians should be aware of associations between certain learning disability syndromes and physical illness (see, for example, Down syndrome, p. 717).

Sensory and motor disabilities, and incontinence are the most important physical disorders in people with learning disability. People with severe learning disability (especially children) usually have one or often several of these problems. Only a third are continent, ambulant, and without severe behaviour problems. A quarter are highly dependent on other people. Among the people with mild learning disability, similar problems occur, but less frequently. Nevertheless, they are important because they determine whether special educational programmes are needed. Sensory disorders add an important additional obstacle to normal cognitive development. Motor disabilities include spasticity, ataxia, and athetosis.

Ear infections and dental caries are common in this population. As children grow older, the likelihood of physical problems increases in people with both mild and severe learning disability. (Cooper, 1999).

Epilepsy Between about 14–24 per cent of people with learning disabilities have a history of epilepsy, compared with 5 per cent in the general population. The prevalence is much higher among those who also have an associated neurological disorder. The rate also increases with the severity of learning disabilities. A lifetime history of epilepsy is present in approximately 7–15 per cent of people with mild to moderate learning disability, 45–67 per cent of those with severe learning disability, and about 50–82 per cent of people with profound learning disability.

Epilepsy is more commonly associated with certain causes of learning disability such as Fragile X syndrome, tuberous sclerosis, Angelman syndrome, Rett syndrome and Neuronal Migration Disorders (NMDs). Certain epilepsy syndromes such as West's syndrome and Lennox-Gastaut syndrome are more common among people with learning disability. The proportion of people with drug-resistant epilepsy is also greater among people with learning disability than in the general population These people tend to have multiple seizure types with an early age of onset and a long duration (for a review see Deb, 2000).

Psychiatric disorders among people with learning disability

In the past, psychiatric disorder amongst the learning disabled was often viewed as different from that seen in people of normal intelligence. One view was that people with learning disability did not develop emotional disorders; another view was that they developed these disorders but that the causes were biological rather than psychosocial. It is now generally agreed that people with learning disability experience psychiatric disturbances similar to those affecting the general population. However, the symptoms are sometimes modified by low intelligence (Deb *et al.*, 2001a). Delusions, hallucinations, and obsessions may not be easily recognized in people who have limited language development and cannot easily describe them. Hence in diagnosing psychiatric disorder among people with learning disability, more emphasis may have to be given to behaviour and less to reports of mental phenomena than would be the case in people of normal intelligence.

The reported **prevalences of psychiatric disorders** among the learning disabled are higher than those in the general population, but because of methodological problems, the range of estimates is wide (Scott, 1994). The problems include the definition and recognition both of the learning disability and of the psychiatric disorder, as well as problems of sampling. The lower the IQ, the greater the difficulty in diagnosing psychiatric syndromes. For a review of these problems among children see Einfield and Tonge (1996); and among adults see Deb *et al.* (2001a, b).

Schizophrenia

The point prevalence of schizophrenia in people with learning disability is about 3 per cent compared with 1 per cent in the general population (Deb *et al.*, 2001b).

In the clinical picture, delusions may be less elaborate than in schizophrenics of normal intelligence, and hallucinations may have a simpler content. When IQ is less than 45, it is difficult to make a diagnosis of schizophrenia with any certainty. Furthermore, some of the symptoms of underlying brain damage such as stereotyped movements and social withdrawal may wrongly suggest schizophrenia. It is always necessary, therefore, to compare behaviour before and after the onset of a suspected psychiatric disorder.

The diagnosis of schizophrenia should be considered as one of several possibilities when intellectual or social functioning worsens without evidence of an organic cause, and especially if any new behaviour is odd and out of keeping with the patient's previous behaviour. (Other possibilities include depressive and anxiety disorders, and abnormal responses to stress.) When there is continuing doubt, a trial of antipsychotic drugs is sometimes appropriate although improvement following medication does not, of course, prove the diagnosis of schizophrenia.

The principles of **treatment** of schizophrenia in people with learning disability are the same as in patients of normal intelligence (see Chapter 12).

Mood disorder

The rate of depressive disorders is similar to that in the general population (Deb *et al.*, 2001a). However people with learning disability are less likely than those of normal intelligence to complain of mood changes or to express depressive ideas. Diagnosis has to be made mainly on an appearance of sadness, changes in appetite and sleep, and behavioural changes of retardation or agitation. Severely depressed patients with adequate verbal abilities may describe hallucinations or delusions. **Mania** has to be diagnosed mainly from overactivity and behavioural signs of excitement, irritability, or nervousness.

The differential diagnosis of mood disorder in people with learning disability includes thyroid dysfunction, which is especially prevalent in people with Down syndrome.

The rate of **suicide** in people with moderate and more severe learning disabilities is lower than in the general population. The rate of deliberate self-harm is less certain because it is difficult to decide the the patient's intentions and knowledge of the likely effects of the injurious behaviour.

The principles of **treatment** of mood disorders among the mentally retarded are the same as among people of normal intelligence (see Chapter 11).

Anxiety disorders and related conditions

Adjustment disorders are common among people with learning disability, occurring when there are changes in the routine of their lives. **Anxiety disorders** are also frequent, especially at times of stress. Phobic disorders may develop but are easily overlooked. **Post-traumatic stress disorders** have been reported in people with learning disability who have suffered physical or sexual abuse (Ryan, 1994). **Obsessive–compulsive disorders** are also found and may be more frequent than in the general population. **Conversion and dissociative symptoms** are sometimes florid, taking forms understandable in terms of the patient's understanding of illness. **Somatoform disorders** and other causes of functional somatic symptoms can result in persistent requests for medical attention.

Treatment is usually directed mainly to bringing about adjustments in the patient's environment reassurance, while counselling, at an appropriate level of complexity, can also be helpful.

Eating disorders

Overeating and unusual dietary preferences are frequent among people with learning disability. Abnormal eating behaviours such as 'pica' (see p. 666) may be more common than was previously thought (Gravestock, 2003) but anorexia nervosa and bulimia appear to be less common than in the general population. Overeating and obesity are features of the Prader–Willi syndrome, a genetic cause of learning disability.

Personality disorder

Personality disorder is common among people with learning disability, but is difficult to diagnose. In this population, there is a considerable overlap between the diagnosis of behaviour disorder and of personality disorder (Corbett, 1979). Sometimes the personality disorder leads to greater problems in management than those caused by the learning disability itself. The general approach is as described on p. 146, though with more emphasis on finding an environment to match the patient's temperament and less on attempts to bring about change through self-understanding.

Delirium and dementia

Delirium may occur as a response to infection, medication, and other precipitating factors. As in people of normal intelligence, delirium in people with learning disability is more common in childhood and old age than at other ages. Disturbed behaviour due to delirium is sometimes the first indication of physical illness. Delirium may also occur as a side-effect of certain drugs (especially antiepileptic, antidepressants, and other psychotropic medication).

Dementia As the life expectation of people with learning disability is increasing, dementia in later life is becoming more common. Alzheimer's disease is more common among people with Down syndrome (see p. 718), and also among learning disabled people over 65 who do not have Down syndrome (Barcikowska *et al.*, 1989). In many of these cases, no cause can be found depite extensive investigation.

Among people with learning disability, a progressive decline in intellectual and social functioning is often the first indication of dementia. Dementia has to be distinguished from conditions such as depression and delirium, which give cause a similar impression of decline - but one that improves with treatment.

Disorders that are usually first diagnosed in childhood and adolescence

Many of the disorders in this category are more frequent in children with learning disability than in the general population and they are more likely to continue into adult life. It is important to be aware that relatively specific developmental disorders of scholastic skills, speech, and language and motor function may occur alongside more global learning disability.

Autism and attention-deficit hyperactivity disorder (ADHD)

Hyperactive behaviour among people with learning disability may be part of the syndrome of learning disability. However, it seems that both autism and ADHD are more common among the people with learning disability than among the general population. These disorders are discussed on pp. 667 and 675, and are not considered further here.

Abnormal movements

Stereotypes, mannerisms, and rhythmic movement disorders (including head banging and rocking) occur in about 40 per cent of children and 20 per cent of adults with severe learning disability. **Repeated self-injurious behaviours** are less common but important. There is a specific association with Lesch–Nyhan syndrome in which the biting away of the corner of a lip is common. Prader–Willi syndrome is strongly associated with a pattern of self-injury where patients pick their skin, and sometimes the subcutaneous tissues. Such clinical observations have given rise to the concept of '**behavioural phenotypes**', in which a behaviour is linked with a specific genotype. However, research increasingly casts doubt on the idea that there are characteristic patterns of behaviour specific to particular genetic abnormalities (see Skuse, 2001).

BOX 25.1 CAUSES OF CHALLENGING BEHAVIOUR

- Pain and discomfort
- Understimulation
- Overstimulation
- Wish to escape an unpleasant situation
- Desire for attention or other reward
- Frustration due to difficulty in communication
- Side-effects of medication
- Psychiatric disorder

Challenging behaviour

The term challenging behaviour is often used to describe behaviour that is of an intensity or frequency sufficient to impair the physical safety of a person with learning disability, to pose a danger to others, or make difficult participation in the community. It is probable that around 20 per cent of learning-disabled children and adolescents and 15 per cent of learning-disabled adults have some form of challenging behaviour. The **causes** of such behaviour are shown in Box 25.1. When possible, the primary cause should be treated. Behaviour modification (see p. 726) carried out in the places in which the behaviour most appears often or, in severe cases, in a residential unit is sometimes helpful. For more information see Emerson (1995) and Deb (2001c).

Forensic problems

People with mild learning disability have higher rates of criminal behaviour than the general population (see Table 26.2, p. 733). The causes of this excess are multiple, but influences in the family and social environment are often important. Impulsivity, suggestibility, vulnerability to exploitation, and desire to please are other reasons for involvement in crime. Compared with the general population, learning-disabled people who commit offences are more likely to be detected and, once apprehended, may be more likely to confess. Among the more serious offences, arson and sexual offences (usually exhibitionism) are said to be particularly common.

Because people with learning disability may be suggestible and may give false confessions, particular care should be taken when questioning them about an alleged offence. In the UK, police interrogation should accord with the Police and Criminal Evidence Act which requires the presence of an appropriate adult to ensure that the person with learning dsiability understands the situation and the questions. Suggestibility can be assessed clinically, although a formal rating scale is available (Gudjonsson, 1992). Once convicted, psychiatric supervision and specialized education may be needed. See Holland (1997) for a review of forensic aspects of learning disability.

Sleep disorders

Serious sleep problems such as obstructive sleep apnoea, excessive daytime sleepiness and parasomnias are not uncommon among people with learning disabilities and can be a source of considerable distress to them and their carers (Brylewski and Wiggs, 2004). Furthermore, sleep disorders may be associated with subsequent challenging behaviours and a worsening of cognitive impairment. The high rate of sleep disorders in this population is accounted for by five factors:

1. coexistent damage to CNS structures important for the sleep–wake cycle.
2. epileptic seizures starting during sleep.
3. epilepsy-related sleep instability which disrupts sleep architecture without causing frank seizures.
4. structural abnormalities in the upper respiratory tract causing sleep apnoea (particularly common among people with Down syndrome).
5. (the most common) inadvertent reinforcement of waking, for example, by giving drinks, allowing the watching of television, and so on.

Treatment is directed to the cause (see p. 372).

Sexual relationships and parenthood

Most people with learning disability develop sexual interests in the same way as other people. Yet although people with learning disability are encouraged to live as normally as possible in other ways, sexual expression is usually discouraged by parents and carers, and sexual feelings may not even be discussed.

In the past, sexual activity by people with learning disability was strongly discouraged because it was feared that such a union might produce disabled children. It is now known that many kinds of severe learning disability are not inherited, and that those that are inherited are often associated with infertility. A second concern is that people with learning disability will not be good parents. A study in Norway found that 40 per cent of 126 children born to parents with learning disability suffered from 'failures of care' (Morch *et al.*, 1997). However, a report from the UK indicates that some people with learning disability can care for a child successfully provided they are strongly supported (Booth and Booth, 1993).

These issues should be considered carefully in each case, and contraception made available where appropriate.

Sexual problems

Some people with learning disability have a child-like curiosity about other people's bodies, which can be misunderstood as sexual. Some expose themselves without fully understanding the significance of their actions.

Effects of learning disability on the family

When a newborn child is found to be disabled, the parents are inevitably distressed. Feelings of rejection are common, but seldom last long and are replaced by feeling of the loss of the hoped-for normal child. Frequently, the diagnosis of learning disability is not made until after the first year of life, and the parents then have to make great changes in their hopes and expectations for the child. They often experience prolonged depression, guilt, shame, or anger, and have difficulty in coping with the many practical and financial problems. They too grieve for the intact child they had hoped and planned for. A few reject their children, some become overinvolved in their care, sacrificing other important aspects of family life (Floyd and Phillippe, 1993), others seek repeatedly for a cause to explain the learning disability. Most families eventually achieve a satisfactory adjustment, although the temptation to over-indulge the child remains. However well they adjust psychologically, the parents are still faced with a long prospect of prolonged hard work, frustration, and social problems. If the child also has a physical handicap, these problems are increased.

There have been several studies on the effect of a child's learning disability on the family. In an influential study, Ann Gath (1978) compared two groups of families, those with a Down syndrome child at home and controls with a normal child of the same age. Gath concluded that:

> despite the understandable emotional reactions to the fact of the baby's abnormality, most of the families in the study have adjusted well, and two years later are providing a home environment that is stable and enriching for both the normal and handicapped children.
>
> (Gath, 1978, p. 116)

However, it seemed likely that siblings were often at some disadvantage because of the time and effort that had to be devoted to the disabled child. These findings have been supported by subsequent research (see Gath, 2000).

More recent studies have found that mothers with a learning-disabled child at home received help from their husbands but little help from other people, and many professionals were seen by the parents as lacking interest and expertise. Many parents report difficulties in obtaining help in looking after the children in school holidays and during weekends or evenings.

As the parents grow older, many fear for the future of their - now adult - disabled son or daughter. They need advice about ways in which they can arrange additional help when they become unable to provide the support that they gave when they were younger; and about ways of helping their son or daughter to remain in the family home after they have died. (See for example, Foundation for Learning Disabilities, 2000.)

For a review of the effects of learning disability on the family see Gath (2000).

Maltreatment and abuse

Many children with learning disability are raised in families characterized by the factors associated, in the general population, with the maltreatment of children (see p. 697). Nevertheless, there is no convincing epidemiological evidence that child abuse is more frequent in families with a learning-disabled child than in other families. When sexual abuse occurs, it may be followed by psychological problems later in life (Sequiera *et al.*, 2003).

Aetiology of learning disability

Introduction

Lewis (1929) distinguished two kinds of mental retardation (as it was then called): subcultural, i.e. the lower end of the normal distribution curve of intelligence in the population, and pathological, i.e. retardation due to specific disease processes. In a study of the 1280 mentally retarded people living in the Colchester Asylum, Penrose (1938) found that most cases were due not to a single cause but to an interaction of inherited and environmental factors. Subsequent research has confirmed the conclusions of these early studies. This is particularly true for mild learning disability which is usually due to a combination of genetic and adverse environmental factors, and which are more common in the lower social classes. Despite advances in knowledge, the cause of learning disability remains unknown in about 50 per cent of cases (Xu and Chen, 2003).

Among **severely learning disabled** people, physical causes are found in 55–75 per cent (Broman *et al.*, 1987). Prenatal causes predominate, as indicated for example by the association with idiopathic cerebral palsy, and epilepsy. Other causes include Down syndrome, fragile X syndrome, and fetal alcohol syndrome. Prenatal genetic causes include single gene defects and quantitative trait loci, which are the accumulating effects of abnormal loci situated in multiple genes that lower the threshold and increases the vulnerability to develop learning disability (Daniels et al., 1998).

Post-natal causes include hypothyroidism, infection, trauma, toxicity. In developed countries these causes

BOX 25.2 SOME SPECIFIC GENETIC SYNDROMES

Six groups of specific genetic syndromes may be recognized:

1. **Dominant conditions** These are rare; examples are the phakomatoses, including neurofibromatosis.
2. **Recessive conditions** This is the largest group of specific gene disorders. It includes most of the inherited metabolic conditions such as phenylketonuria (the commonest inborn error of metabolism), homocystinuria, and galactosaemia.
3. **Sex-linked chromosomal abnormalities** The prevalence of learning disability is 25 per cent greater in males than in females. Lehrke (1972) was the first to suggest that the excess among males might be due to X-chromosome-linked causes. Recent research suggests that up to a fifth of learning disability in males is due to X-linked causes. Many rare specific X-linked syndromes have been identified, for example, glucose dehydrogenase deficiency and the Lesch–Nyhan syndrome. However, in most cases there is no metabolic abnormality, for example, the 'fragile X syndrome' (see p. 718). Sex chromosome abnormalities, such as Klinefelter's syndrome (XXY) and Turner's syndrome (XO), may also cause learning disability.
4. **Autosomal chromosome abnormalities** The most common is Down syndrome (see p. 717).
5. **Conditions with partial and complex inheritance** such as anencephaly. This group is poorly understood.
6. **Neuronal Migrational Disorders (NMDs)** that cause 'cerebral dysgenesis' are associated with severe learning disability and epilepsy. More than 25 genetic syndromes have been identified in relation to NMDs.

are generally less frequent that genetic and perinatal causes, but in developing countries post-natal causes, are important. For a review of aetiology see Deb and Ahmed (2000), and Kaski (2000).

It should be noted that increasing success in identifying specific causes of severe learning disability does not remove the need to **consider all the additional social and other factors in every case**.

Autism which is associated with learning disability is considered in Chapter 24.

Genetic factors

There is good evidence from family, twin, and adoption studies that polygenic inheritance is important in determining intelligence within the normal range, and that much mild mental retardation represents the lower end of the distribution curve of intelligence (Thapar *et al.*, 1994). Fragile X syndrome is the most common known inherited cause of learning disability, and is particularly associated with moderate and mild cases. In severe learning disability, many genetic abnormalities, including about 180 single-gene defects, are responsible for the metabolic disorders and other anomalies that cause the learning disability (see Tables 25.2 and 25.3).

Table 25.2 summarizes the most frequent causes, but it is not exhaustive. Many of these causes are rare, and they are not described in this chapter. Information about some of the less rare conditions is summarized for reference in Table 25.3. Children with these syndromes are more likely to be cared for by paediatricians and geneticists than by psychiatrists. If psychiatrists take over the care of a patient suffering from any of these rare syndromes, they should work closely with the paediatrician and the family doctor, and should acquaint themselves with up-to-date knowledge of the particular syndrome.

For a review of the applications of molecular cytogenetics to learning disability see Xu and Chen (2003). For a review of metabolic causes of learning disability see Kahler and Fahey (2003).

TABLE 25.2 The aetiology of learning disability

Genetic	*With gross disease of the brain*
Chromosome abnormalities	Tuberose sclerosis
Fragile site	Neurofibromatosis
Fragile X syndrome	Cerebral dysgenesis
Trisomy 21	*With brain malformations*
Down syndrome	Neural tube defects
Trisomy 13	Hydrocephalus
Patau's syndrome	Microcephalus
Trisomy 18	**Antenatal damage**
Edwards' syndrome	Infections (rubella, cytomegalovirus, syphilis, toxoplasmosis)
Terminal deletion 5	Intoxications (lead, certain drugs, alcohol)
Cri du chat	Physical damage (injury, radiation, hypoxia)
Microdeletions	Placental dysfunction (toxaemia, nutritional growth retardation)
Williams' syndrome (chromosome 7)	Endocrine disorders (hypothyroidism, hypoparathyroidism)
Prader–Willi syndrome (chromosome 15; often of paternal origin)	**Perinatal damage**
Angelman's syndrome (chromosome 15: often of maternal origin)	Birth asphyxia
Metabolic disorders affecting:	Complications of prematurity
Amino acids (e.g. phenylketonuria, homocystinuria, Hartnup disease)	Kernicterus
The urea cycle (e.g. citrullinuria, aminosuccinic aciduria)	Intraventricular haemorrhage
Lipids (Tay–Sachs, Gaucher's, and Niemann– Pick diseases)	**Postnatal damage**
Carbohydrate (galactosaemia)	Injury (accidental, child abuse)
Purines (Lesch–Nyhan syndrome)	Intoxication (lead mercury)
Mucopolysaccharidoses (Hurler's, Hunter's, Sanfillipo's, and Morquio's syndromes)	Infections (encephalitis, meningitis)
	Impoverished environment

Social factors

Studies of the general population suggest that factors in the social environment may account for variation in IQ of as much as 20 points. The evidence comes from two kinds of enquiry.

Epidemiological studies Low IQ is related to lower social class, poverty, poor housing, and an unstable family environment. Such social factors could be the effects of low intelligence rather than a cause. However, follow-up studies from birth to adolescence have found that psychosocial factors predict IQ (Sameroff *et al.*, 1987).

Improving the environment In one early experiment, children from large and unsatisfactory institutions were transferred to small well-staffed children's homes or given more stimulating education. Twenty years later they were found to have higher IQs than those who, as children, had remained in their original institutions (Skeels, 1966). More recent studies have confirmed that well- and prolonged intervention can be beneficial for socially deprived children (Garber, 1988).

TABLE 25.3 Notes on some causes of learning disability

Syndrome	Aetiology	Clinical features	Comments
Chromosome abnormalities (for Down syndrome and X-linked learning disability, see text)			
Triple X	Trisomy X	No characteristic feature	Mild learning disability
Trisomy 18 (Edwards' syndrome)	Trisomy 18	Growth deficiency, abnormal skull shape and facial features, clenched hands, rocker bottom feet, cardiac and renal abnormalities	
Trisomy 13 (Patau's syndrome)	Trisomy 13	Structural abnormalities of the brain, lip, and palate, polydactyly	Most die within a few weeks of birth
Cri du chat	Deletion in chromosome 5	Microcephaly, hyperteleorism, typical cat-like cry, failure to thrive	Most die in early childhood
Inborn errors of metabolism			
Phenylketonuria	Autosomal recessive causing lack of liver phenylalanine hydroxylase. Commonest inborn error of metabolism	Lack of pigment (fair hair, blue eyes); retarded growth; associated epilepsy, microcephaly, eczema, and hyperactivity	Detectable by postnatal screening of blood or urine; treated by controlling the intake of phenylalanine from the diet during early years of life
Homocystinuria	Autosomal recessive causing lack of cystathione synthetases	Ectopia lentis, fine and fair hair, joint enlargement, skeletal abnormalities similar to Marfan's syndrome; associated with thromboembolic episodes	Learning disability variable; sometimes treated by methionine restriction
Galactosaemia	Autosomal recessive causing lack of galactose 1-phosphate uridyl transferase	Presents following introduction of milk into diet; failure to thrive, hepatosplenomegaly, cataracts	Detectable by postnatal screening for the enzymic defect; treatable by galactose-free diet; toluidine blue test on urine
Tay–Sachs disease	Autosomal recessive resulting in increased lipid storage. (The earliest form of the cerebro-macular degenerations)	Progressive loss of vision and hearing; spastic paralysis; cherry-red spot at macula of retina; epilepsy	Death at 2–4 years
Hurler's syndrome	Autosomal recessive affecting mucopoly-saccharide storage	Grotesque features; protuberant abdomen; hepatosplenomegaly; associated cardiac abnormalities	Death before adolescence
Lesch–Nyhan syndrome	X-linked recessive leading to enzyme defect affecting purine metabolism. Excessive uric acid production and excretion. Gene on short arm of chromosome q26–27	Almost all are normal at birth. Development of choreoathetoid movements, scissors position of legs, and self-mutilation of lips and fingers	Diagnosed prenatally, by sampling amniotic fluid and enzyme estimation. Postnatal diagnosis by enzyme estimation in hair roots. Death in early adult life. Self-mutilation may be reduced by treatment with hydroxytryptophan
Other inherited disorders			
Neurofibromatosis (von Recklinghausen's syndrome)	Autosomal dominant inheritance. Two genes, Nf1 and Nf2	Neurofibromata, café au lait spots, vitiligo; associated with symptoms determined by site of neurofibromata; astrocytomas, meningioma	Learning disability in a minority 50% of cases due to an Nf1 mutation

TABLE 25.3 Notes on some causes of learning disability (*continued*)

Syndrome	Aetiology	Clinical features	Comments
Tuberose sclerosis (epiloia)	Autosomal dominant (very variable penetrance). Caused by two genes, *TSC1* (*hamartin*) on chromosome 9 and *TSC2* (*tuberin*) on chromosome 16	Epilepsy, adenoma sebaceum on face, white skin patches, shagreen skin, retinal phakoma, subungual fibromata; associated multiple tumours in kidney, spleen, and lungs	Learning disability in about 70% (more frequent with *TSC2* gene)
Lawrence–Moon–Biedlsyndrome	Autosomal recessive	Retinitis pigmentosa, polydactyly, sometimes with obesity and impaired genital function	Learning disability usually not severe
Infection			
Rubella embryopathy	Viral infection of mother in first trimester	Cataract, microphthalmia, deafness, microcephaly, congenital heart disease	If mother infected in first trimester, 10–15% infants are affected (infection may be subclinical)
Toxoplasmosis	Protozoal infection of mother	Hydrocephaly, microcephaly, intracerebral calcification, retinal damage, hepatosplenomegaly, jaundice, epilepsy	Wide variation in severity
Cytomegalovirus	Intrauterine infection	Brain damage; only severe cases are apparent at birth	60% of survivors have learning disability
Congenital syphilis	Syphilitic infection of mother	Many die at birth; variable neurological signs, 'stigmata' (Hutchinson teeth and rhagades often absent)	Uncommon since routine testing of pregnant women; infant's tests positive at first but may become negative
Cranial malformations			
Hydrocephalus	Sex-linked recessive; inherited developmental abnormality, e.g. atresia of aqueduct, Arnold–Chiari malformation, meningitis, spina bifida	Rapid enlargement of head. In early infancy, symptoms of raised CSF pressure; other features depend on aetiology	Mild cases may arrest spontaneously; may be symptomatically treated by CSF shunt; intelligence can be normal
Microcephaly	Recessive inheritance, irradiation in pregnancy, maternal infections	Features depend upon aetiology	Evident in up to a fifth of institutionalized patients with severe learning disability
Miscellaneous			
Spina bifida	Aetiology multiple and complex	Failure of vertebral fusion; *spina bifida cystica* is associated with meningocele or, in 15–20%, myelomeningocele; latter causes spinal cord damage with lower limb paralysis, incontinence, etc.	Hydrocephalus in four-fifths of those with myelomeningocele; retardation in this group
Cerebral palsy	Perinatal brain damage; strong association with prematurity	Spastic (common), athetoid and ataxic types; variable in severity	Majority are below average intelligence; athetoid are more likely to be of normal IQ
Hypothyroidism (cretinism)	Iodine deficiency or (rarely) atrophic thyroid	Appearance normal at birth; abnormalities appear at 6 months; growth failure, puffy skin, lethargy	Now rare in UK; responds to early replacement treatment
Hyperbilirubinaemia	Haemolysis, rhesus incompatibility, and prematurity	Kernicterus (choreoathetosis), opisthotonus, spasticity, convulsions	Prevention by anti-rhesus globulin; neonatal treatment by exchange transfusion

TABLE 25.4 Environmental causes of learning disability

Intra-uterine infection – e.g. rubella
Environmental pollutants – e.g. lead
Alcoholism in pregnancy – see p. 437
Severe malnutrition in pregnancy
Iodine deficiency
Excessive irradiation of the uterus

Other environmental factors

Environmental factors are listed in Table 25.4. The timing of these influences is important because there seem to be vulnerable periods of brain development during which damage is particularly likely to follow exposure (Holland, 1994). Malnutrition in the first 2 years of life is probably the most common cause of learning disabilty in the world as a whole, but is much less frequent in developed countries. Iodine deficiency is an important cause in many developing countries.

There is no doubt that severe **lead intoxication** can cause an encephalopathy with consequent intellectual impairment. It is much less certain whether the moderate levels of lead of the kind that result in part from air pollution with lead additives in petrol, can cause intellectual retardation. Because children absorb lead more readily than adults, they are at greater risk from environmental pollution. However, children living in polluted areas are often from lower socioeconomic groups, and it is uncertain how far findings of lower intelligence (compared with children in other areas) are due to the slightly raised lead levels in their blood, and how far to social influences (see Pocock *et al.*, 1994 for a review).

Birth injury

This is an important cause of learning disability. Early studies estimated that clinically recognizable birth injuries accounted for about 10 per cent of learning disability. Pasamanick and Knobloch (1966) suggested a 'continuum of reproductive casualty' in which additional cases of mild intellectual retardation resulted from less obvious brain lesions sustained *in utero* or perinatally. Although prematurity and low birth weight are associated with learning disability (Hack *et al.*, 1994), the theory of a continuum of reproductive casualty is not otherwise supported.

Some specific causes of learning disability

Down syndrome

In 1866, Langdon Down tried to relate the appearance of certain groups of patients to the physical features of ethnic groups. One of his groups had the condition originally called mongolism, and now generally known as Down syndrome. This condition is a frequent cause of learning disability, occurring in 1 in about every 650 live births. It is more frequent among older women, occurring in about 1 in 2000 live births for mothers aged 20–25 and 1 in 30 for those aged 45. The incidence of Down syndrome has decreased because of increased detection of the condition by amniocentesis and subsequent termination of pregnancy.

The clinical picture is made up of a number of features, any one of which can occur in a normal person. Four features together are generally accepted as strong evidence for the syndrome. The most characteristic signs are shown in Table 25.5.

Degree of learning disability IQ is generally between 20 and 50, but in 15 per cent it is above 50. Mental abilities usually develop fairly quickly in the first 6 months to a year of life but then increase more slowly.

Temperament and behaviour Children with Down syndrome are often described as loveable and easygoing, but there is a wide individual variation. Emotional and behaviour problems are less frequent than in forms of learning disability associated with clinically detectable brain damage.

Outcome

In the past, the infant mortality of Down syndrome was high, but with improved medical care survival into adult life is usual. About a quarter of people with Down syndrome now live beyond 50 years of age. In middle

TABLE 25.5 Features of Down syndrome

Moderate or severe learning disability
Placid temperament
Physical features ◆ Slanted eyes and epicanthic folds ◆ Small mouth with furrowed tongue ◆ Flat nose ◆ Flattened occiput ◆ Stubby hands, fingers, and single transverse palmar crease ◆ Hypotonia with hyperextensibility of joints
Associated medical problems ◆ Cardiac anomalies, especially septal defects ◆ Gastrointestinal abnormalities ◆ Atlantoaxial instability ◆ Susceptibility to infection ◆ Impaired hearing
Increased risk of leukaemia, hypothyroidism, autoimmune disorders

life, these people develop Alzheimer-like changes in the brain (Holland *et al.*, 1998), although clinical decline starts later than would be expected from the neuropathological data (Wisniewski *et al.*, 1994).

People with Down syndrome who have lived with their parents may have to leave home when the parents grow old or die. They then face difficult re-adjustments.

Aetiology

In 1959, Down syndrome was found to be associated with the chromosomal disorder of trisomy (three chromosomes instead of the usual two). About 95 per cent of cases are due to trisomy 21. These cases result from failure of disjunction during meiosis and are associated with increasing maternal age. The risk of recurrence in a subsequent child is about 1 in 100. The remaining 5 per cent of cases of Down syndrome are attributable either to translocation involving chromosome 21 or to mosaicism. The disorder leading to translocation is often inherited, and the risk of recurrence is about 1 in 10. Mosaicism occurs when non-disjunction takes place during any cell division after fertilization. Normal and trisomic cells occur in the same person, and the effects on cognitive development are particularly variable (Thapar *et al.*, 1994). Down pathology is presumed to be due to the increased 'dosage' of genes on chromosome 21. This could account for the excess of early-onset Alzheimer's because the APP (amyloid precursor protein) gene is situated in chromosome 21 (see p. 337). The APP leads to deposition of abnormal amyloid in the brain and this is one of the pathways in the cascade leading to Alzheimer's neuropathology (abnormal 'tau' metabolism is the other).

Fragile X syndrome

Fragile X syndrome is the second most common specific cause of learning disability after Down syndrome and is the most common inherited cause. It occurs in around up to 1 in 4000 males and in a milder form in about 1 in 6000 females. It accounts overall for about 10 per cent of those with learning disability.

Physical features There are a number of characteristic but highly variable clinical features, none of which is diagnostic. These features include enlarged testes, large ears, a long face, and flat feet.

Psychological features include abnormalities of speech and language, autistic behaviour and other social impairments, disorders of attention and concentration, and hyperactivity.

Inheritance The inheritance of the condition is unusual and complex, and was difficult to unravel. During recent years a gene referred to as *FMR-1* has been identified. This gene contains an amplified CGG repeat sequence, which constitutes the fragile X anomaly.

TABLE 25.6 Features of fragile X syndrome

About 10 per cent of learning disability
Commoner in males (>2:1)
Learning disability ◆ Variable from mild to profound ◆ Increases late in childhood ◆ Performance IQ affected more than verbal IQ ◆ Poor attention and concentration ◆ Speech repetitive, lacking themes or content ("litany speech")
Behavioural features ◆ Autistic features common
Physical features ◆ Large, protruding ears ◆ Long face with high-arched palate ◆ Flat feet ◆ Lax joints ◆ Soft skin ◆ Large testes (after puberty) ◆ Mitral valve prolapse

Note: All features are particularly variable.

The identification of the genetic abnormality makes it possible to identify affected heterozygous females who are clinically and even cytogenetically normal. These women can be advised of the high risk of affected offspring and the need for prenatal testing. Conversely, many women who are at risk of being carriers can be reassured they do not have the condition. It is possible also to determine whether men are transmitting carriers.

The psychological and psychiatric complications in the syndrome mean that there is a need for regular review of affected people. See Frints *et al.* (2002) for a review of the fragile X syndrome.

Causes of psychiatric disorder and behaviour problems in the learning-disabled

The diversity of psychiatric disorders among the people with learning disability makes it unlikely that they have a single aetiology. As with mental disorder among people of normal intelligence, several causes have to be considered: biological, psychosocial, and developmental (for a review see Deb *et al.*, 2001a). Overall, there is no reason to expect that particular mental disorders comorbid with learning disability have aetiologies which differ from those in people with normal intelligence.

Biological factors include specific associations such as those between the fragile X syndrome and attention-deficit hyperactivity disorder and anxiety disorder; between the Lesch–Nyhan syndrome and self-injury; and between Down syndrome and Alzheimer's disease.

Brain pathology and epilepsy As already noted, people with severe learning disability have some organic brain pathology, as do a smaller proportion of those with moderate and mild learning disability. As mentioned in Chapter 24, psychiatric disorder is associated with brain damage in children of normal intelligence and it is likely, therefore, that some of the psychiatric disorders in people with learning disability are related to brain pathology. Epilepsy and behaviour disorder are associated in people with learning disability (see Deb, 2000) either directly or through the adverse effects of antiepileptic drugs.

Developmental factors include abnormalities of temperament, difficulty in acquiring language and social skills, low self-esteem, and educational failure. These difficulties may discourage the efforts of families and carers, so adding to the disadvantage.

Psychosocial factors such as bereavement or a disrupted family can be causes of mental disorder and behaviour problems in people with learning disability as they are in people of normal intelligence. People with learning disability may develop adjustment disorders or mental disorders when the arrangements for their care are disrupted or if they are treated badly or exploited. Operant conditioning models point to the importance of inadequate environmental reinforcement of adaptive behaviours and the reinforcement of maladaptive behaviours.

Iatrogenic factors can contribute to the causes of psychiatric disorder among people with learning disability. As mentioned above, these include the adverse effects of drugs, especially those used to treat epilepsy, and over- or understimulating environments in the community or within an institution.

Assessment and classification of people with learning disability

Assessment of the learning disabled is directed towards four main areas:

1. cause of the learning disability;
2. associated biomedical conditions;
3. intellectual and social skills development;
4. associated psychiatric disorders and their causes and consequences.

A multiaxial classification is available to record reflect some of this information. (Diagnostic Criteria for psychiatric disorders for use with adults with LD [DC-LD]; Royal College of Psychiatrists, 2001), namely:

Axis I: Severity of learning disability.

Axis II: Cause of learning disability.

Axis III: Psychiatric disorders.

- Level A: Developmental disorders
- Level B: Psychiatric illness
- Level C: Personality disorders
- Level D: Problem behaviours
- Level E: Other disorders.

Severe learning disability can usually be diagnosed in infancy, especially as it is often associated with detectable physical abnormalities or with delayed motor development. Some people with learning disability have specific developmental disorders, i.e. impairment of specific functions greater than would be expected from the general intellectual level. The diagnostic evaluation in childhood includes history taking, physical examination, and cytogenetic and molecular genetic investigations. (See Battaglia and Carey, 2003 for a review.)

The clinician should be cautious in diagnosing less severe learning disability on the basis of delays in development. Although routine examination of a child may reveal signs of developmental delay, suggesting possible learning disability, confident diagnosis often requires specialist assessment.

Full assessment has several stages: history taking, physical examination, examination of the mental state, developmental testing, functional behavioural assessment, analysis of the interaction between the disabled person and the family and the social support systems, and other aspects of adjustment. These stages will be considered in turn. Although this section is concerned mainly with the assessment of children, similar principles apply in adolescence and adult life.

History taking

In the course of obtaining a full history, particular attention should be given to any family history suggesting an inherited disorder and to abnormalities in the pregnancy or the delivery of the child. Dates of passing developmental milestones should be ascertained (see pp. 646–8). A full account of any behaviour disorders should be obtained. Details of any associated medical conditions, such as congenital heart disease, epilepsy, and cerebal palsy, should be documented.

Physical examination

A systematic physical examination should include the recording of head circumference. It is important to be alert for the physical signs suggesting one of the many specific syndromes (see Table 25.2). Neurological examination is important and should include particular attention to impairments of vision and hearing. Neuroimaging studies may be required to supplement the physical examination.

Mental state examination

The approach should be flexible. Many people with learning disability attend and concentrate poorly. Hence, the interview may need to be carried out rather informally while the person is engaged intermittently in some other interest. Questions should be simplified to take account of each person's receptive language and developmental level. Behavioural observations by family, friends, and carers are often most helpful to the obsevations that the assessor is able to make. Clinical assessment can also be supplemented by using standardized scales for the assessment of psychopathology, been adapted for use in patients with learning disability (see the appendix to Deb *et al.*, 2001a).

As in the assessment of patients of normal intelligence, it is important to find out the person's previous baseline state before concluding that an item of current behaviour is evidence of a psychiatric disorder. Some behaviours, such as stereotyped movements or social withdrawal resemble symptoms of psychiatric disorders and may be dismissed as related to the learning disability when they are caused by a disorder – 'diagnostic overshadowing' (Reiss and Szyszko, 1983). However, an increase in a long-standing behaviour may be the first, and sometimes the only, evidence of psychiatric disorder – 'baseline exaggeration' (Sovner and Hurley, 1989).

Developmental assessment

This assessment is based on a combination of clinical experience and standardized methods of measuring intelligence, language, motor performance, and social skills. Although the IQ is the best general index of intellectual development, it is not reliable in the very young or among people who have severe to profound degree of learning disabilities.

Tests used in developmental assessment

Standardized assessment instruments are widely used for screening, diagnosing, and assessing the severity of disorders of psychological development. Many require special training for correct administration but some do not. The choice of test is important because many neuropsychological tests are too difficult for some people with learning disability. The type of test is also important. There are norm-referenced tests such as the Wechsler Adult Intelligence Scale (WAIS) and other IQ measures; criterion-referenced tests which apply to particular skills without reference to population norms; tests of adaptive behaviour in social settings; and assessments of behavioural functioning. An abbreviated version of WAIS, called the Wechsler Abbreviated Scales of Intelligence (WASI) (The Psychological Corporation, 2004) is now available. Another useful, quick method is the use of a Picture Vocabulary test or another non-verbal test such as Raven's Progressive Matrices. Other commonly used instruments are summarized in Box 25.3. The first four provide a general assessment over a range of developmental domains. The others focus, entirely or principally, on specific aspects of development. All have good reliability and validity.

Functional behavioural assessment

The functional assessment of behaviour involves an assessment of events before, during, and immediately after the behaviour takes place. It is based on observations reported by family, carers and members of the clinical team. It is concerned with: abilities related to self-care; social abilities including communication, sensory motor skills, and social relationships. Sometimes key behaviours are counted and recorded on paper or using a palm-top computer.

Assessment of social interaction and adjustment

This assessment is concerned with the interaction between the person with learning disability and people closely involved in care. It is also concerned with opportunities for learning new skills, making relationships, and achieving more choice. If people with learning disability have reasonable language ability, it is usually possible to obtain much of the information from them. When language is less well developed, the account has to be obtained mainly from informants. It is particularly important to obtain a complete description of any

BOX 25.3 COMMONLY USED INSTRUMENTS FOR DEVELOPMENTAL ASSESSMENT

Vineland Social Maturity Scale The Vineland Scale is useful in the assessment of children who do not cooperate in testing since it can be completed by interview with a reliable informant. An overall social age can be derived from the scale, which can be compared with the mental and chronological ages.

The British Ability Scales and Differential Ability Scales These scales measure a range of functions and educational attainments, and can be used to calculate an overall IQ.

The Adaptive Behaviour Scales These scales are probably the most widely used for assessing social functioning in adults with learning disability (Nihira *et al.*, 1975).

The Portage Guide to Early Education This assessment has been adopted for use internationally. It provides a broad developmental assessment including socialization, self-help, language and training is required for the assessor. The test requires the active involvement of the parent or other carer.

Autism Behaviour Check List This questionnaire is completed by the parent or other carer. It is a reliable indicator of problems in the area of autism and delay in social development.

The Disability Assessment Scale This scale focuses on autistic and related social developmental, language disorders, and behavioural problems.

British (Peabody) Picture Vocabulary Test This is a test of language comprehension, suitable for non-speaking children. The test booklet is largely pictorial and the age range covered is 3–19 years. Although professional training is not required, the test is used mainly by psychologists and speech therapists.

Reynell Scales of Language Development These scales assess comprehension and expressive language in the age range 1 month to 6 years. The test is of particular use with non-verbal children.

change from the usual pattern of behaviour. It is often appropriate to ask parents, teachers, or care staff to keep records of behaviours such as eating, sleeping, and general activity so that problems can be identified and quantified. The assessor should keep in mind the possible causes of psychiatric disorder outlined above, including unrecognized epilepsy.

The care of people with learning disability

A historical perspective

Current arrangements for care and the remaining unsolved problems can best be understood in relation to the history of the development of services for people with learning disabilities (see M. Thomson, 1998 for further information).

A review of services can begin usefully in the early years of the nineteenth century. At this time there were numerous reports of improved forms of care, notably by Itard, physician-in-chief at the Asylum for the Deaf and Dumb in Paris, who attempted to train a 'wild boy' found in Aveyron in 1801. This child was thought to have grown up in the wild, isolated from human beings. Itard made great efforts to educate the boy, but after persisting for 6 years he concluded the training had failed. Nevertheless, his work had important and lasting consequences, for it led others to try educational methods. These methods were developed, for example, by Seguin, director of the School for Idiots at the Bicêtre in Paris who, in 1842, published the *Theory and nature of the education of idiots*. Seguin believed that people with learning disability had latent abilities which could be encouraged by special training, involving physical exercise, moral instruction, and graded tasks (Seguin, 1864, 1866).

These ideas were taken up in other countries, particularly Switzerland and Germany. The Swiss physician Guggenbuhl founded the first special residential institution for people with learning disability at Abendberg in 1841. Similar institutions were opened in other parts of Europe to provide a training that would enable their pupils to live as independently as possible while recognizing that many would need long-term care.

At the end of the nineteenth century, several influences led to a more custodial approach to the care of people with learning disability. These influences included the development of the science of genetics, the measurement of intelligence, the beliefs embodied in the eugenics movement, and a general decrease in public tolerance of abnormal behaviour. In England and Wales, such ideas were reflected in the Mental Deficiency Act 1913, which empowered local authorities to provide for the confinement of the 'intellectually and morally defective' and imposed upon the authorities a responsibility to provide training and occupation. In the years that followed, the total number of people of this kind in institution rose from 6000 in 1916 to 50 000 in 1939 and remained at high levels well into the post-war period.

In the 1960s the need for reform was recognized in several developed countries. This was prompted in part by the changes that had already been effected in psychiatric hospitals (see p. 621), and by improved psychological research. However, much of the impetus came from campaigning by groups of parents, and from public concern about the generally poor conditions in which people with learning disabilities were housed. Surveys of hospitals for the 'retarded' showed that the mean IQ of their patients was over 70. Many residents had only mild learning disability, and many did not need hospital care. About the same time, it was shown that training could help many patients, both the mildly and severely learning disabled (O'Connor, 1968). Further research showed the advantages of residential care in small homely units (Tizard, 1964). However, public concern in the UK and other countries was aroused less by the findings of research than by revelations about the scandalously poor conditions in some hospitals for people with learning disabilities.

It is now recognized in all developed countries that people with learning disability should be integrated as far as possible into society. However, there have been divergent views about the best way to achieve greater integration. In the UK, resources have been inadequate and progress slow. In the USA, deinstitutionalization was carried out more quickly, with both successes and failures.

The main current principle of care is 'normalization', an idea developed in Scandinavia in the 1960s. This term refers to the general approach of providing a pattern of life as near normal as possible (Nirje, 1970). Normalization implies that almost all people with learning disability will live in the community, participating in normal activities and relationships, making choices, and having full social opportunities. Children are brought up whenever possible with their families, and adults are encouraged to live as independently as possible. For the few who need special social and health care, accommodation and activities are designed to be as close as possible to those of family life. The concept of normalization has been further developed in the USA and elsewhere, and includes specialist help to enable people to achieve their full potential. Increasingly, disabled people are organizing themselves into advocacy groups, and those who are unable to speak for themselves about the services have advocates to speak for them.

General provisions

The precise model for the care of people with learning disability in a community matters less than the detail in which it is planned and the enthusiasm with which it is carried out. Good planning requires both an estimate of the needs of the population to be served, and a summation of individual assessments of those identified, since each person has individual needs. To achieve this, local case registers and linked developmental records are needed.

The general approach to care is educational and psychosocial. The family doctor and paediatrician are mainly responsible for the early detection and assessment of learning disability. The team providing continuing health care includes also psychologists, speech therapists, nurses, occupational therapists, and physiotherapists. Volunteers can play a valuable part, and it is useful to encourage self-help groups for parents. In the UK, residential provisions for people with learning disability are from several sources: education service, health service, social services, and voluntary organizations.

Specific services

The main elements in a comprehensive service for people with learning disability and their families or carers are:

- the prevention and early detection of learning disability;
- regular assessment of the learning-disabled person's attainments and disabilities;
- advice, support, and practical measures for families;
- provision for education, training, occupation, or work appropriate for each person;
- housing and social support to maximize self-care;
- medical, nursing, and other services for those who require these forms of help as outpatients, day patients, or inpatients;
- psychiatric and psychological services.

Preventive services

Primary prevention depends largely on genetic counselling, early detection of fetal abnormalities during pregnancy, and safe childbirth. **Secondary prevention** aims to prevent the progression of disability by either medical or psychological means. The latter include 'enriching' education and early attempts to reduce behavioural problems. In developed countries, there remains considerable scope for reduction of the genetic causes of severe learning disability, but it is unlikely that it will be possible to affect the incidence of mild learning disability significantly. In developing countries, the incidence of learning disability could be substantially reduced by general measures to improve the health of mothers during pregnancy, and by better perinatal care.

Genetic screening and counselling

These measures begins with assessment of the risk that an abnormal child will be born. Such an assessment is based on study of the family history, on knowledge of the genetics of conditions that give rise to learning disability, and on awareness of the possibilities for genetic screening. The risks of screening are explained to the parents who are encouraged to discuss them. Most parents seek advice only after a first abnormal child has been born. Those who seek advice before starting to have children do so usually because there is a person with learning disability on one or other side of the family. A positive diagnosis of an abnormality leading to termination or indeed a false-positive result of screening causes considerable distress. It is important, therefore, that those involved in screening are alert to psychological issues and have the appropriate counselling skills.

Prenatal care

Prenatal care begins even before conception, with immunization against rubella for girls who lack immunity, and advice on diet, alcohol, and smoking.

Prenatal diagnosis overlaps with genetic screening. It is becoming available for an increasing number of conditions with the aim of providing information to those at risk of having abnormal children, reassurance to others, and appropriate treatment of affected infants through early diagnosis. Amniocentesis, fetoscopy, and ultrasound scanning of the fetus in the second trimester can reveal chromosomal abnormalities, most open neural tube defects, and about 60 per cent of inborn errors of metabolism. Amniocentesis carries a small but definite risk, and so is usually offered only to women who have carried a previous abnormal fetus, women with a family history of congenital disorder, and women over 35 years of age.

Rhesus incompatibility is now largely preventable. Sensitization of a rhesus-negative mother can usually be avoided by giving anti-D antibody. An affected fetus can be detected by amniocentesis and treated if necessary by exchange transfusion. For pregnant women with diabetes mellitus, special care can improve the outlook for the fetus. Further information about these aspects of care will be found in textbooks of obstetrics and paediatrics.

Postnatal prevention

In the UK, all infants are routinely tested for phenylketonuria, and routine testing for hypothyroidism and galactosaemia is becoming increasingly common. Universal screening for elevated levels of lead has been advocated, but recent evidence suggests that it is more appropriate to target screening in areas where lead levels are known to be high (Diermayer *et al.*, 1994). Intensive care units and improved methods of treatment for premature and low-birthweight infants can prevent learning disability in some who would previously have suffered brain damage. However, the methods also enable the survival of some disabled children who would otherwise have died.

Compensatory education

Compensatory education is intended to provide optimal conditions for the mental development of the disabled child. This was the aim of the Head Start programme in the USA, which provided extra education for deprived children. Its methods varied from nursery schooling to attempts to teach specific skills. Many of the results were disappointing (Rutter and Madge, 1976). A more intensive programme with similar aims was carried out in Milwaukee (Garber, 1988). Skilled teachers taught children living in slum areas with mothers who had a low IQ (under 75). This additional education started when the child was 3 months old and continued until school age. At the same time, the mothers were trained in a variety of domestic skills. These children were compared with control children of the same age who came from similar families but who had not received additional education and whose mothers had not been trained. At the age of four-and-a-half, the trained children had a mean IQ 27 points higher than that of the controls. This study can be faulted because the selection of children was not strictly random, and because some of the changes in test scores could have been due to practice. Nevertheless, the main findings probably stand: substantial effort by trained staff can produce worthwhile improvement in children of low intelligence born to socially disadvantaged mothers. The findings indicate the need to train the parents as well as children. Overall, it seems that early interventions can be effective, especially if they are family centred.

However, many uncertainties remain about the components and the delivery of such help (see Murphy, 1994).

Assessment

Severe learning disability is usually obvious from an early stage. Lesser degrees may become apparent only when the child starts school. Family doctors and teachers should be able to detect possible learning disability, but a full assessment may require attendance at a special centre where the child can be observed in many different activities. The methods have been described earlier.

Once learning disability has been diagnosed, regular reviews are required. For children, these reviews are usually carried out by an inter-disciplinary child health team in cooperation with teachers and social workers. The child psychiatrist liaises with the team and sees children referred to him with emotional, behavioural, and psychiatric problems.

It is important to arrange a thorough review before the child leaves school. This review should assess the need for further education, the prospects for employment, unpaid occupation, independent living, and the need for specialist physical and psychological health care. Adults with learning disability need to be assessed regularly to make sure that they are continuing to achieve their potential and still receiving appropriate care. This is usually carried out by a multidisciplinary community team which includes a psychiatrist specializing in the care of the learning disabled.

Help for families

Help for families is needed from the time that the diagnosis is first made. It is not enough to give worried parents a full explanation on just one occasion. They may need to hear the explanation several times before they can absorb all its implications. Adequate time must be allowed to explain the prognosis, indicate what help can be provided, and discuss the part the parents can play in helping their child to achieve full potential. Paediatricians and health visitors are usually involved in this process.

Thereafter, the parents need continuing support. When the child starts school, parents should be kept informed about progress, and feel involved in the planning and provision of care. They should be given help with practical matters, such as day care for the child during school holidays, baby-sitting, or arrangements for family holidays. In addition to practical assistance, the parents need continuing psychological support, which may be provided as a programme for the whole family (Murphy, 1994; Petronko *et al.* 1994).

Families are likely to need extra help when their child is approaching puberty or leaving school. Making the transition from child to adult services is often extremely stressful. Both day and overnight care are often required to relieve carers and to encourage the learning-disabled person to become more independent.

Education, training, and occupation

One aspect of the policy of normalization is that children with learning disability should be educated as far as possible within mainstream schools. The extent to which this is done varies in different countries and different regions of the same country.

Research has consistently shown the value of an early start to the education of children with learning disability, who should attend a play group or nursery class. When school age is reached, the least disabled children can attend remedial classes in ordinary schools. Others need to attend special educational programmes for children with learning disabilities. It is still not certain which learning-disabled children benefit from ordinary schooling. Education in an ordinary school offers the advantages of more normal social surroundings, social integration, and the expectation of progress, but it may have the disadvantage of a lack of special teaching skills and equipment. Also, the methods of teaching emphasizing self-expression are inappropriate for some children with learning disability who need special teaching of language and communication (Howlin, 1994). An advantage in having disabled children in ordinary schools is that other pupils learn to accept that their integration into society is the norm.

Before learning-disabled children leave school, they need reassessment and vocational guidance. Most young people with mild learning disability are able to take normal jobs or enter sheltered employment. Adults with severe disability are likely to transfer to adult day centres, which should provide a wide range of activities if the abilities of each attender are to be developed as much as possible.

Residential care

It is now widely accepted that parents should be supported in caring for their learning-disabled children at home. If care is too heavy a burden for the parents because of their other family commitments, the child with learning disability should, if possible, be in another family. Adults should be supported in ordinary housing, or placed with a family, or lodgings, or in a small residential group home. Studies such as those of

Landesman-Dyer (1981) confirmed that moving learning-disabled children to smaller living units is not itself beneficial. Staff need to encourage the residents to develop their social skills and to live as normally as possible. Also, challenging behaviour is not necessarily reduced by a move to a smaller living unit.

Medical services

People with learning disability should have the same access to general and specialist medical services as other citizens, but they require extra support if they are to obtain full benefit. Children and adults with learning disability often have physical handicaps or epilepsy, for which continuing medical care is needed. This care is usually obtained from the ordinary medical services and this arrangement can work well, provided doctors and nurses are sufficiently aware of how to deal with a person with learning disability and have the time and resources to do so. Families and carers are helped when care is coordinated by a single person so that they do not receive conflicting advice. Specialist nurses have a special role in such coordination. Shared care between neurologists and psychiatrists can improve outcomes for some patients, for example, in the diagnosis and treatment of episodic attacks.

Psychiatric services

Psychiatric care is an essential part of a comprehensive community service for people with learning disability. In some countries this care is provided by the generic mental health services, but in the UK it is generally provided by staff who specialize in the care of people with learning disability.

Treatment of psychiatric disorder and behavioural problems

Treatment of psychiatric disorder in the learning disabled follows the principles described elsewhere in this book, taking account of their special problems.

Psychiatric disorder in people with learning disability usually comes to notice through changes in behaviour. It should be remembered, however, that behavioural change can also result from physical illness or from stressful events, both of which should be carefully excluded. In the most disabled, and especially those with sensory deficits, behavioural disturbance may be due to understimulation and frustration at the inability to communicate wishes and needs. Once the cause is clear, the treatment follows. Physical illness should be treated promptly, stressful events reduced if possible, or a more stimulating environment provided when appropriate. If the disturbed behaviour results from a psychiatric disorder, the treatment is similar in most ways to that for a patient of normal intelligence with the same disorder. Carers are often involved in behavioural assessment and treatment methods and it is important to support them adequately.

The most serious and persistent disorders may require hospital admission for more intensive behavioural management, which may be combined with pharmacotherapy.

Medication

The indications for psychotropic drugs are generally the same as in patients of normal intelligence and the full range of such medication should be available for the learning disabled. However, the psychiatrist has particular responsibility for organizing effective ongoing monitoring, including regular physical examination. The latter is especially important for patients with severe communication impairments who cannot describe adverse effects. Also, neurologically impaired patients may be develop adverse effects at lower doses and suffer from oversedation, delirium, and extrapyramidal symptoms. Antipsychotic and benzodiazepine drugs are often useful in the short-term control of behaviour problems. There are few controlled trials of the efficacy and tolerability of antipsychotic drugs in the longer-term treatment of abnormal behaviour (see Brylewski and Duggan, 2004). Nonetheless, clinical experience suggests that severely behaviourally disturbed patients who do not respond to psychosocial interventions sometimes benefit from prolonged use of medication with frequent monitoring of its effects and adjustment of dosage.

About one-third of patients with learning disability have epilepsy and **antiepileptic drug treatment** is required when the seizures are a significant risk for health, safety, and quality of life. Special care is needed in selecting a drug and dosage that controls seizures without producing unwanted effects. The older antiepileptic drugs sometimes produce oversedation and cognitive blunting. Modern 'first-line' antiepileptic drugs are often carbamazepine and sodium valproate (see pp. 561–2). Some patients with epilepsy that is difficult to treat benefit from one of the 'add-on' antiepileptic drugs but vigilance should be maintained for adverse effects. The choice of drug should usually be made by, or in conjunction with, a specialist in epilepsy.

Psychological treatment

Although limited understanding of language sets obvious limitations to the use of psychotherapy, simple discussion is often helpful. Cognitive therapies can be attempted with some patients with higher verbal ability. Counselling for parents is an important part of treatment. If more formal family therapy is undertaken, families generally prefer structural approaches, which address the problems and solutions relevant for them. Some people with profound learning disability can be helped by the use of play and sensory stimulation to encourage developmental advances (Hewett and Nind, 1998).

Behaviour modification

Behavioural methods are potentially helpful to people with severe learning disability since some of the methods do not require language. Such methods can be used to encourage basic skills such as washing, toilet training, and dressing. Often parents and teachers are taught to carry out the training so that it can be maintained in the patient's everyday environment (Petronko *et al.*, 1994). If the problem is an undesired behaviour, a search is made for any environmental factors that seem regularly to provoke it or reinforce it (functional analysis). If possible, these environmental factors are changed and carers helped to avoid rewarding the behaviour. At the same time, alternative adaptive responses are reinforced. Aggressive behaviour is sometimes dealt with by so-called 'time-out' in which the patient is ignored or secluded until the behaviour subsides. Techniques using negative reinforcement raise important ethical issues, and should not be used (see Matson and Taras, 1989). If the problem is an insufficiency of some socially desirable behaviour, attempts can be made to reinforce such behaviour with material or social rewards, if necessary by 'shaping' the final behaviour from simpler components. Reward should be given immediately after the desired behaviour has taken place (for example, using the toilet). For training in skills such as dressing, it is often necessary to provide modelling and prompting in the early stages, and to reduce them gradually later (Petronko *et al.*, 1994; Spreat and Behar, 1994).

Informing patients

People with learning disablity have the same concerns as other patients about the nature of their disorder, its effects on their lives, and the treatment. These concerns will be formulated in a less complex way, and the answers need to be adapted to the patient's intellectual level and at an appropriate level and expressed in easily understood language.

Special problems

Growing old

Several problems arise more frequently as people with learning disability live longer. When the parents are the carers, they may find care increasingly burdensome as they grow old. Such parents are often concerned about the future of their learning-disabled child when they have died and yet are reluctant to arrange alternative care while they are still alive.

The older person with learning disability also faces special problems. If his parents die first, he faces problems of bereavement. The isolation felt by many of these bereaved people may be increased because other people are not sure how to offer comfort, and because the learning-disabled person may be excluded from the ritual of mourning. These bereaved people should be helped to come to terms with the loss, using the principles that apply generally to grief counselling (see p. 170), but choosing appropriately simple forms of communication (see Hollins and Esterhuyzen, 1997).

A third problem for people with learning disability as they grow old is the onset of dementia. This problem is considered on p. 710.

Exploitation and abuse

People with learning disability are vulnerable to exploitation and to physical and sexual abuse. In the past these problems were associated with poorly managed large institutions, but they can occur also in small community units. Such units need regular supervision, and clinicians should consider abuse as an uncommon but important cause of disturbed behaviour among people with learning disability.

Ethical and legal problems in the care of learning-disabled people

Normalization, autonomy, and the conflict of interests

The policy of normalization encourages learning-disabled people to live as near normal lives as possible. This policy can create conflicts between the interests of the learning-disabled person and those of other people. These conflicts arise because many learning-disabled people require support from carers in some ways, if they are to achieve autonomy in other ways. For example, they may need help with dressing if they are to live away from hospital. Many carers are members of the family of the disabled person and arrangements that are entered into willingly may become burdensome if the needs of the disabled person increase, as the needs of other children increase, or as the parents grow older. It may then be difficult to balance the interests of the disabled person, the carers, and other members of the carers' family. These difficulties can usually be resolved most equitably if they are discussed with the disabled person, the carers, and the other family members, and between the professionals responsible for each of these people.

Normalization can also produce unintended effects. For example, normalization requires that learning-disabled children should be educated in ordinary schools whenever possible. However, in secondary schools, children with special needs were found to be bullied three times more often than other children (Whitney *et al.*, 1994). It could be argued that it is in the immediate interests of an individual child to be educated in a special school where he is less likely to be bullied. However, the long-term interests of learning-disabled children as a group may be advanced more by a policy of education in ordinary schools whilst making strenuous efforts to eradicate bullying. This policy might eventually lead to greater understanding of, and respect for people with learning disability.

Normalization also leads to ethical questions about sexual activity, contraception, and possible conflicts of interest between a learning-disabled mother and her child.

Consent to treatment

The important general issues relating to informed consent for physical and psychiatric treatment are discussed on p. 73–5. Many people with severe learning disability are unable to give informed consent, and it is essential to be aware of local legislation and practice. In the UK, there is no provision for others to give proxy consent for an adult who is not competent in this regard, and the clinical team must proceed in the patient's best interests (though at the time of writing, the matter is under discussion). If there is doubt and inpatient admission is being sought, it is good practice to discuss matters with an approved social worker. Seriously ill patients who refuse potentially life-saving treatments can prove difficult to deal with in general medical settings. If the patient is so intellectually impaired as not to understand the nature of the choice he or she faces and there is a medical emergency, it may be appropriate to proceed with treatment under 'common law'. If there is time, it may be necessary to refer the case for review in court, for example when the question of termination of pregnancy has to be decided.

The reader should discover the legal requirements in the place he is working, and discuss best practice with an experienced practitioner.

Consent to research

Consent to research requires the ability to understand information, to use the information rationally, to appreciate the consequences of situations, and to between alternatives (see Chapter 3). In general, these abilities should be greater as the ratio of risk to benefit of the proposed research increases. The assessment of these abilities among the learning disabled is described in American Psychiatric Association (1998). All people who have agreed to take part in research should understand that they can withdraw consent if they wish. This point should be explained with particular care to the learning disabled. In one study, half the learning-disabled people who understood the purpose of a research project did not understand that they could withdraw from it (Arscott *et al.*, 1998). In general no research should be undertaken involving people who cannot consent, unless the same research cannot be successfully carried out without involving these people. It is important to remember that people with learning disability vary in their capacity to provide informed consent. For example most adults with mild learning disability should be able to provide informed consent but those who have severe and profound disability will not. Some may be able to provide verbal rather than written consent. Some may need sign language, pictures or written information in simple language and large font size in order to understand the research proposal. For some the proposal may have to be discussed repeatedly by a carer before an informed consent could be provided. If it is not possible to obtain informed consent and to exclude the person from research then it is a good practice to have agreement with the carers and the multidisciplinary team members. In every case the research should follow strictly the research governance criteria laid down by organizations such as, in the UK, the Department of Health and the Royal College of Physicians.

Further reading

Deb, S, Matthews, T, Holt, G and Bouras, N (eds) (2001a) *Practice guidelines for the assessment and diagnosis of mental health problems in adults with intellectual Disability.* European Association for Mental Health in Mental Retardation (EAMHMR), www.estiacntre.org. (A user-friendly reference with emphasis on specific manifestation of psychiatric symptoms among adults who have learning disabilities.)

Fraser WI and Kerr, M (eds) (2003) *Seminars in the psychiatry of learning disabilities*. Gaskell, London. (Covers the main topics at a level intended for psychiatric trainees.)

Gelder, MG, López-Ibor, JJ Jr and Andreasen, NC (eds) (2000) *The new Oxford textbook of psychiatry*, Part 10: Mental retardation. Oxford University Press, Oxford. (The 13 chapters in this part of the textbook provide a systematic account of the subject written for the general psychiatrist.)

Hamilton-Kirkwood, L, Ahmed, Z, Allen, D, Deb, S, Fraser, WI, Lindsay, W, McKenzie, K, Penny, E and Scotland, J (Ees) (2001) *Health evidence bulletins Wales: Learning disabilities (intellectual disability)*. NHS Wales, http://www.hebw.uwcm.ac.uk (Health gain recommendations made on the basis of the hierarchy of evidence available.)

NHS Health Scotland (2004) *Health needs assessment report: people with learning disabilities in Scotland*. NHS Health Scotland, Glasgow, www.healthscotland.com. (A comprehensive well-referenced document on the health needs of people with learning disabilities.)

CHAPTER 26

Forensic psychiatry

Chapter contents

Chapter 4 covered general legal and ethical issues in the practice of medicine and psychiatry. This chapter is concerned with other aspects of psychiatry and the law covered by the term **forensic psychiatry**; which is used in two ways:

1. Narrowly, it is applied to the branch of psychiatry that deals with the assessment and treatment of mentally abnormal offenders.
2. Broadly, the term is applied to all legal aspects of psychiatry including the civil law and laws regulating psychiatric practice.

Forensic psychiatrists are concerned with both these issues. In addition, they also assess risk and treat people with violent behaviour who have not committed an offence in law. They have a growing role in the assessment and treatment of victims.

Offenders with mental disorders constitute a minority of all offenders, but they present many difficult problems for psychiatry and the law. These include **legal issues**, such as the relationship between the mental disorder and the crime which may affect the court's determination of responsibility, and **practical clinical questions**, such as whether an offender needs psychiatric treatment and finding the appropriate setting for that treatment.

The psychiatrist therefore needs knowledge not only of the law but also of the relationship between particular kinds of crime and particular kinds of psychiatric disorder. It is also important to be aware that mental health services form only a small part of the social and legal response to criminal deviance; the psychiatrist working with offenders needs to be able to liaise with others in the criminal justice system, such as lawyers, prison staff, and probation officers. Concepts of deviance, guilt, and legality are influenced by legal, political, and social factors, as well as by clinical issues.

In reading this chapter it is important to be aware of the very large differences between countries and jurisdictions which lead to substantial national variations in epidemiology, definitions of crime, legal practice, and the role of the psychiatrist. Readers need to be aware of legal issues and procedures in their jurisdiction. In the following account, the situations and procedures in the UK (and more especially England and Wales) are used as examples to illustrate general themes. Ethical issues are summarized in Box 26.1.

BOX 26.1 ETHICAL ISSUES IN FORENSIC PSYCHIATRY

The principal ethical issues relate to 'boundary problems'. The psychiatrist and others involved need to be clear about accountability to legal authorities, etc., rather than to the individual being assessed and treated. This applies to a variety of activities:

1. Preparation of medico-legal reports. In the UK the responsibility of the psychiatrist is to the Court rather than the patient or their legal representative
2. Assessment of risk. Assessment of the risk to others may be paramount
3. Voluntary and compulsory treatment. The primary reason for treatment may involve decreasing the risk of harm to others. Issues of 'treatability' may arise in patients with personality disorder (see p. 749).

General criminology

There is a very large literature on criminology and many theories of the causes of crime; interested readers are referred to criminology textbooks (see Maguire and Morgan, 2002). Most theories have emphasized the sociological aspects of crime, deviance, and other types of rule-breaking. Social studies have drawn attention to social and economic causes of crime in the family, peer group, and subculture, such as poverty, poor schooling, and unemployment. Since many of the proposed predisposing social and individual factors are interrelated, simple conclusions are not possible. However, it is widely held that such causes of crime are more important than individual psychological factors such as genetics and psychological traits. However, psychological risk factors for offending are the subject of most correctional and forensic mental health programmes, which encourage, for example, the development of coping skills (Dowden *et al.*, 2003).

Prevalence

Prevalence figures must be viewed cautiously because they depend on reporting and much criminal behaviour is unrecorded by the police. This is especially true of violence within the home, such as rape, child abuse, or partner battering. More accurate figures probably come from crime surveys and data from the British Crime Survey are shown in Figure 26.1. Figure 26.2 shows the crimes recorded by the police in England and Wales in 2002–2003, classified by type of offence together with the same data for the British Crime

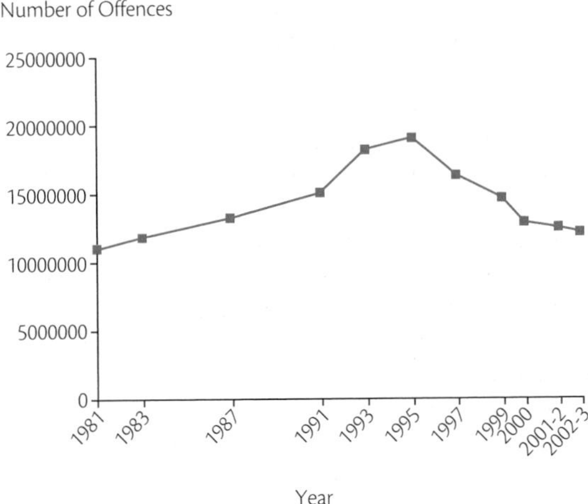

Fig. 26.1 Crimes reported to the British Crime Survey by the public 1981–2003.

Survey (Simmons and Dodd, 2003). In the UK, as in most countries, property offences are the most common type of crime. By contrast, forensic mental health services are most likely to be involved with individuals who have committed crimes of interpersonal violence, apart from instances where repeated property crime may indicate a mental disorder.

National differences

There are large national differences in the rates and patterns of crime. For example, overall rates of reported criminal activity are higher in Australia than in most parts of Europe. Within Europe, overall crime rates in the UK are below those of the Netherlands but above the Scandinavian countries. Crimes of assault are more common in the USA and Australia than in Western Europe (Farrington *et al.*, 2004). Rates and patterns of national statistics are affected by local legislation, the recording of crimes, and by the conduct of legal proceedings.

Gender

In all cultures, crime is predominantly an activity of young men. In England and Wales half of all indictable offences are committed by males aged under 21, and a quarter by males aged under 17. In all cultures surveyed, men make up at least 80 per cent of offenders (Monahan, 1997). In most Western countries, male prisoners outnumber female prisoners by 30:1. This gender difference is reflected in forensic mental health services, where male patients make up the vast majority.

Ethnicity

In most countries, ethnic minority groups are over-represented in prisoner populations. This is usually because minority groups are more likely to be poor, unemployed, and living in poor housing, all of which are risk factors for crime. Minority groups are therefore also more likely to be over-represented in forensic patient populations (Kaye and Lingiah, 2000).

There is considerable concern in many countries as to the extent to which the high rates of arrests and convictions of members of minority groups are also due to

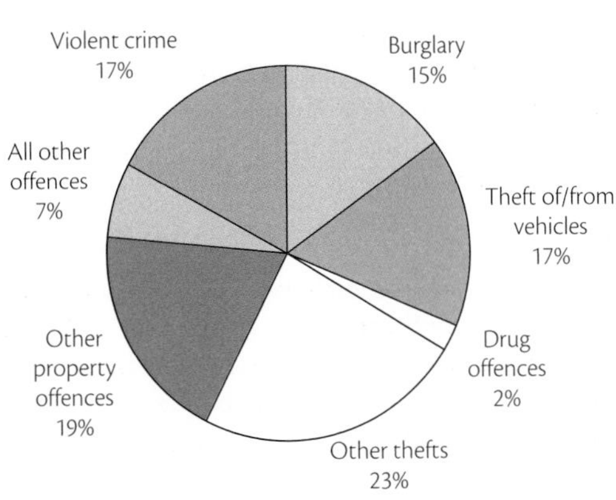

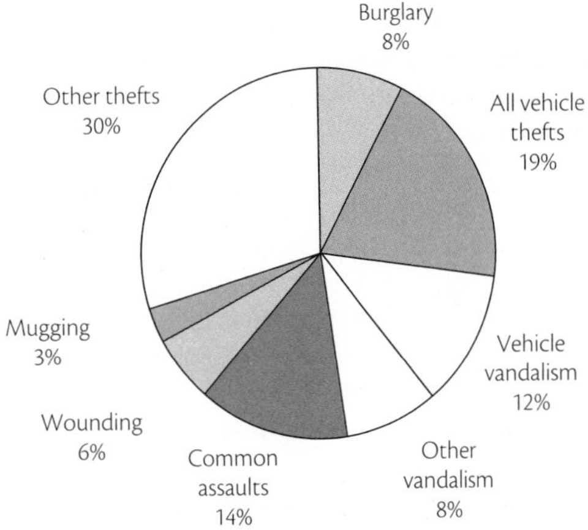

Fig. 26.2 Crimes recorded by the police and those reported to the British Crime Survey by victims of crime 2002–2003. Some of the categories differ and drug offences are not included in the crime survey figures.

discrimination against them at all stages of the criminal justice system: suspicion, stopping and arresting in the street, cautioning and charging, prosecution and trial outcome, and sentencing.

Victims

Most property crime is committed against strangers. By contrast, most serious interpersonal violence (such as rape, homicide, or child abuse) is committed by offenders against people who are known to them. Women are exposed to sexual violence from men in both developed and developing countries. In the latter, women and children are particularly at risk during armed conflicts where about 70 per cent of casualties are non-combatants (Renzetti, 2005).

Victims of crime tend to be disadvantaged groups living in poorer parts of urban communities; on this account we may expect that the mentally disordered are as likely to be victims of crime as perpetrators.

Causes of crime

It is important to distinguish several widely used terms with different meanings.

Criminal behaviour (crime) needs to be distinguished from rule-breaking behaviour; not all rule breaking, or socially unacceptable behaviour is criminal. Thus fire-setting is a behaviour; the crime is called arson. Not all criminal behaviour is violent; in fact the vast majority is not; thus general theories of the causes of crime will not necessarily address the causes of violence.

There is an important distinction between aggression and violence; aggressive behaviour is not always violent, it is constrained by social rules.

Violence is aggressive behaviour that transgresses social norms. An example is street fighting, which transgresses the criminal law, in contrast to boxing, which conforms to social rules.

Multiple factors determine whether an individual is aggressive in a particular situation: personality, the immediate social group, the behaviour of the victim, disinhibiting factors such as alcohol or drugs, general environmental factors such as noise and social pressure, physiological factors such as fatigue, hunger, and lack of sleep, and the presence of mental abnormality. Aggression is not a crime, but violent behaviour generally is because it results in harm defined by the law.

Genetic and physiological factors

Early **studies of twins** suggested that concordance rates for criminality were substantially greater in monozygotic twins than in dizygotic twins (Lange, 1931). **Later adoption studies** in Sweden and in Denmark have confirmed the genetic influence but shown that it is more modest than Lange supposed. It is mainly significant for severe and persistent criminality. Genetic factors are well-established for conduct disorder in children and the continuity in aggressive antisocial behaviour between childhood and adolescence is largely mediated by genetic influences (Eley *et al.*, 2003). The way in which genetic factors might mediate the increased risk of criminal offending is unclear but could involve the hyperactivity and low IQ which are risk factors in children for subsequent adult offending (Rutter, 2005).

The gender difference in offending has raised the question of the influence of either the Y chromosome or testosterone levels on offending. However, there is little evidence that **chromosomal or hormonal abnormalities** are causally associated with criminal behaviour or aggression. As noted previously (Chapter 7) low brain 5-HT function has been associated with impulsive aggression which can be either self or other-directed (Lee and Coccaro, 2001). In addition, there is growing evidence that individuals with sociopathic personalities have long-standing deficits in neuropsychological function, particularly executive processes (Raine *et al.*, 2005).

Psychosocial factors

Individual psychological development interacts with social factors and cultural values to make offending more likely (Table 26.1). Rule-breaking and antisocial behaviour often start in childhood or early adulthood:

- Follow-up studies of delinquent youth show that early patterns of antisocial behaviour are likely to persist into adulthood.
- Delinquency is associated with harsh parenting and poverty.
- Exposure to physical abuse or neglect in childhood significantly increases the risk of violent offending in later life, for both men and women (see Rutter, 2005).

The specific association between childhood adversity and violence may be mediated by a number of factors. First, abused and neglected children may have a heightened perception of threat from others. Second, they may have decreased capacities to make successful interpersonal relationships; perhaps because they have decreased empathy for others, or because they lack the capacity for self-awareness. Individuals who become violent may have decreased capacity to manage arousal or regulate affects such as anger or anxiety; perhaps as a result of being exposed to fear experiences. Of course it is also possible that children and parents may share genetic factors that impair affect regulation or the ability to empathize with others. Finally, it is important to consider the operation of resilience or vulnerability factors, such as temperament (see Rutter, 2005).

Psychiatric causes

There is a small but important group of offenders whose criminal behaviour seems to be partly explicable by specific psychological or psychiatric abnormalities. This group particularly concerns the psychiatrist and is discussed in the next section.

The association between mental disorder and crime

Frequency

One of the few studies of the association between mental disorder and violence in a large community sample, the Epidemiologic Catchment Area Study in the USA, found significant associations between subject's violent behaviour and mental disorder (Swanson *et al.*, 1990). A later study investigated subjects drawn from a birth cohort of individuals born in Denmark between 1944 and 1947 (Brennan *et al.*, 2000). The main findings were:

1. The risk of being arrested for a violent offence was significantly greater in both men (odds ratio 4.6, 95 per cent CI 3.8–5.6) and women (odds ratio 23.2, 95 per cent CI 14.4–37.4) who had been hospitalized for schizophrenia.
2. The risk of being arrested for a violent offence was also greater in men who had been hospitalized for organic psychosis (odds ratio 8.8, 95 per cent CI 7.4–10.0).
3. The increased risk of violent offending in these groups was not explained by demographic factors or comorbid substance misuse.
4. Both men and women with a diagnosis of affective psychosis also showed an increased risk of violent offending; however, in this group the increased risk could be accounted for by alcohol and substance misuse.

An earlier study of the same cohort had shown that alcohol and substance misuse by themselves are associated with a substantially increased risk of violent offending as is antisocial personality disorder (Table 26.2) (Chiswick, 2000).

Research has also focused on the prevalence and association of mental disorder in prisoners but some limitations of this approach need to be appreciated:

- not all criminals are brought to trial and found guilty;
- not all criminals go to prison, so studies of prisoners may result in sampling bias;
- mentally disordered offenders may be diverted away from courts and prisons, or they may not be prosecuted.

Recent work has shown that a significant proportion of prisoners have mental disorders, and this proportion is higher than the general population. In a recent meta-analysis of 62 psychiatric surveys of prisoners, Fazel and Danesh (2002) found that about one in seven prisoners have a treatable psychiatric illness (Table 26.3). A larger number suffer from antisocial personality disorder.

TABLE 26.1 Psychosocial risk factors for offending

Individual factors
Hyperactivity and impulsivity
Low intelligence
Child-rearing – poor supervision, harsh discipline, rejection, teenage mothers
Parental conflict – separations
Criminal parents
Large family size
Social factors
Socioeconomic deprivation
Peer influences
School influences
Community influences

See Farrington (2000).

TABLE 26.2 1944–1947 Danish Birth Cohort Study: relative risk estimates of violent crime between 1978 and 1990

Disorder	Male	Female
Major mental disorder	4.5	8.7
Learning difficulties	7.7	11.5
Antisocial personality	7.2	12.2
Drug misuse	8.7	15.1
Alcohol misuse	6.7	14.9

Source Chiswick (2000).

TABLE 26.3 Meta-analysis of 62 psychiatric surveys of prisoners

Disorder	Male (%)	Female (%)
Psychosis	4	4
Major depression	10	12
Antisocial personality	65	42

The nature of the association

A causal relationship between mental disorder and crime is difficult to show empirically, especially if the type of crime is not defined. The finding that mentally disordered individuals are overrepresented in prison does not necessarily mean that their mental disorder caused them to offend.

Conversely, it must be borne in mind that criminal law-breaking is not an indicator of itself of mental disorder, no matter how heinous or bizarre the behaviour. For example, most sexual violence is not associated with mental disorder in the perpetrator; accounts of sexual violence by invading armies make it clear that some types of violence may have social rather than diagnostic meaning.

Overall, it is important to emphasize that only a small minority of all people who commit violent acts have serious mental illness such as psychosis. The vast majority of patients with psychotic illnesses are no more dangerous than members of the general population, and there is no evidence that homicidal behaviour is becoming more common in people with mental illness (Taylor and Gunn, 1999).

For a review of the association between psychiatric disorder and offending see Chiswick (2000) (Box 26.2).

BOX 26.2 PSYCHIATRIC DISORDER AND OFFENDING

- People with psychotic disorders are more likely than members of the general public to acquire convictions for violent or other crimes (by factors of approximately 8 and 30 respectively).
- This increased likelihood is altered in strength by local factors such as crime rate and sociodemographic variables.
- Antisocial personality disorder and substance misuse disorders have greater associations with offending than does psychotic illness.
- A combination of psychiatric disorders (particularly when one is substance misuse disorder) may be more relevant than any single category of psychiatric disorder.
- Most offending by those with psychiatric disorder is minor in nature; violence when it occurs is likely to be targeted at a family member.

Source Chiswick (2000)

Specific psychiatric disorders

Substance dependence and crime.

There are close relationships between substance abuse and crime which have substantially affected legislation, enforcement, and national policies (Grann and Fazel, 2004).

Alcohol and crime are related in three important ways:

1. Alcohol intoxication may lead to charges related to public drunkenness or to driving offences
2. Intoxication reduces inhibitions and is strongly associated with crimes of violence, including murder
3. The neuropsychiatric complications of alcoholism may also be linked with crime.

An example of this last point is that offences may be committed during alcoholic amnesias or 'blackouts' (periods of several hours or days which the heavy drinker cannot subsequently recall, although at the time they appeared normally conscious to other people and were able to carry out complicated actions). However, the association is complex, and social factors related to drinking may be as important as alcohol itself. See Johns (2000).

Intoxication with drugs may lead to criminal behaviour including violent offences. Drug misusers, especially those dependent on heroin and cocaine, commit repeated offences against both property and people to pay for their drugs. Some of the offences involve violence. Rates of drug abuse are increased among prisoners, and many succeed in obtaining drugs in prison. Involvement in criminal activity and with other criminals may lead to drug usage. For a review of the relationship between drug dependence and crime see Johns (2000).

Learning disability

There is no evidence that most criminals are of markedly low intelligence. However, significantly below average intellectual ability is an independent predictor of offending (Holland *et al.*, 2002).

People with learning disabilities may commit offences because they do not understand the implications of their behaviour, or because they are susceptible to exploitation by other people. While property offences are the most common, sexual offences are also over-represented, particularly indecent exposure by males (Perry *et al.*, 2002). The exposer is often known to the victim and therefore the rate of detection is high. There is also an association between learning disability and arson (Chiswick, 2000).

Mood disorder

Depressive disorder is sometimes associated with shoplifting. Much more seriously, severe depressive disorder may lead to **homicide**. When this happens, the depressed person has usually experienced delusions, for example, that the world is too dreadful a place for him and his family to live in; they may then kill their spouse or children to spare them from the horrors of the world. The killer often commits suicide afterwards. A mother suffering from post-partum disorder may sometimes kill her newborn child or her older children. Rarely, a person with severe depressive disorder may commit homicide because of a persecutory belief, for example, that the victim is conspiring against the patient. Occasionally, ideas of guilt and unworthiness lead depressed patients to confess to crimes that they did not commit.

Manic patients may spend excessively on expensive objects such as jewellery or cars that they cannot pay for. They may hire cars and fail to return them, or steal cars for their own use. They may be charged with fraud, theft, or false pretences. Manic patients are also prone to irritability and aggression, which may lead to offences of violence, though the violence is seldom severe.

Schizophrenia and related disorder

Psychotic illnesses may be associated with violence, especially when paranoid symptomatology is present, or the patient also has a substance abuse problem. Violence may occur because the offender is frightened, and self-control may be reduced by the presence of the psychotic state. Any mental state or disorder in which paranoid psychotic symptoms feature may be associated with an increased risk of violent behaviour.

Epidemiology

Epidemiological studies have strongly suggested that schizophrenia is associated with an increased risk of both violent and non-violent offending (Brennan *et al.*, 2000; Arsenault *et al.*, 2000) (see above). This risk is substantially increased by substance misuse. It is, however, important to put the risk of violent offending in schizophrenia in context because the proportion of violent crime in society attributable to schizophrenia is low, consistently less than 10 per cent (Walsh *et al.*, 2002). A number of clinical risk factors for violence in schizophrenia have been proposed:

- fear and loss of self-control associated with non-systematized delusions
- systematized paranoid delusions including the conviction that enemies must be defended against
- irresistible urges
- instructions from hallucinatory voices (command hallucinations)
- dual diagnosis, particularly substance misuse
- a strong negative affect (depression, anger, agitation).

Risk assessment is discussed on p. 752. However, it is essential to note here that violent threats made by patients with psychosis should be taken very seriously (especially in those with a history of previous violence); most serious violence occurs in those already known to psychiatrists. This is especially true if there is an identifiable victim.

Post-traumatic stress disorder

Post-traumatic stress disorder (PTSD) may be related to offending in three ways:

- Patients with PTSD may abuse substances in ways which increase their risk of criminal behaviour.
- PTSD is associated with increased irritability and decreased affect regulation, which may make angry and aggressive behaviour more likely.
- Rarely, patients with PTSD may experience dissociative episodes in which violence can take place, especially in circumstances resembling their original trauma. This is often hard to determine retrospectively.

PTSD has been the basis for psychiatric defences to homicide, especially in cases where battered women have killed a battering partner. In circumstances where there has been prolonged trauma, occasional acts of retaliatory violence are not uncommon.

Morbid jealousy

The syndrome of morbid (pathological) jealousy (see p. 314) may be associated with several of the above diagnoses. It has been identified in 12 per cent of 'insane' male murderers and 3 per cent of 'insane' women murderers. It is particularly dangerous because of the risk of the offence being repeated with another partner. It may sometimes be hard to distinguish morbid jealousy from culturally accepted beliefs about women held by some subgroups of men. Extreme possessiveness or control of women's behaviour, which may be accompanied by violence, is seen in some cultures and may not be perceived as an indication of mental disorder.

Organic mental disorders

Delirium is occasionally associated with criminal behaviour; usually because of confusion or disinhibition caused by the disorder. Diagnostic problems may arise if the mental disturbance improves before the offender is examined by a doctor.

Dementia is sometimes associated with offences, though crime is otherwise uncommon among the elderly and violent offences are rare. Violent and disinhibited behaviour may also occur after traumatic damage to the brain following **head injury**. It may be hard to distinguish the effects of post-traumatic neurological difficulties from post-traumatic psychological disorder.

Epilepsy

The association between epilepsy and crime is complex and poorly understood. While it has been widely believed that the risk of epilepsy is greater in prisoners than the general population, a meta-analysis of seven studies indicated that this was not the case (Fazel *et al.*, 2002). Violent behaviour is sometimes associated with EEG abnormalities in the absence of clinical epilepsy, but it is doubtful that this indicates a causal relationship.

Epileptic automatisms may, very rarely, be associated with violent behaviour, and subsequent criminal proceedings. Violence is commoner in the post-ictal state than ictally.

Impulse control disorders

DSM-IV contains a rubric for 'impulse control disorders not otherwise classified' which brings together four speculative conditions relevant to forensic psychiatry: intermittent explosive disorder, pathological gambling, pyromania, and kleptomania. (The rubric also contains another condition, trichotillomania, hair pulling). In ICD-10 these conditions are classified under abnormalities of adult personality and behaviour as 'habit and impulse disorders'. Whatever the clinical value of such classifications, none of these conditions has been established as a separate diagnostic entity.

Intermittent explosive disorder

This term is used to describe repeated episodes of seriously aggressive behaviour directed to people or property that is out of proportion to any provoking events and is not accounted for by another psychiatric disorder (for example, antisocial personality disorder, substance abuse, or schizophrenia). The aggression may be preceded by tension and followed by relief of this tension. Later the person feels remorse. If care is taken to exclude other causes, the condition is rare. Many psychiatrists doubt whether this behaviour indicates a distinct psychiatric disorder.

Pathological gambling

Gambling is pathological when it is repeated frequently and dominates the person's life; the gambling persists when the person can no longer afford to pay his debts. The person lies, steals, or defrauds in order to obtain money or avoid repayment and to continue the habit. Family life may be damaged, other social relationships impaired, and employment put at risk.

Pathological gamblers have an intense urge to gamble, which is difficult to control. They are preoccupied with thoughts of gambling, much as a person dependent on alcohol is preoccupied with drink. Often, increasing sums of money are gambled, either to increase the excitement or in an attempt to recover previous losses. If gambling is prevented, the person becomes irritable and even more preoccupied with the behaviour.

Similarities between these patterns of behaviour and those of people dependent on drugs have led to the suggestion that pathological gambling is itself a form of addictive behaviour. Brain imaging studies of pathological gamblers have indicated functional abnormalities in mesolimbic reward pathways that are known to be modified by the processes involved in drug dependence (Goudriaan *et al.*, 2004).

The prevalence of pathological gambling is not known. It is probably more frequent among males. Most gamblers seen by psychiatrists are adults, but there is concern that young people are increasingly being involved, usually with gambling machines in amusement arcades and other places. Pathological gambling may lead to behaviours that bring the gambler to the attention of the courts, for example, fraud or stealing to obtain money to pay for the habit. For a review of pathological gambling see Dickerson and Baron (2000).

Pyromania

Pyromania is one cause of fire-setting (see p. 744). The term pyromania refers to repeated episodes of deliberate fire-setting, which are not carried out for monetary gain, to conceal a crime, as an act of vengeance, for social or political motives, or as a consequence of hallucinations, delusions, or impaired judgement (resulting from intoxication, dementia, or mental retardation, for example). The diagnosis is not made when there is an associated antisocial personality disorder, a manic episode, or (among children or adolescents) a conduct disorder. In this rare condition, the act of fire-setting is preceded by tension or arousal, and is followed by relief of tension. People with pyromania have a preoccupation with fires and firefighting. They enjoy watching fires. They may plan the fire-setting in advance, taking no account of the danger to other people from their actions. When other causes listed above are excluded, pyromania is rare; indeed, some writers doubt its existence.

Kleptomania

The term kleptomania refers to repeated failure to resist impulses to steal objects that are not needed, either for use or for their monetary value. The impulses are not associated with delusions or hallucinations, or with motives of anger or vengeance. Before the act of stealing there is increased tension; after the act there is relief of tension. The diagnosis is not made when there is an associated antisocial personality disorder, a manic episode, or (among children or adolescents) a conduct disorder, nor when the stealing results from sexual fetishism. The objects stolen may be of little value and could have been afforded; they may be hoarded, thrown away, or returned later to the owner. The patient knows that the stealing is unlawful, and may feel guilty and depressed after the immediate pleasurable sensations that follow the act. The disorder occurs more often among women. Associations with anxiety and eating disorders have been described. The behaviour may be sporadic with long intervals of remission, or may persist for years despite repeated prosecutions. When other causes of repeated stealing are excluded, the condition is rare; indeed, some writers doubt its existence as a separate syndrome, pointing out that diagnosis depends on accused persons' descriptions of their own motives. For a review see Marazziti *et al.*, 2003).

Specific offender groups

Females

Women are more law-abiding than men. The most common offence is stealing, with shoplifting accounting for half of all convictions of women for indictable offences. By contrast, violent and sexual offences are uncommon (Heidensohn, 1991). Women are also responsible for forms of antisocial behaviour that are regarded less severely by the law than those for which men are prosecuted, such as soliciting and some forms of social security fraud.

There are differences in the way men and women are treated by the criminal justice system. Women are sentenced more leniently for similar offences and they are more likely to be seen as 'sick'. Psychiatric disorder is frequent amongst women admitted to prison, with personality disorder and substance misuse being especially common (Fazel and Danesh, 2002). Rates for self-harm before and during imprisonment are also high.

The 'premenstrual syndrome' is often suggested as a causative factor by defence lawyers and has occasionally been accepted as such in a number of recent court decisions. It is possible that premenstrual symptoms may complicate or exacerbate pre-existing social and psychological difficulties, but there is no evidence that they are a primary cause of offending.

Young people

National crime statistics show that increasing numbers of people under 18 are becoming involved in criminal behaviour. In Scotland for example, in the year 2000, 34 per cent of young people (aged 12–15) reported committing a criminal offence in the previous year compared to 22 per cent in 1992 (Scottish Executive Central Research Unit, 2002). Most of the offences were minor in nature but 19 per cent reported fighting. Only 2 per cent reported taking illegal drugs (this may be an underestimate because of the self-report nature of the study). Where a young person engages in serious interpersonal violence, the victim is often well known to them, and may be a family member. Serious violence by young people and children is rare and the individuals involved have frequently been the recipient of violence themselves both inside and outside their families (Hamilton *et al.*, 2002).

Ethnic minorities

It is well established that some ethnic groups are overrepresented in the criminal justice system as offenders, and there is some evidence to suggest that this may be so in forensic psychiatric services. Patients from non-Caucasian groups may be more likely to receive mental illness diagnoses, and individual personality difficulties may be overlooked. Different cultural beliefs may be relevant, especially within the family, or to the expression of symptoms of mental illness. As indicated above, people from ethnic minorities may be at risk of negative discrimination by the criminal justice system and also socially stigmatized by having a mental disorder (Kaye and Lingiah, 2000). In the UK, people of African-

Carribean origin have a greater risk of imprisonment but lower rates of psychiatric morbidity while in prison than white prisoners (Coid *et al.*, 2002). The latter contrasts with the excess of African-Carribeans in secure hospitals and may mean that African-Carribeans who have offended while mentally ill are more likely to be admitted to hospital.

Psychiatric aspects of specific crimes

The following sections are concerned with the types of offences that are most likely to be associated with psychological factors: crimes of violence, sexual offences, and some offences against property.

Crimes of violence

Amongst mentally abnormal offenders, violence is more often associated with personality disorder than with major mental illness. It is particularly common in people with antisocial personality traits who misuse alcohol or drugs, or who have marked paranoid or sadistic traits. It is often part of a persistent pattern of impulsive and aggressive behaviour, but it may be a sporadic response to stressful events in 'over-controlled' personalities.

The assessment of dangerousness and the management of violence are discussed on p. 752.

Homicide

Most legal jurisdictions recognize different categories of homicide, depending on the degree of intention and responsibility shown by the perpetrator. For example, in the USA, defendants may be charged with different 'degrees' of murder; in England and Wales, there are three legal categories of homicide: murder, manslaughter, and infanticide.

In England and Wales murder and manslaughter are defined by historical precedent and not by statute. According to a widely quoted definition put forward by Lord Coke in 1797, murder occurs:

> when a man of sound memory and of the age of discretion unlawfully killeth within any country of the realm any reasonable creature in rerum natura under the King's peace with malice aforethought, either expressed by the party or implied by law, so as the party wounded or hit, etc, die of the wound or hit within a year and a day after the same.

Manslaughter is a diverse crime covering all unlawful homicides that are not murder. Various types of homicide fall within this category, but it is customary and useful to divide manslaughter into two main groups, designated 'voluntary' and 'involuntary' manslaughter, respectively. In voluntary manslaughter, the defendant may have malice aforethought of murder but the presence of some defined mitigating circumstances reduces his crime to a less serious grade of criminal homicide. In involuntary manslaughter, there is no malice aforethought; it includes, for example, causing death by gross negligence.

Normal and abnormal homicide

Mental disorders may count as a form of mitigation when an individual is charged with murder, and thus the charge is reduced to manslaughter. It is common practice to divide homicide into 'normal' and 'abnormal' according to the legal outcome. Homicide is 'normal' if there is a conviction of murder or common law manslaughter; it is 'abnormal' if there is a finding of insane murder, suicide murder, diminished responsibility, or infanticide.

'Normal' homicide accounts for half to two-thirds of all homicides occurring in the UK, i.e. the majority of killings. The same is true of other Western countries, such as the USA, where the overall homicide rate is much higher than in the UK. 'Normal' homicide is most likely to be committed by young men of low social class. In the UK, the victims are mainly family members or close acquaintances. In countries with high homicide rates, a greater proportion of killings are associated with robbery or sexual offences. Sexual homicide may result from panic during a sexual offence or may be a feature of a sadistic killing, sometimes committed by a shy man with bizarre sadistic and other violent fantasies.

'Abnormal' homicide accounts for a third to half of all homicides in the UK. It is usually committed by older people. The victims of abnormal homicide are often family members. In those who commit 'abnormal' homicide, the most common psychiatric diagnoses are psychoses, substance use disorder and personality disorder (Fazel and Grann, 2004). Depressive disorder can also be involved especially in those who kill themselves afterwards. Homicide by women is much less frequent than by men; when it occurs and is nearly always 'abnormal' (Shaw *et al.*, 1999).

There is very considerable public concern about dangerousness and homicide amongst mentally ill people. There is no evidence that these problems are increasing or that there is any reason to doubt that, in general principle, the care of mental illness in the community is safe (Taylor and Gunn, 1999). Nevertheless, better care is needed for the very small minority who are dangerous.

A large proportion of all murderers are under the influence of alcohol at the time of the crime and drug misuse is also an important factor.

Multiple homicide

Multiple murders are rare, although they attract great public attention. They include:

- those without mental illness who kill several people at once, sometimes a family killing which is often followed by suicide. Paranoid and grandiose character traits are common (Mullen, 2004).
- killings attributable to a psychotic illness in which the killer aims to save himself or his family from a perceived threat;
- serial killings taking place over a period of time. These may be 'normal' (for example, killings by terrorists), or abnormal (e.g. psychotic, or motivated by sexual sadism or necrophilia).

Homicide followed by suicide

Homicide followed by suicide accounts for about 50 deaths in the UK annually while in the United States, the comparable figure is 1000–1500 (Chiswick, 2000). An epidemiological survey of 327 such deaths (180 victims and 147 perpetrators) in the UK found the following (Barraclough and Harris, 2002):

- 80 per cent of the incidents had one victim and one perpetrator
- 88 per cent of incidents exclusively involved members of the same family
- 75 per cent of the victims were female while 85 per cent of perpetrators were male
- The victims of the male perpetrators were nearly always current or previous female partners and their children while the victims of female perpetrators were predominantly their children
- A few men kill strangers and then themselves. Such individuals may be psychotic or more commonly have paranoid and narcissistic traits and take revenge for trivial or imagined slights or humiliations.

Parents who kill their children

A quarter of all victims of murder or manslaughter in the UK are under the age of 16 and babies under the age of one are at the highest risk of all age groups (Breslin and Evans, 2004). Most children are killed by a parent who is mentally ill, usually the mother. The classification of child murder is difficult, but useful categories are mercy killing, psychotic murder, and killing as the end result of battering or neglect (D'Orban, 1979). This last category is most common.

Infanticide

A woman who kills her child may be charged with murder or manslaughter. Some jurisdictions (such as English law) recognize a special category of child killing called infanticide where the child is under 12 months of age. Infanticide is treated as manslaughter and therefore attracts less harsh penalties. The judge has the same freedom of sentencing for a conviction of infanticide as for a conviction of manslaughter. The English legal concept of infanticide is unusual in that the accused is required to show only that her mind was disturbed as a result of birth or lactation, but not that the killing was a consequence of her mental disturbance.

Infanticide is very rare and fewer than five cases a year are recorded in the UK (Chiswick, 2000). Marks and Kumar (1993) examined records of all infants aged under a year who were victims of homicide during 1982–1988. Infants were most at risk on the first day of life, and the relative risk decreased steadily thereafter until by the final quarter of the first year of life the risk of homicide was the same as that of the general population. Parents were the most frequent perpetrators, mothers on the first day and thereafter fathers were slightly more likely to be recorded as the prime suspect. Mothers received less severe sentences than fathers. Contrary to wide belief, puerperal psychotic illness was a relatively infrequent cause of homicide by the mother, though depression was a factor in some cases. Later infant homicides are usually fatal child abuse. Infanticide was strongly associated with motherhood at a young age. Despite the relative rarity of post-partum psychosis as cause of infanticide, such deaths are potentially preventable which means that the detection and treatment of serious post-partum mental illness should be a priority (Spinelli, 2004).

Family homicide

Another useful way to distinguish homicides is in the context of the relationship between the perpetrator and the victim. Most serious violence takes place within the family. As noted above, a quarter of all homicide victims are aged under 16, and 80 per cent of these are killed by their parents. Most homicide perpetrators know their victims well; half the female victims of homicide are wives or partners of the perpetrator; the rest are often friends or relatives.

Domestic violence

Domestic violence accounts for about a quarter of all violent incidents measured by the British Crime Survey

TABLE 26.4 Ethical and legal issues – domestic violence

Confidentiality is especially important because of the risk of retaliation by the abuser.
Careful records are essential, including documentation of the injuries. Written consent should be obtained for photographs.
Specialist advice should be sought about providing practical and other help to those who wish to end the relationship.
Where the risk of serious violence is believed to be very high, disclosure to the police and other authorities and other persons to provide protection needs to be carefully planned with the maximum collaboration with the victims.

(Mirrlees-Black, 1999). In England and Wales there are about one million incidents of domestic violence annually and about two-thirds of these of are against women. Most batterers do not have either a diagnosable mental disorder or a criminal history. However, heavy drinking is common.

Some people are violent only within their family, whilst others are also violent outside the family. Violence in the family can have long-term deleterious effects on the psychological and social development of the children as well as on the mental health of the partner (see Chapter 8).

Violence in the family may also be directed at children (child abuse is reviewed on p. 696) and to elderly relatives (violence to the elderly is referred to on p. 506). Any of these forms of violence may rarely result in homicide.

Particular alertness to possible domestic violence is required in emergency departments, but also in primary care and in obstetric and paediatric clinics. Intervention is difficult and raises ethical issues (Table 26.4).

Violence to partners

Violence by men towards their wives is much more frequent than violence to husbands, physically more serious, and more often reported. It appears that most of the perpetrators of wife battering are men with aggressive personalities, whilst a few are violent only when suffering from psychiatric illness, usually a depressive disorder. Other common features in the men are morbid jealousy and heavy drinking. Such men may have suffered violence in childhood, and often come from backgrounds in which violence is frequent and tolerated. Although behaviour by the victim may contribute to or provoke (but not justify) violence, this is often hard to assess if only the perpetrator is interviewed; when battering is seen as a 'joint' problem, the batterer may have less incentive to stop the violence. It is vital to bear in mind that repetitive battering, especially in the context of jealousy, is a risk factor for homicide.

Violence in the workplace

Violence is increasing in the workplace and receiving growing attention. As well as physical attacks, it is also being taken to include threats and various forms of harassment (Fletcher *et al.*, 2000). Psychological consequences can be severe. Many organizations have guidelines and training programmes which aim to prevent such problems and to deal with the consequences.

Sexual offences

Sexually violent offences

In the UK, sexual offences account for less than 1 per cent of all indictable offences recorded by the police. Sexual offenders make up a relatively large proportion of offenders referred to psychiatrists, though only a small proportion of people charged with sexual offences are assessed by psychiatrists. Most sexual offences are committed by men; they are rare among women, apart from soliciting for purposes of prostitution.

As a group, sexual offenders are older than other offenders. Reconviction rates of sexual offenders are generally lower than those of other offenders, but a minority of recidivist sexual offenders are extremely difficult to manage (Box 26.2). In the UK, Part 1 of the Sex Offenders Act 1997 requires those convicted or cautioned for relevant sex offences to notify the police of their name and address and any subsequent changes to them. This information is then kept by police on what has become commonly known as the sex offenders register.

The most common sexual offences are indecent assault against women, indecent exposure, and unlawful intercourse with girls aged under 16. Some sexual offences do not involve physical violence (for example, indecent exposure, voyeurism, and most sexual offences involving children); others may involve considerable violence (for example, rape). The nature and treatment of non-violent sexual offences are discussed in Chapter 19, but their forensic aspects are considered here. For a review see Hale *et al.* (2000) and Gordon and Grubin (2004).

The psychological consequences for victims of sexual offences are discussed on p. 745, and sexual abuse of children is discussed below.

Sexual abuse of children

The age of consent varies in different countries. In England and Wales it is illegal to have any heterosexual activity with a person aged under 16, or homosexual activ-

BOX 26.3 SOME FACTORS ASSOCIATED WITH INCREASED RISK OF RE-OFFENDING IN SEX OFFENDERS

- Previous criminal history
- Higher number of sexual offences and more than one type of sexual offence
- Being a childhood victim of sexual abuse
- Violent sexual fantasies
- Negative attitudes to women
- Belief that victims consent or enjoy the act
- Choice of location and occupation to facilitate access to victims
- Use of sadomasochistic or paedophilic pornography
- Substance misuse
- Treatment non-compliance

Source Gordon and Grubin (2004)

ity with people aged under 18. Sexual offences involving children are reported commonly, amounting to over half of all reported sexual offences in the UK. It is probable that many more offences are not reported, particularly those occurring within families. The offences vary in severity from mild indecency to seriously aggressive behaviour, but the large majority do not involve violence.

Adults who commit sexual offences against children may or may not be paedophilic. **Paedophiles** are defined as having a primary sexual interest in prepubertal children. They are almost always male. They may be homosexual or heterosexual, and usually abuse children not previously well known to them. They are rarely mentally ill. Victims are often prepared over a long period of time; some paedophiles may seek work in occupations where they will have access to children who will be left in their care.

It is difficult to classify paedophiles, but the following groups have been recognized:

- the timid and sexually inexperienced
- the learning disabled
- those who have experienced normal sexual relationships but prefer sexual activity with children
- a predatory group who may use violence. In rare cases, paedophile sexual activities end in murder.

However, not all child sex offenders are paedophiles as defined above, because a significant majority of child sex offenders do not have a primary sexual interest in children. Many child sex offenders have 'normal' heterosexual histories and may be involved in such relationships at the time that they offend. Paedophilic child sex offenders typically are strangers to children, or else have gained opportunistic access to children through their chosen work or social activities. However, the majority of child sex offending is carried out by men (usually) who have some familial relationship to the child. Most commonly these are stepfathers or other male members of the extended family circle. These men are typically not primary paedophiles, although it has been argued that some primary paedophiles seek to marry adult women with children in order to access potential victims.

Some researchers have also found that a proportion of men who appear to be primarily attracted to adult women also describe attraction to children. Some theorists have argued that what child sex offenders are excited by is the vulnerability of children and the discrepancy in power between adults and children, rather than the physical qualities of childhood.

Sexual abuse of children by family members is considered on p. 700.

The prognosis is difficult to determine. Among those who receive a prison sentence, the recidivism rate is about one in three. Although most offenders do not progress from less serious to more serious activities, an important minority do progress to violent sexual offences. For this reason psychiatrists may be asked to give an opinion on an offender's dangerousness.

Assessment

Usually, the perpetrator and the victim are assessed separately by different people. Interviewing children after sexual abuse is considered on p. 700; this section considers interviews with the adult. In trying to decide whether an offence is likely to be repeated and whether there is likely to be a progression to more serious offences, the psychiatrist should first consider the depositions and the victim's statement to gain available information about:

- the duration and frequency of the particular sexual activity in the past (remembering that paedophiles often deny their offending);
- the offender's predominant sexual preferences; exclusively paedophile inclinations and behaviour indicate greater risk of repetition. Older paedophiles are less likely to be aggressive.

The interviews should determine:

- previous sexual history;
- whether alcohol or drugs played any part in the offence, and if so whether the person is likely to continue using them;
- regret or guilt;
- stressful circumstances associated with the offence (and the likelihood that these will continue);
- the degree of access to children;
- evidence of any psychiatric disorder or relevant personality features. In drawing conclusions it is important to be aware of the limitations of psychiatric knowledge of this form of behaviour.

Treatment

Treatment is directed towards any associated psychiatric disorder. Direct treatment of the sexual behaviour is difficult. Group therapy run jointly by mental health and probation services may be helpful. A recent systematic review showed some effect of group cognitive behaviour therapy to reduce re-offending at one year (NNT = 6) (Kenworthy *et al.*, 2004). The use of anti-androgens such as cyproterone and medroxyprogesterone has also been advocated but their use is attended by many adverse effects. Luteinizing hormone- releasing hormone agonists are better tolerated but current studies have methodological weaknesses (Briken *et al.*, 2003). In addition, treatment of this nature raises ethical issues.

Indecent exposure

This is the legal term for the offence of indecently exposing the genitals to other people. It is applied to all forms of exposure; exhibitionism is by far the most frequent form, but exposure may also occur as an invitation to intercourse, as a prelude to sexual assault, or as an insulting gesture. Exhibitionism (see also p. 488), is the medical name for the behaviour of those who gain sexual satisfaction from repeatedly exposing to the opposite sex. In England and Wales, indecent exposure is one of the most frequent sexual offences. It is most common in men aged between 25 and 35. Indecent exposers rarely have a history of psychiatric disorder or other criminal behaviour. However, they may have other types of compulsive disorder or substance misuse. However, exhibitionism is listed as a psychiatric disorder in both DSM-IV and ICD-10. Although many do not re-offend, a proportion of offenders are repeated recidivists, and may proceed to more serious sexual violence.

Indecent assault

The term indecent assault refers to a wide range of behaviour from attempting to touch a stranger's buttocks to sexual assault without attempted penetration. The psychiatrist is most commonly asked to give a psychiatric opinion on adolescent boys and on men who have assaulted children. Although many adolescent boys behave in ways that could be construed as 'indecent', more serious indecent behaviour is associated with aggressive personality, ignorance, and lack of social skills and occasionally learning difficulties. Treatment depends on the associated problems.

Stalking

The lay term 'stalking' is usually taken to mean the repeated, unwanted, and intrusive targeting of a particular victim with following and other harassment (see Mullen *et al.* 2000). It implies an intensive preoccupation with the victim. The scope of behaviour is wide:

- following;
- communication by telephone, mail, electronic communication;
- ordering goods and services in the victim's name;
- aggression and threats, including violence, damage to property and false accusations.

Most stalkers are men and victims women. The victims invariably suffer severe distress. Management requires cooperation between forensic psychiatrists and the criminal justice system in assessing risks, treating any associated psychiatric disorder (e.g. erotomania) and protecting and treating the victim. See Mullen (2000) for a review and Chapter 13.

Rape

In English law, a man commits rape if:

- he has unlawful sexual intercourse (whether vaginal or anal) with a woman or man who at the time of the intercourse does not consent to it;
- at the time he knows that she does not consent to the intercourse or he is reckless as to whether she consents to it.

Most jurisdictions define rape in terms of the lack of consent of the victim. Not all jurisdictions recognize male rape or sexual assault. Some countries (such as the USA) additionally define lack of consent by age; so called 'statutory rape'. English law is among the few recognizing rape within marriage.

Rape is a violent act; offenders vary in the degree of aggression which is used, and the extent to which this is instrumental in exerting control, or exciting for its own sake. Most rapists are married or in partnerships; over half fail to perform sexually during the assault. Rapists frequently have previous convictions for non-sexual violent offences.

The act of rape varies in terms of the relationship between the rapist and his victim. Most rapists know their victims and, in contrast to popular belief, stranger rape is a minority. Stranger rapes are more likely to be physically violent and involve the use of weapons; this may reflect the fact that rapists who know their victims may not need to use physical threats to control them. Instead, family members may be threatened. Most rapes take place in the home, another contrast to popular belief (Box 26.4).

Epidemiology

Rape and other forms of sexual aggression towards women are probably much more frequent in the population than the number reported to the police (Box 26.3). Only one-third of reported rapes are proceeded with by the police, and only one-third of those proceeded with will be heard at a higher court. Even then, the alleged rapist has only a one in three chance of being convicted and this is most likely where the rape fits the stereotype of stranger rape. Victims of acquaintance rape (often rightly) assume they will not be believed.

The prevalence of male rape is unknown. It is likely that many male rapes go unreported, since male victims may be reluctant to come forward. As in rape of females, rape of males is associated with a wish to degrade or dominate the other person. Rapists of males tend to be violent heterosexual men; it is likely that they have anxieties about their masculine identity. Some studies have suggested that rape of either men or women is associated with gender identity problems in the rapist (see Dunseith *et al.*, 2004).

Causes

Most explanations of rape are sociocultural in terms of cultural attitudes to women, and social constructions of male and female gender roles. In psychological terms, men who are violent to women often have a rigid and conservative idealized view of the female role, coupled with denigration of any woman who transgresses that role. Rapists frequently blame their victims for the attack, by justifying the rape in terms of the woman's behaviour, e.g. 'she deserved to be raped because she was flirting with X'. Although in many cases the victim is an acquaintance of the rapist, and in a fifth there appears to have been some initial participation by the victim in events leading up to the offence, this should not be confused with voluntary participation in the rape itself. There is little evidence for the frequently expressed view that rape victims encourage the rape itself, or change their minds about having sex.

Rape may be associated with severe mental illness. In these cases it is usually sexual behaviour associated with disinhibition as part of a manic illness, or paranoid delusions in psychotic states. Evidence of current substance abuse is found in at least 50 per cent of rapists. In many cases of rape, both rapists and victim will have been using drugs or alcohol; this may reflect the fact that many rape scenarios begin with both parties being in a social situation. Some men who commit rape, homicide, or other violent offences have considerable sexual problems or suffer sexual jealousy, and these may have contributed to their dangerousness. A small group of men obtain sexual pleasure from sadistic assaults on unwilling partners (see Dunseith *et al.*, 2004).

Prognosis

In the UK, most rapists serve only half their sentence in prison, and are then released on license to be supervised by the probation service. The reconviction rate is 30 per cent. The prison service offers psychological treatment to rapists as part of the Sex Offender Treatment Programme (SOTP) in prisons; the best available data to date suggest that rapists do not make much improvement on this programme (see Marques *et al.*, 2005).

BOX 26.4 **SEXUAL ASSAULT OF WOMEN – FINDINGS FROM THE BRITISH CRIME SURVEY OF 2000**

- About 1 per cent of women said they had been subject to some form of sexual victimization in the last year
- 0.4 per cent of women (leading to an estimated 61,000 victims in the UK) said they had been raped in the previous year
- Current partners (at the time of the attack) were responsible for 45 per cent of rapes. Strangers were responsible for a minority of attacks (8 per cent)
- 18 per cent of sexual assaults were reported to the police

Source Myhill and Allen (2002)

Child abduction

Child abduction is rare. A child may be abducted by one of the parents, by a man with a sexual motive, or by an older child. Babies are usually abducted by women who may have one of three kinds of motives: to achieve comfort, to manipulate another person, and on impulse by psychiatrically disturbed women. Fortunately, most stolen babies are well cared for and are found quickly.

Offences against property

Shoplifting

The vast majority of shoplifting, like other theft, is carried out by people without any mental disorder. Many adolescents admit occasional shoplifting. Both observational studies and the reports of huge losses from shops suggest that shoplifting is common among adults.

A minority of shoplifters suffer from psychiatric disorders. Apart from depressive disorders, various other psychiatric diagnoses may be associated at times with shoplifting (Lamontagne *et al.*, 2000). Patients with all types of mental illness, especially those with 'substance abuse', may steal because of economic necessity. Patients with disinhibiting conditions may be more likely to steal impulsively, and patients with eating disorders may steal food. In other conditions, shoplifting may result from distractibility, for example, organic mental disorders, when the person is confused or forgetful, and panic attacks when the person may run out of the shop without paying.

The **assessment** of a person charged with shoplifting is similar to that for any other forensic problem. If the accused has a depressive disorder at the time of the examination, the psychiatrist should try to establish whether the disorder was present at the time of the offence or whether it developed after the charge was brought. The legal question most often posed is whether the accused had the intention to steal, and if a mental condition could have affected that intention.

Arson

This offence is regarded extremely seriously, not only because it can result in great damage to property, but also because it threatens life. Most arsonists are males. Although the courts refer many arsonists for psychiatric assessment, the psychiatric literature on arson is small. Certain groups can be recognized:

- fire-setters who are free from psychiatric disorder and who start fires for financial or political reasons or for revenge; they are sometimes referred to as motivated arsonists.
- so-called pathological fire-setters, who suffer from learning difficulties, mental illness, or alcoholism. This group accounts for about 10–15 per cent of arsons.
- a third group that meet DSM-IV criteria for pyromania (see p. 736), although the validity of this diagnostic criteria is unsubstantiated. These individuals (who sometimes join conspicuously in firefighting) obtain intense satisfaction and tension relief from fire-setting.

The risks of further offences were assessed in a series of long term follow ups by Soothill *et al.* (2004) who found that while about 10 per cent of offenders were re-convicted for arson, over half were charged with offences of other kinds. An important guideline is that a person convicted of arson a second time is at a much greater risk of further offences.

The factors that point to an increased risk of a further fire setting offence are:

- antisocial personality disorder
- learning difficulties
- persistent social isolation
- evidence that fire-raising was done for sexual gratification or relief of tension.

The scope for psychiatric intervention is limited. Management of arsonists within hospital requires a secure setting and close observation.

Children also present with problems of fire-raising. Sometimes the behaviour represents extreme mischievousness in psychologically normal children, at times as a group activity, and sometimes it springs from psychiatric disturbance, most commonly conduct disorder (Martin *et al.*, 2004). Among children charged with fire-setting, the recurrence rate in the following 2 years is reported to be under 10 per cent.

Psychiatric aspects of being a victim of crime

It is only relatively recently that criminology and society have paid attention to the role and needs of victims (see Mezey and Robbins, 2000, for a review). Surveys of general populations indicate that the experience of being a victim of crime is frequent and is related to geographical area, sex, age, and social habits. Much violence, especially sexual and domestic assaults, is unreported. There are differences between men and women in the experience as victims of crime. Young men are particularly at risk of personal violence by reason of their ways of life, whilst women are more likely to suffer domestic and sexual violence. In the UK, around a sixth of assaults on Asians and Afro-Caribbeans are believed to be racially motivated.

The response of the victim is important in determining whether an offence is reported to the police and whether charges are brought.

Psychological impact

Childhood abuse and experience of violence during childhood may have major consequences in adult life (see p. 171).

Adult crime victims are at risk of a variety of early and late psychological problems. These include the immediate distress following the crime and the subsequent distress associated with investigation and court hearings. Post-traumatic stress disorder (see p. 157) is frequently reported. These consequences are more common and severe immediately after the crime, but they may persist for many years.

Types of crime

Murder

Relatives of victims feel isolation and shame and an inability to share their distress greater than in other kinds of bereavement. The bureaucracy of legal processes increases anger and a feeling of being apart from the world (Rock, 1998).

Rape

There is much evidence that rape victims may suffer long-term psychological effects (Mezey and Robbins, 2000). Recent research has shown very high levels of intrusive thoughts and other post-traumatic symptoms in the week following rape. Serious distress may also be experienced by the partners and families of rape victims.

In the USA, many crisis intervention centres staffed by multidisciplinary teams have been set up for rape victims. Cognitive-behavioural treatment is helpful (see p. 162).

Burglary and robbery

Although the consequences are less severe than those following violent crime, they include adjustment disorder and post-traumatic stress disorder. Victims may become preoccupied with security.

Terrorist crimes

There have been many published reports of terrorist crimes, including shootings, bombings, and hostage-taking. All have reported severe immediate distress with PTSD and other psychiatric consequences, in a minority being persistent.

Other Crimes

Victim distress is also prominent in a number of other offences including domestic violence, workplace violence, and stalking.

Management

The severity and persistence of psychological problems indicate the need for both routine and specialist help for victims. Critical incident debriefing as a sole treatment is not helpful (see Raphael and Wilson, 2000).

Support for victims of crime may be available within the community. For example, in the UK, the Home Office fund the national Victim Support scheme, who routinely contact victims of crime to offer support. A special service is also available to support crime victims who are appearing at the Crown Court. However, these services rely on volunteers who may not be able to offer long-term help and who cannot offer specialist psychiatric intervention. Voluntary groups, such as Rape Crisis, offer support to victims of sexual assault. Compensation is available to crime victims from the Criminal Injuries Compensation Board, and psychiatrists may be asked to provide reports in relation to claims for compensation for psychological distress.

Specialist services

There is a need for access to specialist psychiatric assessment and treatment services with particular experience of the problems suffered by victims. These may be provided within normal community services, within a specialized trauma clinic or, occasionally, in more narrowly defined units such as rape clinics.

Routine psychiatric care

It is important that assessment of routine referrals to psychiatric services includes enquiry about experiences of being a victim as this may be important in both aetiology and planning treatment.

The role of the psychiatrist in the criminal courts

Mental state, intention, and responsibility

Most jurisdictions require evidence of **guilty intention** for an offender to be convicted. Psychiatrists are therefore most often asked to provide opinions about whether psychiatric illness in the accused affected the intent to commit the crime. Underlying the need for psychiatric opinion is the principle that a person should not be regarded as culpable unless they were able to control their own behaviour and to choose whether to commit an unlawful act or not. It follows from this principle that, in determining whether or not a person is guilty, it is necessary to consider their mental state at the time of the act, and especially their intention.

In Anglo Saxon jurisdictions, *mens rea* is a technical term for intention. Intent has various meanings but the main principle is that the person perceives and intends that his act will produce unlawful consequences. Three other forms of intent need consideration:

1. 'Recklessness'. Recklessness is defined as the deliberate taking of an unjustifiable risk. A person is reckless with respect to the consequence of their act, when they foresee it may occur but do not desire it.
2. 'Negligence'. Acting negligently is defined as bringing about a consequence which a 'reasonable and prudent' person would have foreseen and avoided.
3. 'Accident' (or 'blameless inadvertence').

The key issue in responsibility is whether the accused had the mental capacity to form the intention; or whether mental disorder might have affected that capacity. Sometimes it will be beyond psychiatric expertise or evidence to answer this question. A psychiatrist who has been asked to give an opinion on these matters should liaise closely with the lawyers as to the relevant psychiatric contribution.

Children

In most jurisdictions, the age of the accused may be thought to affect their capacity to form the intent to commit crime. Most jurisdictions exclude children under a certain age from criminal prosecution; for example, in English Law, children under 10 are excluded because they are deemed incapable of forming criminal intent (the Latin term for this being *doli incapax*). Children between the ages of 10 and 14 years may be convicted if there is evidence of *mens rea* and that the child knew that the offence was legally or morally wrong.

Competence to stand trial

This issue may arise in relation to any charge. Most jurisdictions require that a defendant must be in a fit condition to defend themselves. In English law, the issue is called 'fitness to plead' and may be raised by the defence, the prosecution, or the judge. It cannot be decided in a magistrates' court, but only by a jury.

It is necessary to determine how far the defendant can:

- understand the nature of the charge;
- understand the difference between pleading guilty and not guilty;
- instruct counsel;
- challenge jurors;
- follow the evidence presented in court.

A person may be suffering from severe mental disorder but still be fit to stand trial.

An individual may be found unfit to plead under the terms of the Criminal Procedures and Insanity (Unfitness to Plead) Act 1991. If an individual is found not fit to plead, then the court will hold a 'trial of the facts' to determine whether the individual carried out the offence. If the offence is not serious, then the court may make an order directing the offender to have treatment, often as an outpatient. In cases where the offence is serious, or carries a mandatory penalty (like murder), the court will direct the offender to be detained in hospital indefinitely. If the person should become fit to plead, they may be returned to court for a trial. Detention after being found unfit to plead (or legally insane – see below) operates in the same way as detention accompanied by a restriction order.

Legal insanity (not guilty by reason of insanity)

This defence may also be raised to any charge. Essentially, in raising the defence, it is argued that the defendant lacked *mens rea* for the charge because they were 'legally insane'. This term has nothing to do with diagnostic terms or classifications such as ICD-10 or DSM-IV. **Legal insanity is defined in different ways in different jurisdictions**, and a finding of insanity usually results in the defendant being admitted for treatment in hospital, as opposed to being sent to prison. In some jurisdictions, a 'not guilty by reason of insanity' verdict may result in more lenient sentencing.

In English Law, insanity is defined in law by the MacNaughten Rules, after the famous case of Daniel MacNaughten who, in 1843, shot and killed Edward Drummond, private secretary to the Prime Minister, Sir Robert Peel. In the trial at the Old Bailey, a defence of insanity was presented on the grounds that MacNaughten had suffered from delusions that he was persecuted by spies. His delusional system gradually focused on the Tory Party, and he decided to kill their leader, Sir Robert Peel (West, 1974). MacNaughten was found not guilty on the grounds of insanity and was admitted to Bethlem Hospital. Because this was a contentious decision, the judges of the time drew up rules which were not enacted in the law but provided guidance. To establish a defence on the ground of insanity, it must be clearly proved that, at the time of committing the act, the party accused was:

> labouring under such a defect of reason, from disease of the mind, as not to know the nature and quality of the act he was doing, or, if he did know it, that he did not know what he was doing was wrong.

Several other jurisdictions (some states in the USA and Australia) have used the MacNaughten Rules as a basis for their own definitions of legal insanity. Many critics have argued that the rules are much too narrow, and that few truly mentally ill offenders would fulfil these criteria. Indeed, it is doubtful whether MacNaughten himself fulfilled them. In some countries, the insanity defence is widely used whenever an individual with a mental illness is charged with an offence, especially crimes of violence like homicide. In English law, the insanity defence is rarely used, mainly because the alternative defence of diminished responsibility (see below) is available.

Diminished responsibility

Some jurisdictions include the concept of diminished responsibility, i.e. an individual's blame worthiness may be reduced by his having a mental illness. In English law, it is *only* available in relation to the charge of murder and is defined as:

> where a person kills or is party to a killing of another, he shall not be convicted of murder if he was suffering from such abnormality of mind (whether arising from a condition of arrested or retarded development of mind or any inherent causes or induced by disease or injury) as substantially impaired his mental responsibility for his acts and omissions in doing or being party to the killing.

There are difficulties with this definition. 'Abnormality of mind' bears no resemblance to any diagnostic category; it is basically anything which the 'reasonable man' would call abnormal. It has been widely interpreted. Successful pleas have been based on conditions such as 'emotional immaturity', 'mental instability', 'psychopathic personality', 'reactive depressed state', 'mixed emotions of depression, disappointment, and exasperation', and 'premenstrual tension'.

The relationship between abnormality of mind and responsibility is not established empirically, and psychiatrists do not necessarily have expertise in this area. Most legal commentators argue that any finding of responsibility is for the jury to decide, and is not a matter of expert evidence. Nevertheless, psychiatrists may be asked to comment on this issue.

Assessment

Most defendants charged with murder undergo extensive psychiatric assessment often from a specialist in forensic psychiatry but sometimes from a general psychiatrist. The defence lawyers often seek independent psychiatric advice. It is good practice for the doctors involved, whether engaged by prosecution or defence lawyers, to discuss the case. Disagreement is unusual. Copies of the reports are distributed to the judge and to the prosecution and defence lawyers. Similar arrangements apply to other offences in which a psychiatric opinion is required.

If the psychiatric evidence is accepted by the court, supporting diminished responsibility, then the defendant will be convicted of manslaughter rather than murder. Whereas a murder conviction results in a mandatory life sentence, a manslaughter conviction can result in a range of sentences; from a suspended sentence to life imprisonment. In other jurisdictions, psychiatric evidence which supports diminished responsibility may affect whether the convicted offender receives the death penalty.

In the UK, offenders who are convicted of manslaughter in this way may be detained in hospital under the relevant mental health law. If the offence is particularly dangerous, and the offender presents a risk to the public, then the court may impose a restriction order, which will then require the Home Office to be involved in decisions about discharge.

Infanticide is a particular form of manslaughter charge, which can only be brought against women who have killed their newly born children (under a year old). If there is psychiatric evidence to show that the woman was mentally ill at the time of the killing, then she will be found guilty of infanticide rather than murder. In this case the court may make a hospital order; restriction orders are rarely applied. This is a rare example of the English law formally recognizing the existence of psychiatric illness as relevant to the commission of an offence; namely post-partum psychosis.

Absence of intention (automatism)

In some cases, it will be argued that the defendant lacked intention altogether for an offence (technically, absence of *mens rea*) – 'automatism'. The paradigm example is acts committed while sleep walking. Automatism is hard to determine retrospectively, and the defence is rarely used. This issue may arise in relation to patients who abuse alcohol or drugs where it may be argued that they were 'intoxicated' and therefore had no intention to commit the crime. The law on intoxication is complicated and specialist legal advice should be sought.

Fitness to be punished

In those jurisdictions which have corporal or capital punishment, psychiatrists may be asked to assess offenders to determine whether they are mentally well enough to be punished. In addition to assessment, psychiatrists may be asked to treat offender patients in order to make them fit to be punished or executed. In countries where this is relevant, such as the USA, there has been considerable debate about the ethical dilemmas raised by this issue. Some authors have argued that it is unethical for psychiatrists to be involved in these procedures.

Other psychiatric issues that may be relevant to the criminal court

Amnesia

Over a third of those charged with serious offences, especially homicide, report some degree of amnesia for the offence and inadequate recall of what happened. It has sometimes been argued that loss of memory should be regarded as evidence of unfitness to plead, but such arguments have been unsuccessful. The factors most commonly associated with claims of amnesia are extreme emotional arousal, alcohol abuse and intoxication, and severe depression. Amnesia has to be distinguished from malingering in an attempt to avoid the consequences of the offence. However, there appear to be instances of true amnesias for offences, just as there is impaired recall by victims and witnesses of offences. Moreover, the factors associated with amnesia are similar in offenders and victims. In the absence of a relevant neuropsychiatric disorder, the presence of amnesia is unlikely to be accepted as having any legal implications (see Johns, 2000).

False confessions

Accounts of trials and other descriptive evidence indicate that false confessions to criminal deeds are sometimes made. However, the frequency of such confessions is unknown. Gudjonsson (1992) suggested that there are three main types of false confession:

1. voluntary
2. coerced–compliant
3. coerced–internalized.

Voluntary confessions may arise from a morbid desire for notoriety, from difficulty in distinguishing fact from fantasy, from a wish to expiate guilt feelings, or from a desire to protect another person. Coerced-compliant confessions result from forceful interrogation and are usually retracted subsequently. Coerced-internalized confessions are made when the technique of interrogation undermines suspects' own memories and recollections so that they come to believe that they may have been responsible for the crime. Factors making a person more likely to make a false confession include a history of substance abuse, head injury, a bereavement, current anxiety, or guilt.

The assessment of possible false confessions is difficult. It requires a thorough review of the circumstances of arrest, custody, and interrogation, as well as an assessment of the personality and the current mental and physical state of the suspect. Usually the assistance of a clinical psychologist will be required to carry out a neuropsychological assessment and in some cases an assessment of suggestibility.

False accusations

Occasionally there are reports of individuals who claim to be the victims of a crime that has not occurred and who make false accusations. Examples are accusations of rape and also of stalking (Pathé *et al.*, 1999). Legal and clinical experience suggests such cases are uncommon and that accusers frequently have severe personality and other problems.

The treatment of offenders with mental disorder

General issues

The **assessment** needs to include as much information as possible from a variety of sources including, if possible, the general practice notes. In forensic cases relatives may not be the most reliable informants; particularly since they have often been victims of interpersonal violence. Careful attention must be paid to both mental illness and personality disorders, as well as histories of substance misuse, which are extremely common.

Forensic psychiatric treatment usually involves treating general psychiatric conditions in specialized settings, such as secure treatment units or hospitals. It may also involve involuntary outpatient care (Swanson *et al.* 2000). Treatment planning involves not only the appropriate medications, but also organization of appropriate psychological interventions. This is particularly true for forensic patients with severe personality disorders. Management of such patients requires specialist training for staff and support by forensic psychotherapists. It also depends upon introducing evidence-based psychiatric care into forensic practice. Many forensic patients suffer from personality disorder; the general principles of management are described in Chapter 7 (see also Bateman and Tyrer, 2004a,b).

Treatability is an issue which is often discussed. Some patients with personality disorder have been excluded from treatment on the grounds of 'untreatability'. This may reflect a lack of familiarity with treatment options available for personality disorder (Bateman and Tyrer, 2004a,b). The notion of 'untreatability' arguably applies equally to patients with severe psychotic illnesses who are 'treatment-resistant' where there may be little evidence of improvement over time. Assessment of treatability is complex and affected by a number of factors (see Box 26.5) (Adshead, 2001). Like risk, treatability assessments may have to be repeated over time.

Settings of treatment

After conviction, an offender may be treated on a compulsory or a voluntary basis. In the UK, special treatment for mentally abnormal offenders is, in principle, provided by the Home Office (the prison medical service and the probation service) and by the Department of Health (special hospitals, specialist forensic services, and general psychiatry services). However, many mentally abnormal offenders do not receive the psychiatric treatment that they require both because of lack of availability of suitable facilities as well as the complex management problems that many such patients pose. Finally there has been a lack of research in forensic psychiatry which means that the evidence base for effective treatment is slender. For a general review of the organization of forensic psychiatric sevices services see Bluglass (2000).

Much work with offenders is carried out by general psychiatrists who assess patients and prepare court reports. General psychiatrists as well as forensic psychiatrists treat offenders given non-custodial sentences. Forensic psychiatrists work in separate units and undertake specialized assessment and court work. In many places there are community forensic services to provide assessment and treatment. Forensic psychiatrists may work to provide care for patients needing security in ordinary psychiatric hospitals.

BOX 26.5 ASSESSMENT OF TREATABILITY

- **The severity of the patient's psychopathology.** Degree of interpersonal dysfunction, multi-agency involvement , record of offending
- **Other aspects of the patient's psychological heath.** Resilience or vulnerability factors. History of positive attachment. Employment record. Motivation to engage in treatment
- **Comorbidity with other disorders.** Treatability is lowered by comorbid psychiatric conditions, particularly substance misuse
- **The availability of appropriate therapy and therapists.** Extent to which treatment is possible only in particularly specialized settings. Availability of such settings.
- **The experience and attitude of the assessor and current evidence base.** Extent of evidence-base for treatment and assessors knowledge of it. However 'palliative care' (support and understanding) is always possible.
- **Timing of assessment.** Patients may be more ready to engage in therapy at some time than at others

The mentally abnormal in prison

Surveys have shown that about a third of sentenced prisoners have a psychiatric disorder and 4 per cent have a psychosis (see Fazel and Danesh, 2002). Most of these disorders can be treated in prison, but a few offenders need transfer to a hospital (Box 26.6).

Prison medical services have to provide psychiatric care under extremely difficult conditions, and it has been argued that there should be a substantial increase in the contribution of psychiatrists to the provision of medical care within prisons. A few prisons offer psychological treatment, usually of personality disorders and sexual offences, as a main part of their work; one such prison is at Grendon Underwood in England. Although there is an undoubted need for psychiatric care within prisons, there would be disadvantages in a system which encouraged the courts to send the mentally abnormal to prison rather than to hospital services.

BOX 26.6 REASONS FOR HOSPITAL TRANSFER OF PRISONERS WITH PSYCHIATRIC DISORDER

- Psychosis
- Failure to improve with medical treatment in prison
- Refusal to have treatment for serious psychiatric illness
- Life threatening self-harm
- Risk of abuse

Offenders in hospital

Most jurisdictions allow for the detention of mentally abnormal offenders in secure psychiatric settings. In England and Wales, a convicted offender may be committed to hospital for compulsory psychiatric treatment under a Mental Health Act hospital order. There is also provision in law for a prisoner to be transferred from prison to a psychiatric hospital. One important point is that hospital orders may have no time limit, whilst most prison sentences are of fixed length. The length of stay in a psychiatric hospital may be shorter than a prison sentence or it may be longer.

Special hospitals and secure units in the UK

In the UK, detention of mentally abnormal offenders may be in a local psychiatric hospital, a medium security unit, or a maximum secure hospital ('special hospital'). In England, the first special provision for the criminally insane was made in 1800. Following a trial in which Hadfield was found not guilty by reason of insanity for shooting at King George III, a special criminal wing was established at the Bethlem Hospital. In 1863, Broadmoor, the oldest of the special hospitals, opened under the management of the then Home Office. There are now four high-security special hospitals in England and Wales.

The detention of patients in special hospitals is usually for an indeterminate length of stay. For those with mental illness (mostly schizophrenia), length of detention is associated with the severity or chronicity of the psychiatric disorder rather than the nature of the offence. By contrast, for patients suffering from psychopathic disorder, the main determinant of length of stay is the assessment of the future risk of offending.

The closure of the larger mental hospitals in the UK has had unforeseen consequences for the care of mentally abnormal offenders. There is less physical security in the new psychiatric wards and hospitals and less willingness by hospital staff and other patients to tolerate severely disturbed behaviour. As a result, it has become increasingly difficult to arrange admission to hospital for offenders, particularly those who are severely disturbed. In addition, length of stay in hospital has shortened, making it more difficult to arrange treatment for patients with chronic disorders and severe behaviour disorder. Two alternative provisions have been developed:

1. well-staffed secure areas in ordinary psychiatric hospitals in which the less dangerous of these patients can be treated;
2. special secure units associated with psychiatric hospitals to provide a level of security between that of an ordinary hospital and a special hospital (medium-secure units). Problems have arisen about the criteria for selecting patients for these special secure units, and about their role in relation to both ordinary psychiatric hospitals and the special hospitals. This is partly because development of the medium secure units in the UK was devolved to local commissioning bodies which in some areas resulted in poorly coordinated service development and inequitable resource allocation (Coid *et al.*, 2001)

Treatment in the community

Offender patients may not pose sufficient risk, or be sufficiently ill, to require treatment in hospital. Courts may also use non-custodial sentences in which the offender-patient may receive support from the probation service as well as psychiatric treatment. On occasions, psychiatric treatment may be made a condition of probation, with which the offender must agree to comply.

The psychiatric treatment provided for a mentally abnormal offender is similar to that for a patient with the same psychiatric disorder who has not broken the law. It is often difficult to provide psychiatric care for offenders with chronic psychiatric disorders who commit repeated petty offences. In the past they would have been long-stay patients in a psychiatric hospital, but now, treated in the community, they may be unwilling to cooperate with treatment and difficult to follow up because they change address or become homeless. Such patients may benefit from Assertive Community Treatment (see p. 636).

The management of violence in health care settings

Violent incidents are not confined to patients with forensic problems, but this is a convenient place to consider their management. Although not frequent, violent incidents in hospitals are increasing. The reasons for this increase appear to include:

- changes in mental health policies that have made dangerousness a relatively more common reason for an admission (since non-violent patients are more likely to be treated in the community)
- overcrowding
- lack of sufficiently experienced staff
- increased use of illicit substances.

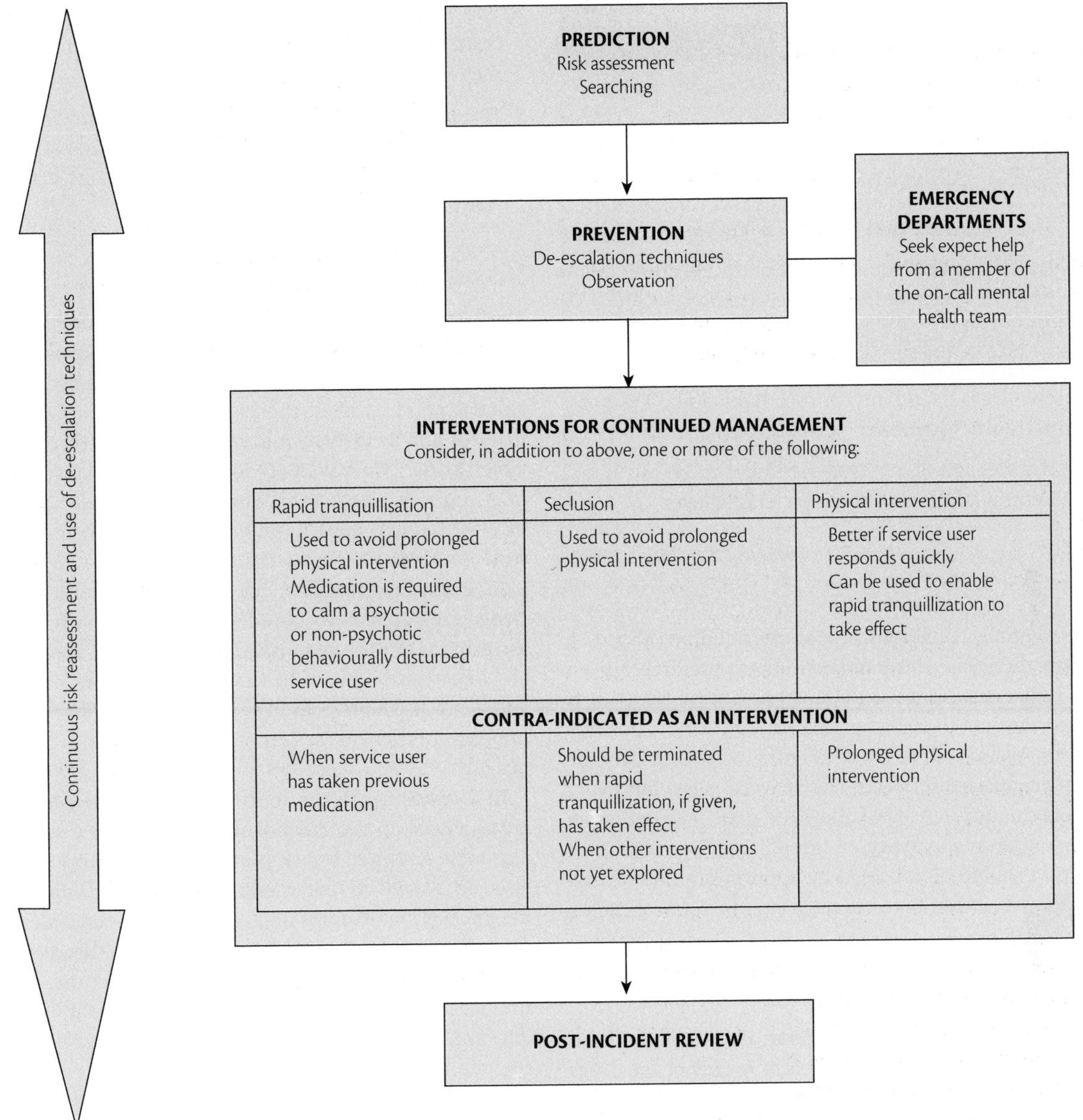

Fig. 26.3 Algorithm for the short-term management of disturbed or violent behaviour in healthcare settings. National Institute for Clinical Excellence (2005c).

All psychiatrists should be familiar with how to manage incidents of violence in inpatient settings. Prior education and training are essential; the National Institute of Clinical Excellence has provided guidelines (National Institute for Clinical Excellence, 2005c) (Figure 26.3). It is important that staff have a clear policy for managing incidents of violence and are trained to carry it out. Such a policy calls for attention to the design of wards, arrangements for summoning assistance, and suitable training of the staff. The general process of risk assessment is described below.

When violence is threatened or occurs, staff should be available in adequate numbers, and emergency medication such as intramuscular lorazapam and haloperidol unobtrusively available. The emphasis should be on the prevention of violence (Box 26.7).

BOX 26.7 DE-ESCALATION TECHNIQUES USED TO PREVENT VIOLENCE

- One staff member should take overall charge of situation
- Move the patient to a suitable room or area to help reduce arousal
- Make sure sufficient staff are available
- Explain to the patient what staff are doing and how they hope to resolve the situation
- Attempt to establish rapport. Show concern and listen attentively. Ask open questions. Monitor own verbal and non-verbal behaviour. Do not patronize the patient or minimize their concerns
- If a weapon is involved ask for it to be put in a neutral location rather than handed over

Source National Institute for Clinical Excellence, 2005

Potentially dangerous people can often be calmed by sympathetic discussion or reassurance, preferably given by someone whom the patient knows and trusts. It is important not to challenge the patient. It is inappropriate to reward violent or threatening behaviour by making concessions in treatment or ward rules, but every effort should be made to allow the patient to withdraw from confrontation without loss of face. The use of medication should be followed by appropriate monitoring (for advice about the use of medications in emergencies, see p. 538).

After an incident has occurred, the clinical team should meet to consider:

- **The future care of the patient.** For mentally disordered patients, there should be a review of the drugs prescribed and their dosage. When violence occurs in a person with a personality disorder, medication may be required in an emergency, but it is usually best to avoid maintenance medication. Other measures include trying to reduce factors that provoke violence or to provide the patient with more constructive ways of managing tension, such as taking physical exercise or asking a member of staff for help.
- **Supportive psychological interventions.** These may be required for patients or staff who have been the victim of a violent assault (see victims of crime, above).
- **Whether the police should be informed.** It should not be forgotten than such assaults are forms of interpersonal violence, which may be criminal.
- **The possible effect on the whole patient group.** Other patients may need support whether or not they were present at the incident.
- **The need for changes in the general policy of the ward.** A violent incident may enable lessons to be learned which are applicable in a general way to ward policies and procedures.

Risk assessment

The change to community care has made both minor criminality and rare violent offences more conspicuous and has resulted in increased public disquiet. Psychiatric services need the resources to minimize difficulties and to identify and manage serious threats of violence. See Mullen (2000) for a review of dangerousness and risk. The psychiatrist may need to assess risk in everyday psychiatric practice and also in forensic work.

In everyday practice, both outpatients and inpatients may appear to be dangerous, and careful risk assessment may be required so that the most appropriate steps can be taken in the interests of the patient and of other people. Risk of serious harm to others is an important criterion for compulsory detention in hospital.

In forensic work the court may ask for the psychiatrist's advice on the defendant's dangerousness so that a suitable sentence can be passed. The psychiatrist may also be asked to comment on offenders who are detained in institutions and who are being considered for release. In both kinds of circumstance there is an ethical dilemma between the need to protect the community from someone who might show violent behaviour and the obligation to respect the human rights of the offender.

There have been two broad approaches to risk assessment:

1. Clinical Psychiatrists have tried to identify factors associated with dangerousness in an individual patient. While some general predictors of violence (for example, antisocial personality disorder and substance misuse) are helpful they, lack specificity in identifying particular individuals at risk (Dolan and Doyle 2000).
2. Actuarial methods have been used to predict future criminal behaviour amongst offenders and amongst other populations, such as psychiatric patients. In general, the low correlations between predicted and observed behaviour have meant they have been

unhelpful in individual predictions. Although some recent instruments have a higher degree of predictive accuracy, they are time-consuming to administer (Monahan *et al.*, 2000).

There are no fixed clinical rules for assessing risk but there are a number of authoritative advisory publications. A thorough review should be made of the history of previous violence, the characteristics of the current offence and the circumstances in which it occurred, and the mental state (Figure 26.4). In making the review, it is helpful to consider certain key questions:

- whether any consistent pattern of behaviour can be discerned;
- whether any circumstances have provoked violence in the past and are likely to occur again in the future;
- whether there is any good evidence that the defendant is willing to change his behaviour;
- whether there is likely to be any response to treatment (Figure 26.4).

Of these predictors, the most useful is a history of past violence (see Mullen, 2000).

Particular difficulties may arise in the assessment of dangerousness in people of antisocial personality or with learning disabilities, both of whom may be poorly motivated to comply with care. Another difficult problem is presented by the person who threatens to commit a violent act such as homicide. Here the assessment is much the same as for suicide threats (p. 414). The psychiatrist should ask the threatener about his intent, motivation, and the potential victim, and should make a full assessment of mental state. Some patients who make threats can be helped by outpatient support and treatment, but sometimes hospital admission is required if the risk is high. It may be necessary to warn potential victims.

TABLE 26.5 Factors associated with dangerousness

Male gender
History
◆ One or more previous episodes of violence
◆ Repeated impulsive behaviour
◆ Evidence of difficulty in coping with stress
◆ Previous unwillingness to delay gratification
◆ Antisocial traits and lack of social support
The offence
◆ Bizarre violence
◆ Lack of provocation
◆ Lack of regret
◆ Continuing major denial
Mental state
◆ Morbid jealousy
◆ Paranoid beliefs plus a wish to harm others
◆ Deceptiveness
◆ Lack of self-control
◆ Threats to repeat violence
◆ Attitude to treatment, poor compliance
Circumstances
◆ Provocation or precipitant likely to recur
◆ Alcohol or drug misuse
◆ Social difficulties and lack of support

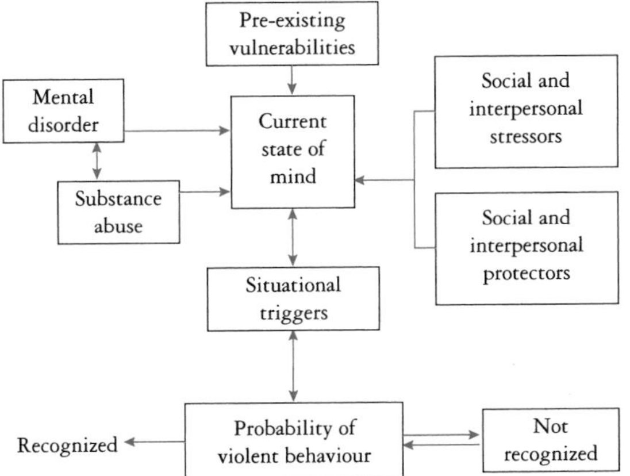

Fig. 26.4 Schematic representation of the issues which should be considered in assessing the probability of violent behaviour. [After Mullen, P. (2000). Dangerousness, risk and the prediction of probability. In *The new Oxford textbook of psychiatry* (eds. M. G. Gelder, J. J. López-Ibor Jr, and N. C. Andreasen), Chapter 11.4.3. Oxford University Press, Oxford. Reproduced with permission]

It is a valuable principle for the psychiatrist not to rely entirely on his own evaluation of dangerousness, but to discuss the problem with other colleagues, including psychiatrists, general practitioners, social workers, and relatives (see Mullen, 2000).

The psychiatric report

A psychiatric report prepared for a major criminal charge is an important document, and should be based on full psychiatric and social examination. It is essential that the psychiatrist read all the depositions by witnesses, statements by the accused, and any previous medical notes and social reports. Family members should be interviewed. When evidence about previous offences is not admissible (as is the case in English Law) the psychiatrist's report should not include these facts. This may cause problems for the psychiatrist, whose opinion is often based in large part on the previous behaviour of the offender. The writing of the court report follows the format described in Box 26.6 and should include an assessment of mental state at the time of the alleged offence and of fitness to plead. The involvement of the psychiatrist at various stages of the legal process in England and Wales is shown in Table 26.6.

The role of the psychiatrist in relation to the court

The psychiatrist's role is to draw on his special knowledge to help the court. He should not attempt to tell the court what to do. In the UK, the duty of the expert medical witness is to the court as a whole; he is not expected to be partisan. It is sometimes hard for psychiatrists to appreciate that they must remain neutral and not provide evidence to order that supports the party instructing them. This is particularly difficult because most psychiatrists use their clinical skills to establish rapport with individuals on whom they are preparing a report.

The psychiatrist should be aware that the court will see the report and that it may be read out in open court. Reports commissioned and paid for by lawyers are the property of the court.

The assessment

When carrying out a psychiatric assessment on a person who is accused of a crime or who has been convicted of an offence, some key points should be kept in mind:

1. Prepare as thoroughly as possible before the interview. Have a clear idea as to the purpose of the examination, and particularly as to any question of fitness to plead. Obtain details of the present charge and past convictions, together with copies of any statements made by the defendant and witnesses. Study any available reports of the defendant's social history; during the subsequent interview go through this report with the defendant and check its accuracy.
2. Begin by explaining to the client the source of the referral and why the referral was made. They should explain that their opinion may be given in court and that the defendant is under no obligation to answer any questions if they choose not to.
3. Make detailed notes, recording any significant comments in the defendant's own words. At some stage in the interview (not necessarily at the start), the alleged crime should be discussed. The defendant may or may not admit guilt but the psychiatrist is not obliged to comment on this.
4. Take a detailed history of physical illnesses, paying particular attention to neurological disorders including head injury and epilepsy.
5. Obtain a careful history of previous psychiatric disorder and treatment. Make a full examination of the present mental state. Special investigations should be requested if suitable. If the defendant's intelligence level is under question, a clinical psychologist should make a separate assessment.
6. If possible, obtain further information from relatives and other informants. If the defendant is remanded in custody, the staff may have long periods of contact with the prisoner and may be able to give particularly useful information.

TABLE 26.6 The involvement of psychiatrists in the stages of the UK legal process

Stage 1 **Arrest**	**Stage II** **Pre-trial**	**Stage III** **At the trial**	**Stage IV** **After the trial**
Removal to a place of safety (police station, hospital, for medical examination)	Court report Remand for inpatient assessment or treatment	Special problems: fitness to plead, diminished responsibility	Treatment under hospital orders or guardianship
Assessment after arrest Court diversion schemes	Transfer from prison for assessment	Advice about subsequent management	Transfer from prison Decisions about release Treatment in the community

BOX 26.8 SOME HEADINGS FOR A COURT REPORT

A statement of the **psychiatrist's full name, qualifications, present appointment** (and, in England and Wales, whether approved under Section 12 of the Mental Health Act).

Where and when the interview was conducted and whether any third person was present.

Sources of information including documents that have been examined.

Family and personal history of the defendant/plaintiff Usually this need not be given in great detail, particularly if a social report is available to the court. The focus should be on information relevant to the diagnosis and disposal.

Present mental state Only the salient positive findings should be stated and negative findings should be omitted. A general diagnosis should be given in the terms of the Mental Health Act (mental illness, mental impairment, or psychopathic disorder). A more specific diagnosis can then be given, but the court will be interested in a categorical statement rather than the finer nuances of diagnosis.

Mental state at the time of the relevant events This is often a highly important issue, especially in criminal cases, and yet it can be based only on retrospective speculation. The assessment can be helped by accounts given by eye witnesses who saw the offender at the time of the crime or soon after. A current psychiatric diagnosis may suggest the likely mental state at the time of the crime. For example, if the accused suffers from chronic schizophrenia or a chronic organic mental syndrome, the mental state may well have been the same at the time of the crime as at the examination. However, if the accused suffers from a depressive disorder (now or recently) or from an episodic disorder such as epilepsy, it is more difficult to infer what the mental state is likely to have been at the material time. To add to the difficulty, even if it is judged that the defendant was suffering from a mental disorder, a further judgement is needed as to his *mens rea* at the time of the crime.

Conclusions A summary of the key findings.

Preparing the report

The preparation of a court report will be affected by the circumstances of the case, and the instructions given by solicitors. Court reports for civil and criminal cases may be very different. A possible outline is given in Box 26.8. More detail is available in Grounds (2000).

In preparing a court report, the psychiatrist should remember that it will be read by non-medical people. Therefore the report should be written in simple English and should avoid jargon. If technical terms are used, they should be defined as accurately as possible. The report should be concise.

Advice on medical treatment

One of the psychiatrist's main functions is to give an opinion as to whether or not psychiatric treatment is indicated. The psychiatrist should make sure that any recommendations on treatment are feasible, if necessary by consulting colleagues, social workers, or others. If hospital treatment is recommended, the court should be informed whether or not a suitable placement is available.

The assessment of risk is important here (see p. 752). The psychiatrist should not recommend any form of disposal other than treatment. However, the court often welcomes respectfully worded comments on the suitability of possible sentences, particularly in the case of young offenders.

The psychiatrist appearing in court

The psychiatrist appearing in court should be fully prepared and should have well-organized copies of all reports and necessary documents. It is helpful to speak to the lawyer involved beforehand, in order to clarify any points that may be raised in court. When replying to any questions in court, it is important to be brief and clear, to restrict the answers to the psychiatric evidence, and to avoid speculation. A number of expert witness training programmes are available, which may be useful for psychiatrists who often give expert evidence.

Further reading

Gelder, MG, López-Ibor, JJ Jr and Andreasen, NC (eds) (2000) *The new Oxford textbook of psychiatry*, Part 11: Forensic psychiatry. Oxford University Press, Oxford.

Maguire, M. Morgan, M and Reiner R (2002) *The Oxford handbook of criminology*, Oxford University Press, Oxford. (An authoritative review of criminology with numerous chapters relevant to forensic psychiatry.)

Gunn, J and Taylor P (2006) *Forensic psychiatry*, Hodder Arnold, London. (A detailed and useful textbook.)

References

Abas M, Broadhead JC, Mbape P, *et al.* (1994). Defeating depression in the developing world. *British Journal of Psychiatry,* **164**, 293–6.

Abel G and Osborn CA (2000). The paraphilias. In MG Gelder, JJ López-Ibor Jr and NC Andreasen, eds. *The new Oxford textbook of psychiatry*, Chapter 4.11.3. Oxford University Press, Oxford.

Abela JR and D'Alessandro DU (2002). Beck's cognitive theory of depression: a test of the diathesis-stress and causal mediation components. *British Journal of Clinical Psychology,* **41**, 111–28.

Abelson JL, Glitz D and Cameron OG (1991). Blunted growth hormone response to clonidine in patients with generalized anxiety disorder. *Archives of General Psychiatry,* **48**, 157–62.

Abou-Saleh MT (2004). Dual diagnosis: management within a psychosocial context. *Advances in Psychiatric Treatment,* **10**, 352–60.

Abrams RC, Alexopoulos GS and Young RC (1987). Geriatric depression and DSM-III-R personality disorder criteria. *Journal of the American Geriatrics Society,* **35**, 383–6.

Abrams RC and Horowitz SV (1996). Personality disorders after age 50: A meta-analysis. *Journal of Personality Disorders,* **10**, 271–81.

Academy of Medical Sciences (2004). *Calling Time. The Nation's drinking as a major health issue.* Academy of Medical S ciences.

Accurso V, Winnicki M and Shamsuzzaman AS (2001). Predisposition to vasovagal syncope in subjects with blood injury phobia. *Circulation,* **104**, 903–7.

Acierno R, Resnick HS and Kilpatrick DG (1997). Health impact of interpersonal violence 1: prevalence rates, case identification, and risk factors for sexual assault, physical assault, and domestic violence in men and women. *Behavioural Medicine,* **23**, 53–64.

Ackerman D and Greenland S (2002). Multivariate meta-analysis of controlled drug studies for obsessive-compulsive disorder. *Journal of Clinical Psychopharmacology,* **22**, 309–17.

Ackerman NW (1958). *The psychodynamics of family life.* Basic Books, New York, NY.

Ackner B and Oldham AJ (1962). Insulin treatment of schizophrenia. A three year follow up of a controlled study. *Lancet,* **1**, 504–6.

AD2000 Collaborative Group (2004). Long-term donepezil treatment in 565 patients with Alzheimer's disease (AD2000): randomised controlled trial. *Lancet,* **363**, 2105–15.

Adams RD, Fisher C, Hakim S, *et al.* (1965). Symptomatic occult hydrocephalus with 'normal' cerebrospinal fluid pressure: a treatable syndrome. *New England Journal of Medicine,* **273**, 117–26.

Adler A (1943). Neuropsychiatric complications in victims of Boston's Coconut Grove disaster. *Journal of the American Medical Association,* **123**, 1098–111.

Adler CM and Strakowski SM (2003). Boundaries of schizophrenia. *Psychiatric Clinics of North America,* **26**, 1–23.

Adshead G (2001). Murmurs of discontentment: treatment and treatability of personality disorder. *Advances in Psychiatric Treatment,* **7**, 407–16.

Afari N and Buchwald D (2003). Chronic fatigue syndrome: a review. *American Journal of Psychiatry,* **160**, 221–36.

Agid O, Kapur S, Arenovich T, *et al.* (2003). Delayed-onset hypothesis of antipsychotic action: a hypothesis tested and rejected. *Archives of General Psychiatry,* **60**, 1228–35.

Ainsworth MDS, Blehar MC, Waters E, *et al.* (1978). *Patterns of attachment: a psychological study of the strange situation.* Erlbaum, Hillsdale, NJ.

Akagi H and House A (2002). The clinical epidemiology of hysteria: vanishingly rare or just vanishing? *Psychological Medicine,* **32**, 191–4.

Aleman A, Kahn RS and Selten JP (2003). Sex differences in the risk of schizophrenia: evidence from meta-analysis. *Archives of General Psychiatry,* **60**, 565–71.

Alexander DA (1972). 'Senile dementia'. A changing perspective. *British Journal of Psychiatry,* **121**, 207–14.

Alexander DA (2005). Early mental health intervention after disasters. *Advances in Psychiatric Treatment,* **11**, 12–18.

Alexander GE and Crutcher MD (1990). Functional architecture of basal ganglia circuits: Neural substrates of parallel processing. *Trends in Neuroscience,* **13**, 266–71.

Alexander JF and Parsons BV (1982). Short-term behavioural interventions with delinquent families: impact on family process and recidivism. *Journal of Abnormal Psychology,* **81**, 219–25.

Alexander PC and Lupfer SL (1987). Family characteristics and long term consequences associated with sexual abuse. *Archives of Sexual Behavior*, **16**, 235–45.

Alexopoulos GS, Meyers BS, Young RC, *et al.* (1997). 'Vascular depression' hypothesis. *Archives of General Psychiatry*, **54**, 915–22.

Allderidge P (1979). Hospitals, madhouses and asylums: cycles in the care of the insane. *British Journal of Psychiatry*, **134**, 321–4.

Alonso J, Angermeyer C, Bernert S, *et al.* (2004). Prevalence of mental disorders in Europe: results from the European Study of the Mental Disorders (ESEMeD) project. *Acta Psychiatrica Scandinavica*, **109**, 21–7.

Alström JE, Nordlund CL and Persson G (1984). Effects of four treatment methods on social phobic patients not suitable for insight-oriented psychotherapy. *Acta Psychiatrica Scandinavica*, **70**.

Althof SE and Seftel AD (1995). The evaluation and management of erectile dysfunction. *Psychiatric Clinics of North America*, **1**, 171–92.

Alwahhabi F (2003). Anxiety symptoms and generalized anxiety disorder in the elderly: a review. *Harvard Review of Psychiatry*, **11**, 180–93.

American Academy of Child and Adolescent Psychiatry (1997a). Practice parameters for the forensic evaluation of children and adolescents who may have been physically or sexually abused. *Journal of the American Academy of Child and Adolescent Psychiatry*, **36**, 37S–56S.

American Academy of Child and Adolescent Psychiatry (1997b). Practice parameters for the assessment and treatment of children, adolescents, and adults with conduct disorder. *Journal of the American Academy of Child and Adolescent Psychiatry*, **36**, 122S–39S.

American Academy of Child and Adolescent Psychiatry (1998a). Summary of the practice parameters for the psychiatric assessment of infants and toddlers (0–36 months). *Journal of the American Academy of Child and Adolescent Psychiatry*, **37**, 127–32.

American Academy of Child and Adolescent Psychiatry (1998b). Practice parameters for the assessment and treatment of children and adolescents with language and learning disorders. *Journal of the American Academy of Child and Adolescent Psychiatry*, **37**, 46S–62S.

American Academy of Child and Adolescent Psychiatry (1998c). Practice parameters for the assessment and treatment of children and adolescents with substance misuse disorders. *Journal of the American Academy of Child and Adolescent Psychiatry*, **36**, 140S–56S.

American Academy of Child and Adolescent Psychiatry (2002). Practice paramenter for the use of stimulant medications in the treatment of children, adolescents and adults. *Journal of the American Academy of Child and Adolescent Psychiatry*, **41**, 26S–49S.

American Diabetes Association, American Psychiatric Association, American Association of Clinical Endocrinologists, *et al.* (2004). Consensus development conference on antipsychotic drugs and obesity and diabetes. *Obesity Research*, **12**, 362–8.

American Psychiatric Association (1994). *Diagnostic and statistical manual of mental disorders.* 4th edn. American Psychiatric Association, Washington, DC.

American Psychiatric Association (1995). *Principles of medical ethics with annotations especially for psychiatry.* American Psychiatric Association, Washington, D.C.

American Psychiatric Association (1998). Guidelines for assessing the decision-making capacities of potential research subjects with cognitive impairment. *American Journal of Psychiatry*, **155**, 1649–50.

American Psychiatric Association (1999). Practice guidelines for the treatment of patients with delirium. *American Journal of Psychiatry*, **156**.

American Psychiatric Association (2000). *Diagnostic and statistical manual of mental disorders.* 4th edn. American Psychiatric Association, Washington, DC.

Anand A and Charney DS (2000). Norepinephrine dysfunction in depression. *Journal of Clinical Psychiatry*, **61**, 16–24.

Anderson C, Connelly J, Johnstone EC, *et al.* (1991). Disabilities and circumstances of schizophrenic patients-a follow-up study. Cause of death. *British Journal of Psychiatry*, **13 (Suppl)**, 30–3, 44–6.

Anderson IM (1999). Lessons to be learnt from meta-analyses of newer versus older antidepressants. In A Lee, ed. *Recent topics from advances in psychiatric treatment*, 45–51. Gaskill Press, London.

Anderson IM (2000). Selective serotonin reuptake inhibitors versus tricyclic antidepressants: a metaanalysis of efficacy and tolerability. *Journal of Affective Disorders*, **58**, 19–36.

Anderson IM (2003). Drug Treatment of depression: reflections on the evidence. *Advances in Psychiatric Treatment*, **9**, 11–20.

Anderson JC, Williams S, McGee R, *et al.* (1987). DSMIII disorder in pre-adolescent children; prevalence from a large sample in the general population. *Archives of General Psychiatry*, **44**, 69–76.

Anderson MC, Ochsner KN, Kuhl B, *et al.* (2004). Neural systems underlying the suppression of unwanted memories. *Science*, 232–5.

Andreasen NC (1999). A unitary model of schizophrenia: Bleuler's 'fragmented phrene' as schizencephaly. *Archives of General Psychiatry*, **56**, 781–7.

Andreasen NC and Hoenck PR (1982). The predictive value of adjustment disorders: a follow-up study. *American Journal of Psychiatry*, **139**, 584–90.

Andreasson S, Allebeck P, Engstrom A, *et al.* (1987). Cannabis and schizophrenia. A longitudinal study of Swedish conscripts. *Lancet*, **2**, 1483–6.

Andrews G, Crino R and Hunt CI (1994). *The treatment of anxiety disorders: clinician's guide and patient manuals.* Cambridge University Press, Cambridge.

Andrews G, Slade T and Peters L (1999). Classification in psychiatry: ICD-10 versus DSM-IV. *British Journal of Psychiatry*, **174**, 3–5.

Angst J (2000). Course and prognosis of mood disorders. In MG Gelder, JJ López-Ibor Jr and NC Andreasen, eds. *The new Oxford textbook of psychiatry*, Chapter 4.5.6. Oxford University Press, Oxford.

Angst J and Dobler-Mikola A (1985). The Zurich Study. VI A continuum from depression to anxiety disorders? *European Archives of Psychiatry and Neurological Sciences*, **235**, 179–86.

Angurlova M, Benkelfat C and Turecki G (2003). A systematic review of association studies investigating genes coding for serotonin receptors and the serotonin transporter: I. Affective disorders. *Molecular Psychiatry*, **8**, 574–91.

Anonymous (1994). Molecules and minds. *Lancet*, **343**, 681–2.

Anonymous (1999). Rehabilitation of persons with traumatic brain injury. *Journal of the American Medical Association*, **282**, 974–83.

Anonymous (2003a). Drugs for disruptive features in dementia. *Drug and Therapeutics Bulletin*, **41**, 1–4.

Anonymous (2003b). Memantine for demntia? *Drugs and Therapeutics Bulletin*, **41**, 73–6.

Anonymous (2004). Managing excessive daytime sleepiness in adults. *Drug Ther Bull*, **42**, 52–6.

Ansbacher H and Ansbacher R (1964). *The individual psychotherapy of Alfred Adler.* Basic Books, New York, NY.

Ansseau M, Dierick M, Buntinkx F, *et al.* (2004). High prevalence of mental disorders in primary care. *Journal of Affective Disorders*, **78**, 49–55.

Appleby L (1993). Parasuicide: features of repetition and the implications for intervention. *Psychological Medicine*, **23**, 13–6.

Appleby L, Shaw J, Sherratt J, *et al.* (2001). *Safety First.* Stationary Office, London.

Arango Y, Huang YY, Underwood MD, *et al.* (2003). Genetics of the serotonergic system. *Journal of Psychiatric Research*, **37**, 375–86.

Aronson R, Offman HJ, Joffe RT, *et al.* (1996). Triiodothyronine augmentation in the treatment of refractory depression. A meta-analysis. *Arch Gen Psychiatry*, **53**, 842–8.

Arscott K, Dagnan D and Kroese B (1998). Consent to psychological research by people with an intellectual disability. *Journal of Applied Research in Intellectual Disability*, **11**, 77–83.

Arseneault L, Cannon M, Witton J, *et al.* (2004). Causal association between cannabis and psychosis: examination of the evidence. *British Journal of Psychiatry*, **184**, 110–17.

Arseneault L, Moffitt TE, Caspi A, *et al.* (2000). Mental disorders and violence in a total birth cohort: results from the Dunedin Study. *Archives of General Psychiatry*, **57**, 979–86.

Ashaye OA, Livingston G and Orrell MW (2003). Does standardized needs assessment improve the outcome of psychiatric day hospital care for older people? A randomized controlled trial. *Aging and Mental Health*, **7**, 195–9.

Asher R (1951). Munchausen's syndrome. *Lancet*, **1**, 339–41.

Ashton H (2004). Benzodiazepine dependence. In PM Haddad, S Durson and B Deakin, eds. *Adverse Syndromes and psychiatric drugs. A Clinical Guide*, 240–59. University Press, Oxford.

Ashworth M and Gerada C (1997). Addiction and dependence-II: Alcohol. *British Medical Journal*, **315**, 358–60.

Asperger H (1944). Die 'Autistischen Psychopathien' Kindesalter. *Archiv für Psychiatrie und Nervenkrankheiten*, **117**, 76–136.

Athwal BS, Halligan PW, Fink GR, *et al.* (2001). Imaging hysterical paralysis. In PW Halligan, C Bass and MJ C., eds. *Contemporary approaches to the study of hysteria: clinical and theoretical perspectives.* Oxford University Press, Oxford.

Audini B, Marks IM, Lawrence RE, *et al.* (1994). Home-based versus out-patient/in-patient care for people with serious mental illness. Phase II of a controlled trial. *British Journal of Psychiatry*, **165**, 204–10.

Auer RN (2004). Hypoglycemic brain damage. *Metabolic Brain Disease*, **19**, 169–75.

Aust R, Sharp C and Goulden C (2002). *Prevalence of drug use: key findings from the 2001/2002 British crime Survey.* Home Office.

Austoker J (1994). Reducing alcohol intake. *British Medical Journal*, **308**, 1549–52.

Aveline M (2001). Very brief dynamic psychotherapy. *Advances in Psychiatric Treatment*, **7**, 373–80.

Babor TF, de la Fuente JR, Saunders J, *et al.* (1989). *AUDIT (the Alcohol Use Disorders Indentification Test) Guidelines for Use in Primary Health Care.* World Health Organization, Geneva.

Bacaltchuk J, Trefiglio RP, Oliveira IR, *et al.* (2000). Combination of antidepressants and psychological treatments for bulimia nervosa: a systematic review. *Acta Psychiatrica Scandinavica*, **101**, 256–64.

Badner JA and Gershon ES (2002). Meta-analysis of whole-genome linkage scans of bipolar disorder and schizophrenia. *Molecular Psychiatry*, **7**, 405–11.

Bailey A, Le Couteur A, Gottesman I, *et al.* (1995). Autism as a strongly genetic disorder: evidence from a British twin study. *Psychological Medicine*, **25**, 63–77.

Bailey A, Palferman S, Heavey L, *et al.* (1998). Autism: the phenotype in relatives. *Journal of Autism and Developmental Disorders*, **28**, 369–92.

Bailey JM and Pillard RC (1991). A genetic study of male sexual orientation. *Archives of General Psychiatry*, **48**, 1089–96.

Bailey S (2000). Juvenile delinquency and serious antisocial behaviour. In MG Gelder, JJ López-Ibor Jr and NC Andreasen, eds. *The new Oxford textbook of psychiatry*, Chapter 9.4.1. Oxford University Press, Oxford.

Bailey S and Aulich L (1997). Understanding murderous 'youth'. In E Welldon and C van Leeson, eds. *Forensic psychotherapy.* Jessica Kingsley, London.

Bailey S and Dolan M (2004). *Forensic Adolescent Psychiatry.* Butterworth, London.

Baird G, Cass H and Slomins V (2003). Diagnosis of autism. *British Medical Journal*, **327**, 488–94.

Bakish D, Hooper CL and Filtreau MJ (1996). A double-blind, placebo-controlled trial comparing fluvoxamine and imipramine in the treatment of panic disorder with and without agoraphobia. *Psychopharmacology Bulletin*, **32**, 135–41.

Bakwin H (1961). Enuresis in children. *Journal of Paediatrics*, **58**, 806–19.

Baldwin DS (2003). Recurrent brief depression – more investigations in clinical samples are now required. *Psychological Medicine*, **33**, 383–6.

Baldwin R, Jeffries S, Jackson A, *et al.* (2004). Treatment response in late-onset depression: relationship to neuropsychological, neuroradiological and vascular risk factors. *Psychological Medicine*, **34**, 125–36.

Baldwin RC (2005). Is vascular depression a distinct sub-type of depressive disorder? A review of causal evidence. *International Journal of Geriatric Psychiatry*, **20**, 1–11.

Baldwin RC, Anderson D, Black S, *et al.* (2003). Guideline for the management of late-life depression in primary care. *International Journal of Geriatric Psychiatry*, **18**, 829–38.

Ball D (2004). Genetic approaches to alcohol dependence. *British Medical Journal*, **185**, 449–51.

Ballard C, Margallo-Lana M, Juszczak E, *et al.* (2005). Quetiapine and rivastigmine and cognitive decline in Alzheimer's disease: randomised double blind placebo controlled trial. *British Medical Journal*, **330**, 874–7.

Ballenger JC (2000). Panic disorder and agoraphobia. In MG Gelder, JJ López-Ibor Jr and NC Andreasen, eds. *The new Oxford textbook of psychiatry*, Chapter 4.7.3. Oxford University Press, Oxford.

Bancroft J (2002). The medicalization of female sexual dysfunction: the need for caution. *Archives of Sexual Behaviour*, **31**, 451–5.

Bancroft JHJ, Skrimshire, A. M., Casson, J., et al. (1977). People who deliberately poison or injure themselves: their problems and their contacts with helping agencies. *Psychological Medicine*, **7**, 289–303.

Bandelow B, Zohar J, Hollander E, *et al.* (2002). World Federation of Societies of Biological Psychiatry (WFSBP) guidelines for the pharmacological treatment of anxiety, obsessive-compulsive and posttraumatic stress disorders. *World Journal of Biological Psychiatry*, **3**, 171–99.

Bandura A (1969). *Principles of behaviour modification*. Holt, Rinehart and Winston, New York, NY.

Barbaresi WJ, Katusic SK, Colligan RC, *et al.* (2005). The incidence of autism in Olmsted County, Minnesota, 1976–1997: results from a population based study. *Archives of Pediatric and Adolescent Medicine*, **159**, 37–44.

Barber TX (1962). Towards a theory of hypnosis: posthypnotic behaviour. *Archives of General Psychiatry*, **1**, 321–42.

Barbui C and Hotopf M (2001). Amitriptyline v. the rest: still the leading antidepressant after 40 years of randomised controlled trials. *British Journal of Psychiatry*, **178**, 129–44.

Barcikowska M, Silverman W, Zigman W, *et al.* (1989). Alzheimer-type neuropathology and clinical symptoms of dementia in mentally retarded people without Down syndrome. *American Journal of Mental Retardation*, **93**, 551–7.

Barja G (2004). Free radicals and aging. *Trends in Neurosciences*, **27**, 595–600.

Barker JC and Barker AA (1959). Deaths associated with electroplexy. *Journal of Mental Science*, **105**, 339–48.

Barlow DH, Esler JL and Vitali BA (1997). Psychosocial treatments for panic disorder, phobias and generalized anxiety disorder. In PE Nathan and JM Gorman, eds. *A guide to treatments that work*, 288–318. Oxford University Press, New York.

Barlow DH, Gorman JM, Shear MK, *et al.* (2000). Cognitive-behavioral therapy, imipramine, or their combination for panic disorder: A randomized controlled trial. *Journal of the American Medical Association*, **283**, 2529–36.

Barnes TR (1989). A rating sclae for drug-induced akathisia. *British Journal of Psychiatry*, **154**, 672–6.

Barnes TR and Spence SA (2000). Movement disorders associated with antipsychotic drugs: clinical and biological implications. In MA Reveley and JFW Deakin, eds. *The psychopharmacology of schizophrenia*, 178–210. Arnold, London.

Barnes TRE, Buckley P and Schulz SC (2003). Treatment-resistant schizophrenia. In S Hirsch and D Weinberger, eds. *Schizophrenia*, Chapter 26. Blackwell Science, Oxford.

Baron M, Gruen R and Ranier JD (1985). A family study of schizophrenic and normal control probands: implications for the spectrum concept of schizophrenia. *American Journal of Psychiatry*, **142**, 447–55.

Baron-Cohen S, Tager-Flusberg H and Cohen DJ (2000). *Understanding other minds: perspectives from developmental cognitive neuroscience*. 2nd edn. Oxford University Press.

Barr LC, Goodman WK, Price LH, *et al.* (1992). The serotonin hypothesis of obsessive compulsive disorder: implications of pharmacologic challenge studies. *Journal of Clinical Psychiatry*, **53**, 17–28.

Barraclough B and Harris EC (2002). Suicide preceded by murder: the epidemiology of homicide-suicide in England and Wales 1988–92. *Psychological Medicine*, **32**, 577–84.

Barraclough BM (1973). Differences between national suicide rates. *British Journal of Psychiatry*, **122**, 95–6.

Barraclough BM, Bunch J, Nelson B, *et al.* (1974). A hundred cases of suicide: clinical aspects. *British Journal of Psychiatry*, **125**, 355–73.

Barraclough BM and Shea M (1970). Suicide and Samaritan clients. *Lancet*, **2**, 868–70.

Barraclough BM and Shepherd DM (1976). Public interest: private grief. *British Journal of Psychiatry*, **126**, 109–13.

Barrowclough C, Johnstone M and Tarrier N (1994). Attributions, expressed emotion, and patient relapse: an attributional model of relatives' response to schizophrenic illness. *Behaviour Therapy*, **25**, 67–88.

Barrowclough C, Lobban F, Hatton C, *et al.* (2001). An investigation of models of illness in carers of schizophrenia patients using the Illness Perception Questionnaire. *British Journal of Clinical Psychology*, **40**, 371–85.

Barsky AJ and Ahern DK (2004). Cognitive-behaviour therapy for hypochondriasis: a randomized controlled trial. *Journal of the American Medical Association*, **291**, 1464–70.

Barsky AJ, Fanta JM, Bailey ED, *et al.* (1998). A prospective 4- to 5-year study of DSM-III-R hypochondriasis. *Archives of General Psychiatry*, **55**, 737–44.

Baruk H (1959). Delusions of passion. In SR Hirsch and M Shepherd, eds. *Themes and variations in European psychiatry*, 375–84. Wright, Bristol (1974).

Basmajian JV (ed.) (1983). *Biofeedback: principles and practice for clinicians*. Williams and Wilkins, Baltimore, MD.

Bass C and Gill D (2000). Factitious disorder and malingering. In MG Gelder, JJ López-Ibor Jr and NC Andreasen, eds. *The new Oxford textbook of psychiatry*, Chapter 5.2.9. Oxford University Press, Oxford.

Bass C and Jack T (2002). Current approaches to chronic pain. *Clinical medicine*, **2**, 505–8.

Bass C, Peveler R and House A (2001). Somatoform disorders: severe psychiatric disorders neglected by psychiatrists. *British Journal of Psychiatry*, **179**, 11–14.

Basson R, McInnes R, Smith MD, *et al.* (2002). Efficacy and safety of sidenafil citrate in women with sexual dysfunction associated with female sexual arousal disorder. *Journal of Women's Health and Gender Based Medicine*, **11**, 367–77.

Bateman A and Fonagy P (1999). Effectiveness of partial hospitalisation in the treatment of borderline personality disorder: a randomised controlled trial. *American Journal of Psychiatry*, **156**, 1563–9.

Bateman A and Fonagy P (2001). Treatment of borderline personality disorder with psychoanalytically oriented partial hospitalization: an 18-month follow up. *American Journal of Psychiatry*, **158**, 36–42.

Bateman A and Fonagy P (2004). *Psychotherapy for borderline personality disorder: mentalisation based treatment.* Oxford University Press.

Bateman A and Tyrer P (2004a). Psychological treatment for personality disorder. *Advances in Psychiatric Treatment*, **10**, 378–88.

Bateman A and Tyrer P (2004b). Services for personality disorder: organization for inclusion. *Advances in Psychiatric Treatment*, **10**, 425–33.

Bateson G, Jackson D, Haley J, *et al.* (1956). Towards a theory of schizophrenia. *Behavioural Science*, **1**, 251–64.

Battaglia A and Carey JC (2003). Diagnostic evaluation of developmental delay/mental retardation: and overview. *American Journal of Medical Genetics*, **117C**, 3–14.

Baucom DH, Shoham V, Muester KT, *et al.* (1998). Empirically supported couple and family interventions for marital distress and adult mental health problems. *Journal of Consulting and Clinical Psychology*, **66**, 53–8.

Bauer M and Döpfmer S (1999). Lithium augmentation in treatment-resistant depression: meta-analysis of placebo-controlled studies. *Journal of Clinical Psychopharmacology*, **19**, 427–34.

Baumgarten M, Hanley JA, Infante-Rivard C, *et al.* (1994). Health of family members caring for elderly persons with dementia. *Annals of Internal Medicine*, **120**, 126–32.

Beard JH, Propst RN and Malamud TJ (1987). The Fountain House model of rehabilitation. *Psychosocial Rehabilitation Journal*, **5**, 47–53.

Beauchamp TL and Childress JF (2001). *Principles of biomedical ethics*. 4th edn. Oxford University Press.

Beautler LE and Moos RH (2003). Coping and Coping styles in personality and treatment planning: Introduction to the special series. *Journal of Clinical Psychology*, **59**, 1045–7.

Bebbington P, Wilkins S, Jones P, *et al.* (1993). Life events and psychosis. Initial results from the Camberwell Collaborative Psychosis Study. *British Journal of Psychiatry*, **162**, 72–9.

Beck A (1988). *Love is never enough*. Harper and Row, New York.

Beck A, Croudace TJ, Singh S, *et al.* (1997). The Nottingham Acute Bed Study: alternatives to acute psychiatric care. *British Journal of Psychiatry*, **170**, 247–52.

Beck A, Schuyler D and Herman J (1974). Development of suicidal intent scales. In A Beck, H Resnik and DJ Lettieri, eds. *The prediction of suicide*, 45–56. Charles, Bowe, MD.

Beck AT (1967). *Depression: Clinical, experimental and theoretical aspects.* Harper and Row, New York.

Beck AT (1976). *Cognitive therapy and the emotional disorders.* International Universities Press, New York, NY.

Beck AT and Freeman A (1990). *Cognitive therapy for personality disorders.* Guildford Press, New York.

Beck AT, Steer RA, Kovacs M, *et al.* (1985). Hopelessness and eventual suicide: a 10-year prospective study of patients hospitalized with suicidal ideation. *American Journal of Psychiatry*, **145**, 559–63.

Beck AT, Ward CH, Medelson M, *et al.* (1961). An inventory for measuring depression. *Archives of General Psychiatry*, **4**, 561–85.

Beck JS (1998). Complex cognitive therapy treatment for personality disorder patients. *Bulletin of the Menninger Clinic*, **62**, 170–94.

Beekman AT, Deeg DJ, Braam AW, *et al.* (1997). Consequences of major and minor depression in later life: a study of disability, well-being and service utilization. *Psychological Medicine*, **27**, 1397–409.

Beekman AT, Geerlings SW, Deeg DJ, *et al.* (2002). The natural history of late-life depression: a 6-year prospective study in the community. *Archives of General Psychiatry*, **59**, 605–11.

Beekman ATFC, Copeland JRM and Prince M (1999). Review of community prevalence of depression in later life. *British Journal of Psychiatry*, **174**, 307–11.

Bellack AS, Gold JM and Buchanan RW (1999). Cognitive rehabilitation for schizophrenia: problems, prospects, and strategies. *Schizophrenia Bulletin*, **25**, 257–74.

Belsky J, Hsieh K-H and Crnic K (1998). Mothering, fathering and infant negativity as antecedents of boys' externalizing problems and inhibition at age 3 years: differential susceptibility to rearing experience? *Developmental Psychopathology*, **10**, 301–19.

Benbow S and Crentsil J (2004). Subjective experience of electroconvulsive therapy. *Psychiatric Bulletin*, **28**, 289–91.

Bender S, Linka T, Wolstein J, *et al.* (2004). Safety and efficacy of combined clozapine-lithium pharmacotherapy. *INternational Journal of Neuropsychopharmacology*, **7**, 59–63.

Bendz H, Aurell M, Balldin J, *et al.* (1994). Kidney damage in long-term lithium patients: a cross-sectional study of patients with 15 years or more on lithium. *Nephrology Dialysis Transplantation*, **9**, 1250–4.

Benjamin H (1966). *The transsexual phenomenon.* Julian Press, New York, NY.

Benjamin RS, Costello EJ and Warren M (1990). Anxiety disorders in a pediatric sample. *Journal of Anxiety Disorders*, **4**, 293–316.

Bennett DA and Holtzman DM (2005). Immunization therapy for Alzheimer disease? *Neurology*, **64**, 10–12.

Bennett DA, Schneider JA, Bienias JL, *et al.* (2005). Mild cognitive impairment is related to Alzheimer disease pathology and cerebral infarctions. *Neurology*, **64**, 834–41.

Bennett DH (1983). The historical development of rehabilitation services. In FN Watts and DH Bennett, eds. *The theory and practice of rehabilitation.* Wiley, Chichester.

Bennett-Levy J, Butler G, Fennell M, *et al.* (eds.) (2004). *Oxford guide to behavioural experiments in cognitive therapy.* Oxford University Press, Oxford.

Berelowicz M and Tarnopolsky A (1993). Borderline personality disorder. In P Tyrer and G Stein, eds. *Personality disorder reviewed*, 90–112. Gaskell, London.

Berg I and Jackson A (1985). Teenage school refusers grow up: a follow-up study of 168 subjects, ten years on average after in-patient treatment. *British Journal of Psychiatry,* **147**, 366–70.

Bergen ALM, Dahl AA, Guldberg C, *et al.* (1990). Langfeldt's schizophreniform psychoses fifty years later. *British Journal of Psychiatry,* **157**, 351–4.

Berger M (1985). Temperament and individual differences. In M Rutter and L Hersov, eds. *Child and adolescent psychiatry: modern approaches*. 2nd edn. Blackwell Scientific, Oxford.

Berger M, van Calker D and Riemann D (2003). Sleep and manipulations of the sleep-wake rhythm in depression. *Acta-psychiatrica-Scandinavica-Supplementum,* **418**, 83–91.

Bergmann K, Foster EM, Justice AW, *et al.* (1978). Management of the demented patient in the community. *British Journal of Psychiatry,* **132**, 441–9.

Berkman LF, Blumenthal J, Burg M, *et al.* (2003). Effects of treating depression and low perceived social support on clinical events after myocardial infarction: the Enhancing Recovery in Coronary Heart Disease Patients (ENRICHD) Randomized Trial. *Journal of the American Medical Association,* **289**, 3106–16.

Berman KF and Meyer-Lindenberg A (2004). Functional brain imaging studies in schizophrenia. In DS Charney and EJ Nestler, eds. *Neurobiology of mental illness*, 311–23. Oxford University Press, Oxford.

Berman RM, Narasimhan M and Miller HL (1999). Transient depressive relapse induced by catecholamine depletion: potential phenotypic vulnerability marker? *Archives of General Psychiatry,* **56**, 395–403.

Bernheim (1890). *Suggestive therapeutics.* 2nd edn. Young J. Pentland, Edinburgh and London.

Bernstein DA and Borkovec TD (1973). *Progressive, relaxation training: a manual for the helpful professions.* Research Press, Champaign, IL.

Bernstein LF (2000). Burn trauma. In A Stoudemier, BS Fogel and DB Greenberg, eds. *Psychiatric care of the medical patient.* Oxford University Press, New York, NY.

Berrios G (2000). Schizophrenia: a conceptual history. In MG Gelder, JJ López-lbor Jr and NC Andreasen, eds. *The new Oxford textbook of psychiatry*, Chapter 4.3.1. Oxford University Press, Oxford.

Berrios GE (1992). Phenomenology, psychopathology and Jaspers: a conceptual history. *History of Psychiatry,* **3**, 303–27.

Berrios GE and Hodges JR (2000). *Memory disorders in psychiatric practice.* Cambridge University Press, Cambridge.

Berrios GE and Kennedy N (2002). Erotomania: A conceptual history. *History of Psychiatry,* **13**, 381–400.

Berson RJ (1983). Capgras' syndrome. *American Journal of Psychiatry,* **140**, 969–78.

Bertram L, Hiltunen M, Parkinson M, *et al.* (2005). Family-based association between Alzheimer's disease and variants in UBQLN1. *New England Journal of Medicine,* **352**, 884–94.

Bhagwanjee A, Parekh A, Petersen PI, *et al.* (1998). Prevalence of minor psychiatric disorders in an adult African rural community in South Africa. *Psychological Medicine,* **28**, 1137–47.

Bhopal RS (1986). The inter-relationship of folk, traditional and Western medicine within an Asian community in Britain. *Social Science and Medicine,* **22**, 99–105.

Bhui K and Sashidharan SP (2003). Should there be separate psychiatric services for ethnic minority groups? *British Journal of Psychiatry,* **182**, 10–12.

Bhui K, Stansfeld S, Hull S, *et al.* (2003). Ethnic variations in pathways to and use of specialist mental health services in the UK. Systematic review. *Br J Psychiatry*, **182**, 105–16.

Bhurgra D and Mastrogianni A (2004). Globalisation and mental disorders: Overview with relation to depression. *British Journal of Psychiatry,* **184**, 10–20.

Bialer P, Wallack J and McDaniel J (2000). Human immunodeficiency virus and AIDS. In A Stoudemire, B Fogel and D Greenberg, eds. *Psychiatric Care of the Medical Patient.* Oxford University Press, New York.

Biederman J (1998). Resolved: mania is mistaken for ADHD in prepubertal children. *Journal of the American Academy of Child and Adolescent Psychiatry,* **37**, 1091–9.

Biederman J, Faraone SV, Keenan K, *et al.* (1992). Further evidence for family-genetic risk factors in attention deficit hyperactivity disorder. *Archives of General Psychiatry,* **49**, 728–38.

Billings JA (2000). Palliative Care. *British Medical Journal,* **321**, 555–8.

Billups KL (2002). The role of mechanical devices in treating female sexual dysfunction and enhancing the female sexual response. *World Journal of Urology,* **20**, 137–41.

Binet A (1877). Le fetishisme dans l'amour. *Revue Philosophique,* **24**, 143.

Binet A and Simon T (1905). Méthodes nouvelles pour le diagnostic du niveau intellectuel des normaux. *L'Année Psychologique,* **11**, 193–244.

Bion WR (1961). *Experiences in groups.* Tavistock Publications,, London.

Bird HR (1996). Epidemiology of childhood disorders in a cross-cultural context. *Journal of Child Psychology and Psychiatry,* **37**, 35–49.

Bird HR, Canino G, Rubio-Stipec M, *et al.* (1988). Estimates of the prevalence of childhood maladjuatment in a community survey in Puerto Rico. *Archives of General Psychiatry,* **45**, 1120–6.

Bird T, Knopman D, VanSwieten J, *et al.* (2003). Epidemiology and genetics of frontotemporal dementia/Pick's disease. *Annals of Neurology,* **54 Suppl 5**, S29–31.

Bishop D (2002). Speech and language difficulties. In M Rutter and E Taylor, eds. *Child and adolescent psychiatry*, Chapter 39. 4th edn. Blackwell, Oxford.

Bittner A, Goodwin RD and Wittchen HU (2004). What characteristics of primary anxiety disorders predict subsequent major depressive disorder? *Journal of Clinical Psychiatry,* **65**.

Black D (2000). The effects of bereavement in childhood. In MG Gelder, JJ López-Ibor Jr and NC Andreasen, eds. *The new Oxford textbook of psychiatry*, Chapter 9.3.5. Oxford University Press, Oxford.

Black D, Harris-Hendriks J and Wolkind S (1998). *Child psychiatry and the law.* 3rd edn. Gaskell, London.

Black DW, Gaffney GR, Schloser S, *et al.* (2003). Children of parents with obsessive-compulsive disorder: a two year follow-up study. *Acta Psychiatrica Scandinavica,* **107**, 305–13.

Blackwell AD, Sahakian BJ, Vesey R, *et al.* (2004). Detecting dementia: novel neuropsychological markers of preclinical Alzheimer's disease. *Dementia and Geriatric Cognitive Disorders,* **17**, 42–8.

Blackwood D (2000). A state and a trait marker in schizophrenia. *Lancet,* **355**, 771–2.

Blair RJR (2003). Neurobiological basis of psychopathy. *British Journal of Psychiatry,* **182**, 5–7.

Blake F, Gath D and Salkovskis PM (1995). Psychological aspects of the premenstrual syndrome: developing a cognitive approach. In R Mayou, C Bass and M Sharpe, eds. *Treatment of functional somatic symptoms.* Oxford University Press, Oxford.

Blanchard R and Hucker SJ (1991). Age, transvestism, bondage, and concurrent paraphilic activities in 117 fatal cases of autoerotic asphyxia. *British Journal of Psychiatry,* **159**, 371–7.

Blanco C and Weissman MM (2005). Interpersonal psychotherapy. In GO Gabbard, JS Beck and J Holmes, eds. *Oxford textbook of psychotherapy*, Chapter 3. Oxford University Press, Oxford.

Blazer DG, Hughes D, K. GL, *et al.* (1991). Generalized anxiety disorder. In LN Robbins and DA Regier, eds. *Psychiatric disorders in America: the epidemiological catchment area study*, 180–203. The Free Press, New York.

Blazer DG and Hybels CF (2005). Origins of depression in later life. *Psychological Medicine,* **36**, 1–12.

Blennow K and Hampel H (2003). CSF markers for incipient Alzheimer's disease. *Lancet Neurology,* **2**, 605–13.

Blessed G, Tomlinson BE and Roth M (1968). The association between quantitative measures of dementia and of senile change in the cerebral grey matter of elderly subjects. *British Journal of Psychiatry,* **114**, 797–811.

Bleuler E (1906). *Affektivität, Suggestibilität, und Paranoia.* Halle, Marhold.

Bleuler E (1911). *Dementia praecox or the group of schizophrenias.* English edn. 1950 edn. International University, New York.

Bleuler M (1974). The long term course of the schizophrenic psychoses. *Psychological Medicine,* **4**, 244–54.

Bloch S (1986). Supportive psychotherapy. In S Bloch, ed. *An introduction to the psychotherapies.* 2nd edn. Oxford University Press, Oxford.

Bloch S (2005). *An introduction to the psychotherapies.* 2nd edn. Oxford University Press, Oxford.

Bloch S and Aveline M (1996). Group Psychotherapy. In S Bloch, ed. *An introduction to the psychotherapies*, Ch 4. 3rd edn. Oxford University Press, Oxford.

Bloch S and Chodoff P (1981). *Psychiatric ethics.* Oxford University Press, Oxford.

Bloch S and Harari E (2005). Family therapy. In GO Gabbard, JS Beck and J Holmes, eds. *Oxford textbook of psychotherapy.* Oxford University Press, Oxford.

Block GJ (1980). *Mesmerism.* William Kaufmann, Los Altos, CA.

Block SD (2000). Assessing and managing depression in the terminally ill patient: ACP-ASIM End of Life Consensus Panel. *Annals of Internal Medicine,* **132**, 209–18.

Bluglass R (2000). Organization of services. In MG Gelder, JJ López-Ibor Jr and NC Andreasen, eds. *The new Oxford textbook of psychiatry*, Chapter 11.9. Oxford University Press, Oxford.

Blum BP and Mann JJ (2002). The GABAergic system in schizophrenia. *INternational Journal of Neuropsychopharmacology,* **5**, 159–79.

Blume SB (1997). Women: Clinical aspects. In JH Lowinson and RB Ruiz, eds. *Substance Abuse: A Comprehensive Textbook.* 3rd edn. Williams & Wilkins, New York.

Boelen PA, van der Bout J and de Keijser J (2003). Traumatic grief as a disorder distinct from bereavement-related depression and anxiety: a replication study with bereaved mental health care patients. *American Journal of Psychiatry,* **160**, 1339–41.

Bogenschutz M and Nurnberg H (2004). Olanzapine versus placebo in the treatment of borderline personality disorder. *Journal of Clinical Psychiatry,* **65**, 104–9.

Bogers JPAM, De Jong JTVM and Komproe IH (2001). Schizophrenia among Surinamese in the Netherlands: High admission rates not explained by high emigration rates. *Psychological Medicine,* **30**, 1425–31.

Boland RJ, Goldstein MG and Haltzman SD (2000). Psychiatric management of behavioural syndromes in intensive care units. In A Stoudemier, BS Fogel and DB Greenberg, eds. *Psychiatric care of the medical patient.* Oxford University Press, New York, NY.

Bollini P and Mollica RF (1989). Surviving without the asylum: an overview of the studies on the Italian Reform Movement. *Journal of Nervous and Mental Disease,* **177**, 607–15.

Bombin I, Arango C and Buchanan RW (2005). Significance and meaning of neurological signs in schizophrenia: two decades later. *Schizophr Bull,* **31**, 962–77.

Bond GR, Drake RE, Mueser KT, *et al.* (1997). An update on supported on the job employment for people with severe mental illness. *Psychiatric Services,* **48**, 335–46.

Bonnet U (2003). Moclobemide: therapeutic use and clinical studies. *CNS Drug Reviews,* **9**, 97–140.

Bonomo Y and Proimos J (2005). ABC of adolescence: substance misuse: alcohol, tobacco, inhalants, and other drugs. *British Medical Journal,* **330**, 777–80.

Booth T and Booth W (1993). Parents with learning difficulties: lessons for practitioners. *British Journal of Social Work,* **23**, 459–80.

Borkovec TD, Newman MG, Pincus AL, *et al.* (2002). A component analysis of cognitive-behavioural therapy for generalized anxiety disorder and the role of interpersonal problems. *Journal of Consulting and Clinical Psychology,* **70**, 288–98.

Borkovec TD and Ruscio AM (2001). Psychotherapy for generalized anxiety disorder. *Journal of Clinical Psychiatry,* **62 (Suppl 11)**, 37–42.

Bosinski HA, Peter M, Bonatz G, *et al.* (1997). A higher rate of hyperandrogenic disorders in female to male transsexuals. *Psychoneuroendocrinology,* **22**, 361–80.

Bouchard TJ and McGue M (2003). Genetic and environmental influences on human psychological differences. *Journal of Neurobiology*, **54**, 4–45.

Bowden CL, Calabrese JR, Bowden C, *et al.* (2003). A Placebo-controlled 18-Month Trial of Lamotrigine and Lithium Maintenance Treatment in Recently Manic or Hypomanic Patients with Bipolar 1 Disorder. *Archives of General Psychiatry*, 392–400.

Bower P, Rowland N and Hardy R (2003). The clinical effectiveness of counselling in primary care: a systematic review and meta-analysis. *Psychological Medicine*, **33**.

Bowlby J (1944). Forty-four juvenile thieves. Their characters and home life. *International Journal of Psychoanalysis*, **25**, 19–53.

Bowlby J (1946). *Forty-four juvenile thieves: their characters and home-life.* Baillière, Tindall and Cox, London.

Bowlby J (1951). *Maternal care and maternal health.* World Health Organization, Geneva.

Bowlby J (1969). Psychopathology of anxiety: the role of affectional bonds. In Studies in Anxiety (ed. M. H. Lader). *British Journal of Psychiatry, Special Publication*, **3**.

Bowlby J (1980). *Attachment and loss.* Basic Books, New York.

Boyer W (1995). Serotonin uptake inhibitors are superior to imipramine and alprazolam in alleviating panic attacks: a meta-analysis. *International Clinical Pharmacology*, **10**, 45–9.

Braak H and Braak E (1991). Neuropathological stageing of Alzheimer-related changes. *Acta Neuropathologica*, **82**, 239–59.

Bradley R, Greene J, Russ E, *et al.* (2005). A Multidimensional Meta-Analysis of Psychotherapy for PTSD. *American Journal of Psychiatry*, **162**, 214–27.

Braid J (1843). *Neurohypnology: or the rationale of nervous sleep, considered in relation with animal magnetism.* Churchill, London.

Bramon E, Rabe Hesketh S, Sham P, *et al.* (2004). Meta-analysis of the P300 and P50 waveforms in schizophrenia. *Schizophrenia Research*, **70**, 315–29.

Bramon E, Walshe M, McDonald C, *et al.*. (2005). Dermatoglyphics and Schizophrenia: a meta-analysis and investigation of the impact of obstetric complications upon a-b ridge count. *Schizophr Res*, **75**, 399–404.

Brandon S (1991). The psychological aftermath of war. *British Medical Journal*, **302**, 305–6.

Brandon S, Cowley P, McDonald C, *et al.* (1985). Leicester ECT trial: results in schizophrenia. *British Journal of Psychiatry*, **146**, 177–83.

Brawman-Mintzer O, Lydiard RB and Emmanuel N (1993). Psychiatric comorbidity in patients with generalized anxiety disorder. *American Journal of Psychiatry*, **150**, 1216–18.

Breakey W (2000). Service needs of individuals and populations. In MG Gelder, JJ López-lbor Jr and NC Andreasen, eds. *The new Oxford textbook of psychiatry*, Chapter 7.2. Oxford University Press, Oxford.

Breen N, Caine D and Coltheart M (2000). Models of face recognition and delusional misidentification: a critical review. *Cognitive Neuropsychology*, **17**, 55–71.

Brennan PA, Mednick SA and Hodgins S (2000). Major Mental Disorders and criminal violence in a Danish birth cohort. *Archives of General Psychiatry*, **57**, 495–500.

Brent DA, Gaynor ST and Weersing VR (2002). Cognitive-behavioural approaches to the treatment of depression and anxiety. In M Rutter and E Taylor, eds. *Child and adolescent psychiatry*, Chapter 54. Oxford.

Breslau N and Prabucki MA (1987). Siblings of disabled children: effects of chronic stress in the family. *Archives of General Psychiatry*, **44**, 1040–6.

Breslin R and Evans H (2004). *Key child protection statistics. Child homicides and deaths.* NSPCC. www.nspcc.org.uk/inform/Statistics/KeyCPstats/4.asp

Bret P, Guyotat J and Chazal J (2002). Is normal pressure hydrocephalus a valid concept in 2002? A reappraisal in five questions and proposal for a new designation of the syndrome as 'chronic hydrocephalus'. *Journal of Neurology, Neurosurgery and Psychiatry*, **73**, 9–12.

Breuer J and Freud S (1893). Studies on hysteria. *The standard edition of the complete psychological works.* Hogarth Press, London (1955).

Brewin C (2000). Recovered memories and false memories. In MG Gelder, JJ López-Ibor Jr and NC Andreasen, eds. *The new Oxford textbook of psychiatry*, Chapter 4.6.3. Oxford University Press, Oxford.

Brewin CR, Andrews B and Rose S (2003). Diagnostic overlap between acute stress disorder and PTSD in victims of violent crime. *American Journal of Psychiatry*, **160**, 783–5.

Brewin CR, Andrews B, Rose S, *et al.* (1999). Acute stress disorder and post-traumatic stress disorder in victims of violent crime. *American Journal of Psychiatry*, **156**, 360–6.

Brewin CR, Wing JK, Mangen SP, *et al.* (1987). Principles and practice of measuring needs in the care of the mentally ill: the MRC Needs for Care Assessment. *Psychological Medicine*, **17**, 971–81.

Bridget C and Polak P (2003). Social systems intervention and crisis resolution. Part I: assessment, and Part II: intervention. *Advances in Psychiatric Treatment*, **9**.

Briken P, Hill A and Berner W (2003). Pharmacotherapy of paraphilias with long-acting agonists of luteinizing hormone-releasing hormone: a systematic review. *Journal of Clinical Psychiatry*, **64**, 890–7.

British Paediatric Association (1992). *Guidelines for the ethical conduct of medical research involving children.* Royal College of Paediatrics and Child Health, London.

Broadhead J, Abas, Sakutukwa GK, *et al.* (2001). Social support and life events as risk factors for depression amongst women in an urban setting in Zimbabwe. *Soc-Psychiatry-Psychiatr-Epidemiol.*, **36**, 115–22.

Broadhead J and Jacoby RJ (1990). Mania in old age: a first prospective study. *International Journal of Geriatric Psychiatry*, **5**, 215–22.

Brock A and Griffiths C (2003). Trends in suicide by method in England and Wales, 1979 to 2001. *Health Statistics Quarterly*, **20**, 7–18.

Brockington I (1998). *Motherhood and mental health.* Oxford University Press, Oxford.

Brockington I (2000). Obstetric and gynaecological conditions associated with psychiatric disorder. In MG Gelder, JJ López-Ibor Jr and NC Andreasen, eds. *The new Oxford textbook of psychiatry*, Chapter 5.4. Oxford University Press, Oxford.

Broman S, Nichols PL, Shaughnessy P, *et al.* (1987). *Retardation in young children: a developmental study of cognitive deficit.* Lawrence Erlbaum, Hillsdale, NJ.

Broome MR, Woolley JB, Tabraham P, *et al.* (2005). What causes the onset of psychosis? *Schizophr Res*, **79**, 23–34.

Brown AS, Begg MD, Gravenstein S, *et al.* (2004). Serologic evidence of prenatal influenza in the etiology of schizophrenia. *Archives of General Psychiatry*, **61**, 774–80.

Brown C and Lloyd K (2001). Qualitative methods in psychiatric research. *Advances in Psychiatric Treatment*, **7**, 350–6.

Brown FW (1942). Heredity in the psychoneuroses. *Proceedings of the Royal Society of Medicine*, **35**, 785–90.

Brown GW and Birley JL (1968). Crises and life changes and the onset of schizophrenia. *Journal of Health and Social Behavior*, **9**, 203–14.

Brown GW, Carstairs GM and Topping GG (1958). *Lancet*, **2**, 685–9.

Brown GW and Harris TO (1978). *Social origins of depression.* Tavistock, London.

Brown GW and Harris TO (1993). Aetiology of anxiety and depressive disorders in an inner-city population. 1 Early adversity. *Psychological Medicine*, **23**, 143–54.

Brown GW, Monck EM, Carstairs GM, *et al.* (1962). Influence of family life on the cause of schizophrenic illness. *British Journal of Preventive and Social Medicine*, **16**, 55–68.

Brown LB and Ott BR (2004). Driving and dementia: a review of the literature. *Journal of Geriatric Psychiatry and Neurology*, **17**, 232–40.

Brown P and Marsden CD (1998). What do the basal ganglia do? *Lancet*, **351**, 1801–4.

Brown P and Pantelis C (1999). Ethical aspects of drug treatment. In S Bloch, P Chodoff and SA Green, eds. *Psychiatric Ethics*, 245–73. 3rd edn. Oxford University Press, Oxford.

Brown RJ (2002). The cognitive psychology of dissociative states. *Neuropsychiatry*, **7**, 221–35.

Brown RJ and Trimble MR (2000). Dissociative psychopathology, non-epileptic seizures, and neurology. *Journal of Neurology, Neurosurgery and Psychiatry*, **69**, 285–9.

Brown TA (1989). Cartesian Dualism and Psychosomatics. *Psychosomatics*, **30**, 322–31.

Brown TM and Boyle MF (2002). Delirium. *British Medical Journal*, **325**, 644–647.

Brown W (1934). *Psychology and psychotherapy.* 3rd edn. Edward Arnold & Co., London.

Bruce M (2000). Managing amphetamine dependence. *Advances in Psychiatric Treatment*, **6**, 33–40.

Bruce M, Scott N, Shine P, *et al.* (1992). Anxiogenic effects of caffeine in patients with anxiety disorders. *Archives of General Psychiatry*, **49**, 867–9.

Bruch H (1974). *Eating disorders: anorexia nervosa and the person within.* Routledge & Kegan Paul, London.

Brudny J, Korein J, Levidow A, *et al.* (1974). Sensory feedback therapy as a modality of treatment in central nervous system disorders of voluntary movement. *Neurology*, **24**, 925–32.

Bryant RA, Harvey AG, Dang ST, *et al.* (1998). Treatment of acute stress disorder: a comparison of cognitive-behaviour therapy and supportive counselling. *Journal of Consulting and Clinical Psychology*, **66**, 862–6.

Brylewski J and Duggan L (2004). *Antipsychotic medication for challenging behaviour in people with learning disability.* 3: CD000377, Cochrane Database of Systematic Reviews.

Brylewski J and Wiggs L (1998). A questionnaire survey of sleep and night-time behaviour in a community-based sample of adults with intellectual disability. *Journal of Intellectual Disability Research*, **42**, 154–62.

Buchanan RW and Heinrichs DW (1989). The Neurological Evaluation Scale (NES): a structured instrument for the assessment of neurological signs in schizophrenia. *Psychiatry Research*, **27**, 335–50.

Bucknill JC and Tuke DH (1858). *A manual of psychological medicine.* John Churchill, London.

Budson AE and Price BH (2005). Memory dysfunction. *New England Journal of Medicine*, **352**, 692–9.

Bughra D (2004). Migration and mental health. *Acta Psychiatrica Scandinavica*, **109**, 243–58.

Buglass D, Clarke J and Henderson AS (1997). A study of agoraphobic housewives. *Psychological Medicine*, **7**, 73–86.

Buka SL, Tsuang MT, Torrey EF, *et al.* (2001). Maternal infections and subsequent psychosis among offspring. *Archives of General Psychiatry*, **58**, 1032–7.

Bunch J (1972). Recent bereavement in relation to suicide. *Journal of Psychosomatic Research*, **16**, 361–6.

Bunney WE, Bunney BG, Vawter MP, *et al.* (2003). Microarray technology: a review of new strategies to discover candidate vulnerability genes in psychiatric disorders. *American Journal of Psychiatry*, **160**, 657–66.

Burgess A and Holmstrom L (1979). Rape: sexual disruption and recovery. *American Journal of Orthopsychiatry*, **49**, 648–57.

Burke MJ and Preskorn SH (1999). Therapeutic drug monitoring of antidepressants - cost implications and relevance to clinical practice. *Clinical Pharmacokinetics*, **37**, 147–65.

Burleigh M (2000). Extinguishing the Ideas of Yesterday: Eugenics and Euthanasia. *The Third Reich. A New History*, Chapter 5, 343–81. Macmillan, London.

Burnett R, Mallett R, Bhugra D, *et al.* (1999). The first contact of patients with schizophrenia with psychiatric services: social factors and pathways to care in a multi-ethnic population. *Psychological Medicine*, **29**, 475–83.

Burns A, Gallagley A and Byrne J (2004). Delirium. *Journal of Neurology, Neurosurgery and Psychiatry*, **75**, 362–7.

Burns A, Lawlor B and Craig S (2002). Rating scales in old age psychiatry. *British Journal of Psychiatry*, **180**, 161–7.

Burns A, Luthert P, Levy R, *et al.* (1990). Accuracy of clinical diagnosis of Alzheimer's disease. *British Medical Journal*, **301**, 1026.

Burns AS, O'Brien J and Ames D (2005). *Dementia.* Hodder and Stoughton, London.

Burns T, Beardsmoore A, Ashok VB, *et al.* (1993). A controlled trial of home-based acute psychiatric services. I: Clinical and social outcome. *British Journal of Psychiatry*, **163**, 49–54.

Burns T, Creed F, Fahy T, *et al.* (1999). Intensive versus standard case management for sever psychotic illness: a randomised trial. *Lancet*, **353**, 2185–9.

Burrow T (1927). The group method of analysis. *Psychoanalytic Review,* **14**, 268–80.

Burrows GD, Stanley R and Bloom P (2002). *International Handbook of Clinical Hypnosis.* John Wiley & Sons Ltd., Chichester.

Burti L (2001). Italian psychiatric reform 20 plus years after. *Acta Psychiatrica Scandinavica,* **104**, 41–6.

Busari JO and Weggerlar M (2005). How to investigate and manage the child who is slow to speak. *British Medical Journal,* **328**, 272–6.

Bushnell JA, Wells JE and Oakley Browne M (1993). Long term effects of intrafamilial sexual abuse in childhood. *Acta Psychiatrica Scandinavica,* **85**, 136–42.

Butler G (1999). *Overcoming social anxiety and shyness.* Robinson, London.

Butler RJ (1994). *Nocturnal enuresis: the child's experience.*

Butler RJ, Forsythe WI and Robertson J (1990). The body worn alarm in treatment of childhood enuresis. *British Journal of Child Psychiatry,* **44**, 237–41.

Butler RW and Braff DL (1991). Delusions: a review and integration. *Schizophrenia Bulletin,* **17**, 633–47.

Bynum WF (1985). The nervous patient in eighteenth and nineteenth-century Britain: the psychiatric origins of British neurology. In WF Bynum, R Porter and M Shepherd, eds. *The anatomy of madness.* Tavistock Publications, London.

Byrne P (2000). Stigma of mental illness and ways of diminishing it. *Advances in Psychiatric Treatment,* **6**, 65–72.

Byrne W and Parsons B (1993). Human sexual orientation. *Archives of General Psychiatry,* **50**, 228–39.

Cade JF (1949). Lithium salts in the treatment of psychotic excitement. *Medical Journal of Australia,* **2**, 349–52.

Cadoret RJ (1978). Psychopathology in adopted-away offspring of biologic parents with antisocial behaviour. *Archives of General Psychiatry,* **35**, 176–84.

Cadoret RJ, Yates WR, Troughton E, *et al.* (1995). Genetic/environmental interaction in the genesis of aggressivity and conduct disorders. *Archives of General Psychiatry,* **52**, 916–24.

Caine D and Watson JD (2000). Neuropsychological and neuropathological sequelae of cerebral anoxia: a critical review. *Journal of the International Neuropsychological Society,* **6**, 86–99.

Calabrese JR, Bowden CL, Sachs GS, *et al.* (1999). A double-blind placebo-controlled study of lamotrigine monotherapy in outpatients with bipolar I depression. *Journal of Clinical Psychiatry,* **60**, 79–88.

Callahan KL, Price JL and Hilsenroth MJ (2004). A review of interpersonal-psychodynamic group psychotherapy outcomes for adult survivors of childhood sexual abuse. *Int J Group Psychother*, **54**, 491–519.

Callicott JH, Mattay VS, Verchinski BA, *et al.* (2003). Complexity of prefrontal cortical dysfunction in schizophrenia: more than up or down. *American Journal of Psychiatry,* **160**, 2209–15.

Campana A, Gambini O and Scarone S (1998). Delusional disorder and eye tracking dysfunction: preliminary evidence of biological and clinical heterogeneity. *Schizophrenia Research,* **30**, 51–8.

Campbell SB (1995). Behaviour problems in preschool children: a review of recent research. *Journal of Child Psychology and Psychiatry,* **36**, 113–49.

Campbell EJ, Scadding JG and Roberts RS (1979). The concept of disease. *Br Med J,* **2**, 757–62.

Campling P (2001). Therapeutic communities. *Advances in Psychiatric Treatment,* **7**, 365–72.

Cantor CH (2000). Suicide in the western world. In K Hawton and K van Heeringen, eds. *The International Handbook of Suicide and Attempted Suicide.* John Wiley and Sons, Chichester.

Cantor-Grae E and Selten JP (2005). Schizophrenia and migration: a meta-analysis and review. *American Journal of Psychiatry,* **162**, 12–24.

Caplan G (1961). *An approach to community mental health.* Tavistock Publications, London.

Caplan HL (1970). *Hysterical conversion symptoms in childhood.*M. Phil. Dissertation. University of London, London. See the account in *Child psychiatry modern approaches*, 2nd edn (ed. M. L. Rutter and L. Hersov). Blackwell, Oxford (1985).

Capuron L and Miller AH (2004). Cytokines and psychopathology: Lessons from interferon-alpha. *Biological Psychiatry,* **56**, 819–24.

Cardno AG and Gottesman II (2000). Twin studies of schizophrenia: From bow-and-arrow concordances to Star Wars Mx and functional genomics. *American Journal of Medical Genetics (Seminars in Medical Genetics),* **97**, 12–17.

Carlson SR, Lacono WG and McgGue M (2002). P300 amplitude in adolescent twins discordant and concordant for alcohol use disorders. *Biological Psychology,* **61**, 203–27.

Carlsson A, Waters N, Holm Waters S, *et al.* (2001). Interactions between monoamines, glutamate, and GABA in schizophrenia: new evidence. *Annual Review of Pharmacology and Toxicology,* **41**, 237–60.

Carmen del rio M, Gomez J and Alvarez FJ (2001–2). Alcohol, illicit drugs and medicinal drugs in fatally injured drivers in Spain between 1991 and 2000. *Forensic Science International,* **127**, 63–70.

Carpenter WT, Jr., Heinrichs DW and Wagman AM (1988). Deficit and nondeficit forms of schizophrenia: the concept. *American Journal of Psychiatry,* **145**, 578–83.

Carr A (1991). Milan systemic family therapy: a review of ten empirical investigations. *Journal of Family Therapy,* **13**, 237–63.

Carroll KM, Fenton LR and Ball SA (2004). Efficacy of disulfiram and cognitive behaviuor therapy in cocaine dependent out-patients; a randomized placebo-controlled trial. *Archives of General Psychiatry,* **61**, 264–72.

Carson AJ, Ringbauer, B., MacKenzie, L., Warlow, C., & Sharpe, M. (2000). Neurological disease, emotional disorder, and disability: they are related: a study of 300 consecutive new referrals to a neurology outpatient department. *Journal of Neurology, Neurosurgery and Psychiatry,* **68**, 202–6.

Caruso S, Agnello C, Intelisano G, *et al.* (2004). Placebo controlled study on the efficacy and safety of daily apomorphine SL intake in premenopausal women affected by hypoactive sexual desire disorder and sexual arousal disorder. *Urology,* **63**, 955–9.

Casey P, Dowrick C and Wilkinson G (2001). Adjustment Disorders. *British Journal of Psychiatry,* **179**, 479–81.

Casey PR and Tyrer PJ (1986). Personality functioning and symptomatology. *Journal of Psychiatric Research*, **20**, 363–74.

Caspi A, Moffitt TE, Newman DL, *et al.* (1996). Behavioural observations at age 3 years predict adult psychiatric disorders. Longitudinal evidence from a birth cohort. *Archives of General Psychaitry*, **53**, 1033–9.

Caspi A, Moffitt TE, Cannon M, *et al.* (2005). Moderation of the effect of adolescent-onset cannabis use on adult psychosis by a functional polymorphism in the catechol-O-methyltransferase gene: longitudinal evidence of a gene X environment interaction. *Biol Psychiatry*, **57**, 1117–27.

Cassano GB, Petracca A and Perugi G (1988). Clomipramine for panic disorder: the first 10 weeks of a long-term comparison with imipramine. *Journal of Affective Disorders*, **14**, 123–7.

Castle D, Der G, Wessely S, *et al.* (1991). The incidence of operationally defined schizophrenia in Camberwell, 1965–84. *British Journal of Psychiatry*, **159**, 790–4.

Castle DJ, McGrath J and Kulkarni J (2000). *Women and Schizophrenia.* Cambridge University Press.

Castle DJ, Scott K, Wessely S, *et al.* (1993). Does social deprivation during gestation and early life predispose to later schizophrenia. *Social Psychiatry in Psychiatric Epidemiology*, **28**, 1–4.

Cattell RB (1963). *The sixteen personality factor questionnaire.* Institute for personality and Ability Testing, Chicago, IL.

Cerletti U and Bini I (1938). Un nuovo metodo di shokterapia; 'Tettroshock'. *Bulletin Accademia Medica Di Roma*, **64**, 136–8.

Chakos M, Lieberman J, Hoffman E, *et al.* (2001). Effectiveness of second-generation antipsychotics in patients with treatment-resistant schizophrenia: a review and meta-analysis of randomized trials. *American Journal of Psychiatry*, **158**, 518–26.

Chalkley AJ and Powell G (1983). The clinical description of forty-eight cases of sexual fetishism. *British Journal of Psychiatry*, **142**, 292–5.

Chamberlain AS (1966). Early mental hospitals in Spain. *American Journal of Psychiatry*, **123**, 143–9.

Chamberlain P (1990). Comparative evaluation of specialized foster-care for seriously delinquent youths: a first step. *International Journal of Family Care*, **2**, 21–36.

Chamberlain SR and Sahakian BJ (2004). Cognition in mania and depression: psycological models and clinical implications. *Current Psychiatry Reports*, **6**, 451–8.

Chambers J, Bass C and Mayou R (1999). Noncardiac chest pain: assessment and management. *Heart*, **82**, 656–7.

Charlton J, Kelly S, Dunnell K, *et al.* (1993). Suicide deaths in England and Wales: trends in factors associated with suicide deaths. *Population Trends*, **71**, 34–42.

Charney DS, Heninger GR and Breier A (1984). Nor-adrenergic function in panic patients. *Archives of General Psychiatry*, **41**, 751–62.

Charney JS and Bremner JD (2004). The neurobiology of anxiety disorders. In JS Charney and EJ Nestler, eds. *The neurobiology of mental illness.* 2nd edn. Oxford University Press, New York.

Chaudron LH and Pies RW (2003). The relationship between postpartum psychosis and bipolar disorder: a review. *Journal of Clinical Psychiatry*, **64**, 1284–92.

Cheeta S, Schifano F, Oyefeso A, *et al.* (2004). Antidepressant-related deaths and antidepressant prescriptions in England and Wales. *British Journal of Psychiatry*, **184**, 41–7.

Cheng ATA and Lee CS (2000). Suicide in Asia and the Far East. In K Hawton and K van Heeringen, eds. *The International Handbook of Suicide and Attempted Suicide*. John Wiley and Sons, Chichester.

Chew-Graham C, Baldwin R and Burns A (2004). Treating depression in later life. *British Medical Journal*, **329**, 181–2.

Chick J (1992). Doctors with emotional problems and how they can be helped. In K Hawton and P Cowen, eds. *Clinical Psychiatry*, 242–52. Oxford University Press, Oxford.

Chick J (2000). Treatment of alcohol dependence. In MG Gelder, JJ López-Ibor Jr and NC Andreasen, eds. *The Oxford Textbook of Psychiatry*, Chapter 4.2.2.4. Oxford University Press., Oxford.

Chick J, Ritson B, Connaughton J, *et al.* (1988). Advice versus extended treatment for alcoholism: a controlled study. *British Journal of Addiction*, **83**, 159–70.

Chilvers C, Dewey M, Fielding K, *et al.* (2001). Antidepressant drugs and generic counselling for treatment of major depression in primary care: randomised trial with patient preference arms. *British Medical Journal*, **322**, 772–5.

Chiswick D (2000). Associations between psychiatric disorder and offending. In MG Gelder, JJ López-Ibor Jr and NC Andreasen, eds. *The New Oxford textbook of psychiatry*. Oxford University Press, Oxford., Oxford.

Chou JC, Solhkhah R and Serper M (2000). Clinical research on antipsychotics in bipolar disorder. *J Psychiatr Pract*, **6**, 310–21.

Chouinard G, Ross-Chouinard A, Annable L, *et al.* (1980). Extrapyramidal symptom rating scale. *Canadian Journal of Neurological Science*, **7**, 233.

Christmas D, Morrison C, Muftah S, *et al.* (2004). Neurosurgery for Mental Disorder. *Advances in Psychiatric Treatment*, **10**, 189–99.

Christodoulou GN (1991). The delusional misidentification syndromes. *British Journal of Psychiatry*, **14**, 65–9.

Ciompi L (1980). The natural history of schizophrenia in the long term. *British Journal of Psychiatry*, **136**, 413–20.

Cipriani A, Barbai C and Geddes J (2005a). Suicide, depression and antidepressants: patients and clinicians need to balance benefits and harms. *British Medical Journal*, **330**, 373–4.

Cipriani A, Pretty H, Hawton K, *et al.* (2005c). Lithium in the prevention of suicidal behavior and all-cause mortality in patients with mood disorders: a systematic review of randomized trials. *Am J Psychiatry*, **162**, 1805–19.

Cipriani A, Wilder H, Hawton K, *et al.* (2005b). Lithium in the prevention of suicidal behaviour and all-cause mortality in patients with mood disorders: a systematic review of randomized trials. *American Journal of Psychiatry*, **in press**.

Citrome L and Volavka J (1999). Schizophrenia: violence and comorbidity. *Current Opinion in Psychiatry*, **12**, 47–51.

Citron M (2004). Strategies for disease modification in Alzheimer's disease. *Nature Reviews Neuroscience*, **5**, 677–85.

Clare AW (1997). The disease concept in psychiatry. In R Murray, P Hill and P McGuffin, eds. *The essentials of postgraduate psychiatry*. Cambridge University Press, Cambridge.

Clark A (2004). Working with Grieving Adults. *Advances in Psychiatric Treatment,* **10**, 164–70.

Clark ANG, Mankikar GD and Gray I (1975). Diogenes Syndrome. A clinical study of gross neglect in old age. *Lancet,* **1**, 366–8.

Clark DM (1986). A cognitive approach to panic. *Behaviour Research and Therapy,* **24**, 461–70.

Clark DM (2000). Cognitive-behaviour therapy for anxiety disorders. In MG Gelder, JJ López-Ibor Jr and NC Andreasen, eds. *The New Oxford textbook of psychiatry*, Chapter 6.3.2.1. Oxford University Press, Oxford.

Clark DM (2001). A cognitive perspective on social phobia. In WR Crozier and LE Alden, eds. *International Handbook of Social Anxiety: Concepts, Research and Interventions.* John Wiley, Chichester.

Clark DM, Ehlers A, McManus F, *et al.* (2003). Cognitive therapy versus fluoxetine in generalized social phobia: a randomized controlled trial. *Journal of Consulting and Clinical Psychology,* **71**, 1058–67.

Clark DM, Salkovskis PM and Hackmann A (1994). A comparison of cognitive therapy, applied relaxation and imipramine in the treatment of panic disorder. *British Journal of Psychiatry,* **164**, 759–69.

Clark DM, Salkovskis PM, Hackmann A, *et al.* (1998). Two psychological treatments for hypochondriasis. A randomised controlled trial. *British Journal of Psychiatry,* **173**, 218–25.

Clark DM and Teasdale JD (1982). Diurnal variation in clinical depression and accessibility of memories of positive and negative experiences. *Journal of Abnormal Psychology,* **91**, 87–95.

Clark L and Harrison J (2001). Assessment instruments. In W Livesley, ed. *Handbook of personality disorders: Theory, research, and treatment.*, 277–306. Guilford Press, New York, NY.

Clarkin JF, Marziali E and Munroe-Blum H (1991). Group and family treatments for borderline personality disorder. *Hospital and Community Psychiatry,* **42**, 1038–42.

Classen C, Koopman C, Hales R, *et al.* (1998). Acute stress disorder as a predictor of posttraumatic posttraumatic stress symptoms. *American Journal of Psychiatry,* **155**, 620–4.

Clayden G, Taylor E, Loader P, *et al.* (2002). Wetting and soiling in childhood. In M Rutter and E Taylor, eds. *Child and adolescent psychiatry*, Chapter 47. 4th edn. Blackwell, Oxford.

Clayton PJ (1979). The sequelae and non-sequelae of conjugal bereavement. *The American Journal of Psychiatry,* **136**, 1530–4.

Cleckley HM (1964). *The mask of sanity: an attempt to clarify issues about the so-called psychopathic personality.* 4th edn. Mosby, St. Louis, MO.

Clomipramine Collaborative Study Group (1991). Clomipramine and the treatment of patients with obsessive-compulsive disorder. *Archives of General Psychiatry,* **48**, 730–8.

Cloninger CR (1986). A unified biosocial theory of personality and its role in the development of anxiety states. *Psychiatric Developments,* **3**, 167–226.

Cloninger CR, Sigvardsson S, Gilligan SB, *et al.* (1988). Genetic heterogeneity and the classification of alcoholism. *Adv Alcohol Subst Abuse*, **7**, 3–16.

Cloninger CR, Svrakic DM and Przybeck TR (1993). A psychobiological model of temperament and character. *Archives of General Psychiatry,* **50**, 975–90.

Coccaro EF and Kavoussi RJ (1997). Fluoxetine and impulsive aggressive behaviour in personalitydisordered subjects. *Archives of General Psychiatry,* **54**, 1081–8.

Coccaro EF, Siever LJ, Clar HM, *et al.* (1989). Serotonergic studies in patients with affective and personality disorders. *Archives of General Psychiatry,* **46**, 587–99.

Cohen BJ, Nestadt G, Samuels JF, *et al.* (1994). Personality disorder in later life: a community study. *British Journal of Psychiatry,* **165**, 493–9.

Cohen HW, Gibson G and Alderman MH (2000). Excess risk of myocardial infarction in patients treated with antidepressant medications: association with use of tricyclic agents. *American Journal of Medicine,* **108**, 2–8.

Cohen Mansfield J (2001). Nonpharmacologic interventions for inappropriate behaviors in dementia: a review, summary, and critique. *American Journal of Geriatric Psychiatry,* **9**, 361–81.

Cohen SD, Monteiro W and Marks IM (1984). Two-year follow-up of agoraphobics after exposure and imipramine. *British Journal of Psychiatry,* **144**, 276–81.

Cohn AH and Daro D (1987). Is treatment too late: what 10 years of evaluative research tells us. *Child Abuse and Neglect,* **11**, 433–42.

Coid J, Petruckevitch A, Bebbington P, *et al.* (2002). Ethnic differences in prisoners. 1: Criminanilty and psychiatric morbidity. *British Journal of Psychiatry,* **181**, 473–80.

Cole JD, Goldberg SC and Klerman GL (1964). Comorbidity of gender dysphoria and other major psychiatric diagnoses. *Archives of General Psychiatry,* **10**, 246–61.

Cole MG, Bellavance F and Mansour A (1999). Prognosis of depression in elderly community and primary care populations: a systematic review and meta-analysis. *American Journal of Psychiatry,* **156**, 1182–9.

College Research Unit of the Royal College of Psychiatrists (1999). *Focus on the use of stimulants in children with attention deficit hyperactivity disorder.* Gaskell, London.

Collighan G, Macdonald A, Herzberg J, *et al.* (1993). An evaluation of the multidisciplinary approach to psychiatric diagnosis in elderly people. *British Medical Journal,* **306**, 821–4.

Collins R, Peto R and Parish S (2003). Large-scale randomized evidence: trials and overviews. In DA Warrell, DJ Weatherall, TM Cox, EJ Benz and JD Firth, eds. *Oxford Textbook of Medicine*, 24–36. Oxford Medical Publications, Oxford.

Collins SJ, Lawson VA and Masters CL (2004). Transmissible spongiform encephalopathies. *Lancet,* **363**, 51–61.

Collishaw S, Maughan B, Goodman R, *et al.* (2004). Time trends in adolescent mental health. *Journal of Child Psychology and Psychiatry,* **45**, 1350–62.

Compton SN, March JS, Brent D, *et al.* (2004). Cognitive-behavioural psychotherapy for anxiety and depressive disorders in childhood: an evidence-based review. *Journal of the American Academy of Child and Adolescent Psychiatry,* **43**, 930–59.

Connell PH (1958). *The treatment of the insane without mechanical restraints.* Oxford University Press, Oxford.

Conwell Y, Duberstein PR and Caine ED (2002). Risk factors for suicide in later life. *Biological Psychiatry,* **52**, 193–204.

Cook JM, Gallagher-Thompson D and Hepple J (2005). Psychotherapy with older adults. In GO Gabbard, JS Beck and J Holmes, eds. *Oxford textbook of psychotherapy*. Oxford University Press, Oxford.

Cook Jr EH, Stein MA, Krasowski MD, *et al.* (1995). Association of attention deficit disorder and the dopamine transporter gene. *American Journal of Human Genetics,* **56**, 993–8.

Coons PM (1998). The dissociative disorders. Rarely considered and underdiagnosed. *Psychiatric Clinics of North America,* **21**, 637–48.

Cooper B (1986). Mental disorder as reaction: the history of a psychiatric concept. In H Katching, ed. *Life events and psychiatric disorder: controversial issues*. Cambrdige University Press, Cambridge.

Cooper JE (2003). Prospects for Chapter V of ICD-11 and DSM-V. *British Journal of Psychiatry,* **183**, 379–81.

Cooper JE, Kendell RE and Gurland BJ (1972). *Psychiatric diagnosis in New York and London.* Oxford University Press, London.

Cooper M, Whitehead L and Boughton N (2004). Eating disorders. In J Bennett-Levy, G Butler, M Fennell, A Hackmann, M Mueller and D Westbrook, eds. *Oxford guide to behavioural experiments in cognitive therapy*. Oxford University Press, Oxford.

Cooper PJ and Murray L (1998). Fortnightly review. Postnatal depression. *British Medical Journal,* **316**, 1884–6.

Cooper SA (1999). The relationship between psychiatric and physical health in elderly people with intellectual disabilities. *Journal of Intellectual Disability Research,* **46**, 54–60.

Copeland JR, Dewey ME, Scott A, *et al.* (1998). Schizophrenia and delusional disorder in older age: community prevalence, incidence, comorbidity, and outcome. *Schizophrenia Bulletin,* **24**, 153–61.

Copeland JRM, Kelleher MJ, Kellett JM, *et al.* (1975). Evaluation of a psychogeriatric service: the distinction between psychogeriatric and geriatric patients. *British Journal of Psychiatry,* **126**, 21–9.

Corbett JA (1979). Psychiatric morbidity and mental retardation. In FE James and RP Snaith, eds. *Psychiatric illness and mental handicap*, 11–25. Gaskell Press, London.

Cormac I, Jones C and Silviera da Mota Neto J (2004). *Cognitive behaviour therapy fro schizophrenia (Cochrane Review).* John Wiley, Chichester.

Correll CU, Leucht S and Kane JM (2004). Lower risk for tardive dyskinesia associated with second-generation antipsychotics: a systematic review of 1-year studies. *American Journal of Psychiatry,* **161**, 414–25.

Coryell W, Noyes R and Clancy J (1982). Excess mortality in panic disorder: comparison with primary unipolar depression. *Archives of General Psychiatry,* **39**, 701–3.

Coryell W and Zimmerman M (1989). Personality disorder in the families of depressed schizophrenic and never-ill probands. *American Journal of Psychiatry,* **146**, 469–502.

Costa PT and McCrae RR (1992). *Revised NEO Personality Inventory (NEO PI-P) and NEO Five Factor Inventory Professional Manual.* Psychological Assessment Resources, Odessa, FL.

Costello E, Angold A, Burns B, *et al.* (1996). The Great Smoky Mountains Study of Youth: functional impairement and serious emotional disturbance. *Archives of General Psychiatry,* **53**, 1137–43.

Cottrell D and Boston P (2002). Practitioner review: the effectiveness of systemic family therapy for children and adolescents. *Journal of Child Psychology and Psychiatry,* **43**, 573–86.

Coulthard M, Farrell M, Singleton N, *et al.* (2002). *Tobacco, alcohol and druguse and mental health.* HMSO.

Courtney C, Farrell D, Gray R, *et al.* (2004). Long-term donepezil treatment in 565 patients with Alzheimer's disease (AD2000): randomised double-blind trial. *Lancet,* **363**, 2105–15.

Cowen PJ (2005). New drugs, old problems. *Advances in Psychiatric Treatment,* **11**, 19–27.

Cowen PJ, Ogilvie AD and Gama J (2005). Efficacy, safety and tolerability of duloxetine 60 mg once daily in major depression. *Curr Med Res Opin,* **21**, 345–56.

Cowie V (1961). The incidence of neurosis in the children of psychotics. *Acta Psychiatrica Scandinavica,* **37**, 37–71.

Cox BJ, Swinson RP, Morrison B, *et al.* (1993). Clomipramine, fluoxetine, and behaviour therapy in the treatment of OCD: a meta-analysis. **24**, 149–53.

Craig T (2000). Mental health services for homeless mentally ill people. In MG Gelder, JJ López-lbor Jr and NC Andreasen, eds. *The new Oxford textbook of pyschiatry*, Chapter 7.10.2. Oxford University Press, Oxford.

Crammer J (1990). *Asylum history: Buckinghamshire County Pauper Lunatic Asylum – St Johns.* Gaskell, London.

Crawford M and Wessely S (1998). The changing epidemiology of deliberate self-harm – implications for service provision. *Health Trends,* **30**, 66–8.

Creamer M, Burgess P and McFarlane AC (2001). PostTraumatic stress disorder: Findings from the Australian National Survey of Mental Health and Well-being. *Psychological Medicine,* **31**, 1237–47.

Creer C and Wing J (1975). Living with a schizophrenic patient. *British Journal of Hospital Medicine,* **14**, 73–82.

Creighton FJ, Hyde CE and Farragher B (1991). Douglas House: Seven years' experience of a community hostel ward. *British Journal of Psychiatry,* **159**, 500–4.

Crimlisk HL, Bhatia K, Cope H, *et al.* (1998). Slater revisited: 6 year follow up study of patients with medically unexplained motor symptoms. *British Medical Journal,* **316**, 582–6.

Crisp AH (ed.) (2004). *Every family in the land: understanding prejudice and discrimination against people with mental illness.* Revised edn. Royal Society of Medicine Press, London.

Crisp AH, Gelder MG, Ricks S, *et al.* (2000). The stigmatization of people with mental illness. *British Journal of Psychiatry,* **177**, 4–7.

Crits-Cristoph P, Siqueland L, Singleton N, *et al.* (2002). Psychosocial treatments for cocaine dependence; National Institute on drug abuse collaborative cocaine treatment study. *Archives of General Psychiatry,* **56**, 493–502.

Cross-National Collaborative Panic Study Second Phase Investigations (1992). Drug treatment of panic disorder: comparative efficacy of alprazolam, imipramine, and placebo. *British Journal of Psychiatry,* **160**, 191–202.

Crow TJ (1985). The two-syndrome concept: origins and current status. *Schizophrenia Bulletin*, **11**, 471–86.

Crow TJ (1994). Aetiology of schizophrenia. *Current Opinion in Psychiatry*, **7**, 39–42.

Crow TJ (2002). Handedness, language lateralisation and anatomical asymmetry: relevance of protocadherin XY to hominid speciation and the aetiology of psychosis. Point of view. *British Journal of Psychiatry*, **181**, 295–7.

Crowe M (1998). Sexual therapy and the couple. In H Freeman, I Pullen, G Stein and G Wilkinson, eds. *Psychosexual disorders*, Chapter 4. Gaskell, London.

Crowe M (2000). Psychotherapy with couples. In MG Gelder, JJ López-Ibor Jr and NC Andreasen, eds. *The new Oxford textbook of psychiatry*, Chapter 6.3.7. Oxford University Press, Oxford.

Crowe M and Ridley J (1990). *Therapy with couples: a behavioural-systems approach to marital and sexual problems*. Blackwells, Oxford.

Crowe RR (1974). An adoption study of antisocial personality. *Archives of General Psychiatry*, **31**, 785–91.

Crowther R, Marshall M, Bond GR, *et al.* (2001). Helping people with severe mental illness to obtain work: systematic review. *British Journal of Psychiatry*, **322**, 204–8.

Csernansky JG, Mahmoud R and Brenner R (2002). A comparison of risperidone and haloperidol for the prevention of relapse in patients with schizophrenia. *New England Journal of Medicine*, **346**, 16–22.

Cummings JL (1993). Frontal-subcortical circuits and human behavior. *Archives of Neurology*, **50**, 873–80.

Cummings JL (2004). Alzheimer's disease. *New England Journal of Medicine*, **351**, 56–67.

Cummings JL and Frankel M (1985). Gilles de la Tourette syndrome and the neurological basis of obsessions and compulsions. *Biological Psychiatry*, **20**, 1117–26.

Cunningham Owens DG and Johnstone EC (2000). Treatment and management of schizophrenia. In MG Gelder, JJ López-Ibor Jr and NC Andreasen, eds. *The New Oxford Textbook of Psychiatry*. Oxford University Press, Oxford.

Curran V and Travill RA (1997). Mood and cognitive effects of 3,4 methylene dioxymethamphetamine (MDMA, 'ecstacy'): weekend high followed by midweek low. *Addiction*, **92**, 821–31.

Curren L, Schmidt U, Treasure J, *et al.* (2005). Time trends in eating disorder incidence. *British Journal of Psychiatry*, **186**, 132–5.

Cutting J (1991). Delusional misidentification and the role of the right hemisphere in the appreciation of identity. *British Journal of Psychiatry. Supplement*, 70–5.

Da Costa JM (1871). An irritable heart: a clinical study of functional cardiac disorder and its consequences. *American Journal of Medical Science*, **61**, 17–52.

Dagleish MR and Nutt DJ (2003). Brain imaging studies in human addicts. *European Neuropsychopharmacology*, **13**, 453–8.

Daniels J, McGuffin P, Owen MJ, *et al.* (1998). Molecular genetic studies of cognitive ability. *Human Biology*, **70**, 281–96.

Daniels N and Sabin JE (1997). Limits to health care: fair procedures, democratic deliberation, and the legitimacy problem for insurers. *Philosophy and Public Affairs*, **26**, 303–50.

Danish University Antidepressant Group (1990). Paroxetine: a selective serotonin reuptake inhibitor showing better tolerance but weaker antidepressant effect than clomipramine in a controlled multicentre study. *Journal of Affective Disorders*, **18**, 289–99.

Dattilio FM (2005). Cognitive-behaviour therapy with couples. In GO Gabbard, JS Beck and J Holmes, eds. *Oxford textbook of psychotherapy.*, Chapter 8. Oxford University Press, Oxford.

David A, Malmberg A, Lewis G, *et al.* (1995). Are there neurological and sensory risk factors for schizophrenia? *Schizophrenia Research*, **14**, 247–51.

David AS (1990). Insight and psychosis. *British Journal of Psychiatry*, **156**, 798–808.

David AS and Busatto G (1999). The hallucination: a disorder of brain and mind. In MA Ron and AS David, eds. *Disorders of brain and mind*, 336–62. Cambridge University Press, Cambridge.

David AS and Prince M (2005). Psychosis following head injury: a critical review. *J Neurol Neurosurg Psychiatry*, **76 Suppl 1**, i53–60.

Davidson JRT, Abraham K, Connor KM, *et al.* (2003). Effectiveness of chromium in atypical depression: A placebo-controlled trial. *Biological Psychiatry*, **53**, 261–4.

Davidson JRT, Foa E, B., Huppert JD, *et al.* (2004). Fluoxetine, comprehensive cognitive behavioural therapy, and placebo in generalized social phobia. *Archives of General Psychiatry*, **61**, 1005–13.

Davidson JRT, Hughes DC, George LK, *et al.* (1993). The epidemiology of social phobia: findings from the Duke Epidemiological Catchment Area Study. *Psychological Medicine*, **23**, 709–18.

Davidson JRT, Weisler RH, Butterfield MI, *et al.* (2003). Mirtazapine vs. placebo in posttraumatic stress disorder: a pilot trial. *Biol Psychiatry*, **53**, 188–91.

Davidson M, Reichenberg A, Rabinowitz J, *et al.* (1999). Behavioral and intellectual markers for schizophrenia in apparently healthy male adolescents. *American Journal of Psychiatry*, **156**, 1328–35.

Davies AM and Fleischman R (1981). Health status and the use of health services as reported by older residents of the Baka neighbourhood, Jerusalem. *Israeli Medical Sciences*, **17**, 138–44.

Davies BM and Morgenstern FS (1960). A case of cysticercosis, temporal lobe epilepsy and transvestism. *Journal of Neurology, Neurosurgery and Psychology*, **23**, 247–9.

Davies G, Welham J, Chant D, *et al.* (2003). A systematic review and meta-analysis of Northern Hemisphere season of birth studies in schizophrenia. *Schizophrenia Bulletin*, **29**, 587–93.

Davis HS and Rockwood K (2004). Conceptualization of mild cognitive impairment: a review. *International Journal of Geriatric Psychiatry*, **19**, 313–9.

Davis JM, Chen N and Glick ID (2003). A meta-analysis of the efficacy of second-generation antipsychotics. *Archives of General Psychiatry*, **60**, 553–64.

Davis JM, Matalon L, Watanabe MD, *et al.* (1994). Depot antipsychotic drugs. Place in therapy. *Drugs*, **47**, 741–73.

Davison K and Bagley CR (1969). Schizophrenia-like psychoses associated with organic disorders of the central nervous system: a review of the literature. In RN Herrington, ed. *British Journal of Psychiatry Special Publication No.4, Current problems in neuropsychiatry*. Headley, Ashford, Kent.

Dawkins S (1961). Non-consummation of marriage. *Lancet*, **2**, 1029–33.

De Amicis LA, C. GD, LoPiccolo J, *et al.* (1985). Clinical follow-up of couples treated for sexual dysfunction. *Archives of Sexual Behaviour*, **14**, 467–89.

de Girolamo G and Dotto P (2000). Epidemiology of personality disorders. In MG Gelder, JJ López-Ibor Jr and NC Andreasen, eds. *The new Oxford textbook of psychiatry*, Chapter 4.12.5. Oxford University Press, Oxford.

De Hert N and Peuskens J (2000). Psychiatric aspects of suicidal behaviour: schizophrenia. In K Hawton and K van Heeringen, eds. *The international handbook of suicide and attempted suicide*, 121–34. JohnWiley & Sons, Chichester.

de la Torre JC (2004). Is Alzheimer's disease a neurodegenerative or a vascular disorder? Data, dogma, and dialectics. *Lancet Neurol*, **3**, 184–90.

de la Tourette G (1885). Etude sur une affection nerveuse characterisée par l'incoordination motrice accompagnee d'écholalie et de coprolalie. *Archives de Neurologie*, **9**, 19–42.

de Pauw K (2000). Depersonalization disorder. In MG Gelder, JJ López-Ibor Jr and NC Andreasen, eds. *The new Oxford textbook of psychiatry*, Chapter 4.9. Oxford University Press, Oxford.

de Wilde EJ (2000). Adolescent suicidal behaviour: a general population perspective. In K Hawton and K van Heeringen, eds. *The International Handbook of Suicide and Attempted Suicide*. John Wiley & Sons, Chichester.

Dean B (2003). The cortical serotonin2A receptor and the pathology of schizophrenia: a likely accomplice. *Journal of Neurochemistry*, **85**, 1–13.

Deb S (2000). Epidemiology and treatment of epilepsy in patients who are mentally retarded. *CNS Drugs*, **13**, 117–28.

Deb S and Ahmed Z (2000). Specific conditions leading to mental retardation. In MG Gelder, JJ López-Ibor Jr and NC Andreasen, eds. *The new Oxford textbook of psychiatry*, Chapter 10.4. Oxford UniversityPress, Oxford.

Deb S, Thomas M and Bright C (2001a). Mental disorder in adults with intellectual disability. 1: Prevalence of functional psychiatric illness among a community-based population aged between 16–64 years. *Journal of Intellectual Disability Research*, **45**, 495–505.

Deb S, Thomas M and Bright C (2001b). Mental disorder in adults with intellectual disability: 2. The rate of behaviour disorder among a community-based population aged between 16–64 years. *Journal of Intellectual Disability Research*, **45**, 506–14.

Deb S, Thomas M and Bright C (2001c). Mental disorder in adults with intellectual disability. 2: The rate of behaviour disorders among a community-based population aged between 16–64 years. *Journal of Intellectual Disability Research*, **45**, 506–14.

Dedman P (1993). Home treatment for acute psychiatric disorder. *British Medical Journal*, **306**, 1359–60.

DeGucht V and Fischler B (2002). Somatization: a critical review of conceptual and methodological issues. *Psychosomatics*, **43**, 1–9.

Dein S (2003). Psychiatric liaison in palliative care. *Advances in Psychiatric Treatment*, **9**, 241–8.

Delgado Escueta AV, Mattson RH, King L, *et al.* (1981). Special report. The nature of aggression during epileptic seizures. *New England Journal of Medicine*, **305**, 711–6.

Den Boer JA and Westenberg HGM (1988). Effect of a serotonin and nor-adrenalin uptake inhibitor in panic disorder: a double blind comparative study with fluvoxamine and maprotiline. *International Clinical Psychopharmacology*, **3**, 59–74.

Denman C (2001). Cognitive-analytic therapy. *Advances in Psychiatric Treatment*, **7**, 243–52.

Department of Health (1996). *Health and personal social services statistics for England*. The Stationery Office, London.

Department of Health (1999). *A national service framework for mental health*. Department of Health, London.

Department of Health (2002). *National suicide prevention strategy for England*. Department of Health Publications, London.

Depp CA and Jeste DV (2004). Bipolar disorder in older adults: a critical review. *Bipolar Disorders*, **6**, 343–67.

Derby IM (1933). Manic-depressive 'exhaustion' deaths. *Psychiatric Quarterly*, **7**, 435–9.

DeRubeis RJ, Hollon SD, Amsterdam JD, *et al.* (2005). Cognitive therapy vs medications in the treatment of moderate to severe depression. *Arch Gen Psychiatry*, **62**, 409–16.

Devanand DP (2002). Comorbid psychiatric disorders in late life depression. *Biological Psychiatry*, **52**, 236–42.

Devereaux PJ, Montori VM, Manns BJ, *et al.* (2002). Double Blind, you have been voted off the Island! *Evidence Based Medicine Health Notebook*, **5**, 36–7.

Devilly GJ and Spence SH (1999). The relative efficacy and treatment distress of EMDR and a cognitive-behavior trauma protocol in the amelioration of posttraumatic stress disorder. *Journal of Anxiety Disorders*, **13**, 131–57.

Di Matteo MR, Lepper HS and Croghan TW (2000). Depression is a risk factor for noncompliance with medical treatment: meta-analysis of the effects of anxiety and depression on patient adherence. *Archives of Internal Medicine*, **160**, 2101–7.

Di Monte DA (2003). The environment and Parkinson's disease: is the nigrostriatal system preferentially targeted by neurotoxins? *Lancet Neurology*, **2**, 531–8.

Dickerson M and Baron E (2000). Contemporary issues and future directions for research into pathological gambling. *Addiction*, **95**, 1145–59.

Dickey CC, McCarley RW and Shenton ME (2002). The brian in schizotypal personality disorder: a review of structural MRI and CT findings. *Harvard Review of Psychiatry*, **10**, 1–15.

Diermayer M, Hedberg K and Fleming D (1994). Backing off universal childhood lead screening in the USA: opportunity or pitfall? *Lancet*, **344**, 1587–8.

Dingemans AE, Bruna MJ and Van-Furth EF (2002). Binge eating disorder: a review. *International Journal of Obesity and Related Metabolic Disorders*, **26**, 299–307.

Dixit AR and Crum RM (2000). Prospective study of depression and the risk of heavy alcohol use in women. *American Journal of Psychiatry*, **157**, 751–8.

Dodel RC, Hampel H and Du Y (2003). Immunotherapy for Alzheimer's disease. *Lancet Neurol*, **2**, 215–20.

Dolan M and Bishay N (1996). The effectiveness of cognitive therapy in the treatment of non-psychotic morbid jealousy. *British Journal of Psychiatry*, **168**, 588–93.

Dolan M, Deakin WJ, Roberts N, *et al.* (2002). Serotonergic and cognitive impairment in impulsive aggressive personality disordered offenders: are there implications for treatment? *Psychological Medicine,* **32**, 105–17.

Dolan M and Doyle M (2000). Violence risk prediction. Clinical and actuarial measures and the role of the Psychopathy Checklist. *British Journal of Psychiatry,* **177**, 303–11.

Dolan RJ (1999). On the neurology of morals. *Nature Neuroscience,* **2**, 927–9.

Doll R, Peto R, Boreham J, *et al.* (2005). Mortality in relation to alcohol consumption:a prospective study among male British doctors. *International Journal of Epidemiology,* **34**, 199–204.

Done DJ, Crow TJ, Johnstone EC, *et al.* (1994). Childhood antecedents of schizophrenia and affective illness: social adjustment at ages 7 and 11. *British Medical Journal,* **309**, 699–703.

Doody RS, Stevens JC, Beck C, *et al.* (2001). Practice parameter: management of dementia (an evidence-based review). Report of the Quality Standards Subcommittee of the American Academy of Neurology. *Neurology,* **56**, 1154–66.

d'Orban PT (1979). Women who kill their children. *British Journal of Psychiatry,* **134**, 560–71.

Dowden C, Antonowiez D and Andrews DA (2003). The effectiveness of relapse prevention with offenders: a mata analysis. *International Journal of Offender Therapy and Comparative Criminology,* **47**, 516–28.

Drake RE, Mercer McFadden C, Mueser KT, *et al.* (1998). Review of integrated mental health and substance abuse treatment for patients with dual disorders. *Schizophrenia Bulletin,* **24**, 589–608.

Drake RE and Mueser KT (2000). Psychosocial approaches to dual diagnosis. *Schizophrenia Bulletin,* **26**, 105–18.

Dreifuss FE, Bancaud J and Henricksen O (1981). Proposal for a revised clinical and electroencephalographic classification of epileptic seizures. *Epilepsia,* **22**, 489–503.

Drevets WL, Gadde KM and Krishnan KR (2004). Neuroimaging studies of mood disorder. In D Chorey and EJ Nestker, eds. *Neurobilogy of mental illness*, 461–90. Oxford University Press,

Dubois P (1909). *The psychic treatment of nervous disorders.* 6th edn. Funk and Wagnalls Company, New York and London.

Dudley M and Gale F (2002). Psychiatrists as a moral community? Psychiatry under the Nazis and its contemporary relevance. *Australian and New Zealand Journal of Psychiatry,* **36**, 585–94.

Dugbartey AT (1998). Neurocognitive aspects of hypothyroidism. *Archives of Internal Medicine,* **158**, 1413–8.

Duman RS (2004). Role of neurotrophic factors in the etiology and treatment of mood disorders. *Neuromolecular Medicine,* **5**, 11–25.

Dunbar HF (1954). *Emotions and bodily changes.* Columbia University Press, New York, NY.

Dunn KM, Croft PR and Hackett TI (1998). Sexual problems: a study of the prevalence and need for health care in the general population. *Good Family Practice,* **15**, 519–24.

Durham RC, Chambers JA, MacDonald RR, *et al.* (2003). Does cognitive therapy influence the long-term outcome of generalized anxiety disorder? An 8–14 year follow-up of two clinical trials. *Psychological Medicine,* **33**, 499–509.

Durkheim E (1951). *Suicide: a study in sociology.* Transl JA Spaulding and G Simpson. Free Press, Glencoe, IL.

Dworkin SF, Turner JA, Mancl L, *et al.* (2002). A randomized clinical trial of a tailored comprehensive care treatment program for temporomandibular disorders. *Journal of Orofacial Pain,* **16**, 259–76.

Dwyer J and Reid S (2004). Ganser's syndrome. *Lancet,* **364**, 471–3.

Eagles JM (2004). Light therapy and the management of winter depression. *Advances in Psychiatric Treatment,* **10**, 234–40.

Eagles JM and Whalley LJ (1985). Decline in the diagnosis of schizophrenia among first admissions to Scottish mental hospitals from 1969–78. *British Journal of Psychiatry,* **146**, 151–4.

Earls F and Mezzacappa E (2002). Conduct and oppositional disorders. In M Rutter and E Taylor, eds. *Child and adolescent psychiatry*, Chapter 26. Blackwell, Oxford.

Earls F, Reich W, Jung K, *et al.* (1988). Psychopathology in children of alcoholic and antisocial parents. *Alcoholism: Clinical and Experimental Research,* **12**, 481–7.

Eaves LJ, Silberg JL, Meyer JM, *et al.* (1997). Genetics and developmental psychopathology: 2. The main effects of genes and environment on behavioural problems in the Virginia Twin Study of Adolescent Behavioural Development. *Journal of Child Psychology and Psychiatry,* **38**, 965–80.

Eckel RH (2002). Obesity: mechanisms and clinical management. *Lancet,* **362**, 105.

Eckhert ED, Bouchard TJ, Bohlen J, *et al.* (1986). Homosexuality in monozygotic twins reared apart. *British Journal of Psychiatry,* **148**, 421–5.

Edelstyn NMJ and Oyebode F (1999). A review of the phenomenology and cognitive neuropsychological origins of the Capgras syndrome. *International Journal of Geriatric Psychiatry,* **14**, 48–59.

Edwards G (1977). Alcoholism: a controlled trial of 'treatment' and 'advice'. *Journal of Studies on Alcohol,* **38**, 1004–31.

Edwards JG and Anderson I (1999). Systematic review and guide to selection of selective serotonin reuptake inhibitors. *Drugs,* **57**, 507–33.

Egan MF, Goldberg EM, Kolachana BS, *et al.* (2001). Effect of COMT Val108–158 Met genotype on frontal lobe function and risk for schizophrenia. *Proceedings of the National Academy of Sciences of the United States of America,* **98**, 6917–22.

Egger M, Davey Smith G, Schneider M, *et al.* (1997). Bias in meta-analysis detected by a simple, graphical test. *British Medical Journal,* **315**, 629–34.

Ehlers A (2000). Post-traumatic stress disorder. In MG Gelder, JJ López-Ibor Jr and NC Andreasen, eds. *The new Oxford textbook of psychiatry*. Oxford University Press, Oxford.

Ehlers A, Mayou RA and Bryant B (1998). Psychological predictors of chronic post-traumatic stress disorder after motor vehicle accidents. *Journal of Abnormal Psychology,* **107**, 509–19.

Ehlers S and Gillberg C (1993). The epidemiology of Asperger syndrome. A total population study. *Journal of Child Psychology and Psychiatry,* **34**, 1327–50.

Ehrhardt AA, Epstein R and Money J (1968). Fetal androgens and female gender identity in the earlytreated adrenogenital syndrome. *Johns Hopkins Medical Journal*, **122**, 160–7.

Einfield SL and Tonge BJ (1996). Population prevalence of psychopathology in children and adolescents with intellectual disability. II Epidemiological findings. *Journal of Intellectual Disability Research*, **40**, 99–109.

Eisenberg L (1986a). Mindlessness and brainlessness in psychiatry. *British Journal of Psychiatry*, **148**, 497–508.

Eisenberg L (1986b). Does bad news about suicide beget bad news? *New England Journal of Medicine*, **341**, 886–91.

Eley TC, Lichtenstein P and Moffitt TE (2003). A longitudinal behavioural genetic analysis of the etiology of aggressive and nonaggressive anti-social behaiviour. *Development and Psychopathology*, **15**, 383–402.

Elkin I, Shea T and Watkins JT (1989). National Institute of Mental Health Treatment of Depression Collaborative Research Programme: general effectiveness of treatments. *Archives of General Psychiatry*, **46**, 971–82.

Ellis HD and Young AW (1990). Accounting for delusional misidentifications. *British Journal of Psychiatry*, **157**, 239–48.

Emerson E (1995). *Challenging behaviour: analysis and intervention in people with learning disabilities*. Cambridge University Press, Cambridge.

Emre M (2003). Dementia associated with Parkinson's disease. *Lancet Neurology*, **2**, 229–37.

Emre M, Aarsland D and Albanese A (2004). Rivastigmine for dementia associated with Parkinson's disease. *New England Journal of Medicine*, **351**, 2509–18.

Emslie G, Rush A, Weinberg W, *et al.* (1997). A double-blind, randomized placebo-controlled trial of fluoxetine in depressed children and adolescents. *Archives of General Psychiatry*, **54**, 1031–7.

Endicott J and Spitzer RL (1978). A diagnostic interview: the schedule for affective disorders and schizophrenia. *Archives of General Psychiatry*, **35**, 837–44.

Endicott J, Spitzer RL, Fleiss JL, *et al.* (1976). The global assessment scale. A procedure for measuring overall severity of psychiatric disturbance. *Archives of General Psychiatry*, **33**, 766–71.

Engel GL (1977). The need for a new medical model: a challenge for biomedicine. *Science*, **196**, 129–96.

Engels GI, Duijsens IJ, Haringsma R, *et al.* (2003). Personality disorders in the elderly compared to four younger age groups: a cross-sectional study of community residents and mental health patients. *Journal of Personality Disorders*, **17**, 447–59.

Enns MW, Cox B and Larsen DK (2000). Perceptions of parental bonding and symptom severity in adults with depression: mediation by personality dimensions. *Canadian Journal of Psychiatry*, **2000**, 263–8.

Enzlin P, Mathieu C, van den Bruel A, *et al.* (2002). Sexual dysfunction in type I diabetes; a controlled study. *Diabetes Care*, **25**, 672–7.

Enzlin P, Mathieu C, van den Bruel A, *et al.* (2003). Prevalence and predictors of sexual dysfunction in patients with type I diabetes. *Diabetes Care*, **26**, 409–14.

Epstein AW (1960). Fetishism: a study of its psychopathology with particular reference to a proposed disorder in brain mechanisms as an etiological factor. *Journal of Nervous and Mental Disease*, **130**, 107–19.

Epstein AW (1961). Relationship of fetishism and transvestism to brain and particularly to temporal lobe dysfunction. *Journal of Nervous and Mental Disease*, **133**, 247–53.

Erkinjuntti T (2000). Vascular dementia. In MG Gelder, JJ López-Ibor Jr and NC Andreasen, eds. *The new Oxford textbook of psychiatry*, Chapter 4.1.9. Oxford University Press, Oxford.

Erkinjuntti T, Roman G and Gauthier S (2004). Treatment of vascular dementia – evidence from clinical trials with cholinesterase inhibitors. *Journal of the Neurological Sciences*, **226**, 63–6.

Ernst A and Zibrak JD (1998). Carbon monoxide poisoning. *New England Journal of Medicine*, **339**, 1603–8.

Ernst E (1999). Second thoughts about safety of St John's wort. *Lancet*, **354**, 2014–5.

Eronen M, Hakola P and Tiihonen J (1996). Mental disorders and homicidal behaviour in Finland. *Archives of General Psychiatry*, **53**, 497–501.

Errera P (1962). Some historical aspects of the concept, phobia. *Psychiatric Quarterly*, **36**, 325–36.

Escobar JI, Waitzkin H, Silver RC, *et al.* (1998). Abridged somatization: a study in primary care. *Psychosomatic Medicine*, **60**, 466–72.

Escriba PV, Ozaita A and Garcia-Sevilla JA (2004). Increased mRNA expressions of alpha2A-adrenoceptors, serotonin receptors and mu-opioid receptors in the brains of suicide victims. *Neuropsychopharmacology*, **29**, 1512–21.

Esquirol E (1845). *Mental maladies, a treatise on insanity.* Transl EK Hunt. Lea and Blanchard, Philadelphia, PA.

Essau CA and Wittchen HU (1993). An overview of the Composite International Diagnostic Interview (CIDI). *International Journal of Methods in Psychiatric Research*, **3**, 79–85.

Essen-Møller E (1971). Suggestions for further improvement of the international classification of mental disorders. *Psychological Medicine*, **1**, 308–11.

Esterson A (1998). Jeffrey Masson and Freud's seduction theory: a new fable based on old myths. *History of the Human Sciences*, **11**, 1–21.

Evans DL, Staab JP, Petitto JM, *et al.* (1999). Depression in the medical setting: biopsychological interactions and treatment considerations. *Journal of Clinical Psychiatry*, **60**, 40–55.

Evans MD, Hollon SD and DeRubeis RJ (1992). Differential relapse following cognitive therapy and pharmacotherapy for depression. *Archives of General Psychiatry*, **49**, 802–8.

Evans M, Morgan H, Hawyard A, *et al.* (1999). Crisis telephone consultation for deliberate self-harm patients: effects on repetition. *Br J Psychiatry*, **175**, 23–7.

Everett CM and Wood NW (2004). Trinucleotide repeats and neurodegenerative disease. *Brain*, **127**, 2385–405.

Eysenck HJ (1970a). *The structure of human personality.* Methuen, London.

Eysenck HJ (1970b). A dimensional system of psychodiagnosis. In AR Mahrer, ed. *New approaches to personality classification*, 169–207. Columbia University Press, New York.

Eysenck HJ and Eysenck SBG (1976). *Psychoticism as a dimension of personality.* Hodder and Stoughton, London.

Fabrega H (2000). Culture, spirituality and psychiatry. *Current Opinion in Psychiatry,* **13**, 525–53.

Faggiano F, Vigna-Taglianti F and Versino E (2003). *Methadone maintenance at different dosages for opioid dependence.* 3: CD002208, Cochrane Database of Systematic Reviews.

Fairburn C (1999). Risk Factors for anorexia nervosa: three integrated case-control comparisons. *Archives of General Psychiatry,* **56**, 468–76.

Fairburn CG (1995). *Overcoming binge eating.* Guilford Press, New York and London.

Fairburn CG, Cooper Z, Doll HA, *et al.* (2000). The natural course of bulimia nervosa and binge eating disorder in young women. *Archives of General Psychiatry,* **57**, 659–65.

Fairburn CG and Harrison PJ (2003). Eating disorders. *Lancet,* **361**, 407–16.

Fairburn CG, Marcus MD and Wilson GT (1993). Cognitive-behavioural therapy for binge eating and bulimia nervosa: a comprehensive treatment manual. In CG Fairburn and GT Wilson, eds. *Binge eating: nature, assessment and treatment,* 361–404. Guilford Press, New York.

Faller KC (1987). Women who sexually abuse children. *Violence and Victims,* **2**, 263–76.

Fallon JH, Opole IO and Potkin SG (2003). The nueroanatomy of schizophrenia: circuitry and neurotransmitter systems. *Clinical Neuroscience Research,* **3**, 77–107.

Falret JP (1854). Mémoire sur la folie circulaire. *Bulletin de l'Academie de Médicine,* **19**, 382–415.

Fanous AH and Kendler KS (2004). The genetic relationship of personality to major depression and schizophrenia. *Neurotoxicity Research,* **6**, 43–50.

Farde L, Wiesel FA, Nordstrom AL, *et al.* (1989). D_1- and D_2-dopamine receptor occupancy during treatment with conventional and atypical neuroleptics. *Psychopharmacology,* **99**, S28–31.

Farington DP, Langan PA and Tonry M (2004). *National crime rates compared.* Bureau of Justice Statistics.

Faris REL and Dunham HW (1939). *Mental disorders in urban areas.* Chicago University Press, Chicago, IL.

Farmer A, Fowler T, Scourfield J, *et al.* (2004). Prevalence of chronic disabling fatigue in children and adolescents. *British Journal of Psychiatry,* **184**, 477–81.

Farmer A, McGuffin P and Williams J (2002). *Measuring psychopathology.* Oxford University Press, Oxford.

Farrell M (2003). Tobacco, alcohol and drug use and cessation of use at follow-up. In N Singleton and G Lewis, eds. *Better or worse: a longitudinal study of the mental health of adults living in private households in Great Britain.* HMSO, Norwich.

Farrington D, Barnes G and Lamberst S (1996). The concentration of offending in families. *Legal and Criminal Psychology,* **1**, 47–63.

Farrington D, Gallagher B, Morley LSL, *et al.* (1988). Are there any successful men from criminogenic backgrounds? *Psychiatry,* **51**, 116–30.

Farrington DP (2000). Psychosocial causes of offending. In MG Gelder, JJ López-Ibor Jr and NC Andreasen, eds. *The new Oxford textbook of psychiatry*, Chapter 11.2. Oxford University Press, Oxford.

Farrington DP (2002). Key results from the first forty years of the Cambridge study in delinquent development. In TP Thornberry and MD Kern, eds. *Taking Stock of Delinquency: an Overview of Findings from Contemporary Longitudinal Studies.* Kluwer/Plenum, New York, NY.

Fawcett J, Scheftner WA, Fogg L, *et al.* (1990). Time-related predictors of suicide in major affective disorder. *American Journal of Psychiatry,* **147**, 1189–94.

Fazel M, Wheeler J and Danesh J (2005). Prevalence of serious mental disorder in 7000 refugees resettled in western countries: a systematic review. *Lancet,* **365**, 1309–12.

Fazel S and Danesh J (2002). Serious mental disorder in 23000 prisoners: a systematic review of 62 surveys. *Lancet,* **359**, 545–50.

Fazel S and Grann M (2004). Psychiatric morbidity among homicide offenders: a Swedish population study. *American Journal of Psychiatry,* **161**, 2129–31.

Fazel S, Hope T, O'Donnell I, *et al.* (2001). Hidden psychiatric morbidity in elderly prisoners. *British Journal of Psychiatry,* **179**, 535–9.

Fazel S, Vassos E and Danesh J (2002). Prevalence of epilepsy in prisoners: systematic review. *British Medical Journal,* **324**, 1495.

Feighner JP, Robins E, Guze SB, *et al.* (1972). Diagnostic criteria for use in psychiatric research. *Archives of General Psychiatry,* **26**, 57–63.

Feinmann C (1999). *The mouth, the face and the mind.* Oxford University Press, Oxford.

Feinstein A (2004). The neuropsychiatry of multiple sclerosis. *Canadian Journal of Psychiatry. Revue Canadienne de Psychiatrie,* **49**, 157–63.

Felt B, Wise CG, Olson A, *et al.* (1999). Guideline for the management of paediatric idiopathic constipation and soiling. *Archives of Paediatric and Adolescent Medicine,* **153**, 380–5.

Fenichel O (1945). *The psychoanalytic theory of neurosis.* Kegan Paul, Trench and Trubner, London.

Fennell M, Bennett-Levy, J. and Westbrook, D. (2004). Depression. In J Bennett-Levy, G Butler, M Fennell, A Hackmann, M Mueller, D Westbrook and K Rouf, eds. *Oxford guide to behavioural experiments in cognitive therapy.*, Chapter 10. Oxford University Press, Oxford.

Fergusson DM, Horwood LJ and Lynskey MT (1993). Prevalence and comorbidity od DSM-III-R diagnoses in a birth cohort of 15 year-olds. *Journal of the American Academy of Child and Adolescent Psychiatry,* **32**, 1127–34.

Ferrier IN (2001). Developments in mood stabilisers. *British Medical Journal,* **57**, 179–92.

Ferrier IN, Tyrer SP and Bell AJ (1999). Lithium therapy. *Advances in Psychiatric Treatment,* **2**, 76–83.

Filley CM (1998). The behavioral neurology of cerebral white matter. *Neurology,* **50**, 1535–40.

Fink P (2000). Somatization disorder and related disorders. In MG Gelder, JJ López-Ibor Jr and NC Andreasen, eds. *The new Oxford textbook of psychiatry*, Chapter 5.2.3. Oxford University Press, Oxford.

Finkelhor D (1984). *Child sexual abuse: new theory and research.* Free Press, London. 53–68.

Finkelhor D (1986). *A sourcebook of child sexual abuse*. Sage, Beverley Hills, CA.

Finlay-Jones R and Brown GW (1981). Types of stressful life event and the onset of anxiety and depressive disorders. *Psychological Medicine*, **11**, 803–16.

First MB and Pincus HA (1999). Classification in psychiatry: ICD-10 v. DSM-IV. A response. *British Journal of Psychiatry*, **175**, 205–9.

First MB, Spitzer RL, Gibbon M, *et al.* (1995). The Structured Clinical Interview for DSMIII-R Personality Disorders (SCID-II), 1: description. *Journal of Personality Disorders*, **9**, 83–91.

Fitzgerald RG and Parkes CM (1998). Blindness and loss of other sensory and cognitive functions. *British Medical Journal*, **316**, 1160–3.

Flakierska N, Lindstrom M and Gillberg C (1988). School refusal: a 15–20 year follow-up study of 35 Swedish urban children. *British Journal of Psychiatry*, **152**, 834–7.

Flament MF and Chabane N (2000). Obsessive-compulsive disorder and tics in children and adolescents. In MG Gelder, JJ López-Ibor Jr and NC Andreasen, eds. *The new Oxford textbook of psychiatry*, Chapter 9.2.6. Oxford University Press, Oxford.

Flaskerud JH and Hu LT (1992). Relationship of ethnicity to psychiatric diagnosis. *Journal of Nervous and Mental Disease*, **180**, 296–303.

Flaum M, Arndt S and Andreasen NC (1991). The reliability of 'bizarre' delusions. *Comprehensive Psychiatry*, **32**, 59–65.

Fleming FM (2003). Brief interventions and the treatment of alcohol use disorders: current evidence. *Recent developments in alcoholism an official publication of the American medical Society on Alcoholism*.

Fleminger S (2000a). The management of dementia. In MG Gelder, JJ López-Ibor Jr and NC Andreasen, eds. *The new Oxford textbook of psychiatry*, Chapter 4.1.14. Oxford University Press, Oxford.

Fleminger S (2000b). Introduction to cognitive disorders. In MG Gelder, JJ López-Ibor Jr and NC Andreasen, eds. *The new Oxford textbook of psychiatry*, Chapter 4.1.1. Oxford University Press, Oxford.

Fleminger S, Oliver DL, Lovestone S, *et al.* (2003). Head injury as a risk factor for Alzheimer's disease: the evidence 10 years on; a partial replication. *Journal of Neurology, Neurosurgery and Psychiatry*, **74**, 857–62.

Fletcher TA, Brakel SJ and Cavanaugh JL (2000). Violence in the workplace: new perspectives in forensic mental health services in the USA. *Br J Psychiatry*, **176**, 339–44.

Flint AJ and Gagnon N (2003). Diagnosis and management of panic disorder in older patients. *Drugs and Aging*, **20**, 881–91.

Flor-Henry P (1969). Psychosis and temporal lobe epilepsy: a controlled investigation. *Epilepsia*, **10**, 363–95.

Floyd F and Phillippe K (1993). Parental interactions with children with and without mental retardation: behavior, management, coerciveness, and positive exchange. *American Journal of Mental Retardation*, **97**, 673–84.

Foa EB, Riggs DS and Gershvny BS (1995). Arousal, numbing and intrusion: Symptom structure of PTSD following assault. *American Journal of Psychiatry*, **152**, 116–20.

Foa EB, Rothbaum BO, Riggs DS, *et al.* (1991). Treatment of posttraumatic stress disorder in rape victims: a comparison between cognitive-behavioural procedures and counselling. *Journal of Consulting and Clinical Psychology*, **59**, 715–23.

Foa EB, Steketee G, Kozak MJ, *et al.* (1987). Imipramine and placebo in the treatment of obsessive compulsives: their effect on depression and on obsessional symptoms. *Psychopharmacology Bulletin*, **23**, 8–11.

Folley DL, Eaves LJ, Wormley B, *et al.* (2004). Childhood adversity, monoamine oxidase A genotype, and risk for conduct disorder. *Archives of General Psychiatry*, **61**, 738–44.

Folstein MF, Folstein SE and McHugh PR (1975). 'Mini-mental state'. A practical method for grading the cognitive state of patients for the clinician. *Journal of Psychiatric Research*, **12**, 189–98.

Fombonne E (1999). The epidemiology of autism: a review. *Psychological Medicine*, **29**, 769–86.

Fombonne E (2003). Epidemiological surveys of autism and other pervasive developmental disorders: an update. *Journal of Autism and Developmental Disorders*, **33**, 365–82.

Fombonne E, Wostead G, Cooper V, *et al.* (2001a). The Maudsley long-term follow-up study of child and adolescent depression.2. Suicidality, criminality and social dysfunction in adulthood. *British Journal of Psychiatry*, **179**, 218–23.

Fombonne E, Wostead G, Cooper V, *et al.* (2001b). The Maudsley long-term follow-up study of child and adolescent depression. 1. Psychiatric outcomes in adulthood. *British Journal of Psychiatry*, **179**, 210–7.

Fonagy P (2000). Psychoanalysis and other long-term dynamic psycotherapies. In MG Gelder, JJ López-Ibor Jr and NC Andreasen, eds. *The new Oxford textbook of psychiatry*, Chapter 6.3.5. Oxford University Press, Oxford.

Fonagy P and Target M (2000). Child psychoanalysis. In MG Gelder, JJ López-Ibor Jr and NC Andreasen, eds. *The new Oxford textbook of psychiatry*, Chapter 9.5.2. Oxford University Press, Oxford.

Ford R, Durcan G, Warner L, *et al.* (1998). One day survey by the Mental Health Act Commission of acute adult psychiatric inpatient wards in England and Wales. *British Medical Journal*, **317**, 1279–83.

Forman MS, Trojanowski JQ and Lee VM (2004). Neurodegenerative diseases: a decade of discoveries paves the way for therapeutic breakthroughs. *Nature Medicine*, **10**, 1055–63.

Forrest GC and Standish E (1984). Supporting bereaved parents after perinatal death. In JE Stevenson, ed. *Recent research in developmental psychopathology*. Oxford.

Fossey MD and Lydiard RB (1990). Placebo responses in patients with anxiety disorders. In R Noyes, M Roth and GD Burrows, eds. *Handbook of anxiety*, 27–56. Elsevier, Amsterdam.

Foster EM, Kay DWK and Bergmann K (1976). The characteristics of old people receiving and needing domiciliary services. *Age and Ageing*, **5**, 345–55.

Foster T (2001). Dying for a drink. Global suicide prevention should focus more on alcohol use disorders. *British Medical Journal*, **323**, 817–8.

Foster T, Gillespie K and McClelland R (1997). Mental disorders and suicide in Northern Ireland. *British Journal of Psychiatry*, **170**, 447–52.

Foulkes SH (1948). *Introduction to group-analytic psychotherapy.* Heinemann, London.

Foulkes SH and Lewis E (1944). Group analysis: a study in the treatment of groups on psychoanalytic lines. *British Journal of Medical Psychology*, **20**, 175–82.

Foundation for Learning Disabilities (2000). *Leaving home, moving on: housing options for people with learning disabilities.* Mental Health Foundation, London.

Foxcroft DR, Lister-Sharp D and Lowe G (1997). Alcohol misuse prevention for young people: a systematic review reveals methodological concerns and lack of reliable evidence for effectiveness. *Addiction*, **92**, 531–7.

Francis PT, Palmer AM, Snape M, *et al.* (1999). The cholinergic hypothesis of Alzheimer's disease. A review of progress. *Journal of Neurology, Neurosurgery and Psychiatry*, **66**, 137–47.

Francks C, Paracchini S, Smith SD, *et al.* (2004). A 77-kilobase region of chromosome 6p22.2 is associated with dyslexia in families from the United Kingdom and from the United States. *American Journal of Human Genetics*, **75**, 1046–58.

Frangou S (2005). Advancing the pharmacological treatment of bipolar depression. *Advances in Psychiatric Treatment*, **11**, 28–37.

Frank E, Kupfer DJ and Perel JM (1990). Three year outcomes of maintenance therapies in recurrent depression. *Archives of General Psychiatry*, **48**, 1053–9.

Frank JD (1967). *Persuasion and healing.* Johns Hopkins Press, Baltimore, MD.

Frankle WG, Lerma J and Laruelle M (2003). The synaptic hypothesis of schizophrenia. *Neuron*, **39**, 205–16.

Frasure-Smith N, Lesperance F, Gravel G, *et al.* (2000). Social support, depression, and mortality during the first year after myocardial infarction. *Circulation*, **101**, 1919–24.

Frasure-Smith N, Lesperance F, Prince RH, *et al.* (1997). Randomised trial of home-based psychosocial nursing intervention for patients recovering from myocardial infarction. *Lancet*, **350**, 473–9.

Frasure-Smith N, Lesperance F and Talajic M (1993). Depression following myocardial infarction. Impact on 6-month survival. *Journal of the American Medical Association*, **270**, 1819–25.

Frederikson M and Furmark T (2003). Amygdaloid regional cerebral blood flow and subjective fear among during symptom provocation in anxiety disorders. *Annals of the New York Academy of Science*, **985**, 341–7.

Freeman W and Watts JW (1942). *Psychosurgery.* Thomas, Springfield.

Freemantle N (2004). Is NICE delivering the goods? *British Medical Journal*, **329**, 1003.

Freemantle N and Geddes J (1998). Understanding and interpreting systematic reviews and meta-analyses. Part 2: meta-analyses. *Evidence-based Mental Health*, **1**, 102–4.

Freud A (1936). *The ego and the mechanisms of defence.* Hogarths Press, London.

Freud A (1966). *Normality and pathology in childhood: assessments of development.* Hogarth Press and Institute of Psychoanalysis, London.

Freud S (1892). *The standard edition of the complete psychological works.* Hogarth Press, London.

Freud S (1893). On the psychical mechanisms of hysterical phenomena. In J Strachey, ed. *The standard edition of the complete psychological works*, 25–42. Hogarth Press, London.

Freud S (1895a). Obsessions and phobias, their psychical mechanisms and their aetiology. In J Strachey, ed. *The standard edition of the complete psychological works.* Hogarth Press, London.

Freud S (1895b). The justification for detaching from neurasthenia a particular syndrome: the anxiety of neurosis. *Neurologisches Zentralblatt*, **14**, 50–66.

Freud S (1911). Psychoanalytic notes upon an autobiographic account of cases of paranoia. (Schreber). *The standard edition of the complete psychological works*, 1–82. Hogarth Press, London.

Freud S (1923). Psychoanalysis. *The standard edition of the complete psychological works*, 235–54. Hogarth Press, London.

Freud S (1927). Fetishism. *International Journal of Psychoanalysis*, **9**, 161–6.

Freud S (1935). *An autobiographic study.* Hogarth Press, London.

Freudenreich O and Goff DC (2002). Antipsychotic combination therapy in schizophrenia. A review of efficacy and risks of current combinations. *Acta Psychiatrica Scandinavica*, **106**, 323–30.

Friedli K, King M and Lloyd M (2000). The economics of employing a counsellor in general practice: analysis of data from a randomised controlled trial. *British Journal of General Practice*, **50**, 276–83.

Friedman M and Rosenman RH (1959). Association of specific behaviour pattern with blood and cardiovascular findings. *Journal of the American Medical Association*, **169**, 1286–96.

Friedman T and Gath D (1989). The psychiatric consequences of spontaneous abortion. *British Journal of Psychiatry*, **155**, 810–30.

Frints SGM, Froyen G, Maryen P, *et al.* (2002). X-linked mental retardation: vanishing boundaries between non-specific (MRX) and syndromic (MRXS) forms. *Clinical Genetics*, **62**, 423–32.

Frith U (1991). Autistic psychopathy in childhood. In U Frith, ed. *Autism and Asperger syndrome*, 37–92. Cambridge University Press, Cambridge.

Frith C (1996). Neuropsychology of schizophrenia, what are the implications of intellectual and experiential abnormalities for the neurobiology of schizophrenia? *British Medical Bulletin*, **52**, 618–26.

Fromm-Reichmann F (1948). Notes on the development of treatment of schizophrenia by psychoanalytic psychotherapy. *Psychiatry*, **11**, 263–73.

Frucht S, Fahn S and Ford B (1999). French horn embouchure dystonia. *Movement Disorders*, **14**, 171–3.

Fryers T (2000). Epidemiology of mental retardation. In MG Gelder, JJ López-Ibor Jr and NC Andreasen, eds. *The new Oxford textbook of psychiatry*, Chapter 10.2. Oxford University Press, Oxford.

Fu CHY, Williams SCR, Cleare AJ, *et al.* (2004). Attenuation of the neural reponse to Sad Faces in Major depression by Antidepressant treatment. *Archives of General Psychiatry*, **61**, 877–89.

Fukuda K, Straus SE, Hickie IB, *et al.* (1994). Chronic Fatigue Syndrome: a comprehensive approach to its definition and management. *Annals of Internal Medicine*, **121**, 953–9.

Fullerton J, Cubin M, Tiwari H, *et al.* (2003). Linkage analysis of extremely discordant and concordant sibling pairs identifies quantitative-trait loci that influence variation in the human personality trait neuroticism. *American Journal of Human Genetics*, **72**, 879–90.

Fulton M and Winokur G (1993). A comparative study of paranoid and schizoid personality disorders. *British Journal of Psychiatry*, **150**, 1363–7.

Furmark T, Tillfors M, Marteinsdottir I, *et al.* (2002). Common changes in cerebral blood flow in patients with social phobia treated with citalopram or cognitive behaviour therapy. *Archives of General Psychiatry*, **59**, 425–33.

Furukawa TA (1999). From effect size into number needed to treat. *Lancet*, **353**, 1680.

Furukawa TA (2004). Meta-analyses and megatrials: neither is the infallible, universal standard. *Evidence Based Medicine Health Notebook*, **7**, 34–5.

Furukawa TA, McGuire H and Barbui C (2002). Meta-analysis of effects and side effects of low dosage tricyclic antidepressants in depression: systematic review. *British Medical Journal*, **325**, 991.

Fyer AJ, Mannuzza S, Chapman TF, *et al.* (1993). A direct interview family study of social phobia. *Archives of General Psychiatry*, **50**, 286–93.

Fyer AJ, Mannuzza S, Chapman TF, *et al.* (1995). Specificity in familial aggregation of phobic disorders. *Archives of General Psychiatry*, **52**, 564–73.

Fyer MR, Frances AJ, Sullivan T, *et al.* (1988). Co-morbidity of borderline personality disorder. *Archives of General Psychiatry*, **45**, 348–52.

Gabbard GO (2000). A neurobiologically informed perspective on psychotherapy. *British Journal of Psychiatry*, **177**, 117–22.

Gabbard GO (2005). Major modalities: psychoanalytic/psychodynamic. In GO Gabbard, JS Beck and J Holmes, eds. *Oxford textbook of psychotherapy*, Chapter 1. Oxford University Press, Oxford.

Gagnon J and Simon W (1973). *Sexual conduct: the social sources of human sexuality.* Aldine, Chicago, IL.

Gaitatzis A, Trimble MR and Sander JW (2004). The psychiatric comorbidity of epilepsy. *Acta Neurologica Scandinavica*, **110**, 207–20.

Games D, Adams D, Alessandrini R, *et al.* (1995). Alzheimer-type neuropathology in transgenic mice overexpressing V717F beta-amyloid precursor protein. *Nature*, **373**, 523–7.

Ganser SJ (1898). Über einen eigenartigen hysterischen Dämmerzustand. *Archiv für Psychiatrie und Nervenkrankheiten*, **30**, 633–40. (British Journal of Criminology **5**, 120–6 (1965))

Garber HL (1988). *The Milwaukee Project: preventing mental retardation in children at risk.* American Association on Mental Retardation, Washington, DC.

Garbutt JC, West SL, Carey TS, *et al.* (1999). Pharmacological treatment of alcohol dependence: a review of the evidence. *Journal of the American Medical Association*, **281**, 1318–25.

Garmezy N and Mastern AS (1994). Chronic adversities. In M Rutter, E Taylor and L Hersov, eds. *Child and adolescent psychiatry: modern approaches*, 191–208. 3rd edn. Blackwell Scientific Publications, Oxford.

Garner J (2003). Psychotherapies and older adults. *Australian and New Zealand Journal of Psychiatry*, **37**, 537–48.

Garrabé J and Cousin F-R (2000). Acute and transient psychotic disorders. In MG Gelder, JJ López-Ibor Jr and NC Andreasen, eds. *New oxford textbook of psychiatry*, Chapter 4.3.9. Oxford University Press, Oxford.

Garralda ME (1994). Primary care psychiatry. In M Rutter, L Hersov and E Taylor, eds. *Child and adolescent psychiatry*, 1055–70. 3rd edn. Blackwell Science, Oxford.

Garralda ME (2000). The relationship between physical and mental health in children and adolescents. In MG Gelder, JJ López-Ibor Jr and NC Andreasen, eds. *The new Oxford textbook of psychiatry*, Chapter 9.3.2. Oxford University Press, Oxford.

Garralda ME and Bailey D (1986). Children with psychiatric disorders in primary care. *Journal of Child Psychology and Psychiatry*, **27**, 611–24.

Garrard P and Hodges JR (2000). Semantic dementia: clinical, radiological and pathological perspectives. *Journal of Neurology*, **247**, 409–22.

Gath A (1978). *Down's syndrome and the family.* Academic Press, London.

Gath A (2000). Families with a mentally retarded member and their needs. In MG Gelder, JJ López-Ibor Jr and NC Andreasen, eds. *The new Oxford textbook of psychiatry*, Chatper 10.8. Oxford University Press, Oxford.

Gath D, Cooper P, Bond A, *et al.* (1982a). Hysterectomy and psychiatric disorder: II. Demographic psychiatric and physical factors in relation to psychiatric outcome. *British Journal of Psychiatry*, **140**, 343–50.

Gath D, Cooper P and Day A (1982b). Hysterectomy and psychiatric disorder: 1. Levels of psychiatric morbidity before and after hysterectomy. *British Journal of Psychiatry*, **140**, 335–42.

Gath D, Cooper P, Gattoni F, *et al.* (1997). *Child guidance and delinquency in a London Borough.* Oxford University Press, London.

Gath D, Hassal C and Cross KW (1973). Whither psychotic day patients? A study of day patients in Birmingham. *British Medical Journal*, **1**, 94–8.

Gaupp R (1974). The scientific significance of the case of Ernst Wagner. In SR Hirsch and M Shepherd, eds. *Themes and variations in European psychiatry.* John Wright and Sons, Bristol.

Gauron EF and Dickinson JK (1966). Diagnostic decision making in psychiatry. *Archives of General Psychiatry*, **14**, 225–32.

Gayford JJ (1981). Indecent exposure: a review of the literature. *Medicine, Science and the Law*, **21**, 233–42.

Gazzaniga MS (2000). Cerebral specialization and interhemispheric communication. Does the corpus callosum enable the human condition? *Brain*, **123**, 1293–1326.

Geddes J (1999). Asking structured and focused clinical questions: essential first step of evidence-based practice. *Evidence based Mental Health*, **2**, 35–6.

Geddes J (2000). From science to practice. In MG Gelder, JJ López-Ibor Jr and NC Andreasen, eds. *The new Oxford textbook of psychiatry*. Oxford University Press, Oxford.

Geddes JR, Burgess S, Hawton K, *et al.* (2004). Long-term lithium therapy for bipolar disorder: systematic review and meta-analysis of randomized controlled trials. *Am J Psychiatry*, **161**, 217–22.

Geddes JR and Carney SM (2003). Relapse prevention with antidepressant drug treatment in depressive disorders: a systematic review. *Lancet*, **361**, 653–61.

Geddes JR and Harrison PJ (1997). Closing the gap between research and practice. *British Journal of Psychiatry*, **171**, 220–5.

Geddes JR, Verdoux H, Takei N, *et al.* (1999). Schizophrenia and complications of pregnancy and labor: an individual patient data meta-analysis. *Schizophrenia Bulletin*, **25**, 413–23.

Gelder MG (1986). Neurosis: another tough old word. *British Medical Journal*, **292**, 972–3.

Gelder MG, López-Ibor Jr JJ and Andreasen NC (eds.) (2000). *New Oxford textbook of psychiatry*. Oxford University Press, Oxford.

Gelder MG, Marks IM and Wolff H (1978). Desensitization and psychotherapy in phobic states: a controlled enquiry. *British Journal of Psychiatry*, **113**, 53–73.

Geller DA, Biederman J, Griffin S, *et al.* (1996). Comorbidity of obsessive compulsive disorder with disruptive behaviour disorders. *Journal of the American Academy of Child and Adolescent Psychiatry*, **35**, 1637–46.

General Medical Council (2004). *Confidentiality: protecting and providing information*. General Medical Council, London.

Gentil V, Lotufo-Neto F, Andrade L, *et al.* (1993). Clomipramine, a better reference drug for panic/agoraphobia. I. Effectiveness comparison with imipramine. *Journal of Pharmacology*, **7**, 316–24.

Gerald MS, Higley S, Lussier ID, *et al.* (2002). Variation in reproductive outcomes for captive male rhesus macaques (Macaca mulatta) differing in CSF 5-Hydroxyindoleacetic acid concentrations. *Brain, Behavior and Evolution*, **60**, 117–24.

Gerard ME, Spitz MC, Towbin JA, *et al.* (1998). Subacute postictal aggression. *Neurology*, **50**, 384–8.

Gijsman HJ, Geddes J, Rendell JM, *et al.* (2004). Antidepressants for bipolar depression: a systematic review of randomized controlled trials. *American Journal of Psychiatry*, **161**, 1537–47.

Gilbert PL, Harris MJ, McAdams LA, *et al.* (1995). Neuroleptic withdrawal in schizophrenic patients. A review of the literature. *Archives of General Psychiatry*, **52**, 173–88.

Gill B, Meltzer H, Hinds K, *et al.* (1996). *Psychiatric morbidity among homeless people*. HMSO, London.

Gill D and Hatcher S (1999). A systematic review of the treatment of depression with antidepressant drugs in patients who also have a physical illness. *Journal of Psychosomatic Research*, **47**, 131–43.

Gill M, Daly G, Heron S, *et al.* (1997). Confirmation of association between attention deficit hyperactivity disorder and a dopamine transporter polymorphism. *Molecular Psychiatry*, **2**, 311–3.

Gill SS, Rochon PA, Herrmann N, *et al.* (2005). Atypical antipsychotic drugs and risk of ischaemic stroke: population based retrospective cohort study. *British Medical Journal*, **330**, 445.

Gillam SJ, Jarman B, White P, *et al.* (1989). Ethnic differences in consultation rates in urban general practice. *British Medical Journal*, **299**, 958–60.

Gilles de la Tourette (1885). Etude sur une affection nerveuse characterisée par l'incoordination motrice accompagnee d'écholalie et de coprolalie. *Archives de Neurologie*, **9**, 19–42.

Gilman K and Whyte I (2004). *Adverse syndromes and psychiatric drug*. Oxford University Press, Oxford.

Gitlin DF, Levenson JL and Lyketsos CG (2004). Psychosomatic medicine: a new psychiatric subspecialty. *Academic Psychiatry*, **28**, 4–11.

Gjessing R (1947). Biological investigations in endogenous psychoses. *Acta Psychiatrica Scandinavica*, **47 (Suppl)**, 93–103.

Glassman AH, O'Connor CM, Califf RM, *et al.* (2002). Sertraline treatment of major depression in patients with acute MI or unstable angina. *Journal of the American Medical Association*, **288**, 701–9.

Global Population Census (2002). *Report WP/02*. Government Printing Office, Washington, DC. http://www.census.gov/ipc/prod/wp02/wp02-1.pdf

Glover G (2000). The minimum data set. At last – information! *Psychiatric Bulletin*, **24**, 163–4.

Glover L and Pearce S (1995). Chronic pelvic pain. In RA Mayou, C Bass and M Sharpe, eds. *Treatment of functional somatic symptoms*, 313–27. Oxford University Press, Oxford.

Goate A, Chartier Harlin MC, Mullan M, *et al.* (1991). Segregation of a missense mutation in the amyloid precursor protein gene with familial Alzheimer's disease. *Nature*, **349**, 704–6.

Godfrey C, Eaton G, McDougal C, *et al.* (2002). *The economic and social costs of Class A drug use in England and Wales*. Study 249, Home Office Research.

Goff DC and Coyle JT (2001). The emerging role of glutamate in the pathophysiology and treatment of schizophrenia. *American Journal of Psychiatry*, **158**, 1367–77.

Goffman E (1961). *Asylums: essays on the social situation of mental patients and other inmates*. Doubleday, New York, NY.

Gold G, Bouras C, Canuto A, *et al.* (2002). Clinicopathological validation study of four sets of clinical criteria for vascular dementia. *American Journal of Psychiatry*, **159**, 82–7.

Gold JM, Queern C, Iannone VN, *et al.* (1999). Repeatable battery for the assessment of neuropsychological status as a screening test in schizophrenia I: sensitivity, reliability, and validity. *American Journal of Psychiatry*, **156**, 1944–50.

Goldberg D (1972). *The detection of psychiatric illness by questionnaire. Maudsley Monograph No. 21*. Oxford University Press, London.

Goldberg D (ed.) (1997). *The Maudsley handbook of practical psychiatry*. Oxford Medical Publications, Oxford.

Goldberg D and Hillier VP (1979). A scaled version of the General Health Questionnaire. *Psychological Medicine*, **9**, 139–45.

Goldberg D and Huxley P (1980). *Mental illness in the community*. Tavistock Publications, London.

Goldberg D and Huxley P (1992). *Common mental disorders: a biosocial model*. Routledge, London.

Goldberg D, Mann A and Tylee A (2000). Psychiatry in primary care. In MG Gelder, JJ López-Ibor Jr and NC Andreasen, eds. *The new Oxford textbook of psychiatry*, Chapter 7.8. Oxford University Press, Oxford.

Goldberg D, Richels J, Downing R, *et al.* (1976). A comparison of two psychiatric screening tests. *British Journal of Psychiatry,* **129**, 61–7.

Goldberg D, Steele J and Smith J (1980). Teaching psychiatric interview techniques to family doctors. *Acta Psychiatrica Scandinavica,* **62**, 41–7.

Goldberg DM, Soleas GJ and Levesque M (1999). Moderate alcohol consumption: the gentle face of Janus. *Clinical Biochemistry,* **32**, 505–18.

Goldberg EM and Morrison SL (1963). Schizophrenia and social class. *British Journal of Psychiatry,* **109**, 785–802.

Goldberg TE, David A and Gold JM (2003). Neurocognitive deficits in schizophrenia. In SR Hirsch and D Weinberger, eds. *Schizophrenia*, 168–84. 2nd edn. Blackwell Publishing, Oxford.

Goldman H and Morrissey JP (1985). The alchemy of mental health policy: homelessness and the fourth cycle of reform. *American Journal of Public Health,* **75**, 727–31.

Goldstein I (1986). Arterial revascularisation procedures. *Seminars in Urology,* **4**, 252–8.

Goldstein RB, Black DW, Nasrallah A, *et al.* (1991). The prediction of suicidesensitivity, specificity, and predictive value of a multivariate model applied to suicide among 1906 patients with affective disorders. *Archives of General Psychiatry,* **48**, 418–22.

Goodman R (1987). The developmental neurobiology of language. In W Yule and M Rutter, eds. *Language development and disorders*, 129–45. MacKeith Press, London.

Goodman R and Scott S (2005). *Child psychiatry.* 2nd edn. Blackwell, Oxford.

Goodman WK, Price LH and Rasmussen SA (1989a). The Yale-Brown obsessive compulsive scale. *Archives of General Psychiatry,* **46**, 1006–11.

Goodman WK, Price LH, Rasmussen SA, *et al.* (1989b). Efficacy of fluvoxamine in obsessive-compulsive disorder. *Archives of General Psychiatry,* **46**, 36–44.

Goodwin GM (1999). Prophylaxis of bi-polar disorder: how and who should we treat in the long term? *European Neuropsychopharmacology,* **9**, S125–9.

Goodwin GM (2003). Evidence-based guidelines for treating bipolar disorder: recommendations from the British Association for Psycopharmacology. *Journal of Psychopharmacology*, 149–73.

Goodwin GM, Bowden CL, Calabrese JR, *et al.* (2004). A pooled analysis of 2 placebo-controlled 18-month trials of lamotrigine and lithium maintenance in bipolar I disorder. *J Clin Psychiatry*, **65**, 432–41.

Goodwin GM and Geddes JR (2003). Latest maintenance data on lithium in bipolar disorder. *European Neuropsychopharmacology,* **13**, S51–5.

Goodwin J (1988). Post-traumatic symptoms in abused children. *Journal of Traumatic Stress,* **4**, 475–88.

Goodyer I (2000). Emotional disorders with their onset in childhood. In MG Gelder, JJ López-Ibor Jr and NC Andreasen, eds. *The new Oxford textbook of psychiatry*, Chapter 9.2.5. Oxford University Press, Oxford.

Goodyer I, Ashby L, Altham PME, *et al.* (1993). Temperament and major depression in 11–16 year olds. *Journal of Child Psychology and Psychiatry,* **34**, 1409–23.

Goodyer I, Kolvin I and Gatzanis S (1985). Recent undesirable life events and psychiatric disorder in childhood and adolescence. *British Journal of Psychiatry,* **147**, 517–23.

Goodyer IM (2001). *The depressed child and adolescent.* 2nd edn. Cambridge Universty Press, Cambridge.

Goodyer IM (2002). Social adversity and mental functions in adolescents at high risk of psychopathology. Position paper and suggested framework for future research. *British Journal of Psychiatry,* **181**, 383–6.

Goodyer IM, Herbert J and Tamplin A (2003). Psychoendocrine antecedents of persistent first-episode major depression in adolescents: a community-based longitudinal enquiry. *Psychological Medicine,* **33**, 601–10.

Goodyer IM, Kolvin I and Gatzanis S (1987). The impact of recent undesirable life events on psychiatric disorders in childhood and adolescence. *British Journal of Psychiatry,* **151**, 179–84.

Goodyer IM, Park RJ, Netherton CM, *et al.* (2001). Possible role of cortisol and dehydroepiandrosterone in human development and psychopathology. *British Journal of Psychiatry,* **179**, 243–9.

Gordon H and Grubin D (2004). Psychiatric aspects of the assessment and treatment of sex offenders. *Advances in Psychiatric Treatment,* **10**, 73–80.

Gorman DG and Cummings JL (1990). Organic delusional syndrome. *Seminars in Neurology,* **10**, 229–38.

Gottesman I (1991). *Schizophrenia genesis: the origins of madness*. W. H. Freeman, New York.

Gottesman II and Gould TD (2003). The endophenotype concept in psychiatry: etymology and strategic intentions. *American Journal of Psychiatry,* **160**, 636–45.

Goudriaan AE, Ossterlaan J, de Beurs E, *et al.* (2004). Pathological Gambling: a comprehensive review of biobehavioral findings. *Neurosciences and biobehavioral reviews.,* **28**, 123–41.

Gould MS, Wallenstein S and Kleinman M (1990). Time-space clustering of teenage suicide. *American Journal of Epidemiology,* **131**, 71–8.

Gould RA, Buckminster S, Pollack MH, *et al.* (1997). Cognitive-behavioral and pharmacological treatment for social phobia: a meta-analysis. *Clinical Psychology: Science and Practice,* **4**, 291–306.

Gournay K (2000). Role of the community psychiatric nurse in the management of schizophrenia. *Advances in Psychiatric Treatment,* **6**, 243–51.

Gournay K and Brooking J (1994). Community psychiatric nurses in primary health care. *British Journal of Psychiatry,* **165**, 231–8.

Gowing L, Ali R and White J (2004). *Buprenorphine for the management of opioid withdrawal.* 4: CD002025, Cochrane Database of Systematic Reviews.

Graham NL, Emery T and Hodges JR (2004). Distinctive cognitive profiles in Alzheimer's disease and subcortical vascular dementia. *Journal of Neurology, Neurosurgery and Psychiatry,* **75**, 61–71.

Graham P (1991). *Child psychiatry: a developmental approach.* 2nd edn. Oxford University Press, Oxford.

Graham P, Turk J and Verhulst F (1999). Motor development and disorders of movement. In P Graham, *et al*., eds. *Child Psychiatry, a developmental approach*, 61. 3rd edn. Oxford University Press, Oxford.

Grahame-Smith DG and Aronson JK (2000). *Oxford textbook of clinical pharmacology and drug therapy.* 3rd edn. Oxford University Press, Oxford.

Grann M and Fazel S (2004). Substance misuse and violent crime: Swedish population study. *British Medical Journal*, **328**, 1233–4.

Grant I and Adams KM (eds.) (1996). *Neuropsychological assessment of neuropsychiatric disorders.* 2nd edn. Oxford University Press, New York, NY.

Grant I and Atkinson JH (2000). Neuropsychiatric aspects of HIV infection and AIDS. In BJ Sadock and VA Sadock, eds. *Comprehensive textbook of psychiatry*. 7th edn. Lippincott, Williams & Wilkins, Philadelphia.

Grant BF, Hasin DS, Stinson FS, *et al.* (2004). Prevalence, correlates, and disability of personality disorders in the United States: results from the national epidemiologic survey on alcohol and related conditions. *J Clin Psychiatry*, **65**, 948–58.

Granville-Grossman K (1993). Mind and body. In MH Lader, ed. *Handbook of Psychiatry*. Cambridge University Press, Cambridge.

Gravestock S (2003). Diagnosis and classification of eating disorders in adults with intellectual disability: the diagnostic criteria for psychiatric disorders for use with adults with learning disabilities/ mental retardation (DC-LD). *Journal of Intellectual Disability Research*, **47**, 72–83.

Gray J, Feldon J, Rawlins J, *et al.* (1991). The neuropsychology of schizophrenia. *Behav Brain Sci*, **14**, 1–84.

Green J (2002). Provision of intensive treatment: inpatient units, day units and intensive outreach. In M Rutter and E Taylor, eds. *Child and adolescent psychiatry*, Chapter 61. 4th edn. Blackwell, Oxford.

Green MF, Kern RS, Braff DL, *et al.* (2000). Neurocognitive deficits and functional outcome in schizophrenia: are we measuring the 'right stuff'? *Schizophrenia Bulletin*, **26**, 119–36.

Green R (1974). *Sexual identity conflict in children and adults.* Duckworth, London.

Green R (1985). Atypical psychosexual development. In M Rutter and L Hersov, eds. *Child and adolescent psychiatry*. 2nd edn. Blackwell Scientific Publications, Oxford.

Green R (1998). Transsexual's children. *International Journal of Transgenderism*, **2**, 1–7.

Green R (2000a). Gender identity disorder in adults. In MG Gelder, JJ López-Ibor Jr and NC Andreasen, eds. *The new Oxford textbook of psychiatry*, Chapter 4.11.4. Oxford University Press, Oxford.

Green R (2000b). Gender identity disorder in children. In MG Gelder, JJ López-Ibor Jr and NC Andreasen, eds. *The new Oxford textbook of psychiatry.*, Chapter 9.2.12. Oxford University Press, Oxford.

Green R and Fleming D (1991). Transsexual surgery follow-up: status in the 1990s. In J Bancroft, C Davis and D Weinstein, eds. *Annual Review of Sex Research*. Society for Scientific Study of Sex, Mt Vernon, IA.

Green RC, Cupples LA, Kurz A, *et al.* (2003). Depression as a risk factor for Alzheimer disease: the MIRAGE Study. *Archives of Neurology*, **60**, 753–9.

Greenberg DM and Lee JW (2001). Psychotic manifestations of alcoholism. *Current Psychiatry Reports*, **3**, 2001–2.

Greicius MD, Geschwind MD and Miller BL (2002). Presenile dementia syndromes: an update on taxonomy and diagnosis. *Journal of Neurology, Neurosurgery and Psychiatry*, **72**, 691–700.

Grice DE, Halmi KA, Fichter MM, *et al.* (2002). Evidence for a susceptibilty gene for anorexia nervosa on chromosome 1. *American Journal of Human Genetics*, **70**, 787–92.

Griesinger W (1867). *Mental pathology and therapeutics.* 2nd edn. Transl C Lockhart Robertson and J Rutherford. New Sydenham Society, London.

Grillon C and Ameli R (2004). Methods of Affective clinical psychophysiology. *Neurobiology of Mental illness*, 127–40.

Grounds A (2000). The psychiatrist in court. In MG Gelder, JJ López-Ibor Jr and NC Andreasen, eds. *The New Oxford Textbook of Psychiatry*, Chapter 11.6. Oxford University Press., Oxford.

Grundy E (1987). Community care for the elderly 1976–84. *British Medical Journal*, **294**, 626–9.

Grunebaum MF, Ellis SP, Li S, *et al.* (2004). Antidepressants and suicide risk in the United States, 1985–1999. *Journal of Clinical Psychiatry*, **65**, 1546–62.

Grunze H, Kasper S, Goodwin G, *et al.* (2003). The World Federation of Societies of Biological Psychiatry (WFSBP) Guidelines for the Biological Treatment of Bipolar Disorders, Part 1: Treatment of Mania. *World Journal of Biological Psychiatry*, **4**, 5–13.

Gudjonsson GH (1992). *The psychology of interrogations, confessions and testimony.* Wiley, Chichester.

Gudjonsson GH, Rabe-Hesketh S and Szmukler G (2004). Management of psychiatric in-patient violence: patient ethnicity and use of medication, restraint and seclusion. *British Journal of Psychiatry*, **184**, 258–62.

Gunnar MR (1998). Quality of early care and buffering of neuroendocrine stress reactions: potential effects on the developing human brain. *Preventative Medicine*, **27**, 208–11.

Gunnell D, Peters T, Kammerling R, *et al.* (1995). Relation between parasuicide, suicide, psychiatric admissions, and socio-economic deprivation. *British Medical Journal*, **311**, 226–30.

Gureje O, Simon GE, Ustun TB, *et al.* (1997a). Somatization in cross-cultural perspective: A World Health Organization study in primary care. *American Journal of Psychiatry*, **154**, 989–95.

Gureje O, Üstün TB and Simon GE (1997b). The syndrome of hypochondriasis: a cross-national study in primary care. *Pyschological Medicine*, **27**, 1001–10.

Gureje O, Von Korff M, Simon GE, *et al.* (1998). Persistent pain and well being: a World Health Organization Study in Primary Care. *Journal of the American Medical Association*, **280**, 147–51.

Gurman AS (2003). *Family therapy: theory practice and research.* Brunner-Routledge.

Gurman AS and Fraenkel P (2002). The history of couple therapy: a millenium review. *Family Process*, **41**, 199–206.

Guthrie E, Kapur N, Mackway-Jones K, *et al.* (2001). Randomised controlled trial of brief psychological intervention after deliberate self poisoning. *British Medical Journal*, **323**, 135–8.

Guthrie E, Moorey J, Margison F, *et al.* (1999). Cost-effectiveness of brief psychodynamic interpersonal therapy in high utilisers of psychiatric services. *Archives of General Psychiatry*, **56**, 519–26.

Gutirriez-Delicado E and Serratosa JM (2004). Genetics of the epilepsies. *Current Opinion in Neurology*, **17**, 147–53.

Guy W (1976). Clinical Global Impressions (CGI). *ECDEU Assessment Manual for Psychopharmacology (revised)*. US Department of Health, Education and Welfare, NIMH, Rockville, MD.

Guze S (1989). Biological psychiatry: is there any other kind? *Psychological Medicine*, **19**, 315–23.

Hachinski V (1999). Stalin's last years: delusions or dementia? *European Journal of Neurology*, **6**, 129–32.

Hachinski V, Lassen NA and Marshall J (1974). Multi-infarct dementia. *Lancet*, **2**, 207–9.

Hack M, Taylor HG, Klein N, *et al.* (1994). School-age outcomes in children with birth weights under 750 g. *New England Journal of Medicine*, **331**, 753–9.

Hackett ML, Anderson CS and House AO (2004). Interventions for treating depression after stroke. *Cochrane Database of Systemic Reviews*, Cd003437.

Hackett TP and Weissman A (1962). The treatment of dying. *Current Psychiatric Therapy*, **2**, 121–6.

Hacking I (1998). *Mad travellers. Reflections on the reality of transient mental illnesses*. Free Association Books, London.

Hackmann A (2004). Panic disorder and agoraphobia. In J Bennett-Levy, G Butler and M Fennel, eds. *Oxford guide to behavioural experiments in cognitive therapy*, Chapter 3. Oxford University Press, Oxford.

Haddock G, Barrowclough C, Tarrier N, *et al.* (2003). Cognitive-behavioural therapy and motivational intervention for schizophrenia and substance misuse. 18-month outcomes of a randomised controlled trial. *British Journal of Psychiatry*, **183**, 418–26.

Häfner H (1987). The concept of disease in psychiatry. *Psychological Medicine*, **17**, 11–4.

Häfner H and an der Heiden W (2003). Course and outcome of schizophrenia. In S Hirsch and D Weinberger, eds. *Schizophrenia*, Chapter 8. 2nd edn. Blackwell, Oxford.

Hale R, Minn C and Zachary A (2000). Assessment and management of sexual offenders. In MG Gelder, JJ López-Ibor Jr and NC Andreasen, eds. *The New Oxford textbook of psychiatry*, Chapter 11.4.2. Oxford University Press, Oxford.

Haley J (1963). *Strategies of psychotherapy*. Grune and Stratton, New York.

Hall JN (2000). Behavioural and observational assessment. In MG Gelder, JJ López-Ibor Jr and NC Andreasen, eds. *The new Oxford textbook of psychiatry*, Chapter 1.10.3.2. Oxford University Press, Oxford.

Hall W and Solowij N (1998). Adverse effects of cannabis. *Lancet*, **352**, 1611–6.

Hallgren B (1960). Nocturnal enuresis in twins. *Acta Psychiatrica Scandinavica*, **35**, 73–90.

Halligan P, Bass C and Marshall J (eds.) (2001). *Contemporary approaches to the study of hysteria. Clinical and theoretical perspectives*. Oxford Medical Publications, Oxford.

Halligan SL, Michael T, Clark DM, *et al.* (2003). Posttraumatic stress disorder following assault: the role of cognitive processing, trauma memory, and appraisals. *Journal of Clinical and Experimental Psychology*, **71**, 419–31.

Halpern JH and Pope HG (2003). Hallucinogen persisting perception disorder: What do we know after 50 years? *Drug and Alcohol Dependence*, **69**, 109–19.

Hamburg DA, Artz P, Reiss E, *et al.* (1953). Clinical importance of emotional problems in the care of patients with burns. *New England Journal of Medicine*, **248**, 355–9.

Hamilton CE, Falshaw L and Browne KD (2002). The Link between recurrent maltreatment and offending behaviour. *International Journal of Offender Therapy and Comparative Criminology*, **46**, 75–94.

Hamilton J, Guthrie E, Creed F, *et al.* (2000). A randomised controlled trial of psychotherapy in patients with chronic functional dyspepsia. *Gastroenterology*, **119**, 661–9.

Hamilton M (1959). The assessment of anxiety states by rating. *British Journal of Medical Psychology*, **32**, 50–5.

Hamilton M (1967). Development of a rating scale for primary depressive illness. *British Journal of Social and Clinical Psychology*, **6**, 278–96.

Hamilton M (ed.) (1984). *Fish's schizophrenia*. 3rd edn. Wright, Bristol.

Hammen C, Brennan PA and Shih JH (2004). Family discord and stress predictors of depression and other disorders in adolescent children of depressed and non-depressed mothers. *Journal of the American Academy of Child and Adolescent Psychiatry*, **43**, 994–1002.

Hardy J, Cookson MR and Singleton A (2003). Genes for parkinsonism. *Lancet Neurology*, **2**, 221–8.

Hardy J and Gwinn-Hardy K (1998). Genetic classification of primary neurodegenerative disease. *Science*, **282**, 1075–9.

Hardy J and Selkoe DJ (2002). The amyloid hypothesis of Alzheimer's disease: progress and problems on the road to therapeutics. *Science*, **297**, 353–6.

Hardy JA and Higgins GA (1992). Alzheimer's disease: The amyloid cascade hypothesis. *Science*, **256**, 184–5.

Hare EH (1959). The origin and spread of dementia paralytica. *Journal of Mental Science*, **105**, 594–626.

Hare EH (1973). A short note on pseudo-hallucinations. *British Journal of Psychiatry*, **122**, 469–73.

Harmer CJ, Shelley NC, Cowen PJ, *et al.* (2004). Increased positive versus negative affective perception and memory in healthy volunteers following selective serotonin and norepinephrine reuptake inhibition. *American Journal of Psychiatry*, **161**, 1256–63.

Harper PS, Gevers S, de Wert G, *et al.* (2004). Genetic testing and Huntington's disease: issues of employment. *Lancet Neurology*, **3**, 249–52.

Harrington R (2001). Developmental continuities and discontinuities. *British Journal of Psychiatry*, **179**, 189–90.

Harrington R (2002). Affective didorders. In M Rutter and E Taylor, eds. *Child and adolescent psychiatry*, Chapter 29. Blackwell, Oxford.

Harrington R, Whittaker J, Shoebridge P, *et al.* (1998b). Systematic review of the efficacy of cognitive-behaviour therapies in childhood and adolescent depressive disorder. *British Medical Journal,* **316**, 1559–63.

Harrington RC, Fudge H, Rutter M, *et al.* (1990). Adult outcomes of childhood and adolescent depression in psychiatric status. *Archives of General Psychiatry,* **47**, 465–73.

Harrington RC, Whittaker J and Shoebridge P (1998a). Psychological treatment of depression in children and adolescents: a review of treatment research. *British Journal of Psychiatry,* **173**, 291–8.

Harris EC and Barraclough B (1997). Suicide as an outcome for mental disorders: a meta-analysis. *British Journal of Psychiatry,* **170**, 205–28.

Harris EC and Barraclough B (1998). Excess mortality of mental disorder. *British Journal of Psychiatry,* **173**, 11–53.

Harris EC and Barraclough BM (1995). Suicide as an outcome for medical disorders. *Medicine,* **73**, 281–96.

Harris JC (1996). Childhood disintegrative disorder. *Developmental Neuropsychiatry,* **2**, 239–43.

Harris L, Hawton K and Zahl D (2005). Value of measuring suicidal intent in the assessment of people attending hospital following self-poisoning or self-injury. *British Journal of Psychiatry,* **186**, 60–6.

Harris T (2001). Recent developments in understanding the psycological aspects of depression. *British Medical Bulletin,* **57**, 17–32.

Harrison G, Hopper K, Craig T, *et al.* (2001). Recovery from psychotic illness: a 15- and 25-year international follow-up study. *British Journal of Psychiatry,* **178**, 506–17.

Harrison G, Mason P, Glazebrook C, *et al.* (1994). Residence of incident cohort of psychotic patients after 13 years of follow-up. *British Medical Journal,* **308**, 813–9.

Harrison G, Owens D, Holton A, *et al.* (1988). A prospective study of severe mental disorder in Afro-Caribbean patients. *Psychological Medicine,* **18**, 643–57.

Harrison PJ (1997). BSE and human prion disease. *British Journal of Psychiatry,* **170**, 298–300.

Harrison PJ (1999). The neuropathology of schizophrenia. A critical review of the data and their interpretation. *Brain,* **122**, 593–624.

Harrison PJ (2000). Dopamine and schizophrenia – proof at last? *Lancet,* **356**, 958–9.

Harrison PJ (2004). The hippocampus in schizophrenia: a review of the neuropathological evidence and its pathophysiological implications. *Psychopharmacology,* **174**, 151–62.

Harrison PJ and Weinberger DR (2005). Schizophrenia genes, gene expression, and neuropathology: on the matter of their convergence. *Molecular Psychiatry,* **10**, 40–68.

Harriss L, Hawton K and Zahl D (2005). Value of measuring suicidal intent in the assessment of people attending hospital following self-poisoning or self-injury. *British Journal of Psychiatry,* **186**, 60–6.

Harry Benjamin International Gender Dysphoria Association (2001). The standards of care for gender identity disorders-sixth version. *International Journal of Transgenderism,* **5**, 1–20.

Hart S, Binggeli N and Brassard M (1998). Evidence for the effects of psychological maltreatment. *Journal of Emotional Abuse,* **1**, 27–58.

Harvey AG and Bryant RA (1998). The relationship between acute stress disorder and post-traumatic stress disorder: a prospective evaluation of motor vehicle accident survivors. *Journal of Consulting and Clinical Psychology,* **66**, 507–12.

Harvey PD (2001). Cognitive and functional impairments in elderly patients with schizophrenia: a review of the recent literature. *Harv Rev Psychiatry,* **9**, 59–68.

Harvey PD and Keefe RS (2001). Studies of cognitive change in patients with schizophrenia following novel antipsychotic treatment. *American Journal of Psychiatry,* **158**, 176–84.

Harwood D, Hawton K, Hope T, *et al.* (2000a). Suicide in older people: mode of death, demographic factors, and medical contact before death. *International Journal of Geriatric Psychiatry,* **15**, 736–43.

Harwood D, Hawton K, Hope T, *et al.* (2000b). Psychiatric disorder and personality factors associated with suicide in older people: a descriptive and case-control study. *International Journal of Geriatric Psychiatry,* **16**, 155–65.

Harwood D and Jacoby R (2000). Suicidal behaviour among the elderly. In K Hawton and K van Heeringen, eds. *The International Handbook of Suicide and Attempted Suicide.* John Wiley and Sons, Chichester.

Haug TT, Blomhoff S, Hellstrom K, *et al.* (2003). Exposure therapy and sertraline in social phobia: 1-year follow-up of a randomized controlled trial. *British Journal of Psychiatry,* **182**, 312–8.

Haw C, Hawton K, Houston K, *et al.* (2001). Psychiatric and personality disorders in deliberate self-harm patients. *British Journal of Psychiatry,* **178**, 48–54.

Hawton K (2000a). Treatment of suicide attempters and prevention of suicide and attempted suicide. In MG Gelder, JJ López-IborJr and NC Andreasen, eds. *The new Oxford textbook of psychiatry*, Chapter 4.15.4. Oxford University Press, Oxford.

Hawton K (2000b). General hospital management of suicide attempters. In K Hawton and K van Heeringen, eds. *The International Handbook of Suicide and Attempted Suicide.* John Wiley and Sons, Chichester.

Hawton K, Arensman E, Townsend E, *et al.* (1998). Deliberate self harm: systematic review of efficacy of psychosocial and pharmacological treatments in preventing repetition. *British Medical Journal,* **317**, 441–7.

Hawton K, Clements A, Sakarovitch C, *et al.* (2001a). Suicide in doctors: a study of risk according to gender, seniority and specialty in medical practitioners in England and Wales, 1979–1995. *Journal of Epidemiology and Community Health,* **55**, 296–300.

Hawton K, Clements A, Simkin S, *et al.* (2000). Doctors who kill themselves: a study of the methods used for suicide. *Quarterly Journal of Medicine,* **93**, 351–7.

Hawton K, Hall S, Simpkin S, *et al.* (2003c). Deliberate self-harm in adolescents: a study of characteristics and trends in Oxford, 1990–2000. *Journal of Child Psychology and Psychiatry,* **44**, 1191–8.

Hawton K, Harriss L, Hall S, *et al.* (2003b). Deliberate self-harm in Oxford, 1990–2000: a time of change in patient characteristics. *Psychological Medicine,* **33**, 987–95.

Hawton K, Harriss L, Hodder K, *et al.* (2001b). The influence of economic and social environment on deliberate self-harm and suicide: an ecological and person-based study. *Psychological Medicine,* **31**, 827–36.

Hawton K, Harriss L, Simkin S, *et al.* (2004c). Self-cutting: patient characteristics ompared with self-poisoners. *Suicide and Life Threatening Behaviour,* **34**, 199–207.

Hawton K, Houston K and Shepherd R (1999a). Suicide in young people: study of 174 cases, aged under 25 years, based on coroner's and medical records. *British Journal of Psychiatry,* **175**, 271–4.

Hawton K, Malmberg A and Simkin S (2004a). Suicide in doctors: a psychological autopsy study. *Journal of Psychosomatic Research,* **57**, 1–4.

Hawton K, Rodham K, Evans E, *et al.* (2002). Deliberate self-harm among adolescents; self-report survey in schools in England. *British Medical Journal,* **325**, 1207–11.

Hawton K, Simkin S, Deeks J, *et al.* (2004b). UK legislation on analgesic packs: before and after study of long term effects on poisonings. *British Medical Journal,* **329**, 1076–9.

Hawton K, Sutton L, Haw C, *et al.* (2005). Schizophrenia and suicide: a systematic review of risk factors. *British Journal of Psychiatry*, in press.

Hawton K and van Heeringen K (eds.) (2000). *The International Handbook of Suicide and Attempted Suicide.* John Wiley and Sons, Chichester.

Hawton K, Zahl D and Weatherall R (2003a). Suicide following deliberate self-harm; long-term follow-up of patients who presented to a general hospital. *British Journal of Psychiatry,* **182**, 537–42.

Hawton KE (1985). *Sex therapy: a practical guide.* Oxford University Press, Oxford.

Hawton KE (1995). Treatment of sexual dysfunctions by sex therapy and other approaches. *British Journal of Psychiatry,* **167**, 307–14.

Hawton KE, Catalan J, Martin P, *et al.* (1986). Long term outcome of sex therapy. *Behaviour Research and Therapy,* **24**, 377–85.

Hawton KE and Oppenheimer C (1983). Women's sexual problems. In A Anderson and A McPherson, eds. *Women's problems in general practice.* Oxford University Press, Oxford.

Hawton KE, Simkin S, Deeks JJ, *et al.* (1999b). Effects of a drug overdose in a television drama on presentations to hospital for self poisoning: time series and questionnaire study. *British Medical Journal,* **318**, 972–7.

Hay P, Bacaltchuk J, Claudino A, *et al.* (2003). *Individual psycotherapy in the out-patient treatment of adults with anorexia nervosa.* 4: CD003909, Cochrane Database of Systematic Reviews.

Hay PJ, Sachdev PS, Cummings S, *et al.* (1993). Treatment of obsessive-compulsive disorder by psychosurgery. *Acta Psychiatrica Scandinavica,* **87**, 197–207.

Haynes B (1999). Can it work? Does it work? Is it worth it? *British Medical Journal,* **319**, 652–3.

Head S, Baker J and Williamson D (1991). Family environment characteristics and dependent personality disorder. *Journal of Personality Disorders,* **5**, 256–63.

Heath AC, Madden PA and Bucholz KK (1999). Genetic differences in alcohol sensitivity and the inheritance of alcoholism risk. *Psychological Medicine,* **29**, 1069–81.

Hecker E (1871). Die Hebephrenie. *Virchows Archiv für Pathologie and Anatomie,* **52**, 394–429. (Virchows Archiv für Pathologie and Anatomie)

Hegarty JD, Baldessarini RJ, Tohen M, *et al.* (1994). One hundred years of schizophrenia: a meta-analysis of the outcome literature. *American Journal of Psychiatry,* **151**, 1409–16.

Heidenssohn F (1991). Women as perpetrators and victims of crime: a sociological perspective. *British Journal of Psychiatry,* **158**, 50–4.

Heim C and Nemeroff CB (2000). The impact of early adverse experiences on brain systems involved in the pathophysiology of anxiety and affective disorders. *Biological Psychiatry,* **46**, 1509–22.

Heiman JR (2002a). Sexual dysfunction: overview of prevalence, etiological factors, and treatments. *Journal of Sex Research,* **39**, 73–8.

Heiman JR (2002b). Psychological treatments for female sexual dysfunction: Are they effective and do we need them? *Archives of Sexual Behavior,* **31**, 445–50.

Heimberg RG, Liebowitz MR, Hope DA, *et al.* (1998). Cognitive-behavioral group therapy versus phenelzine in social phobia: 12 week outcome. *Archives of General Psychiatry,* **55**, 1133–41.

Heinman JR and LoPiccolo J (1983). Clinical outcome of sex therapy. *Archives of General Psychiatry,* **40**, 443–9.

Heinrichs DW and Buchanan RW (1988). Significance and meaning of neurological signs in schizophrenia. *American Journal of Psychiatry,* **145**, 11–18.

Heiser P, Friedel S, Dempfle A, *et al.* (2004). Molecular genetic aspects of attention-deficit hyperactivity disorder. *Neuroscience and Biobehavioural Reviews,* **28**, 625–41.

Helgeland MI and Torgersen S (2004). Developmental antecedents of borderline personality disorder. *Comprehensive Psychiatry,* **45**, 138–47.

Helzer JE and Canino GJ (1992). Comparative analysis of alcoholism in ten cultural regions. In JE Helzer and GJ Canino, eds. *Alcoholism in North America, Europe and Asia,* 289–308. Oxford University Press, Oxford.

Henderson AS (1990). The social psychiatry of later life. *British Journal of Psychiatry,* **156**, 645–53.

Henderson DK (1939). *Psychopathic states.* Chapman & Hall, London.

Henderson DK and Gillespie RD (1930). *Textbook of psychiatry for students and practitioners.* 2nd edn. Oxford University Press, London.

Hendin H and Haas P (1991). Suicide and guilt as manifestations of PTSD in Vietnam combat veterans. *American Journal of Psychiatry,* **148**, 586–91.

Henggeler SW, Rowland MD, Randall J, *et al.* (1999). Home based therapy as an alternative to hospitalization of youths in psychiatric crisis: clinical outcomes. *Journal of the American Academy of Child and Adolescent Psychiatry,* **38**, 1331–9.

Hennen J and Baldessarini RJ (2005). Suicidal risk during treatment with clozapine: a meta-analysis. *Schizophrenia Bulletin,* **73**, 139–45.

Hennessy S, Bilker WB, Knauss JS, *et al.* (2002). Cardiac arrest and ventricular arrhythmia in patients taking antipsychotic drugs: cohort study using administrative data. *British Medical Journal,* **325**, 1070.

Henquet C, Krabbendam L, Spauwen J, *et al.* (2005). Prospective cohort study of cannabis use, predisposition for psychosis, and psychotic symptoms in young people. *British Medical Journal,* **330**, 11–14.

Herbert M (2002). Behavioural therapies. In M Rutter and E Taylor, eds. *Child and adolescent psychiatry*, Chapter 53. 4th edn. Blackwell, Oxford.

Herbert TB and Cohen S (1993). Depression and immunity: a meta-analytic review. *Psychological Bulletin,* **113**, 472–86.

Hermans ML, van Hout HP, Terluin B, *et al.* (2004). The prognosis of minor depression in the general population: a systematic review. *General-hospital-psychiatry,* **26**, 453–62.

Hermelin B and O'Connor N (1983). The idiot savant: flawed genius or clever Hans? *Psychological Medicine,* **13**, 479–81.

Hermens ML, van Hout HP, Terluin B, *et al.* (2004). The prognosis of minor depression in the general population: a systematic review. *Gen Hosp Psychiatry*, **26**, 453–62.

Herrman H, McGorry P, Bennett P, *et al.* (1989). Prevalence of severe mental disorders in disaffiliated and homeless people in inner Melbourne. *American Journal of Psychiatry,* **146**, 1179–84.

Herrmann N, Mamdani M and Lanctot KL (2004). Atypical antipsychotics and risk of cerebrovascular accidents. *Am J Psychiatry*, **161**, 1113–5.

Hersch SM (2003). Huntington's disease: prospects for neuroprotective therapy 10 years after the discovery of the causative genetic mutation. *Current Opinion in Neurology,* **16**, 501–6.

Hershel J, James A, Kaye S, *et al.* (2004). Antidepressants and the Risk of Suicidal Behaviors. *Journal of the American Medical Association,* **292**, 338–43.

Hersov L (1960). Refusal to go to school. *Journal of Child Psychology and Psychiatry,* **1**, 137–45.

Hertlein KM and Ricci RJ (2004). A Systematic Research Synthesis of EMDR Studies: Implementation of the Platinum Standard. *Trauma Violence Abuse,* **5**, 285–300.

Heston LL (1966). Psychiatric disorders in foster home reared children of schizophrenic mothers. *British Journal of Psychiatry,* **112**, 819–25.

Hetherington EM and Stanley Hagan M (1999). The adjustment of children with divorced parents; a risk and resiliency perspective. *Journal of Child Psychology and Psychiatry,* **40**, 129–40.

Hettema JM, Annas P, Neale MC, *et al.* (2003). A twin study of the genetics of fear conditioning. *Archives of General Psychiatry,* **60**, 702–8.

Hettema JM, Neale MC and Kendler KS (2001). A review and meta-analysis of the genetic epidemiology of anxiety disorders. *American Journal of Psychiatry,* **158**, 1568–78.

Hettema JM, Prescott CA and Kendler KS (2004). Genetic and environmental sources of covariation between generalized anxiety disorder and neuroticism. *American Journal of Psychiatry,* **161**, 1581–7.

Heun R, Papassotiropoulos A, Jessen F, *et al.* (2001). A family study of Alzheimer disease and early- and late-onset depression in elderly patients. *Archives of General Psychiatry,* **58**, 190–6.

Hewett D and Nind M (eds.) (1998). *Interaction in action: reflections on the use of intensive interaction.* David Fulton, London.

Heyman I, Fombonne E, Simmons H, *et al.* (2001). Prevalence of obsessive-compulsive disorder in the British nationwide survey of child mental health. *British Journal of Psychiatry,* **179**, 324–9.

Hibell B, Andersson B, Bjarnasson T, *et al.* (2004). *ESPAD report: alcohol and other drug use among students in 35 European countries.* National Research and Development Centre for Welfare and Health (STAKES).

Hickling EJ and Blanchard EB (1999). Current understanding, treatment and law. *The international handbook of road traffic accidents and psychological trauma.* Pergamon, Oxford.

Hickling FW and Rodgers-Johnson P (1995). The incidence of first contact schizophrenia in Jamaica. *British Journal of Psychiatry,* **167**, 193–6.

Higgins ST, Sigmon SC and Wong CJ (2003). Community reinforcement therapy for cocaine-dependent out-patients. *Archives of General Psychiatry,* **60**, 1043–52.

Higgitt A and Fonagy P (1993). Psychotherapy in borderline and narcissistic personality disorder. In P Tyrer and G Stein, eds. *Personality disorder review*, 225–61. Gaskell, London.

Hildyard KL and Wolfe DA (2002). Child neglect: developmental issues and outcomes. *Child Abuse and Neglect,* **26**, 679–95.

Hill J (2003). Early identification of individuals at risk for antisocial personality. *British Journal of Psychiatry,* **44**, S11–4.

Hill J, Pickles A, Burnside E, *et al.* (2001). Child sexual abuse, poor parental care and adult depression: evidence for different mechanisms. *British Journal of Psychiatry,* **179**, 104–9.

Hill K, Mann L, Laws KR, *et al.* (2004). Hypofrontality in schizophrenia: a meta-analysis of functional imaging studies. *Acta Psychiatrica Scandinavica,* **110**, 243–56.

Hiller W, Leibbrand R, Rief W, *et al.* (2002). Predictors of course and outcome in hypochondriasis after cognitive-behavioural treatment. *Psychotherapy and Psychosomatics,* **71**, 318–25.

Hiller W, Zaudig M and Bose MV (1989). The overlap between depression and anxiety on different levels of psychopathology. *Journal of Affective Disorders,* **16**, 223–31.

Hindley P and Kitson N (1999). *Mental health and deafness.* Whurr, London.

Hirsch S and Leff J (1975). *Abnormalities in parents of schizophrenics.* Oxford University Press, London.

Hirsch SR and Weinberger DR (eds.) (2003). *Schizophrenia.* 2nd edn. Blackwell Science, Oxford.

Hirschfeld M (1944). *Sexual anomalies and perversions: physical and psychological development and treatment.* Aldor, London.

Hirschfeld RMA, Allen MH and McEvoy JP (1999). Safety and tolerability of oral loading divalproex sodium in acutely manic bipolar patients. *Journal of Clinical Psychiatry*, 815–8.

Hitchcock N and Pugh P (2002). Management of overweight and obese adults. *British Medical Journal,* **325**, 757–61.

Hjelmeland H, Hawton K, Nordvik H, *et al.* (2002). Why people engage in parasuicide: a cross-cultural study of intentions. *Suicide and Life Threatening Behaviour,* **32**, 380–93.

Ho AK, Sahakian BJ, Brown RG, *et al.* (2003). Profile of cognitive progression in early Huntington's disease. *Neurology,* **61**, 1702–6.

Hobbs M (2005). Brief dynamic psychotherapy. In S Bloch, ed. *An Introduction to the psychotherapies.* 4th edn. Oxford University Press,

Hobson R (1985). *Forms of feeling:the heart of psychotherapy.* Tavistock Publications, London.

Hodges JR (1994). *Cognitive assessment for clinicians.* Oxford University Press, Oxford.

Hodgins S, Kratzer L and McNeil TF (2001). Obstetric complications, parenting, and the risk of criminal behaviour. *Archives of General Psychiatry,* **58**, 746–52.

Hoek HW and van-Hoeken D (2003). Review of the prevalence and incidence of eating disorders. *International Journal of Eating Disorders,* **34**, 383–96.

Hoekstra PJ, Kallenberg CG, Korf J, *et al.* (2002). Is Tourette's syndrome an autoimmune disease? *Molecular Psychiatry,* **7**, 437–45.

Hof PR and Morrison JH (2004). The aging brain: morphomolecular senescence of cortical circuits. *Trends in Neurosciences,* **27**, 607–13.

Hogan DM (1998). Annotation: the psychological development and welfare of children of opiate and cocaine users: review and research needs. *Journal of Child Psychology and Psychiatry,* **39**, 609–20.

Hogarty GE, Flesher S, Ulrich R, *et al.* (2004). Cognitive enhancement therapy for schizophrenia: effects of a 2-year randomized trial on cognition and behavior. *Archives of General Psychiatry,* **61**, 866–76.

Holland AJ (1994). Down's syndrome and Alzheimer's disease. In N Bouras, ed. *Mental health in mental retardation: recent advances and practices,* 154–67. Cambridge University Press, Cambridge.

Holland AJ (1997). Forensic psychiatry and learning disability. In O Russell, ed. *The psychiatry of learning disabilities.* Gaskell, London.

Holland AJ, J. H, Huppert FA, *et al.* (1998). Population-based study of the prevalence and presentation of dementia in individuals with mental retardation. *Journal of Intellectual Disability Research,* **41**, 152–64.

Holland AJ and Oliver C (1995). Down's syndrome and the links with Alzheimer's disease. *Journal of Neurology, Neurosurgery and Psychiatry,* **59**, 111–14.

Holland JC (1998). *Psycho-oncology.* Oxford University Press, Oxford.

Holland T, Clare IC and Mukhopadhyay T (2002). Prevalence of criminal offending by men and women with intellectual disibility and the characteristics of offenders: implications for research and service development. *Journal of Intellectual Disability Research,* **46**, 6–20.

Hollander E, Neville D, Frenkel M, *et al.* (1992). Body dysmorphic disorder. Diagnostic issues and related disorders. *Psychosomatics,* **33**, 156–65.

Hollander E, Tracy KA, Swann AC, *et al.* (2003). Divalproex in the treatment of impulsive aggression: efficacy in Cluster B personality disorders. *Neuropsychopharmacology,* **28**, 1186–97.

Hollingshead AB and Redlich FC (1958). *Social class and mental illness: a community study.* Wiley, New York.

Hollins S and Esterhayzen A (1997). Bereavement and grief in adults with learning disabilities: interventions to support clients and carers. *Journal of Intellectual Disability Research,* **41**, 331–8.

Hollis C (2002). Schizophrenia and allied disorders. In M Rutter and E Taylor, eds. *Child and adolescent psychiatry,* Chapter 37. 4th edn. Blackwell, Oxford.

Hollon SD, DeRubeis RJ, Shelton RC, *et al.* (2005). Prevention of relapse following cognitive therapy vs medications in moderate to severe depression. *Arch Gen Psychiatry,* **62**, 417–22.

Holmes J (2000). Object relations, attachment theory, self-psychology, and interpersonal psychoanalysis. In MG Gelder, JJ López-Ibor Jr and NC Andreasen, eds. *The new Oxford textbook of psychiatry,* Chapter 3.3.2. Oxford University Press, Oxford.

Holmes P and Karp M (1991). *Psychodrama, inspiration and technique.* Tavistock Publications and Routledge, London.

Holmes T and Rahe RH (1967). The social adjustment rating scale. *Journal of Psychosomatic Research,* **11**, 213–8.

Holroyd KA, O'Donnell FJ, Stensland M, *et al.* (2001). Management of chronic tension-type headache with tricyclic antidepressant medication, stress management therapy and their combination: a randomized controlled trial. *Journal of the American Medical Association,* **285**, 2208–15.

Holroyd S (2000). Personality disorders in the elderly. In MG Gelder, JJ López-Ibor Jr and NC Andreasen, eds. *The new Oxford textbook of psychiatry,* Chapter 8.5.6. Oxford University Press, Oxford.

Holsboer F and Kunzel HE (2004). Neurobiology of mental illness. *Clinical Endocrinology,* 155–70.

Holzman PS (2000). Eye movements and the search for the essence of schizophrenia. *Brain Research Reviews,* **31**, 350–6.

Home Office (1999). *Managing dangerous people with severe personality disorder.* HMSO, London.

Home Office Research (2001). *Drug misuse declared in 2000: results from the British Crime Survey.* Study 224, Home Office Research, Development and Statistics Directorate.

Hope T, Hicks N, Reynolds DJM, *et al.* (1998). Rationing and the Health Authority. *British Medical Journal,* **317**, 1067–9.

Hope T, Keene J, Fairburn CG, *et al.* (1999). Natural history of behavioural changes and psychiatric symptoms in Alzheimer's disease. A longitudinal study. *British Journal of Psychiatry,* **174**, 39–44.

Hope T, Savelescu J and Hendrick J (2003). *Medical ethics and the law.* Churchill-Livingstone, Edinburgh.

Hopkins B, Ronalg RG, Michel GF, *et al.* (2004). *The Cambridge Enclyclopaedia of Child Development.* Cambridge University Press, Cambridge.

Horney K (1939). *New ways in psychoanalysis.* Kegan Paul, London.

Horowitz MJ (1986). *Stress Response Systems.* Jason Aronson,N.J.

Hotopf M (2004). Preventing somatization. *Psychological Medicine,* **34**, 195–8.

Hotopf MH, Noah N and Wessely S (1996). Chronic fatigue and psychiatric morbidity following viral meningitis: a controlled study. *Journal of Neurology, Neurosurgery and Psychiatry,* **60**, 504–9.

Hoult J, Reynolds I, Charbonneau-Powis M, *et al.* (1983). Psychiatric hospital versus community treatment: the results of a randomised trial. *Australia and New Zealand Journal of Psychiatry,* **17**, 160–7.

House RM (2000). Transplantation surgery. In A Stoudemier, BS Fogel and DB Greenberg, eds. *Psychiatric care of the medical patient.* Oxford University Press, New York, NY.

Houston F and Royse AB (1954). Relationship between deafness and psychotic illness. *Journal of Mental Science,* **100**, 900–3.

Houston K, Hawton K and Shepperd R (2001). Suicide in young people aged 15–24: a psychological autopsy study. *Journal of Affective Disorders,* **63**, 159–70.

Howard R, Mellers J, Petty R, *et al.* (1995). Magnetic resonance imaging volumetric measurements of the superior temporal gyrus, hippocampus, parahippocampal gyrus, frontal and temporal lobes in late paraphrenia. *Psychological Medicine,* **25**, 495–503.

Howard R, Rabins PV, Seeman MV, *et al.* (2000). Late-onset schizophrenia and very-late-onset schizophrenia-like psychosis: an international consensus. The International Late-Onset Schizophrenia Group. *American Journal of Psychiatry,* **157**, 172–8.

Howard RS and Lees AJ (1987). Encephalitis lethargica. A report of four recent cases. *Brain,* **110**, 19–33.

Howlett AC, Breivogel CS, Childers SR, *et al.* (2004). Cannibinoid physiology and pharmacology: 30 years of progress. *Neuropharmacology,* **47**, 345–58.

Howlin P (1994). Special educational treatment. In M Rutter, E Taylor and L Hersov, eds. *Child and adolescent psychiatry: modern approaches*, 1071–88. 3rd edn. Blackwell Scientific Publications, Oxford.

Howlin P (1998). Practitioner review: psychological and educational treatments for autism. *Journal of Child Psychology and Psychiatry,* **39**, 307–22.

Howlin P (2002). Special educational treatment. In M Rutter and E Taylor, eds. *Child and adolescent psychiatry*, Chapter 68. 4th edn. Blackwell, Oxford.

Howlin P, Goode S, Hutton J, *et al.* (2004). Adult outcomes for children with autism. *Journal of Child Psychology and Psychiatry,* **45**, 212–29.

Hsiao MC, Liu CY, Yang YY, *et al.* (1999). Delusional disorder: retrospective analysis of 86 Chinese outpatients. *Psychiatry and Clinical Neurosciences,* **53**, 575–8.

Hucker SJ (1990). Sexual asphyxia. In P Boeden and R Bluglass, eds. *Principles and practice of forensic psychiatry.* Churchill Livingstone, Edinburgh.

Humphreys M and Johnstone EC (1992). Dangerous behaviour preceding first admissions for schizophrenia. *British Journal of Psychiatry,* **161**, 501–5.

Hunter EC, Sierra M and David AS (2004). The epidemiology of depersonalization and derealization. *Social Psychiatry and Psychiatric Epidemiology,* **39**, 9–18.

Hunter R and MacAlpine I (eds.) (1963). *Three hundred years of psychiatry.* Oxford University Press, London.

Huntington G (2003). On chorea. George Huntington, M.D. *Journal of Neuropsychiatry and Clinical Neurosciences,* **15**, 109–12.

Hyde TM, Ziegler JC and Weinberger DR (1992). Psychiatric disturbances in metachromatic leukodystrophy. Insights into the neurobiology of psychosis. *Archives of Neurology,* **49**, 401–6.

Iancu I, Dannon PN and Zohar J (2000). Obsessive-compulsive disorder. In MG Gelder and JJ López-Ibor Jr, eds. *The new Oxford textbook of psychiatry*, Chapter 4.8. Oxford University Press, Oxford.

Imboden JB, Canter A and Cluff LE (1961). Convalescence from influenza: a study of the psychological and clinical determinants. *Archives of Internal Medicine,* **108**, 393–9.

Ingvar DH and Franzen G (1974). Anomalies of cerebral blood flow distribution in patients with chronic schizophrenia. *Acta Psychiatrica Scandinavica,* **50**, 425–62.

International Molecular Genetic Study of Autism Consortium (1998). A full genome scan for autism with evidence for linkage to a region on chromosome 7q. *Human Molecular Genetics,* **7**, 571–8.

International Multicenter Trial Group on Moclobemide in Social Phobia (1997). Moclobemide in social phobia: a double-blind, placebo-controlled clinical study. *European Archives of Psychiatry and Clinical Neuroscience,* **247**, 71–80.

Ives R (2000). *Disorders relating to the use of volatile substances.* Oxford University Press, Oxford.

Isacsson G, Holmgren P, Wasserman D, *et al.* (1994). Use of antidepressants among peoplecommitting suicide in Sweden. *British Medical Journal,* **8**, 506–9.

Jablensky A (2003). The epidemiological horizon. In SR Hirsch and D Weinberger, eds. *Schizophrenia*, 203–31. 2nd edn. Blackwell Publishing, Oxford.

Jablensky A, Sartorius N, Ernberg G, *et al.* (1992). Schizophrenia: manifestations, incidence and course in different cultures: a World Health Organization 10-Country study. *Psychological Medicine. Monograph Supplement,* **20**, 1–97.

Jackson M and Cawley R (1992). Psychodynamics and psychotherapy on an acute psychiatric ward. The story of an experimental unit. *British Journal of Psychiatry,* **160**, 41–50.

Jacob A, Prasad S, Boggild M, *et al.* (2004). Charles Bonnet syndrome – elderly people and visual hallucinations. *British Medical Journal,* **328**, 1552–4.

Jacobs BW (2002). Individual and group therapy. In M Rutter and E Taylor, eds. *Child and adolescent psychiatry*, Chapter 58. 4th edn. Blackwell, Oxford.

Jacobs BW and Pearse J (2002). Family Therapy. In M Rutter and E Taylor, eds. *Child and adolescent psychiatry*, Chapter 57. 4th edn. Blackwell, Oxford.

Jacobs M (1988). *Psychodynamic counselling in action.* Sage, London.

Jacobs S (1993). *Pathological grief – maladaption to loss.* American Psychiatric Press, Washington D.C.

Jacobs SC, Hansen F and Berkman L (1989). Depressions of ereavement. *Comprehensive Psychiatry,* **30**, 218–24.

Jacobson AM (1996). The psychological care of patients with insulin-dependent diabetes mellitus. *New England Journal of Medicine,* **334**, 1249–53.

Jacobson E (1938). *Progressive relaxation.* Chicago University Press, Chicago.

Jacobson RR (1995). The post-concussional syndrome: physiogenesis, psychogenesis and malingering: an integrative model. *Journal of Psychosomatic Research*, **39**, 675–93.

Jacoby R (2000a). Suicide and deliberate self-harm in elderly people. In MG Gelder, JJ López-Ibor Jr and NC Andreasen, eds. *The new Oxford textbook of psychiatry*, Chapter 8.5.7. Oxford University press, Oxford.

Jacoby R (2000b). Assessment of mental disorder in older patients and of the treatment needs of patients and their carers. In MG Gelder, JJ López-Ibor Jr and NC Andreasen, eds. *The new Oxford textbook of psychiatry*, Chapter 8.4. Oxford University Press, Oxford.

Jagust W (2001). Untangling vascular dementia. *Lancet*, **358**, 2097–8.

Janca A, Üstür TB and Sartorius N (1994). New versions of World Health Organization instruments for the assessment of mental disorders. *Acta Psychiatrica Scandinavica*, **90**, 73–83.

Janet P (1925). *Psychological healing*. Allen and Unwin, London.

Janoff-Bulman R (1985). The aftermath of victimization: rebuilding shattered assumptions. In CR Figley, ed. *Trauma and its wake: the study and treatment of posttraumatic stress disorder*, 15–25. Brunner-Mazel, New York.

Janoff-Bulman R and Frieze IH (1983). A theoretical perspective for understanding reactions to victimization. *Journal of Social Issues*, **39**, 1–17.

Janssen HJEM, Cuisinier MCJ, Hoogduin KAL, *et al.* (1996). Controlled prospective study on the mental health of women following pregnancy loss. *American Journal of Psychiatry*, **153**, 226–30.

Jarquin Valdivia AA (2004). Psychiatric symptoms and brain tumors: a brief historical overview. *Arch Neurol*, **61**, 1800–4.

Jason LA, Richman JA, Rademaker AW, *et al.* (1999). A community-based study of chronic fatigue syndrome. *Archives of Internal Medicine*, **159**, 2129–37.

Jaspers K (1913). *Allgemeine Psychopathologie*. Springer, Berlin.

Jaspers K (1963). *General psychopathology*. 7th, 1959 edn. Transl J Hoenig and MW Hamilton. Manchester University Press, Manchester.

Jaspers K (1968). The phenomenological approach in psychopathology. *British Journal of Psychiatry*, **114**, 1313–23.

Jaycox LH, Zoellner L and Foa EB (2002). Cognitive behaviour therapy for PSTD in rape survivors. *Journal of Clinical Psychology*, **58**, 891–906.

Jeffrey DP, Ley A, McLaren S, *et al.* (2000). *Psychosocial treatment programmes for people with both severe mental illness and substance misuse.*

Jellinger KA (2003). Rett Syndrome – an update. *J Neural Transm*, **110**, 681–701.

Jenike MA (2004). Obsessive-compulsive disorder. *New England Journal of Medicine*, **350**, 259–65.

Jenike MA, Hyman S, Baer L, *et al.* (1990). A controlled trial of fluvoxamine in obsessive-compulsive disorder: implications for a serotonergic theory. *American Journal of Psychiatry*, **147**, 1209–15.

Jenkins JM and Smith MA (1990). Factors protecting children living in disharmonious homes: maternal reports. *Journal of the American Academy of Child and Adolescent Psychiatry*, **29**, 60–9.

Jenkins R, Bebbington P, Brugha TS, *et al.* (1998). British psychiatric morbidity survey. *British Journal of Psychiatry*, **173**, 4–7.

Jenkins R, Lewis G, Bebbington P, *et al.* (1997). The National Psychiatric Morbidity Surveys of Great Britain – initial findings from the Household Survey. *Psychological Medicine*, **27**, 775–89.

Jennings C, Barraclough BM and Moss JR (1978). Have the Samaritans lowered the suicide rate? A controlled study. *Psychological Medicine*, **8**, 413–22.

Jerremalm A, Jansson L and Öst LG (1986). Cognitive and physiological reactivity and the effects of different behavioural methods in the treatment of social phobia. *Behaviour Research and Therapy*, **24**, 171–80.

Jeste DV (2004). Tardive dyskinesia rates with atypical antipsychotics in older adults. *Journal of Clinical Psychiatry*, **65**, 21–4.

Jeste DV, Caligiuri MP, Paulsen JS, *et al.* (1995). Risk of tardive dyskinesia in older patients. A prospective longitudinal study of 266 outpatients. *Archives of General Psychiatry*, **52**, 756–65.

Jilek WG (2000). Traditional non-Western folk healing as relevant to psychiatry. In MG Gelder, JJ López-Ibor Jr and NC Andreasen, eds. *The new Oxford textbook of psychiatry*, Chapter 6.5. Oxford University Press, Oxford.

Johns A (2000). Forensic aspects of alcohol and drug disorders. In MG Gelder, JJ López-Ibor Jr and NC Andreasen, eds. *The New Oxford textbook of psychiatry*, Chapter 11.4.4. Oxford University Press, Oxford.

Johnson J, Cohen P, Brown J, *et al.* (1999). Childhood maltreatment increases risk for personality disorders during early adulthood. *Archives of General Psychiatry*, **56**, 600–6.

Johnson RT (2005). Prion diseases. *Lancet Neurol*, **4**, 635–42.

Johnson W, McGue M, Gaist D, *et al.* (2002). Frequency and heritability of depression symptomatology in the second half of life: evidence from Danish twins over 45. *Psychological Medicine*, **32**, 1175–85.

Johnston D and Reifler BV (2000). The organization and provision of services for the elderly. In MG Gelder, JJ López-Ibor Jr and NC Andreasen, eds. *The new Oxford textbook of psychiatry*, Chapter 8.7. Oxford University Press, Oxford.

Johnstone EC (1991). Disabilities and circumstances of schizophrenic patients: a follow-up study. *British Journal of Psychiatry*, **159 (suppl 13)**, 5–46.

Johnstone EC, Crow TJ, Frith CD, *et al.* (1976). Cerebral ventricular size and cognitive impairment in chronic schizophrenia. *Lancet*, **2**, 924–6.

Johnstone EC, Crow TJ, Frith CD, *et al.* (1988). The Northwick Park 'functional' psychosis study: diagnosis and treatment response. *Lancet*, **2**, 119–25.

Johnstone EC, Macmillan JF and Crow TJ (1987). The occurrence of organic disease of possible or probable aetiological significance in a population of 268 cases of first episode schizophrenia. *Psychological Medicine*, **17**, 371–9.

Jolley AG, Hirsch SR, Morrison E, *et al.* (1990). Trial of brief intermittent neuroleptic prophylaxis for selected schizophrenic outpatients: clinical and social outcome at two years. *British Medical Journal*, **301**, 837–42.

Jones D (2003). *Communicating with vulnerable children: a guide for practitioners.* Gaskell, London.

Jones DPH (2000). Child abuse and neglect. In MG Gelder, JJ López-Ibor Jr and NC Andreasen, eds. *The new Oxford textbook of psychiatry*, Chapter 9.3.1. Oxford University Press, Oxford.

Jones DPH and Alexander H (1978). Treating the abusive family within the family care system. In RE Helfer and RS Kempe, eds. *The battered child*. University of Chicago Press, London.

Jones E, Vermaas RH, McCartney H, *et al.* (2003). Flahbacks and post-traumatic strss disorder: the genesis of a 20th-century diagnosis. *British Journal of Psychiatry,* **182**, 158–63.

Jones K (1992). *A history of the mental health services.* Routledge & Kegan Paul, London.

Jones M (1968). *Social psychiatry in practice.* Penguin Books, Harmondsworth.

Jones P, Rodgers B, Murray R, *et al.* (1994). Child development risk factors for adult schizophrenia in the British 1946 birth cohort. *Lancet,* **344**, 1398–402.

Jones S (2004). Psycotherapy of bipolar disorder: a review. *Journal of Affective Disorders,* **80**, 101–14.

Jorm AF (2000). The ageing population and the epidemiology of mental disorders among the elderly. In MG Gelder, JJ López-Ibor Jr and NC Andreasen, eds. *The new Oxford textbook of psychiatry*, Chapter 8.3. Oxford University Press, Oxford.

Joy CB, Adams CE, Rice K, *et al.* (2004). *Crisis intervention for people with severe mental illnesses.* 4: CD001087, Cochrane Database of Systematic Reviews.

Joyce PR (2000). Epidemiology of mood disorders. In MG Gelder, J López-Ibor, JJ and NC Andreasen, eds. *The new Oxford textbook of psychiatry*, Chapter 4.5.4. Oxford University Press, Oxford.

Joyce PR, Mulder RT, Mckenzie JM, *et al.* (2004). Atypical depression, atypical temperament and a differential antidepressant response to fluoxetine and nortriptyline. *Depression and Anxiety,* **19**, 180–6.

Judd LL, Akiskal HS and Maser JD (1998). A prospective 12-year study of subsyndromal and syndromal depressive symptoms in unipolar major depressive disorders. *Archives of General Psychiatry,* **55**, 694–700.

Judd LL, Akiskal HS, Schettler PJ, *et al.* (2002). The Long-term natural history of the weekly symptomatic status of bipolar I disorder. *Archives of General Psychiatry,* **59**, 530–7.

Judd LL, Rapaport MH, Yonkers KA, *et al.* (2004). Randomized, placebo-controlled trial of fluoxetine for acute treatment of minor depressive disorder. *Am J Psychiatry*, **161**, 1864–71.

Jureidini JN, Doecke CJ, Mansfield PR, *et al.* (2004). Efficacy and safety of antidepressants for children and adolescents. *British Medical Journal,* **328**, 879–83.

Kahlbaum K (1863). *Die Gruppirung der psychichen Krankheiten.* Kafemann, Danzig.

Kahler SG and Fahey MC (2003). Metabolic disorders and mental retardation. *American Journal of Medical Genetics,* **117 C**, 31–4.

Kahn E (1928). Die psychopathischen Personlichkeiten. *Handbuch der Geisteskrankheiten*, 227. Springer, Berlin.

Kallmann FJ (1952). Study on the genetic effects of male homosexuality. *Journal of Nervous and Mental Disease,* **115**, 1283–98.

Kaminen N, Hannula-Jouppi K, Kestila M, *et al.* (2003). A genome scan for developmental dyslexia confirms linkage to chromosome 2p11 and suggests a new locus on 7q32. *Journal of Medical Genetics,* **40**, 340–5.

Kamphuis JH and Emmelkamp PMG (2000). Stalking – a contemporary challenge for forensic and clinical psychiatry. *British Journal of Psychiatry,* **176**, 206–9.

Kampov-Polevoy AB, Eick C, Boland G, *et al.* (2004). Sweet liking, novelty seeking, and gender predict alcoholic status. *Alcoholism, Clinical and Experimental Research,* **28**, 1291–8.

Kandel ER (1998). A new intellectual framework for psychiatry. *American Journal of Psychiatry,* **155**, 457–69.

Kane J, Honigfeld G, Singer J, *et al.* (1988). Clozapine for the treatment-resistant schizophrenic. A double-blind comparison with chlorpromazine. *Archives of General Psychiatry,* **45**, 789–96.

Kane JM (2004). Tardive dyskinesia rates with atypical antipsychotics in adults: prevalence and incidence. *Journal of Clinical Psychiatry,* **65**, 16–20.

Kane RL (1985). Special needs of the elderly. In WW Holland, ed. *Oxford textbook of public health*. Oxford University Press, Oxford.

Kanner AM (2003). Depression in epilepsy: prevalence, clinical semiology, pathogenic mechanisms, and treatment. *Biological Psychiatry,* **54**, 388–98.

Kanner L (1943). Autistic disturbance of affective contact. *Nervous Child,* **2**, 217–50.

Kapczinski F, Lima MS, Souza JS, *et al.* (2003). *Antidepressants for generalized anxiety disorder.* CDSR 2: CD003592, Cochrane Database of Systematic Reviews.

Kapur S (2003). Psychosis as a state of aberrant salience: a framework linking biology, phenomenology, and pharmacology in schizophrenia. *American Journal of Psychiatry,* **160**, 13–23.

Kapur S, Zipursky RB and Remington G (1999). Clinical and theoretical implications of 5-HT_2 and D_2 receptor occupancy of clozapine, risperidone, and olanzapine in schizophrenia. *American Journal of Psychiatry,* **156**, 286–93.

Kasanin J (1994). The acute schizoaffective psychoses. 1933. *American Journal of Psychiatry,* **151**, 144–54.

Kaski M (2000). Aetiology of mental retardation: general issues and prevention. In MG Gelder, JJ López-Ibor Jr and NC Andreasen, eds. *The new Oxford textbook of psychiatry*, Chapter 10.3. Oxford University Press, Oxford.

Katerndahl DA (1993). Lifetime prevalence of panic states. *American Journal of Psychiatry,* **150**, 246–9.

Katon W (1996). Panic disorder: relationship to high medical utilization, unexplained physical symptoms, and medical costs. *Journal of Clinical Psychiatry,* **57 (Suppl 10)**, 11–18.

Katon W, von Korff M, Lin E, *et al.* (1990). Distressed high utilizers of medical care: DSMIII-R diagnoses and treatment needs. *General Hospital Psychiatry,* **12**, 355–62.

Katon WJ, Von Korff M, Lin EH, *et al.* (2004). The Pathways Study: a randomized trial of collaborative care in patients with diabetes and depression. *Archives of General Psychiatry,* **61**, 1042–9.

Katona C and Livingston G (2002). How well do antidepressants work in older people? A systematic review of Number Needed to Treat. *J Affect Disord*, **69**, 47–52.

Katz M, Abbey S, Rydall A, *et al.* (1995). Psychiatric consultation for competency to refuse medical treatment. A retrospective study of patient characteristics and outcome. *Psychosomatics*, **36**, 33–41.

Katzelnick DJ, Kobak KA, Greist JH, *et al.* (1995). Sertraline for social phobia: a double blind, placebo-controlled crossover study. *American Journal of Psychiatry*, **152**, 1368–71.

Kaufman MD (2002). *Clinical neurology for psychiatrists*. 5th edn. WB Saunders, Philadelphia, PA.

Kavka J (1949). Pinel's conception of the psychopathic state. *Bulletin of the History of Medicine*, **23**, 461–8.

Kay DW, Cooper AF, Garside RF, *et al.* (1976). The differentiation of paranoid from affective psychoses by patients' premorbid characteristics. *British Journal of Psychiatry*, **129**, 207–15.

Kay DWK, Beamish P and Roth M (1964). Old age mental disorders in Newcastle-upon-Tyne: 1: a study in prevalence. *British Journal of Psychiatry*, **110**, 146–58.

Kay DWK and Bergmann K (1980). Epidemiology of mental disorder among the aged in the community. In JE Birren and RB Sloane, eds. *Handbook of mental health and ageing*. Prentice-Hall, Englewood Cliffs, NJ.

Kay DWK and Roth M (1961). Environmental and hereditary factors in the schizophrenias of old age ('late paraphrenia') and their bearing on the general problem of causation in schizophrenia. *Journal of Mental Science*, **107**, 649–86.

Kaye C and Lingiah T (2000). *Culture and ethnicity in secure psychiatric practice: working with difference*. Jessica Kingsley, London.

Kaye WH, Frank GK, Meltzer HY, *et al.* (2001). Altered serotonin 2A receptor activity in women who have recovered from bulemia nervosa. *American Journal of Psychiatry*, **158**, 1152–5.

Kazdin AE (1997). Practitioner review: psychosocial treatments for conduct disorder in children. *Journal of Child Psychology and Psychiatry*, **38**, 161–78.

Keel PK, Dorer DJ, Eddy KT, *et al.* (2003). Predictors of mortality in eating disorders. *Archives of General Psychiatry*, **60**, 179–83.

Keller MB, Ryan ND, Strober M, *et al.* (2001). Efficacy of paroxetinein the treatment of adolescent major depression: a randomized controlled trial. *Journal of the American Academy of Child and Adolescent Psychiatry*, **40**, 762–72.

Kelly WF (1996). Psychiatric aspects of Cushing's syndrome. *Quarterly Journal of Medicine*, **59**, 543–51.

Kemp R, Hayward P, Applewhaite G, *et al.* (1996). Compliance therapy in psychotic patients: randomised controlled trial. *British Medical Journal*, **312**, 345–9.

Kempe RS and Goldbloom RB (1987). Malnutrition and growth retardation (failure to thrive) in the context of child abuse and neglect. In RE Helfer and RS Kempe, eds. *The battered child*, 315–35. University of Chicago Press, London.

Kendell RE (1975). *The role of diagnosis in psychiatry*. Blackwell, Oxford.

Kendell RE, Chalmers JC and Platz C (1987). Epidemiology of puerperal psychoses. *British Journal of Psychiatry*, **150**, 662–73.

Kendell R and Jablensky A (2003). Distinguishing between the validity and utility of psychiatric diagnoses. *Am J Psychiatry*, **160**, 4–12.

Kendell RE, Malcolm DE and Adams W (1993). The problem of detecting changes in the incidence of schizophrenia. *British Journal of Psychiatry*, **162**, 212–8.

Kendler KS (1990). Toward a scientific psychiatric nosology. Strengths and limitations. *Archives of General Psychiatry*, **47**, 969–73.

Kendler KS (1997). The diagnostic validity of melancholic major depression in a population-based sample of female twins. *Archives of General Psychiatry*, **54**, 299–304.

Kendler KS (2003). The genetics of schizophrenia: chromosomal deletions, attentional disturbances, and spectrum boundaries. *American Journal of Psychiatry*, **160**, 1549–53.

Kendler KS, Bulik CM, Silberg J, *et al.* (2000). Childhood sexual abuse and adult psychiatric and substance use disorders in women: an epidemiological and cotwin control analysis. *Arch Gen Psychiatry*, **57**, 953–9.

Kendler KS, Gardner CO and Prescott CA (2002). Toward a comprehensive developmental model for major depression in women. *American Journal of Psychiatry*, **159**, 1133–45.

Kendler KS, Gardner CO and Thornton LM (2001). Genetic risk, number of previous depressive episodes, and stressful life events in depicting onset of major depression. *American Journal of Psychiatry*, **158**, 582–6.

Kendler KS and Gruenberg AM (1984). An independent analysis of the Danish adoption study of schizophrenia. VI. The relationship between psychiatric disorders as defined by DSMIII in the relatives and adoptees. *Archives of General Psychiatry*, **41**, 555–64.

Kendler KS, Gruenberg AM and Strauss JS (1981). An independent analysis of the Copenhagen sample for the Danish adoption study of schizophrenia. The relationship between schizotypal personality disorder and schizophrenia. *Archives of General Psychiatry*, **38**, 982–7.

Kendler KS, Kuhn J and Prescott CA (2004). The interrelationship of neuroticism, sex, and stressful life events int he prediction of episodes of major depression. *American Journal of Psychiatry*, **161**, 631–6.

Kendler KS, Masterson CC and Davis KL (1985). Psychiatric illness in first-degree relatives of patients with paranoid psychosis, schizophrenia and medical illness. *British Journal of Psychiatry*, **47**, 524–31.

Kendler KS, McGuire M, Gruenberg AM, *et al.* (1993a). The Roscommon Family Study. III. Schizophrenia-related personality disorders in relatives. *Archives of General Psychiatry*, **50**, 781–8.

Kendler KS, McGuire M, Gruenberg AM, *et al.* (1993b). The Roscommon Family Study. I. Methods, diagnosis of probands, and risk of schizophrenia in relatives. *Archives of General Psychiatry*, **50**, 527–40.

Kendler KS, McGuire M, Gruenberg AM, *et al.* (1993d). The Roscommon Family Study. IV. Affective illness, anxiety disorders, and alcoholism in relatives. *Archives of General Psychiatry*, **50**, 952–60.

Kendler KS, McGuire M, Gruenberg AM, *et al.* (1993c). The Roscommon Family Study. II. The risk of nonschizophrenic nonaffective psychoses in relatives. *Archives of General Psychiatry*, **50**, 645–52.

Kendler KS, Neale MC, Kessler RC, *et al.* (1992b). Childhood parental loss and adult psychopathology in women: a twin study perspective. *Archives of General Psychiatry*, **49**, 109–16.

Kendler KS, Neale MC, Kessler RC, *et al.* (1993e). Panic disorder in women: a population-based twin study. *Psychological Medicine*, **23**, 397–406.

Kendler KS, Neale MC, Kessler RC, *et al.* (1992a). Major depression and generalized anxiety disorder: same genes (partly) different environments? *Archives of General Psychiatry*, **49**, 716–22.

Kendler KS, Neale MC and Walsh D (1995). Evaluating the spectrum concept of schizophrenia in the Roscommon Family Study. *American Journal of Psychiatry*, **152**, 749–54.

Kendler KS and Walsh D (1995). Schizophreniform disorder, delusional disorder and psychotic disorder not otherwise specified: clinical features, outcome and familial psychopathology. *Acta Psychiatr Scand*, **91**, 370–8.

Kendrick T, Burns T and Freeling P (1995). Randomised controlled trial of teaching general practitioners to carry out structured assessments of their long term mentally ill patients. *British Medical Journal*, **311**, 93–8.

Kennard D (1998). *An introduction to therapeutic communities.* 2nd edn. Jessica Kingsley, London.

Kennedy N and Paykel ES (2004). Treatment and response in refractory depression: results from a specialist affective disorders service. *Journal of Affective Disorders*, **81**, 49–53.

Kennerley H (1997). *Overcoming anxiety.* Robinson, London.

Keppel-Benson JM, Oldendick TH and Benson MJ (2002). Post-traumatic stress in children following motor vehicle accidents. *Journal of Child Psychology and Psychiatry*, **43**, 203–12.

Kerkhof A (2000). Attempted suicide; patterns and trends. In K Hawton and K van Heeringen, eds. *The International Handbook of Suicide and Attempted Suicide.* John Wiley and Sons, Chichester.

Kernberg OF (1975). *Borderline conditions and pathological narcissism.* Jason Aronson, New York.

Kerr AM and Stevenson JBP (1985). Rett's syndrome in the West of Scotland. *British Medical Journal*, **291**, 579–80.

Kerr TA, Roth M and Shapira K (1974). Prediction of outcome in anxiety states and depressive illness. *British Journal of Psychiatry*, **124**, 125–31.

Keshavan M, Shad M, Soloff P, *et al.* (2004). Efficacy and tolerability of olanzapine in the treatment of schizotypal personality disorder. *Schizophrenia Research*, **71**, 97–101.

Kessler RC (2004). The epidemiology of dual diagnosis. *Biological Psychiatry*, **56**, 730–7.

Kessler RC, Keller MB and Wittchen HU (2001). The epidemiology of generalized anxiety disorder. *Psychiatric Clinics of North America*, **24**, 13–39.

Kessler RC, McGonagle KA, Zhao S, *et al.* (1994). Life-time and 12-month prevalence of DSM-III-R psychiatric disorders in the United States: results from the National Comorbidity Survey. *Archives of General Psychiatry*, **51**, 8–20.

Kessler RC, Merikangas KR, Berglund P, *et al.* (2003). Mild disorders should not be eliminated from the DSM-V. *Archives of General Psychiatry*, **60**, 1117–22.

Kessler RC, Rubinow DR and Holmes C (1997). The epidemiology of DSM-III-R Bipolar I disorder in a general population survey. *Psychological Medicine*, **51**, 8–20.

Kessler RC, Sonnega A, Bromet E, *et al.* (1995). Posttraumatic stress disorder in the National Comorbidity Survey. *Archives of General Psychiatry*, **52**, 1048–60.

Kessler RC and Walters EE (1998). Epidemiology of DSM-III-R major depression and minor depression among adolescents and young adults in the National Comorbidity Survey. *Depression and Anxiety*, **7**, 3–14.

Kesteren P, Gooren L and Megers J (1996). An epidemiological and demographic study of transsexuals in the Netherlands. *Archives of Sexual Behaviour*, **25**, 589–600.

Kety SS, Rosenthal D and Wender PH (1975). Mental illness in the biological and adoptive families of adopted individuals who have become schizophrenic. In RR Fieve, D Rosenthal and H Bull, eds. *Genetic research in psychiatry*. Johns Hopkins University Press, Baltimore, MD.

Kety SS, Wender PH, Jacobsen B, *et al.* (1994). Mental illness in the biological and adoptive relatives of schizophrenic adoptees. Replication of the Copenhagen Study in the rest of Denmark. *Archives of General Psychiatry*, **51**, 442–55.

Khan A, Khan S, Kolts R, *et al.* (2003). Suicide rates in clinical trials of SSRIs, other antidepressants, and placebo: analysis of FDA reports. *American Journal of Psychiatry*, **160**, 790–2.

Kilbourne EM, Philen RM, Kamb ML, *et al.* (1996). Tryptophan produced by Showa Denko and epidemic eosinophilic-myalgia syndrome. *Journal of Rheumatology*, **23**, 81–8.

Kiloh LG, Smith JS and Johnson GF (1988). *Physical treatments in psychiatry.* Blackwell Scientific Publications, Oxford.

King M and McDonald E (1992). Homosexuals who are twins: a study of 46 probands. *British Journal of Psychiatry*, **160**, 407–9.

King NJ and Bernstein GA (2001). School refusal in children and adolescents: a review of the last ten years. *Journal of the American Academy of Child and Adolescent Psychiatry*, **40**, 197–205.

King R and Apter A (eds.) (2003). *Suicide in children and adolescents.* Cambridge University Press.

Kinsey AC, Pomeroy WB and Martin CE (1948). *Sexual behavior in the human male.* Saunders, Philadelphia, PA.

Kinsey AC, Pomeroy WB, Martin CE, *et al.* (1953). *Sexual behavior in the human female.* Saunders, Philadelphia, PA.

Kipps CM and Hodges JR (2005). Cognitive assessment for clinicians. *J Neurol Neurosurg Psychiatry*, **76 Suppl 1**, i22–30.

Kirby RS (1994). Impotence: diagnosis and management of male erectile dysfunction. *British Medical Journal*, **308**, 957–61.

Kirchmayer U, Davoli M and Verster A (2003). Naltrexone maintenance treatment for opioid dependence. *Cochrane Database Syst Rev*, Cd001333.

Kirkwood TBL (2003). The most pressing problem of our age. *British Medical Journal*, **326**, 1297–9.

Kirmayer LJ and Groleau D (2001). Affective disorders in cultural context. *Psychiatric Clinics of North America*, **24**, 465–78.

Kisely SR and Goldberg DP (1996). Physical and psychiatric comorbidity in general practice. *British Journal of Psychiatry*, **169**, 236–42.

Klein DF (1964). Delineation of two drug-responsive anxiety syndromes. *Psychopharmacologia*, **5**, 397–408.

Klein F, Sepekoff B and Wolf TJ (1985). Sexual orientation: a multiple variable, dynamic process. *Journal of Homosexuality*, **11**, 35–49.

Klein M (1952). Notes on some schizoid mechanisms. In J Jacobs and J Riviere, eds. *Developments in psychoanalysis*. Hogarth Press, London.

Klein M (1963). *The psychoanalysis of children*. Transl A Strachey. Hogarth Press and Institute of Psychoanalysis, London.

Kleinman A (1982). Neurasthenia and depression: a study of somatization and culture in China. *Culture, Medicine and Psychiatry*, **6**, 117–96.

Klerman GL, Budman S, Weissman MM, *et al.* (1987). Efficacy of a brief psychosocial intervention for symptoms of stress and distress among patients in primary care. *Medical Care*, **25**, 1078–88.

Klerman GL, Weissman MM, Rounsaville BJ, *et al.* (1984). *Interpersonal psychotherapy of depression*. Basic Books, New York, NY.

Knapp M and Chisholm D (2000). Economic analysis of psychiatric services. In MG Gelder, JJ López-Ibor Jr and NC Andreasen, eds. *The new Oxford textbook of psychiatry*, Chapter 7.7. Oxford University Press, Oxford.

Knapp M, Mangalore R and Simon J (2004). The global costs of schizophrenia. *Schizophrenia Bulletin*, **30**, 279–93.

Koch JLA (1891). *Die Psychopathischen Minderwertigkeiter*. Dorn, Ravensburg.

Koegel R, Schreibman L, O'Neil RE, *et al.* (1983). The personality and family interactioncharacteristics of parents with autistic children. *Journal of Consulting and Clinical Psychology*, **51**, 683–92.

Koenen KC, Harley R, Lyons MJ, *et al.* (2002). A twin registry study of familial and individual risk factors for trauma exposure and posttraumatic stress disorder. *Journal of Nervous and Mental Disease*, **190**, 209–18.

Koenig HG and Blazer DG (1992). Epidemiology of geriatric affective disorders. *Clinics in Geriatric Medicine*, **8**, 235–51.

Koenigsberg HW, Reynolds D, Goodman M, *et al.* (2003). Risperidone in the treatment of schizotypal personality disorder. *Journal of Clinical Psychiatry*, **64**, 628–34.

Koepp MJ and Duncan JS (2004). Epilepsy. *Current Opinion in Neurology*, **17**, 467–74.

Kohn R, Saxena S, Levav I, *et al.* (2004). The treatment gap in mental health care. *Bull World Health Organ*, **82**, 858–66.

Kolvin I (2000). Speech and language disorders of childhood and psychological mutism. In MG Gelder, JJ López-Ibor Jr and NC Andreasen, eds. *The new Oxford textbook of psychiatry*, Chapter 9.2.11. Oxford University Press, Oxford.

Kolvin I and Fundudis T (1981). Elective mute children: psychological development and background factors. *Journal of Child Psychology and Psychiatry*, **22**, 219–32.

Konradi C and Heckers S (2003). Molecular aspects of glutamate dysregulation: implications for schizophrenia and its treatment. *Pharmacology and Therapeutics*, **97**, 153–79.

Kopelman MD (2000). Amnesic syndromes. In MG Gelder, JJ López-Ibor Jr and NC Andreasen, eds. *The new Oxford textbook of psychiatry*, Chapter 4.1.13. Oxford University Press, Oxford.

Kornfeld DS (2002). Consultation Liaison Psychiatry: Contributions to medical practice. *American Journal of Psychiatry*, **159**, 1964–72.

Kornstein SG, Sholare EF and Gardner DF (2000). Endocrine disorders. In A Stoudemier, BS Fogel and DB Greenberg, eds. *Psychiatric care of the medical patient*. Oxford University Press, New York.

Kovacs M (1996). Presentation and course of major depression during childhood and later years of the lifespan. *Journal of the American Academy of Child and Adolescent Psychiatry*, **35**, 705–15.

Krabbendam L and Aleman A (2003). Cognitive rehabilitation in schizophrenia: a quantitative analysis of controlled studies. *Psychopharmacology*, **169**, 376–82.

Kraepelin E (1904). *Clinical psychiatry: a textbook for students and physicians*. Macmillan, New York, NY.

Kraepelin E (1919). *Dementia praecox and paraphrenia*. Livingstone, Edinburgh.

Kraeplin E (1921). *Manic depressive insanity and paranoia*. Livingstone, Edinburgh.

Krafft-Ebing R (1888). *Lehrbuch der Psychiatrie*. Enke, Stuttgart.

Krafft-Ebing R (1924). *Psychopathic sexuality with special reference to contrary sexual instinct*. 7th German edn. Transl CG Chaddock and FA Davis. Philadelphia, PA.

Kramer M (1969). Cross-national study of diagnosis of the mental disorders: origin of the problem. *Am J Psychiatry*, **10 Suppl**, 1–11.

Kraus L, Augustin R, Frischer M, *et al.* (2003). Estimating prevalence of problem drug use at national level in countries of the European Union and Norway. *Addiction*, **98**, 471–85.

Kreitman N (1961). The reliability of psychiatric diagnosis. *J Ment Sci*, **107**, 876–86.

Kreitman N (ed.) (1977). *Parasuicide*. Wiley, London.

Kretschmer, E. (1927). Der sensitive Beziehungswahn. Reprinted and translated as Chapter 8 in *Themes and variations in European psychiatry* (eds S. R. Hirsch and M. Shepherd). Wright, Bristol (1974).

Kretschmer E (1936). *Physique and character*. 2nd edn. Transl WJH Sprott and KP Trench. Trubner, New York.

Kringlen E (1965). Obsessional neurosis: a long term follow up. *British Journal of Psychiatry*, **111**, 709–22.

Krishnan KR (2002). Biological risk factors in late life depression. *Biological Psychiatry*, **52**, 185–92.

Krishnan KR, Delong M, Kraemer H, *et al.* (2002). Comorbidity of depression with other medical diseases in the elderly. *Biological Psychiatry*, **52**, 559–88.

Kroenke K, Spitzer RL, Williams JB, *et al.* (1994). Physical symptoms in primary care. Predictors of psychiatric disorders and functional impairment. *Archives of Family Medicine*, **3**, 774–9.

Kroenke K and Swindle R (2000). Cognitive-behavioral therapy for somatization and symptom syndromes: a critical review of controlled clinical trials. *Psychotherapy and Psychosomatics*, **69**, 205–15.

Krueger RF (1999). The structure of common mental disorders. *Archives of General Psychiatry*, **56**, 921–6.

Kubler-Ross E (1969). *On death and dying*. Macmillan, New York.

Kurlan R, Como PG, Miller B, *et al.* (2002). The behavioral spectrum of tic disorders: a community-based study. *Neurology,* **59**, 414–20.

Kurtz MM (2005). Neurocognitive impairment across the lifespan in schizophrenia: an update. *Schizophrenia Research,* **74**, 15–26.

Kurz A and Van Baelen B (2004). Ginkgo biloba compared with cholinesterase inhibitors in the treatment of dementia: a review based on meta-analyses by the cochrane collaboration. *Dementia and Geriatric Cognitive Disorders,* **18**, 217–26.

Kuthe A (2003). Phosphodiesterase 5 inhibitors in male sexual dysfunction. *Current Opinion in Urology,* **13**, 405–10.

Kvale G, Berggren U and Milgrom P (2004). Dental fear in adults: a meta-analysis of behavioural interventions. *Community Dentistry and Oral Epidemiology,* **32**, 250–64.

Lachs MS and Pillemer K (2004). Elder abuse. *Lancet,* **364**, 1263–72.

Lachs MS, Williams CS, O'Brien S, *et al.* (1998). The mortality of elder mistreatment. *Journal of the American Medical Association,* **280**, 428–32.

Lader M (1994). Anxiolytic drugs: dependence, addiction and abuse. *European Neuropsychopharmacology,* **4**, 85–91.

Lahiri DK, Sambamurti K and Bennett DA (2004). Apolipoprotein gene and its interaction with the environmentally driven risk factors: molecular, genetic and epidemiological studies of Alzheimer's disease. *Neurobiology of Aging,* **25**, 651–60.

Lambert MV, Sierra M, Phillips ML, *et al.* (2002). The spectrum of organic depersonalization:a review of four new cases. *Journal of Neuropsychiatry and Clinical Neurosciences,* **14**, 141–54.

Lamontagne Y, Boyer R, Hetu C, *et al.* (2000). Anxiety, significant losses, depression and irrational beliefs in first-offence shop-lifters. *Canadian Journal of Psychiatry. Revue Canadienne de Psychiatrie,* **45**, 63–9.

Landesmann-Dyer S (1981). Living in the community. *American Journal of Mental Deficiency,* **86**, 223–34.

Langa KM, Foster NL and Larson EB (2004). Mixed dementia: emerging concepts and therapeutic implications. *Journal of the American Medical Association,* **292**, 2901–8.

Lange J (1931). *Crime as destiny.* Transl C Haldane. George Allen, London.

Langfeldt G (1961). The erotic jealousy syndrome. A clinical study. *Acta Psychiatrica Scandinavica,* **36 (suppl 151)**, 7–68.

Larcher V (2005). ABC of adolescence: consent, competence, and confidentiality. *British Medical Journal,* **330**, 353–6.

Laruelle M and Abi-Dargham A (1999). Dopamine as the wind of the psychotic fire: new evidence from brain imaging studies. *J Psychopharmacol,* **13**, 358–71.

Laruelle M, Kegeles LS and Abi-Dargham A (2003). Glutamate, dopamine, and schizophrenia: from pathophysiology to treatment. *Annals of the New York Academy of Sciences,* **1003**, 138–58.

Lasègue C (1877). Les exhibitionnistes. *Union Medicale,* **23**, 709–14.

Last CG, Hansen C and Franco N (1997). Anxious children in adulthood; a prospective study of adjustment. *Journal of the American Academy of Child and Adolescent Psychiatry,* **36**, 645–52.

Laumann EO, Gagnon JH, T. MR, *et al.* (1994). *The social organization of sexuality.* University of Chicago Press, Chicago, IL.

Launer LJ (2003). Nonsteroidal anti-inflammatory drugs and Alzheimer disease: what's next? *Journal of the American Medical Association,* **289**, 2865–7.

Lauterbach EC (2004). The neuropsychiatry of Parkinson's disease and related disorders. *Psychiatric Clinics of North America,* **27**, 801–25.

Lavori PW (2000). Placebo control groups in randomized treatment trials: a statistician's perspective. *Biological Psychiatry,* **47**, 717–23.

Lawrie SM, Whalley H, Kestelman JN, *et al.* (1999). Magnetic resonance imaging of brain in people at high risk of developing schizophrenia. *Lancet,* **353**, 30–3.

Lazare A (1973). Hidden conceptual models in clinical psychiatry. *N Engl J Med,* **288**, 345–51.

Lazarus RS (1993). Coping theory and research: past, present and future. *Psychosomatic Medicine,* **55**, 234–47.

LeBlanc ES, Janowsky J, Chan BK, *et al.* (2001). Hormone replacement therapy and cognition: systematic review and meta-analysis. *Journal of the American Medical Association,* **285**, 1489–99.

LeCouteur A and Baird G (2003). *National Initiative for Autism: Screening and Assessment (NIASA). National autism plan for children.* National Autism Society, London.

LeDoux J (1998). *The emotional brain.* Weidenfeld & Nicolson, London.

LeDoux JE (2000). Emotion circuits in the brain. *Annual Review of Neuroscience,* **23**, 155–84.

Lee LM, Stevenson RW and Szasz G (1988). Prostaglandin E1 versus phentolamine/papaverine for the treatment of erectile impotence: a double-blind comparison. *Journal of Urology,* **141**, 54–7.

Lee R and Coccaro E (2001). The neuropsychopharacology of criminality and aggression. *Canadian Journal of Psychiatry. Revue Canadienne de Psychiatrie,* **46**, 35–44.

Lee VM, Goedert M and Trojanowski JQ (2001). Neurodegenerative tauopathies. *Annual Review of Neuroscience,* **24**, 1121–59.

Leff J (1981). *Psychiatry around the globe: a transcultural view.* Dekker, New York.

Leff J (1993a). All the homeless people – where do they all come from? *British Medical Journal,* **306**, 669–70.

Leff J (1993b). The Taps Project: evaluating community placement of long-stay psychiatric patients. *British Journal of Psychiatry,* **164**, 1–56.

Leff J (1998). Needs of the families of people with schizophrenia. *Advances in Psychiatric Treatment,* **4**, 277–84.

Leff J, Kuipers L, Berkowitz R, *et al.* (1985). A controlled trial of social intervention in the families of schizophrenic patients: two year follow-up. *British Journal of Psychiatry,* **146**, 594–600.

Leff J and Vaughn C (1981). The role of maintenance therapy and relatives' expressed emotion in relapse of schizophrenia: a two-year follow-up. *British Journal of Psychiatry,* **139**, 102–4.

Leff J, Vearnals S, Wolff G, *et al.* (2000). The London Depression Intervention Trial: Randomised controlled trial of antidepressants v. couple therapy in the treatment and maintenance of people with depression living with a partner: clinical outcome and costs. *British Journal of Psychiatry,* **177**, 95–100.

Lehman AF, Dixon LB, Kernan E, *et al.* (1997). A randomized trial of assertive community treatment for homeless persons with severe mental illness. *Archives of General Psychiatry,* **54**, 1038–43.

Lehman AF, Lieberman JA, Dixon LB, *et al.* (2004). Practice guideline for the treatment of patients with schizophrenia, second edition. *American Journal of Psychiatry,* **161**, 1–56.

Lehmann SW (2003). Psychiatric disorders in older women. *International Review of Psychiatry,* **15**, 269–79.

Lehrke R (1972). A theory of X-linkage of major intellectual traits. *American Journal of Mental Deficiency,* **76**, 611–9.

Leichsenring FaL, E. T. (2003). The effectiveness of pychodynamic therapy and cognitive behavior therapy in the treatment of personality disorders: a meta-analysis. *American Journal of Psychiatry,* **160**, 1223–32.

Lemoine P, Harousseau H, Borteyru JP, *et al.* (1968). Les enfants de parents alcooliques: anomalies observées à propos de 127 cas. *Quest Médical,* **25**, 477–82.

Lenane MC, Swedo SE, Leonard H, *et al.* (1990). Psychiatric disorders in first degree relatives of children and adolescents with obsessive compulsive disorder. *Journal of the American Academy of Child and Adolescent Psychiatry,* **29**, 407–12.

Leonhard K (1957). *The classification of endogenous psychoses.* 8th edn. Transl R Berman. Irvington, New York.

Leonhard K, Korff I and Schultz H (1962). Die Temperamente und den Familien der monopolaren und bipolaren phasishen Psychosen. *Psychiatrie und Neurologie,* **143**, 416–34.

Lesperance F, Frasure-Smith N and Talajic M (1996). Major depression before and after myocardial infarction: its nature and consequences. *Psychosomatic Medicine,* **58**, 99–110.

Lester G, Wilson B, Griffin L, *et al.* (2004). Unusually persistent complainants. *British Journal of Psychiatry,* **184**, 352–6.

Leucht S, Barnes TR, Kissling W, *et al.* (2003). Relapse prevention in schizophrenia with new-generation antipsychotics: a systematic review and exploratory meta-analysis of randomized, controlled trials. *American Journal of Psychiatry,* **160**, 1209–22.

Leucht S, Kissling W and McGrath J (2004). Lithium for schizophrenia revisited: a systematic review and meta-analysis of randomized controlled trials. *Journal of Clinical Psychiatry,* **65**, 177–86.

Leung CM, Chung WS and So EP (2002). Burning charcoal: an indiginous method of suicide in Hong Kong. *Journal of Clinical Psychiatry,* **63**, 447–50.

LeVay S (1991). A difference in hypothalamic structure between heterosexual and homosexual men. *Science,* **253**, 1034–7.

Levin E (1997). Carers. In R Jacoby and C Oppenheimer, eds. *Psychiatry in the elderly*, 392–402. Oxford University Press, Oxford.

Levin RJ (2000). Normal sexual function. In MG Gelder, JJ López-Ibor Jr and NC Andreasen, eds. *The new Oxford textbook of psychiatry*, Chapter 4.11.1. Oxford University Press, Oxford.

Lewis AJ (1934). Melancholia: a clinical survey of depressive states. *Journal of Mental Science,* **80**, 277–8.

Lewis AJ (1936). Problems of obsessional neurosis. *Proceedings of the Royal Society of Medicine,* **29**, 352–36.

Lewis AJ (1953). Health as a social concept. *British Journal of Sociology,* **4**, 109–24.

Lewis AJ (1970). Paranoia and paranoid: a historical perspective. *Psychological Medicine,* **1**, 2–12.

Lewis DA, Hashimoto T and Volk DW (2005). Cortical inhibitory neurons and schizophrenia. *Nat Rev Neurosci,* **6**, 312–24.

Lewis DA and Levitt P (2002). Schizophrenia as a disorder of neurodevelopment. *Annual Review of Neuroscience,* **25**, 409–32.

Lewis EO (1929). *Report on an investigation into the incidence of mental deficiency in six areas 1925–27.* HMSO, London.

Lewis G and Appleby L (1988). Personality disorder: the patients psychiatrists dislike. *British Journal of Psychiatry,* **153**, 44–9.

Lewis G, Hawton K and Jones P (1997). Strategies for preventing suicide. *British Journal of Psychiatry,* **171**, 351–4.

Leys D, Henon H, Mackowiak-Cordoliani M, *et al.* (2005). Poststroke dementia. *Lancet Neurol,* **4**, 752–9.

Lezak MD, Howieson DB, Loring DW, *et al.* (2004). *Neuropsychological assessment.* 4th edn. Oxford University Press, Oxford.

Li SH and Li XJ (2004). Huntingtin-protein interactions and the pathogenesis of Huntington's disease. *Trends in Genetics,* **20**, 146–54.

Liddell MB, Lovestone S and Owen MJ (2001). Genetic risk of Alzheimer's disease: advising relatives. *British Journal of Psychiatry,* **178**, 7–11.

Liddle P and Pantelis C (2003). Brain imaging in schizophrenia. In SR Hirsch and D Weinberger, eds. *Schizophrenia*, 403–17. 2nd edn. Blackwell Publishing, Oxford.

Liddle PF (1987). The symptoms of chronic schizophrenia. A re-examination of the positive-negative dichotomy. *British Journal of Psychiatry,* **151**, 145–51.

Liddle PF, Friston KJ, Frith CD, *et al.* (1992). Patterns of cerebral blood flow in schizophrenia. *British Journal of Psychiatry,* **160**, 179–86.

Lidz T, Fleck S and Cornelison A (1965). *Schizophrenia and the family.* International Universities Press, New York.

Lieberman JA, Phillips M, Gu H, *et al.* (2003). Atypical and conventional antipsychotic drugs in treatment-naive first-episode schizophrenia: a 52-week randomized trial of clozapine vs chlorpromazine. *Neuropsychopharmacology,* **28**, 995–1003.

Lieberman JA, Stroup TS, McEvoy JP, *et al.* (2005). Effectiveness of antipsychotic drugs in patients with chronic schizophrenia. *N Engl J Med,* **353**, 1209–23.

Lieberman MA (1990). A group therapist perspective on self-help groups. *International Journal of Group Psychotherapy,* **40**, 251–77.

Lieberman MA and Yalom I (1992). Brief Group psychotherapy for the spousally bereaved: a controlled study. *International Journal of Group Psychotherapy,* **42**, 117–32.

Lieberman MA, Yalom ID and Miles MB (1973). *Encounter groups: first facts.* Basic Books, New York, NY.

Liebowitz MR, Gorman JM and Fyer AJ (1988). Pharmacotherapy of social phobia: an interim report of a placebo controlled comparison of phenelzine and atenolol. *Journal of Clinical Psychiatry*, **49**, 252–7.

Liebowitz MR, Schneier FR, Campeas R, *et al.* (1992). Phenelzine versus atenolol in social phobia: a placebo controlled comparison. *Archives of General Psychiatry*, **49**, 290–300.

Lilenfeld LR and Kaye WH (1998). Genetic studies of anorexia and Bulimia nervosa. In HW Hoek, JL Treasure and MA Katzman, eds. *Neurobiology in the treatment of eating disorders*. John Wiley, Chichester.

Linde K, Ramirez G, Mulrow CD, *et al.* (1996). St John's Wort for depression – an overview and meta-analysis of randomised clinical trials. *British Medical Journal*, **313**, 253–8.

Lindemann E (1944). Symptomatology and management of acute grief. *American Journal of Psychiatry*, **101**, 141–8.

Lindesay J (2000). Stress-related, anxiety, and obsessional disorders in elderly people. In MG Gelder, JJ López-Ibor Jr and NC Andreasen, eds. *The new Oxford textbook of psychiatry*, Chapter 8.5.5. Oxford University Press, Oxford.

Linehan MM (1993). *Cognitive-behavioral treatment of borderline personality disorder.* Guilford, New York.

Linehan MM, Armstrong HE, Suarez A, *et al.* (1991). Cognitive-behavioral treatment of chronically parasuicidal borderline patients. *Archives of General Psychiatry*, **48**, 1060–4.

Linehan MM, Tutek DA, Heard HL, *et al.* (1994). Interpersonal outcome of cognitive behavioral treatment for chronically suicidal borderline patients. *American Journal of Psychiatry*, **151**, 1771–6.

Linet OI and Ogrinc FG (1996). Efficacy and safety of intracavernosal alprostadil in men with erectile dysfunction. *New England Journal of Medicine*, **334**, 873–7.

Lingford-Hughes AR, Davies SJ, McIver S, *et al.* (2003). Addiction. *British Medical Bulletin*, **65**, 209–22.

Lingford-Hughes AR, Welch S and Nutt DJ (2004). Evidence based guidelines for the pharmacological management of substance misuse, addiction and comorbidity: recommendations from the British Association for Psychopharmacology. *Journal of Psychopharmacology*, **18**, 293–335.

Links P (2000). A lower minimum legal drinking age was associated with increased suicide in youths 18–23 years of age. *Evidence-Based Mental Health*, **3**, 59.

Linnoila MI and Virkkunen M (1992). Aggression, suicidality and serotonin. *Journal of Clinical Psychiatry*, **53**, 46–51.

Linton SJ (2000). A review of psychological risk factors in back and neck pain. *Spine*, **25**, 1148–56.

Liperoti R, Mor V, Lapane KL, *et al.* (2003). The use of atypical antipsychotics in nursing homes. *Journal of Clinical Psychiatry*, **64**, 1106–12.

Lipowski ZJ (1988). Somatization: the concept and its clinical application. *Am J Psychiatry*, **145**, 1358–68.

Lipowski ZJ (1990). *Delirium: acute confusional states.* Oxford University Press, New York.

Lishman WA (1988). Physiogenesis and psychogenesis in the post-concussional syndrome. *British Journal of Psychiatry*, **153**, 460–9.

Lishman WA (1998). *Organic psychiatry: the psychological consequences of cerebral disorder.* 3rd edn. Blackwell Scientific Publications, Oxford.

Livingston G, Johnston K, Katona C, *et al.* (2005). Systematic review of psychological approaches to the management of neuropsychiatric symptoms of dementia. *American Journal of Psychiatry*, **162**, 1996–2021.

Llewellyn S (2003). Cognitive analytic therapy: time and process. *Psychodynamic Process*, **9**, 501–20.

Lloyd CE and Brown FJ (2002). Depression and diabetes. *Current Womens Health Report*, **2**, 188–93.

Lock T (1999). Advances in the practice of electroconvulsive therapy. In A Lee, ed. *Recent topics and advances in psychiatric treatment*, 66–75. Royal College of Psychiatrists, Gaskill Press, London.

Loranger AW, Sartorius N, Andreoli A, *et al.* (1994). The International personality Disorder Examination: the World Health Organization/Alcohol, Drug Abuse and Mental Health Administration International Pilot Study of Personality Disorders. *Archives of General Psychiatry*, **51**, 215–24.

Lord C and Rutter M (1994). Autism and pervasive developmental disorder. In M Rutter, E Taylor and L Hersov, eds. *Child and adolescent psychiatry: modern approaches*, 569–93. 3rd edn. Blackwell Scientific Publications, Oxford.

Lovestone S (2000). Dementia: Alzheimer's disease. In MG Gelder, JJ López-lbor Jr and NC Andreasen, eds. *The new Oxford textbook of psychiatry*, Chapter 4.1.3. Oxford University Press, Oxford.

Lovestone S and McLoughlin DM (2002). Protein aggregates and dementia: is there a common toxicity? *Journal of Neurology, Neurosurgery and Psychiatry*, **72**, 152–61.

Luby JL, Heffelfinger AK, Mrakotsky C, *et al.* (2003). The clinical picture of depression in pre-school children. *Journal of the American Academy of Child and Adolescent Psychiatry*, **42**, 340–8.

Ludman EJ, Katon W, Russo J, *et al.* (2004). Depression and diabetes symptom burden. *General Hospital Psychiatry*, **26**, 430–6.

Lustig SL, Kia-Keating M, Knight WG, *et al.* (2004). Review of child and adolescent refugee mental health. *Journal of the American Academy of Child and Adolescent Psychiatry*, **43**, 24–36.

Luty J (2003). What works in addiction. *Advances in Psychiatric Treatment*, **9**, 280–8.

Luxenberger H (1928). Vorläufiger Bericht über psychiatrische Serienuntersuchungen an Zwillingen. *Zeitschrift für die gesamte Neurologie und Psychiatrie*, **116**, 297–326.

Lyketsos CG, Steinberg M, Tschanz JT, *et al.* (2000). Mental and behavioral disturbances in dementia: findings from the Cache County Study on memory in ageing. *American Journal of Psychiatry*, **157**, 708–14.

Lynch M and Roberts J (1982). *Consequences of child abuse.* Academic Press, London.

Lyness JM (2004). End-of-life care: issues relevant to the geriatric psychiatrist. *American Journal of Geriatric Psychiatry*, **12**, 457–72.

Lyons MJ, R. TW, Eisen SA, *et al.* (1995). Differential hereditability of adult and juvenile antisocial traits. *Archives of General Psychiatry*, **52**, 906–15.

Mace C (2001). All in the mind? The history of hysterical conversion as a clinical concept. In PW Halligan, C Bass and JC Marshall, eds. *Contemporary approaches to the study of hysteria: clinical and theoretical perspectives.*, Chapter 1. Oxford University Press, Oxford.

Mace CJ (1993). Epilepsy and schizophrenia. *British Journal of Psychiatry*, **163**, 439–45.

MacFarlane AB (1985). Medical evidence in the Court of Protection. *Bulletin of the Royal College of Psychiatrists*, **9**, 26–8.

Mackin P and Young AH (2004). Rapid cycling bipolar disorder: historical overview and focus on emerging treatments. *Bipolar Disorders*, **6**, 523–9.

Macritchie K, Geddes JR, Scott J, *et al.* (2003). *Valproate for acute mood episodes in bi-polar episodes.* 1: CD004052, Cochrane Database of Systematic Reviews.

Maden A (1996). Risk assessment in psychiatry. *British Journal of Hospital Medicine*, **56**, 78–82.

Maes HH, Woodard CE, Murrelle L, *et al.* (1999). Tobacco, alcohol and drug use in eight- to sixteen-year-old twins: the Virginia Twin Study of Adolescent Behavioral Development. *Journal of Studies on Alcohol*, **60**, 293–305.

Maguire M and Morgan M (2002). *The Oxford Handbook of Criminology.* Oxford University Press, Oxford.

Mahowald MW, Bornemann MC and Schenck CH (2004). Parasomnias. *Seminars in Neurology*, **24**, 283–92.

Maiden NL, Hurst NP, Lochhead A, *et al.* (2003). Quantifying the burden of emotional ill-health amongst patients referred to a specialist rheumatology service. *Rheumatology*, **42**, 750–7.

Maier W, Lichtermann D, Minges J, *et al.* (1993). Continuity and discontinuity of affective disorders and schizophrenia. Results of a controlled family study. *Archives of General Psychiatry*, **50**, 871–83.

Maier W, Lichtermann D, Minges J, *et al.* (1991). Unipolar depression in the aged: determinants of familial aggregation. *Journal of Affective Disorders*, **23**, 53–61.

Maina G, Forner F and Bogetto F (2005). Randomized controlled trial comparing brief dynamic and supportive therapy with waiting list condition in minor depressive disorders. *Psycotherapy and Psychosomatics*, **74**, 43–50.

Maj M (2000). Dementia due to HIV disease. In MG Gelder, JJ López-Ibor Jr and NC Andreasen, eds. *The new Oxford textbook of psychiatry*, Chapter 4.1.10. Oxford University Press, Oxford.

Maj M (2005). 'Psychiatric comorbidity': an artefact of current diagnostic systems? *British Journal of Psychiatry*, **186**, 182–4.

Major B, Cozzarelli C, Cooper ML, *et al.* (2000). Psychological responses of women after first-trimester abortion. *Archives of General Psychiatry*, **57**, 777–84.

Malaspina D and Coleman E (2003). Olfaction and social drive in schizophrenia. *Archives of General Psychiatry*, **60**, 578–84.

Malizia AL, Cunningham VJ, Bell CJ, *et al.* (1998). Decreased GABA(A) benzodiazepione receptor binding in panic disorder:preliminary results from a quantitative PET study. *Archives of General Psychiatry*, **55**, 715–20.

Mallucci G and Collinge J (2005). Rational targeting for prion therapeutics. *Nature Reviews Neuroscience*, **6**, 23–34.

Malmberg A, Simkin S and Hawton K (1999). Suicide in farmers. *British Journal of Psychiatry*, **175**, 103–5.

Malmberg L and Fenton M (2001). Individual psychodynamic psychotherapy and psychoanalysis for schizophrenia and severe mental illness. *Cochrane Database Syst Rev*, Cd001360.

Malt UF (2000). Psychiatric aspects of accidents, burns and other trauma. In MG Gelder, JJ López-Ibor Jr and NC Andreasen, eds. *The new Oxford textbook of psychiatry*, Chapter 5.3.8. Oxford University Press, Oxford.

Maltby N, Kirsch I, Mayers M, *et al.* (2002). Virtual reality exposure therapy for the treatment of fear of flying: a controlled investigation. *Journal of Consulting and Clinical Psychology*, **70**, 1112–18.

Mann JJ (2003). Neurobiology of suicidal behaviour. *Nature Reviews Neuroscience*, **4**, 819–28.

Marangell LB, Rush AJ, George MS, *et al.* (2002). Vagus nerve stimulation (VNS) for major depressive episodes: one year outcomes. *Biological Psychiatry*, **51**, 280–7.

Marazziti D, Mungai F, Gianotti D, *et al.* (2003). Kleptomania in impulse control disorders. obsessive-compulsive disoreder, and bipolar spectrum disorder: Clinical and therapeutic implications. *Current Psychiatry Reports*, **5**, 36–40.

March J, Silva S, Petrycki S, *et al.* (2004). Fluoxetine, cognitive-behavioral therapy, and their combination for adolescents with depression: Treatment for Adolescents With Depression Study (TADS) randomized controlled trial. *Journal of the American Medical Association*, **292**, 807–20.

Marder SR and Wirshing DA (2003). Maintenance treatment. In S Hirsch and D Weinberger, eds. *Schizophrenia*, 474–88. 2nd edn. Blackwells Science, Oxford.

Markovitz PJ and Wagner C (1995). Venlafaxine in the treatment of borderline personality disorder. *Psychopharmacology Bulletin*, **31**, 773–7.

Markowitz JC (2003). Interpersonal psychotherapy for chronic depression. *Journal of Clinical Psychology*, **59**, 847–58.

Marks IM (1969). *Fears and phobias.* Heinemann, London.

Marks IM (1988). Blood-injury phobia: a review. *American Journal of Psychiatry*, **145**, 1207–14.

Marks IM, Swinson RP and Basoglu M (1993a). Alprazolam and exposure alone and combined in panic disorder and agoraphobia: a controlled study in London and Toronto. *British Journal of Psychiatry*, **162**, 776–87.

Marks IM, Swinson RP, Basoglu M, *et al.* (1993b). Reply to comment on the London/Toronto study. *British Journal of Psychiatry*, **165**, 179–94.

Markus E, Lange A and Pettigrew TF (1990). Effectiveness of family therapy: a meta-analysis. *Journal of Family Therapy*, **12**, 205–21.

Marmar CR, Horowitz MJ, Weiss DS, *et al.* (1988). A controlled trial of brief psychotherapy and mutual help group treatment of conjugal bereavement. *American Journal of Psychiatry*, **145**, 203–9.

Marmor J (1953). Orality in the hysterical personality. *Journal of the American Psychoanalytic Association*, **1**, 527–31.

Marsh JC, D'Aunno TA and Smith BD (2000). Increasing access and providing social services to improve drug abuse treatment for women and children. *Addiction*, **95**, 1237–47.

Marsh L (2000). Neuropsychiatric aspects of Parkinson's Disease. *Psychosomatics*, **41**, 15–23.

Marsh L and Rao V (2002). Psychiatric complications in patients with epilepsy: a review. *Epilepsy Research*, **49**, 11–33.

Marshall EJ and Reed JL (1992). Psychiatric morbidity in homeless women. *British Journal of Psychiatry*, **160**, 761–8.

Marshall J (2000). Alcohol and drug misuse in women. In D Kohen, ed. *Women and Mental Health*, 189–217. Routledge, London.

Marshall M (1994). How should we measure need? Concept and practice in the development of a standardized assessment of need. *Philosophy Psychology and Psychiatry*, **1**, 27–36.

Marshall M (2003). Acute psychiatric day hospitals. *British Medical Journal*, **327**, 116–17.

Marshall M, Almaraz-Serrano AM, Crowther R, *et al.* (2001). *Day hospital versus outpatient care for psychiatric disorders*. 2: CD001089, Cochrane Database of Systematic Reviews.

Marshall M, Hogg L, Lockwood A, *et al.* (1995). The Cardinal Needs schedule: a modified version of the MRC Needs for Care Schedule. *Psychological Medicine*, **25**, 605–17.

Marshall M, Lewis S, Lockwood A, *et al.* (2005b). Association between duration of untreated psychosis and outcome in cohorts of first-episode patients: a systematic review. *Arch Gen Psychiatry*, **62**, 975–83.

Marshall M and Lockwood A (1998). Assertive community treatment for people with psychiatric disorders. *The cochrane Library Issue 2*. Update Software, Oxford.

Marshall M and Lockwood A (2000). *Assertive community treatment for people with severe mental disorders*. 2: CD001089, Cochrane Database of Systematic Reviews.

Marshall M and Lockwood A (2004). *Early Intervention for psychosis*. 2: CD004718, Cochrane Database of Systematic Reviews.

Marshall M, Lockwood A, Zajac-Roles G, *et al.* (2005a). Does a standardised assessment of need enhance the effectiveness of care planning for people with severe mental illness. A cluster-randomised trial. *British Journal of Psychiatry*, in press.

Martin G, Bergen HA, Richarson AS, *et al.* (2004). Correlates of firesetting in a community sample of young adolescents. *Australian and New Zealand Journal of Psychiatry*, **38**, 148–54.

Mason JW, Wang S, Yehudu R, *et al.* (2002). Marked liability in urinary cortisol levels in subgroups of combat veterans with posttraumatic stress disorder during an intensive exposure treatment program. *Psychosomatic Medicine*, **64**, 238–46.

Masters WH and Johnson VE (1970). *Human sexual inadequacy*. Churchill, London.

Mate-Kole C, Freschi M and Robin A (1990). A controlled study of psychological and social change after surgical gender reassignment in selected male transsexuals. *British Journal of Psychiatry*, **157**, 261–4.

Matson JL and Taras ME (1989). A 20 year review of punishment and alternative methods to treat problem behaviors in developmentally delayed persons. *Research in Developmental Disabilities*, **10**, 85–104.

Mattick RP, Breen C, Kimber J, *et al.* (2003a). *Methadone maintenance therapy versus no opioid replacement therapy for opioid dependence*. 2: CD002209, Cochrane Database of Systematic Reviews.

Mattick RP, Kimber J, Breen C, *et al.* (2003b). *Buprenorphine maintenance versus placebo or methadone maintenance for opioid dependence*. 2: CD002207, Cochrane Database of Systematic Reviews.

Mattson MP (2004). Pathways towards and away from Alzheimer's diesease. *Nature*, **430**, 631–9.

Mattson MP, Maudsley S and Martin B (2004). BDNF and 5-HT: a dynamic duo in age-related neuronal plasticity and neurodegenerative disorders. *Trends in Neurosciences*, **27**, 589–94.

Mattson MP and Shea TB (2003). Folate and homocysteine metabolism in neural plasticity and neurodegenerative disorders. *Trends in Neurosciences*, **26**, 137–46.

Maudsley H (1879). *The Pathology of Mind*. Macmillan, London.

Maudsley H (1885). *Responsibility in mental disease*. Kegan Paul and Trench, London.

Maughan B, Gray G and Rutter M (1985). Reading retardation and antisocial behaviour: a follow-up into employment. *Journal of Child Psychology and Psychiatry*, **25**, 741–58.

Maurer K, Volk S and Gerbaldo H (1997). Auguste D and Alzheimer's disease. *Lancet*, **349**, 1546–9.

Mavissakalian M and Perel JM (1992). Clinical experiments in maintenance and discontinuation of imipramine therapy in panic disorder with agoraphobia. *Archives of General Psychiatry*, **49**, 318–23.

Max JE, Lansing AE, Koele SL, *et al.* (2004). Attention-deficit hyperactivity disorder in children and adolescents following traumatic brain injury. *Developmental Neuropsychology*, **25**, 159–77.

May PRA (1968). *Treatment of schizophrenia*. Science House, New York.

Mayer W (1921). Über paraphrene psychosen. *Zentralblatt für die gesamte Neurologie und Psychiatrie*, **71**, 187–206.

Mayou R, Carson A and Sharpe M (2004). Psychological medicine; Obstacles to delivery. *Journal of Psychosomatic Research*, **57**, 217–8.

Mayou R and Farmer A (2002). ABC of psychological medicine: Functional somatic symptoms and syndromes. *British Medical Journal*, **325**, 265–8.

Mayou RA, Bass C and Sharpe M (1995). *Treatment of functional somatic symptoms*. Oxford University Press, Oxford.

Mayou RA, Hawton KE, Feldman E, *et al.* (1991). Psychiatric problems among medical admissions. *International Journal of Psychiatry in Medicine*, **21**, 71–84.

Mayou RA and Sharpe M (1995). Psychiatric illness associated with physical disease. *Ballieres Clinical Psychiatry*, **1**, 201–24.

Mazure CM and Maciejewski PK (2003). A model of risk for major depression: effects of life stress and cognitive style vary by age. *Depression and Anxiety*, **17**, 26–33.

McCabe R, Heath C, Burns T, *et al.* (2002). Engagement of patients with psychosis in the consultation: conversation analytic study. *British Medical Journal*, **325**, 1148–51.

McCann UD, Szabo Z, Scheffel U, *et al.* (1998). Positron emission tomographic evidence of toxic effects of MDMA ('ecstasy') on brain serotonin neurons in human beings. *Lancet*, **352**, 1433–7.

McCarty LM (1986). Mother-child incest: characteristics of the offender. *Child Welfare*, **65**, 447–59.

McClure GMG (2000). Changes in suicide in England and Wales 1960–1997. *British Journal of Psychiatry*, **176**, 64–7.

McClure RK and Lieberman JA (2003). Neurodevelopmental and neurodegenerative hypotheses of schizophrenia: a review and critique. *Current Opinion in Psychiatry*, **16**, S15–28.

McConaghy N (1998). Paedophilia; a review of the evidence. *Australian and New Zealand Journal of Psychiatry*, **32**, 252–65.

McCormack PL and Wiseman LR (2004). Olanzapine: a review of its use in the management of bipolar 1 disorder. *Drugs*, **64**, 2709–26.

McCorry D, Chadwick D and Marson A (2004). Current drug treatment of epilepsy in adults. *Lancet Neurology*, **3**, 729–35.

McDougall (1926). *An Outline of Abnormal psycology*. Methuen, London.

McFarlane AC (1988). The longitudinal course of posttraumatic morbidity. *Journal of Nervous and Mental Disease*, **176**, 30–9.

McGorry PD and Killackey EJ (2002). Early intervention in psychosis: a new evidence based paradigm. *Epidemiologia e Psichiatria Sociale*, **11**, 237–47.

McGrath AM and Jackson GA (1996). Survey of neuroleptic prescribing in residents of nursing homes in Glasgow. *British Medical Journal*, **312**, 611–2.

McGrath JJ and Murray RM (2003). Risk factors for schizophrenia: from conception to birth. In SR Hirsch and D Weinberger, eds. *Schizophrenia*, 232–50. 2nd edn. Blackwell Publishing, Oxford.

McGuffin P, Farmer AE, Gottesman II, *et al.* (1984). Twin concordance for operationally defined schizophrenia. Confirmation of familiality and heritability. *Archives of General Psychiatry*, **41**, 541–5.

McGuffin P, Katz R, Watkins S, *et al.* (1996). A hospital-based twin register of the heritability of DSM-IV. *Archives of General Psychiatry*, **53**, 129–36.

McGuffin P, Rijsdijk F, Andrew M, *et al.* (2003). The heritability of bipolar affective disorder and the genetic relationship to unipolar depression. *Archives of General Psychiatry*, **60**, 497–502.

McGuffin P and Thapar A (1992). The genetics of personality disorder. *British Journal of Psychiatry*, **160**, 12–23.

McGuire H and Hawton K (2003). Interventions for vaginismus. *Cochrane Database of Systematic Reviews*, **1**, CD 001760.

McGuire PK and Frith CD (1996). Disordered functional connectivity in schizophrenia. *Psychological Medicine*, **26**, 663–7.

McIntosh VV, Jordan J, Carter FA, *et al.* (2005). Three psychotherapies for anorexia nervosa: a randomized, controlled trial. *Am J Psychiatry*, **162**, 741–7.

McKeith I, Mintzer J, Aarsland D, *et al.* (2004). Dementia with Lewy bodies. *Lancet Neurology*, **3**, 19–28.

McKeith IG, Galasko D and Korsaka K (1996). Consensus guidelines for the clinical and pathologic diagnosis of dementia with Lewy bodies (DLB). *Neurology*, **47**, 1113–24.

McKenna PJ (1984). Disorders with overvalued ideas. *British Journal of Psychiatry*, **145**, 579–85.

McNally RJ (1994). Choking phobia: a review of the literature. *Comprehensive Psychiatry*, **35**, 83–9.

McNally RJ, Bryant RA and Ehlers A (2003). Does early psychological intervention promote recovery from post-traumatic stress. *Psychological Science in the Public Interest*, **4**, 45–79.

McNeil TF, Cantor Graae E and Weinberger DR (2000). Relationship of obstetric complications and differences in size of brain structures in monozygotic twin pairs discordant for schizophrenia. *American Journal of Psychiatry*, **157**, 203–12.

McShane R, Keene J, Gedling K, *et al.* (1997). Do neurleptic drugs hasten cognitive decline in dementia? Prospective study with necropsy follow up. *British Medical Journal*, **314**, 266–70.

Meadow R (1985). Management of Munchausen syndrome by proxy. *Archives of Diseases of Childhood*, **60**, 385–93.

Mechanic D (1978). *Medical sociology*. 2nd edn. Free Press, Glencoe.

Medford N, Baker D, Hunter E, *et al.* (2003). Chronic depersonalization following illicit drug use: a controlled analysis of 40 cases. *Addiction*, **98**, 1731–6.

Mehlum L, Friis S, Irion T, *et al.* (1991). Personality disorders 2–5 years after treatment: a prospective follow-up study. *Acta Psychiatrica Scandinavica*, **84**, 72–7.

Meichenbaum DH (1977). *Cognitive-behaviour modification*. Plenum, New York.

Meltzer H, Gatward R, Goodman R, *et al.* (2000). *The mental health of children and adolescents in Great Britain*. The Stationery Office, London.

Meltzer HY (2004). What's atypical about atypical antipsychotic drugs? *Current Opinion in Pharmacology*, **1**, 53–7.

Meltzer HY, Alphs L, Green AI, *et al.* (2003). Clozapine treatment for suicidality in schizophrenia: International Suicide Prevention Trial (InterSePT). *Archives of General Psychiatry*, **60**, 82–91.

Mendelson G (1995). 'Compensation neurosis' revisited: outcome studies of the effects of litigation. *Journal of Psychosomatic Research*, **39**, 695–706.

Mendelwicz J, Papadimitiou G and Wilmotte J (1993). Family study of panic disorder: comparison of generalized anxiety disorder, major depression, and normal subjects. *Psychiatric Genetics*, **3**, 73–8.

Menza MA, Kenneth R, Kaufman, *et al.* (2000). Modafinil augmentation of antidepressant treatment in depression. *Journal of Clinical Psychiatry*, 378–81.

Mercer CH, Fenton KA, Johnson AM, *et al.* (2003). Sexual function problems and help seeking behaviour in Britain: national probability sample survey. *British Medical Journal*, **327**, 426–7.

Mercier-Guidez E and Loas G (1998). Polydipsia and water intoxication in psychiatric inpatients: review of the literature. *Encephale*, **24**, 223–9.

Merry S, McDowell H, Hetrick S, *et al.* (2004). *Psychological and/or educational interventions for the prevention of depression in children and adolescents*. 1: CD003380, Cochrane Database of Systematic Reviews.

Merskey H (1999). Ethical aspects of the physical manipulation of the brain. In S Bloch, P Chodoff and SA Green, eds. *Ethical aspects of drug treatment*. 3rd edn. Oxford University Press, Oxford.

Merskey H (2000). Conversion and dissociation. In MG Gelder, JJ López-Ibor Jr and NC Andreasen, eds. *The new Oxford textbook of psychiatry*, Chapter5.2.4. Oxford University Press, Oxford.

Merson S, Tyrer P, Oynett S, *et al.* (1992). Early intervention in psychiatric emergencies: a clinical trial. *Lancet*, **339**, 1311–3.

Mesulam MM (1998). From sensation to cognition. *Brain*, **121**, 1013–52.

Meyer HA, Sinnott C and Seed PT (2003). Depressive symptoms in advanced cancer. Part 1. Assessing depression: the Mood Evaluation Questionnaire. *Palliative Medicine*, **17**, 596–603.

Meyer JH, Houle S, Sagrati S, *et al.* (2004). Brain serotonin transporter binding potential measured with carbon 11-labelled DASB Positron Emission Tomography: Effects of major depressive episodes and severity dysfunctional attitudes. *Archives of General Psychiatry*, **61**, 1271–9.

Meyer JK and Reter DJ (1979). Sex reassignment: follow up. *Archives of General Psychiatry*, **36**, 1010–15.

Meyers WC and Kemph JP (1990). DSMIII-R classification of homicidal youth: help or hindrance? *Journal of Clinical Psychiatry*, **5**, 239–42.

Mezey GC and King MB (1989). The effects of sexual assault on men: a survey of 22 victims. *Psychological Medicine*, **19**, 205–9.

Mezey GC and Robbins I (2000). The impact of criminal victimisation. In MG Gelder, JJ López-Ibor Jr and NC Andreasen, eds. *The New Oxford textbook of psychiatry*, Chapter 11.5. Oxford University Press, Oxford.

Mezzich JE, Kirmayer LJ, Kleinman A, *et al.* (1999). The place of culture in DSM-IV. *Journal of Nervous and Mental Disease*, **187**, 457–64.

Mezzich JE, Olero-Ojeda AA and Lee S (2000). International psychiatric diagnosis. In BJ Sadock and VA Sadock, eds. *The comprehensive textbook of psychiatry*. 7th edn. Lippincott, Williams & Wilkins, Philadelphia.

Michael RT, Gagnon JH, Laumann EO, *et al.* (1994). *Sex in America; a definitive survey*. Little Brown and Company, London.

Michelson D, Dantendorfer K, Knezevic A, *et al.* (2001). Efficacy of usual antidepressant dosing regimens of fluoxetine for panic disorder. *British Journal of Psychiatry*, **179**, 514–8.

Milev P, Ho B-C, Arndt S, *et al.* (2005). Predictive values of neurocognition and negative symptoms on functional outcome in schizophrenia: A longitudinal first-episode study with 7-year follow-up. *American Journal of Psychiatry*, **162**, 495–506.

Miller FG (2000). Placebo-controlled trials in psychiatric research: an ethical perspective. *Biological Psychiatry*, **47**, 707–16.

Miller H (1961). Accident neurosis. *British Medical Journal*, **1**, 919–25, 992–8.

Miller K and Klauber GT (1990). Desmopressin acetate in children with severe primary nocturnal enuresis. *Clinical Therapeutics*, **12**, 357–66.

Miller WR and Rollnick S (1991). *Motivational interviewing: preparing people to change addictive behaviour*. Guildford Press, London.

Miller WR and Wilbourne PL (2002). A methodological analysis of treatments for alcohol use disorders. *Addiction*, **97**, 265–77.

Milne JM, Garrison CZ, Addy CL, *et al.* (1995). Frequency of phobic disorder in a community sample of young adolescents. *Journal of the American Academy of Child and Adolescent Psychiatry*, **34**, 1202–11.

Minuchin S, Rosman B and Baker L (1978). *Psychosomatic families: anorexia nervosa in context*. Harvard University Press.

Mir S and Taylor D (1999). Serotonin syndrome. *Psychiatric Bulletin*, **23**, 742–7.

Mirra SS, Heyman A, McKeel D, *et al.* (1991). The Consortium to Establish a Registry for Alzheimer's Disease (CERAD). Part II. Standardization of the neuropathologic assessment of Alzheimer's disease. *Neurology*, **41**, 479–86.

Mirrlees-Black C (1999). *Domestic violence: Findings from a new British Crime survey self-completion questionnaire*. Home Office, London.

Mishara AL and Goldberg TE (2004). A meta-analysis and critical review of the effects of conventional neuroleptic treatment on cognition in schizophrenia: opening a closed book. *Biological Psychiatry*, **55**, 1013–22.

Mitchell W, Falconer MA and Hill D (1954). Epilepsy with fetishism relieved by temporal lobectomy. *Lancet*, **2**, 626–30.

Moberg PJ, Agrin R, Gur RE, *et al.* (1999). Olfactory dysfunction in schizophrenia: a qualitative and quantitative review. *Neuropsychopharmacology*, **21**, 325–40.

Modestin J, Huber A, Satirli E, *et al.* (2003). Long-term course of schizophrenic illness: Bleuler's study reconsidered. *American Journal of Psychiatry*, **160**, 2202–8.

Mollica R (2000). The special psychiatric problems of refugees. In MG Gelder, JJ López-Ibor Jr and NC Andreasen, eds. *The New Oxford textbook of psychiatry*, Chapter 7.10.1. Oxford University Press, Oxford.

Monaco F and Cicolin A (1999). Interactions between anticonvulsant and psychoactive drugs. *Epilepsia*, **40 Suppl 10**, S71–6.

Monahan J (1997). Clinical and acturial predictions of violence. In D Faigman, D Kaye, M Saks and J Sanders, eds. *Modern scientific evidence: the law and science of expert testimony*, 309. West Publishing, St Paul, MN.

Monahan J, Steadman HJ and Appelbaum PS (2000). Developing a clinically useful actuarial tool for assessing violence risk. *British Journal of Psychiatry*, **176**, 312–9.

Money J, Schwartz M and Lewis VG (1984). Adult herotosexual status and fetal hormonal masculinization and demasculinization: 46 XX congenital virilizing adrenal hyperplasia and 46 XY androgen-insensitivity syndrome compared. *Psychoneuroendocrinology*, **9**, 405–14.

Monk CS and Pine DS (2004). Childhood anxiety disorders: A cognitive neurobiological perspective. In EJ Nestler and DS Charney, eds. *Neurobiology of Mental illness*, 1022–46. Oxford University Press Inc.,

Monteiro W, Marks IM and Ramm E (1985). Marital adjustment and treatment outcome in agoraphobia. *British Journal of Psychiatry,* **146**, 383–90.

Montgomery C (2002). Role of dynamic group therapy in psychiatry. *Advances in Psychiatric Treatment,* **8**, 34–41.

Montgomery SA and Asberg M (1979). A new depression rating scale designed to be sensitive to change. *British Journal of Psychiatry,* **134**, 382–9.

Moore DJ, West AB, Dawson VL, *et al.* (2005). Molecular pathophysiology of Parkinson's disease. *Annual Review of Neuroscience,* **28**, 55–84.

Moran E (2000). Special psychiatric problems relating to gambling. In MG Gelder, JJ López-Ibor Jr and NC Andreasen, eds. *The new Oxford textbook of psychiatry*, Chapter 4.13.3. Oxford University Press, Oxford.

Moran P, Jenkins R, Tylee A, *et al.* (2000). The prevalence of personality.disorder among UK primary care attenders. *Acta Psychiatrica Scandinavica,* **102**, 52–7.

Morano S (2003). Pathophysiology of diabetic dysfunction. *Journal of Endocrinological Investigation,* **26**, 25–9.

Morch WT, Skar J and Andersgard AB (1997). Mentally retarded persons as parents: prevalence and the situation of their children. *Scandinavian Journal of Psychology,* **38**, 343–8.

Morgagni GB (1769). *The seats and causes of diseases investigated by anatomy.* Transl B Alexander. Millar, London.

Morgan C, Mallett R, Hutchinson G, *et al.* (2005). Pathways to care and ethnicity. 1: Sample characteristics and compulsory admission. Report from the AESOP study. *Br J Psychiatry*, **186**, 281–9.

Morimoto K, Miyatake R, Nakamura M, *et al.* (2002). Delusional disorder: molecular genetic evidence for dopamine psychosis. *Neuropsychopharmacology,* **26**, 794–801.

Morin CM, Colecchi C, Stone J, *et al.* (1999). Behavioral and pharmacological therapies for late-life insomnia. *Journal of the American Medical Association,* **281**, 991–9.

Morley S, Eccleston C and Williams A (1999). Systematic review and met-analysis of randomized controlled trials of cognitive therapy and behaviour therapy for chronic pain in adults, excluding headache. *Pain,* **80**, 1–13.

Morris JB and Beck AT (1974). The efficacy of antidepressant drugs. A review of research (1958–1972). *Archives of General Psychiatry,* **30**, 667–74.

Morris JH and Nagy Z (2004). Alzheimer's disease. In MM Esiri, VM Lee and JQ Trojanowski, eds. *The neuropathology of dementia*, 161–206. 2nd edn. Cambridge University Press, Cambridge.

Morris RG (1997). Cognition and ageing. In R Jacoby and C Oppenheimer, eds. *Psychiatry in the elderly*, 37–62. Oxford University Press, Oxford.

Morris RG, Morris LW and Britton PG (1988). Factors affecting the emotional wellbeing of the caregivers of dementia sufferers. *British Journal of Psychiatry,* **153**, 147–56.

Morselli E (1886). Sulla dismorfofobia e sulla tabefobia. *Bolletin Academica Medica,* **VI**, 110–19.

Mortimer AM (2004). Novel antipsychotics in schizophrenia. *Expert Opinion On Investigational Drugs,* **13**, 315–29.

Mount RH, Hastings RP, Reilly S, *et al.* (2000). Behavioural and emotional features of Rett syndrome. *Disability and Rehabilitation,* **23**, 129–38.

Mueller M, Hackmann A and Croft A (2004). Post-traumatic stress disorder. In J Bennett-Levy, G Butler and M Fennel, eds. *Oxford guide to behavioural experiments in cognitive therapy*, Chapter 9. Oxford University Press,

Mueser KT and McGurk SR (2004). Schizophrenia. *Lancet,* **363**, 2063–72.

Mufson L, *et al.* (2004). A randomised effectiveness trial of interpersonal psychotherapy for depressed adolescents. *Archives of General Psychiatry,* **61**, 577–84.

Mukherjee AS, Hollins S, Abou-Saleh M, *et al.* (2005). Low level alcohol consumption and the fetus. *British Medical Journal,* **330**, 375–6.

Mukherjee S, Sackheim HA and Lee C (1988). Electroconvulsive therapy of acute manic episodes: a review of fifty years experience. *Convulsive Therapy,* **4**, 74–80.

Mukherjee S, Sackheim HA and Schnur DB (1994). Electroconvulsive therapy of acute manic episodes: a review of fifty years experience. *American Journal of Psychiatry,* **151**, 169–76.

Mulholland C and Cooper S (2000). The symptom of depression in schizophrenia and its management. *Advances in Psychiatric Treatment,* **6**, 169–77.

Mullen P, Pathé M and Purcell R (2000). *Stalkers and their victims.* Cambridge University Press, Cambridge.

Mullen PD (1997). Compliance becomes concordance. *British Medical Journal,* **314**, 691–2.

Mullen PE (2000). Dangerousness, risk and the prediction of probability. In MG Gelder, JJ López-Ibor Jr and NC Andreasen, eds. *The new Oxford textbook of psychiatry*, Chapter 11.4.3. Oxford University Press, Oxford.

Mullen PE (2004). The Autogenic (self-generated) massacre. *Behaviour Sciences and the Law,* **22**, 311–23.

Mullen PE and Maack LH (1985). Jealousy, pathological jealousy and aggression. In DP Farington and J Gunn, eds. *Aggression and dangerousness.* Wiley, Chichester.

Mullen PE and Martin J (1994). Jealousy: a community study. *British Journal of Psychiatry,* **164**, 35–43.

Mullen PE, Martin JL and Anderson JC (1993). Childhood sexual abuse and mental health in adult life. *British Journal of Psychiatry,* **163**, 35–43.

Muller-Oerlinghausen B, Berghofer A and Ahrens B (2003). The antisuicidal and mortality-reducing effect of lithium prophylaxis: consequences for guidelines in clinical psychiatry. *Canadian Journal of Psychiatry,* **48**, 433–9.

Mundo E, Richter MA, Zai G, *et al.* (2002). 5HT1D receptor gene implicated in the pathogenesis of obsessive compulsive disorder: further evidence from a family based association study. *Molecular Psychiatry,* **7**, 805–9.

Munoz DG, Dickson DW, Bergeron C, *et al.* (2003). The neuropathology and biochemistry of frontotemporal dementia. *Annals of Neurology,* **54 Suppl 5**, S24–8.

Munro A (2000). Persistent delusional symptoms and disorders. In MG Gelder, JJ López-Ibor Jr and NC Andreasen, eds. *The new Oxford textbook of psychiatry*, Chapter 4.4. Oxford University Press, Oxford.

Munroe RL (1955). *Schools of psychoanalytic thought.* Hutchinson Medical, London.

Murphy G (1994). Services for children and adolescents with severe learning difficulties (mental retardation). In M Rutter, E Taylor and L Hersov, eds. *Child and adolescent psychiatry: modern approaches*, 1023–39. 3rd edn. Blackwell Scientific Publications, Oxford.

Murphy GE (1982). Social origins of depression in old age. *British Journal of Psychiatry,* **141**, 135–42.

Murphy GE, Wetzel RD, Robins E, *et al.* (1992). Multiple risk factors predict suicide and alcoholism. *Archives of General Psychiatry,* **49**, 459–63.

Murphy KC (2002). Schizophrenia and velo-cardio-facial syndrome. *Lancet,* **359**, 426–30.

Murray J, Ehlers A and Mayou RA (2002). Dissociation and posttraumatic stress disorder: two prospective studies of road traffic accident victims. *British Journal of Psychiatry,* **180**, 363–8.

Murray J and Williams P (1986). Self-reported illness and general practice consultations in Asian born and British born residents of West London. *Social Psychiatry,* **21**, 139–45.

Murray JB (1998). Psychopharmacological therapy of deviant sexual behaviour. *Journal of General Psychology,* **115**, 101–10.

Murray L and Cooper PJ (1997). Postpartum depression and child development. *Psychological Medicine,* **27**, 253–60.

Murray RM and Lewis SW (1987). Is schizophrenia a neurodevelopmental disorder? *British Medical Journal,* **295**, 681–2.

Murray RM and Reveley A (1981). The genetic contribution to the neuroses. *British Journal of Hospital Medicine,* **25**, 185–90.

Mutanski BS, Chivers ML and Bailey JM (2002). A critical review of recent biological research on human sexual orientation. *Annual Review of Sex Research,* **13**, 89–140.

Mynors-Wallace LM, Gath DH, Day A, *et al.* (2000). Randomized contrlled trial of problem solving treatment, antidepressant medication and combined treatment for major depression in primary care. *British Medical Journal,* **320**, 26–30.

Mynors-Wallace LM, Gath DH, Lloyd-Thomas AR, *et al.* (1995). Randomized controlled trial comparing problem solving treatment with amitriptyline and placebo for major depression in primary care. *British Medical Journal,* **310**, 441–5.

Nadiga DN, Hensley PL and Uhlenhuth EH (2003). Review of the long-term effectiveness of cognitive behavioural therapy compared to medications in panic disorder. *Depression and Anxiety,* **17**, 58–64.

Nagy Z, Esiri MM, Jobst KA, *et al.* (1997). The effects of additional pathology on the cognitive deficit in Alzheimer disease. *Journal of Neuropathology and Experimental Neurology,* **56**, 165–70.

Narrow WE, Rae DS, Robins LN, *et al.* (2002). Revised prevalence estimates in mental disorders in the United States: using a clinical significance criterion to reconcile 2 survey's estimates. *Archives of General Psychiatry,* **59**, 115–23.

Nathan PJ (1999). The experimental and clinical pharmacology of St John's Wort *(Hypericum perforatum L.). Molecular Psychiatry,* **4**, 333–8.

National Institute for Clinical Excellence (2000). *Guidance on the use of methylphenindate for attention deficit-hyperactivity disorder (ADHD) in childhood.* Technology Appraisal Guidance No. 13, National Institute for Clinical Excellence, London. http://www.nice.org.uk

National Institute for Clinical Excellence (2001). *Guidance on the use of donepezil, rivastigmine and galantamine for the treatment of Alzheimer's disease.* Technology Appraisal Guidance No. 19, National Institute for Clinical Excellence, London. http://www.nice.org.uk

National Institute for Clinical Excellence (2002). *Guidance on the use of newer (atypical) antipsychotic drugs for the treatment of schizophrenia.* Technology Appraisal Guidance No. 43, National Institute for Clinical Excellence, London. http://www.nice.org.uk

National Institute for Clinical Excellence (2004a). *Anxiety: management of anxiety (panic disorder, with and without agoraphobia, and generalized anxiety disorder) in adults in primary, secondary and community care.* 22, National Institute for Clinical Excellence, London. http://www.nice.org.uk

National Institute for Clinical Excellence (2004b). *Eating Disorders: Core interventions in the treatment and management of anorexia nervosa, bulimia nervosa and eating disorders.* National Institute for Clinical Excellence, London. http://www.nice.org.uk

National Institute for Clinical Excellence (2004c). *Self-harm: the short-term physical and psychological management and secondary prevention of self-harm in primary and secondary care.* Clinical Guideline 16, National Institute for Clinical Excellence, London. http://www.nice.org.uk

National Institute for Clinical Excellence (2004d). *Depression: management of depression in primary and secondary care.* Clincial Guideline 23, National Institute for Clinical Excellence, London. http://www.nice.org.uk

National Institute for Clinical Excellence (2005a). *Depression in children.* in development, National Institute for Clinical Excellence, London. http://www.nice.org.uk

National Institute for Clinical Excellence (2005b). *Attention-deficit hyperactivity disorder: pharmacological and psychological interventions in children young people and adults.* in development, National Institute for Clinical Excellence, London. http://www.nice.org.uk

National Institute for Clinical Excellence (2005c). *Violence. The short-term management of disturbed/violent behaviour in psychiatric in-patient settings and emergency departments.* Clinical Guideline 25, National Institute for Clinical Excellence, London. http://www.nice.org.uk

National Institutes of Health Consensus Development Panel (1999). Rehabilitation of persons with traumatic brain injury. *JAMA,* **282**, 1974–83.

Nazareth I, Boynton P and King M (2003). Problems of sexual function in people attending London general practioners: a cross sectional study. *British Medical Journal,* **327**, 420–6.

Neary D, Snowden JS, Gustafson L, *et al.* (1998). Frontotemporal lobar degeneration: a consensus on clinical diagnostic criteria. *Neurology,* **51**, 1546–54.

Neary D, Snowden J and Mann D (2005). Frontotemporal dementia. *Lancet Neurol*, **4**, 771–80.

Needleman H, Gunnoe C, Leviton A, *et al.* (1979). Deficits in psychologic and classroom performances of children with elevated dentine lead levels. *New England Journal of Medicine*, **300**, 689–95.

Needleman HL (1998). Childhood lead poisoning: the promise and the abandonment of primary prevention. *American Journal of Public Health*, **88**, 1871–7.

Neeleman J and Wessely S (1997). Changes in classification of suicide in England and Wales: time trends and associations with coroners' professional backgrounds. *Psychological Medicine*, **21**, 467–72.

Neligan G and Prudham D (1969). Norms for four standard developmental milestones by sex, social class and place in the family. *Developmental Medicine and Child Neurology*, **11**, 413–22.

Nelson JC (2003). Managing treatment-resistant major depression. *Journal of Clinical Psychiatry*, **64**, 5–12.

Nestor PJ, Scheltens P and Hodges JR (2004). Advances in the early detection of Alzheimer's disease. *Nature Medicine*, **10 Suppl**, S34–41.

Nettle D (2004). Evolutionary origins of depression: a review and reformulation. *Journal of Affective Disorders*, **81**, 91–102.

Neugebauer R (2005). Accumulating evidence for prenatal nutritional origins of mental disorders. *JAMA*, **294**, 621–3.

Neumann D, Housekamp B, Pollock V, *et al.* (1996). The long-term sequellae of child sexual abuse in women. *Child Maltreatment*, **1**, 6–16.

Neuropathology Group of the Medical Research Council Cognitive Function and Ageing Study MC (2001). Pathological correlates of late-onset dementia in a multicentre, community-based population in England and Wales. *Lancet*, **357**, 169–175.

New AS, Trestman RF, Mitropoulou V, *et al.* (2004). Low prolactin response to fenfluramine in impulsive aggression. *Journal of Psychiatric Research*, **38**, 223–30.

NICHD Early Child Care Research Network (1997). The effects of infant care on infant-mother attachment security: results of the NICHD Study of Early Child Care. *Child Development*, **68**, 860–79.

Nichols DE (2004). Hallucogenics. *Pharmacology and Therapeutics*, **101**, 131–81.

Nigg J and Goldsmith H (1994). Genetics of personality disorders: Perspectives from personality and psychopathology research. *Psychological Bulletin*, **115**, 346–80.

Nihira K, Foster R, Shellhaas M, *et al.* (1975). *AAMD Adaptive Behavior Scale: Residential (ABS-R) American Association on Mental Deficiency (AAMD)*. Washington, DC.

Nillson A (1993). The anti-aggressive actions of lithium. *Reviews in Contemporary Psychopharmacology*, **4**, 269–85.

Nimgaonkar VL, Fujiwara TM, Dutta M, *et al.* (2000). Low prevalence of psychoses among the Hutterites, an isolated religious community. *American Journal of Psychiatry*, **157**, 1065–70.

Nirje B (1970). Normalisation. *Journal of Mental Subnormality*, **31**, 62–70.

Nock MK and Marzuk PM (2000). Suicide and violence. In K Hawton and K van Heeringen, eds. *The International Handbook of Suicide and Attempted Suicide*. John Wiley & Sons, Chichester.

Nolen WA, Van de Putte JJ and Dijken WA (1988). Treatment strategy in depression. 2. MAO inhibitors in depression resistant tricyclic antidepressants: two controlled cross-over studies with tranylcypromine versus 1,5-hydroxytryptophan and nomifensine. *Acta Psychiatrica Scandinavica*, **78**, 676–83.

Nordentoft M, Laursen TM, Agerbo E, *et al.* (2004). Change in suicide rates for patients with schizophrenia in Denmark, 1981–97: nested case-control study. *British Medical Journal*, **329**, 261.

Norman RM and Malla AK (1993). Stressful life events and schizophrenia. I: A review of the research. *British Journal of Psychiatry*, **162**, 161–6.

Nowell PD, Mazumdar S, Buysse DJ, *et al.* (1997). Benzodiazepines and zolpidem for chronic insomnia: a meta-analysis of treatment efficacy. *Journal of the American Medical Association*, **278**, 2170–7.

Noyes R (2000). Hypochondriasis. In MG Gelder, JJ López-Ibor Jr and NC Andreasen, eds. *The new Oxford textbook of psychiatry*, Chapter 5.2.5. Oxford University Press, Oxford.

Nuechterlein KH and Dawson ME (1984). A heuristic vulnerability/stress model of schizophrenic episodes. *Schizophrenia Bulletin*, **10**, 300–12.

Nussbaum RL and Ellis CE (2003). Alzheimer's disease and Parkinson's disease. *New England Journal of Medicine*, **348**, 1356–64.

Nutt D (2001). Neurobiological mechanisms in generalized anxiety disorder. *Journal of Clinical Psychiatry*, **62**, 22–7.

Nutt D and Bell C (1997). Practical pharmacotherapy for anxiety. *Advances in Psychiatric Treatment*, **3**, 79–85.

Nutt D and Lawson C (1992). Panic attacks: a neurochemical overview of models and mechanisms. *British Journal of Psychiatry*, **160**, 165–78.

Nutt D, J and Malizia AL (2004). Structural and functional brain changes in posttraumatic stress disorder. *Journal of Clinical Psychiatry*, **65**, 11–17.

Oates RK, Peacock A and Forrest D (1985). Longterm effects of non-organic failure to thrive. *Paediatrics*, **75**, 36–40.

O'Brien JT, Erkinjuntti T, Reisberg B, *et al.* (2003). Vascular cognitive impairment. *Lancet Neurology*, **2**, 89–98.

O'Brien JT, Lloyd A, McKeith I, *et al.* (2004). A Longitudinal study of hippocampal volume, cortisol levels, and cognition in older depressed subjects. *American Journal of Psychiatry*, **161**, 2081–90.

Ochberg S, Christiansen PE, Benke K, *et al.* (1995). Paroxetine in the treatment of panic disorder: a randomized, double-blind controlled study. *British Journal of Psychiatry*, **167**, 374–9.

O'Connor N (1968). Psychology and intelligence. In M Shepherd and DL Davis, eds. *Studies in psychiatry*. Oxford University Press, London.

O'Connor TG (2002). Attachment disorders in infancy and childhood. In M Rutter and E Taylor, eds. *Child and Adolescent Psychiatry*, Chapter 46. 4th edn. Blackwell Publishing, Oxford.

Ødegaard Ø (1932). Emigration and insanity. *Acta Psychiatrica Scandinavica*, **Suppl 4**.

O'Donnell T, Hegadoren KM and Coupland NC (2004). Noradrenergic mechanisms in the pathophysiology of post-traumatic stress disorder. *Neuropsychobiology*, **50**, 273–83.

Office for National Statistics (2003). Statistics on Alcohol: England. *Statistical Bulletin*.

Offord DR (2000). Epidemiology of psychiatric disorder in childhood and adolescence. In MG Gelder, JJ López-Ibor Jr and NC Andreasen, eds. *The new Oxford textbook of psychiatry*, Chapter 9.1.3. Oxford University Press, Oxford.

Offord DR and Bennett K (2002). Prevention. in child and adolescent psychiatry. In M Rutter and E Taylor, eds. *Child and Adolescent Psychiatry*, Chapter 52. 4th edn. Blackwell Publishing, Oxford.

Offord DR, Boyle MH, Szatmari P, *et al.* (1987). Ontario Child Health Study. I Six month prevalence of disorder and service utilization. *Archives of General Psychiatry*, **44**, 832–6.

Ohayon MM and Lemoine P (2004). Sleep and insomnia markers in the general population. *Encephale*, **2**, 135–40.

Old Age Depression Interest Group (1993). How long should the elderly take antidepressants? A doubleblind placebo controlled study of continuation/prophylaxis therapy with dothiepin. *British Journal of Psychiatry*, **162**, 175–82.

Olney JW and Farber NB (1995). Glutamate receptor dysfunction and schizophrenia. *Archives of General Psychiatry*, **52**, 998–1007.

O'Malley PG, Balden E, Tomkins G, *et al.* (2000). Treatment of fibromyalgia with antidepressants: a meta-analysis. *Journal of General Internal Medicine*, **15**, 659–66.

O'Malley PG, Jackson JL, Santoro J, *et al.* (1999). Antidepressant therapy for unexplained symptoms and symptom syndromes. *Journal of Family Practice*, **48**, 980–90.

Oppenheimer C (2000). Special features of psychiatric treatment for the elderly. In MG Gelder, JJ López-Ibor Jr and NC Andreasen, eds. *The new Oxford textbook of psychiatry*, Chapter 8.6. Oxford University Press, Oxford.

Öst LG (1987a). Age of onset of different phobias. *Journal of Abnormal Psychology*, **96**, 223–9.

Öst LG (1987b). Applied relaxation: description of a coping technique and review of controlled studies. *Behaviour Research and Therapy*, **25**, 397–409.

Öst LG, Alm T, Brandberg M, *et al.* (2001). One versus five sessions of exposure and five sessions of cognitive therapy in the treatment of claustrophobia. *Behaviour Research and Therapy*, **39**, 167–81.

Öst LG and Breitholtz E (2000). Applied relaxation vs. cognitive therapy in the treatment of generalized anxiety disorder. *Behaviour Research and Therapy*, **38**, 777–90.

Ottenbacher KJ and Cooper HM (1983). Drug treatment of hyperactivity in children. *Developmental Medicine and Child Neurology*, **25**, 358–66.

Overall JE and Gorham DR (1962). The Brief Psychiatric Rating Scale. *Psychological Reports*, **10**, 799–812.

Ovsiew F (2004). Antiepileptic drugs in psychiatry. *Journal of Neurology, Neurosurgery and Psychiatry*, **75**, 1655–8.

Owen MJ, Cardno AG and O'Donovan MC (2000). Psychiatric genetics: back to the future. *Molecular Psychiatry*, **5**, 22–31.

Owen MJ, Williams NM and O'Donovan MC (2004). The molecular genetics of schizophrenia: new findings promise new insights. *Molecular Psychiatry*, **9**, 14–27.

Owens D, Horrocks J and House A (2003). Fatal and non-fatal repetition of self-harm: systematic review. *British Journal of Psychiatry*, **181**, 193–9.

Oyefeso A, Ghodse H, Clancy C, *et al.* (1999). Suicide among drug addicts in the UK. *British Journal of Psychiatry*, **175**, 277–82.

Padma-Nathan H, Goldstein I, Payton T, *et al.* (1987). Intracavernosal pharmacotherapy: the pharmacological erection program. *World Journal of Urology*, **5**, 160–5.

Padma-Nathan H, Hellstrom WG, Kaiser FE, *et al.* (1997). Treatment of men with erectile dysfunction with transurethral alprostadil. *New England Journal of Medicine*, **336**, 1–7.

Padwal R, Li SK and Lau DC (2003). Long-term pharmacotherapy for overweight and obesity: a systematic review and meta-analysis of randomized controlled trials. *International Journal of Obesity and Related Metabolic Disorders*, **27**, 1437–46.

Page GP, George V, Go RC, *et al.* (2003). 'Are we there yet?': Deciding when one has demonstrated specific genetic causation in complex diseases and quantative traits. *American Journal of Human Genetics*, **73**, 711–9.

Palazzoli M, Boscolo L, Cecchin G, *et al.* (1978). *Paradox and counterparadox*. Aronson, New York, NY.

Palmer B (2000). Helping people with eating disorders. *A Clinical guide to assessment and treatment*. John Wiley, Chichester.

Palmer BA, Pankratz VS and Bostwick JM (2005). The lifetime risk of suicide in schizophrenia: A reexamination. *Archives of General Psychiatry*, **62**, 247–53.

Palmer R (2004). Bulimia nervosa: 25 years on. *British Journal of Psychiatry*, **185**, 447–8.

Palmer RL (2002). Dialectcal behavior therapy for borderline personality disorder. *Advances in Psychiatric Treatment*, **8**, 10–16.

Pantelis C, Velakoulis D, McGorry PD, *et al.* (2003). Neuroanatomical abnormalities before and after onset of psychosis: a cross-sectional and longitudinal MRI comparison. *Lancet*, **361**, 281–8.

Pantev C, Oostenveld R, Engelien A, *et al.* (1998). Increased auditory cortical representation in musicians. *Nature*, **392**, 811–4.

Pantoni L (2004). Treatment of vascular dementia: evidence from trials with non-cholinergic drugs. *Journal of the Neurological Sciences*, **226**, 67–70.

Pantoni L, Lamassa M and Inzitari D (2000). Transient global amnesia: a review emphasizing pathogenic aspects. *Acta Neurologica Scandinavica*, **102**, 275–83.

Parker G, Roy K, Wilhelm K, *et al.* (2001). Assesing the comparative effectiveness of antidepressants therapies: a prospective clinical practice study. *Journal of Clinical Psychiatry*, **62**, 117–25.

Parkes CM, Benjamin B and Fitzgerald RG (1969). Broken heart: a statistical study of increased mortality among widowers. *British Medical Journal*, **1**, 740–3.

Parkes CM and Brown RJ (1971). The first year of bereavement: a longitudinal study of the reaction of London widows. *Psychiatry*, **33**, 444–6.

Parkes CM and Brown RJ (1972). Health after bereavement: a controlled study of young Boston widows and widowers. *Psychosomatic Medicine*, **34**, 449–61.

Parnas J, Cannon TD, Jacobsen B, *et al.* (1993). Lifetime DSM-III-R diagnostic outcomes in the offspring of schizophrenic mothers. Results from the Copenhagen High-Risk Study. *Archives of General Psychiatry*, **50**, 707–14.

Parnas J, Schulsinger F, Teasdale TW, *et al.* (1982). Perinatal complications and clinical outcome within the schizophrenia spectrum. *British Journal of Psychiatry*, **140**, 416–20.

Parry-Jones B and Parry-Jones WL (1992). Pica: symptom or eating disorder? A historical assessment. *British Journal of Psychiatry*, **160**, 341–54.

Parry-Jones WL (1972). *The trade in lunacy*. Routledge & Kegan Paul, London.

Parsons T (1951). *The Social System*. Free Press, Glencoe.

Pasamanick B and Knobloch H (1966). Retrospective studies on the epidemiology of reproductive casualty: old and new. *Merril-Palmer Quarterly of Behavioral Development*, **12**, 7–26.

Pasmanick B, Scarpitti FR and Lefton M (1964). Home versus hospital care for schizophrenics. *Journal of the American Medical Association*, **187**, 177–81.

Pasquier F, Fukui T, Sarazin M, *et al.* (2003). Laboratory investigations and treatment in frontotemporal dementia. *Annals of Neurology*, **54 Suppl 5**, S32–5.

Patel MX, Smith DG, Chalder T, *et al.* (2003). Chronic fatigue syndrome in children: a cross-sectional survey. *Archives of Disease in Childhood*, **88**, 894–8.

Paterson RJ (2000). *The Assertiveness Workbook: How to Express Your Ideas and Stand Up for Yourself at Work and in Relationships.* New Harbinger Publications.

Pathé M, Mullen PE and Purcell R (1999). Stalking: false claims of victimisation. *British Journal of Psychiatry*, **174**, 170–2.

Pato MT, Zohar-Kadouch R, Zohar J, *et al.* (1988). Return of symptoms after discontinuation of clomipramine in patients with obsessive compulsive disorder. *American Journal of Psychiatry*, **145**, 1521–5.

Patterson GR (1982). *Coercive family process*. Castalia, Eugene, OR.

Patton GC, Coffey C, Carlin JB, *et al.* (2002). Cannabis use and mental health in young people: a cohort study. *British Medical Journal*, **325**, 1195–8.

Paykel ES (1978). Contribution of life events to causation of psychiatric illness. *Psychological Medicine*, **8**, 245–53.

Paykel ES, Prusoff BA and Myers JK (1975). Suicide attempts and recent life events: a controlled comparison. *Archives of General Psychiatry*, **32**, 327–33.

Paykel ES, Scott J, Teasdale JD, *et al.* (1999). Prevention of relapse in residual depression by cognitive therapy. *Archives of General Psychiatry*, **56**, 829–35.

Paykel ES (2000). Not an age of depression after all? Incidence rates may be stable over time. *Psychological Medicine*, **30**, 489–90.

Pearce J, Hawton K and Blake F (1995). Psychological and sexual symptoms associated with the menopause and the effects of hormone replacement therapy. *British Journal of Psychiatry*, **167**, 163–73.

Pedersen CB and Mortensen PB (2001). Family history, place and season of birth as risk factors for schizophrenia in Denmark: a replication and reanaylsis. *British Journal of Psychiatry*, **179**, 46–52.

Pediatric OCD Treatment Study Team (2004). Cognitive-behaviour therapy, sertraline, and their combination for children and adolescents with obsessive-compulsive disorder; the Pediatric OCD Treatment Study (POTS) randomized controlled trial. *Journal of the American Medical Association*, **292**, 1969–76.

Peen J and Dekker J (2004). Is urbanicity an environmental risk-factor for psychiatric disorders? *Lancet*, **363**, 2012–3.

Pelosi AJ and Birchwood M (2003). Is early intervention for psychosis a waste of valuable resources? *British Journal of Psychiatry*, **182**, 196–8.

Penninx BW, Geerlings SW, Deeg DJ, *et al.* (1999). Minor and major depression and the risk of death in older persons. *Archives of General Psychiatry*, **56**, 889–95.

Penrose L (1938). *A clinical and genetic study of 1280 cases of mental deficiency*. HMSO, London.

Perley MJ and Guze SB (1962). Hysteria – the stability and usefulness of clinical criteria. *New England Journal of Medicine*, **266**, 421–6.

Perlis ML, Smith MT, Orff HJ, *et al.* (2002). The effects of an orally administered cholinergic agonist on REM sleep in major depression. *Biological Psychiatry*, **51**, 457–62.

Perls T (2004). Centenarians who avoid dementia. *Trends in Neurosciences*, **27**, 633–6.

Perry DW, Benton C, Walsh M, *et al.* (2002). Mental impairment in the West Midlands: 10 years on. *Medicine, Science and the Law*, **42**, 325–33.

Perry JC, Bannon E and Ianni F (1999). Effectiveness of psychotherapy for personality disorders. *American Journal of Psychiatry*, **156**, 1312–21.

Perry RJ and Miller BL (2001). Behavior and treatment in frontotemporal dementia. *Neurology*, **56**, S46–51.

Peters SD, Wyatt GE and Finkelhor D (1986). Prevalence. In D Finkelhor, ed. *A source book on child sexual abuse*. Sage, London.

Petersen RC, Stevens JC, Ganguli M, *et al.* (2001). Practice parameter: early detection of dementia: mild cognitive impairment (an evidence-based review). Report of the Quality Standards Subcommittee of the American Academy of Neurology. *Neurology*, **56**, 1133–42.

Petronis A (2004). The origin of schizophrenia: genetic thesis, epigenetic antithesis, and resolving synthesis. *Biological Psychiatry*, **55**, 965–70.

Petronko MR, Harris SL and Kormann RJ (1994). Community based behavioral training approaches for people with mental retardation and mental illness. *Journal of Consulting and Clinical Psychology*, **62**, 49–54.

Petry NM and Simcic Jr. F (2002). Recent advances in the dissemination of contingency management techniques: clinical and research perspectives. *Journal of Substance Abuse Treatment*, **23**, 81–6.

Pezawas L, Wittchen HU, fister H, *et al.* (2003). Recurrent brief depressive disorder reinvestigated: a community sample of adolescents and young adults. *Archives of General Psychiatry*, **33**, 407–18.

Pfeffer CR (2000). Suicidal behaviour in children: an emphasis on developmental influences. In K Hawton and K van Heeringen, eds. *The international handbook of suicide and attempted suicide*. John Wiley & Sons, Chichester.

Pfohl B and Blum N (1991). Obsessive-compulsive personality disorder: A review of available data and recommendations for DSM-IV. *Journal of Personality Disorders*, **5**, 363–75.

Pfohl B, Blum N and Zimmerman M (1997). *Structured interview for DSMIV personality disorders*. American Psychiatric Association, Washington, DC.

Pharoah FM, Rathbone J, Mari JJ, *et al.* (2003). *Family intervention for schizophrenia*. 4: CD000088, Cochrane Database of Systematic Reviews.

Phelan M, Slade M, Thornicroft G, *et al.* (1995). The Camberwell Assessment of Need: the validity and reliability of an instrument to assess the needs of people with severe mental illness. *British Journal of Psychiatry*, **167**, 589–95.

Phillips KA (2000). Body dysmorphic disorder. In MG Gelder, JJ López-Ibor Jr and NC Andreasen, eds. *The new Oxford textbook of psychiatry*, Chapter 5.2.8. Oxford University Press, Oxford.

Phillips KA (2004). Psychosis in body dysmorphic disorder. *Journal of Psychiatric Research*, **38**, 63–72.

Phillips ML, Medford N, Senior C, *et al.* (2001). Depersonalization disorder: thinking without feeling. *Psychiatric Research*, **108**, 145–60.

Phipps A and O'Brien J (2002). Memory clinics and clinical governance -a UK perspective. *International Journal of Geriatric Psychiatry*, **17**, 1128–32.

Piacentini J and Langley AK (2004). Cognitive-behavioural therapy for children who have obsessive-compulsive disorder. *Journal of Clinical Psychology*, **60**, 1181–94.

Pichot P (1994). Nosological models in psychiatry. *British Journal of Psychiatry*, **164**, 232–40.

Pickles A, Rowe R, Simonoff E, *et al.* (2001). Child psychiatric symptoms and psychosocial impairement: relationship and prognostic significance. *British Journal of Psychiatry*, **179**, 230–5.

Pilling S, Bebbington P, Kuipers E, *et al.* (2002a). Psychological treatments in schizophrenia: II. Meta-analyses of randomized controlled trials of social skills training and cognitive remediation. *Psychological Medicine*, **32**, 783–91.

Pilling S, Bebbington P, Kuipers E, *et al.* (2002b). Psychological treatments in schizophrenia: I. Meta-analysis of family intervention and cognitive behaviour therapy. *Psychological Medicine*, **32**, 763–82.

Pincus HA, Wakefield Davis W and McQueen LE (1999). 'Subthreshold' mental disorders. *British Journal of Psychiatry*, **174**, 288–96.

Pines M and Schlapobevsky J (2000). Group methods in adult psychiatry. In MG Gelder, JJ López-Ibor Jr and NC Andreasen, eds. *The new Oxford textbook of psychiatry*, Chapter 6.3.6. Oxford University Press, Oxford.

Pinkham AE, Penn DL, Perkins DO, *et al.* (2003). Implications for the neural basis of social cognition for the study of schizophrenia. *American Journal of Psychiatry*, **160**, 815–24.

Pissiota A, Frans O, Michelgard A, *et al.* (2003). Amygdala and anterior cingulate cortex activation during affective startle modulation: a PET study of fear. *European Journal of Neuroscience*, **18**, 1325–31.

Pitts FN and McClure JN (1967). Lacate metabolism in anxiety neurosis. *New England Journal of Medicine*, **25**, 1329–36.

Placidi GP, Ocquendo MA, Malone KM, *et al.* (2001). Aggressivity, suicide attempts, and depression: relationship to cerebrospinal fluid monoamine metabolite levels. *Biological Psychiatry*, **50**, 783–91.

Plasky P (1991). Antidepressant usage in schizophrenia. *Schizophrenia Bulletin*, **17**, 649–57.

Pocock SJ, Smith M and Baghurst M (1994). Environmental lead and children's intelligence: a systematic review of the epidemiological evidence. *British Medical Journal*, **309**, 1189–97.

Pogarell O, Hamann C, Popperl G, *et al.* (2003). Elevated brain serotonin transporter availability in patients with obsessive-compulsive disorder. *Biological Psychiatry*, **54**, 1406–13.

Pollock VE, Briere J, Schneider L, *et al.* (1990). Childhood antecedents of antisocial behavior: Parental alcoholism and physical abusiveness. *American Journal of Psychiatry*, **147**, 1290–3.

Poolsup N, Li Wan Po A and de Oliveira IR (2000). Systematic overview of lithium treatment in acute mania. *J Clin Pharm Ther*, **25**, 139–56.

Pope HG, Jonas JM, Hudson JI, *et al.* (1983). The validity of DSM III borderline personality disorder: a phenomenological, family history, treatment response, and long term follow-up study. *Archives of General Psychiatry*, **40**, 23–30.

Portwich P and Barocka A (1998). Capgras' syndrome and other delusional misidentification syndrome (DMS). *Nervenheilkunde*, **17**, 296–300.

Posener H and Jacoby R (2002). Testamentary capacity. In R Jacoby and C Oppenheimer, eds. *Psychiatry in the elderly*. 3rd edn. Oxford University Press, Oxford.

Post F (1972). The management and nature of depressive illnesses in late life: a follow-through study. *British Journal of Psychiatry*, **121**, 393–404.

Powell GE (2000). Cognitive Assessment. In MG Gelder, JJ López-Ibor Jr and NC Andreasen, eds. *The new Oxford textbook of psychiatry*, Chapter 1.10.3.1. Oxford University Press, Oxford.

Powell J, Geddes J, Deeks J, *et al.* (2000). Suicide in psychiatric in-patients: risk factors and their predictive power. *British Journal of Psychiatry*, **176**, 266–76.

Powers PS and Santana C (2004). Available pharmacological treatments for anorexia nervosa. *Expert Opin Pharmacother*, **5**, 2287–92.

Prager S and Jeste DV (1993). Sensory impairment in late-life schizophrenia. *Schizophrenia Bulletin*, **19**, 755–72.

Pratt JH (1908). Results obtained in treatment of pulmonary tuberculosis by the class method. *British Medical Journal*, **2**, 1070–1.

Press DZ (2004). Parkinson's disease dementia – a first step? *New England Journal of Medicine*, **351**, 2547–9.

Prichard JC (1835). *A treatise on insanity*. Sherwood Gilbert and Piper, London.

Primm AB (1996). Assertive community treatment. In WR Breakey, ed. *Integrated mental health services*. Oxford University Press, New York, NY.

Pringsheim T, Davenport WJ and Lang A (2003). Tics. *Current Opinion in Neurology*, **16**, 523–7.

Prochaska JO and Diclemente CC (1986). Towards a comprehensive model of change. In WR Miller and N Heather, eds. *Treating addictive behaviors: processes of change*, 3–27. Plenum Press, New York.

Protheroe C (1969). Puerperal psychoses: a long term study, 1927–1961. *British Journal of Psychiatry*, **115**, 9–30.

Prudic J, Sackeim HA and Devanand DP (1990). Medication resistance and clinical response to electroconvulsive therapy. *Psychiatry Research*, **31**, 287–96.

Prusiner SB (2001). Shattuck lecture – neurodegenerative diseases and prions. *New England Journal of Medicine*, **344**, 1516–26.

Psychological Corporation (2004). *Wechsler Abbreviated Scales of Intelligence (WASI)*. Harcourt Assessment Co., London.

Pusey H and Richards D (2001). A systematic review of the effectiveness of psychosocial interventions for carers of people with dementia. *Aging and Mental Health*, **5**, 107–19.

Putnam FW and Loewenstein RJ (2000). Dissociative identity disorder. In BJ Sadock and VA Sadock, eds. *Comprehensive textbook of psychiatry*. 7th edn. Lippincott, Williams & Wilkins, Philadelphia.

Pyne JM, Smith J, Fortney J, *et al.* (2003). Cost-effectiveness of a primary care intervention for depressed patients. *Journal of Affective Disorders*, **74**, 23–32.

Quay HC and Werry JS (1986). *Psychopathological disorders of childhood*. 3rd edn. Wiley, New York, NY.

Quincey VL (2003). The etiology of anomalous sexual preferences in man. *Annals of the New York Academy of Sciences*, **989**, 105–17.

Quinn J and Twomey P (1998). A case of auto-erotic asphyxia in a long-term psychiatric setting. *Psychopathology*, **31**, 169–73.

Quitkin FM, Stewart JW, Mcgrath PJ, *et al.* (1993). Columbia atypical depression. A subgroup of depressives with better response to MAOI than to tricyclic antidepressants or placebo. *British Journal of Psychiatry*, **21 (Suppl)**, 30–4.

Rachman J and DeSilver P (1998). *Panic disorder, the facts*. Oxford University Press, Oxford.

Rachman S and Hodgson RJ (1980). *Obsessions and compulsions*. Prentice-Hall, Englewood Cliffs, NJ.

Radke-Yarrow M, Nottelmann E, Martinez P, *et al.* (1993). Young children of affectively ill parents: a longitudinal study of social development. *Journal of the American Academy of Child and Adolescent Psychiatry*, **31**, 68–77.

Raine A, Lencz T, Bihrle S, *et al.* (2000). Reduced prefontal gray matter and reduced autonomic activity in antisocial personality disorder. *Archives of General Psychiatry*, **57**, 119–27.

Raine R, Haines A, Sensky T, *et al.* (2002). Systematic review of mental health interventions for patients with common somatic symptoms: can research evidence from secondary care be extrapolated to primary care? *British Medical Journal*, **325**, 1082.

Rajagopal S (2004). Suicide pacts and the internet. *British Medical Journal*, **329**, 1298–9.

Ralph D and McNicolas T (2000). UK Management guidelines for erectile dysfunction. *British Medical Journal*, **321**, 499–503.

Ramchandani P and Jones DPH (2003). Treating psychological symptoms in sexually abused children: from research findings to service provision. *British Journal of Psychiatry*, **183**, 484–90.

Raphael B (1977). Preventive intervention with the recently bereaved. *Archives of General Psychiatry*, **34**.

Raphael B and Wilson J (2000). *Psychological debriefing. Theory, practice and evidence*. Cambridge University Press, Cambridge.

Rapoport RN (1960). *Community as doctor*. Tavistock Publications, London.

Rapp MA, Dahlman K, Sano M, *et al.* (2005). Neuropsychological differences between late-onset and recurrent geriatric major depression. *American Journal of Psychiatry*, **162**, 691–8.

Rappoport JL and Swedo S (2002). Obsessive Compulsive Disorder. In M Rutter and E Taylor, eds. *Child and adolescent psychiatry*, Chapter 35. Blackwell, Oxford.

Rasmussen SA and Tsuang MT (1986). Clinical characteristics and family history in DSMIII obsessive-compulsive disorder. *American Journal of Psychiatry*, **143**, 317–22.

Ravizza L, Maina G and Bogetto F (1997). Episodic and chronic OCD. *Depression and Anxiety*, **6**, 154–8.

Raz N, Lindenberger U, Rodrigue KM, *et al.* (2005). Regional brain changes in aging healthy adults: General trends, individual differences and modifiers. *Cerebral Cortex*, in press.

Regier DA (2000). Community diagnosis counts. *Archives of General Psychiatry*, **57**, 223–4.

Regier DA, Narrow WE and Rae DS (1994). The *de facto* US mental and addictive disorders service system. *Archives of General Psychiatry*, **50**, 85–94.

Rehm J, Rehn N, Room R, *et al.* (2003). The global distribution of average volume of alcohol consumption and patters of drinking. *European Addiction Research*, **9**, 147–56.

Reich J and de Girolamo G (2000). Diagnosis and classification of personality disorders. In MG Gelder, JJ López-Ibor Jr and NC Andreasen, eds. *The new Oxford textbook of pyschiatry*, Chapter 4.12.4. Oxford University Press, Oxford.

Reineke MA and Shirk SR (2005). Psychotherapy with adolescents. In GO Gabbard, JS Beck and J Holmes, eds. *Oxford textbook of psychotherapy*, Chapter 30. 4th edn. Oxford University Press, Oxford.

Reisberg B, Doody R, Stoffler A, *et al.* (2003). Memantine in moderate-to-severe Alzheimer's disease. *New England Journal of Medicine*, **348**, 1333–41.

Reiss S and Szyszko J (1983). Diagnostic overshadowing and professional experience with the mentally retarded persons. *American Journal of Mental Deficiency*, **87**, 396–402.

Remafedi G, French S, Story M, *et al.* (1998). The relationship between suicide risk and sexual orientation: results of a population based study. *American Journal of Public Health*, **88**, 57–60.

Rendell JM, Gijsman HJ, Keck P, *et al.* (2003). Olanzapine alone or in combination for acute mania. 3: CD004040, *Cochrane Database of Systematic Reviews*.

Resick PA, Nishith P, Weaver TL, *et al.* (2002). A comparison of cognitive-processing therapy with prolonged exposure and a waiting condition for the treatmen of chronic posttraumatic stress disorder in female rape victims. *Journal of Consulting and Clinical Psychology*, **70**, 867–79.

Reyes-Ortiz CA (2001). Diogenes syndrome: the self-neglect elderly. *Comprehensive Therapy*, **27**, 117–21.

Reynolds III CF, Frank E and Perel JM (1999). Nortriptyline and interpersonal psychotherapy as maintenance therapies for recurrent major depression. A randomised controlled trial in patients older than 59 years. *Journal of American Medical Association*, **281**, 39–45.

Rice F, Harold G and Thapar A (2002). The genetic aetiology of childhood depression: a review. *Journal of Child Psychology and Psychiatry*, **43**, 65–79.

Richardson RD and Engel Jr. CC (2004). Evaluation and management of medically unexplained physical symptoms. *Neurologist*, **10**, 18–30.

Richardson SK and Koller H (1992). Vulnerability and resilience in adults who were classified as mildly mentally handicapped in childhood. In B Tizard and V Varma, eds. *Vulnerability and resilience in human development*, 102–23. JKP, London.

Richman N, Stevenson J and Graham P (1982). *Preschool to school: a behavioural study*. Academic Press, London.

Rickles NK (1950). *Exhibitionism*. Lippincott, Philadelphia, PA.

Rimes K and Salkovskis PM (2000). Health screening programmes. In MG Gelder, JJ López-Ibor Jr and NC Andreasen, eds. *The new Oxford textbook of psychiatry*, Chapter 5.5. Oxford University Press, Oxford.

Rimm DC and Masters JC (1979). *Behavior therapy: techniques and empirical findings*. Academic Press, New York, NY.

Ring A, Dowrick C, Humphris G, *et al.* (2004). Do patients with unexplained physical symptoms pressurise general practitioners for somatic treatment? A qualitative study. *British Medical Journal*, **328**, 1057.

Ringel Y, Sperber AD and Drossman DA (2001). Irritable bowel syndrome. *Annual Review of Medicine*, **52**, 319–38.

Ritchie K, Artero S, Beluche I, *et al.* (2004). Prevalence of DSM-IV psychiatric disorder in the French elderly population. *British Journal of Psychiatry*, **184**, 147–52.

Ritchie K and Lovestone S (2002). The dementias. *Lancet*, **360**, 1759–66.

Ritson B (2005). Treatment for alcohol related problems. *British Medical Journal*, **330**, 139–41.

Rivers WH (1920). *Instinct and the unconscious*. Cambridge University Press, Cambridge.

Rivinus TM, Jamison DL and Graham PJ (1975). Childhood organic neurological disease presenting as psychiatric disorder. *Developmental Medicine and Child Neurology*, **23**, 747–60.

Robbins TW and Everitt BJ (1999). Drug addiction: bad habits add up. *Nature*, **398**, 567–70.

Roberts AH (1969). *Brain damage in boxers*. Pitman, London.

Roberts GW, Allsop D and Bruton C (1990b). The occult aftermath of boxing. *Journal of Neurology, Neurosurgery and Psychiatry*, **53**, 373–8.

Roberts GW, Done DJ, Bruton C, *et al.* (1990a). A 'mock up' of schizophrenia: temporal lobe epilepsy and schizophrenia-like psychosis. *Biological Psychiatry*, **28**, 127–43.

Roberts RE, Attkisson C and Rosenblatt A (1998). Prevalence of psychopathology among children and adolescents. *American Journal of Psychiatry*, **155**, 715–25.

Robertson MM (2000). Tourette syndrome, associated conditions and the complexities of treatment. *Brain*, **123**, 425–62.

Robertson MM, Trimble MR and Lees AJ (1988). The psychopathology of the Gilles de la Tourette syndrome. *British Journal of Psychiatry*, **152**, 383–90.

Robin AL, Siegel PT, Moye AW, *et al.* (1999). A controlled comparison of family versus individual therapy for adolescents with anorexia nervosa. *Journal of the Academy of Child and Adolescent Psychiatry*, **38**, 1482–9.

Robins LN (1966). *Deviant children grown up*. Williams & Wilkins, Baltimore, MD.

Robins LN (1993). Vietnam veterans' rapid recovery from heroin addiction: a fluke or normal expectation? *Addiction*, **88**, 1041–54.

Robins LN (2004). Using survey results to improve the validity of the standard psychiatric nomenclature. *Archives of General Psychiatry*, **61**, 1188–94.

Robins LN, Helzer JE, Croughan J, *et al.* (1981). National Institutes of Mental Health Diagnostic Interview Schedule. *Archives of General Psychiatry*, **38**, 381–9.

Robins LN and Price RK (1991). Adult disorders predicted by childhood conduct problems: results from the NIMH Epidemiologic Catchment Area project. *Psychiatry*, **54**, 116–32.

Robins LN and Regier DA (1991). *Psychiatric disorder in America: the epidemiological catchment area study*. Free Press, New York, NY.

Robinson GE (2000). General overview of obstetrics, gynecology and reproductive issues. In A Stoudemier, BS Fogel and DB Greenberg, eds. *Psychiatric care of the medical patient*. Oxford University Press, New York, NY.

Robinson RG (2003). Poststroke depression: prevalence, diagnosis, treatment, and disease progression. *Biological Psychiatry*, **54**, 376–87.

Robson P (2000). Introduction to substance use disorders. In MG Gelder, JJ López-Ibor Jr and N Andreasen, eds. *The new Oxford Texbook of Psychiatry*, Chapter 4.2.3.1. Oxford University Press, Oxford.

Rock P (1998). After homicide: practical and political responses to bereavement. *Clarendon Studies in Criminology*. Oxford University Press, Oxford.

Rockwood K (2004). Size of the treatment effect on cognition of cholinesterase inhibition in Alzheimer's disease. *Journal of Neurology, Neurosurgery and Psychiatry*, **75**, 677–85.

Rodin G and Abbey S (2000). Psychiatric aspects of surgery (including transplantation). In MG Gelder, JJ López-Ibor Jr and NC Andreasen, eds. *The new Oxford textbook of psychiatry*, Chapter 5.3.6. Oxford University Press, Oxford.

Rogers A, Day J, Randall F, *et al.* (2003). Patients understanding and Participation in a trial designed to improve the management of anti-psychotic medication: a qualitive study. *Social Psychiatry and Psychiatric Epidemiology*, **38**, 720–7.

Rohlff C and Hollis K (2003). Modern proteomic strategies in the study of complex neuropsychiatric disorders. *Biological Psychiatry*, **53**, 847–53.

Roman GC (2002). Vascular dementia revisited: diagnosis, pathogenesis, treatment, and prevention. *Medical Clinics of North America*, **86**, 477–99.

Ron M (2001). The prognosis of hysteria/somatization disorder. In PW Halligan, C Bass and JC Marshall, eds. *Contemporary approaches to the study of hysteria: clinical and theoretical perspectives*. Oxford University Press, Oxford.

Ron MA (1989). Psychiatric manifestations of frontal lobe tumours. *British Journal of Psychiatry*, **155**, 735–8.

Room R, Babor T and Rehm J (2005). Alcohol and public health. *Lancet*, **365**, 519–30.

Rooth F (1973). Exhibitionism, sexual violence and paedophilia. *Br J Psychiatry*, **122**, 705–10.

Rosanoff AJ, Handy LM and Rosanoff IA (1934). Criminality and delinquency in twins. *Journal of Criminal Law and Criminology*, **24**, 923–34.

Rose S, Bisson JU and Wessely S (2003). A systematic review of single-session psycholigcal interventions (debriefing). Following Trauma. *Psychotherapy and Psychosomatics*, **72**, 176–84.

Rosen RC and Leiblum SR (1987). Current approaches to the evaluation of sexual desire disorders. *Journal of Sex Research*, **23**, 141–62.

Rosenhan DL (1973). On being sane in insane places. *Science*, **179**, 250–8.

Rosenthal NE, Sack DA and Gillin JC (1984). Seasonal affective disorder: a description of the syndrome and preliminary findings wih light therapy. *Archives of General Psychiatry*, **41**, 24–30.

Ross GW and Bowen JD (2002). The diagnosis and differential diagnosis of dementia. *Medical Clinics of North America*, **86**, 455–76.

Rossler W, Loffler W, Falkenheuer B, *et al.* (1992). Does case management reduce rehospitalization rate? *Acta Psychiatrica Scandinavica*, **86**, 445–9.

Roth AJ, McClear KZ and Massie MJ (2000). Oncology. In A Stoudemier, BS Fogel and DB Greenberg, eds. *Psychiatric care of the medical patient*. Oxford University Press, New York, NY.

Roth M (1955). The natural history of mental disorder in old age. *Journal of Mental Science*, **101**, 281–301.

Roth RM and Saykin AJ (2004). Executive dysfunction in attention-deficit hyperactivity disorder: cognitive and neuroimaging findings. *Psychiatric Clinics of North America*, **27**, 83–96.

Rothbaum BO, Foa EB, Riggs DS, *et al.* (1992). A prospective examination of post-traumatic stress disorder in rape victims. *Journal of Traumatic Stress*, **5**, 455–76.

Rothbaum BO, Hodges L, Anderson PL, *et al.* (2002). Twelve month follow-up of virtual reality and standard exposure therapies for the fear of flying. *Journal of Consulting and Clinical Psychology*, **70**, 428–32.

Rothman D (1971). *The discovery of the asylum*. Little Brown, Boston, MA.

Rouhani M and Holland JC (2000). Psychiatric aspects of cancer. In MG Gelder, JJ López-Ibor Jr and NC Andreasen, eds. *The new Oxford textbook of psychiatry*, Chapter 5.3.7. Oxford University Press, Oxford.

Rouillon F (2004). Long-term therapy for generalized anxiety disorder. *European Psychiatry*, **19**, 96–101.

Rowlands MW (1988). Psychiatric and legal aspects of persistent litigation. *British Journal of Psychiatry*, **153**, 317–23.

Roy A, Nielsen D, Rylander G, *et al.* (2000). The genetics of suicidal behaviour. In K Hawton and K van Heeringen, eds. *The international handbook of suicide and attempted suicide*. John Wiley & Sons, Chichester.

Roy MA, Neale MC, Pedersen NL, *et al.* (1995). A twin study of generalized anxiety disorder and major depression. *Psychological Medicine*, **25**, 1037–49.

Royal College of Physicians (1991). *Physical signs of sexual abuse in children*. Royal College of Physicians, London.

Royal College of Psychiatrists (1993). *Consensus statement on the use of high dose antipsychotic medication*. Royal College of Psychiatrists, London.

Royal College of Psychiatrists (2000). *Good psychiatric practice*. Royal College of Psychiatrists, London.

Royal College of Psychiatrists (2001). *Diagnostic criteria for psychiatric disorders for use with adults with LD [DC-LD]*. Royal College of Psychiatrists, London.

Royal College of Psychiatrists (2005). *The Third Report of the Royal College of Psychiatrists's Special Committee on ECT*. Gaskell Press.

Royal Commission on Long Term Care (1999). *With respect to old age: long term care – rights and responsibilities*. HMSO, London.

Roy-Byrne PP and Cowley DS (1995). Course and outcome of panic disorder: a review of recent studies. *Anxiety*, **1**, 151–60.

Rüdin E (1953). Ein Beitrag zur Frage der Zwangskrankäheit, unsbesondere ihrer hereditaren Beziehungen. *Archiv fur Psychiatrie und Nervenkrankheiten*, **191**, 14–54.

Ruo B, Rumsfeld JS, Hlatky MA, *et al.* (2003). Depressive symptoms and health-related quality of life: the heart and soul study. *Journal of the American Medical Association*, **290**, 215.

Ruschena D, Mullen P, Palmer S, *et al.* (2003). Choking deaths: the role of antipsychotic medication. *British Journal of Psychiatry*, **183**, 446–50.

Rush AJ (2003). Toward an understanding of bipolar disorder and its origin. *Journal of Clinical Psychiatry*, **64**, 4–8.

Rush J, Pincus HA, First MB, *et al.* (2000). *Handbook of psychiatric measures*. American Psychiatric Association, Washington, DC.

Rushton A and Minnis H (2002). Residential and foster care. In M Rutter and E Taylor, eds. *Child and adolescent psychiatry*, Chapter 22. 4th edn. Blackwell, Oxford.

Russell DEH (1984). The prevalence and seriousness of incestuous abuse: stepfathers versus biological fathers. *Child Abuse and Neglect*, **8**, 15–22.

Russell GFM (1979). Bulimia nervosa: an ominous variant of of anorexia nervosa. *Psychological Medicine*, **9**, 429–48.

Russell GFM, Szmulker G, Dare C, *et al.* (1987). An evaluation of family therapy in anorexia nervosa and bulimia nervosa. *Archives of General Psychiatry*, **44**, 1047–56.

Rutter M (1966). *Children of sick parents: an environmental and psychiatric study*. Oxford University Press, Oxford.

Rutter M (1972). Relationships between child and adult psychiatric disorders. *Acta Psychiatrica Scandinavica*, **48**, 3–21.

Rutter M (1985). Resilience in the face of adversity: protective factors and resistance to psychiatric disorder. *British Journal of Psychiatry*, **147**, 598–611.

Rutter M (1995). Clinical implications of attachment concepts: retrospect and prospect. *Journal of Child Psychology and Psychiatry*, **36**, 549–71.

Rutter M (2002). Developmental psychopathology. In M Rutter and E Taylor, eds. *Child and adolescent psychiatry*. 4th edn. Blackwell, Oxford.

Rutter M (2005). Environmentally mediated risks for psychopathology: research strategies and findings. *Journal of the American Academy of Child and Adolescent Psychiatry*, **44**, 3–18.

Rutter M, Bailey A, Bolton P, *et al.* (1993). Autism: syndrome definition and possible genetic mechanisms. In R Plomin and GE McClearn, eds. *Nature, nurture and psychology*, 269–84. American Psychiatric Association, Washington, DC.

Rutter M, Bailey A, Bolton P, *et al.* (1994a). Autism and known medical conditions: myth and substance. *Journal of Child Psychology and Psychiatry*, **35**, 311–22.

Rutter M, Chadwick O and Shaffer D (1983). Head injury. In M Rutter, ed. *Developmental neuropsychiatry*, 83–111. Churchill Livingstone, Edinburgh.

Rutter M, Cox A, Tupling C, *et al.* (1975a). Attainment and adjustment in two geographical areas: I. Prevalence of psychiatric disorders. *British Journal of Psychiatry*, **126**, 493–509.

Rutter M, Giller H and Hagell A (1998). *Antisocial behaviour by young people.* Cambridge University Press, Cambridge.

Rutter M, Graham P and Birch HG (1970a). *A neuropsychiatric study of childhood.* Heinemann, London.

Rutter M, Graham P, Chadwick O, *et al.* (1976a). Adolescent turmoil: fact or fiction. *Journal of Child Psychology and Psychiatry*, **17**, 35–56.

Rutter M and Lockyer L (1967). A five to fifteen year follow-up study of infantile psychosis: I. Description of sample. *British Journal of Psychiatry*, **113**, 1169–82.

Rutter M and Madge N (1976). *Cycles of disadvantage: a review of research.* Heinemann, London.

Rutter M, Maughan B, Mortimer P, *et al.* (1979). *Fifteen thousand hours.* Open Books, London.

Rutter M, Silberg J, O'Connor T, *et al.* (1999). Genetics and child psychiatry: II Empirical research finding. *Journal of Child Psychology and Psychiatry*, **40**, 19–55.

Rutter M and Taylor E (2002). *Child and Adolescent Psychiatry.* 4th edn. Blackwell Publishing, Oxford.

Rutter M, Tizard J and Whitmore K (eds.) (1970b). *Education, health and behaviour.* Longmans, London.

Rutter M, Tizard J, Yule W, *et al.* (1976b). Isle of Wight Studies 1964–1974. *Psychological Medicine*, **6**, 313–32.

Rutter M, Yule B, Quinton D, *et al.* (1975b). Attainment and adjustment in two geographical areas III: Some factors accounting for area differences. *British Journal of Psychiatry*, **126**, 520–33.

Rutter ML (1999). Psychosocial adversity and child psychopathology. *British Journal of Psychiatry*, **174**, 480–93.

Rutter ML, MacDonald H, LeCouteur A, *et al.* (1990). Genetic factors in child psychiatric disorder. II Empirical findings. *Journal of Child Psychology and Psychiatry*, **31**, 39–83.

Rutz W, von Knorring L and Walinder J (1992). Long-term effects of an educational program for general practitioners given by the Swedish Committee for the prevention and treatment of depression. *Acta Psychiatrica Scandinavica*, **85**, 83–8.

Ryan R (1994). Post-traumatic stress disorder in persons with developmental disabilities. *Community Mental Health Journal*, **30**, 45–54.

Ryle A (1990). *Cognitive analytic therapy: active participation in change.* Wiley, Chichester.

Ryle A (1997). The structure and development of borderline personality disorder: a proposed model. *British Journal of Psychiatry*, **170**, 82–7.

Ryle A and Kerr IB (2002). *Introducing cognitive analytic therapy: principles and practice.* John Wiley, Chichester.

Sachdev P (1998). Schizophrenia-like psychosis and epilepsy: the status of the association. *American Journal of Psychiatry*, **155**, 325–36.

Sackeim HA (2003). Electroconvulsive therapy in schizophrenia. In S Hirsch and D Weinberger, eds. *Schizophrenia*, 517–51. 2nd edn. Blackwells Science, Oxford.

Sackett DL (1996). Evaluation of clinical method. In DJ Weatherall, JGG Ledingham and DA Warrell, eds. *Oxford Textbook of Medicine*, 15–21. 3rd edn. Oxford University Press, Oxford.

Sackett DL, Richardson WS, Rosenberg W, *et al.* (1997). *Evidence-based Medicine. How to practice and teach EBM.* Churchill Livingstone, Edinburgh.

Sackheim HA, Prudic J, Devanand DP, *et al.* (1990). The impact of medication resistance and continuation of pharmacotherapy on relapse following response to electroconvulsive therapy in major depression. *Journal of Clinical Psychopharmacology*, **10**, 96–104.

Sackheim HA, Prudic J, Devanand DP, *et al.* (1993). Effects of stimulus intensity and electro placement on the efficacy and cognitive effects of electroconvulsive therapy. *New England Journal of Medicine*, **328**, 839–46.

Sacks O (1973). *Awakenings.* Duckworth, London.

Sainsbury P and Barraclough B (1968). Differences between suicide rates. *Nature*, **220**, 1252–3.

Sakel M (1938). *The pharmacological shock treatment of schizophrenia.* Nervous and Mental Disease Publications, New York.

Salerno SM, Browning R and Jackson JL (2002). The effect of antidepressant treatment on chronic back pain: a meta-analysis. *Archives of Internal Medicine*, **162**, 19–24.

Saletu B, Anderer P, Saletu-Zyhlarz GM, *et al.* (2002). EEG topography and tomography in diagnosis and treatment of mental disorders: evidence for a key-lock principle. *Methods and Findings in Experimental and Clinical Pharmacology*, **24 (Suppl 1)**, 97–106.

Salkovskis P (1997). Obsessive-compulsive disorder. In DM Clark and CG Fairburn, eds. *Science and practice of cognitive behaviour therapy*, Chapter 8. Oxford University Press, Oxford.

Salkovskis P and Bass C (1997). Hypochondriasis. In CG Fairburn and DM Clark, eds. *Science and practice of cognitive behaviour therapy*, Chapter 13. Oxford University Press, Oxford.

Salmon G and West A (2000). Physical and mental health issues related to bullying in schools. *Current Opinion in Psychiatry*, **13**, 381–8.

Salzmann J, Wolfson AN, Schatzenberg A, *et al.* (1995). Effect of fluoxetine on anger in symptomatic volunteers with borderline personality disorder. *Journal of Clinical Psychopharmacology*, **15**, 23–9.

Sameroff A, Seifer R, Barocas R, *et al.* (1987). IQ scores of 4-year-old children: social-environmental risk factors. *Pediatrics*, **79**, 343–50.

Sampson EL, Warren JD and Rossor MN (2004). Young onset dementia. *Postgraduate Medical Journal*, **80**, 125–39.

Sandifer MG, Hordern A, Timbury GC, *et al.* (1968). Psychiatric diagnosis: a comparative study in North Carolina. *British Journal of Psychiatry*, **114**, 1–9.

Sanz EJ, De las Cuevas C, Kiuru A, *et al.* (2005). Selective serotonin reuptake inhibitors in pregnant women and neonatal withdrawal syndrome: a database analysis. *Lancet*, **365**, 482–7.

Saper CB and Scammell TE (2004). Modafinil: a drug in search of a mechanism. *Sleep*, 11–12.

Sar V, Akyuz G, Kundakci T, *et al.* (2004). Childhood trauma, dissociation, and psychiatric comorbidity in patients with conversion disorder. *Am J Psychiatry*, **161**, 2271–6.

Saravanan B, Jacob KS, Prince M, *et al.* (2004). Culture and insight revisited. *British Journal of Psychiatry*, **184**, 107–9.

Sargant W and Dally P (1964). Treatment of anxiety state by antidepressant drugs. *British Medical Journal*, **1**, 6–9.

Sargant W and Slater E (1940). Acute war neuroses. *Lancet*, **2**, 1–2.

Sargant W and Slater E (1963). *An introduction to physical methods of treatment in psychiatry.* Livingstone, Edinburgh.

Sartorius N, Kaelber CT, Cooper JE, *et al.* (1993). Progress toward achieving a common language in psychiatry: results from the field trial of the clinical guidelines accompanying the WHO classification of mental and behavioral disorders in ICD-10. *Archives of General Psychiatry*, **50**, 115–24.

Sartorius N, Ustun TB and Korton A (1995). Progress toward achieving a common language in psychiatry II: results from the International Field Trials of the ICD-10 Diagnostic Criteria for Research for Mental and Behavioral Disorders. *American Journal of Psychiatry*, **152**, 1427–37.

Sarwer DB, Wadden TA, Pertschuk MJ, *et al.* (1998). The psychology of cosmetic surgery: a review and reconceptualization. *Clinical Psychology Review*, **18**, 1–22.

Sashidharan SP (2001). Institutional racism in British psychiatry. *Psychiatric Bulletin*, **25**, 244–7.

Sateia MJ and Nowell PD (2004). Insomnia. *Lancet*, **364**, 1959–73.

Sauer WH, Berlin JA and Kimmel SE (2003). Effect of antidepressants and their relative affinity for the serotonin transporter on the risk of myocardial infarction. *Circulation*, **108**, 32–6.

Saxena S, Bota RG and Brody AL (2001). Brain-behaviour relationships in obsessive-compulsive disorder. *Seminars in Clinical Neuropsychiatry*, **6**, 82–101.

Saxena S, Brody AL, Ho ML, *et al.* (2002). Differential cerebral metabolic changes with paroxetine treatment of obsessive-compulsive disorder vs major depression. *Archives of General Psychiatry*, **59**, 250–61.

Saxena S, Brody AL, Schwartz JM, *et al.* (1998). Neuroimaging and frontal-subcortical circuitry in obsessive-compulsive disorder. *British Journal of Psychiatry*, **173 (Suppl 35)**, 26–37.

Saxena S, Brody AL, Zohrabi N, *et al.* (2004). Cerebral glucose metabolism in obsessive-compulsive hoarding. *American Journal of Psychiatry*, **161**, 1038–48.

Saxena S and Rauch SL (2000). Fuctional neuroimaging and the neuroanatomy of obsessive-compulsive disorder. *Psychiatric Clinics of North America*, 563–86.

Scadding JG (1967). Diagnosis: the clinician and the computer. *Lancet*, **2**, 877–82.

Schachar R (1991). Childhood hyperactivity. *Journal of Child Psychology and Psychiatry*, **32**, 155–91.

Schachar R and Ickowicz A (2000). Attention deficit hyperkinetic disorders in childhood and adolescence. In MG Gelder, JJ López-Ibor Jr and NC Andreasen, eds. *The new Oxford textbook of psychiatry*, Chapter 9.2.3. Oxford University Press, Oxford.

Schanda H, Knecht G, Schreinzer D, *et al.* (2004). Homicide and major mental disorders: a 25-year study. *Acta Psychiatrica Scandinavica*, **110**, 98–107.

Schapira K, Lindsley KR, Linsley A, *et al.* (2001). Relationship of suicde rates to social factors and availability of lethal methods: comparison of suicide in Newcastle upon Tyne 1961–1994. *British Journal of Psychiatry*, **178**, 458–64.

Scharff DE and Scharff JS (2005). Psychodynamic couple therapy. In GO Gabbard, JS Beck and J Holmes, eds. *Oxford textbook of psychotherapy*. Oxford University Press,

Schatzberg AF (2004). Employing pharmaologic treatment. *Journal of Clinical Psychiatry*, **65**, 15–20.

Scheltens P, Fox N, Barkhof F, *et al.* (2002). Structural magnetic resonance imaging in the practical assessment of dementia: beyond exclusion. *Lancet Neurology*, **1**, 13–21.

Schenk D, Barbour R, Dunn W, *et al.* (1999). Immunization with amyloid-β attenuates Alzheimer disease-like pathology in the PDAPP mouse. *Nature*, **400**, 173–7.

Scherder E, Oosterman J, Swaab D, *et al.* (2005). Recent developments in pain in dementia. *British Medical Journal*, **330**, 461–4.

Schernhammer ES and Colditz GA (2004). Suicide rates among physicians: a quantitative and gender assessment (meta-analysis). *American Journal of Psychiatry*, **161**, 2292–302.

Schiffman J, Walker E, Ekstrom M, *et al.* (2004). Childhood videotaped social and neuromotor precursors of schizophrenia: a prospective investigation. *American Journal of Psychiatry*, **161**, 2021–7.

Schimming C and Harvey PD (2004). Disability reduction in elderly patients with schizophrenia. *Journal of Psychiatric Practice*, **10**, 283–95.

Schmideberg M (1947). The treatment of psychopaths and borderline patients. *American Journal of Psychotherapy*, **1**, 45–70.

Schnaider Beeri M, Goldbourt U, Silverman JM, *et al.* (2004). Diabetes mellitus in midlife and the risk of dementia three decades later. *Neurology*, **63**, 1902–7.

Schneider K (1959). *Clinical psychopathology.* Grune and Stratton, New York.

Schneier FR, Goetz D, Campeas R, *et al.* (1998). Placebo controlled trial of moclobemide in social phobia. *British Journal of Psychiatry*, **172**, 70–7.

Schneier FR, Johnson J, Hornig CD, *et al.* (1992). Social phobia: comorbidity and morbidity in an epidemiological sample. *Archives of General Psychiatry*, **49**, 282–8.

Schneier FR, Marshall RD, Street L, *et al.* (1995). Social phobia and specific phobias. In GO Gabbard, ed. *Treatments of psychiatric disorders*. American Psychiatric Press, Washington, D.C.

Schrag A (2005). Driving in Parkinson's disease. *Journal of Neurology, Neurosurgery and Psychiatry*, **76**, 159.

Schrenck-Notzing A (1895). *The use of hypnosis in psychopathia sexualis with special reference to contrary sexual instinct*. Transl CG Chaddock. Institute of Research in Hypnosis Publication Society and the Julian Press, New York, NY (1956).

Schuchter SR and Zisook S (1993). The normal course of grief. In MS Stroebe, W Stroebe and RO Hansson, eds. *Handbook of bereavement*. Cambridge University Press, Cambridge.

Schuckit MA, Smith TL, Anthenellic RA, *et al.* (1993). A clinical course of alcoholism in 636 male inpatients. *American Journal of Psychiatry*, **150**, 786–92.

Schulsinger F (1982). Psychopathy: heredity and environment. *International Journal of Mental Health*, **1**, 190–206.

Schultz JH (1932). *Das autogene training*. Thieme, Liepzig.

Schultz JH and Luthe W (1959). *Autogenic training: a psychophysiological approach*. Grune and Stratton, New York, NY.

Schulz SC, Camlin KL, Berry SA, *et al.* (1999b). Olanzapine safety and efficacy in patients with borderline personality disorder and comorbid dysthymia. *Biological Psychiatry*, **46**, 1429–35.

Schwartz CE, Snidman N and Kagan J (1999). Adolescent social anxiety as an outcome of inhibited temperament in childhood. *Journal of the American Academy of Child and Adolescent Psychiatry*, **38**, 1008–15.

Schwartz J (1994). Low level lead exposure and children's IQ: a meta analysis and search for a threshold. *Environmental Research*, **65**, 42–55.

Schwartz MA and Wiggins OP (1987). Typifications. The first step for clinical diagnosis in psychiatry. *Journal of Nervous and Mental Disorders*, **175**, 65–77.

Schweitzer I, Tuckwell V, O'Brien J, *et al.* (2002). Is late onset depression a prodrome to dementia? *International Journal of Geriatric Psychiatry*, **17**, 997–1005.

Schweizer E and Rickels K (1998). Benzodiazepine dependence and withdrawal: a review of the syndrome and its clinical management. *Acta Psychiatrica Scandinavica*, **393**, 95–101.

Scott A (2005). College Guidelines on electroconvulsive therapy: an update for prescribers. *Advances in Psychiatric Treatment*, **11**, 150–6.

Scott PD (1960). The treatment of psychopaths. *British Medical Journal*, **1**, 1641–6.

Scott S (1994). Mental retardation. In M Rutter, E Taylor and L Hersov, eds. *Child and adolescent psychiatry: modern approaches*, 616–46. Blackwell Scientific Publications, Oxford.

Scott S (2000). Conduct disorders in childhood and adolesence. In MG Gelder, JJ López-Ibor Jr and NC Andreasen, eds. *The new Oxford textbook of psychiatry*, Chapter 9.2.4. Oxford University Press, Oxford.

Scott S (2002). Parent training programmes. In M Rutter and E Taylor, eds. *Child and adolescent psychiatry*, Chapter 56. Blackwell, Oxford.

Scott S, Spender Q, Dolan M, *et al.* (2001). Multicentre controlled trial of parenting groups for child antisocial behaviour in clinical practice. *British Medical Journal*, **323**, 191–4.

Sedler MJ (1995). Delusional disorders. *Psychiatric Clinics of North America*, **18**, 199–425.

Sedman G (1970). Theories of depersonalization: a reappraisal. *British Journal of Psychiatry*, **117**, 1–14.

Seeman MV (1997). Psychopathology in women and men: focus on female hormones. *American Journal of Psychiatry*, **154**, 1641–7.

Seeman MV (2004). Gender differences in the prescribing of antipsychotic drugs. *American Journal of Psychiatry*, **161**, 1324–33.

Seeman P, Bzowej NH, Guan HC, *et al.* (1987). Human brain D1 and D2 dopamine receptors in schizophrenia, Alzheimer's, Parkinson's, and Huntington's diseases. *Neuropsychopharmacology*, **1**, 5–15.

Segal H (1963). *Introduction to the work of Melanie Klein*. Heinemann Medical, London.

Seghorn T, Prensky R and Boucher R (1987). Childhood sexual abuse in the lives of sexually aggressive offenders. *Journal of Child and Adolescent Psychiatry*, **26**, 262–7.

Seguin E (1864). Origin of the treatment and training of idiots. In M Rosen, GR Clark and MS Kivitz, eds. *History of mental retardation*. University Park Press, Baltimore, MD (1976).

Seguin E (1866). *Idiocy and its treatment by the physiological method*. Brandown, Albany, NY.

Seibyl JP, Scanley BE, Krystal JH, *et al.* (2004). Neuroimaging methodologies: utilising radiotracers or nuclear magnetic resonance. In EJ Nestler and DS Charney, eds. *Neurobiology of mental illness*, 190–206.

Seivewright N and McMahon C (1996). Misuse of amphetamines and related drugs. *Advances in Psychiatric Treatment*, **2**, 211–8.

Selten J-P, Veen N, Feller W, *et al.* (2001). Incidence of psychotic disorders in immigrant groups to the Netherlands. *British Journal of Psychiatry*, **178**, 367–72.

Seltzer B, Zolnouni P, Nunez M, *et al.* (2004). Efficacy of donepezil in early-stage Alzheimer disease: a randomized placebo-controlled trial. *Archives of Neurology*, **61**, 1852–6.

Semple DM, McIntosh AM and Lawrie SM (2005). Cannabis as a risk factor for psychosis: a systematic review. *Journal of Psychopharmacology*, **19**, 187–94.

Sensky T, Turkington D, Kingdon D, *et al.* (2000). A randomized controlled trial of cognitive-behavioral therapy for persistent symptoms in schizophrenia resistant to medication. *Archives of General Psychiatry*, **57**, 165–72.

Seong E, Seassholtz AF and Burmeister M (2002). Mouse models for psychiatric disorders. *Trends in Genetics*, **18**, 643–50.

Sequiera H, Howlin P and Hollins S (2003). Psychological disturbances associated with sexual abuse in people with learning disabilities. *British Journal of Psychiatry*, **183**, 451–6.

Serretti A, Mandelli L, Lattuada E, *et al.* (2004). Depressive syndrome in major psychoses: a study on 1351 subjects. *Psychiatry Research*, **127**, 85–99.

Seshadri S, Beiser A, Selhub J, *et al.* (2002). Plasma homocysteine as a risk factor for dementia and Alzheimer's disease. *New England Journal of Medicine*, **346**, 476–83.

Shaffer D (1974). Suicide in childhood and early adolescence. *Journal of Child Psychology and Psychiatry*, **15**, 275–91.

Shaffer D, Pfeffer CR and Gutstein J (2000). Suicide and attempted suicide in children and adolescents. In K Hawton and K van Heeringen, eds. *The International Handbook of Suicide and Attempted Suicide*. John Wiley & Sons, Chichester.

Shapiro F (1995). *Movement desensitization and reprocessing: basic principles, protocols and procedures*. Guilford, New York, NY.

Sharma T and Harvey P (eds.) (2000). *Cognition in Schizophrenia*. Oxford University Press.

Sharpe M (1990). The use of graphical life charts in psychiatry. *British Journal of Hospital Medicine*, **44**, 44–7.

Sharpe M (2002). The English Chief Medical Officer's Working Parties' report on the management of CFS/ME: Significant breakthrough or unsatisfactory compromise? *Journal of Psychosomatic Research*, **52**, 437–8.

Sharpe M (2003). Distinguishing malingering from psychiatric disorders. In PW Halligan, C Bass and DA Oakley, eds. *Malingering and illness deception*. Oxford University Press, Oxford.

Sharpe M and Carson AJ (2001). 'Unexplained' somatic symptoms, functional syndromes, and somatization: do we need a paradigm shift? *Annals of Internal Medicine*, **134**, 926–30.

Sharpe M, Hawton K and Seagroatt V (1994). Depressive disorders in long-term survivors of stroke. Associations with demographic and social factors, functional status, and brain lesion volume. *British Journal of Psychiatry*, **164**, 380–6.

Sharpe M and Mayou R (2004). Somatoform disorders: a help or a hindrance to good patient care? *British Journal of Psychiatry*, **184**, 465–7.

Sharpe M, Strong V, Allen K, *et al.* (2004). Major depression in outpatients attending a regional cancer centre: screening and unmet treatment needs. *British Journal of Cancer*, **90**, 314–20.

Sharpe PC (2001). Biochemical detection and monitoring of alcohol abuse and abstinence. *Annals of Clinical Biochemistry*, **38**, 652–64.

Sharpley M, Hutchinson G, McKenzie K, *et al.* (2001). Understanding the excess of psychosis among the African-Caribbean population in England. Review of current hypotheses. *British Journal of Psychiatry*, **40 (Suppl)**, s60–8.

Shaw C, Abrams K and Marteau TM (1999). Psychological impact of predicting individuals' risks of illness: a systematic review. *Social Science and Medicine*, **49**, 1571–98.

Sheard T and Maguire P (1999). The effect of psychological interventions on anxiety and depression in cancer patients: results of two meta-analyses. *British Journal of Cancer*, **80**, 1170–80.

Sheldon WH, Stevens SS and Tucker WB (1940). *The varieties of human physique*. Harper, London.

Shelton RC, Tollefson GD, Tohen M, *et al.* (2001). A novel augmentation strategy for treating resistant major depression. *Am J Psychiatry*, **158**, 131–4.

Shenton ME, Dickey CC, Frumin M, *et al.* (2001). A review of MRI findings in schizophrenia. *Schizophrenia Research*, **49**, 1–52.

Shepherd M (1961). Morbid jealousy: some clinical and social aspects of a psychiatric symptom. *Journal of Mental Science*, **107**, 687–753.

Shepherd M, Cooper B, Brown AC, *et al.* (1966). *Psychiatric illness in general practice*. Oxford University Press, Oxford.

Shibuya A and Yoshida A (1988). The genotypes of alcohol-metabolising enzymes in Japanese with alcohol liver disease. *American Journal of Human Genetics*, **43**, 744–8.

Shields J (1980). Genetics and mental development. In M Rutter, ed. *Scientific foundations of developmental psychiatry*. Heinemann Medical, London.

Shore JH, Vollmer WM and Tatum EL (1989). Community patterns of post-traumatic stress disorder. *Journal of Nervous and Mental Disease*, **177**, 681–5.

Shorter E (1992). *From paralysis to fatigue. A history of psychosomatic illness in the modern era*. The Free Press, New York.

Shorvon HJ, Hill JDN, Burkitt E, *et al.* (1946). The depersonalization syndrome. *Proceedings of the Royal Society of Medicine*, **39**, 779–92.

Shulman K (2002). Manic illness. In R Jacoby and C Oppenheimer, eds. *Psychiatry in the elderly*. 3rd edn. Oxford University Press, Oxford.

Sibbald B, Addington-Hall J, Brenneman D, *et al.* (1996a). The role of counsellors in general practice: a qualitative study. *Occasional Papers of the Royal College of General Practitioners*, **74**, 1–19.

Sibbald B, Addington-Hall J, Brenneman D, *et al.* (1996b). Investigation of whether on-site general practice counsellors have an impact on psychotropic drug prescribing rates and costs. *British Journal of General Practice*, **46**, 63–7.

Siegert RJ and Abernethy DA (2005). Depression in multiple sclerosis: a review. *Journal of Neurology, Neurosurgery and Psychiatry*, **76**, 469–75.

Sierra M, Phillips ML, Irvin G, *et al.* (2003). A placebo controlled trial of lamotrigine in depersonalization disorder. *Journal of Psychopharmacology*, **17**, 103–5.

Sierra M, Senior C, Dalton J, *et al.* (2002). Autonomic response in depersonalization disorder. *Archives of General Psychiatry*, **59**, 833–8.

Siever LJ, Torgersen S, Gunderson JG, *et al.* (2002). The borderline diagnosis III: identifying endophenotypes for genetic studies. *Biological Psychiatry*, **51**, 964–8.

Silberg J, Meyer J, Pickles A, *et al.* (1996). Heterogeneity among juvenile antisocial behaviours: findings from the Virginia Twin Study of Adolescent Behavioural Development. In G Bock and J Goode, eds. *Genetics of criminal and antisocial behaviour*. Wiley, Chichester.

Silberg J, Rutter M, *et al.* (1999). The influence of genetic factors and life stress on depression among adolescent girls. *Archives of General Psychiatry,* **56**, 225–32.

Silva AJ, Ferrari MM, Leong GB, *et al.* (1998). The dangerousness of persons with delusional jealousy. *Journal of the American Academy of Psychiatry and the Law,* **26**, 607–23.

Silva JA, Derecho DV, Leong GB, *et al.* (2000). Stalking behavior in delusional jealousy. *Journal of Forensic Science,* **45**, 77–82.

Silveira JM and Seeman MV (1995). Shared psychotic disorder: a critical review of the literature. *Canadian Journal of Psychiatry,* **40**, 389–95.

Silverstone T and Cookson J (1982). The biology of mania. In K Granville-Grassman, ed. *Recent advances in clinical psychiatry*. Churchill Livingstone, Edinburgh.

Sim J and Adams N (2002). Systematic review of randomized controlled trials of nonpharmacological interventions for fibromyalgia. *Clinical Journal of Pain,* **18**, 324–36.

Simard M and van Reekum R (2004). The acetylcholinesterase inhibitors for treatment of cognitive and behavioral symptoms in dementa with Lewy bodies. *Journal of Neuropsychiatry and Clinical Neurosciences,* **16**, 409–25.

Simeon D, Knutelska M, Nelson D, *et al.* (2003). Feeling unreal: a depersonalization disorder update of 117 cases. *Journal of Clinical Psychiatry,* **64**, 990–7.

Simmons J and Dodd T (2002/3). *Crime in England and Wales.* Home Office, London.

Simon G (2000). Epidemiology of somatoform disorders and other causes of unexplained medical symptoms. In MG Gelder, JJ López-Ibor Jr and NC Andreasen, eds. *The new Oxford textbook of psychiatry*, Chapter 5.2.2. Oxford University Press, Oxford.

Simon GE, VonKorff M, Piccinelli M, *et al.* (1999). An international study of the relation between somatic symptoms and depression. *New England Journal of Medicine,* **341**, 1329–35.

Simon RI (1997). Video voyeurs and covert videotaping of unsuspecting victims: psychological and legal consequences. *Journal of Forensic Science,* **42**, 884–9.

Simpson HB, Liebowitz MR, Foa EB, *et al.* (2004). Post-treatment effects of exposure therapy and clomopramine in obsessive-compulsive disorder. *Depression and Anxiety,* **19**, 225–33.

Simpson HB, Lombardo I, Slifstein M, *et al.* (2003). Serotonin transporters in obsessive compulsice disorder: a positron emission tomography study with ((11)C)McN 5652. *Biological Psychiatry,* **54**, 1414–21.

Simpson L (1990). The comparative efficacy of Milan Family Therapy for disturbed children and their families. *Journal of Family Therapy,* **13**, 267–84.

Sims A (2003). *Symptoms in the Mind. An introduction to descriptive psychopathology.* 3rd edn. Elsevier Science Ltd., London.

Singer MT and Wynne LC (1965). Thought disorder and family relations of schizophrenics: IV. Results and implications. *Archives of General Psychiatry,* **12**, 201–12.

Singh B, Hawthorne G and Vos T (2001). The role of economic evaluation in mental health care. *Australia and New Zealand Journal of Psychiatry,* **35**, 104–14.

Singh SP, Burns T, Amin S, *et al.* (2004). Acute and transient psychotic disorders: precursors, epidemiology, course and outcome. *British Journal of Psychiatry,* **185**, 452–9.

Singh SP and Lee AS (1997). Conversion disorders in Nottingham: alive, but not kicking. *Journal of Psychosomatic Research,* **43**, 425–30.

Singleton A and Gwinn Hardy K (2004). Parkinson's disease and dementia with Lewy bodies: a difference in dose? *Lancet,* **364**, 1105–7.

Singleton N, Bumpstead R, O'Brian M, *et al.* (2000). *Psychiatric Morbidity among Adults living in Private Households, 2000: Summary Report.* Office for National Statistics, London.

Singleton N, Meltzer H and Gatward R (1997). Psychiatric morbidity among prisoners in England and Wales. *OPCS Surveys of Psychiatric Morbidity in Great Britain.* HMSO, London.

Sink KM, Holden KF and Yaffe K (2005). Pharmacological treatment of neuropsychiatric symptoms of dementia: a review of the evidence. *Journal of the American Medical Association,* **293**, 596–608.

Sipos A, Rasmussen F, Harrison G, *et al.* (2004). Paternal age and schizophrenia: a population based cohort study. *British Medical Journal,* **329**, 1070.

Siris SG, Morgan V, Fagerstrom R, *et al.* (1987). Adjunctive imipramine in the treatment of postpsychotic depression. A controlled trial. *Archives of General Psychiatry,* **44**, 533–9.

Skeels H (1966). Adult status of children with contrasting life experiences: a follow-up study. *Monograph of the Society for Research into Child Development,* **31**.

Skinner BF (1953). *Science and human behaviour.* Macmillan, New York, NY.

Skodal AE, Gunderson JG, Pfohl B, *et al.* (2002a). The borderline disgnosis I: psychopathology, comorbidity, and personality structure. *Biological Psychiatry,* **51**, 936–50.

Skodal AE, Siever LJ, Livesay WJ, *et al.* (2002b). The borderline diagnosis II: biology, genetics, and clinical course. *Biological Psychiatry,* **51**, 951–63.

Skoog G and Skoog I (1999). A 40 year follow-up of patients with obsessive-compulsive disorder. *Archives of General Psychiatry,* **56**, 121–7.

Skoog I (2004). Psychiatric epidemiology of old age: the H70 study – the NAPE lecture 2003. *Acta Psychiatrica Scandinavica,* **109**, 4–18.

Skoog SJ, Stokes A and Turner KL (1997). Oral desmopressin: a randomized double-blind placebo controlled study of effectiveness in children with primary nocturnal enuresis. *Journal of Urology,* **158**, 1035–40.

Skre I, Onstad S, Torgersen S, *et al.* (1993). A twin study of DSMIIIR anxiety disorders. *Acta Psychiatrica Scandinavica,* **88**, 85–92.

Skuse D (1989). Emotional abuse and delay in growth. In R Meadow, ed. *ABC of child abuse*, 23–5. British Medical Association, London.

Skuse D (2001). Endophenotypes and child psychiatry. *British Journal of Psychiatry,* **178**, 395–6.

Skuse D and Bentovim A (1994). Physical and emotional maltreatment. In M Rutter, E Taylor and L Hersov, eds. *Child and adolescent psychiatry: modern approaches*, 209–29. 3rd edn. Blackwell Scientific Publications, Oxford.

Skynner ACR (1991). Open-systems group-analytic approach to family therapy. In AS Gurman and DP Kriskern, eds. *Handbook of family therapy*. Brunner Mazel, New York.

Slade M, Phelan M and Thornicroft G (1998). A comparison of needs assessed by staff and by an epidemiologically representative sample of patients with psychosis.. *Psychological Medicine*, **28**, 543–50.

Slater E (1951). Evaluation of electric convulsion therapy as compared with conservative methods in depressive states. *Journal of Mental Science*, **97**, 567–9.

Slater E (1965). The diagnosis of hysteria. *British Medical Journal*, **1**, 1395–9.

Slater E, Beard AW and Glithero E (1963). The Schizophrenia-like psychoses of epilepsy. *British Journal of Psychiatry*, **109**, 95–150.

Slater E and Shields J (1969). Genetical aspects of anxiety. In MH Lader, ed. *Studies of anxiety*. British Journal of Psychiatry Special Publication,

Small JG, Klapper MH and Kellams JJ (1988). Electroconvulsive treatment compared with lithium in the management of manic states. *Archives of General Psychiatry*, **45**, 727–32.

Smalley SL, Bailey JG, Cantwell DP, *et al.* (1998). Evidence that the dopamine D4 receptor is a susceptibility gene in attention deficit hyperactivity disorder. *Molecular Psychiatry*, **3**, 427–30.

Smith D, Dempster C, Glanville J, *et al.* (2002). Efficacy and tolerability of venlafaxine compared with selective serotonin reuptake inhibitors and other antidepressants: a meta-analysis. *British Journal of Psychiatry*, **180**, 396–404.

Smith DJ (1995). Youth crime and conduct disorders: trends, patterns and causal explanations. In M Rutter and DJ Smith, eds. *Psychosocial disorders in young people: time trends and their causes*. Wiley, Chichester.

Smith Jr GR (1995). Treatment of patients with multiple symptoms. In RA Mayou, C Bass and M Sharpe, eds. *Treatment of functional somatic symptoms*, 175–87. Oxford University Press, Oxford.

Smith Jr GR, Hanson RA and Ray DC (1986). Patients with multiple unexplained symptoms. *Archives of Internal Medicine*, **146**, 69–72.

Smith KA and Cowen PJ (1997). Serotonin and depression. In A Honig and HM van Praag, eds. *Depression: neurobiological, psychopathological and therapeutic advances*, 129–46. John Wiley & Sons Ltd, Chichester.

Smith KA, Morris JS and Friston KJ (1999). Brain mechanisms associated with depressive relapse and associated cognitive impairment following acute tryptophan depletion. *British Journal of Psychiatry*, **176**, 72–5.

Snaith RP, Baugh SJ, Clayden AD, *et al.* (1982). The clinical anxiety scale: an instrument derived from the Hamilton Anxiety Scale. *British Journal of Psychiatry*, **141**, 518–23.

Snider LA and Swedo S (2004). PANDAS: current status and directions for research. *Molecular Psychiatry*, **9**, 900–7.

Snider LA and Swedo SE (2003). Childhood-onset obsessive-compulsive disorder and tic disorders: case report and literature review. *Journal of Child and Adolescent Psychopharmacology*, **13**, S81–8.

Snowling MJ (2002). Reading and other learning difficulties. In M Rutter and E Taylor, eds. *Child and adolescent psychiatry*, Chapter 40. 4th edn. Blackwell, Oxford.

Soloff PH (1994). Is there a drug treatment of choice for borderline personality disorder? *Acta Psychiatrica Scandinavica*, **89**, 50–5.

Soloff PH, George A, Nathan RS, *et al.* (1986). Progress in psychopharmacology of personality disorders: a double blind study of amitriptyline, haloperidol and placebo. *Archives of General Psychiatry*, **43**, 691–7.

Sommer I, Ramsey N, Kahn R, *et al.* (2001). Handedness, language lateralisation and anatomical asymmetry in schizophrenia: meta-analysis. *British Journal of Psychiatry*, **178**, 344–51.

Sonino N and Fava GA (1998). Psychosomatic aspects of Cushing's disease. *Psychotherapy and Psychosomatics*, **67**, 140–6.

Soothill K, Ackerley E and Francis B (2004). The criminal careers of arsonists. *Med Sci Law*, **44**, 27–40.

Soto C (2003). Unfolding the role of protein misfolding in neurodegenerative diseases. *Nature Reviews Neuroscience*, **4**, 49–60.

Sovner R and Hurley AD (1989). Ten diagnostic principles for recognizing psychiatric disorders in mentally retarded persons. *Psychiatric Aspects of Mental Retardation*, **8**, 9–15.

Soyka M, Naber G and Volcker A (1991). Prevalence of delusional jealousy in different psychiatric disorders. *British Journal of Psychiatry*, **158**, 549–53.

Spanagel R (1999). Is there a pharmacological basis for therapy with rapid opioid detoxification? *Lancet*, **354**, 2017–8.

Spataro J, Mullen PE, Burgess S, *et al.* (2004). Impact of Child Abuse on Mental Health. Prospective study in males and females. *British Journal of Psychiatry*, **184**, 416–21.

Spencer MD, Knight RS and Will RG (2002). First hundred cases of variant Creutzfeldt-Jakob disease: retrospective case note review of early psychiatric and neurological features. *British Medical Journal*, **324**, 1479–82.

Spencer TJ, Biederman J, Harding M, *et al.* (1996). Growth deficits in ADHD children revisited: evidence for disorder-associated growth delays? *Journal of the American Academy of Child and Adolescent Psychiatry*, **35**, 1460–9.

Spielberger CD, Gorsuch RL, Lushene R, *et al.* (1983). *Manual for the State-Trait Anxiety Inventory*. Consulting Psychologists' Press, Palo Alto, CA.

Spina E and Scordo MG (2002). Clinically significant drug interactions with antidepressants in the elderly. *Drugs and Aging*, **19**, 299–320.

Spinelli MG (2004). Maternal infanticide associated with mental illness: prevention and the promise of saved lives. *Ameican journal of psychiatry*, **161**, 1548–57.

Spitzer M (1990). On defining delusions. *Comprehensive Psychiatry*, **31**, 377–97.

Spitzer R, First MB and Williams JBW (1992). Now is the time to retire the term 'organic mental disorders'. *American Journal of Psychiatry*, **149**, 240–4.

Spitzer RL and Endicott J (1968). DIAGNO: a computer programme for psychiatric diagnosis utilizing the differential diagnostic procedures. *Archives of General Psychiatry*, **18**, 746–56.

Spitzer RL, Endicott J and Robins E (1978). Research diagnostic criteria: rationale and reliability. *Archives of General Psychiatry*, **35**, 773–82.

Spitzer RL and Wakefield JC (1999). DSM-IV diagnostic criterion for clinical significance: does it help solve the false positives problem? *American Journal of Psychiatry*, **156**, 1856–64.

Spitzer RL, Williams JB, Kroenke K, *et al.* (1994). Utility of a new procedure for diagnosing mental disorders in primary care. The PRIME-MD 1000 study. *Journal of the American Medical Association*, **272**, 1749-56.

Spitzer RL, Williams JBD and Gibbon M (1987). *Structured clinical interview for DSMIV (SCID)*. New York State Psychiatric Institute, New York.

Spitzer RL and Williams JBW (1985). Classification in psychiatry. In HI Kaplan and BJ Sadock, eds. *Comprehensive textbook of psychiatry*. 4th edn. Williams & Wilkins, Baltimore, MD.

Spohr HL, Willms J and Steinhausen HC (1993). Prenatal alcohol exposure and long-term developmental consequences. *Lancet*, **341**, 907–10.

Spreat S and Behar D (1994). Trends in the residential (inpatient) treatment of individuals with a dual diagnosis. *Journal of Consulting and Clinical Psychology*, **62**, 43–8.

Squire LR, Slater PC and Miller PL (1981). Retrograde amnesia and bilateral electroconvulsive therapy. Long-term follow-up. *Arch Gen Psychiatry*, **38**, 89–95.

Srisurapanont M, Jarusuraisin N and Kittirattanapaiboon P (2004). *Treatment for amphetamine dependence and abuse.* Cochrane Database of Systematic Reviews.

Staddon S, Arranz MJ, Mancama D, *et al.* (2002). Clinical applications of pharmacogenetics in psychiatry. *Psychopharmacology (Berl)*, **162**, 18–23.

Stangier U, Heidenreich T, Peitz M, *et al.* (2003). Cognitive therapy for social phobia: individual versus group treatment. *Behaviour Research and Therapy*, **41**, 991–1007.

Stanhope R, Adlard P, Hamill G, *et al.* (1988). Psychological growth hormone secretion during the recovery from psychosocial dwarfism: a case report. *Clinical Endocrinology*, **28**, 335–9.

Starkstein SE and Robinson RG (eds.) (1993). *Depression in neurologic disease.* The Johns Hopkins University Press, Baltimore, MD.

Statham DJ, Heath AC, Madden PA, *et al.* (1998). Suicidal behaviour: an epidemiological and genetic study. *Psychological Medicine*, **28**, 839–55.

Steel J, Sanna L, Hammond B, *et al.* (2004). Psychological sequelae of childhood sexual abuse: Abuse related characteristics, coping strategies and attributional style. *Child Abuse and Neglect*, **28**, 785–801.

Stefanis NC, Hanssen M, Smirnis NK, *et al.* (2002). Evidence that three dimensions of psychosis have a distribution in the general population. *Psychological Medicine*, **32**, 347–58.

Stein A, Gath DH, Bucher J, *et al.* (1991). The relationship between post-natal depression and mother child interaction. *British Journal of Psychiatry*, **158**, 46–52.

Stein DJ, Hollander E and Josephson SC (1994). Serotonin reuptake blockers for the treatment of obsessional jealousy. *Journal of Clinical Psychiatry*, **55**, 30–3.

Stein LJ and Test MA (1980). Alternative to mental hospital treatment. 1. Conceptual model, treatment program and clinical evaluation. *Archives of General Psychiatry*, **37**, 392–7.

Stein MB, Chartier MJ, Hazen AL, *et al.* (1998a). A direct-interview family study of generalized social phobia. *American Journal of Psychiatry*, **155**, 90–7.

Stein MB, Liebowitz MR, Lydiard RB, *et al.* (1998b). Paroxetine treatment of generalized social phobia (social anxiety disorder): a randomized controlled trial. *Journal of the American Medical Association*, **280**, 708–13.

Stein MB, Walker JR and Hazen AL (1997). Full and Partial posttraumatic stress disorder: findings from a community survey. *American Journal of Psychiatry*, **154**, 1114–9.

Stein Z and Susser M (1969). Widowhood and mental illness. *British Journal of Preventative and Social Medicine*, **23**, 106–10.

Steiner H and Lock J (1998). Anorexia nervosa and bulimia nervosa in children and adolescents: a review of the past 10 years. *Journal of the American Academy of Child and Adolescent Psychiatry*, **37**, 352–9.

Stekel W (1953). *Sadism and masochism.* Liveright, London.

Stenager E, N., Madsen C, Stenager E, *et al.* (1998). Suicide in patients with stroke: epidemiological study. *British Medical Journal*, **316**, 1206.

Stenager EN and Stenager E (2000). Physical illness and suicidal behaviour. In K Hawton and K van Heeringen, eds. *The international handbook of suicide and attempted suicide*. John Wiley & Sons, Chichester.

Stengel E (1952). Enquiries into attempted sucide. *Proceedings of the Royal Society of Medicine*, **45**, 613–20.

Stengel E (1959). Classification of mental disorders. *Bulletin of the World Health Organization*, **21**, 601–3.

Stengel E and Cook NG (1958). *Attempted suicide: its social significance and effects.* Chapman & Hall, London.

Stern E and Silbersweig DA (2001). Advances in functional neuroimaging methodology for the study of brain systems underlying human neuropsychological function and dysfunction. *Journal of Clinical and Experimental Neuropsychology*, **23**, 3–18.

Stern RS, Lipsedge MA and Marks LM (1973). Thought-stopping of neutral and obsessional thoughts: a controlled trial. *Behaviour Research and Therapy*, **11**, 659–62.

Stevenson J and Goodman R (2001). Association between behaviour at age 3 years and adult criminality. *British Journal of Psychiatry*, **179**, 197–202.

Stiles WB (1999). Evaluating qualitative research. *Evidence Based Mental Health*, **2**, 99–101.

Stoddard FJ, Sheridan RL, Selter LF, *et al.* (2000). General surgery: basic principles of patient assessment. In A Stoudemier, BS Fogel and DB Greenberg, eds. *Psychiatric care of the medical patient.* Oxford University Press, New York, NY.

Stone JH, Roberts M and O'Grady J (2000). *Faulks basic forensic psychiatry.* Blackwells, Oxford.

Stone M (1985). Shellshock and the psychologists. In WF Bynum, R Porter and M Shepherd, eds. *The Anatomy of Madness*, 242–71. Tavistock Publications, London.

Stone MH, Hurt SW and Stone DK (1987). The PI-500: long term follow-up of borderline inpatients meeting DSMIII criteria. I: global outcome. *Journal of Personality Disorders,* **1**, 291–8.

Stores G (2000). Introduction to sleep-wake disorders. In MG Gelder, JJ López-Ibor Jr and NC Andreasen, eds. *The New Oxford Textbook of Psychiatry*, Chapter 4.14.1. Oxford University Press, Oxford.

Stores G (2001). *A clinical guide to sleep disorders in children and adolescents.* Cambridge University Press, Cambridge.

Storr A (2000). Analytical psychology (Jung). In MG Gelder, JJ López-Ibor Jr and NC Andreasen, eds. *The new Oxford textbook of psychiatry*, Chapter 3.3.1. Oxford University Press, Oxford.

Strain JJ, Rhodes R and Moros DA (2000). Ethical issues in the care of the medically ill. In A Stoudemier, BS Fogel and DB Greenberg, eds. *Psychiatric care of the medical patient.* Oxford University Press, New York, NY.

Strathdee G and Jenkins R (1996). Purchasing mental health care for primary care. In G Thornicroft and G Strathdee, eds. *Commissioning mental health services*, 71–83. HMSO, London.

Stroebe MS and Stroebe W (1993). The mortality of bereavement:. In MS Stroebe and RO Hansson, eds. *Handbook of bereavement*, 175–95. Cambridge University Press, Cambridge.

Stroebel CF (1985). Biofeedback and behavioural medicine. In HI Kaplan and BJ Sadock, eds. *Comprehensive textbook of psychiatry*. 4th edn. Williams & Wilkins, Baltimore, MD.

Strömgren E (1985). World-wide issues in psychiatric diagnosis and classification and the Scandinavian point of view. *Mental disorders, alcohol and drug related problems.* Excerpta Medica, Amsterdam.

Stuart RB (1980). *Helping couples change: a social learning approach to marital therapy.* Guilford Press, New York, NY.

Stulemeijer M, deJong LWA, Fiseler TJW, *et al.* (2005). Cognitive-behaviour therapy for adolescents with chronic fatigue syndrome: randomized controlled trial. *British Medical Journal,* **330**, 14–7.

Stunkard A and Wadden TA (2000). Obesity. In MG Gelder, JJ López-Ibor Jr and NC Andreasen, eds. *The new Oxford textbook of psychiatry*, Chapter 4.10.3. Oxford University Press, Oxford.

Substance Abuse and Mental Health Administration (2004). *Overview of Findings from the 2003 National Survey on Drug Use and Health.* Office of Applied Studies, Substance Abuse and Mental Health Administration, Rockville, MD.

Sullivan H (1953). *The interpersonal theory of psychiatry.* Norton, New York, NY.

Sullivan MD, Katon W, Russo JE, *et al.* (1993). A randomized trial of nortriptyline for severe chronic tinnitus. Effects on depression, disability, and tinnitus symptoms. *Archives of Internal Medicine,* **153**, 2251–9.

Sullivan PF, Bulik CM, Fear JL, *et al.* (1998). Outcome of anorexia nervosa: a case-control study. *American Journal of Psychiatry,* **155**, 939–46.

Sullivan PF, Eaves LJ, Kendler KS, *et al.* (2001). Genetic case-control association studies in neuropsychiatry. *Archives of General Psychiatry,* **58**, 1015–24.

Sullivan PF, Kendler KS and Neale MC (2003). Schizophrenia as a complex trait - evidence from a meta-analysis of twin studies. *Archives of General Psychiatry,* **60**, 1187–92.

Sulloway FJ (1979). *Freud: biologist of the mind.* Fontana, London.

Sultana A and McMonagle T (2000). Pimozide for schizophrenia or related psychoses. *Cochrane Database Syst Rev*, Cd001949.

Suominen K, Henricksson M, Suokas J, *et al.* (1996). Mental disorders and comorbidity in attempted suicide. *Acta Psychiatrica Scandinavica,* **94**, 234–40.

Super M and Postlethwaite RJ (1997). Genes, familial enuresis and clinical management. *Lancet,* **350**, 159–60.

Susser E, Struening EL and Conover S (1989). Psychiatric problems in homeless men. *Archives of General Psychiatry,* **46**, 845–50.

Svenson S and Folstein SE (2000). Psychological aspects and risks of testing for genetic disorders. In A Stoudemier, BS Fogel and DB Greenberg, eds. *Psychiatric care of the medical patient.* Oxford University Press, New York, NY.

Swaab DF and Hoffman MA (1990). An enlarged suprachiasmatic nucleus in homosexual men. *Brain Research,* **537**, 141–8.

Swanson JW, Holzer CE, Ganju VK, *et al.* (1990). Violence and psychiatric disorder in the community: evidence from the Epidemiologic Catchment Area surveys. *Hospital and Community Psychiatry,* **41**, 761–70.

Swanson JW, Swartz MS, Borum R, *et al.* (2000). Involuntary out-patient commitment and reduction of violent behaviour in persons with severe mental illness. *British Journal of Psychiatry,* **176**, 324–31.

Swift W, Copeland J and Hall W (1996). Characteristics of women with alcohol and other drug problems: Findings of an Australian National Survey. *Addiction,* **91**, 1141–50.

Symmers St. CW (1968). Carcinoma of breast in transsexual individuals after surgical and hormonal interference with primary and secondary sex characteristics. *British Medical Journal,* **2**, 83–5.

Szasz TS (1960). The myth of mental illness. *American Psychology,* **15**, 113–18.

Szekely CA, Thorne JE, Zandi PP, *et al.* (2004). Nonsteroidal anti-inflammatory drugs for the prevention of Alzheimer's disease: a systematic review. *Neuroepidemiology,* **23**, 159–69.

Szmukler G (2001). Violence risk prediction in practice. *British Journal of Psychiatry,* **178**, 84–5.

Szmuckler G (2003). Risk assessment: 'Numbers' and 'values'. *Psychiatric Bulletin,* **27**, 205–7.

Szmuckler G and Holloway F (2001). In patient Treatment. In G Thornicroft and G Szmuckler, eds. *Textbook of Community Psychiatry*, Chapter 28. Oxford University Press, Oxford.

Tansella M (1991). Community based psychiatry: longterm patterns of care in South Verona. *Psychological Medicine,* **19**.

Tansella M (2002). The Scientific evaluation of mental health treatments: an historical perspective. *Evidence Based Mental Health*, **5**, 4–5.

Taphoorn MJ and Klein M (2004). Cognitive deficits in adult patients with brain tumours. *Lancet Neurol*, **3**, 159–68.

Target M, Fonagy P, Slade A, *et al.* (2005). Psychosocial therapies with children. In GO Gabbard, JS Beck and J Holmes, eds. *Oxford textbook of psychotherapy*, Chapter 29. Oxford University Press,

Tariot PN, Erb R, Podgorski CA, *et al.* (1998). Efficacy and tolerability of carbamazepine for agitation and aggression in dementia. *American Journal of Psychiatry*, **155**, 54–61.

Tarrier N, Yusupoff L, Kinney C, *et al.* (1998). Randomised controlled trial of intensive cognitive behaviour therapy for patients with chronic schizophrenia. *British Medical Journal*, **317**, 303–7.

Task Force for Psychiatric Measures (2000). *Handbook of psychiatric measures.* American Psychiatric Association, Washington, DC.

Taylor D (1999). Depot antipsychotics revisited. *Psychiatric Bulletin*, **23**, 551–3.

Taylor D, Paton C and Kerwin R (2003). *The Maudsley Prescribing Guidelines 2003.* 7th edn. Martin Dunitz, London.

Taylor E (1991). *Biological risk factors for psychosocial disorders.* Cambridge University Press, Cambridge.

Taylor E (1994). Physical treatments. In M Rutter, E Taylor and L Hersov, eds. *Child and adolescent psychiatry*. Blackwell Scientific Publications, Oxford.

Taylor E and Rutter M (2002). Classification: conceptual issues and substantive findings. In M Rutter and E Taylor, eds. *Child and Adolescent Psychiatry*. 4th edn. Blackwell Publishing, Oxford.

Taylor E, Sandberg S, Thorley G, *et al.* (1991). *The epidemiology of childhood hyperactivity.* Oxford University Press, Oxford.

Taylor FH (1996). The Henderson therapeutic community. In M Craft, ed. *Psychopathic disorders*. Pergamon Press, Oxford.

Taylor FK (1981). On pseudo-hallucinations. *Psychological Medicine*, **11**, 265–72.

Taylor Jr HA (1999). Sexual activity and the cardiovascular patient: guidelines. *American Journal of Cardiology*, **84**, 6N–10N.

Taylor PJ and Gunn J (1999). Homicides by people with mental illness. *British Journal of Psychiatry*, **174**, 9–14.

Taylor PJ, Mahandra B and Gunn J (1983). Erotomania in males. *Psychological Medicine*, **13**, 645–50.

Taylor S, Thordarson DS, Maxfield L, *et al.* (2003). Comparative efficacy, speed, and adverse effects of three PTSD treatments: exposure therapy, EMDR, and relaxation training. *Journal of Consulting and Clinical Psychology*, **71**, 330–8.

Taylor WD and Doraiswamy PM (2004). A systematic review of antidepressant placebo-controlled trials for geriatric depression: limitations of current data and directions for the future. *Neuropsychopharmacology*, **29**, 2285–99.

Teague GB, Bond GR and Drake RE (1998). Program fidelity in assertive community treatment: development and use of a measure. *American Journal of Orthopsychiatry*, **68**, 216–32.

Teasdale JD, Moore RG, Hayhurst H, *et al.* (2002). Metacognitive awareness and prevention of relapse in depression: empirical evidence. *Journal of Consulting and Clinical Psychology*, **70**, 275–87.

Teri L, Gibbons LE, McCurry SM, *et al.* (2003). Exercise plus behavioral management in patients with Alzheimer disease: a randomized controlled trial. *Journal of the American Medical Association*, **290**, 2015–22.

Thapar A, Irving I, Gottesman I, *et al.* (1994). The genetics of mental retardation. *British Journal of Psychiatry*, **164**, 747–58.

Tharyan P and Adams CE (2002). Electroconvulsive therapy for schizophrenia. *Cochrane Database of Systematic Reviews*, Cd000076.

Thase ME and Friedman ES (1999). Is psychotherapy an effective treatment for melancholia and other severe depressive states? *Journal of Affective Disorders*, **54**, 1–19.

Thase ME, Trivedi MH and Rush AJ (1995). MAOIs in the contemporary treatment of depression. *Neuropsychopharmacology*, **12**, 185–219.

Thomas A, Chess S and Birch HG (1968). *Temperament and behaviour disorders in children.* University Press, New York.

Thomas AJ, Kalaria RN and O'Brien JT (2004). Depression and vascular disease: what is the relationship? *Journal of Affective Disorders*, **79**, 81–95.

Thomas P and Bracken P (2004). Critical psychiatry in practice. *Advances in Psychiatric Treatment*, **10**, 361–70.

Thompson A and Pearce J (2000). The child as witness. In MG Gelder, JJ López-Ibor Jr and NC Andreasen, eds. *The new Oxford textbook of psychiatry*, Chapter 9.4.2. Oxford University Press, Oxford.

Thompson C and Briggs M (2000). Support for carers of people with Alzheimer's type dementia. 2: CD000454, *Cochrane Database of Systematic Reviews.*

Thompson D, Lettich L and Takeshita J (2003). Fibromyalgia: an overview. *Current Psychiatry Reports*, **5**, 211–7.

Thompson LW, Gallagher D and Breckenridge JS (1987). Comparative effectiveness of psychotherapies for depressed elders. *Journal of Consulting and Clinical Psychology*, **55**, 385–90.

Thompson WG, Longstreth GF, Drossman DA, *et al.* (1999). Functional bowel disorders and functional abdominal pain. *Gut*, **45**, II43–7.

Thomson M (1998). *The problem of mental deficiency. eugenics, democracy, and social policy in Britain, c.1870–1959.* Oxford University Press, Oxford.

Thornicroft G and Tansella M (2000). Planning and providing mental health services for a community. In MG Gelder, JJ López-Ibor Jr and NC Andreasen, eds. *The new Oxford textbook of psychiatry*, Chapter 7.5. Oxford University Press, Oxford.

Thornley B, Adams CE and Awad G (1997). *Chlorpromazine versus placebo for those with schizophrenia.* Cochrane Database of Systematic Reviews.

Thornley B, Rathbone J, Adams CE, *et al.* (2003). Chlorpromazine versus placebo for schizophrenia. *Cochrane Database of Systematic Reviews*, CD000284.

Tienari P, Wynne LC, Läksy K, *et al.* (2003). Genetic boundaries of the schizophrenia spectrum: Evidence form the Finnish adoptive family study of schizophrenia. *American Journal of Psychiatry*, **160**, 1587–94.

Tienari P, Wynne LC, Sorri A, *et al.* (2004). Genotype-environment interaction in schizophrenia-spectrum disorder. Long-term follow-up study of Finnish adoptees. *British Journal of Psychiatry*, **184**, 216–22.

Tilfors M, Furmark T, Marteinsdottir I, *et al.* (2001). Cerebral blood flow during anticipation of public speaking in social phobia: a PET study. *Biological Psychiatry,* **52**, 1113–19.

Tizard J (1964). *Community services for the mentally handicapped.* Oxford University Press, London.

Toescu EC, Verkhratsky A and Landfield PW (2004). Ca2+ regulation and gene expression in normal brain aging. *Trends in Neurosciences,* **27**, 614–20.

Tollison CD and Adams HE (1979). *Sexual disorders: treatment, theory and research.* Gardner Press, New York.

Tomlinson J (ed.) (2005). *ABC of sexual health.* BMJ Books, London.

Tondo L, Baldessarini RJ, Floris G, *et al.* (1997). Effectiveness of restarting lithium treatment after its discontinuation in bipolar I and bipolar II disorders. *American Journal of Psychiatry,* **154**, 548–50.

Toone B (2000). Epilepsy. In MG Gelder, JJ López-Ibor Jr and NC Andreasen, eds. *The new Oxford textbook of psychiatry*, Chapter 5.3.4. Oxford University Press, Oxford.

Torgersen S (1984). Genetic and sociological aspects of schizotypal and borderline personality disorders: a twin study. *Archives of General Psychiatry,* **41**, 546–54.

Torgersen S, Skre I, Onstad S, *et al.* (1993). The psychometric-genetic structure of DSM-III - R personality disorder criteria. *Journal of Personality Disorders,* **7**, 196–213.

Tost H, Wendt CS, Schmitt A, *et al.* (2004). Huntington's disease: phenomenological diversity of a neuropsychiatric condition that challenges traditional concepts in neurology and psychiatry. *American Journal of Psychiatry,* **161**, 28–34.

Traeen B, Spitznogle K and Beverfjord A (2004). Attitudes and use of pronographyin the Norwegian population 2002. *Journal of Sex Research,* **41**, 193–2000.

Treasure J (2004). Motivational interviewing. *Advances in Psychiatric Treatment,* **10**, 331–7.

Treasure J and Holland A (1989). A Genetic vulnerability to eating disorders: evidence from twin and family studies. *Child and Youth Psychiatry*, 59–68.

Treiman DM (1999). Violence and the epilepsy defense. *Neurologic Clinics,* **17**, 245–55.

Tribe R (2002). Mental Health of Refugees and Asylum Seekers. *Advances in Psychiatric Treatment*, **8**, 240–7.

Trimble MR (1997). Temporolimbic syndromes. In MR Trimble and JL Cummings, eds. *Contemporary Behavioral Neurology.* Butterworth-Heinemann, Boston.

Trinh NH, Hoblyn J, Mohanty S, *et al.* (2003). Efficacy of cholinesterase inhibitors in the treatment of neuropsychiatric symptoms and functional impairment in Alzheimer disease: a meta-analysis. *Journal of the American Medical Association,* **289**, 210–6.

Trost M (2003). Dystonia update. *Current Opinion in Neurology,* **16**, 495–500.

True WR, Rice J, Eisen SA, *et al.* (1993). A twin study of genetic and environmental contributions to liability of posttraumatic stress symptoms. *Archives of General Psychiatry,* **50**, 257.

Trull TJ and Widiger TA (1997). *Structured Interview for the Five-Factor Model of Personality. (SIFFM): professional manual.* Psychological Assessment Resources, Odessa, FL.

Trzepacz P and Dimartini A (2000). *The transplant patient. Biological, psychiatric and ethical issues in organ transplantation.* Cambridge University Press, Cambridge.

Trzepacz PT (2000). Is there a final common neural pathway in delirium? Focus on acetylcholine and dopamine. *Seminars in Clinical Neuropsychiatry,* **5**, 132–48.

Tseng W-S, Asai M, Kitanishi K, *et al.* (1992). Diagnostic patterns of social phobia: comparisons in Tokyo and Hawaii. *Journal of Nervous and Mental Disease,* **180**, 380–5.

Tseng W-S, Kan-Ming M, Hsu J, *et al.* (1988). A sociocultural study of koro epidemics in Guangdong, China. *American Journal of Psychiatry,* **145**, 1538–43.

Tsoi WF and Wong KE (1991). A 15-year follow-up study of Chinese schizophrenic patients. *Acta Psychiatrica Scandinavica,* **84**, 217–20.

Tsuang MT, Stone WS and Faraone SV (2000). Schizoaffective and schizotypal disorders. In MG Gelder, JJ López-Ibor Jr and NC Andreasen, eds. *The new Oxford textbook of psychiatry*, Chapter 4.3.8. Oxford University Press, Oxford.

Tune LE and Salzman C (2003). Schizophrenia in late life. *Psychiatric Clinics of North America,* **26**, 103–13.

Turk DC (1979). The role of psychological factors in chronic pain. *Acta Anaesthesiologica Scandinavica,* **43**, 885–8.

Turkington D, Dudley R, Warman DM, *et al.* (2004). Cognitive-behavioral therapy for schizophrenia: a review. *Journal of Psychiatric Practice,* **10**, 5–16.

Turkington D, Martindale B and Bloch-Thorseen GR (2005). Schizophrenia. In GO Gabbard, JS Beck and J Holmes, eds. *Oxford textbook of psychotherapy*, Chapter 14. Oxford University Press,

Turkington D and McKenna PJ (2003). Is cognitive-behavioural therapy a worthwhile treatment for psychosis? *British Journal of Psychiatry,* **182**, 477–9.

Turner MA, Moran NF and Kopelman MD (2002). Subcortical dementia. *British Journal of Psychiatry,* **180**, 148–51.

Turner S, Iliffe S, Downs M, *et al.* (2004). General practitioners' knowledge, confidence and attitudes in the diagnosis and management of dementia. *Age and Ageing,* **33**, 461–7.

Turner SM, Beidel DC and Jacob RG (1994). Social phobia: comparison of behavior therapy and atenolol. *Journal of Consulting and Clinical Psychology,* **62**, 350–8.

Turner SW, Bowie C and Dunn G (2003). Mental Health of Kosovan Albanian refugees in the UK. *British Journal of Psychiatry,* **182**, 444–8.

Tutte JC (2004). The concept of psychical trauma: a bridge in interdisciplinary space. *International Journal of Psychoanalysis,* **85**, 897–921.

Tyrer P and Bateman AW (2004). Drug treatment for personality disorder. *Advances in Psychiatric Treatment,* **10**, 389–98.

Tyrer P and Davidson K (2000). Management of personality disorder. In MG Gelder, JJ López-Ibor Jr and NC Andreasen, eds. *The new Oxford textbook of psychiatry*, Chapter 4.12.7. Oxford University Press, Oxford.

Tyrer P, Seivewright H and Johnson T (2003). The core elements of neurosis: mixed anxiety-depression (cothymia) and personality disorder. *Journal of Personality Disorders,* **17**, 129–38.

Tyrer P, Tom B, Byford S, *et al.* (2004). Differential effects of manual assisted cognitive behavior therapy in the treatment of recurrent deliberate self-harm and personality disturbance: The POPMACT Study. *Journal of Personality Disorders,* **18**, 102–16.

UK ECT Review Group (2003). Efficacy and safety of electroconvulsive therapy in depressive disorders: a systematic review an meta-analysis. *Lancet,* **361**, 799–808.

Unützer J, Katon W, Callahan CM, *et al.* (2002). Collaborative care management of late-life depression in the primary care setting: a randomized controlled trial. *Journal of the American Medical Association,* **288**, 2836–45.

Ursano RJ and Ursano AM (2000). Brief individual dynamic pyschotherapy. In MG Gelder, JJ López-Ibor Jr and NC Andreasen, eds. *The new Oxford textbood of psychiatry*, Chapter 6.3.4. Oxford University Press, Oxford.

Üstün TB and Sartorius N (1995). *Mental illness in general health care; an international study.* John Wiley, Chichester.

Vaillant GE (1988). What can long-term follow-up teach us about relapse and prevention in addiction? *British Journal of Addiction,* **83**, 1147–57.

Valdimarsdottir U, Helgason AR, Furst CJ, *et al.* (2003). Long term effects of widowhood after terminal cancer: a swedish nationwide follow-up. *Scandinavian Journal of Public Health,* **31**, 31–6.

van Bolkom AJL, de Haan E, van Oppen P, *et al.* (1998). Cognitive and behavioural therapies alone versus in combination with fluvoxamine in the treatment of obsessive compulsive disorder. *Journal of Nervous and Mental Disease,* **186**, 492–9.

Van den Oord EJ, Boomsma DI and Verhulst FC (1994). A study of problem behaviours in 10–15 year old biologically related and unrelated international adoptees. *Behaviour Genetics,* **24**, 193–205.

van der Cammen TJM, Croes EA, Dermaut B, *et al.* (2004). Genetic testing has no place as a routine diagnostic test in sporadic and familial cases of alzheimer's disease. *Journal of the American Geriatrics Society,* **52**, 2110–3.

van der Kolk BA and van der Hart O (1989). Pierre Janet and the breakdown of adaptation in psychological trauma. *American Journal of Psychiatry,* **146**, 1530–40.

Van Kesteren PJ, Asscheman H, Megens JA, *et al.* (1997). Mortality and morbidity of transsexual subjects treated with cross-sex hormones. *Clinical Endocrinology (Oxford),* **47**, 337–42.

Van Kolk BA and Fisler R (1995). Dissociation and the fragmentary nature of traumatic memories: overview and exploratory study. *Journal of Traumatic Stress,* **8**, 505–25.

Van Loon FHG (1927). Amok and latah. *Journal of Abnormal and Social Psychology,* **21**, 434–44.

Van Os J, Gilvarry C, Bale R, *et al.* (1999). A comparison of the utility of dimensional and categorical representations of psychosis. UK700 Group. *Psychological Medicine,* **29**, 595–606.

Van Os J, Hanssen M, Bak M, *et al.* (2003). Do urbanicity and familial liability coparticipate in causing psychosis. *American Journal of Psychiatry,* **160**, 477–82.

Van Tulder MW, Ostelo R, Vlaeyen JW, *et al.* (2002). Behavioural treatment for chronic low back pain: a systematic review within the framework of the Cochrane Back Review Group. *Spine,* **25**, 2688–99.

van Vliet IM, den Boer JA and Westenberg HGM (1994). Psychopharmacological treatment of socialphobia: a double-blind placebo controlled study with fluvoxamine. *Psychopharmacology,* **115**, 128–34.

Van Vreeswijk MF and De Wilde EJ (2004). Autobiographical memory specificity, psychopathology, depressed mood and the use of the Autobiographical Memory Test: a mete-analysis. *Behavior Research & Therapy,* **42**, 731–43.

van Zelst WH, de Beurs E, Beekman AT, *et al.* (2003). Prevalence and risk factors of posttraumatic stress disorder in older adults. *Psychotherapy and Psychosomatics,* **72**, 333–42.

Vaughn CE and Leff JP (1976). The influence of family and social factors on the course of psychiatric illness. A comparison of schizophrenic and depressed neurotic patients. *British Journal of Psychiatry,* **129**, 125–37.

Vauhkonen K (1968). On the pathogenesis of morbid jealousy with special reference to the personality traits of an interaction between jealous patients and their spouses. *Acta Psychiatrica Scandinavica Supplement,* **202**, 2–261.

Veale D (2003). Treatment of social phobia. *Advances in Psychiatric Treatment,* **9**, 258–64.

Veenstra VanderWeele J and Cook EH, Jr. (2004). Molecular genetics of autism spectrum disorder. *Mol Psychiatry*, **9**, 819–32.

Vellutino FR, Fletcher JM, Snowling MJ, *et al.* (2004). Specific reading disability (dyslexia): what have we learned in the past four decades? *Journal of Child Psychology and Psychiatry,* **45**, 2–40.

Verdellen CW, Keijers G, Cath DC, *et al.* (2004). Exposure with response prevention versus habit reversal in Tourette's syndrome a controlled study. *Behaviour Research and Therapy,* **5**, 501–11.

Verhoeff NPLG (1999). Radiotracer imaging of dopaminergic transmission in neuro-psychiatric disorders. *Psychopharmacology,* **147**, 217–49.

Victor M and Adams RD (1953). The effect of alcohol on the nervous system. *Proceedings of the Association of Research in Nervous and Mental Diseases,* **32**, 526–73.

Victor M, Adams RD and Collins GH (1971). *The Wernicke-Korsakoff syndrome.* Blackwell, Oxford.

Viens M, De Koninck J, Mercier P, *et al.* (2003). Trait anxiety and sleep-onset insomnia: evaluation of treatment using anxiety management training. *Journal of Psychosomatic Research,* **54**, 31–7.

Viguera AC and Cohen LS (2000). Psychopharmacology during pregnancy, the postpartum period, and lactation. In A Stoudemier, BS Fogel and DB Greenberg, eds. *Psychiatric care of the medical patient.* Oxford University Press, New York, NY.

Virag R (1982). Intracavernosus injection of papaverine for erectile failure. *Lancet,* **2**, 938.

Volkmar FR and Klin A (2000). Autism and the pervasive developmental disorders. In MG Gelder, JJ López-Ibor Jr and NC Andreasen, eds. *The new Oxford textbook of psychiatry*, Chapter 9.2.2. Oxford University Press, Oxford.

Volkmar FR, Lord C, Bailey A, *et al.* (2004). Autism and pervasive developmental disorders. *Journal of Child Psychology and Psychiatry,* **45**, 135–70.

Volkow ND and Li TK (2004). Drug addiction: the neurobiology of behaviour gone awry. *Nature Reviews Neuroscience*, **5**, 963–70.

Von Economo C (1929). *Encephalitis lethargica: its sequelae and treatment.* Transl KO Newman. Oxford University Press, Oxford.

von Gontard A (1998). Annotation: day and night wetting in children – a paediatric perspective. *Journal of Child Psychology and Psychiatry*, **39**, 439–51.

Von Korff M, Barlow W, Charkin D, *et al.* (1994). Effects of practice style in managing back pain. *Annals of Internal Medicine*, **121**, 187–95.

Von Korff M and Simon G (1996). The relationship between pain and depression. *British Journal of Psychiatry*, **168**, 101–8.

Von Korff R, Eaton WW and Keyl PM (1985). The epidemiology of panic attacks and panic disorder: results in three community surveys. *American Journal of Epidemiology*, **122**, 970-81.

Wade SL, Monroe SM and Michelson LK (1993). Chronic life stress and treatment outcome in agoraphobia with panic attacks. *American Journal of Psychiatry*, **150**, 1491-5.

Waern M, Runeson BS, Allebeck P, *et al.* (2002). Mental disorder in elderly suicides: a case-control study. *American Journal of Psychiatry*, **159**, 450-5.

Wahlbeck K, Cheine M, Essali A, *et al.* (1999). Evidence of clozapine's effectiveness in schizophrenia: a systematic review and meta-analysis of randomized trials. *American Journal of Psychiatry*, **156**, 990–9.

Wakefield JC (1992). The concept of mental disorder. On the boundary between biological facts and social values. *American Psychology*, **47**, 373–88.

Walsh E, Buchanan A and Fahy T (2002). Violence and schizophrenia: examining the evidence. *British Journal of Psychiatry*, **180**, 490–5.

Wampold BE, Minami T, Baskin TW, *et al.* (2002). A meta-(re)analysis of the effects of cognitive therapy versus 'other therapies' for depression. *Journal of Affective Disorders*, **68**, 159–65.

Ward CH, Beck AT, Mendelson M, *et al.* (1962). The psychiatric nomenclature. *Archives of General Psychiatry*, **7**, 198–205.

Ward J, Hall W and Mattick RP (1999). Role of maintenance treatment in opioid dependence. *Lancet*, **353**, 221–6.

Warner J (2004). Clinicians guide to evaluating diagnostic and screening tests in psychiatry. *Advances in Psychiatric Treatment*, **10**, 446–54.

Warner R (2002). Early intervention in schizophrenia: a critique. *Epidemiologia e Psichiatria Sociale*, **11**, 248–55.

Warner RW, Gater R, Jackson MG, *et al.* (1993). Effects of a community mental health service on the practice and attitudes of general practitioners. *British Journal of General Practice*, **43**, 507–11.

Watson JB and Rayner R (1920). Conditioned emotional reactions. *Journal of Experimental Psychology*, **3**, 1–14.

Weaver T, Tyrer P, Ritchies J, *et al.* (2003). Assessing the value of assertive outreach: qualitative study of process and outcome in the UK700 trial. *British Journal of Psychiatry*, **183**, 437–45.

Webster-Stratton C (1991). Annotation strategies for helping families with conduct disordered children. *Journal of Child Psychology and Psychiatry*, **32**, 1047–61.

Wegner DM (1989). *White Bears and other unwanted thoughts: suppression, obsession and the psychology of mental control.* Viking, New York.

Weinberg MS, Williams CJ and Calhan C (1994). Homosexual foot fetishism. *Archives of Sexual Behaviour*, **23**, 611–26.

Weinberger DR (1987). Implications of normal brain development for the pathogenesis of schizophrenia. *Archives of General Psychiatry*, **44**, 660–9.

Weinberger DR (1995). From neuropathology to neurodevelopment. *Lancet*, **346**, 552–7.

Weinberger DR and McClure RK (2002). Neurotoxicity, neuroplasticity, and magnetic resonance imaging morphometry: what is happening in the schizophrenic brain? *Archives of General Psychiatry*, **59**, 553–8.

Weingarten MA, M. P and Leibovici L (2004). Assessing ethics in systematic reviews. *British Medical Journal*, **328**, 1013–4.

Weissman AM, Bland RC, Canino GJ, *et al.* (1996). Cross-national epidemiology of major depression and bipolar disorder. *Journal of the American Medical Association*, **276**, 293–9.

Weissman AM, Levy BT, Hartz AJ, *et al.* (2004). Pooled analysis of antidepressant levels in lactating mothers, breast milk, and nursing infants. *American Psychiatric Association*, **161**, 1066–78.

Weissman MM, Bland RC, Canino GJ, *et al.* (1994). The gross national epidemiology of obsessive compulsive disorder. *Journal of Clinical Psychiatry*, **55**, 5–11.

Weissman MM and Merikangas KR (1986). The epidemiology of anxiety and panic disorders. *Journal of Clinical Psychiatry*, **47**, 11–17.

Wellings K, Field J, Johnson AM, *et al.* (1994). *Sexual behaviour in Britain.* Penguin Books, London.

Wellings K, Nanchalal K, MacDowall W, *et al.* (2001). Sexual behaviour in Britain: early heterosexual experience. *Lancet*, **358**, 1843–50.

Wells A and Butler G (1997). Generalized anxiety disorder. In DM Clark and CG Fairburn, eds. *Science and practice of c ognitive behaviour therapy*, Chapter 7. Oxford University Press, Oxford.

Wender P, Kety S, Rosenthal D, *et al.* (1986). Psychiatric disorders in the biological and adoptive families of adopted individuals with affective disorders. *Archives of General Psychiatry*, **43**, 923–9.

Werneke U, Horn O and Taylor DM (2004). How effective is St John's wort? The evidence revisited. *Journal of Clinical Psychiatry*, **65**, 611–7.

Wertheimer A (2001). *A special scar: the experiences of people bereaved by suicide.* Brunner-Routledge, Hove.

Wertheimer J (1997). Psychiatry of the elderly: a consensus statement. *International Journal of Geriatric Psychiatry*, **12**, 432–5.

Wessely S (1987). Mass hysteria: two syndromes? *Psychological Medicine*, **17**, 109–20.

Wessely S (1990). Old wine in new bottles: neurasthenia and 'M.E.' *Psychological Medicine*, **20**, 35–53.

Wessely S, Hotopf MH and Sharpe M (1998). *Chronic fatigue and its syndromes.* Oxford University Press, Oxford.

Wessely S, Nimnuan C and Sharpe M (1999). Functional somatic syndromes: one or many? *The Lancet*, **354**, 936–9.

West D (1974). Criminology, deviant behaviour and mental disorder. *Psychological Medicine*, **4**, 1–3.

West D and Farrington DP (1973). *Who becomes delinquent?* Heinemann Educational, London.

West D and Farrington DP (1977). *The delinquent way of life.* Heinemann, London.

West MA (1990). *The psychology of meditation.* Clarendon Press, Oxford.

Westen D (1997). Divergences between clinical and other research methods for assessing personality disorders: implications for research and the evolution of Axis II. *American Journal of Psychiatry*, **154**, 895–903.

Westphal C (1872). Die agoraphobie, eine neuropatische Erscheinung. *Archiv fur Psychiatrie und Nervenkrankheiten*, **3**, 209–37.

Wheeler EO, White PD, Reed EW, *et al.* (1950). Neurocirculatory asthenia (anxiety neurosis, effort syndrome, neurasthenia). A twenty year follow up of one hundred and seventy three patients. *Journal of the American Medical Association*, **142**, 878–89.

Whitaker A, Johnson J, Shaffer D, *et al.* (1990). Uncommon troubles in young people: prevalence estimates of selected psychiatric disorders in a nonreferred adolescent population. *Archives of General Psychiatry*, **47**, 487–96.

White PD, Thomas JM, Amess J, *et al.* (1998). Incidence, risk and prognosis of acute and chronic fatigue syndromes and psychiatric disorders after glandular fever. *British Journal of Psychiatry*, **173**, 475–81.

Whitehead C, Moss S, Cardno A, *et al.* (2003). Antidepressants for the treatment of depression in people with schizophrenia: a systematic review. *Psychological Medicine*, **33**, 589–99.

Whiting P, Bagnall A, Sowden A, *et al.* (2001). Interventions for the treatment and management of chronic fatigue syndrome: a systematic review. *Journal of the American Medical Association*, **286**, 1360–8.

Whitley E, Gunnell D, Dorling D, *et al.* (1999). Ecological study of social fragmentation, poverty, and suicide. *British Medical Journal*, **319**, 1037–7.

Whitney I, Smith PK and Thompson D (1994). Bullying and children with special needs. In PK Smith and S Sharp, eds. *School bullying: insights and perspectives*, 213–40. Routledge, London.

Whittington CJ, Kendall T, Fonagy P, *et al.* (2004). Selective serotonin reuptake inhibitors in childhood depression: systematic review of published versus unpublished data. *Lancet*, **363**, 1341–5.

Widiger TA and Clark LA (2000). Toward DSM-V and the classification of psychopathology. *Psychological Bulletin*, **126**, 946–63.

Widiger TA and Costa PT (1994). Personality and personality disorders. *Journal of Abnormal Psychology*, **103**, 78–91.

Wieck A and Haddad PM (2003). Antipsychotic-induced hyperprolactinaemia in women: pathophysiology, severity and consequences. Selective literature review. *British Journal of Psychiatry*, **182**, 199–204.

Wieck A and Haddad PM (2004). Hyperprolactinaemia. In PM Haddad, S Dursun and B Deakin, eds. *Adverse syndromes and psychiatric drugs. A clinical guide.*, 69–88. Oxford University Press, Oxford.

Wild R, Pettit T and Burns A (2003). Cholinesterase inhibitors for dementia with Lewy bodies. *Cochrane Database Syst Rev*, Cd003672.

Wilens TE, Biederman J and Spencer TJ (2002). Attention deficit/hyperactivity disorder across the lifespan. *Annu Rev Med*, **53**, 113–31.

Wilensky DS, Ginsberg G, Altman M, *et al.* (1996). A community study of failure to thrive in Israel. *Archives of Disease in Childhood*, **75**, 145–8.

Wilkinson G, Allen P, Marshall E, *et al.* (1993). The role of the practice nurse in the management of depression in general practice: treatment adherence to antidepressant medication. *Psychological Medicine*, **23**, 229–37.

Williams ER, Guthrie E, Mackway-Jones K, *et al.* (2001). Psychiatric status, somatisation, and health care utilization of frequent attenders at the emergency department: a comparison with routine attenders. *Journal of Psychosomatic Research*, **50**, 161–7.

Williams J, LeFrancois B and Copperman J (2001). *Mental Health Services that Work for Women: Findings of UK Survey.* Tizard Centre, University of Kent, Canterbury.

Williams JMG and Pollock LR (2000). The psychology of suicidal behaviour. In K Hawton and K van Heeringen, eds. *The international handbook of suicide and attempted suicide.* John Wiley & Sons, Chichester.

Willoughby MT (2004). Developmental course of ADHD symptomatology during the transition from childhood to adolescence: a review with recommendations. *Journal of Child Psychology and Psychiatry*, **44**, 88–106.

Wilson B (1999). *Case studies in neuropsychological rehabilitation.* Oxford University Press, New York.

Wilson DN (1997). Psychiatric disorders and mild learning disability. In O Russell, ed. *The psychiatry of learning disabilities*, 125–35. Gaskell, London.

Wilson GT (1993). Behavioral treatment of obesity: thirty years and counting. *Advances in Behaviour Research and Therapy*, **16**, 31–75.

Wilson GT and Fairburn CG (2000). Eating disorders. In PE Nathan and JM Gorman, eds. *Treatments that work*, 559–92. Oxford University Press, New York, NY.

Wilson GT and Fairburn CG (2002). Treatment for Eating Disrders. In PE Nathan and JM Gorman, eds. *A guide to treatment that works.* Oxford University Press, Oxford.

Wilson GT, Fairburn CG and Agras WS (1996). Cognitive-behavioural therapy for bulimia nervosa. In DM Garner and PE Garfinkel, eds. *Handbook of treatment for eating disorders.* Guilford Press,

Wilson M (1993). DSM-III and the transformation of American psychiatry: a history. *Am J Psychiatry*, **150**, 399–410.

Wilson RS, De Leon CF, Barnes LL, *et al.* (2002). Participation in cognitively stimulating activities and risk of incident Alzheimer disease. *Journal of the American Medical Association*, **287**, 742–8.

Wilson S, Roberts L, Roalfe A, *et al.* (2004). Prevalence of irritable bowel syndrome: a community survey. *British Journal of General Practice*, **54**, 495–502.

Wing JK (1994). *Mental illness. In Health care needs assessment.* Radcliffe Medical Press, Abingdon, Oxfordshire.

Wing JK, Beevor AS, Curtis RH, *et al.* (1998). Health of the Nation Outcome Scales (HoNOS). Research and development. *British Journal of Psychiatry*, **172**, 11–18.

Wing JK and Brown GW (1970). *Institutionalism and schizophrenia.* Cambridge University Press, London.

Wing JK, Cooper JE and Sartorius N (1974). *Measurement and classification of psychiatric symptoms; and instruction manual for the PSE and the CATEGO programme.* Cambridge University Press, Cambridge.

Wing JK and Furlong R (1986). A haven for the severely disabled within the context of a comprehensive psychiatric community service. *British Journal of Psychiatry*, **149**, 449–57.

Wing JK and Hailey AM (eds.) (1972). *Evaluating a community psychiatric service.* Oxford University Press, London.

Winstock AR (2000). Disorders relating to the use of ecstacy, other 'party drugs' and Khat. In MG Gelder, JJ López-Ibor Jr and NC Andreason, eds. *Oxford Textbook of Psychiatry*, Chapter 4.2.3.6. Oxford University Press, Oxford.

Winston A, Pollack J, MacCulloch L, *et al.* (1991). Brief psychotherapy for personality disorders. *Journal of Nervous and Mental Disease*, **179**, 188–93.

Winterer G and Weinberger DR (2004). Genes, dopamine and cortical signal-to-noise ratio in schizophrenia. *Trends in Neurosciences*, **27**, 683–90.

Wisniewski HM, Silverman J and Wegiel J (1994). Ageing, Alzheimer disease and mental retardation. *Journal of Intellectual Disability Research*, **38**, 233–9.

Wolfe F, Smythe HA, Yunus MB, *et al.* (1990). The American College of Rheumatology 1990 Criteria for the Classification of Fibromyalgia. Report of the Multicenter Criteria Committee. *Arthritis and Rheumatism*, **33**, 160–72.

Wolff C (1971). *Love between women.* Duckworth, London.

Wolff K, Welch S and Strang J (1999). Specific laboratory investigations for assessments and management of drug problems. *Advances in Psychiatric Treatment*, **5**, 180–91.

Wolff HG (1962). A concept of disease in man. *Psychosomatic Medicine*, **24**, 25–30.

Wolpe J (1958). *Psychotherapy by reciprocal inhibition.* Stanford University Press, Stanford, CA.

Wolpert L (1999). *Malignant Sadness: the anatomy of depression.* 2nd edn. Faber, London.

Wood P (1941). Da Costa's syndrome (or effort syndrome). *British Medical Journal*, **1**, 767–74, 805–11, 846–51.

Woods B and Charlesworth G (2002). Psychological assessment and treatment. In R Jacoby and C Oppenheimer, eds. *Psychiatry in the elderly*. 3rd edn. Oxford University Press, Oxford.

Wooley H, Stein A, Forrest GC, *et al.* (1989). Imparting the diagnosis of life threatening illness in children. *British Medical Journal*, **298**, 1623–6.

World Health Organization (1973). *Report of the International Pilot Study of Schizophrenia.* Vol. 1, World Health Organization, Geneva.

World Health Organization (1978). *Alma-Ata 1978: primary health care.* World Health Organization, Geneva.

World Health Organization (1984). *Mental health care in developing countries: a critical appraisal of research findings.* World Health Organization, Geneva.

World Health Organization (1989). *Composite International Diagnostic Interview (CIDI).* World Health Organization, Geneva.

World Health Organization (1992a). *Glossary: differential definitions of SCAN items and commentary on the SCAN text.* World Health Organization, Geneva.

World Health Organization (1992b). *The ICD-10 classification of mental and behavioural disorders.* World Health Organization, Geneva.

World Health Organization (1998). *Primary prevention of mental, neurological and psychosocial disorders.* World Health Organization, Geneva.

World Health Organization (2004). Prevalence, severity, and unmet need for treatment of mental disorders in the World Health Organization World Mental Health surveys. *JAMA*, **291**, 2581–90.

World Medical Association (2000). *Declaration of Geneva: ethical principles for medical research involving human subjects.* World Medical Association, Edinburgh.

Wright C, Burns T, James P, *et al.* (2003). Assertive outreach teams in London: models of operation. Pan-London Assertive Outreach Study, part 1. *British Journal of Psychiatry*, **183**, 132–8.

Wright IC, Rabe Hesketh S, Woodruff PW, *et al.* (2000). Meta-analysis of regional brain volumes in schizophrenia. *American Journal of Psychiatry*, **157**, 16–25.

Wroblewska AM (1997). Androgenic-anabolic steroids and body dysmorphia in young men. *Journal of Psychosomatic Research*, **42**, 225–34.

Wu G, Lanctot KL, Moosa S, *et al.* (2003). The cost-benefit of cholinesterase inhibitors in mild to moderate dementia: a willingness to pay approach. *CNS Drugs*, **17**, 1045–57.

Wylie K (1994). New approaches to paraphilias. *British Journal of Sexual Medicine*, **21**, 18–21.

Wylie KR, Hallam-Jones R and Walters S (2003). The potential benefit of vacuum devices augmenting psychosexual therapy for erectile dysfunction: a randomized controlled trial. *Journal of Sexual and Marital Therapy*, **29**, 227–36.

Xu J and Chen Z (2003). Advances in molecular cytogenetics for the evalaution of mental retardation. *American Journal of Medical Genetics*, **117 C**, 15–24.

Yalom I, Lieberman MA and Miles MB (1973). *Encounter groups: first facts.* Basic Books, New York, NY.

Yalom ID (1985). *The theory and practice of group psychotherapy.* 3rd edn. Basic Books, New York, NY.

Yang Y, Raine A, Lencz T, *et al.* (2005). Volume reduction in prefrontal gray matter in unsuccessful criminal psychopaths. *Biol Psychiatry*, **57**, 1103–8.

Yatham LN (2004). Newer anticonvulsants in the treatment of bipolar disorder. *The Journal of clinical psychiatry*, 28–35.

Yatham LN, Liddle PF, Shiah IS, *et al.* (2000). Brain serotonin2 receptors in major depression: a positron emission tomography study. *Archives of General Psychiatry*, **57**, 850–8.

Yatham LN, Liddle PF, Shiah IS, *et al.* (2002). PET study of [(18)F]6-fluoro-L-dopa uptake in neuroleptic- and mood-stabilizer-naive first-episode nonpsychotic mania: effects of treatment with divalproex sodium. *Am J Psychiatry*, **159**, 768–74.

Yip PSF, Chao A and Chu CWF (2000). Seasonal variations in suicides:diminished or vanished. Experience in England and Wales 1982–1996. *British Journal of Psychiatry*, **177**, 366–9.

Yonkers KA, Warshaw MG, Massion AO, *et al.* (1996). Phenomenology and course of generalized anxiety disorder. *British Journal of Psychiatry*, **168**, 308–13.

Young AH (2001). Recurrent uni-polar depression requires prolonged treatment. *British Journal of Psychiatry*, **178**, 294–5.

Young J (1999). *Cognitive therapy for personality disorders: A schema-focused approach.* 3rd edn. Professional Resource Exchange Inc, Sarasota, FL.

Young LT, Robb JC, Hasey GM, *et al.* (1999). Gabapentin as an adjunctive treatment in bipolar disorder. *Journal of Affective Disorders*, **55**, 73–7.

Young RC, Biggs JT, Ziegler VE, *et al.* (1978). A rating scale for mania: reliability, validity and sensitivity. *British Journal of Psychiatry*, **133**, 429–35.

Young W, Goy R and Phoenix C (1964). Hormones and sexual behaviour. *Science*, **143**, 212–8.

Yule W (1994). Post-traumatic stress disorders. In M Rutter, E Taylor and L Hersov, eds. *Child and adolescent psychiatry: modern approaches.* 3rd edn. Blackwell Scientific Publications, Oxford.

Yule W and Rutter M (1985). Reading and other learning difficulties. In M Rutter and L Hersov, eds. *Child and adolescent psychiatry: modern approaches.* 2nd edn. Blackwell, Oxford.

Yung PM and Keltner AA (1996). A controlled comparison on the effect of muscle and cognitive relaxation procedures on blood pressure: implications for the behavioural treatment of borderline hypertensives. *Behaviour Research and Therapy*, **43**, 821–6.

Zanarini MC and Frankenburg FR (2001). Olanzapine treatment of female borderline personality disorder patients: a double-blind, placebo-controlled pilot study. *Journal of Clinical Psychiatry*, **62**, 849–54.

Zarei M, Chandran S, Compston A, *et al.* (2003). Cognitive presentation of multiple sclerosis: evidence for a cortical variant. *Journal of Neurology, Neurosurgery and Psychiatry*, **74**, 872–7.

Zeman A, Britton T, Douglas N, *et al.* (2004). Narcolepsy and excessive daytime sleepiness. *BMJ*, **329**, 724–8.

Zhou JN, Hofman MA, Gooren LJ, *et al.* (1995). A sex difference in the human brain and its relation to transsexuality. *Nature*, **378**, 68–70.

Zimmermann P, Wittchen H-U, Hofler M, *et al.* (2003). Primary anxiety disorders and the development of subsequent alcohol use disorders: a 4-year community study of adolescents and young adults. *Psychological Medicine*, **33**, 1211–22.

Zinn S, Stein R and Swartzwelder HS (2004). Executive functioning early in abstinence from alcohol. *Alcoholism, Clinical and Experimental Research*, **28**, 1338–46.

Zitrin CM, Klein DF and Woerner MG (1978). Behaviour therapy, supportive psychotherapy, imipramine and phobias. *Archives of General Psychiatry*, **35**, 307–16.

Zitrin C, Klein D, Woerner M, *et al.* (1983). Treatment of phobias: 1. Comparison of imipramine hydrochloride and placebo. *Arch Gen Psychiatry*, **40**, 125–38.

Zobeck TS, Grant BF, Stinson FS, *et al.* (1994). Alcohol involvement in fatal traffic crashes in the United States: 1979–1990. *Addiction*, **89**, 227–31.

Zoccolillo M, Pickles A, Quinton D, *et al.* (1992). The outcome of childhood conduct disorder: implications for defining adult personality disorder and conduct disorder. *Psychological Medicine*, **22**, 971–86.

Zohar AH, Dina C, Rosolio N, *et al.* (2003). Tridimensional personality questionnare trait of harm avoidance(anxiety proneness) is linked to a locus on chromosome 8p21. *American Journal of Medical Genetics*, **117B**, 66–9.

Zohar J, Kennedy JL, Hollander E, *et al.* (2004). Serotonin-1D hypothesis of obsessive-compulsive disorder: an update. *Journal of Clinical Psychiatry*, **65**, 18–21.

Zohrabian A (2005). The long term effects of and economic consequences of treatments for obesity: work in progress. *Lancet*, **365**, 104–5.

Zucker KJ (2002). Gender identity disorder. In M Rutter and E Taylor, eds. *Child and Adolescent Psychiatry.*, Chapter 44. 4th edn. Blackwell Publishing, Oxford.

Zuger B (1984). Early effeminate behaviour in boys: outcome and significance for homosexuality. *Journal of Nervous and Mental Disease*, **172**, 90–7.

Zwi M and York A (2004). Attention-deficit hyperactivity disorder in adults: validity unknown. *Advances in Psychiatric Treatment*, **10**, 248–59.

Index